KV-637-743

In the Beginning

SECOND EDITION

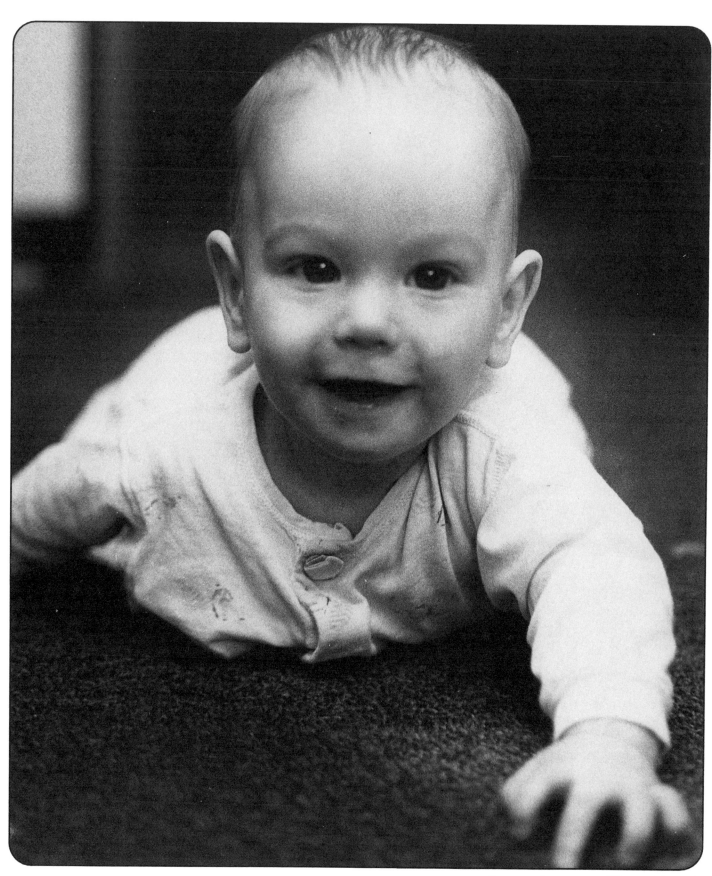

Photograph courtesy of Susan Edmunds.

In the Beginning

DEVELOPMENT FROM CONCEPTION TO AGE TWO

SECOND EDITION

Judy F. Rosenblith

FRANCIS CLOSE HALL
LEARNING CENTRE
UNIVERSITY OF GLOUCESTERSHIRE
Swindon Road
Cheltenham GL50 4AZ
Tel: 01242 532913

SAGE PUBLICATIONS

International Educational and Professional Publisher

Newbury Park   London   New Delhi

Copyright ©1992 by Sage Publications, Inc.

All rights reserved. No part of this book may be reproduced or utilized in any form or by any means, electronic or me-chanical, including photocopying, recording, or by any information storage and retrieval system, without permission in writing from the publisher.

For information address:

SAGE Publications, Inc.
2455 Teller Road
Newbury Park, California 91320

SAGE Publications Ltd.
6 Bonhill Street
London EC2A 4PU
United Kingdom

SAGE Publications India Pvt. Ltd.
M-32 Market
Greater Kailash I
New Delhi 110 048 India

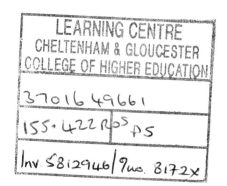

LEARNING CENTRE
CHELTENHAM & GLOUCESTER
COLLEGE OF HIGHER EDUCATION

3701649661

155.422 Ros ps

Inv. 5812946/9no. 8172x

Printed in the United States of America

Library of Congress Cataloging-in-Publication Data

Rosenblith, Judy F.
    In the beginning: development from conception to age two,
second edition / Judy F. Rosenblith
        p.   cm.
    Includes bibliographical references (p.   ) and index.
    ISBN 0-8039-4690-2 (cl)
    1. Infant psychology. 2. Child development. 3. Fetus.
I. Title.
BF719.R67   1992
155.42'2--dc20   92-7965
                              CIP

Photograph acknowledgments: cover and pages xii, 18, 91,196, and 248, ©1989 Mark E. Gibson; page 56, ©1990 Mark E. Gibson; page 146, Jean-Claude Lejeune, Stock, Boston; page 304, Elizabeth Crews, Stock, Boston; page 353, Peter Menzel, Stock, Boston; page 388 Peter Vandermark, Stock, Boston; page 428, Elizabeth Crews, Stock, Boston; page 456, ©1991 Audrey Gibson; and page 502, Michael Dwyer, Stock, Boston.

92 93 94 95 10 9 8 7 6 5 4 3 2 1
Sage Production Editor: Judith L. Hunter

Foreword

A child's early years can build the foundation for a long, healthy life span characterized by curiosity and learning throughout its course. Investments in health and education can be guided by research in biomedical and behavioral sciences in ways likely to prevent much of the damage now being done to children. To bring this potential to fulfillment, we must understand what science can tell us about the first two years of life. These years offer a unique opportunity to construct fundamental building blocks of healthy development. The understanding of childhood casualties and ways to prevent them is illuminated by a developmental perspective. Indeed, the most rapid change and growth in the human life span occurs during the prenatal period through the first two years of life. These are, therefore, years of high vulnerability. Yet they are also times of maximal opportunity for prevention of casualties and promotion of optimal development. Many of the causes of damage to children are interrelated and potentially preventable at reasonable cost. Because such opportunities are heavily concentrated in the first two years of life, this book opens the door to vital but often neglected opportunities.

Is there a research basis for believing that we can affect the long-term course of a child's development by improving his or her environment in the early years? The weight of the available evidence indicates that improvement of damaging environmental conditions can indeed enhance child development, even after a bad start. Such interventions must be constructed on a broad base of firm information and reasonable concepts. A base of this kind cannot be built with a narrow, parochial approach.

This book draws on research and experience in a variety of fields and thereby provides the kind of broad-gauged assessment that is fully adequate to its important task. It is a highly credible and fully intelligible synthesis of existing knowledge about the crucial beginnings of human life. Anyone interested in child development, child health, and the underpinnings of education will find it valuable.

David A. Hamburg, M.D.

Contents

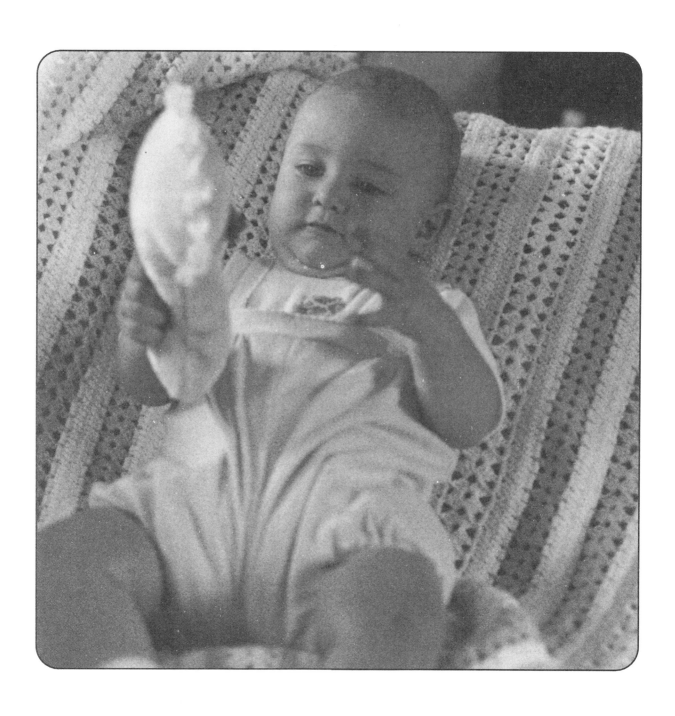

PART I. CONCEPTION THROUGH BIRTH

PART IV. THE SOCIAL CONTEXT

Preface

The study of infants was one of the first areas in which scientific observations of humans were gathered. It has enjoyed several spurts of popularity, most recently from the 1960s to the present, but very few infancy texts were available when the first edition of *In the Beginning* was written in 1985. Because of this paucity, and because we had enjoyed teaching an infancy course together, Judith Sims-Knight and I wrote that book. At the time this revision was in order, Sims-Knight had other responsibilities, hence, except for writing the chapter on cognition (Chapter 10), she has had no responsibility for this edition. As in the first edition, the chapter on language (Chapter 11) is by Paula N. Menyuk. The section on memory in Chapter 7 was drafted by Derek Price.

The text is designed for a broad range of students, including undergraduates with little exposure to psychology. Students using the first edition have ranged from sophomores to seniors and from psychology or biopsychology majors to art, history, and literature majors. I have tried to make the book interesting and relevant to other disciplines, particularly nursing and human development, and have included references that will be informative to this broad spectrum of students. In addition, the comprehensive coverage in the text and its orientation toward evaluation of empirical research make this an appropriate introductory text for graduate students.

This book has two major aims not often seen in textbooks. One is to embed the presentation of current data on and ideas about the functioning of infants in a historical context. In addition to a description of some of the history of the field in Chapter 1, historical studies are considered in the context of specific topics. The second major aim is to present the material in a way that will maximize learning about the process of studying infants as well as the content derived from that study. To do this, I use several techniques.

Research Methods and Issues. One goal of this book is to help students acquire a reading understanding of research methodology. Infancy research continues to grow at a rapid rate, and it is inevitable that facts learned today may be replaced by other facts tomorrow. The most valuable tool students can have is knowledge about how to evaluate new research. Then, when they are faced in later years with new outcomes of research that suggest particular action, they can evaluate the quality of the research and determine whether the new conclusions are reasonable or applicable to their questions. Many curricula leave such learning to methods courses, but it is my feeling that students in those courses often learn rules without developing the ability to apply them. I try to help students develop that ability by using techniques consistent with current understanding of learning. Recent research has demonstrated clearly that people remember material better when they learn it in a meaningful context. Thus research issues are presented here in the context of the research in which they appear. However, memory research also demonstrates that material learned in a specific context is often tied to that context. To solve this problem, a skills theory approach is taken (see Chapter 10). I assume that learning a concept is a skill that develops by combining, differentiating from, and intercoordinating with other skills. Therefore, the methodological points are presented in several contexts and, in the companion manual for this book, are presented in a more general fashion, but related to different instances included in the text. Instructors can choose whether or not to assign those sections, or students can choose whether to read them, assigned or not.

Major Issues or Controversies in Infancy Studies. The strategy for dealing with major issues in infancy studies is similar to that for research. General themes that permeate the study of infancy, such as critical periods or the influences of heredity and environment and their interactions, are presented in each of the several contexts in which they arise. Discussion sections in the manual extract major issues from their contexts and interrelate them.

Practical Implications of Infancy Research. Implications for parenting, and nursing and clinical applications of particular research findings are often noted in the text. They will be dealt with in more detail in the manual.

Theoretical Perspectives. Throughout the text, major theories are discussed in the contexts of the specific issues to which they are relevant. Again, it is my hope that this will be pedagogically more effective than discussion of theories as separable entities.

Vocabulary. Many words that students think are merely vocabulary are considered by instructors to be major concepts. Other words are important because understanding them is necessary to an understanding of a point central to the study of infancy, and others are used with special definitions in infancy research. The student needs to be aware of such words and to have ready access to their definitions. Such words are presented throughout this volume in bold type where they are accompanied by their definitions, be the definitions parenthetical or part of the text. The index carries boldface page numbers for pages on which such terms are defined, so that students can go back to look for definitions as needed.

Many of my colleagues helped me to achieve completion of this edition by commenting on drafts of chapters: Barbara J. Myers for Chapters 1 and 5; Anneliese Korner and Tiffany Field for Chapter 2; Betsy Dyer of Wheaton College's Biology Department for Chapter 3; Dr. Charles Eades, director of obstetrics and gynecology at the Massachusetts Institute of Technology, for Chapter 4; Rachel K. Clifton for several versions of Chapter 7; Derek Price for Chapters 9 and 10; and Kathryn Ann Hirsh-Pasek for Chapter 11. Any errors that remain are solely my fault, or those of the chapter's author. In addition to this help, I am deeply indebted to Marylyn Rands, a former Wheaton College colleague, who patiently edited several drafts of each chapter and helped put the references into proper format.

The addition of a manual for this edition reflects several aims. First, I wanted to add more study hints and recommendations for other readings than could be encompassed in the text. Second, the amount of new material it was necessary to incorporate into the text made it excessively long, even if only the same discussion sections as used last time were to be included.[1] Third, I wanted to be able to include implications for nurses as well as for parents and future parents. Finally, I thought that students might profit from, or even like to have, questions raised for their "prior to examination" thinking. Hence it is my hope that students will opt to use the manual to help them achieve some of the learning goals referred to above.

Judy F. Rosenblith

---

1. Although it is customary to list all authors' names in a first citation of a given work, I have taken the liberty to use et al. for all works authored by three or more people even on a first mention due to the length and complexity of this volume.

NOTE: The author prefers the Latin spelling of Caesarean, however, the publisher decided to use the medical spelling of the term.

Historical and Methodological Introduction

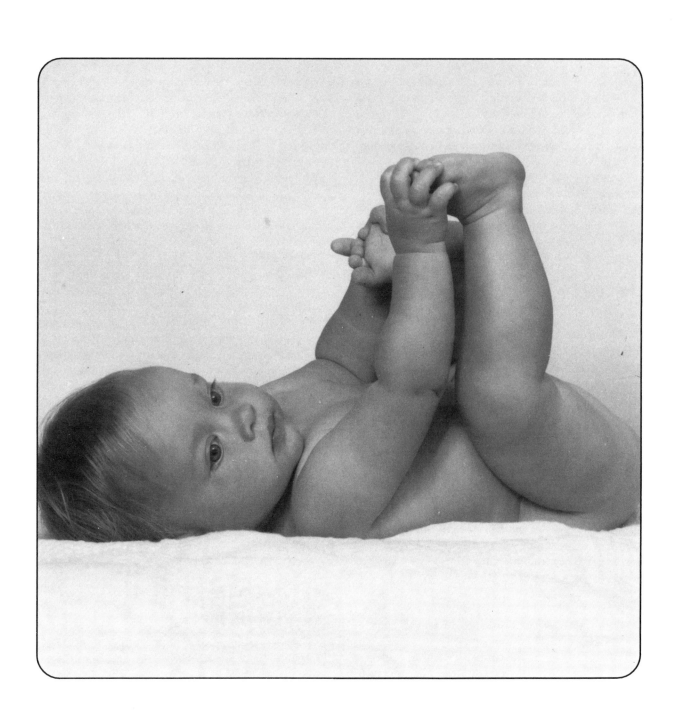

Studying infants has become an extremely popular enterprise in psychology today. Research journals are filled with reports of studies with infants, and one journal is devoted entirely to infancy. Many colleges and universities are introducing courses on infancy into their curricula. Similar excitement over the study of infancy has recurred several times in the history of psychology. A major reason for such intense interest in infancy is that to understand any psychological process fully, one must understand its origins. Fields other than psychology have substantial interests in infancy as well, and research in the field is done by nurses, doctors, and other professionals.

This chapter has two goals. The first is to introduce the reader to the history of the study of infancy, a study that predates the experimental study of humankind. The second is to show how various scientific methods have developed in the course of this research. The chapter begins with a discussion of the reasons for studying infants, as described in the nineteenth century and today. This discussion is followed by descriptions of the various ways in which researchers study infants, in the sequence in which they developed, and the strengths and weaknesses of each approach. The chapter concludes with a discussion of major methodological points.

Reasons for Studying Infants

Infancy is unique in all the ages of humankind in that it marks the beginning of life outside the womb. Through the study of infancy, researchers can explore (a) the roles of heredity and the environment in development; (b) the impact of experiences, particularly the possibly critical early influence of parents, on development; and (c) the impact on parenting of educating parents about the normal course of development. These three themes will recur throughout this book and will be discussed in detail where appropriate.

EARLY INTERESTS

The issues noted above also motivated early researchers. The Department of Education of the American Social Science Association sponsored a group of papers on infant development at their 1881 meeting in Saratoga, New York. They published these papers in the November 1882 issue of the *Journal of Social Science*. Mrs. Emily Talbot (1882), secretary of the department, discussed what is perhaps the all-time favorite issue in infant research, the question of the roles heredity and environment play in development:

That a child does most of his actions by inherited instincts seems to me most plausible. I think, as comparing children with dogs, that, aside from the physical condition, the inherited taste is first shown. Little puppies of a retriever breed will begin to take things hither and thither in their mouths long before puppies of an uneducated ancestry, though there will be a difference in talent and exceptions. In children, besides the natural self-assertion of a young child, there will continually crop out a hint of an inherited facility, which he uses without being taught. Then there is association. Having always seen a dog about, he has no fear of a dog, wants to pull him and roll about with him, does not fear the bark of a dog, though a little startled, if sharp; but of horses he has fear, and a certain fascinated interest—wants to know them, and yet is afraid. (p. 15)

Charles Darwin (1882) focused on some specific issues concerning environmental influences, namely, the role parental influence plays in the development of intelligence and individual differences:

This knowledge [of infants] would probably give a foundation for some improvement in our education of young children, and would show us whether the same system ought to be followed in all cases.

I will venture to specify a few points of enquirry which, as it seems to me, possess some scientific interest. For instance, does the education of the parents influence the mental powers of their children at any age, either at a very early or somewhat more advanced stage?

As observation is one of the earliest faculties developed in young children, and as this power would probably be exercised in an equal degree by the children of educated and uneducated persons, it seems not impossible that any transmitted effect from education could be displayed only at a somewhat advanced age.

It is well known that children sometimes exhibit at a very early age strong special tastes, for which no cause can be assigned although occasionally they may be accounted for by reversion to the taste or occupation of some progenitor; and it would be interesting to learn how far such early tastes are persistent and influence the future career of the individuals. In some instances such tastes die away without apparently leaving any after effect; but it would be desirable to know how far this is commonly the case, as we should then know whether it were important to direct, as far as this is possible, the early tastes of our children. It may be more beneficial that a child should follow energetically some pursuit, of however trifling a nature, and thus acquire perseverance, than that he should be turned from it, because of no future advantage to him. (pp. 6-7)

W. T. Harris (1882), the head of the American Social Science Association, was interested in the role that learning about their infants can play in mothers' abilities to rear them. He believed that through observing her baby,

the mother shall learn to study the growth of her child, and learn what constitutes a stage of progress, and how to discover and remove obstacles to this growth, as well as to afford judicious aid to the child's efforts at mastering the use of his faculties. One intelligent woman who is interested in this subject will kindle an interest which will spread throughout an entire town. The wisdom gained through these observations will extend gradually to all families, and will elevate the character of infant education incalculably.

When the mother becomes observant of the actions of the child as a matter of education, and when there comes to be a stock of generalized experiences on this subject, how much will be done toward correcting evil tendencies upon their first manifestations! It is a trite remark, that the shaping of a tree is an easy affair if undertaken while it is a sapling, but impossible after the tree has attained its growth. The education that goes on within the family is the object which now calls with most importunity on us for our attention as students of social science. (p. 5)

CURRENT INTERESTS

These crucial questions still motivate infant researchers, but a century of research has both narrowed the range of acceptable hypotheses and dramatically increased the precision with which they can be stated. For example, researchers have identified the genetic mechanisms underlying certain disorders and can now examine the ways in which environment interacts with that genetic potential. Even when the specific mechanisms are not known, techniques now exist that enable assessment of whether there is an inherited component to certain behavioral characteristics. Such research has led to the understanding that inheritance always acts through the environment. Thus the important question concerns how heredity interacts with environment, not determination of the relative contributions of each.

Research has also demonstrated that **innate**[1] characteristics (those present at birth) are not purely inherited—that is, that the environment influences individuals long before they are born. For example, it is no longer assumed that a baby an hour old who is very active has inherited a tendency to high activity. Researchers now try to distinguish characteristics that are stable within individuals because they are inherited from those that are stable either because the environment remains stable or because the environment has permanently affected the individual.

A related issue is that of innate ideas. Interest in whether infants are born with some understanding of how the world is organized derives from the philosophical field of **epistemology** (the study of knowledge). The psychological exploration is quite distinct from the philosophical. Because newborn babies have not experienced the world outside the womb, particularly the visual world, they are perfect subjects for the study of innate ideas. If, for example, researchers could show that newborns act as if they know what an object is—that it is three-dimensional, has tactile attributes, and exists independent of the infant—we would have to conclude that humans have innate ideas (a priori synthetic ideas, according to Kant).

Just as research in the last 100 years has led to more complex questions about the influence of heredity, it has led to differentiation among different kinds of environmental influences. Foremost in this domain has been the study of **critical periods**. During a critical period a baby is particularly sensitive to certain kinds of environmental influences. These may be biological influences, such as diseases or drugs taken by the mother during prenatal development, or postnatal environmental influences. For example, learning may take place rapidly and easily during a critical period, but at other times the same environmental events will not have the same effects. The effects of environmental stimulation during critical periods are supposed to be permanent. The timing of a critical period is determined by an individual's biological timetable, and so critical periods represent an interaction between heredity and environment. Critical periods were discovered in **embryology** (the study of biological differentiation from the fertilized egg), but the concept has been applied to many aspects of psychological development as well. For example, Sigmund Freud hypothesized that infancy was a critical period for babies to establish the basic ability to love.

---

1. Throughout this volume, words that are important to understand will appear in boldface when first used, and a definition will be provided in context. In the index, numbers of pages on which such words are first defined appear in bold.

Other kinds of environmental influences also are crucial to development. When and how babies learn by making associations and by imitating are topics that have been of interest to researchers of both the nineteenth and twentieth centuries. Others have focused on learning via cognitive structures. Explicit or implicit in all this research have been the questions of when and how infants' early experiences affect their development.

All of the conceptualizations of the roles of heredity and environment considered together form the basis from which parents' roles in their infants' development can be examined. Researchers no longer ask simply whether a characteristic or a behavior of parents has an effect or not. Rather, they must ask to which of their parents' behaviors do infants respond, and how do parental influences interact with other influences. They have learned that it is especially important to differentiate between immediate effects and long-term effects. It is no longer taken as unassailable truth that parents' influences in infancy determine an offspring's entire life.

Finally, the role that educating parents may have in improving the quality of their parenting is still of vital concern. Researchers no longer assume that it is sufficient simply to expose parents to knowledge of how infants develop, but frequently focus on parents' skills at interacting with their infants.

Thus in infancy research, as in other areas, the more things change the more they remain the same. Although the research has become much more sophisticated, the basic questions remain the same. Likewise, although the answers to basic questions are undoubtedly more accurate today than they were a century ago, they remain tentative. As the famed philosopher Herbert Feigl was fond of saying, answers in science are always true only until further notice (personal communication to Sims-Knight, 1968).

The Beginnings of Behavioral Study of Infants

The history of the psychological study of babies begins with a series of baby biographies in the nineteenth century. The rise of such detailed descriptions of babies was part of the general burst of interest in naturalistic observations. Indeed, Charles Darwin, a naturalist and one of the originators of the theory of evolution, was also an early baby biographer (1877). The first baby biography, however, was published almost 100 years before Darwin's by a German philosopher, Dietrich Tiedemann, in 1787. Several more were published before the "evolutionary" era of the next century. Wilhelm Preyer, a German physiologist, published a somewhat more scientific account of his son's first year of life (Preyer, 1880/1888; see also 1881/1889). It is Preyer, not Tiedemann, who is often credited with being the father of child psychology.

Of the dozens of early naturalistic observations, all but one were of infant development. The exception was the Swiss educator Pestalozzi's diary of his attempts to educate his 4-year-old son. Most of the subjects of these biographies were boys and the authors were their fathers. A notable exception was A. Bronson Alcott's observations of his daughters, especially Anna and Louisa May.

Baby biographies became so popular during the nineteenth century that the Department of Education of the American Social Science Association sponsored a systematic register of baby biographies for the purpose of unlocking "some portion of the secrets of the mental and physical development of infants" (Talbot, 1882, pp. 5-6).

STRENGTHS AND WEAKNESSES OF BABY BIOGRAPHIES

Examination of the early baby biographies can show us both the strengths and the weaknesses of this approach. Lest you think this is only of historical interest, let me hasten to point out that one of the major contributors to our current understanding of infants, Jean Piaget, based his theory of cognitive development on naturalistic observations (baby biographies) of his own three children. Like Preyer, Piaget was highly systematic in making observations and presented his children with numerous informal experimental situations. The baby biography is still a way of achieving scientific insight. The following discussion is presented in the hope that it will both help readers to evaluate existing baby biographies and guide those who wish to write their own. I make use in what follows of many excerpts from baby biographies in order to make methodological points about the study of infants. These are not presented for the reader to learn who said what, or to learn Piagetian psychology (which will come later in the book).

Let us first consider the strengths of such naturalistic observations. Descriptions of behaviors in naturalistic situations provide the starting point of science. There is much to learn about babies from simply watching them, without interfering in their functioning. The following examples from Tiedemann (1787/1927) are descriptions of behaviors that we would today identify as **reflexes** (innate, automatic responses to specific stimuli).

> He had no idea as yet of purposely grasping anything; grasping occurred only by instinctive reflex, by which the fingers, like the leaves of flowers of certain sensitive plants, contract when their inner surfaces are touched by a foreign object. (pp. 207-208)
>
> If he was held in arms and then suddenly lowered from a considerable height, he strove to hold himself with his hands, to save himself from falling; and he did not like to be lifted very high. Since he could not possibly have had any conception of falling, his fear was unquestionably a purely mechanical sensation, such as older persons feel at a steep and unaccustomed height, something akin to dizziness. (p. 216)[2]

Observers can also record newborns' responses to visual, auditory, and tactile stimuli, and thus answer the question of whether newborn babies can see and hear. The first of the following extracts is from Tiedemann's baby biography. The second is from Alcott's letter to the Department of Education of the American Social Science Association for its 1881 meeting. The last two are from the register of baby biographies sponsored by that organization and reported at that meeting.

> It was observed that the boy, when hearing a sound, always turned his face in the direction whence it came; so he had already learned to tell what he heard through the right ear, and what through the left, had also accustomed himself to think of spaces in some sort of relation to his body. (Tiedemann, 1787/1927, p. 217)
>
> During the first days after birth she slept most of the time. As she gradually awoke and was exposed to the light, she opened her eyes as if intent on adjusting these for the purpose of seeing. Luminous objects particularly attracted her notice. While viewing these her hands moved instinctively, her arms were extended and drawn toward the mouth, which also appeared to be sensitive to the stimulus by frequent movements of the lips and tongue. (Alcott, 1882, p. 8)
>
> Medical works give six to ten hours as the earliest time at which hearing is possible, but my boy, born at 1:30, certainly heard, and nervously started at the sound of the cock crowing at 4:30. (Talbot, 1882, p. 12)
>
> He recognized [responded to] the light of a win-

> dow [evidently] at the age of 20 hours, as he was looking at it he was turned round so as to bring the other side towards the window, and at once turned his head towards it. He recognized sounds in a day or two. The younger [twin] recognized light and sound in the same way a day or two later. . . .
>
> . . . (Ten days old) Both evidently noticed a piano played in another room, stopped their incessant baby motions to listen, and put on the same listening look as adults do. This was repeated for a day or two, at times when the piano played; but afterwards as the sound grew familiar they ceased to notice it. (Talbot, 1882, pp. 14-16)

A second achievement permitted by longitudinal observation of one infant or of a group of infants is the plotting of developmental changes over age, such as the disappearance of reflexes and the development of other observable behaviors, such as grasping and language.

The intensive observations of baby biographers can have an advantage over other kinds of studies, both cross-sectional and normative. The changes in development can be charted against the background of the infant's own past, and the behaviors can be placed in the context of the environment and the other behaviors of that infant. Thus the baby biography provides the potential for a rich and full understanding of the meaning of infants' behaviors in a fashion unique to the method. Unfortunately, these same characteristics make baby biographies more vulnerable to misinterpretation and error than are more controlled techniques, as will be explained later.

A good example of the richness of knowledge gleaned from baby biographies can be seen in the following excerpt from Tiedemann's (1787/1927) description of his son's language development:

> On November 29th one could observe a signification of [the] sort that indicated a certain amount of complexity in his ideas, and spoke of some amount of original composition on his part. He had been taught to reply to the question, "How big are you?" ["Wie gross bist du?" in German] by lifting up his hands; now he was required to say the word "grandmama" ["grossmama"] and as the "grand" ["gross"] was too difficult for him to pronounce, he lifted up his hands and at the same time said "mama." (p. 221)

---

2. While the dizziness of older persons does not seem a good analogy, the reflex is an innate automatic response to loss of support. Perhaps a mechanical sensation is appropriate.

Tiedemann was able to describe language development accurately when he was dealing with explicit behaviors that he could clearly observe. Such observations of behaviors and developmental sequences of behaviors are just the first step in the study of infants. The ultimate goal, for both early baby biographers and modern researchers, is to discover the meaning of the behaviors they describe. They want to know, for example, what the infant understands when he says "mama" for the first time. They also want to know how the infant came to be able to say "mama." Was it because his parents had rewarded him for making similar sounds, or was it because his vocal apparatus and brain had matured sufficiently, or were both factors involved?

It is neither straightforward nor easy to assess the meaning of behaviors. Infant investigators, including both some early baby biographers and modern experimentalists, undertake their studies to find out whether their ideas about some aspect of development are correct or not. Unless their investigations are carefully controlled, their expectations are likely to influence their findings. A good example of the power of expectations is found in a study that showed pictures of newborn babies to adults (Rubin et al., 1974). Half the subjects were shown a picture of a baby labeled as a boy, and the others were told the same picture was of a girl. Even though they saw the same picture, subjects described the "girl" baby as cuter, smaller, and quieter and the "boy" baby as larger, stronger, and more vigorous.

Expectations may affect observations in several ways. They may encourage people to see behaviors that do not exist. The above subjects saw not only behavioral differences, but even physical differences that did not exist. Expectations also may cause people to fail to notice behaviors that are there. The best example of this is that psychologists, physicians, nurses, and parents during most of this century believed that newborn babies could not see or hear. Such early developed abilities did not fit the theoretical framework of the times. Behaviors that suggested these abilities were overlooked, or parents' reports of them were said to come from their sentimental biases. The baby biographers' accounts that documented such behaviors, as in the excerpts quoted above, were ignored.

What can be done to control expectations? Much of the scientific methodology developed in the last century has been a response to this problem. Two major strategies can be used in infant biographies or observational studies. First, observers can separate interpretations from descriptions of behaviors observed and can insist that the actual behaviors of the infants provide the basic data of the studies. The second strategy is to develop techniques that can ferret out alternate interpretations and test the validity of each one.

The first strategy can and should always be used, even by parents making baby biographies of their own children. The following example from Tiedemann (1787/1927) demonstrates an observation that does not clearly separate behavior from interpretation:

> Are, then, all the movements of children at this age unintentional? Or could there already be some purpose and acquired knowledge? One circumstance, I think, indicates that even at such an early stage some learning process may occur. The mother was yet unable to offer the child the food which nature intended for him [nursing not established, baby a few days old]; artificial feeding was so far avoided for the reason mentioned above, so he had to suffer some want, and, as he was healthy, some hunger. For the relief he sought to put his own and, if possible, other people's fingers into his mouth in order to suck them, though indeed he did not find his mouth save after many vain attempts. Herein, methinks we can discern something learned, something intentional. (pp. 207-208)

One would be hard-pressed to determine the validity of Tiedemann's statements in this example. It is unknown whether he assumed the baby was suffering or whether the child did something (such as fussing or crying) that was interpretable as suffering. It is unknown what the infant did to make his father think he was intending to put fingers in his mouth for relief, or even why Tiedemann thought they provided relief. Subsequent, more behaviorally based, observations do not support the notion that babies intend to relieve hunger by sucking fingers in the first week of life, although, to be sure, if they find their hands to suck they will be quieted.

Now consider this example from Taine's (1876/1877) baby biography:

> From about ten months, when asked, "Where is grandfather?" she turns to this portrait and laughs. Before the portrait of her grandmother, not so good a likeness, she makes no such gesture, and gives no sign of intelligence. From eleven months when asked "Where is mamma?" she turns toward her mother, and she does the same for her father. I should not venture to say that these actions surpass the intelligence of animals. A little dog, here, understands as well when it hears the word, sugar; it comes from the other end of the garden to get a bit. There is nothing more in this than an association,

for the dog, between a sound and some sensation of taste, for the child between a sound and the form of an individual face perceived; the object denoted by the sound has not as yet a general character.

Here there is a clear differentiation between behaviors (described in the first three sentences) and the interpretation (everything from "I should not venture" to the end of the excerpt). Notice the difference between the excerpt from Taine and this one from Tiedemann (1787/1927) on the same point:

Now he learned also to comprehend a few sentences; on the 14th he knew already what was meant by: "Make a bow," "Swat the fly," which he always accompanied by the appropriate motions. (p. 220)

Tiedemann concluded that his son understood certain phrases ("Make a bow," "Swat the fly") because he always accompanied them by the appropriate motions. The behaviors observed are parallel to those in Taine, but the interpretations differ.

Observations of infants that clearly differentiate behaviors from interpretations provide two advantages over other observations. First, readers know that the infant did something to warrant an interpretation. Second, they can evaluate the reasonableness of the interpretation for themselves.

Once behaviors and interpretations are separated, the observer's interpretation can be evaluated critically. An effective way of doing this within an observational framework is to compare it to alternate interpretations. Once several interpretations are generated, one can see that the original interpretation may be wrong. An example of this procedure for the development of word meaning has just been provided in the above comparison of Tiedemann's conclusions to those of Taine.

Although the early baby biographers rarely did so, it is possible to consider alternate interpretations while doing systematic observations. Piaget's (1945/1962) observations are replete with examples such as the following:

OBS. 1. On the very night after his birth, T. was wakened by the babies in the nearby cots and began to cry in chorus with them. At 0;0 (3) he was drowsy, but not actually asleep, when one of the other babies began to wail; he himself thereupon began to cry. At 0;0 (4) and 0;0 (6) he again began to whimper, and started to cry in earnest when I tried to imitate this interrupted whimpering. A mere whistle and other cries failed to produce any reaction.

There are two possible interpretations of these commonplace observations, but neither of them seems to justify the use of the word imitation. On the one hand it may be that the baby was merely unpleasantly affected by being wakened by the cries of his neighbors, yet without establishing any relation between the sounds he heard and his own crying, whereas the whistle or other sound left him indifferent. On the other hand, it is possible that the crying occurred as a result of its repetition, owing to a kind of reflex analogous to that we saw in the case of suction . . . , but in this case with intensification of the sound through the help of the ear. In this second case, the crying of the other babies would increase the vocal reflex through confusion with his own crying.

Thus in neither case is there imitation, but merely the starting off of a reflex by an external stimulus. (p. 7)[3]

Piaget considered three interpretation—sone claiming the newborn imitated and two claiming it did not—that other processes were involved. This alone helps us to become aware that any one interpretation may be wrong. Notice also that Piaget considered imitation to be an inappropriate interpretation here. He argued that an interpretation of imitation requires the assumption that infants are more advanced (more cognitively complex) than do the other two alternatives. In good scientific tradition, Piaget accepted the simpler explanation, the one that demands the fewest assumptions: that infants respond reflexively to crying. He applied, in scientific terminology, the principle of **parsimony**, known historically as "Occam's razor."

In the comparative example presented earlier, Taine and not Tiedemann applied the principle of parsimony. Taine concluded that infants can respond appropriately to certain words or phrases without necessarily understanding them. The process of associating a motoric response to the verbal stimulus is a simpler one than the process of understanding. Accepting the more parsimonious explanation is often a good strategy, but it is not necessarily always correct. Sometimes more complex interpretations will be supported by later research. Indeed, investigators are still trying to ascertain whether or not the seemingly imitative responses of newborns are truly imitation, as shall be seen in Chapter 9.

Piaget employed two other techniques for deciding

3. The three numbers in Piaget's age notations refer to years of age, months of age, and (days of age). For example, 0;0 (3) describes a 3-day-old infant.

among alternate hypotheses. One was to collect a number of different instances of behavior that were consistent with his favored interpretation. The second was to introduce informal experiments into the observations. In the following example, Piaget (1945/1962) uses both techniques to support his interpretation that babies progress (from the earlier crying example) to a stage in which they truly imitate, but imitate only those actions that are already familiar to them.

> OBS. 9. At 0;6 (25) J. invented a new sound by putting her tongue between her teeth. It was something like pfs. Her mother then made the same sound. J. was delighted and laughed as she repeated it in her turn. Then came a long period of mutual imitation. J. said pfs, her mother imitated her, and J. watched her without moving her lips. Then when her mother stopped, J. began again and so it went on. Later on, after remaining silent for some time, I myself said pfs. J. laughed and at once imitated me. There was the same reaction the next day, beginning in the morning (before she had herself spontaneously made the sound in question) and lasting throughout the day. At 0;7 (11) and on the following days, I only had to say pfs for her to imitate me correctly at once. At 0;7 (13) she imitated this sound without seeing me or realizing where it was coming from. (pp. 19-20)

In this excerpt we see that Piaget was trying to establish that J.'s vocalization was truly imitation. To do so he varied the situation to eliminate other interpretations. He ascertained that J. would imitate both Mommy and Daddy; this demonstration eliminated the hypothesis that the behavior was simply an interactive game with Mommy rather than imitation of a particular behavior. He then found out that J. would imitate even when she had not just made the response herself; this eliminated the hypothesis that J. could reproduce actions only if she was in the midst of repeating them anyway. Finally, he showed that it was not a learned response to Mommy's and Daddy's faces and bodies by demonstrating that J. imitated the sound even when she could not see Daddy.

In this same section Piaget goes on to show that this is not merely a vocal response to one specific vocal stimulus by presenting examples of the imitation of other sounds.

> OBS. 11. At 0;7 (17) J. at once imitated the sounds pfs, bva, mam, abou, hla, and a new phoneme pff which she had been trying out for several days, dif-

ferentiating between them, and without having made them herself immediately before. She was enjoying the imitation, and no longer producing one sound instead of another. (pp. 20-21)

Piaget next provided examples of his infants at the same stage imitating motoric actions, such as sticking out the tongue, opening and closing hands, and "waving." He always gathered as many examples as he could to support his interpretation and did informal experiments to differentiate among hypotheses. The following is a particularly clear example of his use of informal experiments:

> At 0;4 (23) without any previous practice, I showed L. my hand which I was slowly opening and closing. She seemed to be imitating me. All the time my suggestion lasted she kept up a similar movement and either stopped or did something else as soon as I stopped. There was the same reaction when I repeated the experiment at 0;4 (26). But was this response of L. merely due to an attempt at prehension? To test this, I then showed her some other object. She again opened and closed her hand, but only twice, then immediately tried to seize the object and suck it. I resumed the experiment with my hand, and she clearly imitated it, her gesture being quite different from the one she made on seeing the toy. (p. 23)

Although Piaget's techniques were a decided improvement over the more limited ones used by earlier baby biographers, they still have their limitations. The observer/experimenter's biases may still play a large role. For example, we have to take Piaget's word that L.'s gestures were different in the two instances described in the last excerpt. We have to assume that Piaget was not ignoring many behaviors that were nonimitative. For example, J. may have responded pfs to hearing pfs only 35% of the times she heard pfs. Piaget believed she could imitate, and hence may have tended to focus on the instances in which she did imitate and missed the instances in which she did not. If you believed that 7-month-old infants could not imitate, would you consider that imitation in 35% of the instances was sufficient to be called imitation and not chance responding?

Another problem looms larger in baby biographies. Piaget, for example, derived his entire theory of infancy (and three books) from observations of his three children. No three children are an adequate basis from which to **generalize** (i.e., apply the result) to all children. Three children from one family of a brilliant father who are interacted with intensively throughout their infancies provide an even less adequate sample. For these reasons, psychologists in the United States are unwilling to accept research based solely on baby biographies. They insist that such findings as those reported by Tiedemann and Piaget be replicated by well-controlled systematic studies of relatively large groups of infants.

NORMATIVE/DESCRIPTIVE STUDIES

The problem of generalization that is characteristic of baby biographies is solved by **normative/descriptive studies**, which were first developed about 50 years after the first baby biography. In such studies, groups of infants are observed with respect to selected behaviors. The primary goals of such research are to establish that a particular sequence of development occurs and to determine the average age at which each step of the sequence occurs. The former describes development and the latter establishes **norms**, hence the compound name. These studies have an advantage over the infant biographies in that their samples provide a better representation of infants in general than did the beloved offspring of the erudite baby biographers.

The earliest normative study was a thesis, *Observations on the Normal Functioning of the Human Body*, written by Heinrich Feldman, a physician, and published in 1833. The observations of the first 6 pages of this 35-page paper are of walking and speaking in 35 healthy infants. Feldman reported the average age at which babies walked unaided and uttered their first words.

Feldman's infant study was **longitudinal** as well as normative/descriptive; that is, the same children were studied at several ages. Studies that are not longitudinal are **cross-sectional**; that is, different children are studied at each of the ages—a cross section of each age is studied. Baby biographies are by definition longitudinal, but normative/descriptive studies may be either cross-sectional or longitudinal. Early researchers seem to have been more patient than modern investigators; they favored longitudinal studies, while most present-day research is of the more rapidly completed cross-sectional type.

The next landmark normative study, by Kussmaul, another physician, was published in 1859. Although the first pages of this work are devoted to the development of the soul in the first postnatal days, the final two-thirds contains a sophisticated scientific report on findings (Kussmaul's own and those of others) on the functioning of the various senses in the newborn pe-

riod, including taste, smell, touch, pain, sight, and hearing. Kussmaul also included a section on the intelligence of newborns and the responses of **premature** newborns (babies who were born before they were due, or before term).

Many similar studies were done later in the nineteenth century, some of which were intensive studies of a single response, such as the force of sucking. Also in this period we find a doctoral dissertation that repeated many of Kussmaul's earlier experiments, often with large numbers of infants (Genzmer, 1873). This is an early example of a **replication** study, a study designed to test whether previous findings could be obtained again. Replicability is a crucial test of the validity of scientific findings. (By the way, Kussmaul's findings generally did replicate.)

Normative/descriptive studies continue to be an important area of research. Modern normative/descriptive studies of infant physical, motor, and intellectual milestones are described in Chapter 8, which also presents discussion of the meaning and legitimate uses of norms. Other normative/descriptive studies focus on the typical sequence of changes of behaviors rather than on the age at which each kind of behavior is typical. For example, in a descriptive study designed to test Piaget's notions of imitation, one would observe the reactions of a number of babies to adult actions to see if the sequence Piaget described held for children other than his own. Many such studies are described in Chapter 10.

Normative/descriptive studies serve very important practical purposes, including enabling child-care professionals and parents to decide whether a given child is severely delayed in achieving developmental milestones. They also serve as the basis for theoretical interpretations of behaviors, but they do not permit researchers to decide among alternate explanations for the behaviors (or developmental sequences of behaviors). Experiments and correlational studies are necessary for that.

Modern Research Techniques

Since the first psychological laboratories were established in the 1880s and 1890s, much of the history of psychology has involved the development of research methods that permit more probing analyses into questions of age-old interest. This has also been true for studies of infant development. As these techniques have improved, researchers have been better able to test causal hypotheses with respect to developmental sequences.

EXPERIMENTS

Experiments provide the most convincing evidence to be used in judging alternative interpretations. The nature of experiments is perhaps most easily understood in the situation in which the interpretation being tested is whether or not one event directly causes another. For example, Tiedemann noticed that his newborn son struck his face with his hands and did not use them to grasp, so he concluded that the baby did not understand distance. Later, he noticed, his child reached for things accurately. Tiedemann concluded that touching things must "aid sight in forming a conception of external and removed bodies" (distances). The best way to test whether his hypothesis is correct is through an experiment in which one group of babies is prevented from using their hands by **swaddling** (tightly wrapping the baby in such a way that the hands are not free) and another group is allowed to use their hands. If Tiedemann was correct, then the group of babies who used their hands would understand distances (reach more accurately, not strike their faces) at an earlier age than the group who had not used their hands. If the two groups did not differ, the alternative hypothesis (interpretation), that touching is not necessary to form a conception of depth, would be supported.

Since experiments are so important, let us consider their characteristics carefully. The experimenter manipulates the hypothesized cause (the **independent variable**) and measures the consequences on the hypothesized effect (the **dependent variable**). In the example above, experience with the hands is the independent variable and accurate reaching is the dependent variable. Experiments are the one sure way to test causal relations because they are the only studies in which the experimenter has adequate control over the relevant variables.

The experimenter sets up the study so that the only difference between the two groups is the hypothesized cause (use of the hands). This is accomplished by two means. First, the experimenter makes sure that all other conditions (the ages at which the children are tested, the kind of test of reaching they are given, and so forth) are constant. Second, the experimenter assigns subjects to groups **randomly**; that is, subjects are put in particular groups based on pure chance. In the above example, coin tosses could be used to assign subjects to groups. If the coin came up heads, the infant would be in the experimental group (prevented from using hands); if the coin came up tails, the infant would be in the control group (allowed to use hands). Random assignment of subjects to these groups controls for variations among subjects that might result from other techniques of assignment. For example, if differences in the accuracy of their reaching were found and the mothers had been allowed to choose whether or not to swaddle their babies, the differences might result from other maternal behaviors rather than from the experimental restriction of the babies' hands. The mothers who asked that their babies' hands be

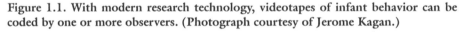

Figure 1.1. With modern research technology, videotapes of infant behavior can be coded by one or more observers. (Photograph courtesy of Jerome Kagan.)

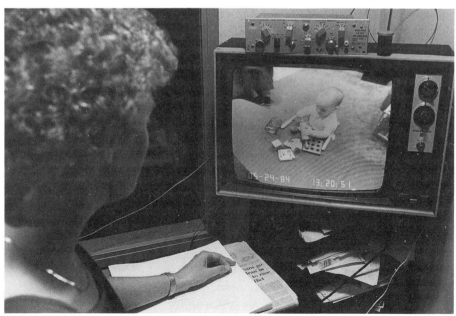

free might be more concerned with the babies' motoric development and might spend more time explicitly training their infants to reach and grasp. If so, and if the nonswaddled group developed motor coordination of their hands more rapidly, the experimenter would not be able to tell whether this was due to the lack of swaddling or to the mothers' training. The mothers' actions are called **extraneous variables** and can be said to have **confounded** the experiment—that is, confounded our ability to find out whether the infants' experience with their hands produced accurate reaching. The confounding occurs because either the independent variable or the extraneous variable, or both, may produce any observed effects.

If infancy researchers could experimentally assess all the issues in which they are interested, they would have much less difficulty in establishing and expanding our knowledge of babies and their development. Unfortunately, many interesting phenomena cannot be studied by the experimental method, especially not with humans. The swaddling study could not actually be done with humans for both ethical and practical reasons. Ethically, the problem is that some parents would be asked to behave toward their babies in ways that deviate from their familial or cultural patterns, thus making them uncomfortable; they would also be asked to make changes in their infant care techniques that might possibly have long-term negative effects on their babies (although we would expect rapid catch-up after swaddling was discontinued). Practically, it would be difficult for parents who were assigned to a condition that did not match their natural inclinations to comply with the experimenter's instructions. This could cause the experimental manipulation to fail. Failure to find a difference between the two groups would then falsely suggest that the treatment had no effect, when, in fact, there had been no "treatment." In these and many other circumstances, different techniques must be used.

CORRELATIONAL STUDIES

Correlational studies, the major alternative to experiments, are studies that indirectly measure a relation between two variables. For example, if the swaddling study discussed above were correlational, the investigator would assess the degree of arm movements babies exhibit in their everyday lives. The researcher might then place the babies into two categories —those with free and those with restricted arm movements—or might give them a range of scores representing the degree of arm movements (from most to least arm movements). The development of the babies'

understanding of distance would be assessed in the same way as in the experiment. The relation between the **predictor variable** (the variable hypothesized to relate to, or predict, the outcome variable—often called the independent variable) and the outcome variable would be assessed statistically, often by a statistic called the **correlation coefficient**. This is a statistic that assesses the degree to which two variables co-relate. A **significant** correlation between the variables indicates that there is a relation between the amount of swaddling and the development of understanding of distance that exceeds what would be found by chance. The size of the correlation (which can vary from 0 to 1.00) determines whether it is significant for the size group on which it was obtained. A correlation can be either positive (the larger one variable is, the larger the other) or negative (the larger one variable is, the smaller the other). It also can be used to determine the strength of the relation. A nonsignificant correlation between the variables indicates that swaddling did not make a difference in the development of understanding of distance.

The limitations of correlational research become apparent when attempts are made to interpret the findings. The causal hypothesis in an experimental study is that the amount of arm movement (the independent or predictor variable) influences the development of perception of distance (the dependent variable). In a correlational study this interpretation or conclusion is not warranted. It could be that the babies' depth perception might have determined how much they moved their arms; that is, babies might move their arms to reach for something once they know it can be reached, hence the more they know, the more they move their arms.

Furthermore, these two exactly opposite conclusions are not the only possibilities. Because participants were not randomly assigned to groups, extraneous subject variables were not controlled. A third, extraneous variable might produce both the amount of arm movements and the perception of distance. For example, mothers who are concerned that their babies receive sensory stimulation are likely both to allow the babies free arm movements and to provide whatever experiences are crucial for development of perception of distance. Thus the mothers' actions to stimulate their babies may cause the variation in both measures and make it look—wrongly—as if the two variables were themselves causally related. Sometimes statistical techniques can be used to help clarify causal relations. And, in some cases, correlational findings can be used to design experimental studies, sometimes with other species.

Although causality cannot be tested directly in a correlational study, there are indirect methods. These are all less convincing than having the results of true experiments, but they do provide valuable ways of assessing the merits of alternative hypotheses.

Correlational studies sometimes try to approximate the equivalence of groups that should result from random assignment of subjects. They do this by establishing that the groups under study do not differ on various extraneous variables the researcher thinks might be relevant to the outcome of the study (age of babies, marital status of mothers, education of mothers, birth weight of babies, and so on). This helps improve confidence in the outcomes, but the researcher may not be aware of all variables that are important to control for. Random assignment of subjects should result in the random distribution of all extraneous variables, including those that are not thought of in advance. Furthermore, random assignment should result in random distributions of combinations of variables (for example, second-born children of mothers under 25 years old) in the groups being compared. Testing for comparability of a list of single variables can never be exhaustive and will never account for such combinations. Several varieties of the indirect method will be discussed throughout this book.

Correlational studies are also used in contexts other than those in which the question of causality (or what leads to what) is of prime importance. One such use is in exploring the stability of individual differences. For example, researchers may wish to know whether height and weight of newborns (or 2-year-olds) relate to the same qualities in adulthood. If the relations are strong (correlations very high), then one can predict the adult characteristic from the infant characteristic. Researchers may wish to know whether complex traits such as intelligence are stable from infancy to later childhood. To find out, they determine the correlations between the given characteristics at the two ages. Issues of stability will be raised throughout this book, and discussion of the broader issue of continuity in development can be found in Chapter 6 of the companion manual.

Research Issues

Methodological issues are discussed in the context of specific studies throughout this book and in the manual. This is done to show how these issues determine the conclusions that can reasonably be drawn from studies, not to subject readers to a study of methodology for its own sake. This approach has the

advantage of making what might otherwise seem dry, abstract, and often difficult material more concrete, meaningful, and alive. For example, it will be easier for the reader to understand what a longitudinal study is if that term is introduced as part of the description of a particular longitudinal study. In this chapter the discussion of research issues is somewhat more extensive and includes more new information than in comparable sections in other chapters.

SAMPLING

A major problem in infant research is that of avoiding biased samples. Participants in one particular study may or may not be representative of all subjects. What baby biographies found about the behaviors of children of highly intelligent, well-educated adults might not be true for children from other life circumstances. This is called the problem of **biased samples.** The word *sample* refers to the participants in a study; a sample is called *biased* when the participants are not representative of a larger group, called a **population,** which often in the case of infant studies is all babies (or all babies in the given society). Modern studies include a broader range of babies than did the baby biographies, but their samples are still rather restricted. Many studies rely on volunteers obtained through notices put up around university areas or through newspaper advertisements. Such volunteers are likely to be highly educated, middle-class, nonworking mothers who have time to bring their babies in for study. Other studies may draw their samples from clinic patients in urban community hospitals. Such samples are likely to be composed primarily of relatively uneducated persons from the lower socioeconomic classes, who are often members of minority groups.

Studies done with biased samples are not useless, because their findings can be applied to the groups that the sample represents. For example, if a study used subjects from a clinic population of a center-city hospital, conclusions could be generalized from that sample to other poor, urban babies. By the same token, it must be kept in mind that those conclusions might not hold for rural, middle-class infants. These are both cases of biased selection of a study group. Within a biased group, subjects may be assigned to experimental conditions in a biased or unbiased (random) way.

The number of subjects in a sample also influences the possibility of its being biased. No matter how carefully a sample of babies is chosen, if there are only a few of them, they may be an unusual group. Simply by bad luck the babies in a sample of 3 or 5 subjects may be all small, or all sleepy, or all advanced in development. As more and more subjects are added, a sample is more likely to include individuals who differ on relevant dimensions. A randomly selected sample with more than 30 members is less likely than smaller samples to be biased by chance. The Department of Education of the American Social Science Association, whose work in the 1880s has been mentioned, was aware of the biasing likely to occur with small samples, and so sponsored the collection of a large number of baby biographies to provide a more representative sample from which to draw conclusions about development.

RESEARCH DESIGN

The **design** of a study depends on what the researcher wants to know and on how much control he or she has over the conditions of the study. Normative/descriptive, correlational, and experimental designs have been introduced in this chapter. Each of these can be used in cross-sectional or longitudinal studies. Normative/descriptive studies chart the developmental sequences and seek to find out when something develops (early or late) and how it develops. Experimental studies try to find out what aspects of development are related or what causes something to develop in a particular way. Experiments investigate at least two variables and typically identify one as the cause (independent variable) and the other as the effect (dependent variable). Correlational studies do not

have independent variables and cannot determine causes, but may explore causal paths using one variable as the predictor variable. Figure 1.2 shows a baby being studied using psychophysiological measures—specifically, of heart rate and respiration—measures that might be used in either experimental or correlational studies.

Because the ultimate goal for many researchers is to find out what causes behavior, or what in the environment determines the course and speed of development, they must always keep in mind the strengths and limitations of each of these kinds of studies. Normative/descriptive studies cannot in themselves tell us what causes behaviors; making causal inferences from descriptive studies is inappropriate because the investigators do not have control over extraneous variables (but correlational analyses are sometimes possible).

To recap, in order to establish that the independent variable causes the behavior of interest, the dependent variable, all other possible causes, called extraneous variables, must be eliminated. This is achieved through two kinds of experimental controls. The first is the attempt to eliminate or control all extraneous variables in the procedures of the study, for example, by treating all participants as much alike as possible, except for the experimental treatment. The second control results from the random assignment of participants to experimental conditions; that is, participants are put into one condition or another by chance and only by chance. Each group will essentially be alike with respect to the distribution of such individual characteris-

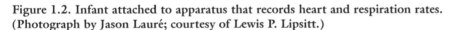

Figure 1.2. Infant attached to apparatus that records heart and respiration rates. (Photograph by Jason Lauré; courtesy of Lewis P. Lipsitt.)

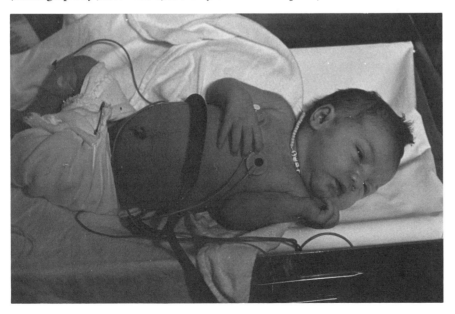

tics as physical and intellectual levels, family backgrounds, and influences of mother, which are potential extraneous variables. If differences are then found between groups, it can be assumed that they are due to the independent variable (provided there are enough subjects, preferably more than 30 in each group). Only experiments with these controls can yield results from which we can be confident that a causal relation exists between the independent and dependent variables.

Some "experiments" are done without random assignment of subjects. They try to compare the groups studied and show that they are alike on possible extraneous variables. But this demands knowledge of all relevant variables, and hence cannot be fully convincing. Correlational studies can try in various ways to approach the controls of experiments, but it is still true that "correlations cannot prove causality."

The second major variation in designs of studies concerns the number of samples and the times at which they are run. Researchers may (a) study one sample at one time, (b) compare two or more samples at one time, or (c) study one or more samples at two or more times. In developmental research comparisons of behavior at two or more ages are often the focus of attention. Such studies may be either cross-sectional (type b) or longitudinal (type c). The number of ages studied is determined by the goals and resources of the particular project. Cross-sectional studies use a different group of children for each age studied (technically a **between**-groups design), and therefore can be completed quite rapidly. In a matter of weeks or months a very large age span (say, newborns, 8-month-olds, and 2-year-olds) can be studied and compared.

All the baby biographies and most early normative studies were longitudinal. They studied the same children at more than one age. Longitudinal studies, which follow the same subjects or groups of subjects (technically a **within**-groups design), must wait for the children in their samples to grow up (2 years in the above example, but 20 years or more in some). This feature poses a new problem for the researcher: The longer the time period studied, the more likely it is that some earlier participants will no longer be available for study. Then conclusions drawn from the research must be tempered by the knowledge that the results are for a portion of the original sample. The higher the proportion who remain, and the more the researcher can show that the dropouts did not differ from those who remained in the study, the surer one can be of the research result.

Cross-sectional studies are often considered a shortcut approach to research that could be done with longitudinal studies. This assumes that two groups of infants at different ages are no different from one group of infants at two ages. Therefore, it is reasoned, it is not necessary to wait for the younger group to grow older to find out how they will behave when they are older. A group of similar babies who have already reached that older age can be substituted. This assumption is valid only if the samples at each age are comparable on all variables other than age (e.g., on sex, race, and social class), including what are called **cohort** variables. Children who grow up at different times are in different cohorts, and may be exposed to unique experiences—for example, to different childbirth practices, to different feeding practices, to TV or not, or to a depression or a famine. Some research questions do not permit the shortcut of a cross-sectional study. For example, if researchers want to explore the effects of early experience on later development, they have to follow the same infants from early infancy to later infancy, childhood, and adulthood, and therefore must do a longitudinal study.

REPLICABILITY

Another important criterion for judging any research is its replicability. **Replication** of a finding means that a study is repeated and the same results or relations are found. (People also talk about replicating a study when they repeat a study but do not find the same results—that is, do not replicate the findings.) Regardless of whether a study is cross-sectional or longitudinal, whether it is normative/descriptive, experimental, or correlational, replicability is the test of its value in predicting or understanding behavior and its development. It may sound like a waste of time to repeat studies, but it is by no means a foregone conclusion that the same results or relations will be obtained. Science provides only an approximate method of discovering truth, and the results of research are always subject to revision when the next study comes along. Because humankind has found no foolproof way of finding truth, scientists and consumers of science have to be satisfied with this approximate method and must be alert to its problems and guard against its errors. One of the best ways to do this is to repeat studies to see if they replicate. If they do, we can have some confidence that methodological flaws are not responsible for the results. If the time span is sufficient, we can have confidence that cultural changes over that time span have not changed the previous relations.

Some methodological flaws that may make a study nonreplicable have been discussed in this chapter. If a sample is biased or different, the findings may not replicate with a new sample. If extraneous variables have not been controlled for, they may differ in the replication study from what they were in the original study and thus lead to nonreplication. Common examples include instances in which the social class of the second sample may differ from that of the original, or the first study may have included only firstborns, whereas the second included many second- and third-born children.

Another type of extraneous variable that may be important resides in the researcher rather than in those studied. One researcher may expect that a study will support a particular hypothesis, and a second investigator attempting to replicate the study may not share that belief. Indeed, the effort to replicate may be based on the experimenter's belief that the previous results are not accurate. Good research methods minimize the role of expectations, both those of the experimenters and those of the subjects. Nevertheless, some evidence, although controversial, suggests that even in the best-controlled situations experimenter expectations may subtly influence results. And while we would not expect infant expectations to influence results, those of parents might play a major role in the behaviors of infants.

Replication studies often add new variations that are designed to test additional hypotheses, such as the influence of particular extraneous variables. For example, a researcher who believes that certain research results were obtained because a sample was largely middle-class might repeat the study with separate middle- and lower-class samples and predict that the results will replicate only for the middle-class sample. A less careful experimenter (or one with limited resources) might replicate the study using only a lower-class sample to compare with the results from the previous study. Such research often fails to control for extraneous variables other than the most obvious, in this case, of social class of subjects being different from the first study.

The time and the place of the replication also may be relevant to the outcome of a replication study. There may be cohort differences. Factors that may affect infant behaviors (feeding practices, the use of anesthesia in childbirth, availability of television) may be different at a given time or place than they were for the original study. In some locales, what seems lower-class according to national standards may seem middle-class. A researcher working in such a community might replicate an original finding for a middle-class group with a "lower-class" sample, although the hypothesis that the result is class linked was correct.

Another reason for repeating studies at a later point in time is to do them using more sophisticated technologies and see if the results are still the same.

Many studies fail to replicate because of methodological flaws or unanticipated confounding variables. Note that a single study, no matter how well done, may in some instances be incorrect. The best way to ferret out such incorrect conclusions is to replicate the research. Note also that even replicated research needs to be replicated again at later times, because extraneous variables may change over time. Unfortunately, the field of psychology tends not to value replication studies unless they contradict original findings. It is extremely hard to get such research published, and therefore it does not help young academics get tenure.

INTERPRETATION OF FINDINGS

Occasionally, two interpretations explain the data of a study equally well, and it is not possible to decide between them on the basis of what is known **empirically** (known through evidence). While some will choose the explanation that fits the theory with which they started the research, the more appropriate way to decide is to invoke the law of parsimony, or Occam's razor. Deciding whether one explanation is more plausible than the other is not possible on scientific grounds, since plausibility is in the judgment of the researcher (in the eye of the beholder). The law of parsimony provides a way of choosing the more plausible explanation if one interpretation is more complex than the other. If a simple explanation can be given for a behavior, then one does not need to invoke a more complex process. For example, if newborns cry when other babies cry, one need not explain the phenomenon as due to the more complex process of imitation if the simpler process of behavioral contagion will cover the data. This is a very important principle in developmental psychology, particularly in work with infants, because researchers are often in the position of having to infer what infants know from their behaviors. Furthermore, it is reasonable to assume that babies progress from simpler to more complex behaviors.

Summary

There have been three general themes in this chapter. One concerns reasons for study of infants, one is historical, and one is methodological. The last two have been entwined in the discussion; methodological points have been made with historical data. The methodological concerns mandate the introduction of a great deal of vocabulary. As has been noted, important vocabulary words throughout this book are printed in bold and defined in context; pages with definitions appear in bold in the index.

The study of infants has fascinated researchers for 200 years. It began in the eighteenth century with baby biographies, which are detailed parental descriptions of infant behavior, usually by fathers. In the nineteenth century biographies became more sophisticated, starting with Preyer and culminating with Piaget in this century. In the late nineteenth century there was an effort to collect biographies from laypersons in order to describe a broader range of children. Such data were seen as providing the mechanism for answering basic questions on (a) the roles of heredity and the environment in development, (b) the impact of early experience on development, and (c) the impact of teaching parents about their infants. The sophistication with which these questions are asked has increased greatly, but the basic interests are the same.

Baby biographies can be useful for describing development if care is taken to make clear distinctions between behaviors and interpretations and to consider alternative interpretations. Aids in distinguishing among alternative interpretations were used by Piaget and include (a) applying the law of parsimony, (b) gathering multiple examples that fit only one alternate interpretation, and (c) introducing informal experiments.

Normative/descriptive studies are an improvement over baby biographies in that they are based on larger, more representative samples. Since they are merely descriptive, they do not provide explanations for behavior patterns, although they do permit us to make broader generalizations about normal development than do baby biographies.

The first psychological laboratories were established at the end of the nineteenth century. Since that time, experiments and correlational studies have become the primary ways of studying infant development. Experiments are controlled situations that enable researchers to determine the effects of an independent variable (the hypothesized cause) on an outcome variable (the dependent variable). When experimental conditions are properly controlled and subjects are randomly assigned to conditions, cause-and-effect relations can be determined.

Correlational studies examine the relations between two or more variables as they naturally exist in a situation. Causality cannot be inferred, although random selection of the subjects studied can increase the generalizability of findings. One good use of correlational studies is to explore the stability of individual differences over time.

Research issues such as sampling, the research design's suitability for answering the questions asked, replicability of findings, and the appropriateness of interpretation will be highlighted throughout the book.

References

ALCOTT, A. B. (1882). Letter to Mrs. Talbot with notes from his diary. *Journal of Social Science, 15*, 8-10.

DARWIN, C. (1877). Biography. *Mind, 2*, 285-294.

DARWIN, C. (1882). Letter to Mrs. Talbot. *Journal of Social Science, 15*, 6-8.

FELDMAN, H. (1833). *Observations on the normal functioning of the human baby.* Bonn: C. Georgia.

GENZMER, A. (1873). Investigations on sensory perception in newborn humans. (National Institute of Health Library No. NIH-74-230c, Trans.). Unpublished doctoral dissertation, University of Halle-Wittenberg.

HARRIS, W. T. (1882). Speech to 1881 meeting of Social Science Association. *Journal of Social Science, 15*, 1-5.

KUSSMAUL, A. (1859). *Untersuchungen über das Seelenleben des neugenborenen Menschen.* Heidelberg: C. F. Winter.

PIAGET, J. (1962). Play, dreams and imitation in childhood (C. Gattegno & F. M. Hodgson, Trans.). New York: W. W. Norton. (Original work published 1945)

PREYER, W. (1888). *The mind of the child: Part I. The senses and the will* (N. W. Brown, Trans.). New York: Appleton. (Original work published 1880)

PREYER, W. (1889). *The mind of the child: Part II. The development of the intellect* (N. W. Brown, Trans.). New York: Appleton. (Original work published 1881)

RUBIN, J. L., Provenzano, F. J., & Luria, Z. (1974). The eye of the beholder: Parents on sex of newborns. *American Journal of Orthopsychiatry, 44*, 512-519.

TAINE, M. H. (1877). Paper on infant development. *Mind, 1*, 252-259. (Original work published 1876)

TALBOT, E. (1882). Papers on infant development. *Journal of Social Science, 15*, 5-23.

TIEDEMANN, D. (1927). Tiedemann's observations on the development of the mental faculties of children (S. Langer & C. Murchison, Trans.). *Pedagogical Seminary and Journal of Genetic Psychology, 34*, 205-230. (Original work published 1787)

PART I

Conception Through Birth

Development From Conception to Birth

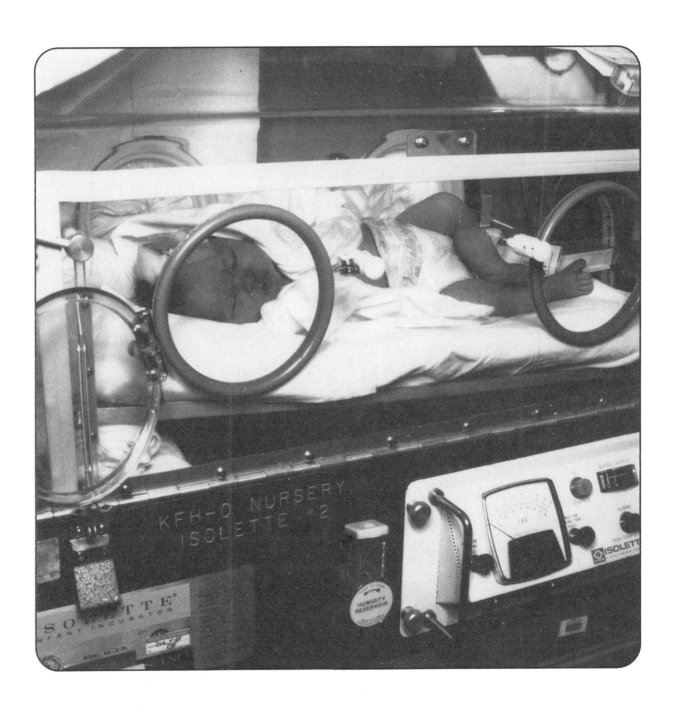

In Western culture birth is celebrated as the beginning of life, but the study of infancy must begin much earlier. Infants at birth are already products of their genetic makeup and the interactions of that genetic makeup with their **prenatal** (before birth) environment. This chapter describes the normal course of prenatal growth and development. It provides the basic information necessary for the student to understand the following three chapters, which describe things that can go wrong genetically, prenatally, and during the birth process.

In addition to acquiring this necessary background knowledge, the student should learn two things about normal development. The first is an appreciation of the many complex and interrelated processes that work together to produce a human infant. The second is the fact that despite this amazing complexity, these processes all work sufficiently well in the vast majority of pregnancies to produce normal, healthy babies. Although students who use this book are not expected to become experts on embryology, this chapter will help them learn something of the basic processes and to have an overview of the development of a few systems. The heart (or circulatory system) and the respiratory system are singled out for more attention than liver or kidneys because they are systems whose functioning undergoes particularly dramatic changes at birth. These changes are crucial to the proper development of the infant and are relevant to later discussion of problems associated with labor and delivery. The sexual system is also described in somewhat more detail than others, both because I assume that it may be of particular interest to students and because it provides such excellent examples of the interaction of genetics and environment. In addition, certain aspects of the development of the organ most crucial to our human functioning—the brain—are described.

Overview of Prenatal Development

It is difficult to know exactly where to begin. We could consider the processes that lead to the formation of the **spermatozoa** (sperm in the male) and the **ovum** (female egg) that is ready for fertilization. Some of what can go wrong with development occurs during these processes. Between the development of the millions of sperm and of the ovum and fertilization, much happens that helps determine whether the ovum will be fertilized and which particular sperm cell will fertilize it. Another set of changes occurs between penetration of the ovum by the sperm (formation of the **zygote**) and the point of the first cleavage division

of the human ovum. Discussion of these changes, however, is more appropriate for biology texts than for this volume. They will not be addressed here.

FERTILIZATION AND EARLIEST DEVELOPMENT (ZYGOTE STAGE)

We shall start at the point at which an ovum and a sperm cell unite (see Table 2.1). Each of these cells has 23 **chromosomes** (see Figure 3.1 in Chapter 3) on which are located the **genes** (the barlike structures in cells that carry all the genetic information). These two cells approach, join, and re-form into a fertilized egg with 46 chromosomes (see Figure 2.1)—a process that takes about 24 hours. Thus this new cell, or zygote, has the same number of chromosomes as all other cells in the body. One might say that the potential for a new human being has then been created. Whether or not this potential is realized depends on many hereditary and environmental influences, as shall be seen. Table 2.1 and the figures showing developing embryos will be helpful for the next sections.

Fertilization normally occurs in the fallopian tubes, through which an ovum passes every month on its trip from the ovaries (where it has ripened) to the **uterus** or womb. It takes 2-3 days for the zygote to reach the uterus. The unfertilized egg is the largest cell in the body, and during its first few days as a zygote it stays the same size, but subdivides several times; that is, after each cell division the cells inside the zygote become smaller (see Figure 2.2). Even at this stage of the first cell divisions environment is important in determining what happens to the genetic message of the **DNA** (deoxyribonucleic acid, the carrier of genetic information in cells). The DNA located in the cell **nucleus** (the part of a cell that governs growth, metabolism, and reproduction) depends upon nutrients in the **cytoplasm** (i.e., protoplasm outside the nucleus) to be able to replicate itself properly.

During the process of so-called **cleavage** divisions, all cells are identical. The original cells had to rely almost entirely on their own reserves for nutrients, but by the time there are 8 cells, they can utilize external nutrients. By the time the zygote has reached the uterus, a journey of 3-4 days, cleavage has proceeded to the point where the zygote has 12 to 16 cells. It now has a new technical name (morula).

By 4 days of age (the number of days counted from conception, commonly called **conceptional age**) the egg mass contains 16 to 64 cells, each about the size of normal cells. They are beginning to change shape and position for the first time, and are called the blastocyst, a substage of the zygote (Figure 2.2, bottom).

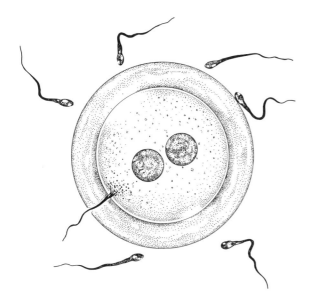

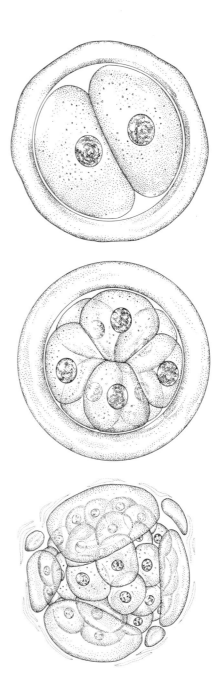

Figure 2.1. The process of fertilization of an ovum by a sperm. One sperm has penetrated the jellylike coating around the egg cell. Its head has detached and swelled as it approached the nucleus of the egg cell (the two circles in the center of the cell are the head of the sperm and the nucleus of the egg). The head of the sperm cell (containing 23 chromosomes from the father) and the nucleus of the egg cell (containing 23 chromosomes from the mother) are now in the position from which they will each release their chromosomes to combine into a new cell with 46 chromosomes. The moment of combination is called fertilization. (Adapted with permission from S. Parker & J. Bavosi, *Life Before Birth: The Story of the First Nine Months.* Cambridge: British Museum [Natural History]/Cambridge University Press, 1979.)

The dividing cells pull away from the center of the mass to form a cavity. The cells separate into two layers, a small inner layer of cells that will form the infant and a large mass of flattened cells on the outside of the cell mass. These flattened cells will form the **placenta** (the structure through which exchange of food, oxygen, and wastes takes place between the mother and the offspring), the **amnion** or **amniotic sac** (which surrounds the infant), and other related structures that will provide for the developing organism. At this time, the blastocyst starts to absorb fluids from the uterine lining, where it is floating.

Figure 2.2. Initial cell division of fertilized egg: (top) after first cell division, (middle) at 8-cell stage, (bottom) at blastocyst stage. There are about 40 cells, and the outer cells are reproducing more rapidly and flattening. (Adapted with permission from S. Parker & J. Bavosi, *Life Before Birth: The Story of the First Nine Months.* Cambridge: British Museum [Natural History]/ Cambridge University Press, 1979.)

Table 2.1

Timetables for Initial Development (Zygote Through Embryonic Stages) and Fetal Development

Name of Stage	Time After Fertilization	Events
Initial development		
Zygote	0-40 hours	Cleavage divisions
Morula	40 hours to 4 days	Reaches uterus; embryonic cell masses develop
Blastocyst	4-8 days	Development of 2-layered (bilaminar) disk; implantation begins; embryonic membranes start to develop
Embryo-Early	12-13 days	Implantation complete
	14 days	Mature placenta begins to develop
	15-20 days	Development of 3-layered (trilaminar) disk; neural tube begins to form; disk becomes attached to uterine wall by short, thick umbilical cord; placenta develops rapidly
	21-28 days	Eyes begin to form; heart starts beating; crown-rump length 5 mm (less than .25 in.); growth rate about 1 mm per day; neural tube closes (otherwise spina bifida); vascular system develops (blood vessels); placental maternal-embryonic circulation begins to function
Embryo-Late	5 weeks	Arm and leg buds form
	7 weeks	Facial structures fuse (otherwise facial defects, e.g., cleft palate)
	8 weeks	Crown-rump length 3 cm (slightly over 1 in.); weight 1 gm (about .03 oz.); major development of organs completed; most external features recognizable at birth are present
Fetal development		
Fetus	8-12 weeks	Movements of arms and legs; startle and sucking reflexes, facial expressions, and external sex organs appear; fingerprints develop; respiratory and excretory systems develop, but are not functional; lanugo develops
	end of first trimester	Length 7.6 cm (about 3 in.); weight 14 g (about .5 oz); simple abortion by curettage no longer possible
	13-16 weeks	Skin and true hair develop; skeleton becomes bony
	17-20 weeks	Length 20 cm (about 8 in.); weight 450 g (less than 1 lb.); movements become obvious to mother ("quickening"); heartbeat can be heard through stethoscope; old cells discarded and replaced by new (hence cells in amniotic fluid)
	25-28 weeks	Begins to acquire subcutaneous fat; terminals of lung and associated blood vessels develop
	end second trimester	Good chance of survival if born prematurely
	by 38 weeks	Fetus becomes plump; lanugo usually shed; testes of male usually descend

IMPLANTATION AND DEVELOPMENT OF
PLACENTA AND RELATED STRUCTURES

Once the two-layered disk has developed sufficiently (about 7 or 8 days after conception), the egg mass begins to implant itself in the wall of the uterus. This requires many complex interactions. Implantation normally takes place in the upper, posterior (back) portion of the uterus. The location of implantation is one of the determinants of the outcome of the pregnancy. The blood supply varies in different parts of the uterus and, in some places, may be inadequate to allow completion of the pregnancy or may result in an undernourished newborn. Furthermore, if the zygote attaches to the bottom of the uterus, the placenta may detach too early (**placenta previa**) or may block delivery. Some placements of the placenta may make it

more difficult to shed after delivery. Inappropriate placements are likely to result in hemorrhage during labor and delivery, which endangers the lives of both mother and child.

The situations described above refer to implantation within the uterus. Sometimes, however, the zygote implants in one of the fallopian tubes or somewhere else in the pelvic cavity (a small gap between the ovaries and fallopian tubes in humans makes such misses possible). Such **ectopic** (outside the uterus) pregnancies usually terminate in the first 2-3 months, either by severe bleeding when the placenta becomes detached or by rupture of the tube, or both. The most common symptoms are abdominal pain and vomiting. Death from loss of blood can result as quickly as 6 hours after symptoms start. There were 78,000 ectopic pregnancies in 1985, or 15/1,000 reported pregnancies, an

11% increase from 1983 (*Morbidity and Mortality Weekly Report*, 1988). However, maternal deaths in the same period dropped to only half as frequent (4.2/10,000).

The Process of Implantation

The outer layer of cells that form the placenta and membranes surrounding the developing organism are also responsible for implantation and for providing nutritional support for the developing organism. These cells thicken and develop amoebalike projections that invade the endometrium or uterine lining, which is made up of tissue, blood, and other fluids. They transport nutrients from the blood and other fluids to the zygote (see Figure 2.3), which takes them in through osmosis (gradual diffusion), because no circulatory system has yet been developed. Human eggs, unlike those of chickens, have no yolks, so the supply of nutrients provided by the ovum is extremely limited. Direct contact between tissue from the zygotic system and the uterine lining provides a supply system to tide the zygote over until the placental system develops.

The Development of Support Structures

During this phase all parts of the embryonic system develop. In the second week after conception, the embryonic membranes begin to develop. The amnion is the "bag" of the phrase *bag of waters*. It contains a clear fluid in which the developing organism floats.

Figure 2.3. Implantation of zygote into uterine wall. The cells on the outside of the ball are absorbing nutrients from the mother's cells; the nutrients, in turn, are absorbed by the internal cells. (Adapted with permission from S. Parker & J. Bavosi, *Life Before Birth: The Story of the First Nine Months*. Cambridge: British Museum [Natural History]/Cambridge University Press, 1979.)

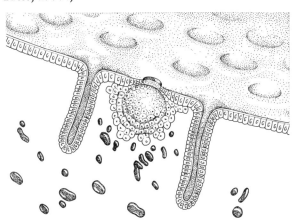

This protects the embryo and later the fetus from blows, bounces, and shakes. The other three membranes—the allantois, chorion, and yolk sac (which develops in humans even though human eggs have no yolks)—play roles in the development of the placenta and the **umbilical cord** (the cord of blood vessels that connects the embryo to the placenta). The **placenta** is a disk-shaped mass of tissues in which small blood vessels from both mother and embryo intertwine without joining (see Figure 2.4). Small molecules can pass from maternal to embryonic and fetal blood vessels and back, but large molecules cannot. Among the substances that can pass the placental barrier are food, oxygen, water, and salts from maternal blood and carbon dioxide and digestive wastes from infant blood. Among the large molecules that cannot pass the placental barrier are red blood cells and many harmful substances, such as most bacteria and a variety of maternal wastes, toxins, and hormones that could damage the developing organism.[1]

The mature placenta starts to develop around the fourteenth day and by the end of the third week after conception it covers 20% of the uterus. Thus the placenta soon takes over the digestive, respiratory, and excretory functions of the embryonic system. The placenta also functions as a gland and produces hormones that are crucial to the proper maintenance of pregnancy. Its role as a source of hormones becomes increasingly important as pregnancy progresses. Both estrogens and progesteronelike hormones are produced and are important not only in the growth of certain systems, but in the maintenance of pregnancy. One hormone's name, progestagen, implies this function: It is pro **gestation** (or pregnancy). Changes in the secretions of hormones probably play an important role in delivery also, but the mechanisms that normally lead to delivery are very little understood.[2]

It is important to remember that some of the placenta and all the fetal membrane systems are derived from the fertilized egg cell and are not structures grown by the mother to help her **conceptus** (product of conception) develop. There are, of course, changes in her uterine lining that help these processes and that are the direct contribution of the maternal organism.

---

1. The whole question of the many mechanisms that govern and control exchange (technically, transport or transfer across the placental barrier) is a highly complex field of study in itself.

2. Hormones play an important role in conception, successful implantation, pregnancy, delivery, and lactation. While many of these roles are fairly well known and understood, many are not. Students who are particularly interested in these questions are referred to the book *Biology of Reproduction* (Hogarth, 1978)

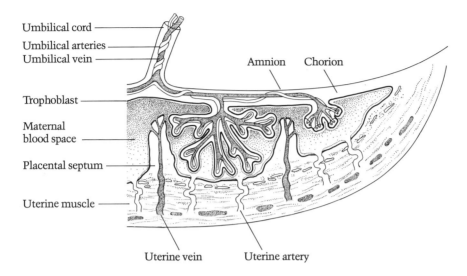

Figure 2.4. Diagram of the placenta attached to the uterine wall. The umbilical cord, at the top of the diagram, takes depleted blood from the developing organism to the placenta, where it disperses through small blood vessels that extend into the maternal blood supply. The placental barrier, which keeps the blood supply of the developing offspring separate from the maternal blood supply, is indicated in this diagram by the dark line labeled the trophoblast. (Adapted with permission from L. B. Arey, *Developmental Anatomy: A Textbook and Laboratory Manual of Embryology* [7th ed.]. Copyright 1965 by W. B. Saunders Company.)

THE EMBRYONIC STAGE OF
DEVELOPMENT

The first stage of development of the conceptus itself is the embryonic stage. This stage is crucial to the normal development of a fetus and is a stage in which environmental damage is most likely to occur, as will be discussed in Chapter 4.

*Initial Differentiation of Embryo
Into Three Layers*

While the egg mass is implanting itself into the uterine wall, the embryonic or original inner cells of the zygote are differentiating into two layers of cells (called **germ** or basic cell layers). The developing organism is now called an **embryo.** The inner layer of germ cells is the precursor of the **endodermal** cells (from *endon,* within, and *derma,* skin) that eventually form the linings of the internal organs, such as the digestive tract, respiratory system, bladder, vagina, and urethra. The outer germ layer gives rise to two kinds of cells: (a) the precursors of the **ectodermal** (outer-covering) cells in the second week after conception, and (b) the precursors of the **mesodermal** (middle-layer) cells in the third week. Ectodermal cells form

the skin, sense receptors (for seeing, hearing, tasting, feeling), nerve cells, mammary and pituitary glands, and the mucus membranes of the mouth and anus. The mesodermal cells eventually form all of the muscles (including heart muscle), connective tissue (such as bone and cartilage), circulatory system (blood vessels and heart), and most of the excretory and reproductive systems.

Every part of the body develops from these three kinds of cells—endoderm, mesoderm, and ectoderm. In general, the endoderm develops into the most internal structures of the body, the mesoderm into the structures surrounding the internal organs, and the ectoderm into the surface structures, as shown in Table 2.2. This characterization is useful, albeit oversimplified.

The ear can be used as an example of the complexity of embryonic differentiation. Figure 2.5 is a diagram of the ear, showing the major structures and their origins. The ectoderm, as the forerunner of external structures, is the origin of most of the structures: the external ear, the outer tympanic membrane (outer part of eardrum), the sense receptors that transform sound into nerve impulses (known collectively as the organ of Corti), and the semicircular canals (structures that have to do with the vestibular system and balance).

Table 2.2
Systems That Develop From the Three Different Layers of the Blastocyst

Ectoderm	Central nervous system: brain and spinal cord
	Peripheral nervous system
	Sensory receivers of ear, nose, eye
	Outer skin layers and associated structures: nails, hair, tooth enamel
	Mammary and pituitary glands
Mesoderm	Circulatory system: heart, blood, lymph
	Skeleton: bone, cartilage
	Muscles and connecting tissues
	Excretory system: kidneys
	Reproductive system
	Inner layer of skin (dermis)
	Outer layers of digestive tube
Endoderm	Respiratory system: lungs
	Digestive system: pharynx, stomach, and intestines

The endoderm forms the inner tympanic membranes (inner part of eardrum) and the eustachian tube (which goes from ear to throat). The mesoderm differentiates into the middle tympanic membrane (the middle part of the eardrum); the hammer, anvil, and stirrup (three small bones in the middle ear that transmit sound); and the mastoid bone (the bone behind the ear). Even though the functions of these various structures may be unfamiliar, one can appreciate the integrated way in which the various parts of the ear differentiate from these basic types of cells into a coordinated, functioning whole.

During this first phase of embryonic differentiation there are a number of spontaneous abortions, often of embryos with major chromosomal defects. They are not aborted earlier because this is the first stage of development that is governed by the genetic material (DNA) of the embryonic cell nucleus. Earlier cleavage divisions are governed by the ribonucleic acid (RNA) that still survives from the original (i.e., the unfertilized) ovum.

The whole process of early differentiation is much more complex than can be described here. Not only do the cells differentiate, but many of them move from one place in the embryo to another along very specific pathways. Some differentiations are apparently self-determined and would happen even if the relevant cells were isolated from the embryo. Other differentiations depend on the chemical actions of their new neighbors and therefore depend on cell migration. Students who are interested in learning more about the details of the process of initial differentiation (which is called *gastrulation*) should consult a good biology text.

*Early Embryonic Development
(3 to 4 Weeks After Conception)*

The differentiation of the mesodermal layer is not all that is happening during the third postconception week. The most critical period of physical development commences then, before most women even know they are pregnant. During the third week the neural tube, destined to become the spinal cord, is developing (Figure 2.6a). At about 21 days, the eyes begin to form. By 24 days the heart, although still just a tube, begins to flutter and then to beat, and the embryo gradually develops a head fold and a tail fold. The prominent part of the head fold is the brain, and the tail bud closes off the spinal cord (Figure 2.6b). These foldings result in an organism with a distinguishable head (crown) and rump, with tail. The embryo's crown-rump length is approximately 5 mm in the fourth week. A severe birth defect called **spina bifida** may occur during this week if the neural tube does not close properly. Victims of this disorder may suffer paralysis, deformity, and/or brain damage (see Figure 2.7).

Also, it is during the fourth week that the first rudiments of the urogenital system are established. Arm and leg buds appear. The heart develops into a four-chambered structure. Primitive blood cells are manufactured and blood vessels start to form. These developments of the vascular system, together with simultaneous ones of the placental system, permit the onset of mature placental functioning. From this point on there is a closed circuit in which embryonic circulation is completely separate from maternal circulation.

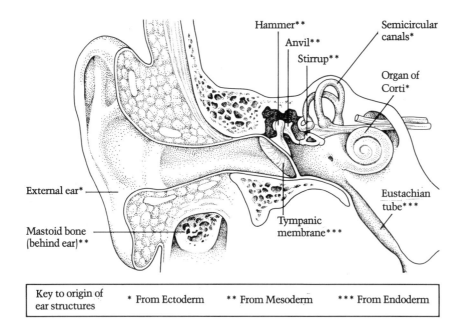

Key to origin of ear structures | * From Ectoderm | ** From Mesoderm | *** From Endoderm

Figure 2.5. Ear structures showing their derivation from the three-layered disk.

*Late Embryonic Development
(5 to 8 Weeks After Conception)*

In the fifth week after conception (Figure 2.6c), the cells inside the arm and leg buds are differentiating into those that will ultimately become muscle, cartilage, or bone cells. In the sixth week (Figure 2.6d) arms and legs are more differentiated and the face has started to form, but is still unrecognizable. During this time, the liver, gallbladder, pancreas, and major divisions of the intestinal tract develop. In the seventh week the facial structures fuse. Errors in this process produce hare lip, cleft nose, cleft chin, and cleft palate. Such errors are very common in the United States, affecting 1 in every 500 births (R. M. Pratt, cited in *NIH Record*, September 28, 1982, p. 6). They often reflect the operation of three factors: genetic predispositions of both the embryo and the mother, and the presence of environmental factors such as drugs, hormones, and chemicals. By the end of 8 weeks the organism weighs about 1 g (.03 oz) and is about 3 cm

(slightly over 1 in.) long. It looks something like a human, although its head is very large due to the rapid development of its brain (Figure 2.6e). By this time, the major steps in the development of the organs are completed and the organism is no longer called an embryo.

The first 8 weeks are called the period of **organogenesis** (the period when organ systems are forming). It is a period of great vulnerability, when many defects of heart, lungs, ears, and other organs can occur.[3]

FETAL STAGE OF DEVELOPMENT
(2 MONTHS TO BIRTH)

During the next 32 weeks of development the organism is known as a **fetus** (see the second part of Table 2.1). The already distinct organs are further differentiated and move to their final positions. They grow to the size and proportions they will have at birth. Growth of crown-rump length, while not steady, averages about 1.5 mm per day.

Third Lunar Month

In the third lunar month (weeks 8-12) the fetus first moves its arms and legs, although its mother may not yet be aware of these movements. The first reflexes appear during this month—first startle and then, by the

---

3. The incredible complexity of these developments during the embryological period can be appreciated by a glance at any chapter of an embryology text describing the growth of any one particular system. Even without knowing the meaning of many of the words used, one can achieve a real sense of the miracle of normal development.

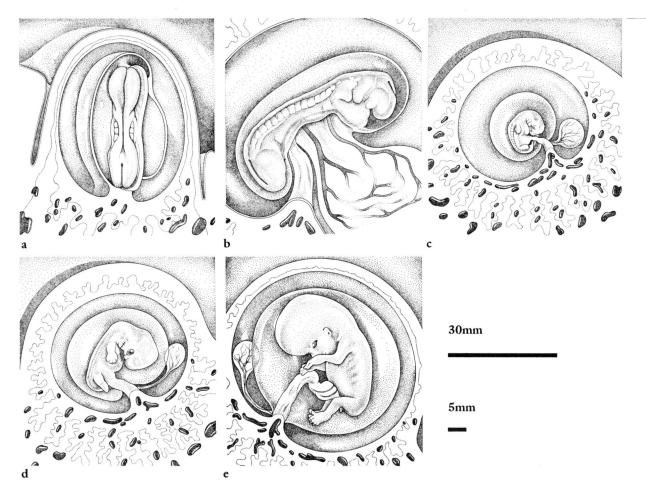

Figure 2.6. The developing embryo (not drawn to scale). In (a) the embryo is less than 5 mm long and in (e) it is 30 mm long. (a) The third week after conception. The two bulges at the top are the brain. The long groove that runs most of the way from the brain to the rump at the bottom is the start of the spinal tube. (b) The embryo a few days later, after the spinal tube has closed. The developing brain, with its three bulges and spinal cord, makes up most of the embryo. The gut and the heart have also been enclosed by the folding together of the head and tail ends. (c) About 5 weeks after fertilization, the arm and leg buds and the tail extending below the leg buds, which developed in the fourth week, are clearly visible. (d) About 6 weeks after fertilization. The opening that looks like a mouth is the developing ear. (e) Two months after fertilization. Organogenesis is complete and the offspring is now called a fetus. (Adapted with permission from S. Parker & J. Bavosi, *Life Before Birth: The Story of the First Nine Months.* Cambridge: British Museum [Natural History]/Cambridge University Press, 1979.)

end of the month, sucking. Facial expressions such as squinting, frowning, and looking surprised appear. External sex organs develop sufficiently in this month to enable identification of sex. The finger, palm, and toe prints are developed enough that the fetus can be identified by them. Respiratory and excretory systems develop greatly but are not yet functional. Part of the fetus is covered by fine hair called lanugo; some of this

hair may still be present at birth. By the end of this month the fetus is 76 mm (3 in.) long, and weighs 14 g (0.5 oz).

This marks the end of the first trimester. All the major organ systems have developed, but the ones that are necessary for survival are not yet functional. During the second trimester (weeks 13 to 26) much of the remaining development of these systems occurs.

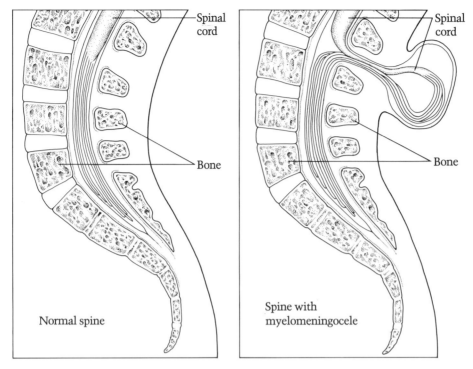

Figure 2.7. Spina bifida. The drawings show a normal spine and a spine with myelomeningocele, the most severe form of spina bifida. (Drawings reprinted by permission from the Spina Bifida Association of America brochure, *Spina Bifida*.)

Second Trimester

In the fourth lunar month (weeks 13 to 16), the first layer of skin and true hair develop. The skeleton becomes bony enough (rather than cartilaginous) to be detected by X rays.

In the fifth lunar month (weeks 17-20), the fetal movements become obvious to the mother and the fetal heartbeat can be heard with a stethoscope. The fetus is now sloughing off skin and respiratory cells and replacing them with new ones. These sloughed-off cells remain in the amniotic fluid and provide the basis for a method of detecting chromosomal abnormalities by a procedure called **amniocentesis**. In this procedure a needle is inserted through the mother's abdominal wall into the amniotic fluid, with care taken to avoid the fetus and placenta, whose position can be determined by **ultrasound** (a technique using inaudible high-frequency sound waves that bounce back from various tissues at different speeds and thereby outline the shape and position of the fetus). A small sample of amniotic fluid is extracted, and the sloughed-off cells of the fetus in it can be cultured and processed to detect chromosomal abnormalities; the fluid

can be processed biochemically to detect products of many genetic defects as well as the presence of excess spinal fluid (or **alpha fetoprotein**), which indicates that the neural tube has not closed and the fetus thus suffers from spina bifida or other neural tube defects. Chromosomal abnormalities, genetic defects, and issues concerning amniocentesis will be discussed more thoroughly in Chapter 3.

During its first 5 lunar months, much of the potential infant's structural development takes place, but it reaches only 10% of its birth weight. At 18 weeks it is still only 203 mm (8 in.) long and weighs less than 450 g (less than 1 lb). Its life-support systems are also still nonfunctional, so it could not live outside its mother's uterus. Much of the fetus's subsequent development is in physical growth and in the final development of the structures necessary for survival on its own.

Third Trimester

In the seventh lunar month (24 to 28 weeks) subcutaneous fat begins to develop, allowing increased weight gain. The infant needs this subcutaneous fat for fuel immediately after birth (breast milk does not start flowing immediately). The terminal portions of the air passages of the lungs and the blood vessel network around them also develop in the seventh month. It is the lack of development of these structures that leads to one of the most serious problems of premature infants, respiratory distress syndrome (RDS).

By the twenty-eighth week the fetus is 20-40 cm (11-16 in.) long and weighs about 1,000 g (about 2.25 lb). The lungs are developed enough that it has a good chance of surviving on its own, especially with the new treatments.

In this last trimester (weeks 27-38) the baby continues to grow rapidly. The number and size of brain cells also expand rapidly. Some research indicates that the protein intake of the mother is particularly important at this time to ensure optimal brain development.

By birth (described in Chapter 5) the fetus has acquired the plump appearance of the normal newborn, its lanugo is usually shed, and, if male, the testes are descended. This entire course of development is summarized in Table 2.1.

TRANSITIONS AT BIRTH

Birth brings about profound changes in the ways many organ systems function, thus placing great demands on the newborn. As examples, the following sections describe the basic changes in the circulatory and respiratory systems.

Circulatory System

In the prenatal circulatory system the umbilical arteries and veins carry blood to and from the placenta, where the fetal blood is oxygenated. There are three "bypasses" or shunts in the prenatal system that must not continue after birth. Complete separation of arterial blood (which is full of oxygen) and venous blood (which has yielded its oxygen to the body, hence is depleted of oxygen) does not occur until birth. The separations that do exist serve to send the most highly oxygenated blood to the upper half of the body, including the brain, while the lower half receives blood with a much lower oxygen content. In fact, the prenatal circulatory system could be called a "make do" situation for the lower half of the body, especially the extremities. Indeed, this poorly oxygenated blood may be a factor in the relatively slow development of the lower body during prenatal growth. This differential development in favor of the upper half of the body is an example of a general principle of development both before and after birth, the principle of

cephalocaudal development. This means that development proceeds from head (*ceph*) to tail (*cauda*), or from top to bottom.

Respiratory System

The other system intimately linked to circulation is the respiratory system (primarily the lungs). Prior to birth, the fetus has received its oxygen from that in the mother's blood by means of the placental and umbilical systems. At birth the walls of the umbilical vessels contract and the umbilical arteries no longer pulsate. How this comes about is not fully known. When the lungs start to operate, the "bypasses" or shunts close rapidly, resulting in full separation of deoxygenated (venous) and aerated (arterial) blood. At first these closings are not anatomical or physical closures. They are what are called physiological or functional closures. Their action depends on a number of factors, including the degree of oxygenation of the fetus. The closures may not always work perfectly in the first hours or even days or weeks of the infant's life. Nevertheless, they normally become structurally closed relatively quickly. Although failures can occur in these processes, as happens in so-called blue babies, it is extraordinary how many complex interactions take place in embryological development and usually do so without producing major problems.

Before birth the lungs themselves are solid but contain fluid. Normally, pressure on the chest during birth expels most of the fluid. Doctors and nurses often give an assist in this process by dangling the baby by the feet, slapping it on the back, or applying gentle suction to draw out more fluid. At birth the respiratory center of the brain is stimulated by impulses from the cold receptors of the skin and by chemoreceptors sensitive to the blood gasses, so that the baby starts to make breathing movements. (Actually, the baby may have made some sporadic breathing movements in utero, which may account for some of the fluid in the lungs.)

If the baby is slow to respond, further stimulation may be used in the form of more slapping of the back, snapping the soles of the feet, or providing oxygen. These measures usually suffice. When breathing starts, the terminal air sacs of the lungs (alveoli) expand and the other vessels (including the lymphatics) open up. However, the majority of the terminal air sacs have not developed by the time of birth. Even among those that are developed, not all suddenly open after the first cry (which serves to bring air and thus oxygen into the lungs). After birth, then, the lungs continue to grow in complexity as well as in size. It has often been said that the lungs provide the real limits to **viability** (the ability to live) outside the uterus.

Interaction of the Circulatory and Respiratory Systems

The complexity of the relations between the respiratory and circulatory systems is illustrated by the interaction between the two systems in closing one of the bypasses mentioned earlier. The expansion of the lungs greatly increases the volume of blood in the lungs, and the pressure from this increased volume of blood distends the left auricle of the heart. Receptors in the wall of the auricle trigger a reflex that leads to closure of a duct that has been important in fetal circulation (the ductus arteriosus). If it were to remain open, it would prevent proper circulation of the blood once the infant is separated from the placental circulatory system. In the normal course of events this biological reflex func-

tions once and once only. If the reflex does not function, the infant will have serious problems because there will be insufficient oxygen for the cells. Because the brain cells are still in a period of rapid growth, they are among those most affected. Today this can usually be corrected surgically.

Development of Organ Systems of Special Interest

SEXUAL DIFFERENTIATION (THE UROGENITAL SYSTEM)

This aspect of embryological development has been chosen for discussion in some detail for three reasons: First, the interactions between heredity and environment are particularly clear-cut for this aspect of devel-

Table 2.3
The Course of Sexual Development

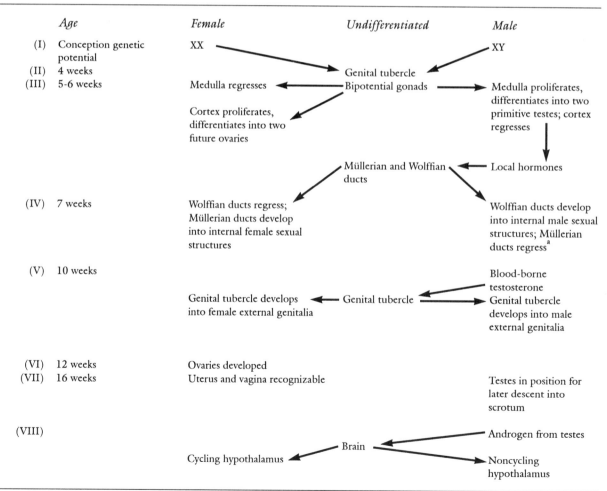

	Age	Female	Undifferentiated	Male
(I)	Conception genetic potential	XX		XY
(II)	4 weeks		Genital tubercle	
(III)	5-6 weeks	Medulla regresses	Bipotential gonads	Medulla proliferates, differentiates into two primitive testes; cortex regresses
		Cortex proliferates, differentiates into two future ovaries		
			Müllerian and Wolffian ducts	Local hormones
(IV)	7 weeks	Wolffian ducts regress; Müllerian ducts develop into internal female sexual structures		Wolffian ducts develop into internal male sexual structures; Müllerian ducts regress[a]
(V)	10 weeks			Blood-borne testosterone
		Genital tubercle develops into female external genitalia	Genital tubercle	Genital tubercle develops into male external genitalia
(VI)	12 weeks	Ovaries developed		
(VII)	16 weeks	Uterus and vagina recognizable		Testes in position for later descent into scrotum
(VIII)			Brain	Androgen from testes
		Cycling hypothalamus		Noncycling hypothalamus

a. But remnant forms prostatic pouch.

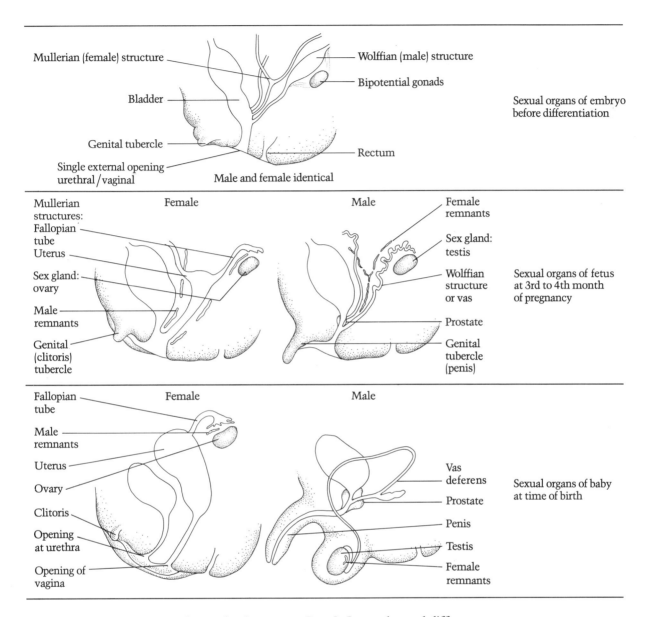

Figure 2.8a. Differentiation of reproductive organs. Part 1: Internal sexual differentiation. Notice the progression from undifferentiated to differentiated states. Most of sexual development is completed in the first trimester. (Reprinted with permission from J. Money & A. Ehrhardt, *Man and Woman, Boy and Girl*. Copyright 1972 by Johns Hopkins University Press.)

opment. Second, there are a number of viable genetic anomalies involving the sex chromosomes (see Chapter 3). Finally, most people are interested in topics related to sex and gender identity. For all these reasons, development of the urogenital system is of particular interest. The course of sexual development is described in Table 2.3 and illustrated in Figure 2.8. Development proceeds from top to bottom in both. In the text, I will refer to the various sections or developmental periods described in the table according to the Roman numerals in the left-hand column.

The process of sexual differentiation is triggered by the genes on the sex chromosomes (see Figure 3.1 in Chapter 3). Female humans have two similar sex chromosomes (symbolized XX) and males have two dissimilar sex chromosomes (symbolized XY). A **gamete**, also called a **germ cell** (i.e., either an egg or sperm cell), has 23 chromosomes, 1 from each of the 23 pairs of chromosomes of the parent. Thus each gamete has one sex chromosome. Since women have two X

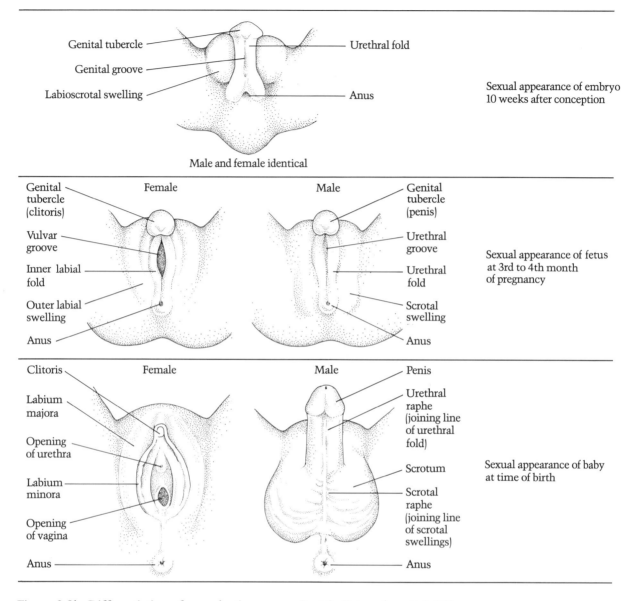

Figure 2.8b. Differentiation of reproductive organs. Part 2: External genital differentiation. Again, notice the progression from undifferentiated to differentiated states. (Reprinted with permission from J. Money & A. Ehrhardt, *Man and Woman, Boy and Girl*. Copyright 1972 by Johns Hopkins University Press.)

chromosomes, the egg will always have an X chromosome regardless of which of the chromosomes is reproduced in the egg. Males, in contrast, contribute an X chromosome to half their sperm and a Y to the other half. If a Y sperm fertilizes the egg, the product is genetically male; if an X sperm fertilizes it, the offspring is genetically female. Therefore, fathers are the sole determiners of children's genetic sex (Figure 2.9).

Sexual determination begins with the genetic potential of the fertilized ovum but is only a potential at that time (see Table 2.3, section I). In the time that elapses

between the fertilization of the ovum and its implantation in the uterine wall (the period of the zygote), no physical differences can be detected as a result of the genetic difference. Also, in early embryological development, three undifferentiated sexual structures develop in which no differences between male or female forms can be detected. They are (a) the genital tubercle, which eventually develops into the external genitalia (it develops at section II and differentiates at section V of Table 2.3); (b) the bipotential gonad, which develops into ovaries or testes (see section III of

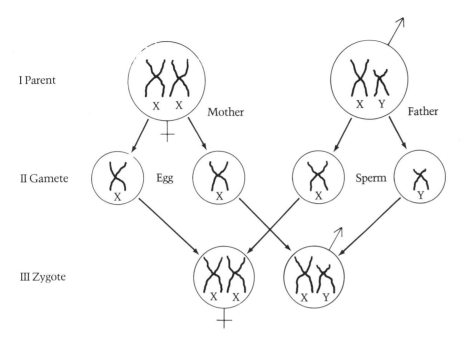

Figure 2.9. Meiosis. During this type of cell division, a maternal cell produces two eggs, both of which have the X chromosome, and a paternal cell produces two sperm cells (or spermatozoa), one with an X chromosome and one with a Y. If an X sperm fertilizes an egg, the zygote has the female sex chromosome combination (XX); if a Y sperm fertilizes an egg, the zygote is male (XY).

Table 2.3); and (c) the Müllerian and Wolffian ducts, which differentiate into the internal sexual structures (sections III and IV of Table 2.3). All of these undifferentiated structures are bipotential; that is, they can develop into either male or female structures.

The sexual differentiation of each of the primordia (precursor) sexual structures occurs at different times during organogenesis. Thus there is a repeated pattern of going from an undifferentiated form to a sexually differentiated form. This pattern is emphasized in Table 2.3 by the arrows that radiate from the center column (the undifferentiated states) to the two side columns (which represent the differentiated male and female forms).

The first primordial structure to differentiate sexually is the bipotential gonad, which starts differentiating at 5-6 weeks after conception (section III of Table 2.3). Because the female can be considered the basic sex in humans (as will become clear), female development is described here first. The surface, or cortex, of the bipotential gonad or genital gland begins to proliferate and the internal part, or medulla, begins to regress. The single structure differentiates into two parts, each of which will become an ovary. At 7 weeks after conception, the internal sexual structures begin to differentiate. In females the Müllerian ducts de-

velop into internal female structures and the Wolffian ducts start to regress (section IV of Table 2.3).

This course of development is governed by the X chromosomes. If the embryo has a Y chromosome, an additional step takes place that changes the development radically. At 5-6 weeks the central part of the genital gland (medulla) starts to proliferate and the surface portion (cortex) regresses (section III of Table 2.3). When the genital gland differentiates into two primitive testes, these testes secrete fetal androgen (a male hormone similar to the testosterone produced by adult male testes) and another hormone that has not yet been identified. The androgen acts to stimulate the development of the Wolffian ducts and the unidentified hormone acts to suppress the development of the Müllerian ducts, that is, to change the course of development (section IV of Table 2.3). This initial action of the hormones is local—that is, limited to the region that is adjacent to the testes—because there is as yet no circulatory system. If the testis on one side is removed but that on the other side left, the ducts will undergo the changes that make them masculine on the side with the testis, but will become like those of the female on the castrated side. Female is said to be the basic sex because if androgen is removed from an embryo with male genes, it will develop female structures. I will return to this point after completing the description of the developmental sequence.

A similar pattern of development produces the external genitalia (clitoris, labia, and so on in females; penis, scrotum, and so on in males). At 10 weeks after conception the single genital tubercle, which appeared at 4 weeks, develops a vertical groove (which separates it into two urethral folds), a urogenital slit, and two labioscrotal swellings. All of these structures are still bipotential (see Figure 2.8). In the female, who does not receive stimulation from male hormones, the tubercle itself will regress in size and become the clitoris. In the male, in whom male hormones are produced, it will grow to become the penis. In the female the two urethral folds will remain two separate structures and develop into the labia minora (the minor or inner lips surrounding the vagina). In the male, the two folds will fuse to form the urethra and scrotal pouch. In the female, the two labioscrotal swellings will develop into the two labia majora (the major or outer lips) and the single mons. In the male they will fuse to form the scrotum. The single urogenital slit will deepen in the female to form the vestibule and opening portion of the vagina.

In females the ovaries are developed by 12 weeks (section VI of Table 2.3), while the urethra, prepuce (foreskin), and penile (or urethral) meatus (opening) are still forming in the male. By the sixteenth week the differentiation of the sexual structures of the human male is complete (section VII of Table 2.3).

I would like to return now to the statement that female is the basic sex. What is true for early gonadal development is true throughout sexual differentiation. If genetically male mammals such as rats and guinea pigs are denied androgen by castration during sexual differentiation, they will not develop male organs appropriately. They will show signs of those aspects of female physiology that develop after that time. In adulthood, if given female hormones, they will even develop some of the appropriate female sexual behaviors, although they will be sterile. We know that the prenatal absence of male hormones has produced this potential for female sexual behavior, because male rats castrated after adulthood will not develop female sexual behaviors even if given female hormones.

The reverse can also happen. If genetic females are injected with male hormones at the time of sexual differentiation, they will develop dwarfed ovaries and some masculine physiology. At adulthood they will not exhibit normal female sexual behaviors, even if given large doses of female hormones. There is an unfortunate human analogue to this research on the masculinizing of genetic females by hormones. For a time,

androgens were given to pregnant women as part of a medical treatment. Their girl babies were often born with partially developed male organs and inadequately developed female organs. Genetically female infants developing in mothers with conditions that cause the adrenals to secrete large quantities of male hormones may also be physically masculinized.

To summarize the major points from this research: Sexual differentiation occurs at particular points in development. If no male hormones are present in the first of these, the organism develops female internal sexual characteristics. If male hormones are present, the organism develops male internal sexual characteristics. This happens even when the hormonal situation does not match the genetic sex. The same thing happens slightly later with respect to external sexual characteristics. The hormones, and not the testes themselves, are known to cause the differentiation, because injecting androgen is as effective as transplanting testes into the female. The resulting sexual differentiation (whether or not it matches genetic sex) produces permanent changes that cannot be reversed by hormone treatment after birth.

Sexual differentiation does not end with the development of the physical sexual structures. Appropriate sexual behaviors also become physiologically encoded in the brain (section VIII of Table 2.3). One of the major differences between male and female rat sexual behavior is its cyclicity. Females are cyclical, males are not. The female cycle is produced by regular changes in levels of several different hormones (both gonadal and pituitary) that are regulated by the hypothalamus, a center in the brain close to the pituitary gland. The cyclical pattern in females produces an ovulatory period followed by a nonovulatory period. Female mammals typically are most receptive sexually around the time they ovulate, and they are then said to be "in heat." In many nonhuman species nonovulatory female mammals will reject sexual advances.

Other sexual behaviors of both males and females appear to be at least partially set in the brain. For example, injecting the female hormone estrogen into male rats results in *male*, not female, sexual behaviors (Fisher, 1967).

The degree to which brain structures and behaviors related to them become permanently differentiated is still a controversial area of research. Behaviors thought to be sexually differentiated are aggression, including rough-and-tumble play, and spatial reasoning. Structurally the brain differs in lateralization, which is assumed also to affect function.[4] Sufficient evidence does not exist to demonstrate convincingly to all experts in the field that these are biologically based sex differences. (For an excellent review of the research to that date, see Reinisch, 1974.)

All of these aspects of behavior are multiply determined. Any one individual can show both "masculine" and "feminine" behaviors, and many people are more like the other sex than their own (e.g., many males are less aggressive than many females and many females are better spatial reasoners than many males). For these reasons I shall refrain from further consideration of sex differences in relation to brain differentiation.

THE CENTRAL NERVOUS SYSTEM (BRAIN AND SPINAL CORD)

Development of the central nervous system is discussed here because the brain is crucial for the intelligent behavior that marks humans. That is only part of its importance. The **central nervous system (CNS)**, including the spinal cord, governs all of our bodily functions. The brain structures begin to develop shortly after conception, when the neural tube develops from specialized ectodermal cells. Before the neural tube closes in the fourth week postconceptional age (or sixth week postmenstrual age, as researchers in this field are likely to say), the neural cells have proliferated into many layers. At first these cells appear to be all alike, but some of them, the future motor neurons, soon send fibers beyond the neural tube to surrounding tissues. After the neural tube closes, three bulges appear at the head end of the tube (see Figure 2.6b). These are the precursors of the three main divisions of the brain: the forebrain, midbrain, and hindbrain. At this time the extraordinary proliferation of cells in the CNS has already started. From the time the bulge at the head of the neural tube appears, the head of embryo and fetus is very large in proportion to the rest of the body.

Cell Growth

Neurons, also called nerve cells, are the basic unit by which messages are sent throughout the brain, spinal cord, and peripheral nerves. The adult brain contains one million, million neurons (1,000,000,000,000). Neurons are not the only cells in the brain, however. About half the cellular volume of the brain is made up of neuroglia or **glial cells**, which serve a supportive role for the neurons. They transmit food (glucose and amino acids) from the blood supply to the neurons, some probably serve as scaffolding, and others manufacture **myelin** (the fatty insulating sheath that is deposited around the neurons and that is necessary for the proper conduction of nerve impulses in many

nerves). In the development of each kind of cell, there is an initial phase during which there is rapid proliferation of the number of cells. This is followed by a period in which the previously formed cells increase in size or die, while new ones continue to develop. In the final phase cells continue to increase in size and in myelination, but no new cells develop.

The neurons first develop between the eighth and sixteenth week after conception. They originally consist only of their nuclei and a bare minimum of cytoplasm (the part of the cell surrounding the nucleus) and hence continue to grow in size for some time. The process of cell division to produce new cells probably stops earlier for neurons in the cortex than for most other cell types (by 28 weeks postconception). The glia develop later than the neurons. They start to form at about 13 weeks postconception, have their peak of cell division from 18 weeks after conception to 4 months after birth, and cease to form new cells by 15 to 24 months postnatally. In summary, then, most cells in the brain are formed during the fetal period and first 2 years of life.

This should not, however, be construed to mean that no further development occurs after this age. The development of axons and dendrites, those processes that connect one neuron to another, is extremely rapid during the first three years of life, and then gradually slows down to reach its adult rate by puberty, but never stops. The development of the myelin sheath, necessary for normal functioning of the CNS, continues after neuron cell division has stopped. Much of the helplessness of newborns stems from the lack of myelination of their nervous systems. Their more efficient systems (sucking and swallowing) are controlled by nerves that are completely myelinated at birth. Myelin's importance is dramatically illustrated by what happens in multiple sclerosis (MS), in which the myelin sheath is damaged. MS victims gradually lose functioning of various parts of the CNS, resulting in paralysis, numbness, blindness, deafness, unsteady gait, impairment of speech, and mental changes.

Myelination develops in different brain areas at different times. Functional rather than geographical units determine the timetable for myelination. The nerve fibers carrying impulses from the senses to specific cortical areas myelinate at the same time as those carrying motor impulses from those areas to the periphery. For example, the neurons to and from the auditory system begin to myelinate in the sixth prenatal month and

---

4. An excellent book reviewing all aspects of cerebral lateralization and its implications for child development is *Brain Lateralization in Children* (Molfese & Segalowitz, 1988).

myelination continues until age 4. In the visual system the sensory and motor neurons start to myelinate just before birth, but complete the process rapidly. The neurons that connect the cerebellum (the center of coordination and balance) to the cortex or forebrain (the part of the brain that governs higher processing) only begin to myelinate after birth and the process continues until 4 years of age. The efficiency of these connections that myelination brings about is necessary for the precise control of voluntary movement. Other structures continue to myelinate until puberty or beyond. These examples of myelination timetables demonstrate that each neural system has its own specific timetable, which may differ from others in nature, in time of onset, and in course.

An overall view of the phenomenal early growth of the brain is provided by charting overall brain weight. From early fetal life, the brain's weight is closer to its adult weight than is any other organ (except perhaps the eye, which is partly an outgrowth of the brain, as we shall see shortly). By birth, the brain weighs one-fourth as much as in adulthood. Its rate of growth during infancy continues to be phenomenal, even though neurons cease to increase in number. By 6 months it weighs half as much as an adult brain, and at 2 years (when it has tripled its weight since birth) it achieves three-fourths of its adult weight. This is by far the most rapid growth in the body, which explains why the heads of embryos, fetuses, and young babies always look so large in relation to the rest of their bodies. Compare this rapid growth with the much slower growth of overall body weight. At birth a baby weighs about 5% of its adult weight, and does not reach half of adult weight until about 10 years of age.

Despite this early growth of the brain, there is one feature of brain development that is different from that of other organs. Not all is growth. Neurons normally die off in vast quantities, perhaps as many as half of those formed. Also, axons not only develop (grow), but also retract. This aspect of brain development is reviewed by Janowsky and Finlay (1986). (A good brief overview of the development can be found in Kolb, 1989.)

Development of the Cortex

The cortex, or forebrain, is of particular interest because it is the seat of our higher intellectual processes. Its growth has been painstakingly mapped by Conel (1939-1967) at 6, 7, and 8 months (postmenstrual), at birth, and at 5 ages between 1 and 24 months. It is first identifiable 6 weeks after conception, and by 24 weeks it has the beginnings of the six-layered structure

typical of the adult organ. The primary motor areas, whose cells govern most movements, are earliest to develop. Within them, those controlling the upper limbs and trunk develop first and appear quite mature and functional by 1 month after birth. This is another example of the cephalocaudal course of development. By 3 months all of the primary motor areas are relatively mature.

Next to develop are the primary sensory areas. The area for touch is first, followed by the visual area, and then the auditory area. Cells in the visual area show the most rapid rate of maturation a few weeks before birth. All of the association areas, with their integrative functions, lag behind these primary areas, but they develop in relation to them and in the same order. Maturation of structure is closely linked to function. As Tanner (1978) has said, "The stages of mental functioning described by Piaget and others [see our Chapter 10] have many of the characteristics of developing brain or body structure and the emergence of one stage after another is probably dependent on (i.e., limited by) progressive maturation and organization of the cortex" (p. 111).

Development of the Eyes

The development of the eyes illustrates the complex interaction between the CNS and other bodily structures (in this case, ectoderm) that occurs during development. The beginnings of eye development occur at 3½ weeks postconception, right after the first bulges of the top of the neural tube develop (see Figure

Figure 2.10. Embryological development of the eye. The optic vesicle has migrated to the surface, which has caused the ectodermal tissue to separate from the ectoderm and thicken into a lens vesicle. (Adapted with permission from F. Beck, D. B. Moffat, & J. B. Lloyd, *Human Embryology and Genetics*. Oxford: Blackwell Scientific Publications, 1973.)

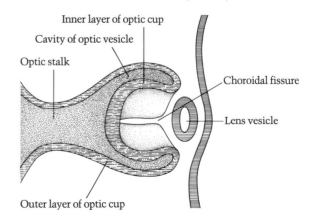

Inner layer of optic cup
Cavity of optic vesicle
Optic stalk
Choroidal fissure
Lens vesicle
Outer layer of optic cup

2.6a). Two spherical bulges, called the optic vesicles, appear on each side of the forebrain. They enlarge until they reach the surface (or ectodermal layer). This contact causes the latter to thicken and change into a circular depression that ultimately separates from the surface and becomes the lens vesicle (see Figure 2.10). The latter will, in turn, develop into the lens of the eye, whereas each optic vesicle will form the optic nerve and pigmental layers of the retina.

The interaction between the optic vesicle and the lens vesicle provides another classic example of the importance of local environments in determining normal differentiation of organs. An earlier example was the local action of testicular hormones producing appropriate internal male organs. Here, local chemical effects in the optic vesicle induce the lens to form. If the optic vesicle is removed, no lens will form. If it is transplanted at the appropriate developmental stage (say, to a leg) a lens will be formed from the ectoderm at the site of the transplant. The chemicals produced by the optic vesicle induce the leg ectoderm to form a lens.

HOW DO WE KNOW ABOUT PRENATAL DEVELOPMENT?

How have researchers learned all this about the development of organisms that are shielded from our view by women's bodies and that cannot be probed or manipulated without running the risk of maiming or killing them? Much of the existing knowledge comes from studies of other mammals, particularly rats, guinea pigs, and pigs. The gains in knowledge and practical help to humans are believed by most persons involved to offset the unpleasant realities of sacrificing the animals to study embryological and fetal development. However, animal experimentation, although necessary and invaluable, is not enough by itself. Differences between any two species are enormous, and even with our closest relatives, chimpanzees and gorillas, physical and psychological systems may differ markedly. It is dangerous to generalize from one species to another; therefore, we always need to **corroborate** (verify or make sure of the adequacy of the generalization) animal observations with studies of humans.

The products of spontaneous abortions have been used as subjects of corroborating studies. This does not give us a very good view of normal development, however, since many of these abortions are of abnormal embryos or fetuses (as already mentioned and as will be further discussed in Chapter 3). It would be better to study the products of elective abortions, because a large proportion of these organisms are normal.

Before the Supreme Court ruled in 1973 that women might legally have abortions even if not in severe physical or emotional danger, legal abortions were rare and often undergone in cases where the fetus might not be normal. Many medical and psychological researchers and practitioners hoped that the change in abortion laws would allow the useful side benefit of promoting research in prenatal development, but this has not happened. All research in this area was stopped for a period while representative groups of concerned persons debated the ethics of such research. It is not yet clear what the long-term outcome of this debate will be, although some types of research are now permitted in some states.

PRENATAL BEHAVIOR

A new field of study has arisen since the advent of **ultrasound**, a noninvasive technique for imaging the developing fetus (further description appears in Chapter 3). Researchers at Prechtl's laboratory in Holland have done some of the most systematic work studying patterns of movement. They have identified 16 different patterns, all of which existed by 15 weeks postmenstrual age (de Vries et al., 1982). The fetus changed position more frequently after 10 weeks, reaching a peak at 13 to 15 weeks and declining after 17 weeks. Different movements had different courses of development (de Vries et al., 1985). Breathing movements change from occurring every 2 to 3 seconds at 10 weeks to every second at 19 weeks (de Vries et al., 1986). Given the early stability of definite movement patterns (de Vries et al., 1988), these researchers have proposed their usefulness for assessing development of the CNS in normal and abnormal conditions. This theme has been further elaborated by Prechtl (1988). The quality of general fetal movements in early pregnancy (by 20 weeks) and the organization of behavioral states in the near-term fetus appear most useful. This group has also warned against use of vibroacoustic stimuli in studying the fetus, as it appears to induce abnormal behavioral states that last for prolonged periods (Visser et al., 1989).

Variants of Prenatal Development

The above discussion has described the typical course of prenatal development, but the development of many babies varies from this normative description in various ways. The following sections discuss two relatively common variations, twinning and prematurity.

They are placed here because these phenomena are best understood when contrasted with typical prenatal development.

TWINNING

Twinning is a common variant of prenatal development; it occurs in 1 in every 80 pregnancies. There are two basic types of twins: identical or **monozygotic** (MZ) twins, who share the same genetic blueprint, and fraternal or **dizygotic** (DZ) twins, who do not. Identical twins come from a single ovum fertilized by a single sperm (one zygote). In the zygote stage of cell division, the cells split off into two separate organisms. Most MZ twins result from division of the inner mass at the blastocyst stage, when the organism is implanting in the uterine wall and the embryonic membranes are starting to develop. These twins have only one placenta and chorion (the outermost membrane surrounding the developing organism) but usually have two umbilical cords and amniotic sacs (see Figure 2.11a).

In perhaps 20-30% of cases the split occurs prior to the zygote stage, during cleavage divisions, and the

two organisms implant separately and have two chorions and two placentas. This results in dichorionic MZ twins. This condition enables blood transfer between the two, which can result in weight differences, differences in anemia, and, in the extreme, the death of the donor twin (for a review, see O'Brien & Hay, 1987).

The separation of an embryo into two units sometimes takes place still later and does not result in complete separation. Such twins are called Siamese twins because a pair of them who were widely exhibited in sideshows in the nineteenth century happened to be from Siam. Such twins may be joined at various parts of their bodies and share various organ structures. Whether they can be surgically separated to enable one or both to live and/or lead normal lives depends on the degree of sharing and the particular structures shared.

Fraternal twins result from the fertilization of two different ova by two different sperm, hence the name dizygotic. Each zygote implants separately and develops a separate placenta, chorion, and so on (see Figure 2.11b). DZ twins are simply siblings, and share the genetic characteristics of their parents to the extent that any nontwin brothers and sisters do. In fact, there has

Figure 2.11. Twins in utero. (a) These twins could be fraternal or identical; they have individual placentas, amniotic sacs, and chorions. (b) These identical twins have a single placenta and chorion, but individual amniotic sacs. The amnions are the thin white lines, the chorions are the black lines, and the endometrium is the thick white line surrounding the chorion. (Adapted with permission from L. B. Arey, *Developmental Anatomy: A Textbook and Laboratory Manual of Embryology* [7th ed.]. Copyright 1965 by W. B. Saunders Company.)

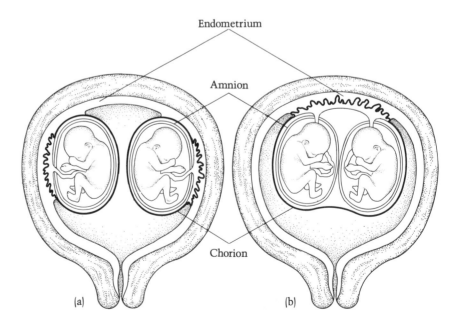

been at least one documented case in which DZ twins were half brothers rather than full brothers. This fact was obvious because the two fathers were of different races. DZ twins develop from both different ova and different sperm. The latter means that fraternal twins may be of different sexes, while identical twins, who develop from the same fertilized ovum, are always the same sex.

The mechanisms that produce twins also produce multiple births involving more than two offspring. The base rate for these has been 1 in 6,400 for triplets and 1 in 512,000 for quadruplets. Such multiples may be fraternal or identical or a combination. In recent history the numbers of fraternal multiple births have increased markedly, primarily as a result of the use of hormones in treating infertility. These hormones stimulate ovulation, and sometimes they work too well. The woman releases many mature egg cells, and a number of them may be fertilized and develop at the same time. In *in vitro* fertilization (that done outside the body, in a glass container), several fertilized eggs are usually implanted into the uterus. This is done so that there is more than one chance that at least one will attach itself and develop well, but the practice often results in multiple births. Since a uterus is of finite size, and since the number of extra organisms a mother's body can support is finite, the more developing babies there are, the more likely they are to be born early, to have very low birth weights (or both), or to die in utero.

The intrauterine environments for sets of twins are not identical either for MZ or DZ twins. For those with separate placentas, one may implant at a more favorable spot than the other. Those who share a placenta are competing for limited resources, and one may get less nourishment than the other. Growth appears to be about equal and not retarded for either twin prior to 30 weeks gestational age (Naeye et al., 1966). The different survival, health, and nutritional status of members of twin pairs appears to be related to their birth order. Numerous studies have found a wide assortment of differences that favor firstborn and heavier twins. The perinatal mortality rate for firstborn twins is 48.8/1,000, compared with 64.1/1,000 for second-borns and 10.4 for singletons in a major study of twins born in the 1980s (Spellacy et al., 1990). Twins with similar birth weights had similar mortality rates. Differences between first- and second-born twins and between lighter and heavier twins need to be examined in relation to whether one went home before the other. This can affect parent-infant relations and have lasting effects on behavior (Hay & O'Brien, 1984).

Because MZ twins have the same genetic makeup, they are of interest to individuals who wish to study the roles of heredity and environment in development and behavior. Fraternal twins provide a nice control group, since they have no more in common genetically than any other siblings, but share the experience of being twins. Nontwin siblings provide another important control. And cousins make useful controls for children in the family who may be affected by the stresses caused by the presence of twins. These comparisons provide an experiment of nature, albeit one with flaws. (See Hay & O'Brien, 1984, for a review of the problems in twin research. The same issue of *Child Development* in which their article appears presents a number of important twin studies in 16 articles devoted to developmental behavioral genetics.)

BABIES BORN TOO SOON (PREMATURES) OR TOO SMALL

Babies are born at different weights, and not all have been gestating for 40 weeks, which is normally taken as the end of fetal development. Those born too early in fetal development, or born very small, have difficulty surviving. The systems that must radically change their function at birth are not yet sufficiently developed. Although remarkable strides have been made in providing care that enables these infants to live, their survival is still highly dependent on the degree of development at birth, as well as on the availability of sophisticated medical care (see Figure 2.12). Prematurity may affect future development, both directly and indirectly, because the very aspects of intensive care that help to ensure survival may themselves have good or bad effects on later development.

The prevention of premature and **low birth weight** (**LBW**) births (those under 2,500 g, or 5.5 lb) is widely considered to be the most important factor in improving neonatal health. Progress was made between 1971 and 1977, when the rate declined from 7.8% to 7.1% of births, which is approximately what it is now (although the rate is 10-20% in some minority groups). Almost 250,000 LBW babies were born in the United States in 1979 (Institute of Medicine, 1982).

Technically, *prematurity* refers to babies born prior to 38 weeks after conception, but it has also been defined in terms of birth weight. This results in confounding babies who have suffered intrauterine growth retardation with those who are gestationally premature. It is possible to distinguish between premature (preterm) babies and those who are small for their gestational age (**SGA**; sometimes called small for dates,

SFD). The distinction is relevant inasmuch as there are differences between these two groups in the degree to which they are at risk and in the kinds of problems they face. Older studies assessed neither prematurity nor size in relation to gestational age, but used a birth weight of just under 2,500 g (less than 5.5 lb) as the **operational definition** (the definition that operates, or is used in the study) of prematurity. This was largely because doctors did not trust mothers' reports of the time of conception or even of the time of onset of the last menstrual period.

Schemes were developed to determine the gestational age of the baby. The best known are those of Dubowitz et al. (1970), and the simplification of that scheme by Ballard and colleagues (1977), and of Lubchenco and colleagues (Lubchenco, 1970; Lubchenco et al., 1966). Recent studies use these

schemes or reliable maternal reports, or both, to separate premature from SGA babies. (For a review of these distinctions, see Rosen in Institute of Medicine, 1982.) Because many early studies did not make such distinctions, we sometimes use the term *premature* when all we really know is that the baby was small.

Causes of Prematurity or Low Birth Weight

There are many causes of LBW, premature, and SGA births. Some of them are genetic and will be dealt with in Chapter 3. Many are due to maternal problems or to exposures to teratogenic or toxic substances, topics that will be covered in Chapter 4. Also discussed in Chapter 4 are fetal conditions that do not lead to early abortion or miscarriage, but that may result in LBW, premature, or SGA births. Failure of the placenta to attain adequate size and structure, which may itself be caused by some of the above, but also by problems of the site of implantation, is another cause. Twins and other multiple births are likely to be born prematurely or SGA, because they must compete for limited resources. The larger the number, the smaller and more premature the infants are apt to be. In addition, a number of factors that may not be directly causal are correlated with the likelihood of prematurity and low birth weight. Examples are socioeconomic status (**SES**), race, and lack of prenatal care.

Figure 2.12. (left) A relatively healthy premature baby who is still wired to some monitoring apparatus. Note that the baby is still quite small compared with a woman's hand. (Photograph courtesy of the Office of Research Reporting, National Institute of Child Health and Human Development, Washington, DC.) (right) A smaller, sicker premature being monitored for many functions, and on oxygen by mask. (Photograph courtesy of Tiffany Field.)

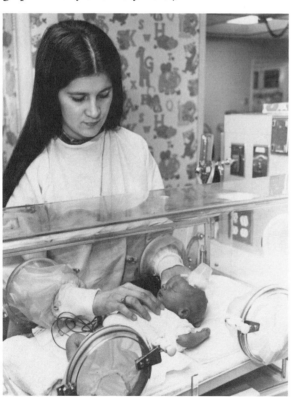
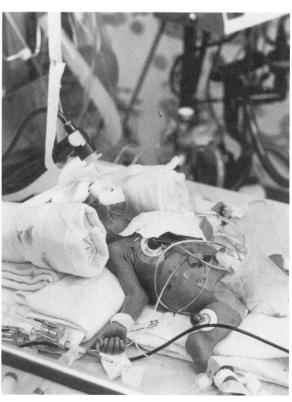

Part of the difficulty in studying the effects of prematurity stems from this multiplicity of established and possible causes. Some causes may be more dangerous or harmful to later development than others.

Factors Associated With Prematurity or Low Birth Weight

Much of the research on prematures has focused on assessing later outcomes for those who had nothing wrong with them other than the fact that they were premature. However, in real life prematures often do have other things wrong with them. Whatever caused their prematurity or low birth weight may have affected them in other ways, particularly neurologically. These babies are also more prone to damage in the birth process and postbirth period, and such damage may have its own effects. They are more likely to suffer from **anoxia** (lack of oxygen) and **hyperbilirubinemia** (too much bilirubin, which leads to jaundice and, in the extreme, to kernicterus, which damages the brain). Anoxia and hyperbilirubinemia have been shown (in a sample of low-SES blacks) to be related to degree of impairment, where prematurity itself was not (Braine et al., 1966). These findings have been corroborated by subsequent research (Goldstein et al., 1976). Higher bilirubin levels have been related to poorer visual functioning and longer periods of active sleep in black prematures a full month after levels were clinically imperceptible, and after controlling for other medical risk factors (Friedman et al., 1987).

Because their lungs are immature, prematures may have respiratory distress syndrome, a condition in which assistance is needed for breathing. Greater effectiveness in treating this problem is responsible for much of the improvement in survival rates. **Surfactant**, a liquid (surface active, like soap) that reduces surface tension of pulmonary fluids, thus contributing to the elastic properties of the pulmonary tissue, is becoming a principal treatment to supplement ventilation. Human surfactant is derived from amniotic fluid recovered in the performance of cesareans, and is in very short supply. Trials with bovine surfactant appear promising, as do efforts to synthesize it. Surfactant decreases the amount of oxygen needed and the length of time it is necessary to use a mechanical ventilator. The latter can lead to bronchopulmonary dysplasia (**BPD**), a much more serious lung disease with lasting medical and developmental consequences (Clark, 1988; Myers et al., 1991), including a high incidence (15%) of cerebral palsy (Skidmore et al., 1990).

Brain hemorrhages of several different types, all given different abbreviations (ICH, IVH, PIVH), are more frequent in prematures than in full-term infants. Ultrasound examination, a technique described more fully in Chapter 3, can provide a picture of the brain and the damage. It has been used since the late 1970s to determine the numbers of prematures affected and to quantify the degree of damage (Stewart et al., 1987). The rate of some types is affected by whether delivery is vaginal or by cesarean and, if the latter, whether labor occurred prior to the cesarean (Tejani et al., 1984). Studies indicate that 30-65% of **very low birth weight** (**VLBW**) babies (those weighing less than 1,500 g) have evidence of bleeding (Williams et al., 1987). According to research conducted by Hopkins et al. (1990), babies with ICH do less well than controls on both the Bayley Mental Development Index (MDI) and Psychomotor Development Index (PDI) (see Chapter 8) at 4 months; those with severe hemorrhages do less well than those with mild ones on the PDI. This research showed that temperament and interaction with mothers were unaffected by ICH or its severity, but were affected by the side on which the ICH occurred.

Cerebral palsy (CP) is more frequent in prematures, and the rate of its occurrence has not seemed to be much affected by the new treatments for prematures (Shields & Schifrin, 1988; Stanley & English, 1986). Rates vary in studies from 4% (Powell et al., 1988a, 1988b) to 10% (Bozynski et al., 1988), to 15% (Harris, 1987), or 24% for surviving infants weighing 500 to 2,000 g (Stanley & English, 1986). Different types of CP are related to different factors. Spastic diplegia, a severe form of CP in which muscles are hypertonic or stiff (spastic) and both sides of the body are affected, is related to gestational age, to bruising at birth, and to some form of respiratory disease in the first week of life. In contrast, spastic hemiplegia, in which only one side is affected, is more related to birth weight than to gestational age, and then to the length of time oxygen was needed, one form of serious brain hemorrhage, and triplet pregnancy (Powell et al., 1988a, 1988b). Spastic CP in general is related to being SGA (Blair & Stanley, 1990).

Prematures are more likely to develop retrolental fibroplasia (**RLF**), a condition that can lead to blindness, as a result of too much oxygen. When the cause of RLF became known, practitioners ceased to expose premature babies to such high concentrations of oxygen, and this cause of blindness greatly decreased. Now that we are keeping younger prematures alive, however, it has become necessary to use higher concentrations of oxygen, and cases of RLF, now called retinopathy of prematurity, are becoming more frequent. RLF is also associated with lower **IQ** or intelligence quotient (a standard means where 100 is average—see Chapter 8) than that found for infants of equivalent birth weight (Genn & Silverman, 1964).

Effects of Prematurity or Low Birth Weight

The problems of measuring the effects of prematurity are as difficult as those of determining its causes. Three related problems are of particular concern. First, the presence of short-term effects does not mean there will necessarily be long-term effects. This problem will reappear in later chapters (as, for example, in the discussion of the effects of drugs used during childbirth). Premature and SGA babies are initially retarded in many areas of development, but most catch up.

Second, because premature infants are, in fact, conceptionally younger than full-term infants born on the same day, a lag would be expected in behaviors that depend largely on physiological maturity. Thus to say that developmental retardation has occurred one would have to determine that the prematures are farther behind than their conceptional age would indicate. A baby who is 4 weeks premature and is 4 weeks behind developmentally is not retarded. To indicate that a handicap is caused by prematurity, one must show a developmental lag that is greater than the amount of prematurity (e.g., 6 weeks behind developmentally, but only 4 weeks premature). Developmental lags are difficult to detect in very young infants, because only a limited number of developing behavior systems can be measured (see Chapter 8). Furthermore, such developmental lags as are measured may be only temporary. Slowly developing babies often catch up to more rapidly developing babies. Prematures would be expected to catch up from their developmental lags, unless they also suffer from some specific damage such as inadequate brain cell development or mild brain damage.

This brings us to our third problem: how to detect long-term deficits. Many researchers use as their dependent measure average performance on some scale, such as on a motor test or IQ test. They then examine the average difference in IQ between premature and term children. This difference between the two groups may be very small. But averages mask the potentially most important effect of prematurity: that prematures are at greater risk for serious defects than are full-term babies. If the researchers had instead measured the frequency of occurrence of different levels of IQ, they might have found a disproportionate number of low IQs in the premature group. A study that found just that will serve as a good example. Wiener and colleagues (1968) found an average difference at 8 to 10

years of age between the IQs of prematures and term infants of only about 5 points. This was after eliminating all infants with IQs below 50. Despite the similar averages, there were twice as many prematures with IQs between 50 and 80 (the two least retarded categories of retardation). There are several problem areas in infancy (also in other aspects of psychology and in medicine) where the number of persons seriously handicapped by a given condition may be more relevant than the average difference between those with the condition and those without.

A fourth problem concerns the fact that one must separate studies evaluating the outcomes for premature babies according to the time period in which the study was done. The neonatal care available to keep small prematures alive changed markedly in the 1970s. A much larger percentage of prematures survive now, although the degree of prematurity that is viable (that allows the baby to live) has not changed much. Adequate means of tube feeding and more adequate ideas of nutritional requirements make it less likely that prematures will be undernourished. Pneumonia as a result of inhaling formula due to immaturity of swallowing and breathing mechanisms is avoided. Warming to compensate for poor temperature regulation is better controlled. Better methods of monitoring physiological functioning have been developed, enabling doctors to catch problems more rapidly and to take actions that may prevent not only death, but permanent damage. Since 1965 bilirubin (see Chapter 4) has been kept at lower levels (and by less drastic steps subsequently); since 1970 hypoglycemia (low blood sugar level) has been better controlled. These changes should lead to lowered possibility of brain damage. Nevertheless, problems still remain. For example, finding the optimal level of oxygen to administer to avoid causing RLF and still provide enough for normal brain growth is difficult, even though oxygenation of the brain appears to be less important in preterm babies (Rosensheim et al., 1978) than for those born at 40 weeks, because the brain is undergoing a growth spurt at the normal time of birth (Gluck, 1977).

One direct comparison of survival and outcome before and after current practices of neonatal intensive care units (**NICUs**) found a 37% survival rate for those born from 1966 to 1970 at less than 1,500 g, but 68% survival for those born from 1980 to 1982 (Kitchen et al., 1986). Survival improved for all except those weighing less than 700 g. At first glance it appeared that, at age 2, the Mental Development Index (**MDI**) scores on the Bayley test of those who had survived were improved. However, compared with controls, and taking account of SES differences, they were not better off. In one study only 40% of infants born at extremely low birth weight (**ELBW**; below 1,000 g) were alive at age 2 (Portnoy et al., 1988), but only 19% in a study of those born between 1976 and 1979 (Lefebvre et al., 1988). Only one-third of the survivors had no significant problems in school. In a later study 70% lived, but only 54% of those from 500 to 750 g (Edmunds et al., 1990).

Behavior, not just survival, has changed over time. Visual and auditory orienting responses are better for prematures born after 1984 than for earlier cohorts, especially for the younger, higher-risk group (25-34 weeks gestation; Riese, 1989).

Immediate Effects. It is clear that low birth weight babies are more likely than those of normal weight to die in their first hours, days, or weeks (see Table 2.4). The smaller the neonate, the greater the risk. Babies born too soon or too small often lack the necessary physiological development to enable the circulatory and respiratory systems to function properly. They may be unable to make the rapid and extensive changes at birth to allow adequate breathing and blood circulation.

Those who withstand the stresses and survive may still have suffered some insult. To determine whether such damage exists is one of the goals of outcome research. This is often coupled with research designed to try to determine ways to optimize outcomes.

Short-Term Behavioral Effects. In the short term, general developmental retardation is clear. Premature infants are likely to lack sleep-wake cycles, to attend to visual stimuli differently (while still preterm), to lack normal neonatal reflexes, and to be retarded in sensorimotor development. They start to catch up in many of these areas (such as sleep-wake cycles and basic visual attention) by the time they reach the age at which they would have been born (Kopp & Parmelee, 1979; Parmelee & Sigman, 1976). One group of black prematures observed in detail were awake more, changed state more often, and fussed and cried more than full-term controls when both were at normal term age and neither was being stimulated. When stimulated by auditory and tactile stimuli, the preterms responded in the same ways as healthy term neonates, but when aroused to a crying state, they were more difficult to soothe (Friedman et al., 1982; Jacobs et al., 1979). (For a good description of preterm behaviors in the immediate postnatal period, see Tronick et al., 1990.)

Long-Term Effects. Long-term effects are to be found in a variety of outcomes ranging from physical size to school performance.

Physical size. One correlate of low birth weight that is long term is physical size. A study of 10-year-olds who had been very small at birth (less than 1,500 g, or 3.33 lb) found that 41% weighed less and 47% were shorter than 90% of other children their age (Lubchenco et al., 1963; see also Drillien, 1964). More recent studies have corroborated these long-term physical effects, using SGA rather than birth weight as their measure (for example, see Kopp & Parmelee, 1979). Furthermore, VLBW girls have been found to give birth to LBW babies (Thomson, 1959; Thomson & Billewicz, 1963).

Intelligence. Findings with respect to long-term effects on intellectual ability are probably the most controversial, because the conclusions vary with (a) the time period in which the study was done, (b) the measures used, (c) how prematurity and LBW were defined, and (d) the sample studied (including type of nursery care, SES, and whether severely damaged babies were excluded). Nevertheless, studies tend to be consistent in finding that there is greater intellectual impairment among those with very low birth weights (e.g., Caputo & Mandell, 1970; Rantakallio & von Wendt, 1985). If the measure of long-term effects used is the rate of moderate to severe intellectual impairment or neurological problems, then prematurity (or low birth weight, or both) is a serious disability. Depending on the study, 5-40% of such children were later moderately or severely impaired.

Data on all children born in one area of Finland in

Table 2.4

Survival and Degree of Impairment of Low Birth Weight Infants as a Function of Birth Weight and Year Born (in percentages)

	Low Birth Weight			Very Low Birth Weight		
	1960	1971-1975	1976	1960	1971-1975	1976
Died	72	54	33	92	80.5	50
Severely abnormal	6.7	4.5	7.6	2.3	2.8	5.7
Moderately abnormal	14	23.5	10.5	4.0	3.2	7.3
Normal	7.2	17.8	48.6	1.7	13.5	36.5

SOURCE: Adapted from Budetti et al. (1981).

1966 show that the percentage of those with IQs below 86 (primarily measured in adolescence) increases steadily with lower birth weight, going from 2.5% for those who weighed more than 2,500 g at birth to 20% for those who weighed less than 1,500 g (Rantakallio & von Wendt, 1985). In some studies, Bayley scores in the first 2 years do not seem to distinguish sharply LBW or VLBW babies from controls, especially if only those with no neurological problems are compared (Vohr et al., 1988); however, in others they do (Bradley et al., 1987). In the latter study, MDIs at 18 months were only 76. They correlated with the 5-minute Apgars and with the variety of stimuli and organization of the environment at home. Lower IQs of VLBW infants at age 3 were related to the perinatal complications of prematurity, to SES, and to being male (Crisafi & Driscoll, 1989). The sex difference has been found in other studies. SES interacts with birth weight and sex in determining outcomes, and it becomes more important with increasing age.

Recently, more attention has been paid to outcome measures other than IQ and obvious neurological impairment. School performance, language development, and visual processing or visual-motor behaviors have received special scrutiny. Socioemotional development is beginning to be looked at. At 6 and 9 years, after controlling for IQ, VLBW children have been reported by their parents to be less compliant and less socially mature, and to have more learning problems (Zelkowitz et al., 1991). They have been rated by teachers as less aggressive at age 6 and as more withdrawn at age 9.

Language development. A number of studies indicate that language development may be especially affected in LBW children. Decreased vocalization that lasted beyond 14 months of age differentiates prematures from well-matched controls (Crawford, 1982). In a sample in which many had hearing deficits, delayed verbal expression and vocabulary skills persisted through 6½ years, despite normal intelligence and relatively normal achievement of developmental milestones (Richman, 1980). In a study in which hearing was not assessed, language comprehension at 3 years was related to birth weight for both VLBW and term infants (Siegel, 1982). In a study conducted at the University of California, Los Angeles, language abilities at 22 months in one sample were more retarded than would be expected on the basis of conceptional age, but not at 3 years (Ungerer & Sigman, 1983). However, at age 8 the prematures were again less verbally competent, had lower verbal IQs, and were more distractible (Cohen et al., 1986, 1988).

Studies of LBW babies born more recently also show language problems. Language development at age 5 was delayed, and negatively correlated with both birth weight and gestational age, even for prematures who were neurologically unimpaired, but not in term infants (Largo et al., 1986). An ELBW group differed at age 2 only on the Verbal Scale of the McCarthy examinations (Portnoy et al., 1988). At 2 years VLBW infants (both AGA and SGA), some of whom had had RDS, were lower on both receptive and expressive language (Vohr et al., 1988). About 30% of them, but none of the controls, were more than 1.5 standard deviations below the standardization mean. Finally, a study that compared later outcomes for those born in the mid-1970s to outcomes for those born in the late 1970s found that birth weight was not related to outcomes at 12 or 14 years for the former group, but was related at 8 and 10 years for the latter group (Boussy et al., 1990). These intriguing differences were a result of the data from the VLBW group. The later behaviors of the LBW group improved, but those of the VLBW were much worse than for the earlier cohort. It is tempting to think of this in terms of survival of the fittest having operated for the earlier cohort.

School performance. School performance seems to be more affected than IQ per se. In a group studied at UCLA, at age 8, 20% of the English-speaking and 30% of the Spanish-speaking LBW children were in special education settings and 5% had been retained in their grades. Even in those with IQs of 80 or above, 25% had learning problems (Cohen et al., 1986). In a study of 45 VLBWs, 22% performed poorly in school, compared with 2% for their controls (Lloyd et al., 1988). If one looks at different birth weights within the VLBW category, findings indicate that 22% of the 1,251-1,500 g group have trouble by age 8, but 75% of the 500-750 g group does (Edmonds et al., 1990).

Studies done earlier show similar findings. Rubin et al. (1973) found that a wide variety of school-related measures in grades 1 to 5 were poor for LBW children, but not for prematures as such. Drillien et al. (1980) found problems in school at age 6 to 7 for LBW infants (here, less than 2,000 g) born between 1966 and 1977. Two-thirds of the LBW males and over half of all SFD children had problems that led to special educational placement or the need for special services in school. The figures were not as high in children born a few years later (Drillien et al., 1980). And Swedish data for LBW children born in 1955 show both poorer school performance and lower IQ (Lagerström et al., 1989).

Other. Other types of differences between premature and term babies include poorer visual information processing at 1 year (Rose, 1983) and at 3 years (Ungerer

& Sigman, 1983), poorer performance on a task requiring visual-motor integration as assessed by copying forms at 5 years (Siegel, 1983), and poorer scores on the Rutter Scale of Behavior Problems for VLBW children (Lloyd et al., 1988). Play and personal-social interactions might be expected to be more affected by postnatal experience and less by biological maturity. It is therefore interesting to note that clear effects of conceptional age on these behaviors are present at 13½ months and some at 22 months (Ungerer & Sigman, 1983). An interesting finding is that poor performance at age 5 predicts trouble at age 8 for prematures (Edmonds et al., 1990).

Conclusions regarding long-term effects. From the studies cited above and many others, it is possible to conclude that LBW children are more likely to have language and school problems than they are to have lowered IQs. Most LBW and even VLBW babies develop to be within the normal range on IQ and have no obvious impairments. Whether these apparently normal children have suffered some intellectual impairment is a more difficult question; whether their IQs are as high as those of their siblings and parents is not specified in most studies.

Methodological problems. One methodological problem that complicates interpreting the studies is that many include all premature/LBW children regardless of the causes or factors associated with the prematurity or its treatments. Among the postnatal factors, the presence and degree of RDS and of brain hemorrhages need to be taken into account. Researchers have been able to find some consistency by considering two factors—the presence of neurological damage and how low the birth weight is. While neurological damage is not easy to assess (see the section on neurological testing in Chapter 8), two studies (each using a different technique to assess neurological damage) have found birth weight to be unrelated to later IQ when those with neurological damage were eliminated from the sample (McDonald, 1964; Wiener et al., 1965). Furthermore LBW babies below 2,000 g born between 1966 and 1970 who were neurologically normal during the first year did not differ from controls at 6 to 7 years of age (Drillien et al., 1980).

Head circumference, a crude measure of brain growth, appears to be a good indicator of the degree of later neurobehavioral problems (Lipper et al., 1981). Growth in head circumference is related both to more medical problems in the NICU and to poorer outcomes (Eckerman et al., 1985). Attentional deficits, which are thought to have a CNS basis, when present at age 2 are related to a lower IQ at age 5, accounting for 29% of the variance (Astbury et al.,

1987). Also, distractibility at ages 8 and 12 was higher for the prematures in the UCLA study mentioned above.

Another complication in dealing with the data is that of sex differences. For example, one study found no sex differences in the objective test performances of children, but LBW preterm males had a higher proportion of negative outcomes (Rubin et al., 1973). Next to preterm boys, SGA infants were most at risk regardless of their gestational age at birth. Sex differences in outcomes occur in many studies, and boys are always more disadvantaged than girls (see, e.g., Largo et al., 1986; Portnoy et al., 1988). Boys born at 1,500 g or less are much more likely to suffer brain hemorrhages than girls (72% versus 28%), probably due to slower maturation of the cerebral vascular system in boys (Amato et al., 1987).

Causes of the Effects of Prematurity or Low Birth Weight

What is it about prematurity or LBW that produces long-term effects? The answer is crucial to understanding why some babies seem much more at risk than others. Answers could lie in what it was that caused prematurity or LBW in the first place (biological) or in factors associated with the birth (biological) or the immediate postbirth environment (in the NICU), which could cause biological or social problems. Finally, the long-term effects could be caused by the interaction of biological and postnatal environmental factors.

Biological. First, let us summarize the biological causes to highlight their complexity. Prematurity and low birth weight or low birth weight for gestational age may be caused by many different fetal, placental, and maternal conditions. Some of these surely can have a direct effect on the offspring independent of the prematurity they may cause. To give just one example, a fetal infection transmitted from the mother may lead to small size and to neurological damage of the fetus, which may lead to early birth and to most, if not all, subsequent deficits. Other conditions that may lead to retarded prenatal growth and premature birth (or both) may retard brain growth and lead to permanent deficit. Genetic defects (see Chapter 3) may result in small size or prematurity and in later defects. Many conditions or exposures of the embryo or fetus during pregnancy may affect birth weight and prematurity and may damage the CNS (see Chapter 4).

At the time of birth the shock to the baby's biological systems of being born too early may be greater than the infant is able to recover from fully. In addition, the stresses of extrauterine life on the immature systems of the premature may cause lasting effects.

Whether prematurity or retarded prenatal growth can themselves cause permanent damage, especially if not accompanied by neurological damage, is a very controversial question. For heavier LBW babies the evidence suggests that prematurity or retarded growth (or both) does not itself give rise to permanent intellectual deficits. The long-term effects found for very small or very premature babies are likely to be caused by associated neurological damage or other correlated factors, or even by later events in the infants' lives. For example, fetal hypoxia, respiratory complications, and infection have all been shown to relate to the probability of deficits at age 1 (Low et al., 1985).

Immediate Postnatal Environment. In addition to all the above ways that premature or LBW infants may have been biologically damaged, one must ask: What are the possible effects of life in the NICU? On theoretical grounds the damaging effects of such an environment have been suggested with respect both to biology and to handicaps to the mother-infant relationship. A review of this topic that provides an excellent picture of life in the NICU can be found in Wolke (1987). Mother-infant relations are discussed in Chapter 5, but effects on the infant of NICU life will be examined here.

NICUs are usually characterized by constant light and lots of sounds. Such an environment tends to deprive the newborn of patterned stimulation, while at the same time overstimulating. The lack of day/night variation in NICUs may affect physiological organization. The longer an infant remains in this environment, the more likely it will suffer a lasting biological effect. Infants in more brightly lit units have been found to keep their eyes closed a larger proportion of the time than other babies, a self-protective device that may, however, interfere with cognitive processing (Lawson & Turkewitz, 1986).

Such factors could help account for differences in sleep patterns that look more mature than those of term babies (which might be expected on the basis of the premature's longer independence from the maternal system) in some aspects, but less mature in others (Booth et al., 1980; Parmelee et al., 1967). The lesser maturity could be ascribed to the lack of normal light/dark cycles or of patterned stimuli generally.

Sleep behaviors still differ at age 3 (Walker, 1989).

Prematures exposed to patterned kinesthetic and auditory stimulation have shown better sleep organization, as well as fewer abnormal reflexes, another sign of greater neurological organization. Prematures have been found to be less mature motorically and to have more deviant reflexes and less varied states than either sick babies in intensive care or healthy babies kept in the hospital (not in intensive care) because of the illness of their mothers (Holmes et al., 1982). These infants were more like sick term infants than like healthy ones. Their behavior was not related to their gestational age, but to their illnesses, sex, obstetric complications, and the length of time they had been hospitalized. The longer the prematures had been in the hospital, the more their physiological organization was affected. In contrast, the longer babies who had been ill were in the hospital, the more their ability to interact with others was affected.

In addition, the NICU baby is exposed to a great many aversive procedures in a day (234 for VLBW babies according to research cited by Wolke, 1987). These interfere with sleep, cause episodes of **apnea** (temporary cessation of breathing) and other undesirable physiological reactions, and are rarely timed to fit the babies' needs.

Posthospital Environment. It has long been known that the effects of prematurity depend in part on the kind of postnatal environment in which the infant was raised. Most research on the social causes of poor outcomes of prematurity has focused on crude measures of environment such as SES, race, or maternal education. In some cases the environment has been assessed more directly, as, for example, by the HOME scales.[5] In others, mother-infant interactions have been assessed according to the protocols of the specific study. In all cases there is concern with specifying particular aspects of maternal and home stimulation that can help children avoid deficits resulting from prematurity.

Studies consistently find that although conditions around the time of birth (perinatal factors) are important predictors of short-term problems, later social or environmental factors are the best predictors of long-term outcome (for a review of this literature, see Kopp & Parmelee, 1979). High-SES prematures appear able to overcome their early developmental retardation, but those from lower-SES homes frequently suffer long-term deficits. A recent large-scale study addressing these issues found that decreases in mental status did not occur between ages 2 and 4 or 5 for children whose mothers had completed college, but did for all other educational levels, and did not occur for whites,

---

5. HOME, an Inventory of Home Stimulation (Bradley & Caldwell, 1977), examines maternal-infant interaction and the home environment using both direct observation and questioning of the mother.

but did for blacks and Hispanics (Resnick et al., 1990). While decreases occurred between ages 1 and 2 for all birth weight categories, further declines to age 4-5 were significant only for those weighing less than 1,000 g. In the UCLA study cited previously, infants whose mothers were socially responsive to them in infancy were superior on cognitive performance throughout the first 5 years. By age 8, both a higher-SES home and a responsive mother were needed for good intellectual competence (Beckwith & Cohen, 1987).

Such findings reflect an **interaction** effect, which means that two independent variables (class and prematurity in this case) influence each other as to how each influences the outcome (or dependent variable). To confirm such interactions statistically, we would need to find both (a) no difference between premature and full-term middle-class children and (b) a difference between premature lower-class and full-term lower-class children. Such interactions have been found in numerous studies (including Bakeman & Brown, 1980; Douglas, 1956; Drillien, 1964; Werner et al., 1967). However, at least one well-done early study found no such interaction (Wiener et al., 1965). Inconsistencies in the outcomes of methodologically sound research usually occur because not all of the important factors have been identified. For example, even within lower-SES groups, mothers' IQs and educations consistently predict their infants' later IQs. Thus Wiener and colleagues (1965) may have failed to find SES differences because their lower-class population may have been less disadvantaged on IQ, education, or other stimulants for intellectual development. In short, SES is too crude an index and includes no specific behaviors, hence it would be wise to look for more exact aspects of the environment that protect the vulnerable child.

I have mentioned race in addition to SES as an environmental factor. Blacks are more likely than others to have premature and low birth weight babies, whether as a result of biological predisposition or their exposure to more negative factors (such as less and poorer-quality prenatal care, or less adequate diet) before and during pregnancy is not fully known.

When actual characteristics of the home environment are examined, there is the possibility of determining the importance of specific variables and whether they are the same for premature and term infants. This question has been examined by Siegel (1982). All six subscales of HOME administered at 12 months were significantly related to IQ at 3 years of age for preterms, but only two scales were related for term infants. The total HOME score was highly corre-

lated with IQ and language comprehension for preterm infants ($r = .66$ and $r = .55$). HOME was not significantly correlated with either variable for full-term infants. This was true regardless of SES or developmental level for the prematures. Relations between HOME and outcomes for full-term infants occurred only for those who were developmentally delayed. Schraeder and colleagues (1987) have also shown that environmental variables account for about half of the variance in developmental outcome at 3 years.

These data could lead to the conclusion that all aspects of the home environment are important for the development of infants at risk, but that they are not particularly relevant to the outcomes of "normal" children. Such a conclusion finds further support in data showing that the number of neonatal complications did not affect IQ in responsive environments, but did affect it in less responsive environments (Cohen et al., 1982).

Several studies that have measured specific mother-infant interactions at different ages have found that mothers of preterm babies were more responsive than mothers of term babies during early infancy (for example, Bakeman & Brown, 1980; Beckwith & Cohen, 1978; Beckwith et al., 1976). Bakeman and Brown (1980), however, found that outcomes at 3 years (social ability in a day camp and IQ) were not predicted by these early social interactions, but by the mother's responsiveness when the baby was 20 months. This sample of preterm infants was not very biologically handicapped, but they and their controls were socially disadvantaged. The influence of maternal interactions on IQ was only moderate and not operative in early infancy.

It may be that generalizations based on the above studies will not hold for prematures with different levels of postbirth illness. Mothers of prematures who were healthy or had RDS or bronchopulmonary dysplasia were compared at 4 and 8 months in a teaching task (Jarvis et al., 1989). Mothers of infants with bronchopulmonary dysplasia (the sickest) were less sensitive, less responsive to their infants' distress, and showed less fostering of social and emotional growth. Furthermore, they showed a decline in those behaviors from 4 to 8 months.

Prediction of Outcomes. It is clear that both parents and doctors would like to be able to predict which premature infants are likely to have long-term problems and which are not. Much of the discussion thus far is relevant to this question, but I now want to address it specifically.

First, it is commonly accepted that the smaller,

more premature, or smaller for gestational age the infant, the more likely there will be problems. This conclusion is challenged by some data for prematures (Cohen & Parmelee, 1983; Cohen et al., 1982) and for SGA infants (Hawdon et al., 1990). Hawdon et al. (1990) found that SGA infants born in the mid-1970s were not handicapped in IQ, reading, or educational attainment at ages 10 to 11 in relation to the degree of their smallness. The authors feel that this was likely the result of better dietary management at birth compared with earlier study samples. The best predictors of these infants' later status were their mothers' IQs and their ordinal positions. In contrast, a Finnish study of infants born in the early 1970s found SGA to be the strongest predictor of poor outcomes at age 9 (with neonatal neurological symptoms next, and then SES) (Lindahl et al., 1988). That SES would be a predictor in that much more homogeneous society is interesting.

Second, in the effort to determine the deleterious effects of prematurity without other complications, researchers have established that the presence and degree of neurological damage are important determinants of outcome.

An opportunity to examine multifactorial determinants of outcome is provided by the UCLA prospective study of cognitive development in prematures already referred to several times. It started in 1972, when neonatal care units were already quite sophisticated (for a description, see Parmelee et al., 1976). The sample studied was diverse in ethnic and SES makeup, in the degree of prematurity (25 to 37 weeks), and in birth weight (800 to 2,495 g). Two characteristics of prematures identified by this group (and others) to differ from those of term infants were visual attention (at term date) and sleep patterns (at term date and 3 months later). The caregiving environment was assessed at 1, 8, and 24 months, and an index of caregiving in the first 2 years was developed.

Both visual fixation at term and the index of responsiveness affected outcomes, but the effects of the caregiving environment were greater than those of the neurological organization of visual attention at term (40 weeks). The average IQs of the 5-year-olds who had short fixation times at term and relatively responsive caregiving were 19 points higher than those who had long fixation times at term and less responsive caregiving in the first 2 years (Beckwith, 1976; Beckwith & Parmelee, 1983). Nevertheless, the amount of variation in the outcomes means that individual prediction would still be hazardous. (For a similar view of interaction in a longitudinal study, see Meyer-Probst et al., 1983.)

The maturity of the quiet sleep pattern at term appeared to be a more potent biological indicator of trouble (Beckwith & Parmelee, 1983, 1984). By itself it made a 10-point difference in IQ at age 5. Sleep pattern, together with responsive caretaking, accounted for a 23-point difference. When the maturity of active sleep at 3 months was examined, it made as big a difference as the responsiveness of caregiving (13 and 14 points). The best combination was 19 points better than the poorest. This biological indicator of neurological organization appears to be a powerful factor in relation to later IQ. Nevertheless, the power of the environment is shown by the fact that no infant from the group with responsive mothers had an IQ below 100. IQs ranged from 80 to 134 for those with more mature sleep patterns, and from 40 to 138 for those with less mature sleep patterns. Thus we see that good physiological status cannot protect all from some deficit, while responsive mothering can apparently assure normality.

Another aspect of physiological status is found in the degree to which state patterns are consistent, with inconsistency indicating a risk for developmental problems (Thoman et al., 1981). An index of stability of sleep-wake patterns from one neonatal observation to another correlated with the infant's performance on the **Newborn Behavior Assessment Scales (NBAS, or Brazelton** scales; see Chapter 8), with medical problems, and with later mental and motor development (Tynan, 1986). It might be used as a nonintrusive technique for assessment.

These data offer real hope that someday researchers will be able to find a group of indicators that will be reasonably good predictors of the chances for normal development. However, the IQs found in this study were rather high, mostly normal or above. It cannot be assumed that this is typical for all prematures. The families in this study had more than the usual amounts of support for dealing with their premature infants. This takes us to our next question. Are there steps that can be taken to reduce any adverse effects of prematurity?

Intervention Studies

Two types of interventions will be examined here: short-term interventions (during the hospital stay) and long-term interventions (focused on the mother). All of the interventions to be discussed are behavioral, not medical.

Hospital Interventions. Hospital interventions began because premature infants are likely to receive care that is different from the care mature newborns receive and to receive it for relatively long periods. This may affect the baby directly, or it may affect parent-infant interaction and hence the later development of the child.

Traditionally the premature has been placed in an incubator or isolette immediately after birth (see Figure 2.12). In these devices, temperature, oxygen level, and humidity can be controlled. The infant is often hooked to monitoring devices and sometimes to tubes for feeding. In general, the infant is separated from its parents for a considerable period after birth. Until recently parents were not encouraged to visit their premature babies, and may even have been discouraged. (For an excellent review of the issues of changing beliefs and practices relating to the stimulation of premature infants, see Korner, 1990.)

Nurses often handle premature infants less than they do others, but doctors and nurses subject them to stressful maneuvers. As mentioned above, prematures are exposed to constant light and noise (the nursery is kept well lighted so that observation is easy, and the incubator or isolette machinery makes a considerable amount of noise). This deprivation of normally patterned sensory experience may itself have negative effects on babies (Caputo & Mandell, 1970), as has been shown in animals (see Chapter 7).

Concern with the effects of these environmental variables on premature infants has led many workers in hospitals to provide extra stimulation: handling, stroking, or rocking. It has been shown that the handling of newborn rats allows them to cope with later stress more effectively, and Knudtson (1978) found a similar result for human infants. She gave sick and well prematures a total of 30 minutes of stroking, spread throughout the day. She measured their physiological reactions to stress (by measuring variations in a chemical, cortisol, that is involved in stress reactions) and their behavioral organization (using the Brazelton Neonatal Scale). The stroked infants had consistently better adaptation to stress and better behavioral organization. Three months after the infants left the hospital, Knudtson gave them the Bayley and Gesell infant development tests (described in Chapter 8). The stroked infants scored significantly higher on the mental, but not the motor, part of the Bayley. They were also superior on sensory responsiveness and fine motor development. These findings are corroborated by those of a smaller study that also found effects at 7 to 8 months of age (Solkoff et al., 1967).

Rocking motion is another form of stimulation to which the normally gestating in utero baby is exposed and that the premature lacks. Several studies have shown that rocking in the isolette leads to better weight gain and organization of behavior in the immediate newborn period (Korner, 1979; Korner et al., 1975; Neal, 1968). The long-term effects are not known, however, since relevant follow-up studies were not done. Nevertheless, many people have become concerned about the kind of neonatal care prematures receive. They feel that if such minor interventions can produce such strong short-term effects, more drastic changes could lead to even more important changes.

A group of investigators from Albert Einstein College of Medicine combined tactile stimulation (massage) with rocking (Rose, 1980; Rose et al., 1980; Schmidt et al., 1980). They were interested in whether this would improve preterm infants' responsivity to stimulation. For the intervention group, both behavioral and heart rate responses to tactile stimuli were between those of term infants and those of comparable prematures who had not received the extra stimulation (Rose et al., 1980). The effects of the same stimulation was studied using cardiac and motor responses to the sound of a heartbeat and to tactile stimulation during sleep, but the results were extremely complex (Schmidt et al., 1980). At 6 months of age, when infants normally prefer a novel to a familiar stimulus, the three groups were tested for their preference (Rose, 1980). The routinely cared-for preterms did not prefer the novel stimulus, but both the term babies and the stimulated preterms did in two out of three problems.

Babies provided patterned kinesthetic and auditory stimuli (Barnard & Bee, 1983) showed improved organization during the hospital period, and markedly better (16 to 33 points higher than controls) Bayley MDI scores at 2 years, although there had been no differences at 8 months.

It is clear from these studies that preterm babies can profit from receiving some of the experiences that they would naturally have if they were in a home environment. This has led to a reform movement oriented toward providing handling, rocking, and enriched sensory stimulation. The reform already has some counterreaction, with doctors warning about the dangers of overstimulation, especially of the poorly developed skin.[6] Another reform movement in the making concerns the provision of sucking for the premature; this is discussed in Chapter 6. The reform movement oriented toward mother-infant interactions in the hospital is discussed in Chapter 5.

---

6. For an excellent review of the issues of changing beliefs and practices regarding the stimulation of premature infants, see Korner (1990). For a review of the methodological issues related to intervention with high-risk infants, see Korner (1987).

Social Interventions During Infancy. The basis for early social intervention was discussed as early as 1971 (Wright, 1971). This pioneering study looked at intervention primarily directed toward mothers or families (described in Bromwich & Parmelee, 1979). A later study looked at intervention with a population triply at risk (premature infants of lower-SES teenaged black mothers) (Field et al., 1980). Half of the 60 mothers who volunteered were randomly assigned to intervention and half to a control group. In addition, 30 fullterm infants of teenage mothers and 30 preterm and 30 term infants of adult mothers were assessed as control groups. The intervention consisted of half-hour visits (twice a week for 4 months and monthly thereafter) designed (a) to educate the mothers about normal development and child-rearing practices, (b) to teach them age-appropriate exercises and stimulation methods, and (c) to facilitate mother-infant interactions in the hope of promoting both communication skills and harmonious mother-infant relations. The infants were assessed at birth and at 4 and 8 months.

When adult preterm and teen preterm control mothers were compared, the teens had less realistic expectations and less desirable child-rearing attitudes at 4 months, and they rated their infants' temperaments as more difficult at both 4 and 8 months. At 8 months their infants had lower Bayley mental scores. These data suggest that the target group needed the kind of intervention the experimental group was receiving.

Compared with preterm controls, preterm intervention infants did better at four months. They had higher scores on the Denver Developmental Screening Test, weighed more, and were taller. Their mothers also differed. They had more realistic expectations and more desirable child-rearing attitudes, and rated their babies' temperaments as less difficult. Although feeding interactions generally did not differ for the two groups, both mothers and infants in the intervention group were rated as more optimal in face-to-face interactions. At 8 months the intervention group babies had higher Bayley mental scores (110 versus 101), the mothers received higher ratings on emotional and verbal responsivity and involvement with their infants (on the HOME scales), and rated their infants as having easier temperaments (being more adaptable and more persistent, and having more optimal thresholds on the Carey Infant Temperament Questionnaire, or ITQ).

Although the research on how the environment compensates for problems associated with prematurity has only begun to unravel the mysteries of the subject, practical applications are easy to make. Optimizing the environment of prematures is important. Special services in the first 3 years of life are being explored in a large-scale, multi-institution study using randomized selection of prematures to receive the education or to be controls who receive lesser (but still greater than normal) services: home visits, a developmental curriculum, parent groups. So far, IQ at age 3 has been shown to be 15 points higher for the heavier group, and 8 points higher for the under 2,000 g group. In the Boston branch of the study, where more services were available to everyone and the educational level was higher, both experimentals and controls improved about equally ("Early Intervention Shown Beneficial," 1991).

We know that such factors as mother's education, positive attitudes, and caregiving behaviors, as well as the home's middle-class status, are related to higher IQ. Enrichment day care can also help compensate for general SES disadvantages (see Chapter 13). Providing help to parents who need it may not be sufficient to erase all risk associated with prematurity, but it is likely to help and unlikely to hurt.

Summary

In 9 months a single cell grows and differentiates into an amazingly complex being who can survive on his or her own, and also gives rise to a number of structures that help support this development. The egg is fertilized while still in the fallopian tubes, and it has already reproduced itself several times by the time it reaches the uterus. By the fourth day the cell mass has 16 to 64 cells and has begun to differentiate into two layers, one of which will eventually be a baby if all goes well, and the other of which will provide the placenta and other support structures. By 14 days, which is approximately when the mother misses her first period, implantation is complete and the cells are differentiating into endoderm, mesoderm, and ectoderm. In the third week the first precursor structure—the neural tube—and the placenta begin to develop. During the next 6 weeks, the period of organogenesis, all the organs of the body take form and some of them, such as the heart and circulatory system, actually function, though not in the same fashion they will after birth. By this time (8 weeks after conception) such external features as eyes, ears, and hands are recognizable. In the third month the fetus first moves its arms and legs and exhibits reflexes. The external sex organs are sufficiently developed to identify sex. This marks the end of the first trimester. The fetus is still so small that its mother does not yet look pregnant, and does not feel its movements. Nor can it survive if removed from her body.

In the fifth lunar month (weeks 17-20) the fetus's movements become obvious to the mother. This time historically has been called the time of quickening; according to Thomas Aquinas, this is when the soul enters the body. The fetal heartbeat is strong enough to be heard through a stethoscope placed on the mother's abdomen. The fetus sloughs off skin and respiratory cells into the amniotic fluid, which allows doctors to gather (amniocentesis) and process them to detect many chromosomal, genetic, and developmental abnormalities.

In the last half of its time in the womb, the fetus develops greatly in size and weight. The organ systems develop to the point that they become able to function and hence to allow the fetus to have a chance to survive if born prematurely. The brain develops rapidly.

SEXUAL DEVELOPMENT

Embryos start to develop structures characteristic of their genetic sex at 5 weeks after conception. For each stage of sexual differentiation (i.e., of the gonads or sex glands, the internal sexual structures, the external genitalia, and the brain) development proceeds from undifferentiated primordia. These structures have the potential to develop into either male or female forms. In each case the female form develops unless hormones produced by male gonads intervene and change the course of development.

CIRCULATORY SYSTEM

Before birth the fetal blood receives oxygen from maternal blood via the placenta (not from the fetal lungs). At birth, when the lungs first draw air and the respiratory system begins functioning, the circulatory system changes reflexively so that venous and arterial blood are separated. The lungs then function to provide oxygen. Immature respiratory development and malfunctions in the transition from fetal to infant respiratory and circulatory systems create many of the problems faced by premature newborns.

CENTRAL NERVOUS SYSTEM

The neural tube, the primordium of the central nervous system, is one of the first structures visible in the embryo. It develops earlier and more rapidly than most other organ systems. The first brain cells (neurons) develop at 8 weeks after conception. Brain cells increase in number until about 24 months after birth, when glial cells stop reproducing. Development of the myelin sheath and of neuron processes and connec-

tions, necessary for proper functioning of the brain, continues long after cell division has ceased. The areas of the cortex develop in a regular and integrated sequence. The primary motor areas develop before the sensory and association areas, and their order of development follows the cephalocaudal sequence. Next, the primary sensory areas of the cortex develop in the order of touch, vision, and audition. Association areas develop last.

SOURCE OF KNOWLEDGE

Knowledge of early prenatal development comes primarily from embryological studies of other species, but in other countries studies of the products of abortion add to our knowledge. Behavior of the latter stages of development is now accessible to study via ultrasound.

TWINS

Twins are an interesting variant on normal prenatal development. Because they can either be genetically identical or merely siblings conceived simultaneously (or nearly so), they offer a testing ground for looking at genetic and environmental contributions to development. There are, however, many methodological and even statistical problems in such studies.

PREMATURITY

Prematurity, or being born too soon, is one of the most common variants of development and is a major neonatal health problem. Its effects are much studied, as are those of being SGA (that is, having suffered prenatal growth retardation). Low birth weight or prematurity can be caused by problems in the fetus, in the placenta, or in the mother (poor health, nutrition, and other factors to be discussed). Prematures are at risk for other medical problems, including respiratory distress, neurological deficits, anoxia, hyperbilirubinemia, and death. Prematures have short-term lags in many aspects of development. Their long-term physical growth is compromised. The degree of neurological and intellectual handicap is less certain, and depends in part on neonatal care practices at the time of birth. Language development and school performance may be more affected than IQ. There is no good evidence for long-term effects on social development.

Are long-term effects of prematurity a result of biological insults (prenatal or even from the environment of the neonatal intensive care unit) or of social and environmental handicaps after discharge from the hospital? Or do they depend on a combination or interaction of both? Environmental factors appear more important in determining the outcomes for children at risk than for normal-term infants, but medical risk factors other than prematurity (for example, serious brain hemorrhage and bronchopulmonary dysplasia) also affect outcomes.

Intervention studies focused on providing appropriate stimulation of prematures while they are in the hospital and on helping mothers and prematures subsequent to discharge have been shown to be effective in a number of ways, including raising intelligence test scores in later infancy and preschool years.

Overall, it appears that the outlook is favorable for prematures who are not neurologically damaged or who do not suffer the negative effects of the prolonged mechanical ventilation that kept them alive. Intervention may allay the effects for these infants, too.

Embryology Sources

Some understanding of embryology is necessary for an understanding of the complexities of the constitution of the newborn, but thorough coverage of this subject is clearly beyond the scope of this book. Consequently, the section of this chapter that deals with embryology is not referenced in the conventional way. The books used most in the writing of this portion of the chapter are listed below. In addition, numerous other sources have influenced the ways I have used these materials, as well as my feeling for the importance of this period of life.

AREY, L. B. (1965). *Developmental anatomy: A textbook and laboratory manual of embryology* (7th ed.). Philadelphia: W. B. Saunders.

BECK, F., Moffat, D. B., & Lloyd, J. B. (1973). *Human embryology*. Oxford: Blackwell Scientific Publications.

EHRHARDT, A. A., & Baker, S. W. (1974). Fetal androgens, human animal nervous system differentiation, and behavioral sex differences. In R. C. Friedman, R. M. Richart, & R. L. Vande Wiele (Eds.), *Sex differences in behavior*. New York: John Wiley.

HAINES, R. W., & Mohiuddin, A. (1968). *Human embryology* (4th ed.). Edinburgh: E. & S. Livingston.

HOGARTH, P. (1978). *Biology of reproduction*. New York: John Wiley.

MONEY, J., & Ehrhardt, A. (1972). *Man and woman, boy and girl*. Baltimore: Johns Hopkins University Press.

SPRINGER, S. P., & Deutsch, G. (1981). *Left brain right brain*. San Francisco: Freeman.

TANNER, J. M. (1978). *Fetus into man*. Cambridge, MA: Harvard University Press.

References

AMATO, M., Howald, H., & von Muralt, G. (1987). Fetal sex and distribution of peri-intraventricular hemorrhage in preterm infants. *European Neurology, 27*, 20-23.

ASTBURY, J., Orgill, A. A., & Bajuk, B. (1987). Relationship between two-year behavior and neurodevelopmental outcome at five years of very low-birthweight survivors. *Developmental Medicine and Child Neurology, 29*, 370-379.

BAKEMAN, R., & Brown, J. V. (1980). Early interaction: Consequences for social and mental development at 3 years. *Child Development, 51*, 437-447.

BALLARD, J. L., et al. (1977). A simplified assessment of gestational age. *Pediatric Research, 11*, 374.

BARNARD, K. E., & Bee, H. L. (1983). The impact of temporally patterned stimulation on the development of preterm infants. *Child Development, 54*, 1156-1167.

BECKWITH, L. (1976). Caregiver-infant interactions and the development of the high-risk infant. In T. Tjossem (Ed.), *Intervention strategies for high-risk infants and young children*. Baltimore: University Park Press.

BECKWITH, L., & Cohen, S. E. (1978). Preterm birth: Hazardous obstetrical and postnatal events as related to caregiver-infant behavior. *Infant Behavior and Development, 1*, 403-411.

BECKWITH, L., & Cohen. S. E. (1987). Social interaction with the parent during infancy and later intellectual competence in children born preterm. *Early Child Development and Care, 27*, 239-254.

BECKWITH, L., Cohen, S. E., Kopp, C. B., Parmelee, A. H., & Marcy, T. G. (1976). Caregiver-infant interaction and cognitive development in preterm infants. *Child Development, 47*, 579-587.

BECKWITH, L., & Parmelee, A. H. (1983, July). *Preterm infants from birth to five years: Social factors and cognitive development.* Paper presented at a symposium on follow-up studies of children born at risk, at the meeting of the International Society for the Study of Behavioral Development, Munich.

BECKWITH, L., & Parmelee, A. H. (1984, April). *Infant sleep states, EEG patterns, caregiving and 5 year IQs of preterm children.* Paper presented at a symposium on sleep at the International Conference on Infant Studies, New York.

BLAIR, E., & Stanley, F. (1990). Intrauterine growth and spastic cerebral palsy. *American Journal of Obstetrics and Gynecology, 162*, 229-237.

BOOTH, C. L., Leonard, H. L., & Thoman, E. B. (1980). Sleep state and behavior patterns in preterm and full term infants. *Neuropediatrics* (formerly *Neuropediatrie*), *11*, 354-364.

BOUSSY, C. A., Scott, K. G., & Swales, T. P. (1990, March). *Changes in outcome for high risk infants.* Paper presented at the Conference on Human Development, Richmond, VA.

BOZYNSKI, M. E. A., Nelson, M. N., Genaze, D., Rosati-Skertich, C., Matalon, T. A. S., Vasan, U., & Naughton, P. M. (1988). Cranial ultrasonography and the prediction of cerebral palsy in infants weighing 1200 grams *Developmental Medicine and Child Neurology, 30*, 342-348.

BRADLEY, R. H., & Caldwell, B. M. (1977). Early home environment and changes in mental test performance in children from 6 to 30 months. *Developmental Psychology, 12*, 93-97.

BRADLEY, R. H., Caldwell, B. M., Rock, S. L., Casey, P. M., & Nelson, J. (1987). The early development of low-birthweight infants: Relationship to health, family status, family context, family processes, and parenting. *International Journal of Behavioral Development, 10*, 301-318.

BRAINE, M. D. S., Heimer, B., Wortis, H., & Friedman, A. M. (1966). Factors associated with impairment of the early development of prematures. *Monographs of the Society for Research in*

Child Development, 31 (4, Serial No. 106).

BROMWICH, R. M., & Parmelee, A. H., Jr. (1979). An intervention program for pre-term high-risk infants and their parents. In T. M. Field, A. M. Sostek, S. Goldberg, & H. H. Shuman (Eds.), *Infants born at risk*. New York: Spectrum.

BUDETTI, P., McManus, P., Barrand, N., & Heinen, L. U. (1981, August). *The implications of cost-effectiveness analysis of medical technology: Case study no. 10. The costs and effectiveness of neonatal intensive care* (U.S. Congress, Office of Technology Assessment, Publication No. 341-844/1016). Washington, DC: Government Printing Office.

CAPUTO, D. V., & Mandell, W. (1970). Consequences of low birth weight. *Developmental Psychology, 3*, 363-383.

CLARK, A. J. (1988). Human surfactant as prophylactic treatment of respiratory distress syndrome in newborns. *Research Resources Reporter, 12*, 1-4.

COHEN, S. E., & Parmelee, A. H. (1983). Prediction of five-year Stanford-Binet scores in preterm infants. *Child Development, 54*, 1242-1253.

COHEN, S. E., Parmelee, A. H., Beckwith, L., & Sigman, M. (1986). Cognitive development in preterm infants: Birth to 8 years. *Journal of Developmental and Behavioral Pediatrics, 7*, 102-110.

COHEN, S. E., Parmelee, A. H., Sigman, M., & Beckwith, L. (1982). Neonatal risk factors in preterm infants. *Applied Research in Mental Retardation, 3*, 265-276.

COHEN, S. E., Parmelee, A. H., Sigman, M., & Beckwith, L. (1988). Antecedents of school problems in children born preterm. *Journal of Pediatric Psychology, 13*, 493-507.

CONEL, J. (1939-1967). *The postnatal development of the human cerebral cortex* (Vols. 1-7). Cambridge, MA: Harvard University Press.

CRAWFORD, J. W. (1982). Mother-infant interaction in premature and full-term infants. *Child Development, 53*, 957-962.

CRISAFI, M. A., & Driscoll, J. M. (1989, April). *Intellectual development at 3 years of age in very low birth weight infants*. Paper presented at the annual meeting of the Society for Research in Child Development, Kansas City, MO.

DE VRIES, J. I., Visser, G. H., & Prechtl, H. F. (1982). The emergence of fetal behavior: I. Qualitative aspects. *Early Human Development, 7*, 301-322.

DE VRIES, J. I., Visser, G. H., & Prechtl, H. F. (1985). The emergence of fetal behavior: II. Quantitative aspects. *Early Human Development, 12*, 99-120.

DE VRIES, J. I., Visser, G. H., & Prechtl, H. F. (1986). Fetal behavior in early pregnancy. *European Journal of Obstetrics, Gynecology and Reproductive Biology, 21*, 271-276.

DE VRIES, J. I., Visser, G. H., & Prechtl, H. F. (1988). The emergence of fetal behavior: III. Individual differences and consistencies. *Early Human Development, 16*, 85-103.

DOUGLAS, J. W. B. (1956). Mental ability and school achievement of premature children at eight years of age. *British Medical Journal, 1*, 1210.

DRILLIEN, C. (1964). *The growth and development of the prematurely born infant*. Edinburgh: E. & S. Livingston.

DRILLIEN, C., Thomson, A., & Burgoyne, K. (1980). Low birth weight children at early school age. *Developmental Medicine and Child Neurology, 22*, 26-47.

DUBOWITZ, L. M., Dubowitz, V., & Goldberg, C. (1970). Clinical assessment of gestational age in the newborn infant. *Journal of Pediatrics, 77*, 1-10.

Early intervention shown beneficial for low-birth-weight children. (1991, January). *Harvard Medical Area Focus*, pp. 1, 5-7.

ECKERMAN, C., Sturm, L., & Gross, S. (1985). Different developmental courses for very-low-birthweight infants differing in early head growth. *Developmental Psychology, 21*, 813-827.

EDMONDS, J. E., Keith, E. P., & Szymonowicz, W. M. (1990, April). *School performance of very low birthweight (VLBW) preterm children at 8 years of age*. Paper presented at the International Conference on Infant Studies, Montreal.

FIELD, T. M., Widmayer, S. M., Stringer, S., & Ignatoff, E. (1980). Teenage, lower-class, black mothers and their preterm infants: An intervention and developmental follow-up. *Child Development, 51*, 426-436.

FISHER, A. E. (1967). Chemical stimulation of the brain. In *Psychobiology: The biological basis of behavior*. San Francisco: Freeman.

FRIEDMAN, S. L., Jacobs, B. S., & Werthmann, M. W., Jr. (1982). Preterms of low medical risk: Spontaneous behavior and soothability at expected date of birth. *Infant Behavior and Development, 5*, 3-10.

FRIEDMAN, S. L., Zahn-Waxler, C., Waxler, M., & Werthmann, M. W. (1987). Effects of physiologic jaundice on behavioral function in low-risk preterm infants. *Journal of Applied Developmental Psychology, 8*, 53-66.

GENN, M. M., & Silverman, W. A. (1964). The mental development of ex-premature children with retrolental fibroplasia. *Journal of Nervous and Mental Disease, 138*, 79-86.

GLUCK, L. (Ed.). (1977). *Intrauterine asphyxia and the developing fetal brain*. Chicago: Year Book Medical Publishers.

GOLDSTEIN, K. M., Caputo, M. M., & Taub, H. B. (1976). The effects of prenatal and perinatal complications on development at one year of age. *Child Development, 47*, 613-621.

HARRIS, S. (1987). Early neuromotor predictors of cerebral palsy in low-birthweight infants. *Developmental Medicine and Child Neurology, 29*, 508-519.

HAWDON, J. M., Hey, E., Kolvin, I., & Fundudis, T. (1990). Born too small: Is outcome still affected? *Developmental Medicine and Child Neurology, 32*, 943-953.

HAY, D. A., & O'Brien, P. J. (1984). The role of parental attitudes in the development of temperament in twins at home, school and in test situations. *Acta Genet Med Gemellol, 33*, 191-204.

HOGARTH, P. (1978). *Biology of reproduction*. New York: John Wiley.

HOLMES, D. L., Nagy, J. N., Slaymaker, F., Sosnowski, R. J., Prinz, S. M., & Pasternak, J. F. (1982). Early influences of prematurity, illness, and prolonged hospitalization on infant behavior. *Developmental Psychology, 18*, 744-750.

HOPKINS, J., Heller, W., & Cox, S. (1990, April). *Effects of intracranial hemorrhage on infant socioemotional development*. Paper presented at the International Conference on Infant Studies, Montreal.

Institute of Medicine. (1982). Summary of workshop on low birth weight infants. In Institute of Medicine, *Infants at risk for developmental dysfunction*. Washington, DC: National Academy Press.

JACOBS, B. S., Friedman, S. C., & Werthmann, M. W., Jr. (1979, April). *A comparison of temperament in pre-term, full-term, and post-term infants*. Paper presented at the annual meeting of the Eastern Psychological Association, Philadelphia.

JANOWSKY, J. S., & Finlay, B. L. (1986). The outcome of perinatal brain damage: The role of normal neuron loss and axon retraction. *Developmental Medicine and Child Neurology, 28*, 375-389.

JARVIS, P. A., Myers, B. J., & Creasey, G. L. (1989). The effects of infants' illness on mothers' interactions with prematures at 4 and 8 months. *Infant Behavior and Development, 12*, 25-35.

KITCHEN, W. H., Rickards, A. L., Ryan, M. M., Ford, G. W., Lissenden, J. V., & Boyle, L. W. (1986). Improved outcome to two years of very low-birthweight infants: Fact or artifact? *Developmental Medicine and Child Neurology, 28,* 579-588.

KNUDTSON, F. W. (1978). *Effects of tactile stimulation on responsivity to stress in high-risk premature infants.* Paper presented at the Invited Symposium: Effects of Early Experience on Infant Development, Western Psychological Association, San Francisco.

KOLB, B. (1989). Brain development, plasticity, and behavior. *American Psychologist, 44,* 1203-1212.

KOPP, C. B., & Parmelee, A. H. (1979). Prenatal and perinatal influences on infant behavior. In J. D. Osofsky (Ed.), *Handbook of infant development* (pp. 29-75). New York: John Wiley.

KORNER, A. F. (1979). Maternal rhythms and waterbeds: A form of intervention with premature infants. In E. B. Thoman (Ed.), *Origins of the infant's social responsiveness.* Hillsdale, NJ: Lawrence Erlbaum.

KORNER, A. F. (1987). Preventive intervention with high-risk newborns: Theoretical, conceptual and methodological perspectives. In J. D. Osofsky (Ed.), *Handbook of infant development* (2nd ed., pp. 881-912). New York: John Wiley.

KORNER, A. F. (1990). Infant stimulation: Issues of theory and research. *Clinics in Perinatology, 17,* 173-184.

KORNER, A. F., Kraemer, H. C., Haffner, M. E., & Cosper, L. M. (1975). Effects of flotation on premature infants: A pilot study. *Pediatrics, 56,* 361-367.

LAGERSTRM, M., Bremme, K., Eneroth, P., & Magnusson, D. (1989). *School performance and IQ-test scores at age 13 as related to birth weight and gestational age* (Report No. 699). Stockholm: University of Stockholm, Department of Psychology.

LARGO, R. H., Molinari, L., Comenale Pinto, L., Weber, M., & Duc, G. (1986). Language development of term and preterm children during the first five years of life. *Developmental Medicine and Child Neurology, 28,* 333-350.

LAWSON, K. R., & Turkewitz, G. (1986). [Letter to the editor]. *New England Journal of Medicine, 314,* 449.

LEFEBVRE, F., Bard, H., Veilleux, A., & Martel, C. (1988). Outcome at school age of children with birthweights of 1000 grams or less. *Developmental Medicine and Child Neurology, 30,* 170-180.

LINDAHL, E., Michelsson, K., Helenius, M., & Parre, M. (1988). Neonatal risk factors and later neurodevelopmental disturbances. *Developmental Medicine and Child Neurology, 30,* 571-589.

LIPPER, E., Lee, K., Gartner, L. M., & Grellong, B. (1981). Determinants of neurobehavioral outcome in low-birth-weight infants. *Pediatrics, 67,* 502-505.

LLOYD, B. W., Wheldall, K., & Perks, D. (1988). Controlled study of intelligence and school performance of very low-birthweight children from a defined geographical area. *Developmental Medicine and Child Neurology, 30,* 36-42.

LOW, J. A., Galbraith, R. S., Muir, D. W., Broekhoven, L. H., Wilkinson, J. W., & Karchmar, E. J. (1985). The contribution of fetal-newborn complications to motor and cognitive deficits. *Developmental Medicine and Child Neurology, 27,* 578-587.

LUBCHENCO, L. O. (1970). Assessment of gestational age and development at birth. *Pediatric Clinics of North America, 17,* 125-145.

LUBCHENCO, L. O., Hansman, C., & Boyd, E. (1966). Intrauterine growth in length and head circumference as estimated from live births at gestational ages from 26 to 42 weeks. *Pediatrics, 37,* 403-408.

LUBCHENCO, L. O., Horner, F. A., Reed, L. H., Hix, I. E., Jr., Metcalf, D., Colig, R., Elliot, H. C., & Bourg, M. (1963). Se-

quelae of premature birth. *American Journal of Diseases of Children, 106,* 101-115.

McDONALD, A. D. (1964). Intelligence in children of very low birthweight. *British Journal of Preventive and Social Medicine, 18,* 59-74.

MEYER-PROBST, B., Rosler, H.-D., & Teichmann, H. (1983). Biological and psychosocial risk factors and development during childhood. In D. Magnusson & V. L. Allen (Eds.), *Human development: An interactional perspective.* New York: Academic Press.

MOLFESE, D. L., & Segalowitz, S. J. (Eds.). (1988). *Brain lateralization in children: Developmental implications.* New York: Guilford.

Morbidity and Mortality Weekly Report. (1988). Vol. 37, p. 637.

MYERS, B. J., Jarvis, P. A., Creasey, G. L., Kerkering, K. W., Markowitz, P. I., & Best, A. M. (1991). *Prematurity and respiratory illness: Brazelton scale (NBAS) performance of preterm infants with bronchopulmonary dysplasia (BPD), respiratory distress syndrome (RDS), or no respiratory illness.* Manuscript submitted for publication.

NAEYE, R. L., Benirschke, K., Hagstrom, J. W. C., & Marcus, C. C. (1966). Intrauterine growth of twins as estimated from live birth weight data. *Pediatrics, 37,* 409-416.

NEAL, M. V. (1968). Vestibular stimulation and developmental behavior of the small premature infant. *Nursing Research Report, 3,* 1, 3-5.

O'BRIEN, P. J., & Hay, D. A. (1987). Birthweight differences, the transfusion syndrome and the cognitive development of monozygotic twins. *Acta Genet Med Gemellol, 36,* 181-196.

PARKER, S., & Bavosi, J. (1979). *Life before birth: The story of the first nine months.* Cambridge: British Museum (Natural History)/Cambridge University Press.

PARMELEE, A. H., & Sigman, M. (1976). Development of visual behavior and neurological organization in pre-term and full-term infants. In A. D. Pick (Ed.), *Minnesota Symposia on Child Development* (Vol. 10). Minneapolis: University of Minnesota Press.

PARMELEE, A. H., Sigman, M., Kopp, C. B., & Haber, A. (1976). Diagnosis of the infant at high risk for mental, motor, and sensory handicaps. In T. Tjossem (Ed.), *Intervention strategies for high risk infants and young children.* Baltimore: University Park Press.

PARMELEE, A. H., Wenner, W. H., Akijama, Y., Schultz, M. S., & Stern, E. (1967). Sleep states in premature infants. *Developmental Medicine and Child Neurology, 9,* 70-77.

PORTNOY, S., Callias, M., Wolke, D., & Gamsu, H. (1988). Five-year follow-up of extremely low-birthweight infants. *Developmental Medicine and Child Neurology, 30,* 590-598.

POWELL, T. G., Pharoah, P. O. D., Cooke, R. W. I., & Rosenbloom, L. (1988a). Cerebral palsy in low-birthweight infants: I. Spastic hemiplegia: Associations with intrapartum stress. *Developmental Medicine and Child Neurology, 30,* 11-18.

POWELL, T. G., Pharoah, P. O. D., Cooke, R. W. I., & Rosenbloom, L. (1988b). Cerebral palsy in low-birthweight infants: II. Spastic diplegia: Associations with fetal immaturity. *Developmental Medicine and Child Neurology, 30,* 19-25.

PRECHTL, H. F. (1988). Developmental neurology of the fetus. *Bailliere's Clinical Obstetrics and Gynaecology, 2,* 21-36.

RANTAKALLIO, P., & von Wendt, L. (1985). Prognosis for low-birthweight infants up to the age of 14: A population study. *Developmental Medicine and Child Neurology, 27,* 655-663.

REINISCH, J. M. (1974). Fetal hormones, the brain, and sex differences: A heuristic, integrative review of the recent literature. *Archives of Sexual Behavior, 3,* 51-90.

RESNICK, M. B., Stralka, K., Carter, R. L., Ariet, M., Bucciarelli, R. L., Furlough, R. R., Evens, J. H., Curran, J. S., & Ausbon, W. W. (1990). Effects of birth weight and sociodemographic variables on mental development of neonatal intensive care unit survivors. *American Journal of Obstetrics and Gynecology, 162*, 374-378.

RICHMAN, L. C. (1980, August). *General intellectual and specific language development of low birth weight children.* Paper presented at the annual meeting of the American Psychological Association, Montreal.

RIESE, M. L. (1989, April). *Preterm infants' orienting responses: Improvements over time.* Paper presented at the annual meeting of the Society for Research in Child Development, Kansas City, MO.

ROSE, S. A. (1980). Enhancing visual recognition memory in preterm infants. *Developmental Psychology, 16*, 85-92.

ROSE, S. A. (1983). Differential rates of visual information processing in full-term and preterm infants. *Child Development, 54*, 1189-1198.

ROSE, S. A., Schmidt, K., Riese, M. L., & Bridger, W. H. (1980). Effects of prematurity and early intervention on responsivity to tactual stimuli: A comparison of preterm and full-term infants. *Child Development, 51*, 416-425.

ROSENSHEIM, J. J., Davidson, P. W., Reuter, S. H., Walters, C. P., & Walk, R. D. (1978, August). *The visual placing response in oxygen deprived infants.* Paper presented at the annual meeting of the American Psychological Association.

RUBIN, R. A., Rosenblatt, C., & Balow, B. (1973). Psychological and educational sequelae of prematurity. *Pediatrics, 52*, 352-363.

SCHMIDT, K., Rose, S. A., & Bridger, W. H. (1980). The effect of heartbeat sound on the cardiac and behavioral responses to tactual stimulation in sleeping, premature infants. *Developmental Psychology, 16*, 175-184.

SCHRAEDER, B. D., Rappaport, J., & Courtwright, L. (1987). Preschool development of very low birthweight infants. *Image: Journal of Nursing Scholarship, 19*, 174-178.

SHIELDS, J. R., & Schifrin, B.S. (1988). Perinatal antecedents of cerebral palsy. *Obstetrics and Gynecology, 71*, 899-905.

SIEGEL, L. S. (1982). Reproductive, perinatal, and environmental factors as predictors of the cognitive and language development of preterm and full-term infants. *Child Development, 53*, 963-973.

SIEGEL, L. S. (1983). Correction for prematurity and its consequences for the assessment of the very low birthweight infant. *Child Development, 54*, 1176-1188.

SKIDMORE, M. D., Rivers, A., & Hack, M. (1990). Increased risk of cerebral palsy among very low birth-weight infants with chronic lung disease. *Developmental Medicine and Child Neurology, 32*, 325-332.

SOLKOFF, N., Yaffe, S., & Weintraub, D. (1967). Effects of handling on the subsequent development of premature infants. *Developmental Psychology, 1*, 765-768.

SPELLACY, W. N., Handler, A., & Ferre, C. D. (1990). A case-control study of 1253 twin pregnancies from a 1982-1987 perinatal data base. *Obstetrics and Gynecology, 75*, 168-171.

STANLEY, F. J., & English, D. R. (1986). Prevalence of and risk factors for cerebral palsy in a total population cohort of low-birthweight (<2000) infants. *Developmental Medicine and Child Neurology, 28*, 559-568.

STEWART, A. L., Reynolds, E. O. R., Hope, P. L., Hamilton, P. A., Baudin, J., Costello, A. M. de L., Bradford, B. C., & Wyatt, J. S. (1987). Probability of neurodevelopmental disorders estimated from ultrasound appearance of brains of very preterm infants.

Developmental Medicine and Child Neurology, 29, 3-11.

TANNER, J. M. (1978). *Fetus into man.* Cambridge, MA: Harvard University Press.

TEJANI, N., Rebold, B., Tuck, S., Ditroia, D., Sutro, W., & Verma, U. (1984). Obstetric factors in the causation of early periventricular-intraventricular hemorrhage. *Obstetrics and Gynecology, 64*, 510-515.

THOMAN, E. B., Denenberg, V. H., Sievel, J., Zeidner, L. P., & Becker, P. T. (1981). State organization in neonates: Developmental inconsistency indicates risk for developmental dysfunction. *Neuropediatrics, 12*, 45-54.

THOMSON, A. M. (1959). Maternal stature and reproductive efficiency. *Eugenics Review, 51*, 157-162.

THOMSON, A. M., & Billewicz, W. Z. (1963). Nutritional status, maternal physique, and reproductive efficiency. *Proceedings of the Nutrition Society, 22*, 55.

TRONICK, E. Z., Scanlon, K. B., & Scanlon, J. W. (1990). Protective apathy: A hypothesis about the behavioral organization and its relation to clinical and physiologic status of the preterm infant during the newborn period. *Clinics in Perinatology, 17*, 125-154.

TYNAN, W. D. (1986). Behavioral stability predicts morbidity and mortality in infants from a neonatal intensive care unit. *Infant Behavior and Development, 9*, 71-79.

UNGERER, J. A., & Sigman, M. (1983). Developmental lags in preterm infants from one to three years of age. *Child Development, 54*, 1217-1228.

VISSER, G. H., Mulder, H. H., Wit, H. P., Mulder, E. J., & Prechtl, H. F. (1989). Vibro-acoustic stimulation of the human fetus: Effect on behavioral state organization. *Early Human Development, 19*, 285-296.

VOHR, B. R., Coll, C. G., & Oh, W. (1988). Language development of low-birthweight infants at two years. *Developmental Medicine and Child Neurology, 30*, 608-615.

WALKER, J. (1989). The behavior of 3-year-old children who were born preterm. *Child Care, Health and Development, 15*, 297-313.

WERNER, E., Simonian, K., Bierman, J. M., & French, F. E. (1967). Cumulative effect of perinatal complications and deprived environment on physical, intellectual, and social development of preschool children. *Pediatrics, 39*, 480-505.

WIENER, G., Rider, R. V., Oppel, W. C., & Harper, P. A. (1965). Correlates of low birth weight: Psychological status at 6-7 years of age. *Pediatrics, 35*, 434-444.

WIENER, G., Rider, R. V., Oppel, W. C., & Harper, P. A. (1968). Correlates of low birth weight: Psychological status at 8-10 years of age. *Pediatric Research, 2*, 110-118.

WILLIAMS, M. L., Lewandowski, L. J., Coplan, J., & D'Eugenio, D. B. (1987). Neurodevelopmental outcome of preschool children born preterm with and without intracranial hemorrhage. *Developmental Medicine and Child Neurology, 29*, 243-249.

WOLKE, D. (1987). Environmental and developmental neonatology. *Journal of Reproductive and Infant Psychology, 5*, 17-42.

WRIGHT, L. (1971). The theoretical and research base for a program of early stimulation care and training of premature infants. In J. Hellmuth (Ed.), *The exceptional infant: Studies in abnormalities* (Vol. 2). New York: Brunner/Mazel.

ZELKOWITZ, P., Papageorgiou, A., Allard, M., & Weiss, M. J. S. (1991, April). *Behavioral adjustment and self-concept in very low birthweight and normal birthweight children.* Paper presented at the annual meeting of the Society for Research in Child Development, Seattle.

Genetic Abnormalities

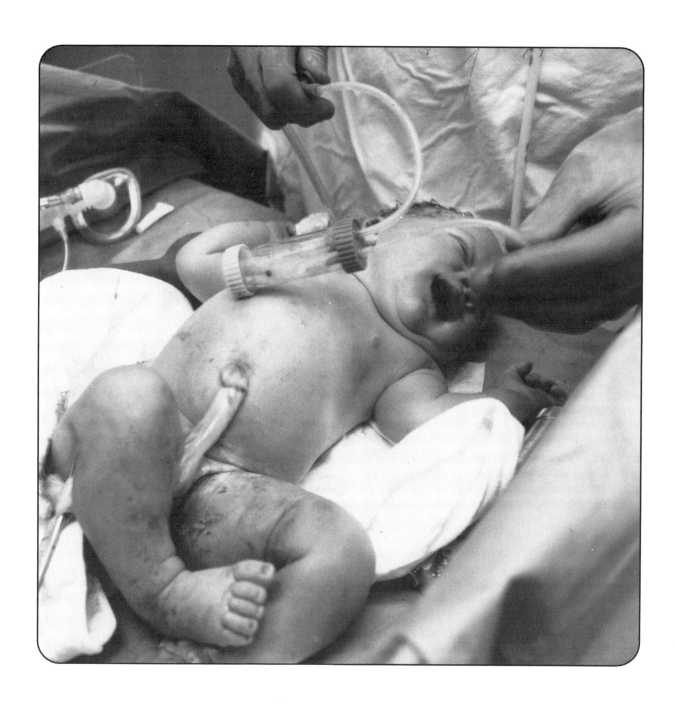

Having examined the history of infancy studies and study methods, as well as prenatal growth and development of infants, we turn now to examination of a number of genetic factors. Genetics affects development before and after birth.

Heredity, Environment, and Constitution

The set of biological and behavioral characteristics babies have at birth is called their constitution. Many of its aspects are inherited; that is, they are transmitted from parents to offspring through the genes. Some characteristics may be genetic in that they result from mutations that were not inherited, but that may be passed on. The environment prior to birth may also affect the constitution, a matter to be considered in Chapter 4. Every baby is born with a constitution that is the product of both heredity and environment. Developmental problems arising from defects in genes and chromosomes will be discussed in this chapter.

Rather than describe every known chromosomal or genetic abnormality, I have selected examples that allow for a discussion of issues relevant to genetic counseling, to detection prior to birth or in infancy, or to treatment during infancy. Many of the defects chosen as examples, like other chromosomal and genetic defects, involve mental retardation, but there are instances of physical and medical disorders as well.

BACKGROUND INFORMATION ABOUT GENETICS

To help the student understand the discussion of these issues, a brief review of some basic concepts of genetics is offered in this section, along with descriptions of some techniques by which genetic defects can be identified.

The **genotype** is the basic genetic makeup of an individual, transmitted from parents to their offspring. The **phenotype** refers to the observable characteristics of an organism, both biological and behavioral. The phenotype always results from the interaction of the genotype with the environment.

The basic units that transmit the information of heredity are the **genes**. They are arranged in linear order on the **chromosomes**, long, threadlike structures in cell nuclei. Humans have 46 chromosomes, 23 from each parent, which form pairs in the fertilized egg (see Figure 3.1). In 22 of these pairs, both members have the same structure; these are called **autosomal** pairs. All genes on them are also paired, one on each member. The combination of the pairs of genes

determines the genotype. The twenty-third pair consists of the sex chromosomes (discussed in Chapter 2), where all genes are not paired, thus leading to "sex-linked" genetic disorders.

The first technique developed to study the actions of genes was the observation of the inheritance patterns of traits. In the 1800s, Gregor Mendel, a monk of peasant origins, first demonstrated that inherited characteristics are carried from generation to generation as discrete units. By careful, extensive experiments with pea plants, he discovered that a number of characteristics, such as the color and form of seeds, flowers, and pods, all varied in subsequent generations in predictable proportions. For example, if red-flowered plants are bred with white-flowered plants, all offspring have red flowers, but if a red-flowered plant that has one dominant R gene and one recessive r (white results from rr) gene, half of the resulting plants are red and half white. Such a pattern is characteristic of traits determined by a dominant gene (here for red) and a recessive gene (here for white). There are different frequency patterns of transmission for traits that are governed by a single recessive gene, by a single dominant gene, or by single genes on a sex chromosome (the most common of which are X-linked). Mendel's ratios can be used to trace genetic mechanisms in humans as well as in peas.

Tracing family histories or pedigrees to determine frequencies of occurrence of diseases identified many human genetic defects. In the case of sex-linked or **X-linked** diseases, males who inherit an abnormal gene on their X chromosome are affected by the disease, whereas females who inherit an abnormal gene on one X chromosome have a normal gene on the other X and are "carriers"—that is, they may pass the abnormal gene to their offspring. For example, hemophilia (bleeder's disease) was shown to be sex linked by its pattern of occurrence in the descendants of Queen Victoria of England, who was a carrier. Only phenotypic traits were observed in family histories prior to the development of modern genetic techniques. The presence and nature of genotypes were inferred from the distributions, among relatives, of the phenotypic trait. Phenylketonuria (PKU), which is not a sex-linked trait, but determined by an abnormality in both copies of one gene, was originally identified as a genetic trait from a study of a family history.

As scientists learned more about genetic mechanisms, they discovered that many genetic defects resulted in missing or defective enzymes. Indeed, what genes do is to code for production of proteins such as enzymes. **Enzymes** are substances that help the body convert one substance to another, as, for example, in

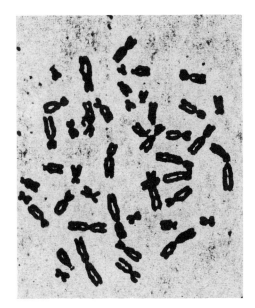 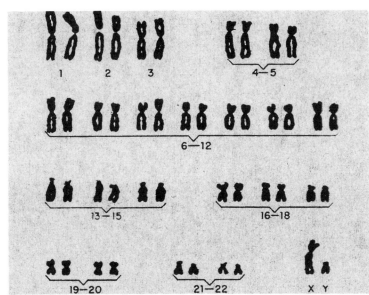

Figure 3.1. Analysis of a human chromosome complement. The part of the figure at left shows the spread-out chromosomes from a cell. The part at right shows the chromosomes arranged into a standard karyotype, numbered as shown. The sex chromosomes, labeled X and Y, are at the lower right. (Original furnished by Dr. J. J. Biesele, from H. E. Sutton, *An Introduction to Human Genetics.* New York: Holt, Rinehart & Winston, ©1965. Used by permission of the publisher.)

the transformation of food to chemicals usable by the cells. A defect in, or absence of the production of, an enzyme leads to unusual levels of particular chemicals in the body. Levels of either the enzyme itself or related chemicals can often be detected by laboratory analysis. An unusual amount of a particular chemical in the body is a phenotypic trait that can be used to infer the associated genotype or genetic trait. Most inborn errors of metabolism appear to be the result of the action of a single pair of genes.

This method of determining genetic traits provides several advantages over studying pedigrees. It not only eliminates the necessity of tracking down relatives, but it can lead to detection before the more overt phenotypic expression of the trait develops. For instance, the chemical imbalance associated with PKU can be detected before overt signs of abnormal behavior occur, thus allowing doctors to intervene before the defects (retardation and hyperactivity in the case of PKU) develop. There is hope that this kind of prevention may be achieved in other so-called inborn errors of metabolism. In many cases, amniocentesis or chorionic villus sampling (to be discussed later) can be used to detect an inborn error prenatally, allowing the option of abortion and a new pregnancy attempt.

Geneticists are currently making tremendous advances in understanding the biochemistry of genes and genetic transmission. New techniques for identifying genetic disorders are being developed, and ultimately new treatments, including actual modification of the genes, are likely to be possible. At present it is worth noting that when we are concerned with behavior rather than physical defects, it is rarely possible to find more than half of the phenotypic variance accounted for by genetic variance (Plomin, 1990). (For a more thorough account of genetic mechanisms, see Plomin et al., 1990, especially chaps. 1-7. Emery & Mueller, 1988, is a good source of information on medical genetics.)

CHROMOSOMAL DISORDERS

Many known disorders are defects in the chromosomes rather than in one gene or gene pair on a chromosome. Chromosomal defects can be detected by means of a procedure called **karyotyping**, in which cells are obtained from a person, grown in a culture medium, then chemically stopped in the middle of cell division and treated and stained. The chromosomes are then photographed, enlarged, and arranged according to shape and banding patterns. Figure 3.1 shows a typical karyotype. Many chromosomal abnormalities can be detected by inspection of such karyotypes. However, a picture of chromosomes is not a picture of the genotype.[1]

The state of the chromosomes in the developing embryo and fetus is a joint outcome of heredity and development to that point. Irradiation, certain drugs, and long-term effects on the aging of eggs (which are already present in a female's body by the time she is born) may lead to chromosomal abnormalities. Thus even chromosomes are affected by the environment, and this means they are phenotypic, not genotypic or purely determined by heredity. *Genotype*, then, refers only to the inherited potential of individuals, and its manifestation is always mediated by the environment. Environmental influences affect sperm and ova before an egg is fertilized, and they continue to act throughout development. As we saw in Chapter 2, during early differentiation of the embryo, the immediate chemical environment of the cells influences whether and how they will differentiate. In Chapter 4, examples are given of foreign substances that affect both early stages of differentiation and later prenatal development. In short, every aspect of a baby's constitution is a result of the interaction between heredity and environment.

IMPORTANCE OF GENE AND CHROMOSOME DISORDERS

Before discussing some of the terrible things that can go wrong even before a baby is born, I would like to reassure you that the percentage of babies born with serious genetic defects is *very small*. Major chromosomal abnormalities affect 0.5%, which is about the same proportion as that for aneuploid cases (Robinson et al., 1984); gene defects affect 1-2% of the general population of living adults in the United States. As many as half of all conceptions involve such abnormalities, but only about 1 in 200 fetuses that survives to be born might have some form of chromosomal anomaly (President's Commission for the Study of Ethical Problems, 1983). Many of these die in the first months or years of life. Survivors often have abnormalities of the sex chromosomes, which are not as serious in their effects as are those of other chromosomes.

However, these figures underrepresent the importance to society of genetic and chromosomal abnormalities for the following reasons:

(1) Many are spontaneously aborted early in pregnancy or die before birth or in early childhood, and therefore are not represented in statistics for

the general population, although they may have had a great impact on the families.

(2) Sizable proportions of patients in hospitals and institutions for the retarded have gene or chromosome abnormalities.

(3) Certain genetic effects are much more frequent in particular racial and ethnic groups, and hence are a greater source of worry for members of those groups.

The first two of these reasons will be considered in the following section; the third will be alluded to in the later discussions of Tay-Sachs disease, beta thalassemia, and sickle-cell anemia.

INCIDENCE AND MORTALITY (BEFORE, DURING, AND AFTER BIRTH)

Determining prenatal mortality from any one cause is not at all straightforward. Every stage of pregnancy contributes to pregnancy loss. Spontaneous abortions and miscarriages are detected in about 10% of conceptions. This is only a fraction of the total rate, however, because spontaneous abortions early in pregnancy are reabsorbed (**resorbed**) into the mother's body rather than aborted, so even if the mother thinks she was pregnant, she has no way of determining that she has lost her potential offspring. Estimates of the proportion of human conceptions that are spontaneously aborted run as high as 40-60% (Boue & Boue, 1974; Boué et al., 1975; Little, 1988).

A sense of these early losses can be gained by considering some estimates of mortality due to defective eggs at various stages (Hertig & Rock, 1949; Witschi, 1970; see also D. H. Carr, 1963, 1971). According to these estimates, 16% of bad eggs in contact with sperm fail to fertilize, and an additional 15% that have been fertilized are lost at the cleavage stage, prior to implantation. Another 27% are lost by the second week, or about when the first menses are missed (in the implantation stage), and another 8% by the second missed menses (in the embryological stage). These are all absorbed into the mother's body. Thus, of the potentially grossly abnormal infants that might result from bad eggs, 66% have been lost before most women even know they are pregnant.

It is estimated that 30% of conceptions perish before implantation (Opitz et al., 1987). Japanese researchers, who are not prohibited from studying the products of planned abortions, examined 37 embryos aborted in the early stages of implantation (14 to 24 days postconception); 32% were either grossly abnor-

---

1. New cytogenetic techniques enable much finer analysis of chromosomal defects that have identified chromosomal damage as causes of a number of previously known syndromes (Punnett & Zakai, 1990).

mal or already degenerating prior to the abortion (Shiota et al., 1987).

A recent technique enables evaluation of losses after the first week. Even in healthy young women, 22% of pregnancies ended spontaneously in the first month and another 9% after the pregnancies were diagnosed (Wilcox et al., 1988). At present, pregnancy losses in the first week are not determinable, but failures of *in vitro* fertilization offer a hint. Chromosome imbalance may often be the cause, as shown by the fact that 21% of 251 fertilized eggs that failed to implant were **aneuploid** (did not have double the number of gametic chromosomes; i.e., had an extra or a missing chromosome), with 13% having less and only 8% having more chromosomal material than normal (Bongso et al., 1988). The average age of the women in this study was over 36 years, and higher than that of those who had no aneuploidy.

How many later prenatal losses are due to gene and chromosome abnormalities? From 50% to 60% of the spontaneous abortions in the first three months of pregnancy have chromosomal abnormalities, as determined by karyotyping. Chromosomal anomalies are 100 times more frequent in spontaneous abortions than in live births. These rates are quite stable in various parts of the world, giving credence to the notion that this is a very basic biological error rate. It is fortunate that most conceptions with such abnormalities die before birth.

Amniocenteses provide an upwardly biased estimate of the prevalence of chromosomal problems inasmuch as they are usually done on women at risk because of age, previous pregnancy result, or family history. A 2.5-2.8% rate is found in Canadian and U.S. studies, based on thousands of cases (Allanson et al., 1983; Epstein & Golbus, 1977; Naber et al., 1987). An English study randomly assigned more than 4,500 women, aged 25 to 34 and not at risk, to have or not have amniocenteses. Of these, 1% had chromosomal abnormalities (Tabor & Phillip, 1987). (For an excellent overview of chromosomal causes of fetal deaths, with clear explanations of mechanisms, see Warburton, 1987.) By birth the rates of chromosomal abnormalities have reached the low level noted earlier. Among unselected newborns, 0.5-0.75% have some chromosomal abnormality.

Comparable rates for specific gene disorders are much more difficult to determine because a single clear test such as karyotyping is not available. Nevertheless, estimates are possible. Lubs (1977) has estimated that 1-2% of all infants born alive suffer from a single gene defect. An additional 1-2% of newborns have some condition related to genetics, involving

Table 3.1

Relation of Birth Defects to Infant Mortality in the United States in 1915 and 1976

	1915	1976
Overall infant mortality (per 10,000 live births)	1,000	150
Infant deaths due to birth defects (per 10,000)	64	26
Contribution of birth defects to death rate (%)	6.4	17.3

SOURCE: National Institutes of Health (1979).

multiple genes or interactions between genes and the environment or both. These conditions include club foot, cleft lip and palate, and neural tube defects (National Institutes of Health, 1979). Thus 3-5% of liveborn infants in the United States, or 100,000 to 150,000 newborns each year, are affected by genetically based defects.

Infants with physical birth defects, detectable at birth, constitute about 6% of all infants born alive (Shapiro et al., 1965). They are more likely to have genetic problems: Approximately 20% have defects of known genetic transmission and another 3-5% have defects due to chromosomal abnormalities.

The fetus with chromosomal abnormalities or gene defects who makes it to birth (3-5% of all live births) is more likely to die during infancy. Such infants accounted for 17.3% of infant deaths in 1976, compared with 6.4% in 1915 (see Table 3.1). In fact, as sanitation, nutrition, antibiotic therapy, and obstetric care have improved, there has been, until recently, an overall decline in infant mortality. As a result, the *percentage* of infant deaths due to congenital malformations has increased. It is likely that genetic defects account for 20% of infant deaths, being exceeded only by immaturity and birth injuries.

Genetic defects are the second most common cause of death in the 1-4 age range, and the third cause in the 15-19 age group. (The figures given here are from 1978 data from the National Center for Health Statistics.) People die at all ages from primarily genetic causes. Some genetic conditions, such as cystic fibrosis and galactosemia, may not be identified early in life, although they may cause death in infancy or later. Others, such as Huntington's disease, surface only in mid-life and cause death in mid- to late life.

FREQUENCY OF GENETIC AND
CHROMOSOMAL DISORDERS IN
SPECIAL POPULATIONS

Genetic-related disorders are far more prevalent in
the hospitalized and among residents in institutions
for the mentally retarded than among the general population. Conditions with genetic origins (single-gene
disorders, chromosomal and developmental anomalies
and malformations, and multifactorial traits) occur in
6% of live births. More than half are multifactorial
traits that account for almost one-third of all admis-
sions to pediatric inpatient services and childhood
deaths (Rosenberg, 1986-1987; see also World Health
Organization, 1972).

Figures for mental retardation are similar. Of
210,000 individuals institutionalized for mental retardation in 1970, approximately 20-25% of the cases
could be ascribed to genetically influenced factors; the
proportion is higher among the most severely retarded. At least 40% of those with IQs below 50 (the
most severe retardation) have chromosomal disorders,
single gene defects, or severe developmental malformation syndromes such as spina bifida. The institutionalization of individuals whose retardation is caused
or influenced by genetic factors cost $315 million per
year in 1970, which is $967 million in 1990 dollars or
more than $1.25 billion in medical cost dollars.

Specific Disorders

It is important to remember the following points:

(1) The problems of genes and chromosomes described in this chapter, and the environmentally
caused constitutional defects described in the
next, are all negative. Information regarding the
genetics of interesting positive characteristics,
such as high intelligence and positive personality
traits, is sparse.
(2) Although we can make a long catalog of unpleasant outcomes of pregnancy, most babies who survive the newborn period do not have these
afflictions.

_____

2. A thorough survey of many aspects (genetic, health, and
intervention, for example) of Down syndrome can be found in
Pueschel et al. (1987).
3. The chromosomal cause of Down syndrome was suggested
as early as 1932, but was proven only in 1959, after the development of appropriate staining techniques enabled identification of
the chromosomes.

(3) Not all birth defects are as dramatic and devastating as those described here, and some, such as
cleft palate and club foot (both surgically correctable), can be either hereditary or nonheredi-
tary (see Chapter 4).

There are several ways to organize material in the
area of genetics. This discussion begins with defects of
the chromosomes and proceeds to those of the genes,
which are located on the chromosomes and which determine the inheritance of specific traits.

CHROMOSOMAL ABNORMALITIES

Chromosomal defects can be inherited or can result
from **mutations**—permanent changes in the chromosomes that are heritable. Chromosomal changes usually
are incompatible with life, and affected conceptuses
(products of conception) are often resorbed or
aborted early. Those that survive to be born are likely
to have a large number of abnormalities produced by
the disruption of gene functions. Chromosomal abnormalities usually involve either an extra or a missing
chromosome or part of a chromosome, as will be explained for Down syndrome.

Down Syndrome

Down syndrome (DS) or trisomy 21 is a good
starting point for the discussion of chromosomal abnormalities for a number of reasons: (a) It is one of
the most frequent chromosomal abnormalities (affecting 1 in 700 newborns), (b) it demonstrates several
genetic complexities, (c) it is one of the most common
causes of mental retardation, and (d) it provides a
good example for discussion of some of the social issues involved in dealing with abnormalities.[2]

Characteristics. Down syndrome used to be called
Mongolism because most persons afflicted with it have
flat faces and upward-slanting eyes with an epicanthic
fold on the eyelid similar to that of Asians or Mongols,
and there may be a yellowish cast to the skin. This
term is now avoided because of its spurious negative
reference to an ethnic group. Instead, it is called
Down syndrome or trisomy 21, after the man who
originally described it in 1866 or descriptive of its
most frequent cause.[3] Other **stigmata** (physical defects) that may be present include an enlarged tongue,
a wide space between the first and second toes, and
finger ridge and palm line patterns that differ from
those in normal babies. An example of the latter is the
so-called simian crease, a line that goes straight across

the palm like the line on the palm of a monkey or ape rather than curving down as it does in 90% of humans. Figure 3.2 shows a child with a relatively mild case of Down syndrome.

In addition to these externally visible signs, there are internal problems. Congenital heart disease is common, and many Down syndrome babies die in the first few years from cardiac complications. Eye defects, frequent hypothyroidism in adulthood, numerous metabolic and biochemical problems, and a high risk for leukemia are frequently found. Of particular importance are immunological problems that lead to a high level of susceptibility to infections. Taken together, these problems led to an average life expectancy of 9 years in 1929 and 15 years in the 1940s. After the advent of antibiotics, heart surgery, and better metabolic diagnosis and treatment, the life expectancy increased to 30 years, with 25% living to age 50 (Patterson, 1987). British Columbian data show that 50% of those with heart anomalies, and 79% of those without, live to age 30 (Baird & Sadovnick, 1987). The longer life span led to findings that DS cases often suffer early deterioration that may be linked to Alzheimer's disease. The brains of 35-year-old DS cases contain the same kinds of amyloid plaques as those of Alzheimer victims, and the gene for making amyloid is on chromosome 21 (Goldgaber et al., 1987). But clinical evidence of Alzheimer's is lower (10-45%) than one would expect from the prevalence of the plaques (Thase, 1987; for a review, see Oliver & Holland, 1986), and sharp IQ (intelligence quotient, a standard measure of intelligence, where 100 is average) drops were found only after age 50 (Brown et al., 1990).

Another aspect of the brain that seems to be affected by DS is the speed of myelination of the brain. Wisniewski and Schmidt (1989) found it to be slower for DS children than for others who died between 2 months and 6 years of age. There is some correlation between delay in myelination and that in developmental milestones.

The most prominent behavioral characteristic of DS is mental retardation. From 10% to 20% of all moderately and severely retarded children (the second and third most severe categories of retardation) are Down cases. In India, for example, 14% of a mentally retarded group were DS cases (Krishnan et al., 1989). IQs vary between 20 and 80, with the majority between 45 and 55 (Robinson et al., 1984). This will be discussed further below, in connection with social issues.

Language usage is even more handicapped than IQ in many instances. For example, when DS adolescents

and young adults are matched to same-age controls with the same degree of mental retardation (average IQ 40), they perform similarly on vocabulary and simple grammatical constructions, but are less able to deal with grammatically more difficult sentences (Marcell, Croen, & Sewell, 1990). DS cases also differ in their ability to imitate sentences, and short-term memory is implicated in the differences (Marcell, Sewell, & Croen, 1990). The nonverbal communication of 18- to 48-month-old DS infants also differs from that of controls matched on mental age (MA). They have strengths in social interaction skills compared with MA-matched normals, and weakness in requesting help or objects compared even with MA-matched retarded children (Mundy et al., 1988). The weakness is related to their later expressive language skills.

The long-time description of Down children as having pleasant, placid dispositions may not be accurate. Mothers filling out Carey's Infant Temperament Questionnaire did not describe their DS infants as easier than did mothers of normal infants; indeed, a greater percentage were in the more difficult range (Bridges & Cicchetti, 1982). Fewer than half of the DS infants scored in the same category in ratings made 6 months later, which shows that their temperaments were not immutably fixed by their chromosomal abnormality. Furthermore, a longitudinal study of family-reared DS children studied from birth showed that, at 8 to 9 years of age, 11 of the 22 survivors had serious behavior problems. These were concentrated in boys with very limited or no language skills (Gath, 1985).

DS infants demonstrate less frequent and less intense affective expression, but no more negative behaviors than normal infants (Bridges & Cicchetti, 1982; Emde et al., 1978; Landry & Chapieski, 1990). They shift affect expression more frequently than MA-matched nonretarded children, and look more at social partners' faces (Kasari et al., 1990). They are similar to MA controls in various aspects of play behaviors, but not in social play and interaction (Beeghly et al., 1989). Compared with age-mates or mental age-mates, they have been found to be less contingently responsive to their mothers, to initiate fewer social interactions, and to engage in less structured turn-taking social games. The more positive affect displayed toward people and the shorter the average length of their looks at partners' faces, the higher their verbal skills (Kasari et al., 1990).

Frequency. DS is the most frequent chromosomal anomaly, occurring in 1 in 700 births (Fraser, 1984; National Institutes of Health, 1979; Patterson, 1987),

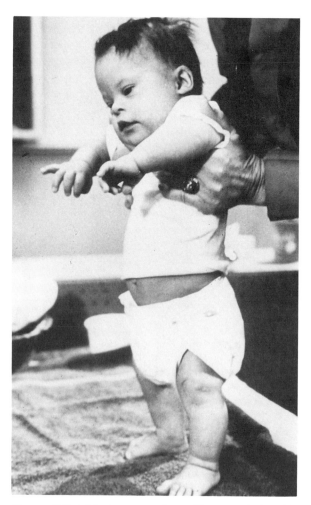

Figure 3.2. This is a very "good" Down baby. Although the baby needs more support in maintaining an erect posture than would be expected at this age, the child displays few of the physical traits that usually characterize a Down infant. (Photograph courtesy of the Office of Research Reporting, National Institute of Child Health and Human Development, Bethesda, MD.)

but possibly in 1 in every 200 conceptions (Polani, 1966). Thus some 75% of trisomy 21 zygotes may be spontaneously aborted. More females than males have DS, possibly due to the greater vulnerability of males prenatally, which allows more female fetuses with the syndrome to survive to be born.

The frequency data need to be broken down by age of the mother in order for the risks to be understood properly. DS babies are rarely born to young mothers (1 in 2,400 live births for mothers under 20), but the rates start to rise dramatically after the mother reaches 30, reaching about 1 in 109 live births for mothers 40-45. If one includes both live born and those prenatally

diagnosed, this figure rises to about 1 in 50 pregnancies (Hook, 1982). Although the rate is higher for older mothers, the number of cases is greater for younger mothers, since they have many more babies. Fathers are the source of the extra chromosome in 25% of the cases (Plomin et al., 1990); however, paternal age does not appear to be related to the frequency of occurrence.

Forms and Mechanisms. The complexities of genetic mechanisms are well illustrated by the several forms of DS. Although all forms have some abnormality involving the twenty-first chromosome, their natures and causes vary. The most common cause, called **nondisjunction** (failure to divide properly), accounts for 95% of all cases. Nondisjunction occurs during **meiosis**, the cell division that results in the formation of gametes (ova and spermatozoa). When a pair of chromosomes fails to separate during meiosis, a gamete may receive both chromosomes or no chromosome of a given pair. When the abnormal germ cell from one parent joins a normal gamete from the other parent, the resulting zygote (fertilized egg) has 1 or 3 chromosomes. In DS, chromosome number 21 failed to separate, and the individual in question got the gamete with 3 number 21s.[4]

Nondisjunction is rarely inherited, in part because few DS cases reproduce. After a chromosomally normal mother has a child with a nondisjunction, her risk of having another is about the same as that for any mother of her age. Nondisjunction is markedly affected by the age of the mother, as are some other chromosomal anomalies.

A rarer form of DS, which accounts for less than 4% of all cases, is the result of a mechanism called **translocation**, in which the chromosome breaks during meiosis and a piece becomes attached to another chromosome or wrongly attached to its own chromosome (Hook, 1982). In the case of DS, extra material from the twenty-first chromosome is relocated or attached to some other chromosome, or wrongly attached to chromosome 21; for example, tops and bottoms may be inverted. One-third of these cases are inherited; the others, like the cases of nondisjunction, result from spontaneous errors in the formation of the egg or sperm.

Women who carry a translocated chromosome 21

---

4. The technical description of the karyotype for such people is 47,XX,21+ or 47,XY,21+ (for females and males, respectively). The three parts of the description identify the total number of chromosomes (47, not the normal 46), which sex chromosomes are present (XX or XY), and the chromosome pair that has become a triplet (pair 21).

may be normal, but about 1 in 5 of their offspring will have DS (the rates vary from 1 in 1 to 1 in 60, depending on which other chromosome has the extra material attached to it). Other offspring will appear normal, but may be carriers like their mothers. When a young woman gives birth to a DS child, she is twice as likely as her husband to be the carrier. This is thought to be because spermatozoa with an aberrant chromosome complement are less likely to succeed in fertilizing an egg. Karyotyping of the DS infant can help the parents make plans about future childbearing, since the risks of having another Down child differ for nondisjunction and translocation.

A third chromosomal abnormality called **mosaicism** accounts for 2% of DS cases. Normally all cells (except the germ cells) have the same chromosomal makeup. In some persons, some cells have the normal number of chromosomes and others do not; they vary, as do the stones in a mosaic. Mosaicism can result from nondisjunction occurring after fertilization. If it is prior to embryogenesis, the descendants of even one abnormal cell would be distributed widely throughout the body. Mosaicism exists for other chromosomes, but if it involves the twenty-first chromosome it may result in DS. Individuals who are mosaic for DS tend to have fewer symptoms than trisomic or translocation cases. They may suffer less severe retardation and may even appear normal in intelligence. However, it should be noted that the only top-level functioning DS person in a large-scale longitudinal study in Australia was a trisomy 21, not a mosaic (Gunn et al., 1991). When a known mosaic mother of any age is pregnant, it is a good idea to determine the fetus's status, as is done for older mothers. (For a full discussion of the genetics of DS, see Plomin et al., 1990.)

Social Issues. Institutionalization versus home care for Down syndrome children is a major issue. In the past, many DS infants were institutionalized at or shortly after birth inasmuch as, even without genetic analyses, they could usually be diagnosed at birth on the basis of physical characteristics. Because of the poor prognosis for intellectual development, parents were often advised to institutionalize them quickly in order to avoid becoming too attached and to prevent problems for present or anticipated brothers and sisters.

More recently, experts have encouraged parents to keep their afflicted babies at home as long as possible. Advocates of home rearing were impressed by the data indicating that home-reared DS cases had IQs as much as 15 points higher than institution reared cases. A relatively large proportion of home-reared children (13%

to 34%, depending on the study) are only mildly retarded (have IQs of 50 to 69), whereas only 1-4% of institutionalized cases have IQs that high. This difference may be less impressive than it looks due to the fact that the more seriously retarded children were more likely to have been institutionalized. Further, at least one recent retrospective study has found no differences in IQs between home- and institution-reared DS persons (Brown et al., 1990).

IQs of DS children usually decrease with age. Several studies of both home- and institution-reared DS persons have shown that early stimulating intervention programs can prevent early decreases in IQ and adaptive functioning (Connolly et al., 1984; Hayden & Dmitriev, 1975; Stedman & Eichorn, 1964). However, a large-scale Australian study that has investigated two cohorts, one of which had ample access to early intervention programs and the other of which, an earlier one, did not, found no significant difference in their overall progress (Gunn et al., 1991). This same study did not find the plateau in intellectual development by adolescence that others have reported. This is in agreement with the findings of a three-nation study conducted by Rauh et al. (1991).

The pendulum of advice may have swung too far. It is all well and good to advise parents to keep a child with DS at home and to provide a maximally stimulating environment for that child. However, some parents are not equipped to deal with the stresses involved in home care for such children or to provide a stimulating environment. Some parents react to these children's handicap by providing lots of tender loving care, but make few demands and do not really stimulate. Strong demands accompanied by love may be needed for optimal development. Most communities lack adequate support systems to help parents cope with either the psychological stresses or the practical work of providing stimulation for DS children. Parents' guilt feelings may be increased if they find they cannot cope with the problems and later need to institutionalize their children.

Keeping a DS infant at home has been found to lead to marital problems in the first 2 years, a finding similar to that for parents of prematures reported in Chapter 2 (Gath, 1978), but not over a longer time span (J. Carr, 1988; Gath, 1978). Minor psychiatric illness and physical health problems have been found to be more common for both fathers and mothers of DS children than for those of controls (J. Carr, 1988; Gath, 1985). Furthermore, Gath found that three-fourths of the siblings of Down children had behavior problems, but Carr (1988) reports that sibs do not suffer a major disadvantage.

Problems of home rearing increase with age. In middle childhood 50% of DS children have been found to have behavior problems (Gath, 1985). At adolescence, sexuality and pregnancy pose new problems. The parents get older and may find it more difficult to cope, and other family members are seldom ready and willing to assume the responsibility. Brown et al. (1990) found that the social-adaptive functioning of older DS persons declines less in the institutionalized than in the home reared; the researchers attribute this finding to the inability of older parents to provide stimulation and to cope generally, together with their earlier tendency to assume responsibilities that might have been given to the DS child or adolescent.

What is to be done when parents can no longer cope? Will adults with DS adapt to institutions as readily as they would have as children? Will parental guilt about institutionalizing their offspring be any less after the years of interdependency? I know of no research undertaken to address these questions. Parents who have a choice must weigh the potential stress that coping with these problems might create for themselves and other family members against the potential advantages for the afflicted child.

Home rearing is not a panacea. Marked retardation is still the norm. A majority in one study were moderately or severely retarded (IQs between 24 and 49) (Cornwell & Birch, 1969). IQs of both home-reared and institutionalized children decline with age; those whose IQs were in the middle 50s in preschool years may be in the 30s by their teens. In a prospective longitudinal study of 30 cases, the IQs of the 22 available at 8 to 9 years of age ranged from below 20 to 80, with a mean of 48, and all but 2 were in British special schools (Gath & Gumley, 1984). Home rearing may well make the difference between complete dependency in adulthood and being able to function in a sheltered workshop, especially for relatively bright DS individuals. Home rearing in settings where there is good available schooling for stimulating the child and relieving the parent of some responsibility is clearly much more desirable than home rearing in settings where the society, through the schools, does not offer adequate programs.

Institutions could provide stimulating environments and improve intellectual performance in their DS children if adequately funded. In one state hospital, workers undertook training with a group of 8-year-olds hospitalized in early infancy with current mental ages of 2 or 3 years. The workers stressed language skills and dealt with the children both individually and in groups of five. The IQs of these children stopped dropping, they began to talk and use names, and some even learned to read (Stedman & Eichorn, 1964). Whether institutions can equal homes in intellectual stimulation is unknown and not likely to be discovered in an era when most state institutions are inadequately funded and, indeed, will not accept any but the worst DS cases.

Research has focused on intellectual development. Emotional development of those reared in institutions and in group-care homes should also be compared with that of those reared at home. Although people might assume that the loving warmth of a family is the only adequate environment for emotional well-being, it is not clear that living in institutions is necessarily worse for the emotional well-being of DS children. It appears that many, although not all, adapt well to institutional life. Adaptation may depend in part on age at institutionalization, as well as on the nature of the institution. Quality of institutional and home-care facilities varies widely and needs to be taken into account. Home life, which is usually less regular or predictable than institutional life, may lead to emotional problems, particularly if there is tension stemming from resentment of some family members toward the child. Again, I know of no research on these questions.

I have referred above to the kind of support available in the community to help DS children and their parents. There is also the problem of dealing with DS adults, especially when their parents are no longer able to assume responsibility for them. The success of home rearing for a DS child depends in part on the kind of support the primary caretaker, usually the mother, has. Some families have relatives who provide help with care; others can afford to hire adequate help. But many must depend on society, which, overall, does not have a good record of providing such care. Some communities have good public school facilities and sheltered apartments, homes, and workshops for older DS persons, but many locales lack such services. Community placement of formerly institutionalized individuals can be at various levels of care, and, as in all such matters, quality can vary widely.

Another kind of societal support is found in preschool programs designed to enable DS children to reach their optimal levels of functioning. One such program at the University of Washington Model Preschool Center in Seattle started almost at birth. It had four levels: (a) an Infant Learning Program that met once a week for 30 minutes of parent training in early motor and sensory development (children from 5 weeks through 18 months), (b) an Early Preschool Program (18 months to 3 years), (c) an Advanced

Preschool Program for children from 3 to 5, and (d) a kindergarten for those 4½ to 6 (Hayden & Dmitriev, 1975).

It is not possible to reach any firm conclusions based on Hayden and Dmitriev's (1975) small sample composed of children widely varied in age when they entered the program and when studied. The early results appeared impressive, but long-term outcomes are not clear. The developmental lag on the Peabody Picture Vocabulary Test for children already in the program was about 6.5 months, compared with 21 months for children of the same ages who had just entered the program. However, children in the program were still showing IQ gains rather than losses, and the average IQ was in the low 80s, which is high for those with DS. The children lagged more in language than in other areas, but some were making progress in learning to read. A very different effect was that parents in the program who left the area started similar programs in their new communities. It has served as a model for programs in other places as well.

Sheltered workshops, preschool programs, and other sorts of community support for home-reared retarded people do, of course, cost money. However, because the cost of institutionalizing a single DS victim for an entire lifetime is high and likely to increase as life expectancy increases, it is likely that community support that would allow more families to keep their DS children at home would cost society less in the long run.[5] In Great Britain it has been reported that the longer life expectancy of those with DS is resulting in much greater pressure for more societal provisions. It is clear that society could provide a good deal of support for parents at much lower cost than that of institutionalization. In Australia, which has good support programs, the extra expenses of caring for a Down syndrome compared with a normal child have been shown to be considerable, but hardly in the range of the $160 per day estimated for institutional care there (Gunn & Berry, 1987).

The best environment for a given DS child depends, of course, on individual circumstances. Perhaps one of the most important things to remember from the research is that DS cases cannot be described as a group; they are all individuals (see, e.g., Hayes & Gunn, in press). Their outcomes depend on their characteristics; the psychological strengths of the parents, other family members, and children in the family; the financial capability to provide caretakers; and the community's resources. For many DS children and their families the best solution might still be an institution, but in most states only the worst cases would be admitted or kept there. Most of those who became wards of the state would be placed in homes of varied quality with a small number of other mentally handicapped individuals.

The handling of infants with DS has been discussed in detail here because it illustrates the more general issues that apply to a number of the severe problems seen at birth or in infancy. Clearly, these issues are present beyond infancy, and often become greater as the child grows older. A good source of material on the development of Down persons from 6 weeks to 21 years, and the burden carried by their mothers, can be found in J. Carr (1988). (A recent edited volume on Down is that of Cicchetti & Beeghly, 1990.)

Other Abnormalities of Autosomal Chromosomes

If Down conceptuses had 3 chromosome 21s, what about the other egg cell that received no chromosome 21 at all and would, if fertilized, result in a person with a missing chromosome? Monosomic zygotes, except for those missing one sex chromosome, do not survive embryonic life. Some babies (1 in 45,000 live births) are born with a substantial portion of the short arm of chromosome 4 or 5 missing. They have a very high pitched and monotonic cry, hence the condition is called *cri du chat* (cry of the cat) syndrome. They are usually **microcephalic** (have a less-than-normal-sized cranial cavity) and severely retarded (see Figure 3.3); they account for 1% of the institutionalized with an IQ of less than 35.

If trisomy 21 causes Down syndrome, what about trisomies of other chromosomes? All trisomic conceptions have high intrauterine mortality, and only those involving the smaller chromosomes (see Figure 3.1) survive to be born with any frequency. Trisomy 13 occurs in about 1 in 6,000 births; 50% die in the first month of life (Plomin et al., 1990). The next most frequently **viable** (mature enough and functioning well enough to live outside the womb) is trisomy 18. It is the most frequent chromosomal abnormality among late-pregnancy abortions and fetal deaths during labor and delivery, occurring in over 25% of such cases (Bauld et al., 1974). The frequency of trisomy 18, like that of trisomy 21, increases greatly with maternal age. It occurs in fewer than 1% of infants born to mothers under 20 years of age, but in 30-40% of infants whose mothers are over 40.[6]

---

5. Unfortunately, long-run savings often fail to compete with short-run savings when it comes to spending tax dollars.

6. For a brief description and pictures of the other gross chromosomal anomalies, see Fraser (1984), and for a catalog of unbalanced chromosome aberrations in humans, with their courses and outcomes, see Schinzel (1983).

Abnormalities of Sex Chromosomes

Abnormalities of the sex chromosomes occur in several forms. The one viable case of a **monosomic** person (one with a totally missing chromosome) is a person with a single sex (X) chromosome. This anomaly is called Turner's syndrome, and the karyotype is 45,X0 (the zero stands for the missing chromosome). Some fetuses with this abnormality survive, although an estimated 95% of all such conceptions are spontaneously aborted. There are also individuals with extra sex chromosomes. These nondisjunction problems include 47,XXX, 47,XXY, and 47,XYY, and sometimes even more Xs. The more Xs, the greater the problems. Extra Xs appear to be more viable than other extra chromosomes, presumably because all Xs in excess of 1 become inactive by the third week after conception. While not fully confirmed, this appears likely. The inactive chromosome shows as a chromatin or Barr body and there is always one less Barr body than there are X chromosomes. This enables a simpler determination of X chromosome anomalies (from any body cell) than karyotyping.

Although abnormal complements of sex chromosomes do not create treatment problems in infancy, they are included here because they are detected during karyotyping. As prenatal karyotyping becomes increasingly common, more and more parents will learn of their offspring's chromosomal anomalies before birth. It is thus important to understand the implications of these disorders for development. Most abnormalities of the sex chromosomes affect reproductive functioning and physical development. Intellectual deficiency or behavioral problems have been found, but in methodologically inadequate studies of individuals brought to the attention of the medical establishment because they have physical, intellectual, or behavioral problems.

Prior to the 1960s and 1970s, knowledge of characteristics of those with chromosomal anomalies was biased by the fact that those who had no problems other than a chromosomal abnormality would not be studied. Those typically studied were already adolescents or adults, so that many of the abnormal group might have died, been put into institutions for the retarded, or been lost from the population under study in other ways. To ascertain whether a given chromosomal anomaly actually plays a role in a given problem, one must determine that people with that anomaly are more likely to have that problem than a comparable sample of chromosomally normal individuals. This can be done only in a **prospective study**, in which the subjects are selected for longitudinal study before any

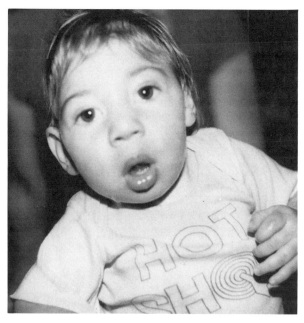

Figure 3.3. This picture of a microcephalic child shows the disproportion between the facial part of the head and the part of the skull that contains the brain. (Photograph courtesy of the Kennedy-Donovan Center.)

problem manifests itself.

Large-scale screening of newborns for sex chromosome anomalies began in the 1960s (Bell & Corey, 1974; Court-Brown, 1969; Robinson & Puck, 1967). A total of 200 infants with sex chromosome abnormalities were found among the 140,000 screened. Fewer problems were found when these cases were followed than in the studies that started with persons already in trouble. The results demonstrate that children with the same karyotype vary widely in the degree of their deficits or problems. Furthermore, Bender et al. (1987) found that genotype and postnatal environment interact to determine the degree of developmental problems shown. These authors followed 46 children with sex chromosome abnormalities (too few of any one type to consider separately) identified in the screening of 40,000 newborns. They found that language, motor, psychosocial, and school impairment occurred much more frequently in them (if not mosaic) than in their siblings. However, family dysfunction influenced the outcome markedly for those with anomalies, but only psychosocial and language impairment were affected for controls. Bender et al. called special attention to the cases with genetic anomalies who did not appear handicapped, emphasizing the importance of studying such cases.

The following sections discuss specific syndromes

resulting from abnormalities of the sex chromosomes using data that come both from studies of special populations and from prospective studies.

Turner's Syndrome. The 2% of conceptions with a 45,X0 chromosomal complement (monosomy) that survive to be born appear to be normal females at birth. Estimates of prevalence vary, but Lubs (1970), using data from a group of studies with appropriate newborn sampling procedures, concludes that 1 in 2,500 births is the most likely rate, a rate accepted by Plomin et al. (1990). The frequency of births of Turner's babies does not increase with maternal age.

Turner's girls often come to medical attention during childhood because of early sexual development (called infantile sexual development), yet they never commence menstruation. At maturity they are shorter than average, have webbed necks, and poor mammary development and immature external genitalia, conditions often treated with female hormones. Internally, either they lack ovaries or whatever tissue there is fails to produce ova, so that they are sterile. Most Turner's individuals have normal intelligence and no neurological defects, but they tend to have visual-spatial problems, as shown by data from a prospective study (Pennington et al., 1982; see also Pidcock, 1984). The prospective study showed they were lower on performance IQ than verbal, and exhibited problems with handwriting in school.[7]

Turner's syndrome girls often have psychological difficulties due to their appearance and to parental attitudes. These are called **indirect effects** because the chromosomal abnormality does not directly cause the psychological problems; rather, it causes some other problem (such as unattractive appearance) that in turn leads to psychological problems.

Trisomy X. Females with three X chromosomes (47,XXX) are relatively frequent—1 per 1,000 births (Plomin et al., 1990). They do not appear to have the physical abnormalities typical of other sex chromosome abnormalities, although Lubs (1970) found major physical anomalies in 2 of 9 cases from a large group of unselected karyotyped infants. The sexual structures of trisomy X females, unlike those of Turner's females, develop normally and permit fertility. Menstrual irregularities and early menopause have been reported, but there is no good evidence of a difference from normal XX women.

Intellectual development appears to be affected by trisomy X. Lubs (1970) reports that 3 of his 9 cases had borderline IQs. The 11 cases found in the Pennington et al. (1982) study tended to show global delay in intellectual development and a need for speech therapy in school, but not actual retardation. Nevertheless, the incidence of trisomy X females in institutions for the retarded is 39 per 1,000, compared with 14 per 1,000 for those without chromosomal anomalies (McClearn & DeFries, 1973). Reports conflict concerning the relation of frequency of trisomy X to parental age.

Klinefelter's Syndrome. Males born with an extra X chromosome (47,XXY) have **Klinefelter's syndrome**, which is somewhat more frequent than Turner's, occurring in from 1 in 1,000 to 1 in 2,200 births, according to the prospective studies cited by Lubs (1970), but in 2 per 1,000 births according to Plomin and colleagues (1990). Like most nondisjunction syndromes, it increases in frequency with maternal age, and it occurs with about equal frequency in blacks and whites. Males with Klinefelter's have small and immature testes, and are sterile. At maturity they lack adequate male hormones and hence have little facial or body hair and lack other secondary sexual characteristics. They also have femalelike breast development.

Mental retardation appears to be associated with this syndrome. A particularly large and impressive chromosomal study of tall Danish men in the army found that Klinefelter's men had significantly lower intelligence scores and less education than tall men with no chromosomal anomalies (Witkin et al., 1976).[8] Whether the Klinefelter's cases simply had a higher proportion of mentally retarded individuals, or most had somewhat lower than average intelligence, but in the normal range, or whether they differed on related skills that can affect test scores is not clear. In nonrandomly selected groups, rates of retardation of from 25% to 50% have been found. However, Lubs's (1970) review of prospective data found that only 1 in 15 cases (6-7%) was below normal in intelligence as measured by standard IQ tests. As a group, the 15 cases found by Pennington and colleagues (1982) had higher performance than verbal IQ, attention problems, and reading difficulties, and tended to need speech therapy.

---

7. It has been hypothesized that spatial ability is influenced by a major recessive allele on the X chromosome. This was thought to explain the greater spatial ability of males. The hypothesis has been rejected on other grounds (Plomin, 1990), but it is interesting that females, with only one X, should have had greater, not less, spatial ability according to the hypothesis.

8. Tall men were chosen because of the linkage of XYY and aggression with being tall.

Klinefelter's syndrome has also been associated with a variety of personality and emotional problems. For example, Jarvik et al. (1973) found that XXY men constituted a higher proportion of residents in mental hospitals than their proportion in the general population, based on data from several earlier reports. Such data do not necessarily lead to the conclusion that the chromosomal abnormality produced the psychological abnormalities. Many such problems are likely to be a result of indirect effects of physical appearance on individuals' adjustment.

As with Turner's syndrome, sex hormones can be used therapeutically for those with Klinefelter's syndrome. Androgen can be used to stimulate development of secondary sex characteristics, thereby alleviating some of the indirect effects due to the negative influence of appearance.

XYY Anomaly. This chromosomal defect, with its extra Y chromosome, attracted a great deal of controversy in the 1970s. It was discovered accidentally in 1961, when a man was karyotyped because he was the father of a child with Down syndrome. Subsequent accidental discoveries occurred when males with some sort of physical abnormality (often undescended testes or genital abnormalities) were examined. Being tall and possibly having a relatively large proportion of genital anomalies are the only physical characteristics associated with XYY.

In 1965, 7 men who were XYY and 1 who was XXYY were found among a group of 197 hard-to-manage retarded men. The XYY pattern was subsequently found to occur rather frequently among highly aggressive, tall criminals in penal institutions. Even though there were no data at that time to demonstrate that the XYY rate was higher in these aggressive populations than in the general population, many people concluded that an extra Y chromosome causes abnormally high aggressiveness. This conclu-

sion was widely disseminated by the press despite several articles on the methodological problems of this research (Kessler & Moos, 1970; Kivowitz, 1972). An Australian court of law even ruled that an XYY murderer could not be held responsible for his actions and should not receive the maximum penalty. Presumably the extra Y chromosome should have!

The first step in evaluating such claims is to determine the **base rate** (the rate of occurrence in the general population). Early estimates of frequency of XYY males in the general population varied from 1 in 250 to 1 in 2,000. The combined data from newborn screening studies showed an incidence of approximately 1 per 1,000 (Jarvik et al., 1973), a rate that is still accepted (Plomin et al., 1990) if all numbers of extra Ys are included. The evidence is contradictory as to whether the base rates are the same for different ethnic groups. Walzer et al. (1969) reported a frequency of 1 in 862 among 10,817 Caucasians, but no cases among 2,756 blacks, but another study reported no race difference in newborn rates. No differences were found according to socioeconomic status or maternal age in a large-scale study (Walzer & Gerald, 1975). The rate for institutionalized males is much greater (19 per 1,000 based on 18 studies with 5,342 males) than that for the population at large (Shah, 1970). Nevertheless, fewer than 1 in 100 XYY males is institutionalized (Kessler, 1975).

Let us look at the central issue of aggression. Jarvik and colleagues (1973) found 25 studies of XYY males in criminal populations. When all the samples were considered together (5,066 subjects), the total frequency of XYY was 1.9%, which is 15 times that found in either newborn males or the general adult male population.[9] The chromosomal study of more than 4,000 tall men in the Danish army referred to above revealed that 42% of the 12 XYYs found had criminal records, compared with 19% of the 16 XXYs and 9% of the XY men (Witkin et al., 1976). The three groups did not differ in the frequency with which they committed violent crimes; indeed, only one XYY man had committed a crime that involved aggression.

The Danish XYY men, like their XXY counterparts, performed significantly below normal on an army intelligence test and had not achieved educational levels as high as had chromosomally normal men. This agrees with Jarvik et al.'s (1973) pooled data. An excess of XYY karyotypes among mentally subnormal tall men who are antisocial to the extent of needing to be restrained was found by Casey et al. (1969). These data suggest that any disturbance in the XY chromosome balance predisposes an individual to intellectual and emotional difficulties. However, such difficulties

---

9. Racial differences in the incidence of XYY types have been found among highly aggressive populations. A report issued in 1974 showed that whites in institutional "security settings" were three times as likely as blacks in the same settings to have XYY karyotypes. This would presumably be congruent with an interpretation that genetics plays a greater role in this type of crime for whites than for blacks. It would obviously also be tempting to conclude that social or environmental forces play a greater role in this type of crime for blacks. But it is difficult to come to any conclusion about the reasons for this reported race difference in the incidence of XYY among criminals until we know for sure whether there are race differences in the frequency of XYY in the general population.

Table 3.2

Summary of Frequency of Chromosomal Anomalies

	Type of Anomaly	Incidence	Symptoms
Autosomal anomalies			
Edward's syndrome	Trisomy 18	1 in 5,000	Early death; many congenital problems
D-trisomy syndrome	Trisomy 13	1 in 6,000	Early death; many congenital problems
Cri du chat	Deletion of part of short arm of chromosome 4 or 5	1 in 10,000	High-pitched, monotonous cry; severe retardation
Down syndrome	Trisomy 21; 5% involve translocation	1 in 700	Congenital problems; retardation
Sex chromosomal anomalies			
Turner's syndrome	X0 or XX-X0 mosaics	1 in 2,500	Some physical stigmata and hormonal problems; specific spatial deficit
Females with extra X chromosomes	XXX, XXXX, XXXXX	1 in 1,000	For trisomy X, no distinctive physical stigmata; perhaps some retardation
Klinefelter's males	XXY, XXXY, XXXXY, XXYY, XXXYY	2 in 1,000	For XXY, sexual development problems; tall; perhaps some retardation
Males with extra Y chromosomes	XYY, XYYY, XYYYY	1 in 1,000	Tall; perhaps some retardation

SOURCE: Plomin et al. (1990). Reprinted by permission.

may also result from indirect effects or from interactions of constitutional phenotype with postnatal environment. If there is an increase in aggressiveness in XYY men, it might be because the extra Y causes men to be tall and of low intelligence. Their lower intelligence might make it less likely that they would use reasoning to solve conflicts; their height might result in their being more effective at using physical force than short men, thus they may receive more reinforcement for using aggression. This would increase their tendency to use force, and their lower intelligence would make it more likely that they would be caught if they committed crimes. Later research indicates that the characteristics of impulsiveness, inability to delay gratification, and failure to learn from past punishment might be more appropriate foci for further research in this area.

I conclude this section on chromosomal anomalies by summarizing the major anomalies, their cause, frequency, and associated symptoms (see Table 3.2).

Methodological Issues. The data presented above on the relation of height, antisocial behavior, and XYY provide an example of one of the major problems of correlational research. The research itself does not tell us about causation. Subjects cannot be randomly assigned to be XY or XYY; supporting data that would make causal inference more reasonable are lacking; and even the base rate of XYY for tall men who are not in institutions (other than the Danish army) is unknown. Without such evidence, there is no way to decide between direct-cause and indirect-cause interpretations.

A study from birth of the development of XYY and closely matched XY boys could resolve the controversy. If the XYY boys were aggressive as babies, before having much exposure to their postnatal environments, or if virtually all XYY infants were aggressive, we might conclude that the extra Y chromosome caused the aggressive behavior or antisocial personality. If only an excessive number of XYYs were aggressive, we might talk about the predisposing role of an extra Y. If aggressiveness or antisocial personality were to develop later (and was shown to be totally unrelated to child rearing) the role of the extra Y would be more certain. We would still need a control group of boys with extra chromosomal material from different chromosomes to establish aggression as a specific effect of an extra Y, rather than simply a result of any extra chromosomal material.

Ethical Issues. By a curious twist of fate, a study designed to answer these questions was aborted as a result of a challenge to its ethics. Although much of the challenge was based on a false understanding of the procedure, the publicity of the challenge made it possible for parents to determine that their boys were in the study, hence invalidating the research, since a self-fulfilling prophecy, in which parents expected their boys to become aggressive and treated them in ways that encouraged them to do so, might have been created. To create such an expectation would be unethical, although in this case it was done by the protectors, not the researchers. The parents had originally been told that the researchers did not know what if any effect a "broken" chromosome would have.

Ethical debate regarding the rights of those studied

(and their families) is repeated over and over in various areas of research with humans (and sometimes even more vigorously for other species).

Fragile X. Some persons (1 in 2,000 live births) have what is called a **fragile X site, or fra(X)**. This is a thin area on the X chromosome of either a male or a female that may lead to breakage or translocations of a portion of the chromosome. The number of cells showing the fragile X site varies widely (a mosaic). Fragile sites on other chromosomes do not appear to be clinically relevant. Fragile X males are short and have large heads, hands, feet, and, according to some studies, testes (Nussbaum & Ledbetter, 1986). Gaze aversion was prevalent in one sample, and 50% were hyperactive (Pueschel & Finelli, 1985). Both males and females with fragile X have long ears (Thake et al., 1987).

Mental retardation, usually moderate, is associated with fra(X). The degree of retardation may or may not be related to the number of cells showing fra(X) (Ho et al., 1988). IQs may decline with age, but further evidence is needed. Fragile X accounts for at least 2% of male residents of institutions for the retarded (Neri et al., 1988) and 8% (10% of girls and 6% of boys) of the mildly retarded without known etiology. It is exceeded only by Down syndrome as a chromosomal cause of retardation.

In general, the fra(X) syndrome has an X-linked inheritance pattern but lacks the expected X-linked inheritance pattern in which female heterozygotes or carriers are spared. About a third of heterozygote fra(X) females have a significant degree of intellectual impairment, although their IQs are higher than those of fra(X) boys (Ho et al., 1988; Thake et al., 1987). Those who are impaired tend to have a larger proportion of cells with fra(X) sites, according to research cited in Plomin et al. (1990). About 20% of males who have fra(X) appear to be unaffected in terms of IQ, although they often have specific learning disabilities. They, too, serve as carriers and pass on fra(X) to their offspring (Sherman et al., 1985).

The risk for a brother of a fra(X) being retarded is 1 in 2, and for a sister it is 1 in 4. The degree of retardation appears to be similar for siblings (Thake et al., 1987). This risk of recurrence makes it important to assess whether fra(X) is involved in a family that has had a retarded child. (Further information on this topic can be found in a highly readable book by Hagerman & McBogg, 1983.)

There is currently an effort in 12 centers to link fra(X) with autism (Brown et al., 1986). Results differ among the centers, but the largest study found 13% of 183 autistic males to have fra(X). It is estimated that

12% of fra(X) males are autistic, and autismlike characteristics have been found in 90% of 50 fra(X) males. As with retardation, it would seem important to evaluate fra(X) among autistic males for purposes of genetic counseling. There are some indications that treatment with folic acid may have beneficial effects, but the data are inconclusive (Ho et al., 1988).

ABNORMALITIES RESULTING FROM GENE DEFECTS

Now that we have surveyed several problems resulting from chromosomal abnormalities, let us turn to problems that are caused by specific genes. **Genes** are the units of the chromosomes that carry specific genetic information. While there are only 46 chromosomes, there are an estimated 50,000 to 100,000 genes (McKusick, 1986). Genes code for sequences of amino acids that constitute proteins and enzymes, which serve as catalysts for all the biochemical reactions in the body and regulate their timing.

More than 2,000 single-gene defects are known. Single-gene recessive traits are the most frequent of the known disorders. Some traits are carried by dominant genes, some are carried on the sex chromosomes and have their own pattern of inheritance (called X-linked), and some traits (called **polygenic**) are determined by the actions and interactions of several genes. Indeed, most traits in which psychologists are interested are probably polygenic. Traits with single recessive inheritance patterns have been the source of much of our current understanding of genetic mechanisms. Many of them are related to the lack of some enzyme that is crucial for a particular metabolic function. The diagram in Figure 3.4 includes the examples to be discussed here, and shows where some treatment efforts using enzymes might lie. Other types of treatment will be addressed later, in the discussion of genetic counseling.

Most gene defects discussed here are caused by a single autosomal recessive gene. The word *autosomal* indicates that the problem lies on one of the 22 paired chromosomes rather than on the sex chromosomes. Genes work in pairs, both members of a pair at the same site on its chromosome. Each site can be in one of two or more states (technically, one of two or more **alleles**). If one state or allele is dominant, it will be expressed in the phenotype even if present in only one copy (i.e., on one chromosome); the other allele is said to be **recessive**.

A **recessive** trait will be expressed in the phenotype only when both genes in the pair have the recessive allele. Because one chromosome comes from the

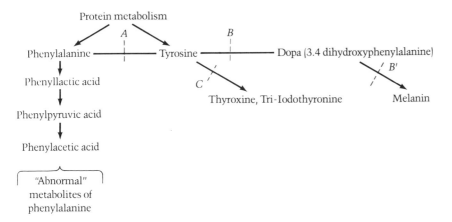

Figure 3.4. Steps in the metabolism of the amino acids phenylalanine and tyrosine. Blocks at the lettered points result in certain disorders. A block at A, caused by an enzyme deficiency, results in a buildup of phenylalanine and the resulting mental retardation syndrome known as phenylketonuria (PKU). The column extending downward from phenylalanine represents other chemicals that result when the normal metabolic pathway is blocked. A block at B or B′ prevents the formation of melanin, the pigment that gives color to hair, skin, and eyes, and thus produces albinism. A block at C leads to a low level of the hormones thyroxine and tri-iodothyronine, which produces goiterous cretinism, with its associated mental retardation and small stature. (After Fig. 4.6 [p. 223] in *Genes, Environment, and Behavior: An Interactionist Approach*, by Jack R. Vale. Copyright © 1980 by Harper & Row, Publishers, Inc. By permission of the publisher.)

mother and one from the father, both parents must have contributed a germ cell with a recessive allele to an afflicted baby. In the gene defects discussed below, the parents are **heterozygous carriers**. This means that they both have a dominant gene that is normal, and hence rarely suffer from the defect themselves, although detectable effects sometimes occur. They both had one recessive (nonnormal) gene, which they passed on to their offspring in the sperm or ovum.

Phenylketonuria (PKU)

Phenylketonuria (PKU) is a particularly interesting disease to examine, not only because its effects are dramatic, but also because it was the first inborn error of metabolism to be understood and to be controlled by environmental manipulation.[10] Like most inborn errors of metabolism, PKU is inherited as a simple autosomal recessive characteristic. Its locus appears to be on chromosome 12. The problem stems from the liver's inability to produce an enzyme that is crucial for the proper metabolism of **phenylalanine**, an amino acid that is a constituent of natural proteins, including that in milk. PKU infants build up large concentrations of phenylalanine and other abnormal metabolic products (see Figure 3.4). These abnormal metabolites

affect the central nervous system, especially the brain, in ways that are not fully understood. Heterozygotes are less protected from the effects of the troublesome gene than in some recessive traits. They do not convert or metabolize phenylalanine as well as normal homozygotes, and they may have lower IQs (Bessman et al., 1978).

The primary symptoms of the disease are severe retardation, often accompanied by hyperactivity and other behavioral problems. PKU used to account for substantial numbers of institutionalized retarded. In general, the infant appears normal at birth and shows normal progress for the first 1 to 3 months. Between 3 and about 6 months the infant is likely to become either unresponsive and listless or extremely irritable. Developmental milestones, such as sitting up and turning over, are not achieved on schedule, and there is progressive retardation. By 4 years of age afflicted children are characteristically very retarded. The primary stigmata involve lack of pigmentation in the skin, hair, and eyes, which is not very obvious early in infancy. However, the abnormal odor of the urine is

_____

10. A good review of nutritional therapy for a number of inborn errors of metabolism can be found in Levy (1989).

what often led to discovery. Some PKU infants tend to have vomiting or other feeding difficulties; some show excessive irritability or overactivity early, but others develop these symptoms more slowly (Berry, 1976). An atypical or mild form is not associated with retardation, but infants with the classical type rarely have normal intelligence unless treated (Levy et al., 1970).

Screening. PKU is the most prevalent metabolic disorder and is most often tested for in genetic screening programs. After evidence began to accumulate that its effects could be controlled environmentally, its early detection became important in order to avoid wasted lives, parental heartbreak, and the costs of institutionalization. There was then wide-scale pressure to make neonatal screening for PKU mandatory. Massachusetts had the first law in 1963; as of 1980, 47 states had laws requiring it, and the other 3 had voluntary programs. Initially the error rate was high because the urine test used then did not become accurate until a few weeks after birth, when the infant's metabolism has been separated from the maternal system. The blood test now used is accurate earlier, but also depends on the infant's processing of its postnatal food intake.

Many infants would be lost to testing in the United States if it were not done during the brief hospital stay after birth. Massachusetts provides mothers with a filter paper that they are to soak in the urine on a diaper when the baby is 4 to 6 weeks old and mail in for repeat testing. This practice successfully screens 97-98% of babies. This specimen can be used to test for a wide range of defects in amino acid metabolism (Levy et al., 1970), and Massachusetts is 1 of 5 states that tests for 5 or more conditions. In Great Britain, every baby is seen at home within 14 days of birth by a health visitor who tests any babies that were not born in the hospital or who left the hospital prior to 7 days of age.

Northern European and British populations have about 1 PKU case in 10,000 live births (Kidd, 1987; Smith & Wolff, 1974), as did Massachusetts (Levy et al., 1970). In contrast, in Japan, where more than 6 million neonates have been screened, cases of PKU are fewer than 1 in 100,000 (Tada et al., 1984).

Dietary Treatment. Putting the infant on a low phenylalanine diet sounds simple, but in practice it is not. The diet is highly restrictive, because of the large number of foods that contain phenylalanine. It is also expensive (the special protein formula costs about $400 per month), and it needs to be monitored carefully so that the level of phenylalanine is not only kept low, but it is also kept high enough to prevent stunt-

ing growth (Smith et al., 1973; Smith & Wolff, 1974; Steinhausen, 1974).

Dietary treatment, whether of PKU or of other inborn errors of metabolism, poses other issues and problems. The Committee on Nutrition of the American Academy of Pediatrics has noted that dietary treatment of any hereditary metabolic disease, including PKU, is simpler in theory than in fact (Lowe et al., 1967). Before dietary treatment for any given disorder is instituted, the committee states that three questions must be answered:

(1) Is the untreated disease harmful?
(2) Is the treatment useful?
(3) Can the dietary treatment itself cause harm either to persons with the disease or to those treated by mistake? ·

Each of these questions is considered in turn below (see National Academy of Sciences, 1975, chap. 3).

Answers to the first and second questions are easy in the case of PKU. The effects of not treating PKU are strong and undesirable. Research has demonstrated the effectiveness of proper dietary treatment, although some children with genetic PKU on normal diets have been found to have normal intelligence (e.g., Hsia, 1968). What about effectiveness? The age at which the diet is started is crucial for the outcome. There is a critical or sensitive period for the effects on the brain of the inappropriate metabolic products found in PKU (see the review in Kaplan, 1962). To be maximally effective, the diet should be started in the first or second month of life (Berman et al., 1966; Hudson et al., 1970; Steinhausen, 1974). Infants treated prior to 6 months of age had IQs in the range of 70 (borderline retardation) to 100 (normal). This means that almost all of these children are able to attend normal schools (Smith & Wolff, 1974). Those who were started on the diet at 7 to 18 months of age had IQs in the 50 to 70 range (mild and borderline retardation), and those who were not started until after 2 years had IQs below 30 (severe or profound retardation). Late treatment has some positive effects, in that it reduces the aggressive and listless behaviors that are found in PKU children.

Although IQ seems reasonably protected by the diet, PKU children still differ from their non-PKU siblings. In one study, parents rated their PKU 3- to 7-year-olds as more predictable (rhythmic) and intense, and less persistent than their sibs (Schor, 1983). Their 8- to 12-year-old children (who were no longer on the diet) were rated as less persistent, predictable, and intense, and as more distractible (Schor, 1984). Some evidence suggests that complex spatial visualization is depressed relative to sibling controls in a well-monitored group ranging in age from 6 to 23 years (Brunner et al., 1987). It also appears that EEGs show abnormalities even in treated cases, and that these abnormalities increase with age and are independent of IQ levels (Pietz et al., 1988). Adolescents on unrestricted diets show neuropsychological deficits beyond what would be suggested by their IQs, deficits that are at least partially reversible by a return to the diet (Clarke et al., 1987). The practice of stopping the diet at about 6 years, when most brain growth is complete, has come into general question (see, e.g., Holtzman et al., 1986). Preliminary evidence indicates that administering large neutral amino acids may improve neuropsychological functioning in PKU cases (Jordan et al., 1985).

Is it the dietary treatment or something else that accounts for the better outcomes for babies treated early? PKU babies are not randomly assigned to dietary treatment or no-treatment groups (which would be unethical if evidence favors the efficacy of the diet), hence it could be that parents who choose the diet are more effective in general and contribute to the higher IQs of the treated group. This alternative explanation is unlikely, however (Smith & Wolff, 1974). In families in which one PKU child (born after treatment became available) was treated early and an older sibling had not been, the untreated or late-treated siblings had lower IQs (range 10-110, median 65) than those treated early (range 65-120, median 100). Such sibling control studies are particularly convincing.

The question of whether the treatment itself can cause harm is important. It is necessary to avoid overrestricting phenylalanine (an essential building block), because growth would then be impaired. Errors in identification of PKU are unavoidable, because some babies who have elevated levels of phenylalanine do not have PKU. Since these babies cannot initially be distinguished from PKU babies who will suffer irreparable harm, it was originally thought that all must be given the diet. However, since starting treatment in the second month appears to be as effective as starting in the first month, there is time to allow confirmation of diagnosis.

Social Implications. Since treatment started, a large proportion of PKU babies are growing up to be productive members of society *and* to reproduce. Their potential for reproduction raises two problems for the next generation. First, **eugenicists** (persons who argue that genetic weaknesses should be eliminated from the population by preventing reproduction in genetically

inferior people, for example, by sterilization) are concerned that the gene pool is weakened if persons with genetic defects are allowed to reproduce. Fortunately, this movement is not currently prevalent. Should it arise in the future, however, one needs to be aware that sterilizing PKU persons would not eliminate PKU. This is true because (a) it occurs about as frequently as a result of spontaneous mutations of the genes as it does from inheritance, and (b) there is a high frequency of carriers (from 1 to 2 per 100 persons). Even extreme eugenicists would not wish to sterilize all carriers.

Second, treated PKU women who reproduce are almost certain to have mentally retarded children, even if the children do not inherit the second defective gene from the father. Lenke and Levy (1980) reviewed worldwide data covering 524 pregnancies of 155 women successfully treated for PKU. If maternal phenylalanine levels were high, virtually all of their offspring were retarded, 73% were microcephalic, and congenital heart defects were prevalent. If maternal levels were low, fewer infants were retarded, but even at very low levels 25% were microcephalic. Restarting the low phenylalanine diet helps to keep levels low, but ideally it should be started prior to or at the very start of pregnancy (Drogari et al., 1987). This is proving difficult to manage for a variety of social reasons; PKU young adults are less socially mature, less informed about birth control, more often live at home, and are more swayed by parental attitudes toward birth control than their peers ("Study Tracks the Pregnancies," 1989). Keeping women on the diet into their adulthood is being proposed. Even close compliance with the diet before and during pregnancy may not ensure normality (Lenke & Levy, 1982).

Tay-Sachs Disease

Like PKU, **Tay-Sachs disease** is inherited as an autosomal recessive characteristic. It results in an inability to produce a crucial enzyme, hexosamidase A, and this causes various fatty substances to build up in body cells, including those of the brain. Tay-Sachs infants appear normal at birth, but their nervous systems are gradually destroyed because of the effects of the missing enzyme. The effects are seen starting at around 3 to 6 months after birth. Tay-Sachs babies gradually lose motor abilities, such as sitting up and rolling over, and deteriorate intellectually. They become deaf, blind, and paralyzed. Death is inevitable, usually occurring by 2 years. The psychological tragedy of watching what was an apparently healthy baby deteriorate and die in this fashion can hardly be exaggerated.

In addition to the psychological costs, the medical costs of caring for one of these children during its brief lifetime can be staggering.

Tay-Sachs disease is rare in general, but not equally so in all ethnic groups. Among non-Jews it occurs in 1 out of 300,000 pregnancies. Among Ashkenazic Jews (those from Eastern Europe, which includes about 90% of American Jews), 1 in 30 persons is a carrier. This means that the likelihood that both parents will be carriers is 1 in 900, and because it is an autosomal recessive trait, 1 of every 4 offspring of two carriers will have the disease. Therefore, an average of 1 in every 3,600 pregnancies among Ashkenazic Jews will result in a Tay-Sachs child. In mixed marriages this frequency becomes 1 in 30,000.

Fortunately, the level of the enzyme hexosamidase A can be measured in both carriers and fetuses. Carriers have only about half the amount of hexosamidase A as healthy or homozygous dominant individuals, thus permitting Ashkenazic couples to know prior to conception whether they are both carriers. (The fact that they appear normal is testimony to the built-in safety factors of our biological systems.) Prospective parents who are both carriers will know that they have a 25% chance of giving birth to a Tay-Sachs baby. They can decide not to conceive; they can decide to conceive and abort the fetus if it has Tay-Sachs, and then conceive again; or they can conceive and fail to abort but try to prepare themselves psychologically for the trauma they face. This screening has significantly lowered the number of infants born with Tay-Sachs, from 50-100 infants per year to 13 as of 1980 (President's Commission for the Study of Ethical Problems, 1983).

Cystic Fibrosis

Cystic fibrosis (CF), another autosomal single recessive trait, is a disease of the secretory epithelia that affects their ability to transport salt and water. This can lead to heavy, dehydrated mucus in the airways that must be expelled. In the United States, this is done by pounding on the chest wall; in Europe, breathing exercises are taught prior to development of the cough reflex. Persons with CF are subject to chronic bacterial infections, and digestive problems may also occur due to blockage of the pancreatic ducts. CF occurs in about 1 in every 2,500 live births (Lemna et al., 1990) and 1 in 25 white Americans possesses one gene for this trait (is a carrier).

Children with CF used to have a life expectancy of only 9 or 10 years, but early detection and antibiotic treatments have extended this. However, many of the bacteria become resistant to antibiotics, and the thick-ness of the mucus, plus structural damage done over time, may inhibit their ability to act. Nevertheless, the current median life span for individuals with CF is slightly more than 20 years, and one-third of the more than 15,000 patients listed in the registry of the North American National Cystic Fibrosis Foundation are older than 21 years of age (Colten, 1990). Inasmuch as the homozygous cases do not normally reproduce, there is strong selection pressure against the homozygous recessive state. Perhaps the heterozygous state has some advantage that we do not yet understand.

Recent discovery of the gene that causes CF makes it possible to determine whether a given pregnancy carries a normal, a carrier, or a CF fetus. More than 60% of a small sample of families prenatally diagnosed as carrying a CF fetus chose to abort. In Belgium, 65% of 105 families with a CF child did not become pregnant again within 5 years (Evers-Kisbooms et al., 1988), and 85% of those who had not been sterilized intended to have prenatal diagnosis if they became pregnant.

Cretinism

Cretinism is a mental retardation syndrome produced by hypothyroidism, which is caused by several different mechanisms. One form, familial goiterous cretinism, is inherited as a single recessive trait, but through several possible metabolic dysfunctions, one (block at C) is diagrammed in Figure 3.4. Other forms are environmentally caused or of unknown origin. Whatever the cause of the insufficiency of thyroid hormones, the results for the baby are the same (see also Chapter 4).

The signs appear within a few weeks of birth. Growth is stunted; the body is short, but the head is relatively large; the neck is short and thick; the hands are broad and short; the abdomen is enlarged. The face takes on a characteristic pattern of low forehead; puffy, wrinkled eyelids; scant eyebrows; large, depressed nose; thick lips; and large, protruding tongue. The skin is dry, the body is flabby, and the baby is inactive and slow to respond. Motor and language development are delayed, and intellectual retardation is severe. It is possible to prevent cretinism by providing iodine to mothers prior to conception and in the first half of pregnancy (Delong et al., 1985). It is also possible to treat an affected infant with a substitute for thyroid hormone (desiccated thyroid substance). If treatment is started early in infancy and continued with regularity, many of the characteristics of this disorder can be avoided. Treatment later in life is only palliative. Before these measures were available, cre-

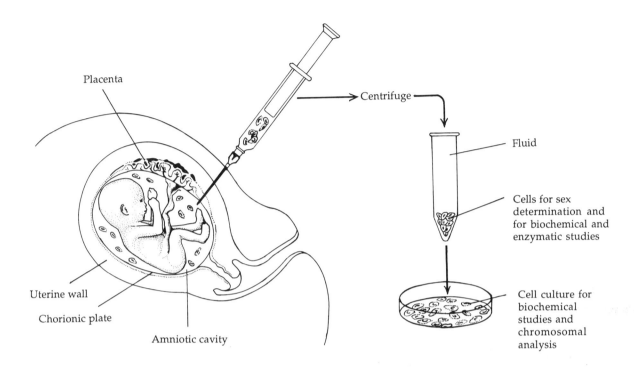

Figure 3.5. Amniocentesis. A needle is used to withdraw a small amount of fluid containing fetal cells from the amniotic cavity. The cells and fluid are separated in a centrifuge and the cells are cultured for a variety of tests.

tinism accounted for sizable numbers of institutionalized mentally retarded in the United States, as it still does in some parts of the world.

Other Gene Disorders

Only a few of the most common gene disorders have been discussed here, those that are of particular relevance to infancy or infancy-related issues, such as prevention and treatment of retardation. Those that are relatively frequent but that are not associated with retardation have not been considered. The other retardation syndromes identified by neonatal screening are much less frequent than PKU (Levy et al., 1970). In addition to defects caused by autosomal recessive genes, there are autosomal dominant gene defects and defects carried on the X sex chromosome.

Mutant genes cause five different genetic disorders, each of which causes a different deficiency, but all of which lead to accumulation of toxic levels of ammonium, which can cause seizures, brain damage, and death. Normally, ammonium would be transformed into urea and excreted in the urine. About 1 in 2,500 newborns has one of these five disorders, and most die

within a year. A group of Johns Hopkins researchers pioneered an attempt to treat them using dietary therapy to reduce the accumulation of ammonium. In that study, 24 cases who survived an early coma were treated, and 92% survived at least 1 year. However, their mean IQ at 12 to 74 months was 43 (Msall et al., 1984). If early diagnosis and therapy were available, perhaps rather than achieving only a brief prolongation of life, we might prevent brain damage.

X-Linked Traits. We turn now to the **X-linked traits,** which were the first disorders to be analyzed by amniocentesis (see Figure 3.5). Such defects occur when a particular recessive gene from the mother is carried on the X chromosome of an ovum fertilized by a sperm carrying a Y chromosome. In such cases the gene on the X chromosome passed to the son from the mother does not have a balancing one from the Y chromosome from the father, hence the trait will be expressed even though it is recessive.

The mother is a heterozygous carrier and therefore the dominant gene on her other X chromosome (the one she did not pass on to her affected son) protects her from the defect. Sons of a carrier mother and normal father have a 50/50 chance of having the trait, since each gene has a 50/50 chance of being the one in the ovum that is fertilized. Daughters of carrier mothers and normal fathers (who have a dominant gene on their X chromosomes) will be normal, inasmuch as the recessive and aberrant gene must be on both X chromosomes. They might, however, receive the recessive gene from their mothers and be carriers.

Hemophilia. Perhaps the best known sex-linked traits are color blindness and hemophilia, the "bleeder's disease" familiar to students of history. Hemophilia is caused by a deficiency of the substances that lead to blood clotting. Because hemophiliacs are at risk of bleeding to death from even the most minor injuries, they must lead extremely restricted lives. There are treatments that enable a less restricted life, but they are difficult, expensive, and involve transfusions of blood or blood products; these have led to a considerable number of infections with HIV, the virus that causes AIDS.

The incidence of hemophilia in males is about 1 in 10,000 births. For females, who would have to inherit two recessive genes, the incidence is 1 in 50 million births. Detection of carrier females is more than 90% accurate, but 25% of new cases are caused by mutations, not by inheritance. A precise blood test exists for detecting the deficiency as early as the sixteenth week after conception (Firshein et al., 1979).

Lesch-Nyhan syndrome. **Lesch-Nyhan syndrome** is an X-linked trait that essentially affects only males. The gene defect leads to the absence or inactivity of an enzyme controlling purine metabolism, which has its highest activity in the basal ganglia of the brain. The result is a neurological condition that develops in infancy, typically prior to 1 year of age. Mental retardation, cerebral palsy, and spasmodic, involuntary motor movements are followed, by age 3, by the behavioral syndrome of compulsive biting and self-mutilation of the lips and hands, head banging, and aggressive behavior toward others. The self-mutilation occurs despite apparent normal response to pain, as evidenced by screaming in response to self-injury. Most of these boys show severe retardation, little language development, and poor motor development. They die before reaching adulthood.

Analyses to detect the abnormal levels of enzymes and uric acid that characterize Lesch-Nyhan are now possible. They can determine whether the mother is a carrier (again, carrier mothers have lower levels of the enzyme than normal women) and, using amniocentesis, whether the fetus is affected. Previously all male fetuses of carrier mothers had to be aborted if they wanted to avoid bringing to life a child who would die

soon and miserably. Now only affected males need be aborted. This disorder is fortunately quite rare (1 in 50,000).

BALANCED POLYMORPHIC SYSTEMS

There is also something geneticists call a **balanced polymorphic system**. In such a system one gene carries a negative characteristic, but it also carries a characteristic that can be positive in some circumstances. Sickle-cell disease is the only definitive example of such a system. The gene responsible for PKU is relatively frequent in Northern Europeans, among whom only two mutations account for most cases, and among Yemenite Jews, where a different few account for it (DiLella et al., 1987; Kidd, 1987). This suggests that the carrier status might have some advantage, and in the Irish and West Scottish groups it appears to lower the spontaneous abortion rate (Woolf, 1985).

Sickle-Cell Anemia

Sickle-cell anemia is a hemoglobinopathy (disorder of the blood's hemoglobin or oxygen-carrying molecules). It too is an autosomal recessive trait that must be inherited from both parents, but cases also arise as a result of new mutations. The homozygous person is said to have sickle-cell anemia and the heterozygote to have sickle-cell trait. In this disorder the red blood cells contain a form of hemoglobin (HbS) that crystallizes when there is inadequate oxygen, as happens at high altitudes or with overexertion. The pain of an attack is excruciating. The red blood cells are shaped like sickles and tend to clump together, and thus may block off blood vessels. These cells live only half as long as normal red cells (those with HbA). Victims suffer from reduced growth, delayed puberty, neurological impairment, and blindness, as well as damage to many other organ systems. Infections are a problem, and one function of screening may be to allow preventive use of antibiotics to reduce the frequent deaths from pneumonia. The importance of early screening is obvious when one considers that, in Nigeria, 70% of the 78,000 sickle-cell anemia sufferers born per year die by 5 years of age (Akinyanju, 1989).

Sickling is rather frequent among blacks (8% of black Americans have the trait) and peoples in parts of the world with high malaria rates. In some parts of northern Greece and central India, 20-30% of the population is affected. The incidence is increasing in Europe. Although estimates vary from study to study, they converge around a figure of 1 in 500 persons having a gene for the trait in the United States (President's Commission for the Study of Ethical Problems, 1983; Rowley, 1989).

While exact mortality and morbidity rates for the United States are not known, Scott estimated in 1970 that 50% of persons with sickle-cell anemia did not reach the age of 20, and most did not live to 40 years. Survival rates are improving, and about 15% of the participants in a major current study are over 30 years of age (Smith, 1989).

Since victims often do not live long enough to reproduce, and since male fecundity is lowered, it is reasonable to ask why these selection pressures do not result in the trait's disappearing by natural selection. One reason may be that sickled cells are poor hosts for the malaria parasite that spends part of its life cycle in red blood cells. Therefore, the sickle-cell person is protected from malaria in the critical years when he or she has lost some immunity provided by the mother's system and has not yet developed his or her own. But, more important for the next generation, heterozygous carriers, who have only 20-40% of their red blood cells sickle shaped, are less likely than persons with no gene for sickling to contract malaria. Unless subjected to extreme environmental pressures (such as flying in a nonpressurized plane, overexerting themselves at high altitudes, or extreme overexertion), they are less likely to develop the serious problems of those with two genes for sickling. Thus it is an advantage to be a heterozygote in areas of the world that have malaria, even though some of your offspring will develop sickle-cell anemia if you are a heterozygote and mate with a carrier or a person having the disorder.

This system is called polymorphic because there are two possible consequences of the presence of the gene, sickle-cell anemia and malaria resistance. It is balanced because the biological advantage of malaria resistance offsets the maladaptiveness of sickling in those parts of the world (such as equatorial Africa) where malaria exists. Sickling genes are not needed in temperate climates, and nonblack, non-Mediterranean citizens of the United States rarely have them. If a population that has the sickling gene moves to a temperate climate, the advantage of the gene should disappear and its frequency should drop. The time span for such a genetic response is not known, but North American blacks do have a markedly lower incidence of sickle-cell anemia than is found in equatorial Africa. Whether selection pressure or mixing of black with white genotypes plays the principal role in bringing this about is far from clear. In the case of the increase in frequency in Europe, it has to be the result of population shifts, ethnic mixing, or both.

Despite this downward shift in incidence, sickle-cell anemia is one of the most important genetic problems in the United States. It is much more frequent than PKU or cystic fibrosis. Many infants born with the disease do not show signs of it until after 2 years of age, but they are at risk for developing a potentially life-threatening blood infection, which can be prevented by doses of oral penicillin if started by 4 months of age.

Although diagnostic tests have been available for 15 years, sickle-cell has not been routinely screened for in newborns. New York state has had mandatory newborn screening for a while, and programs are currently being set up in Massachusetts, Rhode Island, Connecticut, and at least 25 other states. The lack of a cure and the relative rarity of genetic or pregnancy screening in the United States may partially account for this delay. However, racial politics are another reason. In the 1970s blacks feared screening lest they be sterilized or otherwise prevented from bearing children, thus leading to genocide. Currently this attitude appears to have changed. The consequences of screening in the United States differ from those in Europe. There, more than 90% of diagnosed fetuses are aborted. In the United States, parents who have had one child with sickle-cell anemia tend to avoid pregnancy or to ask for screening, but if the fetus is diagnosed to have sickle-cell disease, only 39% terminate the pregnancy (Rowley, 1989).

Infants are also indirectly affected by having mothers with sickle-cell. These mothers are more likely to die in childbirth or to become physically unable to care for their infants or to die while they are still infants. In Memphis, Tennessee, in a hospital serving a virtually all-black population, only 1 in 2,000 obstetric patients has sickle-cell anemia, but these account for 1 in 6 patient deaths. Only 50% of the sickle-cell mothers who survive have live babies to take home with them. Some progress has been made in reducing the perinatal death rate in Nigeria. There, conservative treatment in pregnancy, including blood transfusions if necessary, has lowered the infant death rate to 114 per 1,000 and the maternal death rate to 28 per 1,000 (Akinyanju, 1989). Carrier women, who have only a minority of their cells sickled, are not at greater risk for perinatal mortality, but they tend to have more premature births and more babies who are low in birth weight for their gestational age.

Thalassemias (Alpha and Beta)

Thalassemias, like sickle-cell disease, are disorders of the hemoglobin. They are caused by at least 50 different gene variants. Both alpha and beta types lead to hemoglobin deficiency, which leads to insufficient oxygen being delivered to the cells. Alpha thalassemia is particularly frequent and severe in Asians; however, people who have both alpha thalassemia and sickle-cell anemia have milder cases of the latter (Embury, 1989). The high frequency of thalassemia has led some to suggest that it might be a balanced polymorphic system.

Beta thalassemia is most frequent in Mediterranean countries. The homozygous condition is catastrophic (Glader, 1984). Treatment requires blood transfusions every three weeks, together with therapy to prevent the buildup of iron, which used to cause death by heart attack prior to age 20. Bone marrow transplants appear to offer hope for survival, and even event-free survival, if done before liver damage occurs (Lucarelli et al., 1990).

Like sickle-cell, these syndromes can be detected prenatally (Leonard & Kazazian, 1978). Active screening programs for them exist in Italy and in England (for immigrant populations). For example, prior to the availability of prenatal diagnosis, Greek Cypriots in London who were at risk for beta thalassemia had much lower birthrates than Greek Cypriots not at risk. Subsequent to the availability of screening they have the same birthrate as other Greek Cypriots (Rowley, 1989). Among Asian Muslims, the knowledge of their child's being a carrier affects the parents' choice of a marital partner, so that school-age screening would offer considerable advantage, especially because first-cousin marriages are preferred (Elton et al., 1989). The best guess is that in those areas with screening (the northeastern United States and parts of the Mediterranean basin) cases have dropped 50%, and that it can be eliminated (Kuliev, 1986). Parents in areas with screening have more pregnancies and more completed pregnancies. (For further information on any aspect of the thalassemias, see Bank, 1990.)

RH FACTOR: A COMPLEX
GENE-ENVIRONMENT INTERACTION

This discussion of the **Rh factor** appears after the section on genetics and ahead of the chapter on environmental effects on the fetus for a very good reason.

The fetus does not inherit a defect, but a factor in the makeup of its blood that may create an environmental problem for it. Another way of looking at this problem is to view it as an interaction between the genetics of the mother and that of the fetus. Some people have red cell antigens in their blood. This factor is called Rh because rhesus monkeys have it. Humans who have the antigen are called Rh positive (Rh+) and those who do not are called Rh negative (Rh-). When a mother is Rh-, her baby may inherit Rh+ blood from the father. Because Rh+ is dominant, the baby's chance of inheriting Rh+ is 100% if the father is homozygous, 50% if he is heterozygous.[11] If the baby is Rh+ and the blood of the baby and mother mix while the baby is in the uterus, the mother's body will consider the Rh+ factor a foreign substance and will produce antibodies.[12] Those antibodies cross the placenta and in effect attack the baby's blood, which produces a chemical substance called bilirubin, which causes the baby to be severely jaundiced (look very yellow). When bilirubin levels are high for some time they can cause **kernicterus**, a form of brain damage that may result in death.

As is often the case with hereditary traits, Rh- is unequally distributed in the world. The Rh- genotype occurs in 15% of Caucasians and 5% of blacks in the United States. It is rare or absent in many populations, especially in eastern Asia, the Pacific, and among natives of the Americas.

The first Rh+ baby of an Rh- mother will usually be spared, inasmuch as the placental circulation system keeps the mother's blood separate from that of the fetus. A first baby has problems only if there has been a previous abortion or tubal pregnancy or an injury during pregnancy that has led to the mixing of fetal and maternal blood (possibly from the process of implantation itself), or the mother has had a previous transfusion with Rh+ blood. In the birth process itself, however, some mixing usually occurs, and the mother's body starts to produce antibodies, leading to a problem for the next child. The severity would depend on the number of antibodies the mother had developed, which in turn depends on the amount of maternal and infant blood that has mixed. Each succeeding baby would be more likely to be affected, to be more severely affected, and finally the effects would be so severe that the mother would not be able to carry a live fetus to term. (See Figure 3.6 for an illustration of what happens to the brains of such babies.)

The first efforts to conquer this disorder involved testing the prospective mother and father to determine whether there was an incompatibility—that is, whether the mother was Rh- and the father was Rh+. If so,

---

11. Actually, the rhesus blood group is not the result of a single gene, but rather of multiple genes, which produce 36 possible combinations in the new organism. Nevertheless, the two combinations relevant to our discussion (Rh+ and Rh-) account for 91% of persons in Western Europe and North America.

12. This is the same basic mechanism that is involved in the rejection of skin grafts or organ transplants.

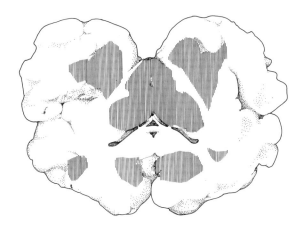

Figure 3.6. Cross sections of the brain of a baby who had kernicterus. The shaded portions show the damaged parts of the brain, which actually are yellow. (From Gellis & Feingold, 1968.)

they could decide to limit their family size. It then became possible to test the mother to determine her antibody level during later stages of pregnancy. If it was high and the fetus was viable, it could be delivered then, before it became more affected. Next came exchange transfusions. At birth, a longer section of umbilical cord than usual was left attached to the baby and whole blood genetically compatible with its own was pumped in until all the baby's blood, with its damaging bilirubin, had been replaced. It might be necessary to do this several times in the newborn period. Development of a technique to do exchange transfusions while the fetus was still in the uterus further improved treatment. By the 1950s, third-trimester amniocentesis enabled a direct assessment of the blood type of the fetus and of the amount of bilirubin in the fluid, which indicated the severity of the effects of incompatibility. The outcome of these tests helps doctors determine whether prenatal blood transfusions are necessary or whether to deliver the baby prior to term. In utero transfusions have been greatly aided by the use of ultrasound.

Before effective diagnosis and treatments such as these were developed, some 10,000 babies born in the United States each year either died or suffered brain damage because of Rh incompatibility. By the middle 1960s about 95% of these babies were saved from death by postnatal exchange transfusions, although some had residual brain damage because it can commence in utero, and there is some question of the transfusion having an adverse effect. Of those who would otherwise die in utero, 40% could be saved by

prenatal exchange transfusions. Thus by the 1960s most victims of Rh incompatibility could survive with proper medical treatment. However, hospitals varied in their ability to provide such treatment.

These were not cures, since they did not prevent the attack by the maternal antibodies on the blood of the fetus. Later, a treatment that does just that was developed: Rhogam injections given to Rh- mothers within 72 hours after the birth of their first child prevent her developing Rh+ antibodies that could attack her next fetus.[13]

Rh incompatibility is particularly interesting because it demonstrates that a normal hereditary trait can become maladaptive when the fetus is exposed to a destructive environment. The next chapter will offer additional examples of subtle interactions between genetics and the environment. Moreover, effective treatment modes for babies with Rh incompatibility could be developed only to the extent that the basic mechanisms of the disorder were understood. Thus the key to dealing with this disorder was basic research into the nature of the problem rather than applied research on various trial-and-error treatments.[14]

Genetic Diagnosis

PRIOR TO BIRTH

Knowledge about genetic disorders has become increasingly important as our ability to diagnose them prior to birth has improved. At first, knowing that family history put you at risk for having abnormal offspring gave you the option of not having children. Then we became able to tell the sex of a fetus and later still to diagnose many things about chromosomal and gene-caused disorders. This new knowledge has opened many options for family planning and genetic counseling. I have continually referred to diagnostic

13. This does not mean that there are no babies with unsafe levels of bilirubin. Other problems can cause this condition, some of which are also related to blood incompatibilities, for example, ABO incompatibility. A transfusion team must still always be on call. Milder levels of kernicterus are often treated by placing the baby under lights, the effectiveness and side effects of which are still controversial. Recent studies indicate that this may well be safely done at home, thus saving longer hospital stays and the associated costs.

14. Anyone interested in learning all that we know about the location on chromosomes of various human genes can get "The Human Genome Map" from *Science*, published by the American Association for the Advancement of Science (Stephens et al., 1990). A similar map is also found in *NIH Research*.

techniques above; it seems reasonable at this point to provide an overview of the techniques used.

Amniocentesis

The process of doing amniocentesis was described in Chapter 2, together with the rationale. It was only in the 1960s that tissue culture techniques included cultivation of fetal tissue. Then it became possible to use amniocenteses done in the fifteenth to nineteenth weeks of pregnancy to detect: (a) chromosomal abnormalities (by karyotyping), (b) by-products of inborn errors of metabolism (by automated biochemical analyses), and (c) the presence of alpha fetoprotein. More than 190 metabolic defects and congenital disorders can be diagnosed prenatally, in addition to an increasing number of chromosomal aberrations (President's Commission for the Study of Ethical Problems, 1983).

In a series of more than 6,000 amniocenteses done in the late 1960s and early 1970s, 5% of the fetuses were shown to be genetically abnormal (National Institutes of Health, 1979). A history of amniocenteses done on women over 35 in Ohio from 1972 to mid-1984 showed only 2.5% with abnormal chromosomes (Naber et al., 1987). Thus a primary function of this diagnostic tool is to reassure parents at risk for having a child with one of the detectable disorders that they need not fear that outcome. It is interesting to note that while population density affected utilization of diagnostic services in the Ohio study, religion did not.

Are there risks associated with fetal diagnosis using amniocentesis? Nationwide studies conducted in the United States and Canada to ascertain fetal damage, spontaneous abortion, and maternal infection or hemorrhage found no significant increase in problems. Prenatal deaths; birth weights; birth defects; problems of labor, delivery, and the newborn period; and development at one year did not differ for controls and those who had had amniocenteses. In cases where large needles were used or more than one insertion was required, there was an increase in problems. An even larger, but methodologically flawed, study in Great Britain found an increase, which disappeared after correcting only for different maternal ages in the controls (National Institutes of Health, 1979). Current studies examining maternal anxiety in the period of waiting for results are not sufficiently large or controlled to enable discussion of psychological stress (or relief) as outcomes.

Chorionic Villus Sampling

In **chorionic villus sampling** (**CVS**) cells are re-

moved from the projections on the chorionic membrane (see Figure 2.4 in Chapter 2). This can be done either through the cervix with a catheter or through the abdomen with a needle as in amniocentesis. It can be done at 9 to 11 weeks postconception, thus enabling much earlier diagnosis of the serious disorders for which one would contemplate abortion. This could reduce both the physical and the psychological trauma of an abortion.

While it is becoming increasingly popular, there are more restrictions on CVS than on amniocentesis. The catheters used in the cervical approach are classified by the FDA as experimental, and only a few centers and doctors are allowed to use them. In addition, in the case of amniocentesis, the practice that doctors need to become expert in the technique was obtained on women about to undergo abortion; such practice cannot be obtained that way for chorionic villus sampling in many states, because of laws banning research on fetuses.

The safety of CVS is less well documented than that of amniocentesis. Recent reports of a seven-center study with more than 6,000 cases in the United States indicate that pregnancy loss was only .8% higher than for amniocentesis, but assignment was not random, hence one cannot place faith in this result (Rhoads et al., 1989); however, Canadian figures for a randomly assigned group were .6% higher. There were no significant maternal problems. Italian data indicate no significant effects on fetal growth, premature delivery, congenital defects, or fetal loss (Brambati et al., 1990). No errors in diagnosis were found when both direct study and long-term cultures were used (Ledbetter et al., 1990).

Other Diagnostic Techniques

Several other techniques are used to diagnose genetic problems, including some used postnatally.

Detection of Alpha Fetoprotein. Alpha fetoprotein can be detected using maternal or infant blood samples. High levels of this fetal protein suggest the presence of neural tube defects (spina bifida or anencephaly), which affect 1 in 1,000 births. If a high level is found, sonograms from ultrasound should be used to picture the fetus or an amniocentesis done to assess more accurately the amounts given off by the fetus.

Low levels of alpha fetoprotein are associated with higher risk of chromosomal disorders. This could be very useful in identifying Down cases in mothers under 35, an age at which an amniocentesis would not normally be justified, even though 80% of Down births are to younger mothers. The blood test could be followed by amniocentesis in suspect cases. At least one state, California, requires that doctors offer this test to pregnant women. Since there are no risks associated with the test, there is no reason not to have it, unless abortion would not be contemplated under any circumstance.

Blood samples can also be used to determine the sex of the fetus, hence they can be a first screen for X-linked traits.

Ultrasound. Computerized video images of the fetus and its internal organs (and those of the mother) are produced from the echoes of high-frequency sound waves. The procedure is both painless and apparently risk free. In addition to being an adjunct to other techniques, it can be used to diagnose structural abnormalities, including not only spina bifida, but heart conditions. Early diagnosis of such problems makes it possible to have the equipment and personnel ready to start treatment shortly after birth. Measurements of skeletal and facial features made using this noninvasive technique can also be used to identify cases that might have Down syndrome, who could be then be tested using amniocentesis for accurate diagnosis. Ultrasound can also be used to study fetal behavior, as noted in Chapter 2.

Direct Gene Testing. Since 1980 it has been possible to test the genes using so-called restriction enzymes, which cut the DNA. When a mutation has altered the sequence of the subunits of DNA (adenine, guanine, cytosine, and thymine, or AGCT) the cut pieces of DNA are different. This technique can be used early in pregnancy to detect a gene defect, but unless ethnicity or family history tells which gene defect to look for, this is not a help. One cannot just start testing for the 3,000 single-gene defects that are known.

Postnatal Screening. Postnatal screening for inborn errors of metabolism can identify PKU, cretinism, and other conditions not discussed here that are now treatable. In time, perhaps still more will be identifiable. At least a dozen conditions of mental retardation associated with abnormal metabolism of amino acids have been identified in addition to PKU. They are all rarer than PKU and less well understood.[15]

In all of these disorders there are variations in the number and severity of symptoms that are modifications of the basic genetic patterns. As our knowledge expands, we will probably find that some of these differences are linked with genetic or chromosomal differences. Enzymatic deficiencies that are now grouped

as a single syndrome will be traceable to various genetic abnormalities (for example, gene deletion, mutation, absence of cell receptors or of activators for the enzyme, or inhibitors to enzyme action).

In order to start treatments early when available and to improve genetic counseling, various states have adopted mandatory screening tests.

Limits on Our Knowledge

All of these advances in diagnosis have not led to an ability to account for most birth defects. Remember that 65-70% of all birth defects are of unknown origin. Why should that figure be so high? First, the vast number and rarity of genetically based disorders make them hard to diagnose. More than 3,000 human diseases caused by defects in the content or expression of the genetic code have been identified, and most of them are very rare. This rarity means that the average doctor or hospital has little or no experience in recognizing these defects, hence correct diagnosis is difficult. Centralized computer systems are being developed so that doctors can provide information about an infant to a computer. It can then request further observations about the baby. This back-and-forth dialogue continues until the computer, on the basis of all the information programmed into it, can match the doctor's description with a probable diagnosis. If there is no match, the computer reports that the doctor's description does not fit any diagnostic description in the program.

A second difficulty in detecting the sources of genetic disorders is that the disorders are extremely complex, reflecting in part the complexity of development itself. For example, in Chapter 2, discussion of the embryological development of the ear showed the structures of the human ear and the complex way in which they develop from the three primary germ layers (endoderm, mesoderm, and ectoderm). It is obvious that in this complex process there are many ways that development could go wrong. Hearing loss has been found in nine known genetic syndromes, in addition to occurring in trisomies of chromosomes 21-23, 13-15, and 17-18 (Gluck, 1971). There are, moreover, more than 60 types of hereditary deafness (Konigsmark, 1971). In addition, 17 severe neural deafness syndromes with unknown origins account for more

---

15. For an overall look at the techniques, potential, and problems associated with prenatal diagnosis, there are two excellent reviews written for the nonspecialist: Epstein and Golbus (1977) and Fuchs (1980).

than half of all cases of congenital deafness. These syndromes may result from dominant, recessive, or sex-linked transmission. They may or may not be associated with other disorders, and, if associated, the particular systems that have defects vary.

A third difficulty in studying genetically related characteristics is that many of the traits that most of us (students, parents, or researchers) are interested in, such as intellectual and temperamental traits, are polygenic. The role of genetic variation and the action of the causative genes are difficult to detect in the phenotypic traits. Polygenic traits lead to widespread individual variability due to the combined action of two or more genes that, in turn, interact with variations in the environment to determine the final phenotypic expression. Such traits are usually continuously distributed in the familiar form of the bell-shaped curve. Because the action of the genes in producing the phenotypic variation is unknown, it is difficult to determine when two people differ genetically on a trait.

I cannot leave this topic without calling attention to the fact that the U.S. government is currently funding an endeavor called the Human Genome Project, which is aimed at identifying all human genes and their locations on the chromosomes. The U.S. Congress has published an Office of Technology Assessment (1988) report in which the chapters on applications to research and on social and ethical considerations are relevant to all students. Other chapters would be relevant to those with a medical or biological focus.

Genetic Counseling

As noted earlier, the lowered perinatal mortality that accompanied better prenatal care and delivery services resulted in the genetic component in the remaining mortality becoming greater. Can genetic counseling reduce the incidence of genetic abnormalities that lead either to death or to some of the crippling disorders surveyed here? I have already answered this question for some of the conditions discussed; however, let me summarize and expand.

Genetic counseling is not new. Modern genetic counseling began when a method for detecting sex from cells in the amniotic fluid developed. In 1949, Barr determined that female, but not male, cells have a piece of chromosomal material on the membranes of the cell nucleus that stains darkly (now called Barr bodies). Thus if the mother's family had a history of an X-linked disease, the parents could decide to abort male fetuses and raise only girls. Such abortions were

legal in most states even after abortion had become illegal (and before the Supreme Court's constitutional interpretation that allowed abortions as a matter of maternal choice). It was argued that having a child with some of the X-linked disorders could affect the mother's mental health, which was a reason for legal abortion.

When more precise tests for some X-linked traits made it possible to identify whether a particular fetus had the trait, it became possible to keep unaffected male fetuses until term. Recently, it has been reported that a London hospital is using *in vitro* fertilization in order to implant only female embryos in mothers who are carriers for genetic diseases that are fatal to boys (*Boston Globe*, July 31, 1990).

In the case of non-sex-linked disorders, knowledge of the sex of the fetus is of no help in avoiding the birth of seriously handicapped children. This may account for the fact that parents in this category often receive less adequate genetic counseling. Parents of cystic fibrosis children have frequently not received adequate counseling with respect to the risks for future children (Wright et al., 1979).

The new gene technologies are changing the possibilities. According to Lemna et al. (1990), with the recent discovery of the gene that causes CF, screening that will identify 95% of carriers should be possible within a year. If two carriers are married, these authors recommend adoption, artificial insemination from a noncarrier, or conceiving and testing for CF in the fetus with the option to abort. Many parents of CF children have opted not to have any more children rather than run the risk of having another CF child. This was the only option open to them prior to the possibility of genetic testing of the fetus, which allows the option of aborting an affected fetus.

Genetic counseling with respect to Down syndrome is complicated by the fact that so few of the cases are inherited, but eased by the option of prenatal testing with the option to abort for those to whom that is acceptable.

A Finnish study of 4,691 women randomly assigned to early ultrasound screening compared with 4,619 randomly assigned to the usual practices of their physicians showed no differences in birth weights or labor inductions (Saari-Kemppainen et al., 1990). However, the perinatal mortality in the routinely screened group was half that in the normal practices group (4.6 versus 9 per 1,000). This was primarily due to early detection of major malformations that led to induced abortions. The early detection of twins led to a lower perinatal mortality rate for them.

It is not possible to do justice to the topic of genetic

counseling in a few paragraphs. However, it is clear that, with the explosion of genetic knowledge, we must remember that thorough and intelligent research is needed before the development of widespread practical application based on partial knowledge.

Summary

Genetic and chromosomal disorders account for a number of problems that affect infants. Although most abnormal conceptuses do not survive to be born, or die shortly after birth, about .5% of newborns have chromosomal abnormalities and 3-5% have some genetic defect. This small proportion of infants accounts for a large proportion of hospitalizations of infants and children, and for staggering sums in hospital costs.

CHROMOSOMAL ABNORMALITIES

Chromosomal abnormalities usually involve an extra or missing chromosome (or piece of one) and are detectable by karyotyping. Down syndrome, the most frequent chromosomal disorder, and one of the most common causes of mental retardation, is usually caused by a third chromosome 21. This can be caused by nondisjunction occurring during gamete cell division and by translocation, where an extra piece of 21 attaches to either the 21 or another chromosome. Translocation accounts for only 4% of Down cases, but one-third are inherited. Mosaicism, in which nondisjunction has occurred after conception, is another cause. Mothers over 40 years of age are at much greater risk for trisomy 21.

The degree of retardation and the number and severity of physical defects vary widely. Life expectancy is increasing. The benefits and hazards of home versus institutional care have been presented, and the question of whether society provides adequate support systems to help families cope with Down children has been raised.

Trisomies other than Down occur, but most are spontaneously aborted during the embryonic stage. One that sometimes survives is trisomy 18. It accounts for many deaths in late pregnancy and around childbirth, and is related to maternal age. Monosomies, other than that of a single X, do not survive, but one syndrome (cri du chat) that is much more devastating than Down involves a missing piece of chromosome 4 or 5.

Most syndromes involving abnormal numbers of sex chromosomes are caused by nondisjunction during meiosis of either sperm or egg cells. Turner's syndrome (45,X0) is the only viable case of a totally missing chromosome. Extra X chromosomes are found in two syndromes, XXX (trisomy X) and XXY (Klinefelter's syndrome). Sexual systems are abnormal in varying degrees and behavior and intelligence may be somewhat affected. Treatment with sexual hormones may improve the appearance of those with Turner's and Klinefelter's syndromes.

An extra Y chromosome is found in the XYY syndrome. Men with this syndrome are tall, often have genital anomalies, and are relatively low in intelligence. Behavioral consequences have been the subject of much debate, especially the claim (based on inappropriate samples) that these men are more aggressive than normal.

Fragile X is an inherited condition in which there is a thin area on some of the X chromosomes (i.e., it is a mosaic) that may break or translocate. It is second only to Down as a chromosomal cause of retardation.

DISORDERS CAUSED BY GENES

Genes provide the codes for the production of all body substances, including the enzymes used in all biochemical processes. Genetic problems can frequently be diagnosed by biochemical testing. Most common and best known are the defects that are autosomal recessive traits that are expressed only when each parent contributes the defective gene to the new organism. PKU, Tay-Sachs disease, cystic fibrosis, and some forms of cretinism are of this type. The severity of the disorders varies; some are fatal early in life (Tay-Sachs), some later in life (cystic fibrosis), and some are not fatal. Those that are not fatal often produce substantial mental retardation, as do PKU and cretinism. The phenotypic expression of mental retardation in both PKU and cretinism can be controlled by environmental intervention, hence it is important to diagnose these conditions early. In cretinism the appropriate therapy is administration of thyroid; in PKU it is a diet low in phenylalanine started very early in life and continued for a number of years (and resumed in the event of pregnancy). The control of the phenotypic expression is not perfect. Mothers treated for PKU may have retarded children whether or not they inherit the defect. It is not yet clear whether reinstituting dietary control can prevent this.

Another autosomal recessive trait is sickle-cell anemia, which arises frequently as a result of mutations. It has been described as being part of a balanced polymorphic system, in which being a carrier has an advantage. Mediterranean and black populations in parts of the world with high rates of malaria are frequently carriers. This is a life-threatening condition in which red blood cells clump at low oxygen levels or with extreme exertion. The clumping can lead to further oxygen loss in organs or tissues served by the blood vessels. It is possible to determine carrier status as well as to diagnose fetally.

Other disorders affecting blood and oxygen supply are alpha and beta thalassemias, which are caused by many different gene variants. The former is prevalent among Asians and the latter among Mediterranean people. These are life threatening, pose great medical problems during life, and can be effectively screened for. There is some hope for effective treatment.

X-linked traits are the other long-known and well-understood class of genetic disorders. They stem from a recessive gene that is present only on the X chromosome. Since the woman has another X chromosome she will never have the trait, but is called a carrier, and her male offspring who get the gene from the "wrong" chromosome will develop the trait. Hemophilia (bleeder's disease) is such a trait, the royal pedigree of which was well known before modern genetics. Treatment includes blood transfusions, hence the current tragedy of AIDS among hemophiliacs. Lesch-Nyhan syndrome is a tragic and fortunately rare example of an X-linked trait in which the central nervous system is destroyed by the abnormal metabolic chain. Carriers and male fetuses can be diagnosed.

Rh factor provides an interesting interaction of genetic and environmental influences. If a baby inherits the dominant Rh+ blood type from its father and its mother has the recessive Rh-, then the mother's blood, if and when it mixes with that of her fetus, produces antibodies that attack the baby's blood cells, causing them to produce bilirubin that not only turns the skin and whites of the eyes yellow, but can damage the brain and even kill the fetus. The history of increasingly successful efforts to avoid this source of damage has been detailed.

GENETIC DIAGNOSIS AND COUNSELING

Genetic diagnosis has progressed from following family trees to being able to detect carriers and whether or not a fetus has certain genetic abnormalities. Prenatally, amniocentesis permits karyotyping of cells to determine the normality of fetal chromosomes; chorionic villus sampling makes it possible to do this earlier in gestation; alpha fetoprotein levels in blood can reveal the possibility of neural tube defects and of Down syndrome, which can then be checked by other techniques; ultrasound can be used to assess

structural abnormalities; and biochemical analysis of fluid obtained in amniocentesis can detect many gene defects. Direct study of genes can be done if one knows which genes to study. Postnatally, tests can be used to detect PKU and other defects for which treatment is possible.

Genetic counseling moved from advice not to have children if a family tree had certain disorders to being able to determine the sex of a fetus from the Barr bodies. This allowed mothers with a family history of X-linked diseases such as hemophilia to choose to abort male fetuses. The new techniques allow determination of whether a male fetus is actually affected, hence making it possible for such mothers to have normal male children. Tay-Sachs, cystic fibrosis, and Down syndrome can all be detected prenatally, allowing parents to make informed decisions. The use of antenatal diagnosis combined with abortion of affected fetuses actually operates to allow many parents who would not otherwise have children to do so.

Unlike the case for chromosomal abnormalities and those arising from defects in single genes, most of the human characteristics in which psychologists and parents are interested are polygenic, and the mechanisms of their inheritance are not understood.

References

AKINYANJU, O. O. (1989). A profile of sickle cell disease in Nigeria. In C. F. Whitten & J. F. Bertles (Eds.), Sickle cell disease [Special issue]. *Annals of the New York Academy of Sciences, 565.*

ALLANSON, J. E., McGillivray, B. C., Hall, J. G., Shaw, D., & Kalousek, D. K. (1983). Cytogenetic findings in over 2,000 amniocenteses. *Canadian Medical Association Journal, 129,* 846-848.

BAIRD, P. A., & Sadovnick, A. D. (1987). Life expectancy in Down syndrome. *Journal of Pediatrics, 110,* 849-854.

BANK, A. (Ed.). (1990). Sixth Cooley's anemia symposium [Special issue]. *Annals of the New York Academy of Sciences, 612.*

BAULD, R., Sutherland, G. R., & Bain, A. D. (1974). Chromosome studies in investigation of stillbirths and neonatal deaths. *Archives of Disease in Childhood, 49,* 782-788.

BEEGHLY, M., Weiss-Perry, B., & Cicchetti, D. (1989). Structural and affective dimensions of play development in young children with Down syndrome. *International Journal of Behavioral Development, 12,* 257-277.

BELL, A. G., & Corey, P. N. (1974). A sex chromatin and Y body survey of Toronto newborns. *Canadian Journal of Genetics and Cytogenetics, 16,* 239-250.

BENDER, B., Linden, M., & Robinson, A. (1987). Environment and developmental risk in children with sex chromosome abnormalities. *Journal of the American Academy of Child Psychiatry, 26,* 499-503.

BERMAN, P. W., Waisman, H. A., & Graham, F. K. (1966). Intelligence in treated phenylketonuric children: A developmental study. *Child Development, 37,* 731-747.

BERRY, H. K. (1976). Hyperphenylalaninemias and tyrosinemias. *Clinics in Perinatology, 3,* 15-40.

BESSMAN, S. P., Williamson, M. L., & Koch, R. (1978). Diet, genetics, and mental retardation—interaction between phenylketonuric heterozygous mother and fetus to produce nonspecific diminution of IQ: Evidence in support of the justification hypothesis. *Proceedings of the National Academy of Sciences, 78,* 1562-1566.

BONGSO, A., Chye, N. S., Ratnam, S., Sathananthan, H., & Wong, P. C. (1988). Chromosome anomalies in human oocytes failing to fertilize after insemination in vitro. *Developmental Medicine and Child Neurology, 30,* 844-845.

BOUE, A., & Boue, J. (1974). Chromosome abnormalities and abortion. *Basic Life Sciences, 4,* 317-339.

BOUE, J., Boue, A., & Lazar, P. (1975). Retrospective and prospective epidemiological studies of 1,500 karyotyped spontaneous human abortions. *Teratology, 12,* 11-26.

BRAMBATI, B., Lanzani, A., & Tului, L. (1990). Transabdominal and transcervical chorionic villus sampling: Efficiency and risk evaluation of 2,411 cases. *American Journal of Medical Genetics, 35,* 160-164.

BRIDGES, F. A., & Cicchetti, D. (1982). Mothers' ratings of the temperament characteristics of Down syndrome infants. *Developmental Psychology, 18,* 238-244.

BROWN, F. R., III, Greer, M. K., Aylward, E. H., & Hunt, H. H. (1990). Intellectual and adaptive functioning in individuals with Down syndrome in relation to age and environmental placement. *Pediatrics, 85,* 450-452.

BROWN, W. T., Jenkins, E. C., Cohen, I. L., Fisch, G. S., Wolf-Schein, E. G., Gross, A., Waterhouse, L., Fein, D., Mason-Brothers, A., Ritvo, E., Ruttenberg, B. A., Bentley, W., & Castells, S. (1986). Fragile X and autism: A multicenter study. *American Journal of Medical Genetics, 23,* 341-352.

BRUNNER, R. L., Berch, D. B., & Berry, H. (1987). Phenylketonuria and complex spatial visualization: An analysis of information processing. *Developmental Medicine and Child Neurology, 29,* 460-468.

CARR, D. H. (1963). Chromosome studies in abortuses and stillborn infants. *Lancet, 2,* 603-606.

CARR, D. H. (1971). Chromosome studies in selected spontaneous abortions and early pregnancy loss. *Journal of Obstetrics and Gynecology. 37,* 570-574.

CARR, J. (1988). Six weeks to twenty-one years old: A longitudinal study of children with Down's syndrome and their families. *Journal of Child Psychology and Psychiatry, 29,* 407-431.

CASEY, M. D., Blank, C. E., & Street. (1969). [Letter]. *Lancet, 2,* 859-860.

CICCHETTI, D., & Beeghly, M. (Eds.). (1990). *Children with Down syndrome: A developmental perspective.* New York: Cambridge University Press.

CLARKE, J. T., Gates, R. D., Hogan, S. E., Barrett, M., & MacDonald, G. W. (1987). Neuropsychological studies on adolescents with phenylketonuria returned to phenylalanine-restricted diets. *American Journal on Mental Retardation, 92,* 255-262.

COLTEN, H. R. (1990). Screening for cystic fibrosis: Public policy and personal choices. *New England Journal of Medicine, 322,* 328-329.

CONNOLLY, B. H., Morgan, S., & Russell, F. F. (1984). Evaluation of children who participated in an early intervention program: Second follow-up study. *Physical Therapy, 64,*

1515-1518.

CORNWELL, A. C., & Birch, H. G. (1969). Psychological and social development in home-reared children with Down's syndrome (Mongolism). *American Journal of Mental Deficiency, 74,* 341-350.

COURT-BROWN, W. M. (1969). Sex chromosome aneuploidy in man and its frequency, with special reference to mental subnormality and criminal behavior. *International Review of Experimental Pathology, 7,* 31-97.

DELONG, G. R., Stanbury, J. B., & Fierro-Benitez, R. (1985). Neurological signs in congenital iodine deficiency disorder (endemic cretinism). *Developmental Medicine and Child Neurology, 27,* 317-324.

DiLELLA, A. G., Marvit, J., Brayton, K., & Woo, S. L. C. (1987). An amino acid substitution involved in phenylketonuria is in linkage disequilibrium with DNA haplotype 2. *Nature, 327,* 333-336.

DROGARI, E., Smith, J., Beasley, M., & Lloyd, J. K. (1987). Timing of strict diet in relation to fetal damage in maternal phenylketonuria. *Lancet, 2,* 927-930.

ELTON, P. J., Baloch, K., & Evans, D. I. K. (1989). The value of screening for beta thalassemia trait amongst Asian Muslim schoolchildren. *Journal of Reproductive and Infant Psychology, 7,* 51-53.

EMBURY, S. H. (1989). Alpha thalassemia: A modifier of sickle cell disease. In C. F. Whitten & J. F. Bertles (Eds.), Sickle cell disease [Special issue]. *Annals of the New York Academy of Sciences, 565.*

EMDE, R., Katz, E., & Thorpe, J. (1978). Emotional expression in infancy: Early deviations in Down's syndrome. In M. Lewis & L. Rosenblum (Eds.), *The development of affect.* New York: Plenum.

EMERY, A. E. H., & Mueller, R. F. (1988). *Elements of medical genetics* (7th ed.). Edinburgh: Churchill Livingston.

EPSTEIN, C. J., & Golbus, M. S. (1977). Prenatal diagnosis of genetic diseases. *American Scientist, 65,* 703-711.

EVERS-KISBOOMS, G., Denoyer, L., Cassiman, J. J., & Van den Berghe, H. (1988). Family planning decisions after the birth of a cystic fibrosis child: The impact of prenatal diagnosis. *Scandinavian Journal of Gastroenterology, 143*(Suppl.), 38-46.

FIRSHEIN, S., Hoyer, L., Lazarchick, T., Forget, B., Hobbins, J., Clyne, L., Pitlick, F., Muir, W. A., Merkatz, I., & Mahoney, M. (1979). Prenatal diagnosis of classic hemophilia. *New England Journal of Medicine, 300,* 937-941.

FRASER, F. C. (1984). Gross chromosomal aberrations. In M. E. Avery & H. W. Taeusch, Jr. (Eds.), *Schaffer's diseases of the newborn* (5th ed.). Philadelphia: W. B. Saunders.

FUCHS, F. (1980). Genetic amniocentesis. *Scientific American, 242,* 47-53.

GATH, A. (1978). *Down's syndrome and the family: The early years.* London: Academic Press.

GATH, A. (1985). Parental reactions to loss and disappointment: The diagnosis of Down's syndrome. *Developmental Medicine and Child Neurology, 27,* 392-400.

GATH, A., & Gumley, D. (1984). Down's syndrome and the family: Follow-up of children first seen in infancy. *Developmental Medicine and Child Neurology, 26,* 500-508.

GELLIS, S. S., & Feingold, M. (1968). *Atlas of mental retardation syndromes.* Washington, DC: U.S. Department of Health, Education and Welfare.

GLADER, B. E. (1984). Erythrocyte disorders in infancy. In M. E. Avery & H. W. Taeusch, Jr. (Eds.), *Schaffer's diseases of the*

88   CONCEPTION THROUGH BIRTH

newborn (5th ed.). Philadelphia: W. B. Saunders.

GLUCK, L. (1971). *Neurosensory factors in newborn hearing.* Paper presented at the Conference on Newborn Hearing Screening, California State Department of Public Health, San Francisco.

GOLDGABER, D., Lerman, M. I., McBride, O. W., Saffioti, U., & Gajdusek, D. C. (1987). Characterization and chromosomal localization of a cDNA encoding brain amyloid of Alzheimer's disease. *Science, 235,* 877-880.

GUNN, P., & Berry, P. (1987). Some financial costs of caring for children with Down syndrome at home. *Australia and New Zealand Journal of Developmental Disabilities, 13,* 187-193.

GUNN, P., Hayes, A., Crombie, M., Jobling, A., & Cuskelly, M. (1991, July). *Variation and variability in persons with Down syndrome: A longitudinal study of a population.* Paper presented at the meeting of the International Society for the Study of Behavioral Development, Minneapolis.

HAGERMAN, R. J., & McBogg, P. M. (Eds.). (1983). *The fragile-X syndrome.* Dillon, CO: Spectra.

HAYDEN, A. H., & Dmitriev, V. (1975). An intervention program for atypical infants. In B. Z. Friedlander, G. H. Sterritt, & G. E. Kirk (Eds.), *Exceptional infant: Vol. 3. Assessment and intervention.* New York: Brunner/Mazel.

HAYES, A., & Gunn, P. (in press). Developmental assumptions about Down syndrome and the myth of uniformity. In C. J. Denholm (Ed.), *The adolescent with Down syndrome.* Victoria, BC: University of Victoria, School of Child and Youth Care.

HERTIG, A., & Rock, J. (1949). A series of potentially abortive ova recovered from fertile women prior to the first missed menstrual period. *American Journal of Obstetrics and Gynecology, 58,* 968-993.

HO, H.-Z., Glahn, T. J., & Ho, J.-C. (1988). The fragile X syndrome. *Developmental Medicine and Child Neurology, 30,* 257-261.

HOLTZMAN, N. A., Kronmal, R. A., Van Doorninck, W., Azern, C., & Koch, R. (1986). Effect of age at loss of dietary control on intellectual performance and behavior of children with phenylketonuria. *New England Journal of Medicine, 314,* 593-598.

HOOK, E. B. (1982). Epidemiology of Down syndrome. In S. M. Pueschel & J. E. Rynders (Eds.), *Down syndrome: Advances in biomedicine and the behavioral sciences.* Cambridge, MA: Ware.

HSIA, D. Y.-Y. (1968). Nutritional management in hereditary metabolic disease [Annotations]. *Developmental Medicine and Child Neurology, 10,* 103-104.

HUDSON, F. P., Mordaunt, V. L., & Leahy, I. (1970). Evaluation of treatment begun in first three months of life in 184 cases of phenylketonuria. *Archives of Disease in Childhood, 45,* 5-12.

JARVIK, L. F., Klodin, V., & Matsuyama, S. S. (1973). Human aggression and the extra Y chromosome. *American Psychologist, 28,* 674-682.

JORDAN, M. K., Brunner, R. L., Hunt, M. M., & Berry, H. (1985). Preliminary support for the oral administration of valine, isoleucine and leucine or phenylketonuria. *Developmental Medicine and Child Neurology, 27,* 33-39.

KAPLAN, A. R. (1962). Phenylketonuria: A review. *Eugenics Quarterly, 9,* 151-160.

KASARI, C., Mundy, P., Yirmiya, N., & Sigman, M. (1990). Affect and attention in children with Down syndrome. *American Journal of Mental Retardation, 95,* 55-67.

KESSLER, S. (1975). Extra chromosomes and criminality. In R. R. Fieve, D. Rosenthal, & H. Brill (Eds.), *Genetic research in psychiatry.* Baltimore: Johns Hopkins University Press.

KESSLER, S., & Moos, R. H. (1970). The XYY karyotype and criminality: A review. *Journal of Psychiatric Research, 7,* 153-170.

KIDD, K. K. (1987). Phenylketonuria: Population genetics of a disease. *Nature, 327,* 282-283.

KIVOWITZ, J. (1972). The XYY syndrome in children: A review. *Child Psychiatry and Human Development, 2,* 186-194.

KONIGSMARK, B. W. (1971). *Hereditary and congenital factors affecting newborn sensorineural hearing.* Paper presented at the Conference on Newborn Hearing Screening, California State Department of Public Health, San Francisco.

KRISHNAN, B. R., Ramesh, A., Kumari, M. P., & Gopinath, P. M. (1989). Genetic analysis of a group of mentally retarded children. *Indian Journal of Pediatrics, 56,* 249-258.

KULIEV, A. (1986). Thalassaemia can be prevented. *World Health Forum, 7,* 286-290.

LANDRY, S. H., & Chapieski, M. L. (1990). Joint attention of six-month-old Down syndrome and preterm infants: I. Attention to toys and mother. *American Journal of Mental Retardation, 94,* 488-498.

LEDBETTER, D. H., Martin, A. O., Verlinsky, Y., Pergament, E., Jackson, L., Yang-Feng, T., Schonberg, S. A., Gilbert, F., Zachary, J. M., Barr, M., Copeland, K. L., et al. (1990). Cytogenetic results of chorionic villus sampling: High success rate and diagnostic accuracy in the United States collaborative study. *American Journal of Obstetrics and Gynecology, 162,* 495-501.

LEMNA, W. K., Feldman, G. L., Kerem, B., Fernbach, S. D., Zevkovich, E. P., O'Brien, W. E., Riordan, J. R., Collins, F. S., Tsui, L., & Beaudet, A. L. (1990). Mutation analysis for heterozygote detection and the prenatal diagnosis of cystic fibrosis. *New England Journal of Medicine, 322,* 291-296.

LENKE, R. R., & Levy, H. L. (1980). Maternal phenylketonuria and hyperphenylalinemia: An international survey of untreated and treated pregnancies. *New England Journal of Medicine, 303,* 1202-1208.

LENKE, R. R., & Levy, H. L. (1982). Maternal phenylketonuria: Results of dietary therapy. *American Journal of Obstetrics and Gynecology, 142,* 548-553.

LEONARD, C., & Kazazian, H. (1978). Prenatal diagnosis of hemoglobinopathies. *Pediatric Clinics of North America, 25,* 631-642.

LEVY, H. L. (1989). Nutritional therapy for selected inborn errors of metabolism. *Journal of the American College of Nutrition, 8*(Suppl.), 54-60.

LEVY, H. L., Karolkewicz, V., Houghton, S. A., & MacCready, R. A. (1970). Screening the "normal" population in Massachusetts for phenylketonuria. *New England Journal of Medicine, 282,* 1455-1458.

LITTLE, A. B. (1988). There's many a slip 'twixt implantation and the crib. *New England Journal of Medicine, 319,* 241-242.

LOWE, C. R., Coursin, D. B., Heald, F. P., Holliday, M. A., O'Brien, D., Owen, G. M., Pearson, H. A., Scriver, E. R., Filer, L. J., & Kline, O. L. (1967). Nutritional management in hereditary metabolic disease. *Pediatrics, 40,* 289-304.

LUBS, H. A. (1970). Cytogenetic problems in antenatal diagnosis. In M. Harris (Ed.), *Early diagnosis of human genetic defects: Scientific and ethical considerations* (HEW-NIH Publication No. 72-25). Washington, DC: Government

Printing Office.

LUBS, H. A. (1977). Applications of quantitative karyotypy to chromosome variation. In P. Jacobs, W. Price, & P. Law (Eds.), *Human population cytogenetics*. Baltimore: Williams & Wilkins.

LUCARELLI, G., Galimberti, M., Polchi, P., Angelucci, E., Baronciani, D., et al. (1990). Bone marrow transplantation in patients with thalassemia. *New England Journal of Medicine, 322,* 417-421.

MARCELL, M. M., Croen, P. S., & Sewell, D. H. (1990, March). *Language comprehension in Down syndrome and other trainable mentally handicapped individuals.* Paper presented at the Conference on Human Development, Richmond, VA.

MARCELL, M. M., Sewell, D. H., & Croen, P. S. (1990, March). *Expressive language in Down syndrome and other trainable mentally handicapped individuals.* Paper presented at the Conference on Human Development, Richmond, VA.

McCLEARN, G. E., & DeFries, J. C. (1973). *Introduction to behavioral genetics.* San Francisco: Freeman.

McKUSICK, V. A. (1986). *Mendelian inheritance in man* (8th ed.). Baltimore: Johns Hopkins University Press.

MSALL, M., Batshaw, M., Suss, R., Brusilow, S., & Mellits, E. D. (1984). Neurologic outcome in children with inborn errors of urea synthesis: Outcome of urea-cycle enzymopathies. *New England Journal of Medicine, 310,* 1500-1505.

MUNDY, P., Sigman, M., Kasari, C., & Yirmiya, N. (1988). Nonverbal communication skills in Down syndrome children. *Child Development, 59,* 235-249.

NABER, J. V., Huether, C. A., & Goodwin, B. A. (1987). Temporal changes in Ohio amniocentesis utilization during the first twelve years (1972-1983), and frequency of chromosome abnormalities observed. *Prenatal Diagnosis, 7,* 51-65.

National Academy of Sciences. (1975). *Genetic screening: Programs, principles, and research.* Washington, DC: Author.

National Institutes of Health. (1979). *Antenatal diagnosis: Report of a consensus development conference* (Publication No. 79-1173). Bethesda, MD: U.S. Department of Health, Education and Welfare.

NERI, G., Opitz, J. M., Mikkelsen, M., Jacobs, P. A., Daviews, K., & Turner, G. (Eds.). (1988). X-linked mental retardation 3 [Special issue]. *American Journal of Medical Genetics, 30*(1-2).

NUSSBAUM, R. L., & Ledbetter, D. H. (1986). Fragile X syndrome: A unique mutation in man. *Annual Review of Genetics, 20,* 109-145.

OLIVER, C., & Holland, A. J. (1986). Down's syndrome and Alzheimer's disease: A review. *Psychological Medicine, 16,* 307-322.

OPITZ, J. M., FitzGerald, J. M., Reynolds, J. F., Lewin, S. O., Daniel, A., Ekblum, L. S., & Phillips, S. (1987). The Montana Fetal Genetic Pathology Program and a review of prenatal death in humans. *American Journal of Medicine and Genetics, 3*(Suppl.), 93-112.

PATTERSON, D. (1987). The causes of Down syndrome. *Scientific American, 257,* 42-48.

PENNINGTON, B. F., Bender, B., Puck, M., Salbenblatt, J., & Robinson, A. (1982). Learning disabilities in children with sex chromosome anomalies. *Child Development, 53,* 1182-1192.

PIDCOCK, F. S. (1984). Intellectual functioning in Turner syndrome. *Developmental Medicine and Child Neurology, 26,* 539-545.

PIETZ, J., Benninger, C., Schmidt, H., Scheffner, D., & Bickel, H. (1988). Long term development of intelligence (IQ) and EEG in 34 children with phenylketonuria treated early. *European Journal of Pediatrics, 147,* 361-367.

PLOMIN, R. (1990). The role of inheritance in behavior. *Science, 248,* 183-188.

PLOMIN, R., DeFries, J. C., & McClearn, G. E. (1990). *Behavioral genetics: A primer* (2nd ed.). New York: W. H. Freeman.

POLANI, P. E. (1966). Chromosome anomalies and abortions. *Developmental Medicine and Child Neurology, 8,* 67-70.

President's Commission for the Study of Ethical Problems in Medicine: Biomedical and Behavioral Research. (1983). *Screening and counseling for genetic conditions* (Library of Congress No. 83-600502). Washington, DC: Government Printing Office.

PUESCHEL, S. M., & Finelli, P. V. (1985). *Neurological investigation in patients with fragile-X syndrome.* Paper presented at the annual meeting of the American Academy of Cerebral Palsy and Developmental Medicine. (Abstracted in *Developmental Medicine and Child Neurology, 27,* 95-96)

PUESCHEL, S. M., Tingey, C., Rynders, J. E., Crocker, A. C., & Crutcher, D. M. (Eds.). (1987). *New perspectives on Down syndrome.* Baltimore: Paul H. Brookes.

PUNNETT, H. H., & Zakai, E. H. (1990). Old syndromes and new cytogenetics [Annotation]. *Developmental Medicine and Child Neurology, 32,* 820-831.

RAUH, H., Rudinger, G., Bowman, T. G., Berry, P., Gunn, P. V., & Hayes, A. (1991). The development of Down's syndrome children. In M. E. Lamb, H. Keller (Eds.) *Infant development: Perspectives from German speaking countries.* Hillsdale, NJ: Erlbaum.

RHOADS, G. G., Jackson, L. G., Schlesselman, S. E., de la Cruz, F. F., Desnick, R. J., Golbus, M. S., Ledbetter, D. H., Lubs, H. A., Mahoney, M. J., Pergament, E., Simpson, J. L., Carpenter, R. J., Elias, S., Ginsberg, N. A., Goldberg, J. D., Hobbins, J. C., Lynch, L., Schiono, P. H., Wapner, R. J., & Zachary, J. M. (1989). The safety and efficacy of chorionic villus sampling for early prenatal diagnosis of cytogenetic abnormalities. *New England Journal of Medicine, 320,* 609-617.

ROBINSON, A., Goodman, S., & O'Brien, D. (1984). Genetic and chromosomal disorders, including inborn errors of metabolism. In C. H. Kempe, H. K. Silver, & D. O'Brien (Eds.), *Current pediatric diagnosis and treatment* (8th ed.). Los Altos, CA: Lange Medical.

ROBINSON, A., & Puck, T. (1967). Studies on chromosomal nondisjunction in man, II. *American Journal of Human Genetics, 19,* 112-129.

ROSENBERG, L. E. (1986, December-1987, January). Gene therapy for inherited diseases. *News Report, National Academy of Sciences,* pp. 12-14.

ROWLEY, P. T. (1989). Prenatal diagnosis for sickle cell disease: A survey of the United States and Canada. In C. F. Whitten & J. F. Bertles (Eds.), Sickle cell disease [Special issue]. *Annals of the New York Academy of Sciences, 565.*

SAARI-KEMPPAINEN, A., Karjalainen, O., Ylostalo, P., & Heinonen, O. P. (1990). Ultrasound screening and perinatal mortality: Controlled trial of systematic one-stage screening in pregnancy. The Helsinki Ultrasound Trial. *Lancet, 336,* 387-391.

SCHOR, D. P. (1983). PKU and temperament: Rating children three through seven years old in PKU families. *Clinical Pediatrics, 22,* 807-811.

SCHINZEL, A. (1983). *Catalogue of unbalanced chromosome*

aberrations in man. Berlin: Walter de Gruyter.

SCHOR, D. P. (1984). PKU and temperament in eight twelve-year-old children. *Developmental Medicine and Child Neurology, 26,* 110.

SCOTT, R. B. (1970). Health care priority and sickle cell anemia. *Journal of the American Medical Association, 214,* 731-734.

SHAH, S. A. (1970). *Report of the XYY chromosomal abnormality* (U.S. PHS Publication No. 2103). Washington, DC: Government Printing Office.

SHAPIRO, S., Ross, L. J., & Levine, H. S. (1965). Relationship of selected prenatal factors to pregnancy outcome and congenital anomalies. *American Journal of Public Health, 55,* 268-282.

SHERMAN, S. L., Jacoby, P. S., Morton, N. E., Froster-Iskenius, U., Peebles, P. N., et al. (1985). Further segregation analysis of the fragile X syndrome with special reference to transmitting males. *Human Genetics, 69,* 289-299.

SHIOTA, K., Uwabe, C., & Nishimura, H. (1987). High prevalence of defective human embryos at the early postimplantation period. *Teratology, 35,* 309-316.

SMITH, I., Lobascher, M., & Wolff, O. H. (1973). Factors influencing outcome in early treatment of phenylketonuria. In J. W. T. Seakins, R. A. Saunders, & C. Toothill (Eds.), *Treatment of inborn errors of metabolism*. London: Churchill Livingston.

SMITH, I., & Wolff, O. H. (1974). Natural history of phenylketonuria and influence of early treatment. *Lancet, 2,* 540-544.

SMITH, J. A. (1989). The natural history of sickle cell disease. In C. F. Whitten & J. F. Bertles (Eds.), Sickle cell disease [Special issue]. *Annals of the New York Academy of Sciences, 565.*

STEDMAN, D. J., & Eichorn, D. H. (1964). A comparison of the growth and development of institutionalized and home-reared mongoloids during infancy and early childhood. *American Journal of Mental Deficiency, 69,* 391-401.

STEINHAUSEN, H. C. (1974). Psychological evaluation of treatment in phenylketonuria: Intellectual, motor, and social development. *Neuropaediatrie, 5,* 146-155.

STEPHENS, J. C., Mador, M. L., Cavanaugh, M. L., Gradie, M. I., & Kidd, K. K. (1990). The human genome map. *Science, 250*(Suppl.), 1-4.

STICKLE, G. (1971). *Health is indivisible*. Paper presented at the National Foundation of the March of Dimes Conference for Community Leaders, Boston.

Study tracks the pregnancies of PKU mothers. (1989, December 7). *Harvard Medical Area Focus,* pp. 1, 6-8.

SUTTON, H. E. (1965). *An introduction to human genetics*. New York: Holt, Rinehart & Winston.

TABOR, A., & Phillip, J. (1987). Incidence of fetal chromosome abnormalities in 2264 low-risk women. *Prenatal Diagnosis, 7,* 355-362.

TADA, K., Tateda, H., Arashima, S., Sakai, K., Kitagawa, T., Aoki, K., et al. (1984). Follow-up study of a nation-wide neonatal metabolic screening program in Japan: A collaborative study group of neonatal screening for inborn errors of metabolism in Japan. *European Journal of Pediatrics, 142,* 204-207.

THAKE, A., Todd, J., Webb, T., & Bunday, S. (1987). Children with the fragile X chromosome at schools for the mildly mentally retarded. *Developmental Medicine and Child Neurology, 29,* 711-719.

THASE, M. E. (1987). The relationship between Down syn-
drome and Alzheimer's disease. In L. Nadel (Ed.), *The psychobiology of Down syndrome*. Cambridge: MIT Press.

U.S. Congress, Office of Technology Assessment. (1988). *Mapping our genes: The Genome Projects: How big, how fast?* (Publication No. OTA-BA-373). Washington, DC: Government Printing Office.

VALE, J. R. (1980). *Genes, environment, and behavior: An interactionist approach*. New York: Harper & Row.

WALZER, S., Breau, G., & Gerald, P. S. (1969). A chromosome survey of 2,400 normal newborn infants. *Journal of Pediatrics, 74,* 438-448.

WALZER, S., & Gerald, P. S. (1975). Social class and frequency of XYY and XXY. *Science, 190,* 1228-1229.

WARBURTON, D. (1987). Chromosomal causes of fetal death. *Clinical Obstetrics and Gynecology, 30,* 268-277.

WILCOX, A. J., Weinberg, C. R., O'Connor, J. F., Baird, D. D., Schlatterer, J. P., Canfield, R. E., Armstrong, E. G., & Nisula, B. C. (1988). Incidence of early loss of pregnancy. *New England Journal of Medicine, 319,* 189-194.

WISNIEWSKI, K. E., & Schmidt, S. G. (1989). Postnatal delay of myelin formation in brains from Down syndrome infants and children. *Clinical Neuropathology, 8,* 55-62.

WITKIN, H. A., Mednick, S. A., Schulsinger, F., Bakkestrom, E., Christiansen, K. O., Goodenough, D. R., Hirschhorn, K., Lundsteen, C., Owen, D. R., Philip, J., Rubin, D. B., & Stocking, M. (1976). Criminality in XYY and XXY men. *Science, 193,* 547-555.

WITSCHI, E. (1970). Teratogenic effects from overripeness of the egg. In F. C. Fraser & V. A. McKusick (Eds.), *Proceeding of Third International Conference of Congenital Malformations* (Excerpta Medica International Congress Series 204). Amsterdam: Excerpta Medica.

WOOLF, L. I. (1985). The heterozygote advantage in phenylketonuria [Letter to the editor]. *Developmental Medicine and Child Neurology, 27,* 773-774.

World Health Organization. (1972). *Genetic disorders: Prevention, treatment, and rehabilitation* (Report of World Health Organization Scientific Group, Technical Report Series No. 497). Geneva: Author.

WRIGHT, L., Schaefer, A. B., & Solomons, G. (1979). *Encyclopedia of pediatric psychology*. Baltimore: University Park Press.

Influence of Prenatal Environment
on Constitution

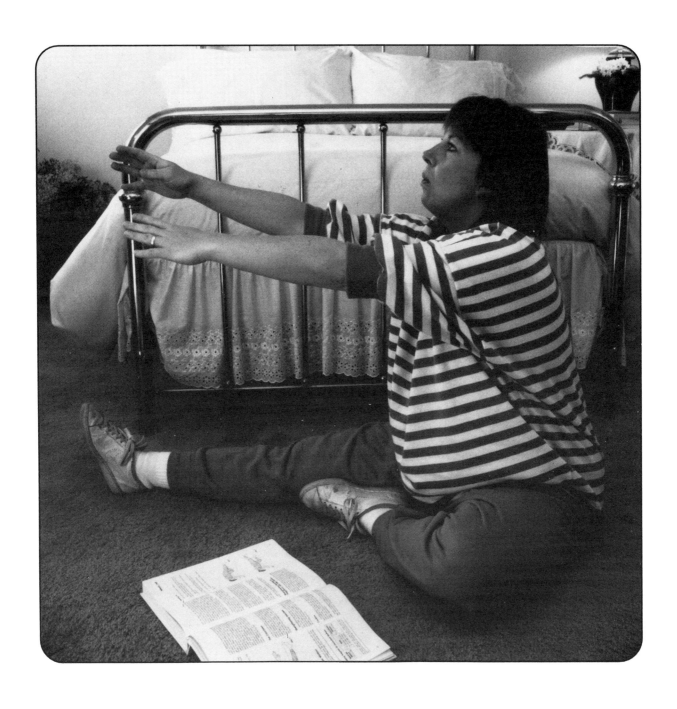

What aspects of the environment affect the growth and development of the embryo and fetus and hence help to determine the constitution of the infant at birth? As was true in the discussion of genetic effects, the answers to the questions posed here are based primarily on investigations of problems. Something goes wrong and scientists look for preceding events or influences that could have caused the problem. Babies with no problems or with good constitutions are not studied. Today it is known that, in at least some cases, diseases, drugs, radiation, and maternal stresses can affect fetal development and cause **congenital** defects (those present at birth, or constitutional). Blood incompatibilities were mentioned in Chapter 3 as an interesting case of prenatal influence that involves an interaction between genetics and the environment. Further study may show that the effects of increasing maternal age are in fact caused by some environmental agent, such as radiation. Very young maternal age is also associated with higher risks to the fetus in ways that will be discussed in this chapter. It is likely that some of these risks also stem from environmental causes.

Birth defects, one of the principal causes of death, disease, and disability in infancy and childhood, have both genetic and environmental causes. As the term *environment* is used here, it includes not just exogenous substances taken in by the mother, but her health, nutrition, and diseases, some of which may result in the release of endogenous substances (such as hormones and drugs) that may act in toxic ways. However, the causes of 60% of birth defects are unknown (Kalter & Warkany, 1983). Thus a perfect baby is not guaranteed even if all environmental agents and conditions known to produce birth defects are avoided and no known hereditary problem is present.

For many years, doctors and psychologists tried to convince mothers that the old wives' tales about "marking" the unborn infant were false, as indeed they were. If you are pregnant and frightened by a horse, your baby will not be marked by a horse-shaped birthmark because of it; nor will it have a hare lip if you are startled by a rabbit; nor will attendance at concerts during pregnancy cause your baby to be musical or even a music lover. This is not to say that musical ability and interest do not run in families. They do, but probably for reasons other than prenatal exposure. Mothers who expose their unborn children to music may carry genes that predispose to musical ability, and they are likely to provide a **postnatal** (after birth) environment that offers many opportunities for the development of their children's musical talent.[1]

We now know that the protection provided by pla-

cental exchange is not complete. As Beck et al. (1973) have written: "There is no doubt that covert extrinsic factors (probably multiple) in combination with a genetic predisposition (in many cases polygenic) are able to push the developing organism beyond a critical threshold in the direction of malformation" (p. 292).

Extrinsic environmental factors that can damage the embryo or fetus can be put into several broad categories: (a) maternal diseases or conditions, (b) malnutrition and oxygen deprivation, (c) drugs, (d) irradiation, and (e) stress. Some of these are called **teratogens** (substances that produce congenital malformations). This chapter is partly concerned with **teratology** (the science of studying the causes of abnormal structural development). This is a relatively young field of science that received great impetus from the thalidomide episode. Teratology has been broadened to include behavioral deficits as well as congenital malformations; this is called *behavioral teratology*. For a review of this field, see Voorhees and Mollnow (1987). The field has grown and diversified rapidly, and there is a current move to restrict the concept of a teratogen to those things that cause **dysmorphogenesis** (gross structural malformations). Other compounds that produce alterations in the normal sequence of developmental processes are beginning to be studied under the heading of **developmental toxicology**, a topic dealt with here either under this name or still as behavioral teratology (see Hutchings, 1989).

Before discussing different teratogens and toxic factors and other harmful conditions, I wish to outline the types of outcomes used to measure their effects. A common measure is death rates. This includes losses early in pregnancy through **resorption** (assimilation of structures previously produced by the body—that is, reabsorption of zygotes, blastulas, or embryos), spontaneous abortions, deaths later in pregnancy (miscarriages or stillbirths), and deaths after delivery (neonatal or newborn). Until recently it has been thought that injuries sustained prior to implantation were always fatal. This view is being challenged (Iannaccone et al., 1987). When all prenatal deaths and stillbirths are combined into one overall measure, it is called **pregnancy wastage**.

Babies who die as a result of a teratogen or toxic factor are either those who have been exposed to the most massive doses or at a critical period or those who are most vulnerable, a condition affected by heredity. Babies who survive may well be harmed, but in less obvious ways that are difficult to determine. Large-scale malformation registries are needed if we are to be able to search for teratogenic risks in humans (Kallen, 1987).

Dysmorphogenesis can occur due to harmful substances, especially during the embryonic period, when differentiation of structures is taking place, and may not be incompatible with life.[2] Many factors in the fetal period can result in growth retardation and low birth weight. Babies who are small for their gestational age (**SGA**) are said to suffer from **intrauterine growth retardation** (**IUGR**). Small babies, whether SGA or LBW (less than 5.5 lb, but not necessarily SGA), seem to be more vulnerable to a variety of postnatal problems, but with many individual exceptions (see Chapter 2). Low birth weight babies account for 70% of all neonatal deaths. Hence any environmental factor that increases the probability of having a low birth weight infant is undesirable.

Functional deficits (those related to nervous system function) must be assessed after the relevant function develops. Minor ones are difficult to assess and a prebirth cause is hard to determine. Small head circumference at birth was related to neurological problems in a sample of more than 4,500 who had been members of the Boston sector of the National Collaborative Perinatal Project (NCPP), but neurological deficits at age 7 do not seem related to IUGR itself, unless there were indications of anoxia (Berg, 1989). A frequently used outcome measure is intelligence as measured by IQ. IQ can be measured reliably only some years after birth, hence it can have been influenced by a large number of postnatal factors. Nevertheless, an amazing array of teratogens and toxic factors affect IQ. It is hypothesized that this is because the brain experiences its greatest growth prenatally. Vulnerability continues into postnatal life, especially for the nervous system. Other measures of function will be discussed in relation to particular studies. A review of animal data, together with a discussion of possible mechanisms, can be found in Grimm (1987).

Maternal Diseases

Two kinds of maternal diseases can affect the embryo, fetus, or newborn: infectious diseases and noninfectious chronic diseases. Both types are discussed below.

INFECTIOUS DISEASES THAT ACT PRENATALLY

The mother may contract a disease during pregnancy or may have one when she starts the pregnancy that can affect the fetus.

Rubella

An early demonstration that the placenta does not provide an impregnable barrier against infections was the discovery of the effects of **rubella** (German measles). Congenital deafness used to occur in spurts, often in such numbers as to be virtual epidemics. This led medical investigators in the mid-1960s to search for an environmental event that occurred in similar spurts. They found rubella, a disease so mild that many mothers of congenitally deaf infants were not aware of having been ill.

With more intense study of the infants, it became clear that deafness was not their only handicap. They were likely to have been SGA, and a larger proportion than normal had heart defects, cataracts, abnormal retinas, neuromotor defects, and immunological defects that left them prone to unusual infections; many were retarded and autistic (McIntosh, 1984). Doctors refer to such a cluster of problems as a **syndrome**. When rubella was confirmed as the cause of these problems, they became known as the rubella syndrome. As more and more defects were identified, it became the "expanded rubella syndrome." It is important to note that in 85% of cases the defects are not detected in the immediate postbirth period.

This syndrome provides examples of critical periods in embryological development. The negative effects of rubella are most frequent and most profound during organogenesis, but they continue into the second trimester. The organ systems affected differ according to when in pregnancy the infection occurred. Growth is most likely to be permanently stunted if infection was in the first 8 weeks; cataracts occur only if infection was prior to day 60; and heart defects and deafness occur up to 11 weeks. Half of the fetuses that survive the mother's infection in the first month of pregnancy are damaged, but the figure for the entire first trimester is 15-25%.

Deafness and disorders of the retina can occur in either the first or the second trimester, but only 10% of fetuses are affected in the second. Deafness occurs as a result of damage to both structures of the ear (organ of Corti) and the central nervous system (see, for example, the review by McIntosh, 1984). Rubella epidemics posed a significant threat to developing offspring that in the mid-1960s left some 20,000-30,000 damaged infants, 16,000 of whom were deaf.

---

1. For other ways in which prenatal exposure to music may have an effect, see Chapter 7

2. For an overall picture of minor morphological variants and their role in syndromes of importance, see Mehes (1987).

In 1983 Gallaudet College for the Deaf had to greatly expand its facilities to deal with the influx of students.

Now that the dangers of rubella in early pregnancy are known, extensive attempts to control it are made. Immunization of women prior to reproductive age is desirable. It should not occur when there is a chance of pregnancy, because maternal infection in the month prior to pregnancy can affect the fetus. Unfortunately, this does not always prevent defects when the immunized mother is exposed to rubella. Every effort should be made to protect women who have not had rubella from exposure. If a pregnant woman is exposed, a serum antibody test can help assess the risk to the fetus (McIntosh, 1984). If the results are unclear, amniocentesis can determine whether the rubella virus reached the amniotic fluid, and the woman can decide whether to have an abortion. All these measures together have reduced cases of rubella syndrome in the United States to between 23 and 77 per year during the 1970s (a rate of 1.33 per 100,000 live births). This is a real epidemiologic success story. (**Epidemiology** is the science that deals with the incidence, distribution, and control of disease.)[3] However, progress did not affect all portions of society equally, leaving blacks and Hispanics at much greater risk (Kaplan et al., 1990). Also, there are indications that rubella may be beginning to be more frequent again.

Syphilis

Most bacteria, unlike viruses, are too large to cross the placental barrier. However, the bacterium that produces syphilis (*Treponema pallidum*, also called *Spirocheta pallida*) can. Transmission of this venereal disease to the fetus is more likely later in pregnancy. It appears that syphilis affects the potential baby only *after* the sixteenth to eighteenth week of gestation. Thus it is not associated with defects in organogenesis, but with destructive **lesions** (abnormal changes in structure) of already-developed organs. Lesions have been found on the cornea of the eye, producing blindness, and on the skin and mucous membranes. As many as 34% die before birth, and substantial numbers of those born alive die early in life. Those that survive are likely to be growth retarded and to suffer problems with their livers, inflammation of the lining of the abdomen (peritonitis), anemia, central nervous system

problems, and pegged teeth (Ricci et al., 1989). It is possible that some effects may be indirect or result from hormonal changes that appear to occur in both mother and fetus during pregnancies of syphilitic women (Parker & Wendel, 1988). An excellent survey of the effects of syphilis on the maternal-fetal dyad, and of the current status of the problem, can be found in Fletcher and Gordon (1990).

Antibiotics became available to the public after World War II, and the Public Health Service aggressively pursued policies to eradicate venereal diseases. As a result, syphilis virtually disappeared in the 1950s and 1960s. Unfortunately, the Public Health Service budgets implementing these policies were cut shortly before the "sexual revolution" of the late 1960s, and the number of cases has increased since the early 1970s. Syphilis is again a significant problem. Fortunately, most states require that all pregnant women reporting to doctors or hospitals be given the simple blood test that detects syphilis. If the disease is detected and cured by antibiotics before the sixteenth to eighteenth week of gestation, serious defects to the fetus will be avoided, although some of the long-term effects, such as the **stigmata** (plural of **stigma**, or mark) affecting the skin and teeth may still occur. If all women received adequate prenatal care, the effects of syphilis on the unborn could be largely eliminated. Unfortunately, many women do not get adequate prenatal care, and those most at risk are the ones least likely to get it. One inner-city hospital serving an impoverished population reported 18.4 syphilis cases per 1,000 for a 2½-year period in the mid-1960s (Ricci et al., 1989; for English and Australian data, respectively, see also Bowell et al., 1989; Garland & Kelly, 1989).

Human Immunodeficiency Virus and AIDS

The human immunodeficiency virus (HIV) is the current hot issue among maternal infections that are transmitted to a fetus. Pediatric AIDS was first recognized in 1982. The National Association of Children's Hospitals estimates that 3,000 infants are infected with HIV each year, 80% of them born to drug abusers. The virus may be transmitted in utero, during delivery, or through breast milk. Women who have no symptoms may transmit the virus. The proportion of babies who contact it from the mother varies in different studies from 30% to 65% (Enkin et al., 1989). Data from San Francisco and Los Angeles show that 30-50% of infants born to infected women develop AIDS. Figures are so variable because there is no clear diagnostic test for neonates (see "Maternally Transmitted HIV Infection," 1990). The rates of AIDS births are

---

3. Great Britain attempted only selective, not universal, vaccination as in the United States, and there is still a substantial problem there (Enkin et al., 1989). Since they do not confirm hearing loss there until almost 1 year, which is late for starting therapy, the problem is even greater (Wild et al., 1989).

12.9 and 9.6 per 10,000 in the two cities, and is 12 times as high for blacks as for whites (California Department of Health Services, 1989).

If contracted in utero, HIV is a teratogen that produces frequent dysmorphic features. Many HIV babies are born preterm or SGA, but whether this is due to AIDS or associated risk factors such as drug abuse is unknown. After birth the babies have frequent infections, especially persistent and recurrent thrush, and often are characterized by failure to thrive. (A survey of the problems is found in Iannetti et al., 1989.) A large majority of the cases (78-90%) develop neurological complications (including impaired brain growth) as a result of active infection of the brain (Epstein et al., 1986) and viral and bacterial infections accompanying AIDS (Iannetti et al., 1989). Onset may be anytime between 2 months and 5 years. Behaviorally, this leads to a loss of developmental milestones, intellectual deficits, and generalized weakness, especially of the legs (Byers, 1989; Ultman, 1988).

These children are likely to have parents who are unable to care for them adequately due to their own AIDS or to their drug habits, and are often abandoned at the hospitals where they are born.

ORGANISMS THAT AFFECT THE BABY AT BIRTH

The following sections discuss four infections that are transmitted primarily at the time of delivery. While that is a **perinatal** event (one that takes place around the time of birth), the resulting problems are not directly related to the birth process. They are discussed here to stress the point that environmental agents act at various times during development.

Cytomegalovirus and Herpes Virus Hominis

The first two, cytomegalovirus (CMV) and herpes virus hominis (HVH), are both members of the herpes simplex virus family and both produce chronic or recurrent infections that are frequently reactivated in pregnancy.

CMV affects the mother's genitalia, breasts, or urinary tract (singly or together), but usually does not produce symptoms about which the woman complains. It becomes latent, but frequently is reactivated during pregnancy. It most often affects the **cervix** (the opening from the uterus to the vagina), hence the infant contracts it when passing through the cervix during birth. Although 60% of all women have antibodies to CMV, it is especially prevalent in the sexually active, the young, and the poor. It is active or reactivated in

3% of women in their first trimester and in about 12% near term (McIntosh, 1984). A large prospective study found that half of the mothers with primary infections had congenitally infected babies, but three-fourths of mothers infected in the third trimester (Kumar et al., 1984). Fetal damage was lower, however, for those whose mothers were infected later in pregnancy. It appears that only 25% of congenitally affected infants got CMV from a reactivated infection (Preece et al., 1984). Overall, it is the most common cause of congenital infection in the United States (Grose & Weiner, 1990).

Relatively few fetuses are afflicted with CMV prior to delivery, and only some of those have obvious symptoms. The evidence for the few that do have symptoms at birth is depressing. One-fourth are dead by 3 months of age and two-thirds of the remainder are developmentally or intellectually impaired. CMV has also been implicated in 7% of a series of 70 deaths from congenital heart disease occurring shortly after birth. Those who do not have obvious symptoms or defects may be at risk with respect to hearing and intellectual development. CMV is said to be the leading infectious cause of mental retardation and congenital deafness in the United States. There are currently no effective treatments for either infant or mother (Avery & Taeusch, 1984). However, it appears that vaccination would produce immunity and be very cost-effective (Porath et al., 1990).

Worldwide, CMV occurs in 9 per 1,000 live births. About 0.5-1.5% of newborns in the United States are infected, and 5-10% of these may later be found to be deaf or mentally retarded (Sever et al., 1979). Overall, severe damage from CMV occurs in from 1/5,000 to 1/20,000 live births.

HVH is less prevalent than CMV, but in 1974 it occurred in 1% of obstetric patients in the practices of some doctors or hospitals (Alford et al., 1974). It is the type of herpes that is primarily transmitted venereally. It usually affects the vagina or cervix, and, if active at the time of birth, may infect the fetus. HVH is found more frequently among women who are sexually active, poor, and young. Since the 1974 figures were gathered, the epidemic nature of herpes has become more serious, and it now affects more middle-class persons. Figures indicate 300,000 new cases per year. Babies can become infected as they pass through the cervix and vagina during the birth process, or even through skin breaks caused by the scalp electrodes used for fetal monitoring. Infection is a rare (1/2,500 to 1/10,000 births) but very serious occurrence (Enkin et al., 1989). If the mother's infection is in the active stage (i.e., if she has symptoms), 50% of exposed babies will contract the virus. Of these, 15% will have localized infections that are not serious. The death rates for the remaining 85% vary according to the type of infection. Of those with a localized type that involves the CNS, 50% will die; of those who develop whole-body infections, 90% will die. These death rates can be lowered to 10% and 50%, respectively, through proper diagnosis and treatment, but half of the survivors will develop microcephaly, spasticity, paralysis, seizures, deafness, or blindness (Whitly et al., 1980, cited in McIntosh, 1984).

Whether HVH affects earlier prenatal development is not clear. Signs of fetal disease are rare, but there may be an increased spontaneous abortion rate in early pregnancy among women with genital herpes, perhaps because the virus crosses the placenta. If so, the rates of fetal disease may be low only because many HVH victims have already died.

Preventing infection of babies is not easy, because in two-thirds of the cases of maternal infection there are no active lesions. There is no cure for HVH, but the chances of active lesions during late pregnancy can be reduced by medications currently available. When a mother is diagnosed as having an active case close to delivery time, a cesarean section prior to or shortly after the breaking of the waters can be used with reasonable success to protect the fetus. There are currently no effective treatments.

Gonorrhea

The third infectious agent transmitted primarily at the time of delivery is the gonococcus (plural gonococci), the bacterium that produces gonorrhea. Gonorrhea is a venereal disease in which symptoms may be very mild in women, so that they often do not seek medical attention, resulting in the risk that they may be unaware of their infection. It used to account for a large proportion of congenitally blind infants. Laws have long been in effect in 48 states that mandate the use of silver nitrate or penicillin in the eyes of newborns. The antibiotics are probably more effective than silver nitrate.[4] These will destroy the organisms (gonococci) that cause gonorrhea, thus preventing infection and subsequent blindness. Other surfaces of the newborn do not provide a sufficiently warm, moist environment to permit the organisms to live long enough to cause infection. (For a good current survey, see Fletcher & Gordon, 1990.)

------

4. Antibiotics are also effective against another genitally transmitted parasite, *Chlamydia trachomatis*, which can affect the eyes and cause pneumonia (Enkin et al., 1989).

Group B Streptococcus

The fourth infectious agent transmitted primarily during birth is group B streptococcus. These bacteria cause life-threatening infections in nearly 11,000 babies each year, with 55% of premature and 15% of full-term babies dying. Treatment of the mother during pregnancy with antibiotics leads to a lower death rate for the infants. However, treatment of the infants at birth is often counterproductive, with increased deaths from sepsis caused by organisms resistant to antibiotics (Enkin et al., 1989). A vaccine for pregnant women that will protect the fetus is currently under study.

Other Infectious Diseases

Most prevalent among other infectious agents is **toxoplasmosis**, an infection caused by the simplest animal, the protozoan *Toxoplasma gondii*. Contact with cats, particularly with cat feces, and eating raw or poorly cooked meat are the most frequent source of the disease in humans. Countries such as France and Belgium, where raw and very rare meats are more often eaten, routinely screen for it (it is estimated that 80% of the French population are positive for this organism). Even in Florence, Italy, the rate is estimated to be 11% among pregnant women, with 4% fetal infection (Calabri et al., 1989). The timing of the mother's infection is important. The baby is more likely to be affected if the mother is infected late in pregnancy, but the effects are more severe if she had it early. In one study, severe disease occurred in 14% of first-trimester infections, but in no third-trimester cases. French workers advocate abortion for first-trimester cases and treatment with antiprotozoan drugs where that solution is rejected. Drugs have not been very effective or safe (Dutton, 1989; Enkin et al., 1989), but there is recent evidence, not yet confirmed, of a more effective regime (Hohlfeld et al., 1989).

Toxoplasmosis has been tentatively linked to epidemics of congenital hydrocephalus (Carter, 1965). It is also linked to **microcephaly** (abnormal smallness of the head) and damage to eyes, brain, lungs, and liver (Sever et al., 1985), and possibly to neuroendocrine disturbances, especially of the pituitary system (Massa et al., 1989). Its frequency varies from 1 to 24 per 10,000 live births. In the United States it is estimated that the related special education and institutional costs exceed $116 million and may exceed $2.5 billion (Roberts & Frenkel, 1990). Medical costs are estimated at $42,000 per case.

Viruses that are suspect but have not been proven damaging are Epstein-Barr and hepatitis B. Treatment for hepatitis B, which is very prevalent in some parts of the world, is possible for the infant, and vaccines are being developed. Hence it is not of great importance *if* compliance to treatment regimes is achieved (Jonas et al., 1990). The infectious hepatitis rates over a 12-year period in Victoria, Australia, showed a strong relation to the rates of Down syndrome (Collman & Stoller, 1962), a finding for which I know of no replication.

Finally, the most common viral infection, influenza, may affect prenatal development. Its earlier postulated relation to anencephaly has not been borne out (Saxen et al., 1990). It has been implicated in a fivefold increase in childhood leukemia (Fedrick & Alberman, 1972). Spontaneous abortions, intrauterine growth retardation, and premature deliveries are more frequent in pregnancies of women who had severe influenza (Dumont, 1989). There are conflicting data about its possible relation to later schizophrenia (Kendell & Kemp, 1989). In all events, pregnant women with a tendency to respiratory or pulmonary disease might well consider vaccination. (For a recent review of the effects of viral infections and the mechanisms of their action, see Dickinson & Gonik, 1990.)

IMPLICATIONS OF OUR KNOWLEDGE OF INFECTIOUS AGENTS

Most bacteria, which are usually much larger than viruses, cannot cross the placental barrier. Hence investigations of the influence of infectious diseases on prenatal development have focused on viral diseases, which affect approximately 5% of pregnancies. It is thought that in all the diseases discussed above, placental infection is a precursor to fetal infection.

Timing is important in fetal infections. Rubella is harmful only when it reaches the fetus at the time the vulnerable organ is developing. Syphilis does its damage after organogenesis. CMV, HVH, and gonorrhea are dangerous at the time of birth, as is group B streptococcus.

The practical applications of such knowledge are obvious. With good prenatal care, starting even before pregnancy, most of the dangers discussed here can be prevented or alleviated. Since the causes of most birth problems are currently unknown, future research is likely to find other infectious agents that are capable of harming the embryo, fetus, or newborn. Also, new infectious agents can arise, as AIDS has.

Chronic Conditions of the Mother

We turn now to noninfectious chronic diseases, or conditions a woman may have that may affect the fetus.

HORMONAL DISORDERS

Hormonal disorders are one class of chronic maternal condition that can affect the development of a growing fetus. Three common hormonal diseases are discussed below: hypothyroidism, hyperthyroidism, and diabetes.

Hypothyroidism

Hypothyroidism is a condition in which not enough thyroid hormone is produced. If the mother has it, she can be treated with hormones to replace or supplement her own. Unfortunately, not all mothers are adequately treated, and this may pose problems for their pregnancies or for their surviving offspring. Such mothers have a high incidence of spontaneous abortions (50% in a large-scale French study by Mida et al., 1989), premature deliveries, stillbirths, and infants with major anomalies (Jones & Man, 1969). Those infants that escape more serious problems are likely to have poorer-than-average development in infancy and beyond. Both mental and motor development at 8 months are lower for infants whose mothers had inadequate treatment than for those whose mothers had adequate treatment (Man & Jones, 1969). These children are still deficient at 4 and 7 years (Man, Holden, & Jones, 1971; Man, Jones, et al., 1971). In the study conducted by Man and colleagues, the average IQ at age 4 of the normal controls was 100 and that of offspring of adequately treated mothers was 103, compared with 94 for those whose mothers were inadequately treated. Fortunately, management for thyroid deficiency makes it possible to avoid many of the problems.

The importance of sibling controls in research is illustrated by data from three mothers who had two pregnancies during the above-cited study, with adequate treatment in only one. The 4-year IQs of the three pairs were as follows: Pair 1, 92 treated versus 72; Pair 2, 100 treated versus 76; and Pair 3, 117 treated versus 101 (Man & Serunian, 1976). These three pairs illustrate an important methodological problem. If one were to look only at the treated member of Pair 1, one might conclude that treatment does not result in full normality; the untreated case in Pair 3 might lead one to believe that maternal abnormality does not lead to a problem for the infant. In fact, all three pairs show that adequate treatment of hypothyroid mothers leads to significantly higher IQs (16 to 24 points higher) in the children compared with siblings born when the mothers were not adequately treated. This example shows the dangers of reasoning from individual cases, or **case studies**. It also reaffirms the importance of adequate control groups.

Hyperthyroidism

An overactive maternal thyroid also affects the fetus, but much less than hypothyroidism. The problems found in a study of 41 pregnancies (31 women) included 5 fetal deaths, 3 cases with goiter, and cases of hypothyroidism, hyperthyroidism, Down syndrome, undescended testes (Burrow, 1965), and heart problems (Ellert et al., 1989). Experiments with rats confirm these findings (Kumar & Chadhuri, 1989). Unlike the situation for hypothyroidism, the drugs used for treatment of hyperthyroidism cross the placental barrier, and may themselves be harmful to prenatal development. The effects of the disease cannot be separated from those of the drug, and neither can be separated from those of genetic inheritance, which contributes to thyroid problems.

Diabetes

This is another hormonal disease that can affect fetal development. Women with diabetes frequently have spontaneous abortions or miscarriages, and they have a relatively high incidence of stillbirths. Even now the spontaneous abortion rate in women with insulin-dependent diabetes is as high as 30%, or twice that of the normal population (Miodovnik et al., 1990). Prior to the introduction of insulin in the 1920s, a third of pregnant diabetic women died and 60% of their pregnancies ended in death. By 1960, 80% of the babies survived, and today it is 97-98%, with near 100% survival for the mothers. Prematurity remains a problem; Greene, Hare, Krache, et al. (1989) found the rate at one major treatment center to be 26% (compared with 10% overall for the hospital). It was usually linked to preeclampsia, and the researchers conclude that preventing high blood pressure should be the focus of preventive efforts, not further control of diabetes.

Surviving infants of diabetic mothers have been much more likely to suffer nontrivial abnormalities than infants of nondiabetic mothers—four times as likely in older data (Kitzmiller et al., 1981; Pederson et al., 1964) and twice as likely in newer data from a large sample (McCarter et al., 1987). The abnormalities include cardiac, neural tube, skeletal, and kidney problems, defects that occur during the highly vulnerable first 8 weeks of gestation (Kitzmiller et al., 1981), which is usually before the mother seeks medical care. The rate of serious defects in offspring is estimated to be 2-3% for nondiabetics, 4-5% for controlled diabetics, and 30-40% for those with poorly controlled diabetes. McCarter et al. (1987) raise the question as to whether diabetes is itself teratogenic or whether it enhances the effects of other teratogens (i.e., serves as a **coteratogen**). Insulin that has crossed the placental barrier and magnesium deficiency, which is often found in diabetics, are two possible factors other than sugar levels (Miodovnik et al., 1990).

One project tried to contact every diabetic woman in New England who was interested in pregnancy. Those who agreed to participate were taught to monitor their body temperature to determine probable pregnancy and to seek early confirmation. The pregnant women were hospitalized immediately so they could be taught home use of two new technological advances (a glucose meter and a portable insulin pump) designed to maintain a steadier biochemical state than the usual insulin injections. Both intensive therapy, monitored 6 to 7 times per day by the glucose meter, and continuous insulin pump therapy had good birth outcomes (Coustan et al., 1986). A German study cited by Avery and Taeusch (1984) has shown that not a single offspring with a congenital anomaly was born to more than 200 women who had vigorous control started prior to and continued throughout pregnancy. However, a fairly broad range of control has been found to be satisfactory for keeping abortions and infant malformations to a minimum (Greene, Hare, Cloherty, et al., 1989). The only randomized trial of degree of control found that tight control was more beneficial than either very tight or only moderate control (Enkin et al., 1989).

Even with tight control the fetal development of motor behavior is delayed in the first trimester (studied using ultrasound), but parallel to slower growth (Visser et al., 1986). The development of behavioral states near term is also affected by diabetes in first pregnancies (Mulder et al., 1987).

The stage of the mother's diabetes is also important to fetal development. Vascular complications of diabetes lead to three times as many major abnormalities as in infants of normal mothers. Infants of mothers whose disease had progressed to affect the kidneys or the **retina** (the part of the eye that transforms light into nerve impulses) had eight times as many major abnormalities. These findings raise the question as to whether it is diabetes itself or the other problems associated with it that cause some teratogenic effects.

Diabetics are also at greater risk of giving birth to both SGA babies and very heavy or so-called macrosomic babies that are maturationally retarded. Babies weighing 10 to 13 pounds are not infrequent among diabetic mothers; hence diabetics are often delivered by cesarean. With current care, it should be possible to eliminate many of these cesarean deliveries (Enkin et al., 1989).

It is reassuring to note that a 5-year follow-up of Swedish children born to diabetic mothers showed them all to have normal physical and neurological development. Most had above-average IQs, and their IQs were not related to maternal or birth factors. Unfortunately, the 17% of children who did not participate in the follow-up had had more perinatal complications, and we do not know what their outcomes would be (Persson & Gentz, 1984).

All of these effects are poorly understood. They appear to be environmental rather than genetic, inasmuch as diabetes in the father is not related to them. The National Institute of Child Health and Human Development is supporting major efforts to learn more about how these problems are caused and how they can be avoided.

NONHORMONAL DISORDERS

Women who suffer from heart disease, high blood pressure (hypertension), and kidney disorders are themselves at risk during pregnancy, as are the infants they carry. Such women have a greater chance of giving birth to SGA infants, possibly due to placental abnormalities. A woman who has a severe case of one of these diseases may opt for abortion to protect her health. If she decides to continue the pregnancy, the baby is sometimes delivered early by cesarean section, either to avoid further strain on the mother or because there are indications that the fetus is having problems and has developed sufficiently to be more likely to survive on its own.

MATERNAL AGE

Another condition of the mother that affects pregnancy outcome is her age. Increasing maternal age is related to a sharp increase in chromosomal abnormalities, as discussed in Chapter 3. However, recent data on almost 4,000 first pregnancies (almost 800 over age 35) show that although older mothers have higher rates of complications, their risk of poor neonatal out-

come is not appreciably increased (Berkowitz et al., 1990). The women in this study were private patients, and hence not suffering from serious social disadvantage. A recent survey of the medical literature by Mansfield (1988) points to the flaws in most studies suggesting higher risk.

Babies of very young mothers are also at much greater risk than those of mothers in their 20s, but primarily for being premature, SGA, or both, rather than for having chromosomal abnormalities. It had been thought that adolescent mothers were physiologically too immature to provide a proper growing environment for the embryo and fetus, but if young mothers receive good diets and good prenatal care, their infants are not at risk for prematurity or LBW. Thus the associated factors of poor prenatal care and diet appear to be the causal factors in the increased risk for prematurity and LBW in this group. However, a good diet and good prenatal care are not the norm for pregnant adolescents in our society, especially not for those from underprivileged environments. To avoid these handicapping conditions, ways of improving prenatal diets and health care for pregnant adolescents must be found. In addition, we must find ways of addressing the social, economic, and psychological disadvantages of teenage pregnancy, and the risk to a baby of being raised by an immature parent or parents.

Other Possible Factors

Fetal malnutrition and oxygen deprivation are caused by varied factors that need separate consideration. We will start with maternal malnutrition.

MATERNAL MALNUTRITION

The developing baby is entirely dependent upon the mother's blood for its nutrition and oxygen. Thus maternal nutrition is an important factor in the nutrition of the developing embryo and fetus. Contrary to the old wives' tale (often supported by doctors) that the fetus will rob the mother to further its own development, the fetus is far from a perfect parasite.

Nutritional status is not determined by any single aspect of diet. The principal components used to assess it are total number of calories, number and type of protein calories, and appropriate amounts of various vitamins and important minerals. Good nutrition consists of a proper balance of all of these elements. Needs for specific ingredients (such as vitamin A) may differ for marginally undernourished mothers (Hussein et al., 1988). Poor nutrition may result from a lack of or from an inability to utilize any one class of substance.[5] The latter means that malnutrition may occur because of the woman's metabolic system rather than because of a poor diet.

The nutritional status of a woman affects all aspects of her reproductive life, from the age of onset of menstruation to the onset and regularity of ovulation and likelihood of conception.[6] Both chronic and acute malnutrition have their effects. The effects of acute malnutrition are startling: loss or marked disruption of menstrual cycles, failure to become pregnant even when no birth control is practiced, high spontaneous abortion rates, high fetal and neonatal death rates, and high proportions of premature and SGA babies. These effects are well documented for war-imposed famine conditions, as, for example, in the long-term siege of Leningrad during World War II. When short-term acute famine occurs in a population that is well nourished before and after, as it did in Holland during World War II, the long-range effects on surviving offspring are minimal (Stein et al., 1975). Even then, neurological consequences have been found for those whose acute malnutrition occurred early in pregnancy (Stein & Susser, 1975a, 1975b; Stein et al., 1975).

The increase in neurological consequences as a result of malnutrition is consistent with research on the development of the brain. Rat data indicate that malnutrition in utero and up to 17 days after birth, when some parts of the brain are developing rapidly (rats are less mature at birth than humans), leads to an apparently permanent decrement in the number of brain cells (Winick, 1969; Winick & Noble, 1966). Bedi (1987) finds that not all of the effects are permanent. The most severe cell decreases occur in rat pups deprived both before and after birth (Winick, 1976). Human data obtained by the same brain assay techniques indicate that the brains of children who died of malnutrition in the first year had fewer cells than those of children the same ages who died accidental deaths (Winick & Rosso, 1969).

Data on infants' performance on psychological tests in the first 3 years of life also indicate that pregnancy

---

5. Serious reading of studies in this field demands that one carefully differentiate between lack of sufficient calories and lack of sufficient (and appropriate) protein calories. Most of the work on vitamin deficiencies is less available to students than that on calorie or protein calorie deficiencies. That on the relevance of trace elements such as zinc, manganese, and copper is even less available (and less well documented).

6. A list of references documenting these relations can be found in many sources. The 1975 National Academy of Sciences booklet *Nutrition and Fertility* is an excellent example.

and lactation appear to be the crucial times to supplement diets (Klein et al., 1976; Werner, 1979). This should probably be considered to be at least through the first year (Galler et al., 1984). Practically speaking, of course, most women cannot choose when they will suffer malnutrition. Chronic malnutrition before, during, and after pregnancy is a common problem in large parts of the world, including sizable segments of the population of the United States (see, for example, Naeye et al., 1973).

Even if chronically deprived mothers obtained adequate nutrition during pregnancy and nursing through prenatal and "well baby" programs, malnutrition effects would not be eliminated. The outcome of a pregnancy is related to prior nutritional status as well as to that during pregnancy. Even the birth weights of mothers are related to their pregnancy outcomes (Hackman et al., 1983). Poverty and malnutrition operate over more than one generation and are usually confounded with sociocultural disadvantage. Shipping or awarding food to those in need does not always solve the problem of later achievement for children being born (see, for example, Grantham-McGregor et al., 1987).

Children who are sufficiently malnourished suffer permanent growth retardation that becomes a pregnancy risk factor for females when they reach adulthood. For example, in a Scottish study of 26,000 births, decreasing stature was related to increasing rates of perinatal deaths, prematurity, and delivery complications (Thomson & Belliwicz, 1963). These outcomes were all affected by **parity** (number of infants born to a particular mother), age of mother, and social class, but decreasing stature affected the rates of problems independent of the other factors. Findings are similar for such different ethnic groups as Japanese, Filipino, and Polynesian, and populations with different expected genetic heights (Werner, 1979). As Werner (1979) summarizes, "Women whose growth environment has been poor are at a greater risk in childbearing than are those whose opportunities for growth and development have been adequate" (p. 39).

Adequate nutrition can be attained by those from cultures with very different dietary habits and needs. For example blacks, Asians, and Hispanic-Americans, who are more likely than whites to be lactose intolerant, can, with proper care, receive alternative sources of calcium. Pregnant vegetarians can get adequate iron supplements and calcium intake. Fad diets are rarely concerned with adequate nutritional balance. Their popularity may be responsible for the increased frequency with which neonatologists are seeing vitamin and trace mineral deficiencies in newborns (National Academy of Sciences, 1975).

Because the outcome of a pregnancy is related to maternal nutritional status before, as well as during, pregnancy and even to maternal (and possibly grand-maternal) birth weight, those concerned with infant health have a large stake in advocating adequate nutrition. Indeed, the recent National Research Council report on weight gain during pregnancy advocates a gain of 28-40 pounds except for the obese, compared with the limit of 25 pounds proposed in 1970. This may be even more important now that more low birth weight babies survive to become future parents. Unfortunately, programs to promote adequate nutrition for pregnant women and babies (such as WIC) have been cut back in the United States, and it is not clear that the 1991 proposals will alter this. This is likely to prove very costly in the long run. Nevertheless, while emphasizing the importance of nutrition, we must not lose sight of the importance of environmental stimulation in relation to it. A study in Colombia clearly demonstrated that more food by itself helped to only a minor degree, while food supplementation combined with behavioral stimulation produced major improvements in later intellectual performance (Sinisterra, 1987).

A discussion of specific dietary components is not possible here, but one element of extreme importance, iodine, deserves mention. Iodine is intimately related to thyroid function, and its lack can lead to cretinism, which used to be a major cause of mental retardation in the United States. In the Western world, thanks to iodized salt, iodine deficiency is no longer a problem. However, as late as 1985, UNICEF reported on the basis of research by the Indian Council of Medical Research that in North India and Nepal iodine deficiency affects from 4% to 15% of babies born, reducing their mental capacities and fine motor capabilities even if they are not cretins.[7] Effects are irreversible unless there is intense hormone therapy in the first year of life.

PRENATAL INFANT MALNUTRITION AND OXYGEN DEPRIVATION

Poor nutrition of the infant can result from factors other than poor nutrition of the mother. Several aspects of development discussed in Chapter 2 affect the nutrition of the developing organism. Some causes of poor nutrition for the fetus include implantation at a part of the uterus where the blood supply is not good; placental inadequacy, which may occur even in well-nourished mothers; and multiple fetuses to be nourished. Some of the maternal diseases that affect prenatal development do so by cutting down on nutri-

ents and/or oxygen to the fetus. Regardless of the source, intrauterine malnutrition has lasting consequences, even where overall nutrition and medical care are good. A 12- to 14-year follow-up of clinically malnourished infants in a middle- to upper-SES Swedish group showed a lower IQ (104, compared with 121 for controls) and a greater need for special education (Hill et al., 1984).

This discussion will concentrate on the role of multiple births and maternal diseases. Twins, triplets, and larger groups require more nutrients than a single fetus. All multiple births are more likely than singletons to be premature (the more fetuses, the more premature). This may be due, at least in part, to the mother's inability to meet the nutritional demands placed on her system. In general, multiple-birth babies are also SGA. Identical twins who share a single placenta are particularly affected, and often one is much more stunted in growth than the other. In extreme cases the smaller of the two may not survive. For twins who have two placentas, one may have attached in a more favorable location than the other, which can lead to quite different birth weights. In the case of identical twins, these nutritional differences can produce environmental differences in persons of identical genetic makeup. The neonatal differences in weight and strength often persist, even into adulthood. Lighter twins are often more handicapped in school (Lis, 1989). Constitutional differences due to nutrition are one source of phenotypic differences between genetically identical individuals. This is another example of the effect of environmental events or circumstances on the phenotype.

The location of implantation, placental inadequacy, and multiple fetuses are all conditions that interact with the mother's nutritional status in affecting the fetus. The well-nourished mother is better able to nourish two or more fetuses than is the poorly nourished mother. A poorly located implantation in a well-nourished mother may result in a better outcome than a well-located implantation in a mother who is a long-term victim of malnutrition.

Some of the maternal diseases that affect prenatal development do so by cutting down on the nutrients or oxygen available to the fetus. Heart, kidney, lung, and gastrointestinal diseases, anemia, and hypertension are all associated with intrauterine growth retardation (Carlson, 1988). Maternal diseases may interfere with the normal growth of the placenta, or the blood sup-

---

7. In some villages in Bhutan, one-third of the population are cretins.

ply may be affected directly, as happens in high blood pressure or in severe, prolonged toxemia. One or more factors may limit the ability of the fetus to grow, especially toward the end of gestation. The most important nutrient limited by blood flow problems may be oxygen, which, although different from protein, vitamins, and total caloric energy, is extremely important for prenatal development.

There are serious effects of oxygen deprivation that are independent of, but parallel to, the effects of nutritional deprivation. One demonstration of such effects is seen in babies born at different altitudes. Numerous studies have found that babies born to mothers who live at high altitudes during pregnancy tend to be LBW or SGA. For example, nearly 24% of babies in Lake County, Colorado (3,200 m, or about 10,000 ft, above sea level) were low in birth weight. This rate is far above that for other areas of the United States. However, in areas where people have lived for many generations at these altitudes, the effects do not appear to be as great, despite the fact that diet and prenatal care may be worse than in Lake County. For example, in Cuzco (3,416 m above sea level) babies are about 400 grams heavier than those in Lake County, and only 10% of the infants are of low birth weight (Haas, 1970). Biological responses acquired as a result of lifelong residence at high altitudes or as a result of genetic selection may account for these differences.

Despite the smaller effects in some populations, those living at high altitudes have consistently lower birth weights than those of the same ethnic group living at a lower altitude in the same country. Social class, maternal smoking, parity, and parental stature have been controlled for in some of these studies, making it likely that oxygen levels account for the results (Haas, 1970, 1973). Rat pups exposed in utero to altitudes of 33,000 to 46,000 ft have lower birth weights (Vierck et al., 1966). These data have led to some concern about the effects of travel to extremely high altitudes for pregnant women who are not adapted to such an environment. Anoxia in newborn rats (a time approximately equivalent to the end of the second trimester in humans) causes behavioral deficits in both males and females (Grimm, 1987). Both nutrition and oxygen may well be important mediators of some of the effects of drugs that will be discussed shortly. It is also true that drugs, including hormones, may mediate the stressful effects of oxygen deprivation.

HYPERTHERMIA

Hyperthermia can operate as a teratogen. High heat, usually caused by maternal illness, has the po-

tential of altering brain growth, especially in early pregnancy. Animal data make this clear (see Shiota & Kayamura, 1989; Shiota et al., 1988). They also demonstrate the power of various substances to interact in producing an effect. Mice exposed to both alcohol and hyperthermia, but at doses too low for either to have a teratogenic effect, showed that the combination does produce a teratogenic effect (Shiota et al., 1988).

Hyperthermia has been hypothesized to lead to mental retardation in humans (Upfold & Smith, 1988). However, human data clearly indicate that the sauna as used by the Finns does not act as a teratogen or even affect fertility in males (Waha & Erkkola, 1988). An excellent review that cautions about the lack of any human evidence is found in Warkany (1986), and a counterargument appears in Smith et al. (1986).

Effects of Nonpsychotropic Drugs

Another class of substances that produce developmental abnormalities is drugs, including prescribed, over-the-counter, and illegal drugs. Many drugs, in large doses, are known to cause malformations in animals. In November 1961, Warkany and Kalter's review of the teratogenic effects of viral and bacterial infections, anoxia, and irradiation appeared. It warned that despite the possible inaccuracies when extrapolating from animals to humans, drugs might cause teratogenic risk in humans. This was at about the time the thalidomide disaster surfaced.

THALIDOMIDE

As was the case for rubella, the effects of thalidomide were discovered because of an epidemic of children born with a well-defined set of developmental abnormalities. The most publicized of these were arms, legs, or both that were "flipperlike" or almost totally absent. Medical detective work found that the mothers of these infants all had taken a mild sedative, thalidomide, prescribed by their doctors or simply purchased to treat morning sickness, anxiety, or sleeplessness. Few cases occurred in the United States, because thalidomide had not been licensed for use here, but some 4,500 thalidomide babies (not counting the one-third who died soon after birth) were born in West Germany.

After thalidomide was identified as the cause of the limb abnormalities, other effects were discovered: malformations of the eyes, ears, heart, intestines, and urogenital tract. Both mental subnormality and epilepsy were more frequent in thalidomide babies than in the population at large, thus indicating that the central nervous system was affected (McFinn & Robertson, 1973; Stephenson, 1978).

There is a critical period for the action of thalidomide between the twentieth and thirty-fifth days after conception. This is a time when mothers are likely to suffer from morning sickness and hence to have taken this supposedly mild drug. Taking it for only a few days, or even for only one day at the most sensitive period, can produce defects. The number and seriousness of the defects vary, perhaps depending on when within the sensitive period the mother took the drug. Indeed, it has been said that the thalidomide syndrome is really a series of syndromes that depend on the developmental stage at the time of taking the drug (Fraser, 1984).

The psychological and financial problems of having a thalidomide baby were great. In England, parents won a lawsuit holding the drug company responsible for many of the expenses, but only long after the birth of these babies. Physicians, psychologists, and therapists of many types, together with parents, were faced with the challenge of how to allow these children maximum interaction with their world. Engineers developed arm and leg devices for these children. The Institute of Mechanical Engineers in London published a special supplemental volume titled *Basic Problems of Prehension, Movement, and Control of Artificial Limbs*, in which several of the papers were especially directed toward the thalidomide child. The thalidomide story led to the establishment of international registries of birth defects to provide a base line to enable determination of when excess cases are occurring.

How did medical authorities let such a powerful teratogen get licensed?[8] The answer to that question attests to the complexity of doing research on new drugs. New drugs are usually tried on animals before they are given to humans, but often on only one species or one strain of one species. If the animals are not harmed, large-scale, well-controlled trials with humans, called **clinical trials**, follow. Clinical trials are basically nonexperimental, because the drug is given only to appropriate patients, who are not a random sample of the population. Good clinical trials have an experimental component, in that patients of equivalent status are randomly assigned to treatment and control groups. Other standard drugs or a **placebo** (nonactive substance) may be given to the control group or groups. It would be unethical to give people with severe medical problems a placebo unless no drug of proven value exists against which to compare the experimental drug.

To ensure that a new drug has no teratogenic effects, tests need to be conducted on pregnant females of several species, including humans. Effects may not be the same in different species, and may differ for embryos or fetuses and adults. For example, neither aspirin nor thalidomide harms adult rats or humans. However, aspirin is highly teratogenic in rats, but not clearly teratogenic in humans, whereas thalidomide is teratogenic in humans, but not in rats.

In the thalidomide disaster many Western European countries licensed thalidomide as an over-the-counter drug before clinical trials of its teratogenic effects were conducted. While this seems negligent from our current point of view, remember that in those far-off days (the 1960s) many experts still thought that the placental barrier was complete. The thalidomide episode made the safety of drugs taken during pregnancy a nonacademic question. "The placenta was finally dethroned as a 'barrier' " (Hutchings, 1978, p. 197).

Even when effects in animals differ from those in humans, well-controlled studies with lower animals can uncover the mechanisms by which teratogens act. For example, they can determine whether teratogens such as viruses or given types of drugs act through the mother on the embryo or fetus, or affect the maternal-fetal interchange, or affect the unborn infant directly. The more we know about the mechanisms, the better we can predict the effects of new drugs and ferret out potentially harmful environmental agents.

STEROID HORMONES

Steroid hormones include the sex hormones and those produced by the adrenal glands. Some of this class of drugs are known to be teratogens.

Sex Hormones

As long as 30 years ago, it was recognized that treating pregnant mammals (including monkeys) with male sex hormones could produce **pseudohermaphroditism**, a condition in which the sex of a female offspring is not clear from external characteristics. This occurs in human infants as a result of certain medical conditions. It was also shown as early as 1960 that female infants of pregnant women given

---

8. A new effort to obtain restricted licensing of thalidomide is likely. It appears to be useful for treating graft-host disease in bone marrow transplants, in avoiding severe complications of Hanson's disease (leprosy), and possibly for treating rheumatoid arthritis. It even appears that it might be useful in treating HIV infections.

androgenic (male) hormones for the treatment of breast cancer prior to the twelfth week of pregnancy were masculinized. This means that differentiation of the sexual organs are affected. That is definite.

Critical periods for neural differentiation appear clear in animal work (see Goy & McEwen, 1980). The question of whether or to what degree human brain and behavior differentiation are affected by prenatal exposures to sex hormones, to what degree that is likely to occur when one is not experimentally manipulating exposure, is far from settled. Also unclear are exactly what effects different hormones have. Inasmuch as the steroid hormones are very similar to each other chemically, and one can be metabolized to yield others, it is difficult to be sure that the drug administered is the one that has the effect.

We return now to the effects of androgen in a study with rhesus macaque monkeys that is both well controlled and follows the animals longitudinally (Goy et al., 1988). Pregnant macaques received androgen either early or late in pregnancy. Their offspring (and normal controls) were followed in their social groups so that their interaction with peers and adult females could be assessed. Those with early exposure (EE) were physically masculinized. They had scrotal and penile development similar to that of males, no vaginal opening, and their menarche was delayed 6 months. Those with late exposure (LE) did not have these effects, as we would expect from our knowledge of sexual differentiation (Chapter 2). Sexual mounting behaviors were more frequent for both androgenized female groups than for normal females, but lower than for males (except abortive mounts about equal for the early group). Mothers did more genital inspection of males and EE females and both mounted the mother more. Play behaviors (rough play and play initiation) showed a quite different pattern, in that it was the LE females that were more like males, while the EE females were like the normals. Such differences might be affected by the ways the infants were treated. Males in the colony treated the masculine-appearing EEs like females, but they treated the normal-appearing LEs like males. Mounting and rough play were also differently affected by weaning. There is evidence that these behaviors are mediated by different brain structures. The researchers conclude that understanding causal factors in "the development and expression of masculine behavior will be advanced by research which can elucidate both social factors and neuroendocrine mechanisms that mediate each behavioral dimorphism of the total constellation." While human data cannot be as well controlled, play behavior appears to af-

fected in the same direction as in other mammals (Meyer-Bahlburg et al., 1988).

Diethylstilbestrol (DES) is a synthetic estrogen given during pregnancy to avoid miscarriages. It has been widely publicized because of the occurrence of cancer in the female offspring of women who received it. Its use was banned in 1971, long after randomized trials showed it to be ineffective in preventing miscarriage, stillbirth, neonatal death (or all of these combined), or premature deliveries (Enkin et al., 1989). In fact, DES increased the rate of fetal death, miscarriage, and premature birth (Avery & Taeusch, 1984).

Males were also affected, with an estimated 30% being infertile (Avery & Taeusch, 1984). Testicular as well as ovarian germ cell cancers are related to use of hormones in pregnancy (Preston, 1989). (Agents that are teratogenic are often carcinogenic. Which effect occurs may depend on the susceptibility of target organs at the time of exposure.) Behavioral as well as physiological effects have been shown in the guinea pig, where prenatal exposure to DES both masculinizes behavior and defeminizes it (Hines et al., 1987).

The female hormone progesterone has been used for the last 40 years to treat pregnant women who show signs of aborting or who have a history of previous spontaneous abortions, and to avoid toxemia. Evidence for its efficacy is scant, though the hormone may reduce prematurity. A synthetic version is now used. Progestins are a major component of birth control pills and are sometimes used to bring on late menstruation. Continued use of birth control pills when a woman is pregnant but does not realize it, or using progestin to bring on a late menstruation when pregnant, can result in accidental exposure of an embryo or fetus. Hence some millions of infants have been exposed to some dosage of either natural or synthetic progestins. Fetal development is adversely affected according to some studies, but not others, and sexual differentiation is affected according to some poorly controlled studies.

The effects of natural progesterone differ from those of the synthetics. Natural progesterone antagonizes the masculinizing action of testosterone in infrahuman animals, while the synthetics appear to have some androgenic potential, as indicated by the masculinization of the genitalia in a small percentage of female offspring of mothers who took them during pregnancy. Behavioral effects, especially tomboyism and high IQ, are indicated by some studies, but problems of sample selection and controls make the results inconclusive (e.g., see Dalton, 1968; Ehrhardt & Money, 1967). The fact that effects were dependent on dosage and related to the time of administration in

Dalton's study adds credence to the findings. In a later study, Dalton (1976) found that children of mothers given progesterone, usually to avoid toxemia, were more likely to gain entry into university, a very competitive matter in England. They had higher entry rates than offspring of normal pregnancies or of mothers who had toxemia but were not treated with progesterone.

Infants exposed to synthetic progestin (or it together with estrogen or DES) were compared with nonexposed siblings in a blind study (Reinisch, 1977; Reinisch & Karow, 1977). Exposed children were more independent, individualistic, self-assured, and self-sufficient, both as tested and as reported by their mothers, than their siblings, but had the same IQs (121 versus 120). Many factors could account for IQ not being affected, including a ceiling effect because the IQs are already so high.

A more recent study with well-selected control subjects found that play behaviors in both boys and girls (after controlling for the effects of pregnancy complications) were somewhat less masculine and somewhat more feminine (Meyer-Bahlburg et al., 1988; this contains a good review as well). However, the differences were very modest. The authors conclude that at this stage of knowledge prenatal hormone exposures cannot be dismissed as a potential contributor to the development of sex differences in behavior.

The human studies are inconclusive with respect to effects of hormones on intelligence and personality. However, all studies have found effects of exogenous hormones on human fetuses.

Adrenal Hormones or Corticosteroids

These hormones, too, have been used in the treatment of a number of medical conditions (especially rheumatic, allergic, and endocrine disorders) and have been used to induce ovulation and support pregnancy.[9] Cortisone and prednisone (five times as potent), the synthetic compounds, were considered suspect for use in pregnant women because in mice they produced high rates of resorptions, stillbirths, and prematurity. Human evidence did not bear out such dire effects. The higher dosage levels used in animal studies compared with those used in human treatments or species differences might account for the different results. Exposed infants have been found more likely than their nonexposed siblings to be SGA (Reinisch et al., 1978). Also, exposed infants who are not SGA are smaller at birth than their nontreated siblings. These effects on the developing fetus may be direct effects on growth inasmuch as corticosteroids

cross the placental barrier readily. Prednisone has also been shown to produce placental abnormalities, so the effects could result from them, hence be indirect. However, the fact that we know that young children treated with corticosteroids for asthma show severe growth retardation makes it plausible that growth may be directly affected.

Corticosteroids are also given to mothers prenatally to prevent respiratory distress syndrome in their infants who are going to be born prematurely. An extremely sound study with random assignment to drug or placebo has followed such offspring to 10-12 years of age. No differences have been found between the groups in intellectual or motor development, school achievement, or behavioral disturbances (Schmand et al., 1990).

The available research makes it clear that excessive doses of corticosteroids are dangerous to humans, even though adequate amounts are necessary for proper development of the embryo and fetus. Better evaluation of particular effects and the dosages that produce them is still needed.

ASPIRIN

Aspirin is teratogenic in animals when high doses are given. Humans do not typically take such high doses. In humans, as in other animals, aspirin acts in conjunction with benzoic acid (a widely used preservative in such foods as catsup) to increase the level of teratogenic effects. Several retrospective studies have found more malformed infants among those mothers who took aspirin in the first trimester than among control groups. More cardiac defects have also been found (Werler et al., 1989). Behavioral effects are still unclear. One study has found the frequent use of aspirin (but not of acetaminophen) in the first half of pregnancy to be related to lower IQ at age 4 (at least for girls) as well as deficits in several fine motor performances (see, respectively, Streissguth et al., 1987; Barr et al., 1990). Aspirin use in the first 20 weeks has been shown in another study to be unrelated to IQ at age 4 (Klebanoff & Berendes, 1988).

Aspirin diminishes the clotting ability of the blood, which normally is low in newborns, especially in pre-

---

9. Corticosteroids are also given to mothers about to give birth to premature infants. They are effective in reducing respiratory distress syndrome and other causes of neonatal mortality if given between 1 and 7 days prior to delivery. Not only are deaths reduced, but neurological and intellectual functioning appear to be better than in controls, despite their lower gestational age (Enkin et al., 1989).

matures. Hence aspirin taken shortly before delivery could be dangerous for the baby. Physicians often recommend that pregnant women avoid aspirin unless it is absolutely necessary because of possible teratogenesis in early pregnancy and blood clotting problems in late pregnancy. However, there is recent evidence from both Israel and England that aspirin in the last trimester may help prevent toxemia in pregnant women at risk (Emond, 1990).

EXCESS VITAMINS

Vitamins can be considered in the same category as drugs. An excess of certain vitamins has teratological effects. An excess of vitamin A leads to defects of closure of structures: of facial structures, resulting in cleft palate, or of the neural tube, resulting in spina bifida. An excess of vitamin D has also been shown to cause congenital defects (Seelig & Roemheld, 1969).

ANTIEPILEPTIC DRUGS

Antiepileptic drugs, such as valproic acid, are known to cause chromosome breakage after long-term treatment of children (Curatolo et al., 1986). International cooperative monitoring programs have shown them to increase the risk of spina bifida and other major and minor anomalies (Lammer et al., 1987). These are thought to act primarily by being a folic acid antagonist, as will be explained in the next section.

FOLIC ACID ANTAGONISTS AND FOLIC ACID DEFICIENCY

Folic acid antagonists produce a severe deficiency in folic acid that almost always kills the embryo in laboratory animals. Consequently, they were used experimentally to produce abortions in humans in the 1950s and early 1960s. The figures for several studies combined indicate that about 70% of women treated with one of these compounds (usually aminopterin) did abort. Of the fetuses that did not abort and were born at a viable age, between 20% and 30% had defects. There was no one pattern of malformations, which may mean that the drug has different effects at different gestational ages. Which organs are affected would depend on which critical period was disrupted.

Folic acid deficiency due to improper diet or to anticonvulsant drugs apparently predisposes the fetus to malformation, especially of the CNS (Gordon, 1968). Dietary manipulation of folic acid in animals can produce teratogenic effects, especially **hydrocephalus** (literally, "water head" or "water on the brain"), a

syndrome resulting in a very large head and severe brain damage (Kalter, 1968). In humans, folic acid deficiency may increase the risk of neural tube defects such as spina bifida, which can cause hydrocephaly. There is suggestive evidence (not based on random clinical trials) that giving folic acid during pregnancy to women who have had babies with neural tube defects may reduce the likelihood of their having another such child. Cuban data substantiate the role of folic acid supplement prior to pregnancy in reducing neural tube defects (Vergel et al., 1990). One study of 123 mothers found no cases among 44 treated mothers, but 6 cases among 79 untreated ones (Laurence, 1985). In a study of almost 27,000 pregnancies, neural tube defects were 3.5 times more frequent among women who took no vitamin supplements during pregnancy as among those who took vitamins containing a folic acid supplement in their first 6 weeks of pregnancy (Milunsky et al., 1989). Those who took other vitamins or who started the supplemented vitamins after 7 weeks of pregnancy were not much helped.

Neural tube defects have declined sharply in certain areas of the world in recent years (e.g., by 50% in South Wales), perhaps because women in these areas are eating more green vegetables (a primary source of folic acid) and eating them for larger portions of the year. Pregnant women taking anticonvulsants and those planning pregnancy should discuss folic acid supplementation with their physicians.

INHALANT ANESTHETICS

Long-term exposure to the inhalant anesthetics used in operating rooms may have led to pregnancy wastage, especially when inhalants were administered by mask. Exposed operating-room nurses have been shown to have more miscarriages (30%, compared with less than 9% for general-duty nurses; Cohen et al., 1971). Their miscarriages also tended to occur earlier in pregnancy (at 8 compared with 10 weeks). More recently, an increase in late, but not early, spontaneous abortions has been found in operating-room nurses whose jobs not only expose them to anesthetics, but are physically and psychologically stressful as well (McDonald et al., 1988). Women physicians whose practices were limited to anesthesiology had a 38% loss over a 6-year period, compared with 10% for other women doctors (Katz et al., 1988). There is also some evidence that there are increased abortion rates and more congenital defects when the father has worked around inhalant anesthetics (Gunderson & Sackett, 1982).

Infants born to mothers who received anesthetics for dental work or minor surgery during pregnancy have been shown to look almost 50% longer at visual patterns than similar infants not exposed (Blair et al., 1984). Such longer looking times have also been found in prematures.

OTHER POSSIBLE TERATOGENIC DRUGS

Additional drugs may be teratogenic, but conclusive evidence does not yet exist. Antibiotics are suspect. Some studies have shown elevated pregnancy wastage or defects, whereas other studies have not. Both ampicillin and tetracycline have been found to be associated with a sixfold increase in heart defects (Zierler & Rothman, 1985). The effects of tetracycline may be prevented by increasing vitamin B. But these are animal data, and the evidence on whether tetracycline is teratogenic in humans is not clear. Streptomycin and kanamycin are associated with eighth cranial nerve damage, which affects hearing (Holdiness, 1987).

Quinine was long used by laypersons to produce abortions, albeit with uncertain success. In the high dosages used for such purposes (but not in the lower dosages used to combat malaria) there is some questionable evidence for visual or auditory defects in humans. In animal studies death and retardation of growth are found, but few malformations.

Several drugs used to treat psychological difficulties are suspect. Imiprimine and other antidepressants have been implicated with a form of limb deformity not unlike that caused by thalidomide, but the evidence is quite tenuous. Both sexes of young rat pups (comparatively in the third trimester) exposed to Zimelidine, another antidepressant, have shown learning deficits (Grimm, 1987). The antischizophrenic drug phenothiazine lowers birth weight and results in behavioral changes as measured on the Brazelton scale (Coles et al., 1990). Insulin was formerly used in large doses to produce shock in psychiatric patients. When this was done in the first 14 weeks of pregnancy, the effects were quite startling. In one study of 14 cases, 4 deaths, 4 malformed infants, and 2 mentally defective children resulted. Electrical stimulation has replaced insulin as a way of inducing shock in psychiatric patients, so this danger seems past.

Other drugs used for the treatment of specific diseases may possibly be teratogenic. The following drugs are suspect at this time: oral hypoglycemic drugs (not insulin) used in the treatment of diabetes, alkylating agents used in the treatment of cancer, and drugs used in the treatment of tuberculosis. Also suspect is the flavor enhancer monosodium glutamate. On the other hand, it has been said that current chemotherapies are well tolerated by the fetus (Willard, 1989). Establish-

ing the teratogenic effects of drugs is very difficult. Animal studies do not provide conclusive evidence for humans. Drugs that may harm a fetus cannot ethically be given to a woman unless she has the disorder for which the drug is relevant. Therefore, it is very difficult to separate the effects of the drug from the those of the disorder. A more detailed review of the effects of environmental agents, such as drugs, other chemicals, and radiation, can be found in Voorhees and Mollnow (1987).

Another class of substances to which people are exposed by work or residential location are pesticides. These contain a number of drugs, the damaging effects of which on the fetus are not yet clear, but they do reach the fetus at least as early as 22 weeks. Maternal self-reported exposure is related to an increase in stillbirths and in SGA infants (Savitz et al., 1989). Even paternal exposure leads to a small increase in stillbirths. Both prenatal and postnatal exposure to PCBs affect weight, and infants breast-fed for over 1 year with high levels in maternal milk have lower activity levels at 4 years (Jacobson et al., 1990a). Jacobson et al. (1990b) have also reported poorer short-term memory on both verbal and quantitative tests at 4 years for those exposed prenatally, but no cognitive differences related to nursing.

Other substances in the environment, such as agricultural agents and household cleansers, are under suspicion, but adequate data from which to draw any firm conclusion are lacking. In J. C. McDonald et al.'s (1987) study of 301 infants with defects, matched individually to an equal number without defects, gastrointestinal and urinary tract abnormalities were more frequent in the offspring of women whose work exposed them to aromatic solvents in early pregnancy. Those women in the sample of 56,067 who worked in service and manufacturing, some of which were jobs that involved exposure to various potentially damaging chemicals, had an excess of births with congenital defects. They also had an excess of low birth weights. An excess of late abortions has been found in agricultural and horticultural workers and in leather workers (McDonald et al., 1988). While physical stress might be a major factor in the agricultural group, it seems likely that chemical exposures might be more important for those who work in horticulture and leather.

The Problems of Psychotropic Drugs and Their Study

Psychotropic drugs are those that people take for the psychological effects they produce. Examples include both legal and illegal drugs such as heroin, methadone, lysergic acid diethylamide (LSD), marijuana, amphetamines, cocaine, and alcohol. Psychotropic drugs receive the most publicity because of what amounts to an epidemic of drug abuse among pregnant women.

THE PROBLEM

A 1988 survey by the National Association for Perinatal Addiction Research and Education of 36 hospitals across the United States, in both urban and suburban areas and serving all socioeconomic groups, showed that 11% of women had used illegal drugs during pregnancy. This would suggest that 375,000 newborns each year would face possible health damage from drug abuse. However, other estimates are as low as 30,000 per year for crack cocaine. In New York City, the number of babies with health complications from prenatal drug abuse doubled in a single year (from 1986 to 1987, when it was 2,521). Given the magnitude of the problem, efforts to determine the effects of these drugs have continued in spite of the methodological difficulties. (An excellent brief overview of the problems can be found in Brown, 1991.)

THE RESEARCH PROBLEM

It is difficult to assess the factors that cause problems in offspring of drug abusers, because (a) drug abusers typically take many drugs, (b) the drugs they take are often impure, (c) abusers are more likely to be malnourished, and (d) abusers are less likely to seek or receive adequate prenatal care. It is even possible that the drugs given infants to treat postnatal withdrawal could contribute to the later behavioral difficulties of exposed infants. One or more of these factors may contribute to the babies' problems, and we do not have the data to tell which ones or which combinations are crucial. The possibility of different genetic sensitivities must also not be overlooked (Hutchings, 1985).

When babies are followed longitudinally to determine the long-term effects of drug exposure, there is usually considerable loss of sample, especially from the addict groups. Some studies report on babies of mothers who, although on drugs, received good prenatal care, and others concentrate on those whose mothers received little or no prenatal care. Some of the babies have been reared in their biological families and others have not. Interpretation of results is therefore extremely difficult. In a survey of longitudinal studies of

children born to methadone-maintained mothers, Kaltenbach and Finnegan (1984) conclude:

> Methadone outcome studies have been based on a main effects model of development which assumes a cause and effect relationship between a specific risk factor and outcome. . . . the underlying assumption is that any impairment or dysfunction is the result of the biological insult of narcotic exposure. . . . [This is a possible model right after birth, but] any long term effects are not so easily determined. . . . development is highly dependent not only on the characteristics of the infant, but the care-taking environment, and their mutual influence upon each other. . . . biological risk is either attenuated or potentiated by the child's social environment. (p. 274)

Given the magnitude of the problem, efforts to determine the effects of these drugs have continued in spite of the methodological difficulties. This discussion begins with drugs that are legal.

Legal Psychotropic Drugs

The first psychotropic drug we shall consider is alcohol. Next to cigarettes (whose psychotropic qualities are less clear), alcohol is the most likely drug to be consumed and abused in U.S. society.

ALCOHOL

Alcohol can cross the placental barrier. Critical periods during development, when its effects are maximal, are suggested but not well documented by current research. Binge drinking as well as chronic consumption may have effects. Withdrawal may play a role in the effects, but because it is mild it may go unnoticed. The effects of alcohol appear to interact with genetic characteristics of the embryo or fetus to determine whether and to what degree it is affected. This discussion will first consider fetal alcohol syndrome and fetal alcohol effects, pregnancy loss, decreased size, lowered intelligence, and behavioral effects. The effects of moderate and heavy drinking will then be compared, and other factors associated with alcohol consumption that may contribute to negative effects will be considered.

Fetal Alcohol Syndrome and Fetal Alcohol Effects

Doctors and psychologists have identified what is called the **fetal alcohol syndrome** (**FAS**). The characteristics include (a) pre- and postnatal growth deficiencies, (b) dysmorphic characteristics (facial asymmetries, short palpebral fissures, small cheekbones, congenital heart defects, anomalies of the joints and limbs), and (c) CNS manifestations (microcephaly, EEG abnormalities, behavioral and cognitive problems). A diagnosis of FAS requires problems in each of the three areas and high exposure to alcohol in utero (see Figure 4.1). **Fetal alcohol effects (FAE)** is the diagnosis when there are fewer and milder symptoms. Prior to U.S. research interest, which started in the 1970s, the French and Germans had called attention to FAS (Heuyer et al., 1957; Lemoine et al., 1968; Uhlig, 1957).

In dramatic contrast to the earlier neglect of FAS in the United States, it is now seen by some as one of the most common congenital neurological disorders (together with Down syndrome and spina bifida). It has been said to occur in some degree in 1 of every 750 infants born in the United States (Mukherjee & Hodgen, 1982). Full-blown FAS has various estimates for prevalence (from .4 to 3.1 per 1,000 live births), but may be as high as 20 per 1,000 in some American Indian tribes (Abel, 1981). FAE is estimated at between 1.7 and 5.9 cases per 1,000 live births. FAS/FAE has been described as probably the "most frequent known teratogenic cause of mental deficiency in the Western world" (Clarren & Smith, 1978, p. 1066). Kalter and Warkany (1983), however, conclude that these views "have been widely publicized and uncritically accepted by many individuals and organizations, including government agencies" (p. 492). A similar viewpoint has been expressed by Abel (1985), who also warns that recommending abstinence to mothers may cause stress-related effects in the newborn similar to those the warning was intended to avoid. One careful reviewer states that it is currently recognized that full-blown FAS occurs only in offspring of chronic alcoholics (Hutchings, 1987). (Recent data may make it necessary to add "or to binge drinkers.") Even among heavy drinkers only a small proportion have babies characterized by FAS (Rosett et al., 1983), for example, in only 2 among 140 alcoholics and binge drinkers (Ioffe & Chernik, 1988).

Methodologically adequate animal studies clearly show that prenatal administration of alcohol produces both dysmorphogenesis and long-term neurobehavioral problems in many species (for reviews, see Abel, 1980a, 1981, 1984; Meyer & Riley, 1986; Petrakis, 1987; West, 1986). The animal studies rule out factors other than alcohol as causes for the problems seen. They also point to damage to the hippocampus as a likely cause (see Hutchings, 1982; West, 1986). Peak

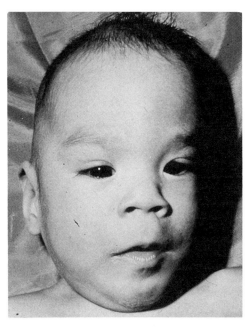

Figure 4.1. This FAS baby exhibits facial asymmetry and unusual shape of the eyes. (Photograph courtesy of Dr. Ann P. Streissguth.)

blood alcohol levels appear to be crucial for producing microcephaly (Pierce & West, 1986a, 1986b). The doses needed for various effects are less clear for humans.

A teratological drug that can result in a problem such as FAS may have negative effects other than FAS/FAE. A number of these are discussed below.

Pregnancy Loss

Spontaneous abortions and miscarriages are related to the use of alcohol. One massive study has shown marked increases in spontaneous second-trimester abortions for regular, but not for occasional, drinkers (Harlap & Shiono, 1980). Another large prospective study found increased risk of abortion at a level of drinking 1 oz of absolute alcohol twice a week (Kline et al., 1980). Mothers who drink during pregnancy are also more likely to have had previous pregnancy losses (S. W. Jacobson et al., 1984).

The mechanisms that produce these effects are not clear. On the one hand, these studies suggest that the effects are due to alcohol's acting as a poison, not as a teratogen. This is because the timing of abortions found in both studies fails to support the conclusion that they were a result of malformations. On the other hand, McLaren (1985) demonstrated that female mice given alcohol prior to ovulation produced more monosomic and trisomic ova than normal. Because such ova are more likely to be aborted, chromosomal abnormalities might be the mechanism by which alcohol produces abortions. Kalter and Warkany (1983), in their extensive review, call for caution in accepting pregnancy loss as an effect of alcohol consumption for any but heavy drinkers, in view of the conflicting evidence.

Low Birth Weight and Prematurity

As with other teratologic agents, data from both human and animal studies indicate that prenatal growth may be affected by prenatal alcohol exposure. Indeed, growth problems are part of the definition of FAS.

In rats, the greater the amount of alcohol to which they are exposed, the greater the slowing of growth (Brown et al., 1979). In humans the effects of the alcohol cannot be so clearly separated from those of associated factors, such as nutritional disturbances and deficiencies and smoking. These extraneous factors can also produce malformations of the central nervous system and growth retardation (Abel, 1984).

Two large-scale studies have found effects on birth weight that were statistically independent of maternal nutritional variables such as anemia, weight, and weight gain. Sokol et al. (1980) found effects on birth weight regardless of preterm status. A large-scale prospective study in Germany that controlled for a number of relevant variables, including smoking, found shorter gestations in mothers who were moderate or heavy drinkers (Mau & Netter, 1974). Not all studies agree with these. Alcohol use was not related to birth weight in one prospective study with a low-SES sample (Rosett et al., 1983). In a study of older mothers, alcohol consumption prior to pregnancy was not related to birth weight or height (O'Connor et al., 1986). Alcohol, together with the mother's prepregnancy weight, race, smoking habits, and education, and the baby's sex accounted for only 11% of the variance in birth weights. Other large-scale studies have failed to find growth retardation after controlling for relevant variables (Brooke et al., 1989; Ernhart et al., 1985; Kline et al., 1987). Overall, this somewhat confusing evidence would seem to indicate that alcohol is not an important factor in relation to birth weight *if* other factors, especially smoking, are controlled for.

However, an additive relation between smoking and alcohol consumption, similar to that for pregnancy loss, has been found for both SGA and prematurity (Sokol et al., 1980). Compared with mothers who neither drank nor smoked, those who abused alcohol had 24 times as many SGA infants, those who smoked had

18 times as many, and those who did both had 39 times as many. Other studies have found similar patterns, both for chronic alcoholics and for moderate drinkers (Kaminski et al., 1978; Little et al., 1976; Streissguth, 1977). After controlling for the effects on birth weight of smoking, alcohol still has some effect in smokers (Brooke et al., 1989).

Behavioral and CNS Effects

Here again, studies do not agree. One group has found that prenatal alcohol exposure results in poorer habituation and operant learning, two primary response systems that allow newborns to take in information about their world (see Chapter 9) (Martin et al., 1977; Streissguth et al., 1983). Other studies have failed to confirm differences in habituation and have generally found no effects on neonatal test performance (Ernhart et al., 1985; Richardson & Day, 1986). Newborns of mothers who drank during pregnancy have also been found to have generally lower levels of arousal, less vigorous bodily activity, more frequent state changes (see Chapter 6), and disturbed sleep states (Landesman-Dwyer et al., 1978; Rosett et al., 1979; Streissguth et al., 1983). But this combination of findings is somewhat contradictory, given that "lower levels of arousal" means easier to console, not excitable, and easily self-quieting.

A variety of other behavioral effects have been linked to prenatal exposure to alcohol, but the evidence for each is sparse and inconclusive. It has been linked to state regulation in the newborn by some researchers (Rosett et al., 1978), but not by others (Ernhart et al., 1985; Richardson & Day, 1986). In a well-controlled study of 441 cases, the development of the EEG at from 30 to 40 weeks gestation was abnormal, especially for binge drinkers (Ioffe & Chernik, 1988). Patterns in both REM and quiet sleep were affected. It has also been linked to the rather vague group of disorders labeled "childhood hyperactivity" or "minimal brain dysfunction," which are characterized by high levels of activity, difficulty in concentrating, and distractibility. Data supporting these linkages are less compelling than those for impaired intelligence or for newborn behavioral effects.

Mental retardation is now seen as the most serious defect, as well as the most sensitive indicator, of alcohol abuse. In his review covering France, Belgium, and Germany, as well as the United States, Abel (1984) notes that nearly all studies of FAS report retardation. The severity of retardation is not known, because of the relatively small number of children who have been followed systematically.

In a prospective study of 500 children selected from 1,500 pregnant women and followed to age 7, the IQs of 56 cases diagnosed as FAS averaged 65, and those of 26 cases diagnosed as FAE averaged 80 (Streissguth, Sampson, & Barr, 1989). The degree of retardation appears to be somewhat related to the severity of the physical signs of FAS, but the numbers are small (Streissguth et al., 1978a). The ages of the cases in this study varied widely, with the result that several different IQ tests had to be used.

It is important to remember that all studies using IQ measure it some years after birth, and hence are potentially confounded by the effects of postnatal environment. Alcoholics are apt to provide less-than-ideal environments for their children. In a study of alcohol use by 25 older women pregnant for the first time, it was found that heavier drinkers spent less time with their infants, and that the amount of time spent by the mother was related to the 1-year-old's Mental Development Index (O'Connor et al., 1986). In this study of educated women getting good medical care, mothers' intelligence was not related to the infants' Mental Development Index (MDI) at 1 year as one would expect. However, the MDI was related to the mothers' alcohol consumption, as was the discrepancy between the mothers' IQs and the infants' MDIs. MDIs were 115 for infants of abstinent and light-drinking mothers and about equal to their mothers' IQs. MDIs were 8 points below their mothers' IQs (108) for infants of light to moderate drinkers, and 21 points below (99) for those of moderate to heavy drinkers.

Studying the effects of postbirth environment is important as a guide for social action. If the IQs of FAS children improve when they are raised by someone other than their mothers, it would suggest that social service agencies should provide such alternative care. The data on the effects of home environment are scarce and contradictory. One study found IQ to be 10 points lower for 6 children who had lived with their alcoholic mothers at least part of the time (74) than for 6 with other living arrangements (Jones et al., 1974). In another study, however, the IQs of 17 cases of FAS who did not live with an alcoholic mother averaged only 66, failed to improve over a 4-year time span, and were not related to the care situation (Streissguth et al., 1978b). These data are difficult to interpret because of the extreme range of ages, use of different IQ tests, and small numbers of subjects. Streissguth, Sampson, and Barr (1989) report that among the primarily American Indian FAS/FAE group they studied, the problems of intellectual and adaptive behavior found in the adolescents and adults

occurred despite the fact that many of them were reared in foster or adoptive homes for much of their lives.[10] In contrast, a West German study showed improvement in most aspects of functioning (not hyperactivity and distractibility) over a 3- to 4-year period (Spohr & Steinhausen, 1987).

Moderate Versus Heavy Drinking

Most of the effects described above were found in babies of chronic alcoholics, heavy drinkers, or binge drinkers. Does moderate or light drinking also affect the embryo or fetus? Evidence from studies done in France, Germany, and the United States shows that moderate drinking is related to somewhat lower birth weight. In a study of several hundred pregnant women in a prepaid health plan in Seattle, this effect remained even when factors known to be related to birth weight (mother's age, height, parity, and smoking, and the sex of the infant) were controlled (Streissguth et al., 1981). Several studies in humans (Ernhart et al., 1989; Harlap & Shiono, 1980; Rosett et al., 1976; Rosett & Sander, 1979) and one in dogs (Ellis & Pick, 1980) indicate no excess of anomalies or of growth retardation in offspring of mild or occasional drinkers. Graham and colleagues (1988) showed that 20% of heavier drinkers had babies with effects at 4 years of age, compared with 9% for those of lighter drinkers.

A study to determine effects on different outcomes found that for physical anomalies the proportion of days on which drinking occurred was related to the number of anomalies, but the quantity taken at a given time was not (Ernhart et al., 1985).

A prospective study that identified 163 high-risk cases from pregnancy interviews indicated that low dosages may produce effects similar to those found in FAS (Hanson et al., 1978). In this study, 11 problem cases were found and 9 were from the high-risk group. Only 2 were severely affected enough to be classed as FAS, and both of their mothers were heavy drinkers. The 7 more mildly affected babies had mothers who drank 1 oz or more of absolute alcohol per day in the month prior to recognition of pregnancy. In another study, 18 infants whose mothers had had one or more drinks per day in the first trimester had different sleep and arousal behaviors from 13 whose mothers abstained (Scher et al., 1988). Smoking was controlled for. The Ottawa Prenatal Prospective Study (OPPS) of a relatively low-risk population found social levels of

---

10. For an account of one adopted Indian child, see *The Broken Cord* by Dorris (1989).

drinking related to lower cognitive scores at ages 2 and 3, but not at age 4 (Fried & Watkinson, 1990). At age 3 cigarettes and alcohol had a potentiating effect that was no longer present at age 4.

If we look at the data the other way around to define the risk for the potential mother having a baby with a detectable problem, it appears to be almost 10% if she drank 1 to 2 oz of absolute alcohol per day, but 19% if she drank 5 oz. Estimates for chronic alcoholics are 40%. Unfortunately, the long-term significance of detectable problems that are less severe than those labeled FAS is not known (Oullette et al., 1977; Rosett et al., 1976). (Rosett's 1980 editorial gives a reasonable review of the topic.)

Factors Other Than In Utero Alcohol Exposure

Smoking, nutrition, and abuse of other substances are possible confounding variables in the relation between alcohol consumption and poor infant outcomes, as is the time at which alcohol is consumed.

Other In Utero Exposures. We will consider the combination of smoking and drinking first, both because it is so frequent and because a number of studies have found the combination to have worse effects than either alone. Studies have found that from 36% (Cahalan et al., 1969) to 60% (Rosett et al., 1976) of the women categorized as heavy drinkers smoke more than a pack of cigarettes a day. An increase in stillbirths has been reported for women who both smoked and drank, compared with those who drank the same amounts but did not smoke (Kaminski et al., 1978). Behavioral differences in newborns have also been demonstrated (Landesman-Dwyer et al., 1977; Martin et al., 1977, 1978). These range from those of clear importance, such as sucking inefficiency and poor learning, to those whose meaning is unclear (e.g., atypical sleeping postures). Behavioral differences were also found for infants whose mothers smoked but only drank moderately. Clearly the amount smoked must be controlled for in any attempts to assess the effects of alcohol, and vice versa. The combination of alcohol and other drugs and medicines also needs to be studied. Alcohol abusers frequently abuse other drugs as well.

---

11. Paternal effects on developmental outcomes have been studied for other agents and for genetic contributions, but do not allow clear-cut conclusions. Students wishing to pursue this topic are referred to Gunderson and Sackett (1982).

Prepregnancy Parental Alcohol Use. Factors that might affect outcome, other than in utero exposure to alcohol from the mother, have been identified. One is the possible effect of alcohol consumption by the father on his genetic contribution to the embryo. The second is the prepregnancy alcohol consumption of the mother.

The possible role of the sperm has been seriously studied only in animals. This is unfortunate, because in many families there is a tendency for both parents to drink (or not drink). Thus the father's drinking is a potential confounding or contributing factor to effects found for maternal drinking. Although animal studies have not addressed directly the relative roles of father's and mother's alcohol consumption, they have isolated the effects of males' alcohol consumption by mating them to healthy non-alcohol-consuming females. Early studies indicated that offspring of chronically intoxicated male guinea pigs (from alcohol fumes) were frequently abnormal and had "grandchildren" that were less often viable (Stockard, 1913; Stockard & Papanicolaou, 1916; see also Heuyer et al., 1957). Male mice injected with alcohol and mated with normal females produced more resorptions and stillbirths (Badr & Badr, 1975). The mates of rat males who drank alcohol for their liquid had fewer pups (more resorptions) than the mates of those who drank water (Pfeifer et al., 1977). Their pups were actually slightly heavier (common with smaller litter size) but became lighter at a later age. Rat pups with "alcoholic" fathers were less likely to survive than those of water-drinking fathers (78% compared with 93%). There were pronounced sex differences, with females being more affected than males. Furthermore, the female offspring of alcohol-drinking fathers preferred higher concentrations of alcohol when they were older. Male offspring showed the opposite tendency.

If we extrapolate to the human case, it would seem possible that differences in the occurrence of FAS and related symptoms in babies whose mothers consumed a given level of alcohol may be related to paternal drinking habits.[11] There is one study at least that shows that the prepregnancy drinking of fathers is related to the birth weight of the offspring independent of maternal drinking and after ruling out maternal smoking, maternal caffeine consumption, and other drug use as influences (Little & Sing, 1987).

The second factor, prepregnancy drinking by the mother, has already been alluded to. It has been noted that prepregnancy drinking can usually not be separated from that done early in pregnancy, making it difficult to draw conclusions about the importance of this factor. A critical period for teratogenicity at around the time of conception is suggested (Ernhart et al., 1987; Ernhart & Wolf, 1987). It is too bad that the animal studies have not manipulated both paternal and maternal prepregnancy alcohol exposure in ways that allow a clear-cut separation of their effects.

Extrapolation from the mouse data would indicate that the third week of gestation might be a critical period of influence. Since several studies found that drinking before knowledge of pregnancy was most related to outcome, these data would argue for planned pregnancies in which drinking is lowered prior to becoming pregnant and during early pregnancy.

Genetic Characteristics of the Conceptus. The third factor concerns the role of genetic susceptibility and its interaction with exposure to alcohol and other drugs. These effects are dramatized by the occasional findings of differences in the effects on fraternal twins, in one case a marked sex difference (Riese, 1989). One twin may be affected so slightly that it might not have been detected had the other twin not been an obvious victim of FAS (Christoffel & Salofsky, 1975). Similar differences between twins have been found for other drugs, including thalidomide (Lenz, 1966; Loughnan et al., 1973). A genetic difference in susceptibility seems likely. However, one pair of monozygotic twins have been seen who did not exhibit identical characteristics of FAS, although both had it (Palmer et al., 1974). This cannot be caused by genetic differences, hence differences in prenatal environment need to be examined. They are most likely to relate to factors of placental exchange.

The data make it mandatory that studies measure the prepregnancy alcohol intake of both father and mother if the teratologic potential of alcohol is to be understood. In addition, they mandate careful consideration of sex differences in findings. Most studies, at least in the United States, have not had large enough samples to do this. Finally, the role of genetic susceptibility of the offspring needs to be considered, although current techniques allow only rough methods of studying it in humans.

Mechanism of Action

Studies with pregnant monkeys suggest a possible mechanism for the action of maternal alcohol intake on the fetus (Mukherjee & Hodgen, 1982). Five monkeys in the third trimester of pregnancy, operated on to allow direct examination of umbilical and placental functioning, were injected with alcohol solutions. In all cases the blood vessels in the umbilical

cord collapsed within 15 minutes, with gradual recovery during the next hour. All five fetuses developed severe oxygen deficiency (hypoxia) and acidosis (another indication of abnormality). Such changes were not seen in any controls. Although changes in the placenta do not appear to be permanent (Sokol et al., 1980), repeated episodes could have a damaging effect on the brain, which is in a stage of marked growth in the third trimester. Such research is, of course, impossible to do with humans. Nevertheless, there is some indication that factors related to the placental exchange system do operate in humans.

The possible role of hormonal changes as a result of alcohol exposure needs further exploration. Animal data suggest that adrenocortical function may be affected (Weinberg, 1989; Zimmerberg & Reuter, 1989). The effects of exposure to alcohol in utero appear to be caused, at least partly, by hypothyroid function, and might be avoided by early hormone replacement (Gottesfeld & Silverman, 1990). If thyroid or other hormonal function is a mechanism of action, the possibility of ameliorative treatment is raised. Zinc deficiency results from alcohol abuse, and has been shown to potentiate the effects of thalidomide as a teratogen in rats as well as to be a teratogen in humans. Again, we have a possible mechanism for the operation of alcohol as well as one lending itself to correction by use of dietary zinc supplementation (Flynn et al., 1981).

CIGARETTE SMOKING

The effects of smoking are included here in the legal psychotropic drug category despite the fact that neither the psychotropic nature of nicotine nor its being a direct cause of problems is clear. Changes in oxygen and carbon monoxide levels, poorer nutrition, or other associated life-style variables may contribute to the effects that have been attributed solely to cigarette smoking. There are even data that question whether smoking per se has any effect. These are not very often cited now that there are more studies linking smoking to negative outcomes and smoking is, appropriately, under heavy attack for general health reasons.

First, the data that link maternal smoking to negative outcomes of pregnancy are described. Second, the issue of causality is addressed through descriptions of some data that suggest that smoking itself is not the causal factor, as well as some that suggest it is. Finally, discussion is presented concerning what other differences between smokers and nonsmokers might influence or account for the correlations between smoking and infant problems.

What Problems Are Correlated With
Smoking During Pregnancy?

When a pregnant woman smokes, it affects her fetus's heart rate (Sontag, 1941), its breathing and movements (Thaler et al., 1980), and possibly the placenta (Naeye, 1978, 1979a). What are the consequences of smoking on offspring?

Physical Problems. Birth weight and prematurity have been the most studied outcomes. Both have consistently been found to be related to smoking. The U.S. Department of Health, Education and Welfare (1979) has reported more than 45 studies that confirmed the relation of smoking to birth weight or prematurity (see Silverman, 1977). This relation has been found in prospective as well as retrospective studies, in studies of blacks as well as of whites, of lower-class as well as middle-class subjects, and in representative samples. A massive retrospective study has shown that the effects of smoking on birth weight and preterm delivery are

Figure 4.2. This poster, widely distributed by the American Cancer Society, dramatizes the dangers of smoking during pregnancy. (Courtesy of the American Cancer Society.)

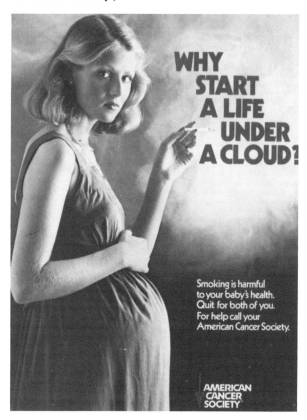

relatively minor for babies of young mothers, but great for those over 35 (Wen et al., 1990). This could be due to the cumulative effect of smoking on the mother's circulatory system, with resulting decreased uteroplacental blood flow. Effects have been found to be greater for males than for females (Wertelecki et al., 1987). Studies have failed to agree on whether (a) prematurity or SGA is the more important result, (b) LBW babies of smoking mothers are as likely as those of nonsmoking mothers to die, or (c) there are long-lasting disadvantages for those who survive.

Having thus summarized the complex evidence, let us look at some of it in more detail. Perhaps the first prospective study was done in Baltimore (Frazier et al., 1961). The sample was 2,736 black women seen at city prenatal health clinics and delivered of single live infants in city hospitals. The rate of births under 5.5 lb went from 11.2% for nonsmokers to 18.4% for smokers, with the increase proportional to the amount smoked. Fetal and neonatal death rates were higher for infants of smokers than of nonsmokers, despite the fact that the mothers were comparable in age, education, and work history. The study found that nervousness was not related to low birth weight in nonsmokers, but was related in smokers (23% LBW babies of nervous smoking mothers, 17% for the rest). However, this study did not examine many variables that other studies have found to be correlated with smoking (e.g., drinking).

Another prospective study by Yerushalmy (1971) was larger and dealt with a broader sample of mothers in a prepaid health care plan, who might be expected to have better health and nutrition. There were 9,793 whites and 3,290 blacks in the sample. The data confirm that smoking is related to lower birth weight, with twice as many LBW babies among smokers, *but* the increase in mortality that would be expected with low birth weights was not found. Indeed, LBW babies born to smoking mothers were only about half as likely to die as those born to mothers who never smoked (Yerushalmy, 1964). A still larger study, Britain's Birthday Trust Prenatal Survey, followed all babies born in the United Kingdom in one week in March 1958 (16,000) and found lower birth weights for babies of smoking mothers (Davie et al., 1972). Unfortunately, the study did not examine mortality according to birth weight. In addition, at least one study has reported lower birth weight for babies whose mothers were exposed to passive smoking, especially for those in the lower classes (Rubin et al., 1986).

More recent studies confirm the role of smoking in reducing birth weight (Barr et al., 1984; Butler & Golding, 1986; Dowler & Jacobson, 1984; Kline et al., 1987), but in one study of middle-class women, smoking accounted for less than 6% of the variance in birth weight and no infants were SGA (Dowler & Jacobson, 1984). In the British study cited above, the social class relationship to low birth weight was found to be entirely explained by the differences in amounts smoked and the size of the mothers (Butler & Golding, 1986). Most studies find differences of 150 to 200 g, not a major difference unless in a premature baby. Barr and the Seattle group (1984) found weight differences at birth, but not at 8 months. At 3 years, children of mothers who quit smoking during pregnancy were taller and heavier than those of mothers who continued. The effect for height remained after adjustment for maternal smoking after birth (Fox et al., 1990).

Infants are more likely to die both before and around birth if their mothers smoked, although not as likely as other LBW babies. This effect of smoking is very dependent on the race of the mother. An analysis of 6 studies and 60,000 births in the United States found a significantly greater risk of mortality for blacks whose mothers smoked, but not for whites (Singleton et al., 1986). The most dramatic increase was for black babies whose mothers had smoked more than a pack per day.

Although the data are not as clear-cut as the "don't smoke when pregnant" ads would like us to believe, babies of smoking mothers are apt to have other problems, such as more malformations of the heart and other organs, and to suffer respiratory and prenatal infections. Finally, deaths from **sudden infant death syndrome** (**SIDS**, or "crib death"), the leading cause of death from 1 month to 1 year, were 52% more frequent among infants whose mothers had smoked (Naeye, 1979b). Such data do not enable control for other relevant factors, since the occurrence of SIDS is only 2-3 per 1,000. In Sweden, where the SIDS rate is only .7 per 1,000, smoking doubles the SIDS risk, and the more that is smoked, the greater the risk (Haglund & Cnattingius, 1990).

Behavioral Problems. Smoking by pregnant women has been shown to affect newborn behavior, but the effects have not been very consistent from one study to another. On the Brazelton examination, babies have been shown to be less irritable (J. L. Jacobson et al., 1984), to have poorer habituation (Picone et al., 1982; Richardson & Day, 1986), to differ in auditory responses (Picone et al., 1982; Sexton, 1978), and to have poorer orientation (Richardson & Day, 1986). Cigarette smoking in the first trimester has been found to be significantly negatively correlated with the habit-

uation, orientation, motor, and state clusters on the NBAS (Richardson & Day, 1986). However, the highest correlations were only in the .26-.28 range (for habituation and orientation) and the others were less than .15. Hence no meaningful amount of variance is accounted for in any of these behaviors. Third-trimester smoking was related to only one variable at a very low level ($r = .11$).

Long-Term Outcomes. Some outcomes associated with smoking occur later in infancy or childhood. This means that the problem of inferring that the prenatal exposure was causal is great. Nevertheless, long-range outcomes are of great interest.

The most frequently used outcome measure is IQ. In a very large prospective study (50,000 pregnancies of predominantly lower-class women), the Collaborative Perinatal Research Project (CPRP), Naeye (1979b) found no IQ differences in babies of smoking mothers compared with those of nonsmoking mothers. Hardy and Mellits (1972) found no IQ differences, nor did a small retrospective study of middle-class children (Lefkowitz, 1981). The latter study showed that, at 11 years of age, the offspring of smokers did not differ from those of carefully matched nonsmokers on (a) height, (b) weight, (c) four measures of intellectual status including reading and IQ (determined by figure drawing), (d) five measures of happiness or depression, or (e) five measures of personal and social functioning (including one of movement assessment). Although Lefkowitz relied on mothers to report their smoking during long-ago pregnancies, their reliability seems plausible because mothers who reported smoking had infants whose birth weights were lower in the expected amount (196 g). Longitudinal data gathered before the pressure on mothers not to smoke also show no effects on IQ at age 4 after adjusting for alcohol and other relevant variables (Barr et al., 1990). There appeared to be a relation between smoking and motor development at age 4, but when the two 3½-pack-a-day smokers were removed from the heavy smoking group this no longer held (Barr et al., 1990). Other studies have found lower cognitive and language scores at 3 years (Fried, 1989b) and lowered cognitive scores for children whose mothers continued to smoke compared with those whose mothers quit (Sexton et al., 1990). The role of postnatal exposure to smoke was not controlled for in the latter study.

Most studies have found that smoking during pregnancy does not result in decreased IQ, and the differences between them and those that have found such effects need to be understood. One factor might be the nature of the population studied. Broman and Nichols (1981), analyzing data from the CPRP, found that for higher-IQ children there was a negative correlation between maternal smoking during pregnancy and later IQ. The IQ scores decreased in relation to the amount of maternal smoking. Other data from the project showed that minimal brain damage at age 7 was related to the length of time the mother had smoked prior to pregnancy (Nichols & Chen, 1981).

Other studies suggest that smoking during pregnancy does result in long-term outcomes for the offspring. Britain's massive Birthday Trust Survey found negative outcomes (Davie et al., 1972). At age 7, the offspring of mothers who had smoked heavily during pregnancy were a half inch shorter and were 4 months behind the average reading level, less well adjusted at school, generally clumsy, and had apparent spatial problems (were in the bottom 10% of their class on copying simple designs). The OPPS data showed different relations between smoking and outcomes at different ages. Smokers' babies had lower cognitive scores (and auditory measures) at 1 year, but not at 2 years, after controlling for home environment (neither cognitive nor language scores). Verbal aspects of cognitive behavior at 3 and 4 years of age were lower for smokers' babies after controlling for home environment. In a sample that was stratified both for alcohol use and amount smoked, IQ at age 4 was not related to smoking after controlling for alcohol use and sociodemographic variables (Streissguth, Barr, et al., 1989) or to motor development (Barr et al., 1990), although it had been related to poorer orientation and attention at age 4 (Streissguth et al., 1984).

A retrospective study using a composite measure called the Morbidity Ratio (MR), which measures the occurrence of any handicapping condition, also found differences related to smoking (Stott & Latchford, 1976). The handicaps included malformations, physical defects, neurological symptoms, retardation in developmental milestones, behavior disturbances, and nonepidemic illness. Offspring of smokers (N = 439) had a 55% higher MR than those of nonsmokers (N = 739), who, in turn, had fewer handicapping conditions than would be expected from population figures. The researchers also report that the MR rose with the amount the mother smoked. A recent review marshals a good deal of evidence in support of these findings (Stevens et al., 1988).

It is difficult to draw conclusions from these studies and especially difficult to interpret those using the Morbidity Ratio where smoking in the household after the child's birth might cause some of the problems. Recent data confirm the greater likelihood of infectious diseases in children who live with a smoker (Overpeck & Moss, 1991). Overall, it appears that prenatal maternal smoking does not affect the IQ of the offspring, although it may affect verbal behavior for low-risk children and IQ for higher-IQ children. Evidence for other long-term effects must be considered inconclusive because the findings on reading level, adjustment, and spatial problems differed in the two studies in which they were measured. Lefkowitz (1981), Naeye (1979b), and Hardy and Mellits (1972) agree that if the perinatal period is survived, there are no harmful long-term effects on growth or intellectual functioning.

Does Smoking (or Nicotine) Cause These Problems?

The research just described is all correlational, and correlations do not prove causality. Correlations between smoking and infant problems do not prove that smoking causes the difficulties. It would be impossible to conduct an experiment in which pregnant women were randomly assigned to smoking and nonsmoking conditions. We therefore need to find indirect ways of assessing causality. One such way is to allow women to serve as their own controls. This can be done by finding women who smoked during one pregnancy and did not smoke during another. If smoking is the causal factor, then the offspring exposed to smoking prenatally should differ from those who were not. Yerushalmy's (1972) large sample yielded 210 white infants born to mothers who had not yet started to smoke and who had another baby after starting to smoke. The percentage of low birth weight infants was substantially the same whether the mothers were not yet smoking (9.5%) or smoking (8.9%). The same similarity in the proportions of low birth weight infants held when comparing infants of mothers who had an infant while smoking and had another after quitting. Yerushalmy concludes:

> These findings raise doubt and argue against the proposition that cigarette smoking acts as an exogenous factor which interferes with the intrauterine development of the fetus. Rather, the evidence appears to support the hypothesis that the higher incidence of low birth weight infants is due to the smoker, not the smoking. (p. 283)

The data on mothers' switching needs to be evaluated in terms of the fact that older women have a higher risk of infant mortality, and possibly of other problems. Infant mortality is greater for a nonsmoking mother 35 or over than for a smoking mother of the same parity but under 35 (Butler & Alberman, 1969). A more recent study has found small weight losses for those who switched to smoking and marked gains for those who switched in the opposite direction (Wainwright, 1983).

The type of evidence provided by the MR as the dependent measure of infant problems does show that giving up smoking helps (Stott & Latchford, 1976). When the mother gave up smoking when she became pregnant, the health risk for her infant was like that of infants whose mothers had not smoked and was much lower than that for babies whose mothers smoked during pregnancy.

Clearly we have a problem that is not yet resolved. Yerushalmy has unusually good data in that he is comparing a relatively large number of offspring of mothers when they smoked and when they did not. He finds the same results regardless of whether the women went from nonsmoking to smoking pregnancies or from smoking to nonsmoking pregnancies. This is important because mothers who change in one direction are unlikely to share relevant characteristics with women who moved in the other direction (other than the fact that both will be older for the second pregnancy). Women who smoked in an earlier but not in a later pregnancy are likely to be health conscious, and hence may have made special efforts to ensure good prenatal care even in the pregnancy during which they smoked. Those efforts might have compensated for the harmful effects of smoking. It is unlikely that women who started smoking in a later pregnancy did so because they were concerned about health. Thus any extraneous variables that might explain the results for women who became nonsmokers would not likely explain the finding for women who became smokers.

I do not mean to argue that Yerushalmy's data are right and others are wrong. The seemingly contradictory findings of Yerushalmy and Stott may really not be inconsistent. The dependent measures used were very different. Yerushalmy used low birth weight. Stott and Latchford's MR is a composite measure of a variety of outcomes, present anywhere from the neonatal period through 4 years. Such a composite would be more sensitive than a single measure. If smoking has very small effects on a number of infant problems, each one alone might not be detectable, but when all are put together, a measurable effect might be obtained. But the validity of the MR can be questioned because it can be influenced by experiences after birth. In addition, some measures included in it do not have known relevance. A resolution of these discrepant findings would require research beyond

that of Wainwright, which unfortunately is not being done. It is unclear whether researchers have lost interest or the medical and political establishments have made up their minds and no longer support such research.

Possible Extraneous Variables

As is the case for alcohol, with smoking one needs to look at other variables that may be affecting the outcomes.

Nutrition. Despite our uncertainty as to whether smoking itself is deleterious, there are factors associated with smoking that may contribute to the observed difficulties of infants. One such factor is maternal weight gain, which in turn may reflect malnutrition. Mothers who smoke during pregnancy gain less weight; the more they smoke, the less weight they gain (Rush, 1973, 1974). A lower maternal weight gain is associated with lower birth weight of the offspring, and, to a lesser extent, with shorter length and smaller head circumference at birth (Luke et al., 1981). The effects found for smoking could be malnutrition effects. Other social habits associated with smoking might also tend to decrease the adequacy of nutrition.

Placental Abnormalities. Naeye (1978, 1979a), in the massive CPRP study referred to above, found that **placenta previa** (an abnormal implantation of the placenta near the opening of the cervix, so that it tends to precede the baby at birth, causing severe maternal hemorrhage) was more common in smokers and in women who had previously smoked than in nonsmokers. Other placental problems were strongly implicated in Meyer et al.'s (1976) data, especially for women who smoked more than a pack a day. Placental abnormalities can result in decreased nutrition and poorer oxygen supplies to the fetus. Animal data indicate that carbon monoxide exposure is a more likely cause of damage than is oxygen deprivation. Chronic exposure to moderate levels of carbon monoxide may disrupt neuronal proliferation and possibly even affect neurochemical transmission (Fechter, 1987).

These correlational findings do not tell us whether it is smoking or some other characteristic of women who smoke that produces the placental abnormalities, which in turn produce the negative outcomes. To decide whether smoking itself produces the abnormalities would again require studies that use mothers as their own controls. Light could be shed on the issue by appropriate animal research. Until researchers can isolate the exact cause of the placental abnormalities, it is useful to know that women who smoke are at increased risk for them so that their doctors can determine whether their smoking patients experience placental insufficiency during pregnancy.

To summarize the arguments presented thus far: Fetal malnutrition, including oxygen deprivation, caused by placental abnormalities or low maternal weight gain, or both, have been suggested as correlates of smoking. Both are known to lead to low birth weights and short gestations. Therefore, it is thought that these factors may produce the negative outcomes for babies of smoking mothers. What is not known is whether smoking directly produces the placental abnormalities and low maternal weight gain or whether these are indirect effects.

Paternal Smoking. It is clear that paternal smoking is an important variable for any outcomes, such as the MR, that can be affected by exposure to smoke after birth, but preliminary data have also implicated paternal smoking prior to birth in an increased risk of certain childhood cancers (leukemia, lymphoma, and brain cancer). If confirmed, these data should lead to research on the question of whether this results from a genetic effect on the sperm prior to conception (Overpeck & Moss, 1991).

Other variables. Two variables known to be related to smoking are lead accumulation and twinning. Again, however, the causal role of smoking is not clear. It is known that various stresses are related to increased lead levels in pregnant women (Rothenberg et al., 1989). Cigarette smoking is related to an increased accumulation of lead in both mother and fetus among urban dwellers in industrial areas. This increase is sufficient to inhibit production of an enzyme that helps the red blood cells make hemoglobin, which is essential for the nutrition and oxygenation of the fetus. While lead levels are lower in fetal than in maternal blood, they rise in direct proportion to those of the mother. It is not known what other effects the raised lead levels might have and whether they are sufficient to cause brain damage (Kuhnert et al., 1977). Mexican data suggest decreased ability to self-quiet and to be consoled in the first month if lead levels have risen late in pregnancy, even though they are not at high levels. Three U.S. and one Australian study indicate that low levels of lead exposure impair neurobehavioral development, but have less effect than postnatal exposure (Davis & Svendsgaard, 1987), whereas the Sydney Lead Study found that low levels are not associated with mental or motor deficits in the preschool years (Cooney et al., 1989).

The twinning rate is twice as high in smokers as in nonsmokers (Yerushalmy, 1972), but varies markedly according to race. White women had to smoke only 5 or more cigarettes a day to be at increased risk of twinning, but black women had to smoke 15 or more. Because twinning itself leads to an increased risk of prematurity and low birth weight, and because twin births are often excluded in studies of the effects of smoking, it is quite possible that research data underestimate the overall effects of smoking on birth weight and prematurity.

Other differences between smoking and nonsmoking pregnant women might contribute to their infants' problems. In Yerushalmy's (1971) sample, a higher proportion of smoking mothers consumed beverages higher in alcohol and caffeine (coffee, beer, and whiskey) and a lower percentage drank milk. Alcohol we know to cause problems, and caffeine is under suspicion. Smoking mothers also were less likely to use contraceptives or to plan their pregnancies. In short, smoking pregnant women seem less health conscious and planful.

What Should Smoking Women Do During Pregnancy?

Should women stop smoking during pregnancy or not? Should they smoke less? If so, how much less? Each woman who is faced with the prospect of giving up a very strong habit for the sake of her unborn child must make that decision herself. It is easy to say that it is better to be safe than sorry and to recommend that all women completely give up smoking while pregnant. That is what most obstetricians recommend. Smoking is related to serious health problems for women, and birth weight is lower for offspring of smokers, whether at a meaningful level or not, and whether or not smoking itself is the cause.

However, one should also consider the fact that a pregnant woman who gives up smoking may also create problems for the fetus. She may be resentful of the pregnancy, and this may carry over to the offspring. There may be physiological or psychological concomitants of giving up smoking that future research will find to be harmful to the infant. A compromise solution might be for the woman to cut down on smoking and to make sure that her prenatal medical care and nutrition are good so as to help eliminate other possible risks. How much to cut down on smoking is also a difficult question. The amount of smoking that appears to be related to the poorest outcomes differs in different studies and for blacks and whites. Overall, it appears that a total of fewer than 14 cigarettes per day if black and fewer for whites might be helpful. For women who decide to continue smoking during pregnancy, greater weight gain during pregnancy may help to compensate for the growth retardation and thus decrease the risk of low birth weight. (Those seriously interested in this topic should read *Smoking for Two* by Fried & Oxorn, 1980.)

CAFFEINE

In the mid-1970s people became concerned about the possible teratogenic effect of caffeine. The Arthur D. Little Company did a series of reviews of literature and studies on the topic at the behest of the National Coffee Association. By the late 1970s there were still few human data. The difficulties of separating caffeine intake from smoking and alcohol are as great as the reverse. Smokers are often heavy coffee drinkers, which may be related to the fact that they clear caffeine from the system 50% more rapidly than nonsmokers. Animal data are contradictory, but caffeine leads to cleft palate and extra digits in rodents, and to learning deficits in male rats (Grimm, 1987). In 1980 the U.S. Food and Drug Administration issued a warning based on the rodent data for consumption equivalent to 50 to 70 cups of coffee per day in humans.

What Do We Actually Know?

Caffeine has effects on fertility. It can affect spermatogenesis. Animal data show an increase in sterile or infertile matings, followed by both pre- and postimplantation losses not explainable on a genetic basis (Weathersbee et al., 1977). In human data it is hard to interpret findings on the spermatozoa, because caffeine used by the female could affect the motility of the sperm. An early retrospective study found near total reproductive loss for those drinking more than eight cups per day (Weathersbee et al., 1977). However, there are many methodological difficulties with this study. Caffeine has also been implicated in lower birth weight, but some studies find no effect (Berger, 1988). Extensive testing of motor performance at 4 years yielded very few and partially contradictory effects of caffeine exposure in early pregnancy (Barr et al., 1990).

Higher congenital malformation rates have been found in only one study of women who reported they drank more than eight cups of coffee per day. There was no control for their use of other possibly injurious substances.

Behavioral effects of caffeine occur at very similar dosages (per unit weight) across many species as does

acute toxicity. Caffeine has been shown to affect brain growth in rats (Tanaka et al., 1987). Brain stem and cortical serotonin levels are raised by caffeine.

Caffeine is used to treat neonates with severe apnea spells. It appears to increase sensitivity to carbon dioxide and thus to increase central respiratory drive.

I conclude by quoting the conclusion of Berger (1988), the author of an excellent recent review of the human data: "Until more information is available, it might be prudent to limit caffeine intake to approximately 300 mg per day during pregnancy in view of decreases in birth weight that might occur at or above that level of consumption" (p. 953).

Illegal Psychotropic Drugs

Illegal drugs, unlike alcohol, which is a true teratogen, primarily affect the behavior and physiological functioning of the baby rather than produce structural defects. They provide the clearest instances of behavioral teratogens or developmentally toxic compounds. We know most about the effects of heroin and methadone, which is often used to replace heroin, but our knowledge about cocaine, or crack, like its use, is growing rapidly.

HEROIN AND METHADONE
(THE OPIATES OR OPIOIDS)

Heroin passes the placental barrier, so that infants of addicted women are born addicted. The withdrawal symptoms they suffer after birth can kill them. Only after doctors came to recognize that this was what was wrong with relatively large numbers of babies did they learn to manage them appropriately and to spare their lives. Heroin-exposed babies are shorter and have smaller head circumferences than other high-risk babies or babies of the same SES (Wilson et al., 1979). Survivors suffer from a number of behavioral difficulties (for example, in motoric behaviors, soothability, and sleep cycles).

Of the estimated 500,000 heroin addicts in the United States, some 70,000 have been treated by switching them to methadone maintenance, which is legal. This avoids maternal infections from contaminated needles and having the fetus exposed to repeated intrauterine withdrawal when the mother cannot get her "fix." Inasmuch as women on methadone maintenance often abuse other drugs, we cannot evaluate the effects of methadone itself, even in these samples. However, its effects on the newborn appear to be almost as bad as those of heroin. The babies are subject to high perinatal mortality (Finnegan et al., 1977; Zelson et al., 1973). Withdrawal symptoms usually start by 72 hours, but peak at 3 to 6 weeks and may be prolonged in nursing babies. The babies suffer more seizures and have more severe elevation of bilirubin levels (hyperbilirubinemia), hence have more potential CNS damage. The breathing responses of newborns whose mothers were on methadone are altered for some 20 to 40 days after methadone can no longer be detected in their systems. This could contribute to the high rate of sudden infant deaths (SIDS) among babies of methadone-maintained mothers (Ostrea et al., 1975). The severity of withdrawal from methadone is less than that for heroin. Also, intrauterine growth appears to be enhanced by methadone, but retarded by heroin (Kendall et al., 1976; see Hutchings, 1982, for a review).

It is reasonable to suspect some CNS damage even in those methadone babies who do not have seizures, because they have been exposed daily while in utero to an increased level of carbon dioxide and, therefore, to a decreased level of oxygen. CNS difficulties affect motoric maturation. Methadone babies at 1 day and at 1 month of age are much more likely than well-defined controls to exhibit poor motoric maturity, but are not likely to have generally poor state (Johnson et al., 1984; Marcus et al., 1982; Ostrea et al., 1975). Tremors, agitation, restlessness, and sleep disturbances persist for 4 to 6 months (Chasnoff et al., 1980; Hans, 1989). Research with monkeys supports the interpretation of CNS problems as a cause of the difficulties.

Researchers disagree on whether methadone alters state behaviors or produces decreased visual alerting (Marcus et al., 1982; Strauss et al., 1975, 1976). Several studies have found the sexes to be affected differently, with males being more affected than females.

One study of long-term outcomes for both heroin- and methadone-exposed infants compared both of them with unexposed infants raised by addicted parents (Wilson, 1989). The two groups did not differ in average mental test performance in the first 2 years or at 3 to 5 years. This suggests that being reared by addicts is the potent factor. However, 24% of the heroin-exposed children tested as retarded, compared with 2.5% of the controls.[12] A General Cognitive Index at 3 to 5 years was related to (a) the obstetric prenatal risk score, (b) the amount of prenatal care,

and (c) the quality of the home environment. Motor incoordination was 2.9 times as frequent in children treated for newborn narcotic withdrawal as in those who had no or only mild (untreated) withdrawal. Despite a thread of results relating drug exposure to motor or visual-motor problems, IQ was most related to home environment ($r = .40$). In contrast, the Bender Gestalt Test, which is supposed to reflect neurological damage, was most related to the severity of maternal drug abuse ($r = .37$). A 2-year follow-up of methadone-exposed children whose mothers had good prenatal care and who were raised by their parents shows similar results (Hans, 1989).

MARIJUANA

The prenatal effects of marijuana have not been well studied in humans, despite the long history of its use (see Abel, 1980b). A handful of animal studies suggest that it may have a teratogenic effect. Its active ingredient can cross the placental barrier in rats (Vardaris et al., 1976), and thus it has teratogenic potential. Abnormally high fetal loss has been produced by high doses of the active ingredient of marijuana (THC) in rhesus monkeys (Sassenrath et al., 1979), perhaps as a result of problems in chromosome segregation during cell division.

Although no conclusive evidence of teratogenicity exists for humans, some evidence points to the possibility of subtle effects on birth weight, body length, and length of gestation—all effects that could be mediated by retardation in placental development caused by THC (Zuckerman, Frank, et al., 1989). A city hospital population showed lower birth weights for babies whose mothers used marijuana prior to and during pregnancy (Zuckerman, Frank, et al., 1989). However, the size of the effect differed for different ethnic groups, with little effect for whites and the largest effects for Hispanics and immigrant blacks (Amaro et al., 1986). But, after adjusting for other risk factors, only whites were at increased risk for delivering a low birth weight, SGA, or premature infant, and occasional use was not related to any of these outcomes (Hatch & Bracken, 1986). Similarly, offspring of mothers who used only marijuana were not more apt to be premature (Witter & Niebyl, 1990). The complex ethnic differences and interactions with maternal weight prior to pregnancy demonstrate the importance of knowing the nature of the sample studied in interpreting results of studies.

One possible reason for different results in different studies is maternal nutrition. Rat data show a strong interaction between the amount of protein in the ma-

---

12. It is often important to look at the percentages at extremes, rather than at average differences.

ternal diet and the effects of marijuana smoke (Charlebois & Fried, 1980). When it was combined with low protein in the maternal diet there were an excess of stillbirths, litter destruction, and postnatal deaths. Delayed developmental milestones were more marked in the adequate diet group than in the extra protein group.

Marijuana users did not differ in miscarriage rates, Apgars, frequency of complications, or major physical anomalies at birth compared with controls matched for alcohol and cigarette usage and income in a relatively low-risk population (Fried, 1989a, 1989b). Prevalence of congenital anomalies was also not related to marijuana in 5% of persons for whom it was the only drug used (Witter & Niebyl, 1990).

Neurobehavioral effects have been found in the first days of life using the Brazelton scale (Fried & Makin, 1987). The effects were increased tremors and exaggerated and lengthy startles to mild or no stimuli, unaccompanied by other signs that characterize narcotic withdrawal. Poorer visual, but not auditory, habituation was also found in the OPPS study (Fried, 1989a, 1989b) and in an earlier study with monkeys (Golub et al., 1981). Similar findings occurred in neurological examinations at 9 and 30 days, but visual differences were not significant (Fried, 1989a, 1989b; Fried et al., 1987). Sleep and motility were affected in a relatively small sample of marijuana-exposed infants regardless of the trimester of exposure (Scher et al., 1988).

Analyses of data on the OPPS children at 12 and 24 months that controlled for other variables showed no unique contribution of marijuana history to mental or motor development or language scores or a composite visual behavior score. At 3 years, quantitative scores on the McCarthy were lower for children of heavy users, but not after controlling for confounding factors. At this age they also had superior motor performance. However, at 4 years both memory and verbal measures were negatively associated with heavy prenatal marijuana exposure, even after controlling for confounding factors (Fried, 1989a, 1989b). At later ages the greater demands on the children may make subtle differences more obvious, a possibility predicted by Fried.

Another health risk from smoking marijuana may be similar to that from smoking cigarettes. Marijuana contains 70% more benzopyrene and more tars, both cancer-causing agents, than cigarettes. Marijuana also reduces the antibacterial defense systems of the lungs. Given the widespread use of this drug, further studies to either establish or rule out negative effects are very much needed (Institute of Medicine, 1982).

COCAINE

As recently as 1982 an obstetric text stated that cocaine was not known to have any deleterious effect on the fetus. However, animal work on the detrimental effects of cocaine had started in 1980. Isolated reports of problems in human pregnancies began to appear in 1983, and in 1985 a report based on small samples showed high rates of spontaneous abortion, of abruptio placentae (which compromises the life of both mother and infant), and of neonatal neurobehavioral deficiencies (Chasnoff et al., 1985). The Chasnoff expanded sample had similar results (Chasnoff et al., 1987). A 38% rate of miscarriage was noted. Premature births, lower birth weights, more abruptio placentae, and more stillbirths from abruptio placentae have been found by many (Bingol et al., 1987; Karmel et al., 1990; Little et al., 1989; MacGregor et al., 1987; Mastrogiannis et al., 1990; Neerhof et al., 1989; Oro & Dixon, 1987). A higher rate of malformations, especially of the urinary tract, have been found (Bingol et al., 1987; Chavez et al., 1989), suggesting cocaine may be a true teratogen. As in other studies of abnormal outcomes, the figures for the proportions that are abnormal (here below 2,500 g, or SGA) are more interesting than the average weight differences for the groups compared.

Markedly higher rates of SIDS have been found (15% for cocaine babies, 4% for methadone babies, and .3% for nonexposed; see Chasnoff et al., 1987, 1989). Riley and his colleagues (1988) found 10 to 20 times the average national incidence. However, a larger prospective study failed to find a higher rate of SIDS (Bauchner et al., 1988).

Poorly regulated states are already found in the fetal period, using ultrasound techniques to score behaviors (Hume et al., 1989). Tremors and problems in motor and visual-motor development, muscle hypertonicity, irritability, and attention spans are frequently found after birth (Chasnoff et al., 1985, 1987; Karmel et al., 1990). In addition, cocaine-exposed babies have visual preferences that are less affected by arousal levels than "normal" NICU babies (Karmel et al., 1990). Whereas normal infants prefer a slower rate of presentation when aroused and a faster one when less aroused, cocaine-exposed babies tend to prefer the faster frequencies even when they are more aroused. They also are less affected by stressors (Karmel et al., 1990). When stressed to the point of crying, normal-weight cocaine babies had higher-pitched, longer-lasting, and more variable cries (Lester et al., 1991). The LBW cocaine babies took longer to cry, had fewer cries, and cried less loudly. The problems of cocaine babies are such that they are likely to interfere with the mother-infant relationship, which is already handicapped by the mother's drug use.

A specific research study is presented to illustrate the complexities of research efforts. Chasnoff and Griffith (1989) compared 23 infants whose mothers had stopped using cocaine in the first trimester (Group 1) with 52 who used it throughout pregnancy (Group 2). The proportions who were of different ethnic groups and who used alcohol or marijuana were similar for the two groups.

Group 1 infants did more poorly on the motor cluster of the Brazelton and almost half never reached an alert state in order to be tested for orientation, compared with one-fourth for Group 2. In addition, Group 1 infants were more fragile and less able to complete the exam, had greater imbalances in motor tone, and were judged lower in reinforcement value than the infants exposed throughout pregnancy. Group 2 infants were, however, born at a lower gestational age and were more likely to be low birth weight or SGA. The groups did not differ on rates of abruptio placentae. Both groups (after excluding prematures) demonstrated impaired orientation, motor ability, and state regulation, and increased abnormal reflexes on the Brazelton. The differences in favor of Group 2 are counterintuitive and need to be replicated; the role of withdrawal effects needs to be looked at. If confirmed, these results would indicate the need for different counseling than users now receive.

It is hardly reassuring to note that rat data indicate that adult brain metabolism is altered by neonatal exposure at a stage roughly comparable to the third trimester in humans (Dow-Edwards et al., 1988). Brain metabolism is affected in humans both at the time of administration and subsequently. Females are more affected than males. The fetus shows cardiovascular changes, including small strokes, prenatally. In one study more than a third of infants born addicted to cocaine had evidence of brain damage attributed to tiny stokes prenatally (Dixon & Bejar, 1989). Brain and behavioral effects are found at doses where little general toxicity occurs. (For data and further references, see Dow-Edwards et al., 1988; Woods et al., 1989.)

While follow-up data are not extensive, they are discouraging as far as postnatal improvement is concerned. Emotional and social behaviors seem to be affected, and cognitive behaviors are either directly affected or affected because of other problems, such as emotionality and inability to concentrate (Beckwith, 1988; Howard, 1989; Howard et al., 1989).

With the alarming increase in the number of cocaine babies being born (10% to 20% or more of births in some hospitals), more understanding of problems and possible treatments is of the utmost importance.[13] To obtain a good picture of the correlates of cocaine use, it is mandatory that large samples be studied and appropriate statistical models be used to control for other variables (Frank et al., 1988).

OTHER ILLEGAL DRUGS

Another well-known psychotropic drug is LSD. There has been a great deal of discussion about whether this drug causes chromosomal damage to those who take it, and whether this damage could be transmitted to offspring. A comprehensive review of more than 100 articles on the subject concludes that moderate doses of pure LSD do not produce chromosomal damage (Dishotsky et al., 1971). Because LSD has not been the drug of choice since the 1960s, there are few current studies. However, some reports indicate the use of LSD may be increasing.

PCP (angel dust) was a popular street drug in the 1970s that also had dire effects on the fetus. In addition to withdrawal, problems with later sleep, temperament, and attachment have been noted (Wachsman et al., 1989). Crystal methamphetamine (ice) is a current worry in Hawaii and on the West Coast. Its mechanisms of action are very similar to those of cocaine. Like cocaine, ice often results in hemorrhages in the brain (Dixon & Bejar, 1989). There is some evidence that it might become the street drug of the 1990s. Amphetamine addiction during pregnancy also has been shown in a Swedish study to have negative consequences for the child's peer relations and aggression at age 8 (Eriksson et al., 1989). Perhaps even more startling is the fact that only 21 of 65 children in this study were in the custody of their biological mothers at age 8.

In a study reported by Sandrock et al. (1990), substance abuse (substance unspecified) was related to lower birth weight and younger gestational age, accounting for 33% and 25% of the variance, respectively, in well-screened and matched samples of abusers and nonabusers. In addition, infants of abusers were more apt to have low Apgars, neurobehavioral symptoms such as irritability, tremors, and hypertonicity, and cardiopulmonary problems.

13. For a good brief review, see Pitts and Weinstein (1990). For an account of ways of trying to treat infants' various symptoms, see Lewis et al. (1989).

Direct Effects of External Environment

All of the prenatal effects of drugs and diseases discussed have touched the infant by way of the mother and the placenta. The harmful agent crosses the placenta, or an insufficiency in the mother results in something not being passed through the placenta, or the functioning of the placental interchange system itself is affected adversely. Hence the mother's being startled by a rabbit could affect an offspring only if it produced a physiological reaction in the mother that could do this, or if the baby could see it and was startled.

Because embryos and fetuses are cut off from the environment outside their mothers' bodies, they are generally well protected from direct environmental effects. Nevertheless, there are direct effects. The only firmly established example is radiation, which passes through the mother's body to affect the egg, embryo, or fetus directly. Noise and very strong blows to the abdomen may also directly affect the fetus. Environmental factors such as heavy physical labor or extreme grief may result in maternal stress sufficient to alter hormonal and other physiological responses sufficiently to affect the fetus. These effects are, like those of other teratogens, mediated by physiological reactions in the mother.

RADIATION

Radiation is often called the "universal teratogen." In animals it has been shown to produce malformations or improper development in all organ systems, including the central nervous system. In addition, it can change susceptibility to various cancers. The effects depend upon level of dosage, length of exposure, and timing of exposure. The pattern of effects is not necessarily the same in different species, or in different studies of the same species. Effects can result from exposure prior to conception, prior to implantation, or during embryological and fetal development.

Effects induced prior to fertilization could result from chromosomal damage from irradiation to either ova or sperm cells. Both chromosomal breakage and translocations may occur. The mother is likely to be the crucial parent, because effects on her ova are cumulative over time. Since her ova are present even prior to her own birth, they are particularly vulnerable to the effects of long-term low levels of radiation. Her ova are affected by every X ray she receives and perhaps even by the background radiation where she lives. Indeed, this may be part of the reason older mothers have increased numbers of offspring with genetic

problems involving the chromosomes.

In contrast to the situation with the female, the male produces new sperm cells throughout his life. Any effects of irradiation (below the dosage that damages the whole sperm-production mechanism) are very short term unless an affected sperm results in a pregnancy. Children of men who work at nuclear plants, particularly those who received high radiation doses in the 6 months prior to the conception, appear to be at increased risk of having leukemia compared with those of men in other jobs (Beral, 1990; Gardner et al., 1990). Among the effects of both high single dosages and chronic low doses of X rays are lowered fertility both for males and females. This may in part represent failure of damaged cells to give rise to conception or the likelihood of early abortion or miscarriage.

There are confusing data from Norway that show a marked increase in miscarriages after the Chernobyl incident, out of proportion to the amount of radiation to which people were exposed (Ulstein et al., 1990). The authors speculate about possible factors such as radiation in food that could account for the data. Gofman (1990) summary of existing data concludes there is no safe level of radiation as far as cancer is concerned, and this might provide a basis for this type of finding. While Gofman's conclusions are highly controversial in the scientific community (see Chandler, 1990), a number of scientists feel they should not be dismissed.

Most of the teratogenic effects of X-irradiation appear to be due to the irradiation of the ovum, embryo, or fetus. Some 30 anomalies, many of which involve the central nervous system, have been reported following fetal irradiation. Microcephaly, often seen in mental retardation, is most frequent, but hydrocephaly and other brain malformations, skull defects, and Down syndrome are all increased. Clearly, human experiments using X rays or other irradiation cannot be done to test the validity of these case study results.

Unfortunately, it is the case that we have corroborating data on humans from the "natural experiment" resulting from the atomic bombings of Hiroshima and Nagasaki during World War II. Women in those areas who were pregnant at the time the bombs were dropped showed an enormous increase in the likelihood their offspring would have one or more birth defects. There was also a dose relation, in that the closer the pregnant women were to the places the bombs dropped, the higher the probability of birth defects (Blot & Miller, 1973). Moreover, there was evidence of critical periods. A reanalysis of the radiation data from Japan (Snow, 1985) showed that those exposed in the first 2 weeks after conception had infants with small heads who were not retarded, whereas those who were 8 to 16 weeks into gestation at exposure had babies who were severely retarded. Intelligence was lowered by about 30 IQ points by 1 Gy (a measure of dosage equal to 100 rad)[14] if received in the eighth to fifteenth week. Before the eighth week or after the twenty-fifth week this amount had no effect (Vos, 1989). Long-term follow-up shows that those exposed prenatally to relatively small doses (.30 Gy) develop adult-type cancers earlier than those not exposed until adulthood (Kato et al., 1989). There is now a dramatic increase of adult cancers among prenatally exposed survivors of the atomic bombing (Nomura, 1989).

Data from naturally occurring levels of radiation, such as that given off by certain rock formations, also exist. Pregnant women who live near such rock formations have a greater probability of giving birth to malformed babies (Gentry et al., 1959). In India, Down syndrome and other genetic forms of severe mental retardation have been found to be four times as high in an area of relatively high background radiation levels as in the control population. Similar findings exist for parts of Brazil (Mauss, 1983).

The relation between irradiation and Down has been further documented by a study of 216 families with a Down infant and a comparable control group of families with normal children of the same sexes born in the same hospital at the same time. The Down mothers had had seven times as much exposure to radiation. The fathers also had had more exposure to radar, which involves low-level irradiation (Cohen & Lilienfeld, 1970). Contradictory findings regarding irradiation and increases in Down syndrome are cited in Pueschel (1983).

Another effect of X-irradiation that can be found in rats and mice is reduced learning ability. A report on human victims of in utero exposure to atomic radiation from the Hiroshima and Nagasaki bombs shows that, in general, the risk of mental retardation rose directly with increasing dose (Blot & Miller, 1973).

One of the classic books on teratology states:

Prenatal irradiation produces death, decreased size, and congenital malformations. Preimplantation, pre-organogenetic, and undifferentiated embryos are killed or retarded in growth, but not usually malformed, whereas those undergoing differentiation or organogenesis are malformed as well as stunted and killed. (Kalter, 1968, p. 137)

These findings imply that it is unwise to have *unnecessary* X rays, especially during one's childbearing years and during pregnancy. Frivolous usage, such as for fitting children's shoes or determining pelvic size in pregnancy, could raise total exposure of women at childbearing age to harmful levels.[15] Dental usage has improved, and even for less careful usage, technicians are probably more at risk than their patients. Many states that once required chest X rays for employment in positions that require contact with many young people (e.g., teachers) now mandate X rays only if the skin test is positive (a sign of previous exposure, not current disease). Thus the primary source of X-irradiation strong enough to be a major teratogen today is its therapeutic, not its diagnostic, use. A major source of radiation effects on conception is preconceptional or gestational exposure to radiation used to treat cancer in the mother. Recent statistical data indicate that children have good outcomes if no radiation is given *during* pregnancy (Willard, 1989).

Other forms of irradiation, such as those from microwave ovens and from electrical fields resulting from power lines or from household wiring, have been considered suspect. Computer terminals have been exonerated (Schnorr et al., 1991). There are few existing data on this subject, and what data exist are flawed. There seems no real reason to suspect such sources, although a thoroughly prudent approach might be to not use electric blankets during pregnancy. If they are used to warm the bed, they should be unplugged afterward, not just turned off (Morgan, 1989).[16]

OTHER POSSIBLE EXTERNAL AGENTS

Other direct effects of the environment are possible. Although floating in the amniotic fluid protects fetuses from many blows, jars, and sounds, they can hear very loud sounds and they can be affected by very strong blows. It is known that very strong blows can bring on premature labor, and it is even possible that such events in early development might be responsible for club feet. No research has yet demonstrated unequivocally that environmental events outside the mother's

---

14. The Gy (abbreviation for Gray) is the official international unit for absorbed dose that takes account of body weight.

15. Although formerly almost routine, use of X rays to determine whether pelvic size would permit vaginal deliveries never made sense. The female pelvis is built to stretch during delivery, and an X ray cannot determine stretchability. Today ultrasound imaging has replaced X rays in determining the relation of the fetus to the mother's structure. There are no known negative effects, but its long-term safety is not yet fully documented.

16. This booklet provides excellent examples of scientific writing for the nonexpert, but the degree of caution lacks any research base.

body (other than radiation) affect the developing embryo or fetus.

There are possible effects of extreme noise. If they turn out to exist, they would have far-ranging implications for the general issue of whether the external environment can directly affect prenatal development. Let us look at the evidence. It has long been known that fetal activity level changes after exposure to loud sounds. There is also evidence that infants born to mothers who have lived near a jet airport during their pregnancies are more likely to be stillborn or to have relatively low birth weights (Ando & Hattori, 1970, 1973; Horner, 1972) and more birth defects (Jones & Tauscher, 1978). It is possible that airplane noises do not directly affect the fetus in utero, but that effects are mediated through the mother, either by her hormonal reactions to the stress of the noise or her transmission of air pollutants from jet exhaust through the placental exchange system.

There is suggestive evidence that infants born to mothers who lived in airport noise throughout their pregnancies react less to the noise than those whose mothers moved near a jet airport late in pregnancy or after the infant was born. If these impressionistic data are correct, we need to find out why such differences occur. It may be that the infants, while still in utero, suffer hearing loss from long-term exposure in the same way that people of any postnatal age do when they are exposed repeatedly to loud noises (jets, rock music, noisy factories, and so on). Alternatively, the offspring of long-term residents may become habituated—that is, become used to hearing the airplane noises—while in utero and so do not respond to this very familiar noise. (The process of habituation is discussed in Chapters 7 and 9.)

If the effects of prenatal exposure to airplane noise on auditory responses after birth are verified and found to be due to noise itself, not to the mother's reactions to it, they would constitute another known agent with a direct effect on the baby. This would be particularly clear-cut because infants' responses to auditory stimulation are direct responses to the independent variable, the airplane noise, rather than a nonspecific effect, such as low birth weight, which has many disparate causes. When effects are measured after birth, the mothers' hormonal and physiological responses to stress are no longer transmitted to their offspring, hence cannot influence the babies' responses.

Although this is an intriguing line of research, the basic phenomenon is not firmly established. The Committee on Hearing, Bioacoustics, and Biomechanics of the National Research Council (1982) examined all available evidence and concluded, "There is no conclusive evidence of detrimental effects of high-intensity sound in higher mammals" (p. 10). With respect to human data, the committee notes the limited amounts of data, inadequate samples, and lack of appropriate control populations. Nevertheless, the committee suggests that "until better information is available it would appear prudent for pregnant women to avoid exposures of long duration (several hours per day) to loud noises" where loud noises are defined as sounds above 90 dB sound pressure level (p. 10).

The brevity of this section on direct effects accurately reflects the limited body of knowledge. The only direct effects of external environment on the embryo or fetus that are firmly established are those of radiation.

Prenatal Stress

Although the prenatal environmental factors discussed so far could be said to produce stress, there are other conditions more commonly given the label of stress. These can be either physical or psychological.

PHYSICAL STRESS

The role of physical work during pregnancy is one that has long interested people. The degree to which pregnant women are treated with tender loving care and protected from physical labors changes with time and place. In pioneer days, society could ill afford to lose the work done by its women; hence they worked throughout most of their pregnancies. This is true in many cultures, or portions of cultures, where most people live under substandard conditions.

In the United States and many other Western societies, the period of this century prior to the 1960s or 1970s was generally characterized by what we might now consider overprotection of pregnant women. For example, in the 1940s, when I was having my children, mothers were advised not to swim after 6 or 7 months or to drive a car after 7 months. I did talk my doctor into allowing me to drive for 8 months, and actually drove (in a blizzard) the night before my delivery at full term. In the 1970s most doctors had a more moderate outlook on the physical stresses pregnant women could safely undergo; for example, a colleague of mine was allowed to pursue running during her pregnancy until it became painful (in her ninth month). A recent review states that although more research is needed, the majority of published studies indicate that fitness-type conditioning does not jeopardize fetal well-being in healthy, well-nourished women (Wolfe et al., 1989) and may lead to easier childbirth. The article gives a prudent set of guidelines to follow in the absence of further scientific data. Exercise in late pregnancy is thought to be a possible trigger of premature labor. The rowing ergometer, recumbent bicycle, and upper-arm ergometer produce the least uterine activity in the last trimester of pregnancy (Durak et al., 1990).

Older studies reported greater numbers of malformations and problems in infants of mothers who worked at extremely hard jobs. These included jobs that led to the mother's suffering from toxemia (often combined with her generally poor physical condition) and frequently involved exposure to various chemical pollutants and frequent illness on the job. Hence it is hard to determine the effect of the physical labor itself.

Stott (1972), whose work was cited above in relation to smoking, also studied the effects of work. In his random Glasgow sample he found 153 mothers who worked hard and 26 who did heavy work at which they had to stand a great deal and who complained of feelings of tiredness. As a measure of effects he used his Morbidity Ratio (MR). There were no effects on the children of the mothers' hard work, but the 26 mothers with the greatest degree of physical stress had children at greater risk for high morbidity. A 30% increase in the MR was found for those who stood nearly all day and carried heavy loads (Stott & Latchford, 1976). Much earlier work had found that mothers who did heavy pulling or carried heavy loads during pregnancy had infants with a significant increase in congenital defects, as well as a greater incidence of prematurity and perinatal death. Women who do such work are likely to have many other characteristics, such as poor nutrition, poor living conditions, and illnesses, that operate to make their childbearing more hazardous. However, recent data show a significant association between standing on the job and preterm births, but not low birth weight, even after statistical controls for parity, smoking, education, caffeine and marijuana use, race, and marital status (Teitelman et al., 1990). A. D. McDonald et al. (1987) interviewed a massive sample (more than 56,000 women with more than 104,000 pregnancies) about their social and personal characteristics, and examined several outcomes of their pregnancies. While the researchers did not define occupational groups with sufficient detail to make possible an adequate assessment of the degree of physical (or chemical) stress, this study's use of statistical controls for many possible confounding variables (e.g., smoking, alcohol, ethnicity, education, height) and its sample size make it worth reporting. The outcomes examined were spon-

taneous abortion, stillbirth (without defect), congenital defects, and birth weight below 2,500 g. Those in sales and in service occupations, both of which are likely to involve being on one's feet a great deal, had more spontaneous abortions. An excess of stillbirths without defects were found for those who worked in agriculture, horticulture, leather work, and certain sales occupations. The first three all involve exposure to chemical agents. Low birth weight was more frequent in occupations characterized by their employment of low-SES people. While the differences are small, they are statistically significant because of the large sample. Jobs that involve a lot of standing led to more premature births (7.7% compared with 4.2% for sedentary jobs). The rate was even lower, 2.8%, for women with active jobs (Teitelman et al., 1990). In this large sample low birth weight was not affected after controlling for confounding factors.

Work environments may have teratogenic effects due to chemical or other exposures (including X rays) that are known to be capable of harming the embryo or fetus. More often, workers may be exposed to substances or conditions that are thought to have the potential to harm, for example, pesticides or high levels of noise, as in textile factories. There is simply not enough evidence yet to tell us which substances actually are dangerous and how dangerous they are. None of the evidence indicates that holding a job during pregnancy, in itself, threatens the well-being of the developing organism.

Little attention has been paid to the possible role of the father's work. Recent evidence that the risk for Down syndrome varies in some paternal occupation groups needs further study (Olshan et al., 1989).

PSYCHOLOGICAL STRESS

Through the ages, magical mechanisms have been thought to account for effects of what we would call psychological stress. Actually, there are biologically sound mechanisms by which psychological stress might be transmitted to the offspring. Stress elicits hormonal reactions, and the hormones may pass the placental barrier and have an effect on development. Even anxiety about and during labor and delivery may cause stress that could increase the risk of complications that can affect the infant (see Chapter 5). The influence of psychological stress during pregnancy on the physiological and behavioral responses of human offspring was first investigated by Sontag and his colleagues in the 1930s and 1940s (for a summary, see Sontag et al., 1969). In the late 1950s experimental studies of such effects were conducted using animal models.

Animal Studies

Early research on prenatal psychological stress was begun by Thompson and his collaborators (Thompson, 1957; Thompson et al., 1962). They used animals to enable control of variables that are impossible to control in humans. Female rats were trained to avoid shock when a conditioned stimulus (CS) was presented. After training they were mated, and during their pregnancies the CS, but no shock, was presented. They could not make the response that had previously permitted them to avoid the shock. Thus the experimenters could create stress in the pregnant rats without giving them shocks that might have a direct effect on their fetuses or on the fetal-maternal system. Hence any effects on the fetuses could be presumed to result from the *psychological* stress.

The effects of prenatal exposure to maternal anxiety were separated from those of being reared by an anxious mother who might care for her pups in an atypical way, a control that would be impossible in human studies. The shock-escape-trained rats were mated at the same time as rats that had not been trained (or shocked). Then, when the rats gave birth, half of the pups from the trained ("anxious") rat mothers (dams) were given to the nonanxious dams and vice versa (a procedure known as **cross-fostering).**

There were behavioral differences between those pups that gestated in the "anxious" and those that gestated in the "normal" dams, regardless of which they had been reared by. When placed in an open field, which arouses fear in rats, rats from the anxious dams had increased defecation and decreased activity, and took longer to start to run, all signs of emotionality. These differences were relatively long lasting (Hockman, 1961; Thompson, 1957; Thompson et al., 1962). The prenatal treatment also affected the dam's behavior after her pups were born, thus underscoring the importance of cross-fostering. Stressed dams have been shown to produce different effects in offspring and stressed pups to elicit different maternal behaviors from unstressed dams than do nonstressed pups (Moore & Power, 1986).

Later researchers added controls for some, but not all, extraneous influences. The chief unanswered criticism is that the loud buzzer used as a CS might itself be aversive. If so, it could have affected the pups directly. Subsequent studies have used a large variety of stressors: handling and saline injection (Peters, 1982), restraint and light exposure (Ward, 1984), crowded housing (Crump & Chevins, 1989; Moore & Power, 1986), and direct injection of ACTH (Stylianopoulou, 1983). Monkey studies have shown that shining light into the cages of pregnant females, jumping up and down in front of

them, and daily handling all produce stress responses in the fetus (Morishima et al., 1978; Myers & Myers, 1979). The continued stress of daily handling leads to placental insufficiency and low birth weight (Myers & Myers, 1979).

Recent studies have tended to look at adult sexual behaviors in the offspring of the stressed dams. A number of the stressors studied show deficits in these behaviors for males (Crump & Chevins, 1989; Stylianopoulou, 1983; Takahashi et al., 1987; Ward, 1984).

Taken in their totality, these studies raise another question of great interest concerning the role of genetic differences generally, not just sex differences. Some of the early replications of Thompson's work failed to obtain the same results. It turned out that either different species (mice instead of rats) or different strains of rats had been used in these studies. It is possible that there are differences among strains in both hormonal and behavioral reactions to stressful experiences. It is also possible that the same maternal disturbance could have different effects on fetuses with different genotypes. In fact, it is likely that the maternal and fetal genotypes would interact and that the genotypes of both, as well as their interaction, would lead to phenotypic differences. Unfortunately, experiments that have examined strain crosses in ways that would help to separate these effects have neglected to use the necessary control of cross-fostering. It is necessary not only for the reasons cited above, but because research has shown that the rearing practices of mothers of different strains or species affect the phenotypic behaviors of the young.

Strain and species differences are of particular relevance to the issues of this book, because they may be highly analogous to individual differences in humans. Even in such a direct treatment condition as injecting ACTH in the pregnant dams, there are litter differences (Stylianopoulou, 1983). Research with strain crosses shows that the effect of any given stress or strain on a particular organism depends both on the genotype of the mother exposed to the stress and the genotype of the infant exposed to the mother's stress reactions during intrauterine life.

On the basis of animal work, Frida and Weinstock (1988) have concluded that prenatal stress induces permanent changes that might cause the increased reactivity to anxiety-provoking situations that prenatally stressed rats show.

Human Studies

Much of the available research on humans has studied women who have children with some abnormality and who have reported on their pregnancy histories from memory. Such retrospective studies almost invariably show more unusual or abnormal factors or stresses than one would expect. Mothers of children with severe problems such as cerebral palsy or retardation may seek a plausible explanation by selectively remembering (or inventing) events in their past histories. In contrast, mothers whose children have no abnormalities may have forgotten similar untoward events given their lack of consequence. Because of these problems, the results of **prospective** studies (studies that commence prior to knowledge of the outcome) that start with pregnant women and determine the stresses they are subject to prior to giving birth are much more convincing. No long-term memory is required and the mother has no outcome to try to explain. Unfortunately, the outcomes measured in prospective studies are not always meaningful.

In research conducted by Davids and colleagues, women ($N = 53$) who seemed accepting of and unstressed by their pregnant state (based on responses to projective tests administered during pregnancy) were less likely to have assorted complications of delivery or abnormalities (Davids & DeVault, 1962; Davids et al., 1961). Greek and British data show that high psychological stress scores, measured by questionnaires, are related to obstetric complications (Georgas et al., 1984; Newton, 1985). Indian data suggest that women with threatened abortions during pregnancy are more likely to have such stresses as economic problems, family illness, and adjustment to in-laws than those with normal pregnancies (Jahan, 1987a, 1987b).

Davids and DeVault (1962) also measured maternal anxiety using the Taylor Manifest Anxiety Scale, and related it to later development of the infant. Infants of anxious mothers scored lower on the Bayley test at 8 months of age (102.5 versus 109.5 on mental and 100.5 versus 107.5 on motor performance). However, postbirth factors could account for this inasmuch as the mothers differed in a variety of ways (higher maternal irritability, hostility, and control) (Davids et al., 1963).

Another prospective study administered an anxiety test to mothers in each trimester of pregnancy (Ottinger & Simmons, 1964). Babies of mothers in the high-anxiety group cried more when hungry than babies of mothers in the low-anxiety group. Since they did not cry more after feedings, the interpretation was that babies stressed by maternal anxiety during pregnancy were less able to cope with the stress of hunger. However, more crying may not be maladaptive, because it might serve to get food more quickly.

Stott (1973) found that stress was related to infant outcomes only when it involved personal tension in the mother. Deaths, illnesses in the family, and similar

events led to higher morbidity scores only if the circumstances were traumatic and involved direct participation of the pregnant woman—for example, helping an accident victim or helping after an attempted suicide. Czechoslovakian findings of Cepicky and Mandys (1989) show that birth weight is not affected by being widowed during pregnancy. Situational stresses led to higher morbidity scores only when they included personal tensions, and then the relation was particularly high when the stress was continuous, likely to erupt at any time, or incapable of resolution. When unfavorable surroundings or low socioeconomic status were not accompanied by personal tensions, they were only slightly related to child morbidity. Every single aspect of child morbidity, except physical defects, was associated with personal tensions during pregnancy. A case-by-case analysis of the 14 mothers who had been high on personal tensions during pregnancy showed that 10 of their infants had one or more indications of congenital hyperactivity, and twice as large a proportion of their infants were late or poor walkers as in the group at large. In today's world one has to remember that women under tension are more likely to use and abuse drugs and gain less weight, all factors that could lead to negative outcomes for their fetuses (Zuckerman, Amaro, et al., 1989).

Stott engaged in extensive comparisons and analyses to bolster the conclusion that postnatal factors could not account for the relations found. Hence, although his study was correlational, he considered it plausible to consider personal tensions to be the causal factor. Stott and Latchford's (1976) larger, but retrospective, study confirmed many of these findings. Temporary physical stresses such as operations, accidents, and falls were not related to morbidity. However, morbidity was increased by moving to a new locale in what appeared to be direct relation to the personal tensions associated with the move. The MR was increased 20% by moves in the same locale, 31% by those to new localities, and 47% by those that both took the family away from the mother's mother and were reported as disturbing. Fear of job loss had more deleterious effects than actual job loss, and economic worries, such as a husband out of work or being in debt during pregnancy, were related to morbidity. The effects of illnesses and deaths during pregnancy were small compared with those related to tensions with husbands, family members, or outsiders. The MR increased 57% for those whose mothers reported fears about their marriages, 94% for marital discord, and 137% for being short of money but having husbands who spent freely. Inasmuch as these sorts of personal tensions continue during the child's postnatal life, and inasmuch as children in such families do not get assigned to rearing by nonanxious mothers, prenatal effects cannot be separated from postnatal.

The data from one study that is not quite prospective and yet not really retrospective are worth citing (Cohen, 1981). Mothers responded to a standardized interview after giving birth but before they had had any extended contact with their infants. The interview was scored for physical, psychological, and total stress during pregnancy. The mothers also rated themselves on their anxiety in general and their anxiety during pregnancy. All infants had previously been assessed on the Graham/Rosenblith neonatal tests (see Chapter 8), and all were judged healthy to the degree that they were not receiving any special care in the nursery. Low psychological stress scores were related to low irritability during the neonatal examination, and moderate physical stress scores were related to good motor performance. Mothers' self-reports on their degree of stress during pregnancy were less related to their babies' behaviors than were the scores derived from the interviews about actual happenings during pregnancy. Mothers rated low on anxiety during pregnancy were more likely to have babies with optimal scores on the neonatal subtest most related to outcomes at 4 and 7 years of age (Rosenblith, 1979, 1990). Although the above data are based on only 32 mother-infant pairs, they are not only significant, but impressive. Of the 8 babies whose mothers scored in the lowest quartile for psychological stress during pregnancy, 7 were in the lowest quartile on irritability. At the other extreme, of the 7 babies whose mothers were in the highest quartile, only 1 was in the lowest quartile on irritability.

One short-term stress, anxiety while waiting for an amniocentesis to detect possible genetic abnormalities, increases maternal scores on an anxiety questionnaire (Rossi, 1987). Fetal motor activity during the preliminary ultrasound examination is increased compared with those whose mothers are undergoing routine ultrasound examination. Fetal activity has also been shown to be modified by artificially induced maternal emotions (Van-den-Bergh et al., 1989).

One form of possible prenatal stress that is of special interest is that occasioned by premarital conception and/or illegitimate birth. Stewart (1955) showed that there was twice as much prematurity and three times as many perinatal deaths in such groups, even though three-fourths of the infants were born in wedlock. In fact, the proportion of fetal deaths was higher among the premaritally conceived than among the illegitimate. A Czechoslovakian study showed that babies born to unmarried mothers had lower birth weights then those born to married women or women wid-

owed during pregnancy (Cepicky & Mandys, 1989). Stott and Latchford (1976) showed a 44% increase in the MR for the illegitimate or premaritally conceived. Among those illegitimate infants who were adopted (a form of cross-fostering) the MR was only 37% higher, but it was 66% higher for those kept by their mothers. Although the data are biased in favor of those adopted by the fact that unhealthy babies had a poorer chance of being adopted, the question of postnatal influence again looms large.

The sort of stress that results from unwelcome pregnancy is not limited to premarital or illegitimate pregnancies. Those mothers in Stott and Latchford's (1976) study who reported that they had not intended the pregnancy had children with a 24% increase in MR, and children whose mothers reported feeling desperate about the pregnancy had a 46% increase. Premarital and unwanted pregnancies showed greater effects in families that were also inadequately housed. These data are compatible with Czechoslovakian data on the offspring of parents who had twice been denied a requested abortion, hence had given birth to unwanted children. These children continue to differ from controls throughout childhood and adolescence in ways that reflect lower psychological health (Matejcek et al., 1985).

Stott did not present data on deaths or pregnancy loss. Drillien et al. (1966) had shown earlier that there are increased prenatal deaths in pregnancies when the mother is emotionally distressed. Because boys are more likely to die prenatally, this finding provides a possible explanation for the fact that families with high amounts of stress have more girls than boys (Eckhoff et al., 1961). There are other data that make this speculation plausible, though it is still unproven. A recent review of studies on the effects of maternal psychosocial stress on prematurity and delivery complications found such relations, but not relations to birth weight (Levin & DeFrank, 1988).

Several studies recently have looked at one stressful occupation, that of physician, in relation to obstetric complications and pregnancy outcomes. Women physicians have usually not differed in complications from control groups or their age groups, with the possible exception of having an excess of premature births (Osborn et al., 1988; Phelan, 1988).

A prospective Swedish study interviewed 532 mothers with regard to 41 stress factors and divided them according to levels of psychosocial stress (Nordberg et al., 1989). The children (452 of them) were followed for the first year to year and a half of life. Of the 90 (20%) who were below average in development, 32% came from homes with serious psychosocial stress and

29% from homes with mild stress. Of the 9 children with really low scores on a developmental test, 7 came from homes with psychosocial stress. Unfortunately, it is not possible to tease out the purely psychological from the social stresses in these data.

The effects of stress on the prenatal maternal and embryonic/fetal systems are presumably mediated by hormonal reactions in the mother. Earlier in this chapter we saw that excess hormones, either administered exogenously (from outside) or produced by a mother with a hormonal disorder (endogenous) are harmful to the developing embryo and fetus. It should also be added that those produced by the fetus itself may play a role. In the case of psychological stress, the increased levels of hormonal production are presumably lower than those required to produce obvious damage, but great enough to have some deleterious effects on the embryo or fetus. A recent Japanese study looked directly at women's hormonal reactions to two potentially stressful situations, working when pregnant and living with their parents. The hormonal outputs of both groups indicated that they were under considerable stress (Hiraoka, 1989).

As can be seen from the animal data, long-range effects on adult sexual behavior need to be examined. There are some human data, albeit inadequate, that indicate a weak influence of stress in the second trimester on sexual orientation (Ellis et al., 1988). Better prospective studies and prospective studies linked with hormonal studies are necessary if we are to understand the role of psychological stress during pregnancy more fully. As techniques of hormonal assay improve, it will be possible to deal directly with hormonal levels during pregnancy in relation both to psychological stressors and to outcomes for infants. Genetic differences in reactions to stress (discussed in relation to the animal work) may be mediated by differential reactivity of the hormonal systems. Such differences in both the maternal and fetal genotype may be important.

OVERVIEW

The methodological difficulties, the relative sparseness, and the noncomparability of studies of psychological stress during pregnancy make it difficult to decipher the research in this area (see McAnarney & Stevens-Simon, 1990, for a recent brief review). Nonetheless, considering both the relatively well-controlled experimental animal research and the human studies with all their problems, it seems likely that babies of women who are tense/anxious/stressed during pregnancy are adversely affected. Exactly how is diffi-

cult to tell, because the dependent measures vary greatly across studies. If we put the effects into three major classes—emotionality, physical outcomes, and sexual behaviors of males—we can find consistencies across variations in experimental designs and operational definitions. Increased emotionality is a major effect found in animal research and may be roughly comparable to the measures of irritability and crying when hungry that have been found to correlate with psychological stress in the human studies. Birth complications and the Morbidity Ratio have been used to assess physical outcomes, and correlations with psychological stress during pregnancy have been found for both. Animal data point to differences in adult sexual behaviors of males as a result of many types of maternal prenatal stresses.

One must also remember the effects of stress on other behaviors that can affect the fetus. One group who works with inner-city pregnant women has pointed out that educating women about the harmful effects on their fetuses of various drugs they take may be futile if there are no programs to help them deal with the stresses in their lives. Stress in their patients was related to use of cigarettes, alcohol, and cocaine (Zuckerman, Amaro, et al., 1989).

The positive conclusions derived from this analysis need to be tempered by the knowledge of the inadequacies of the research. Prospective rather than retrospective studies, cross-fostering to control for experiences after birth (adoption or foster homes in humans), hormonal assays to measure directly the hormonal concomitants of stress, new and better manipulation of stress in animal research, and clearly defined outcome measures are needed. The research to date is more tantalizing than conclusive.

Issues in Teratology

Teratology is the study of the causes of congenital malformations. It could have been discussed in Chapter 3, because teratologists also study problems with genes and chromosomes that cause congenital defects. In strict usage, teratology is concerned with major congenital malformations (Kalter & Warkany, 1983). However, the concept has been broadened by some to include more minor malformations and behavioral differences (see Fein et al., 1983; Hutchings, 1978, 1989; Werboff & Gottlieb, 1963).

I agree with the behavioral teratologists or developmental toxicologists that behavioral differences are important and may exist for more agents and with less exposure than gross malformations. I also agree with

Kalter and Warkany (1983) when they say that "the ascertainment of minor structural blemishes and aberrations, which are usually of little or no medical importance, of reduced birth weight at term, spontaneous abortion, and of mental retardation is often liable to biases" (p. 425).

The study of teratology in its broader conceptualization is important if it meets the following criteria: (a) The outcomes studied are of long-term importance for the medical or psychological functioning of the child, as would be the case for mental retardation; and (b) close attention is paid to the methodological problems. I fear that research that does not meet these criteria is publicized and made the basis for policies of mothers, doctors, and even federal agencies.

COMPLEXITIES OF TERATOLOGY

We have seen that a given teratological agent may have very different effects depending on timing, dosage (or severity), genotype, and unknown factors. Another way of trying to make clear the complexities of teratology is to examine all of the different teratological agents or events that have been accused of leading to one single problem. For illustration, hearing impairment will be discussed here.

Hearing impairment may be genetically caused or caused by prenatal or perinatal environmental events. Maternal diseases, diseases contracted by the baby during delivery, and drugs may all affect the newborn's hearing. Rubella in the mother is a frequent cause of hearing problems, and so are diabetes and syphilis (5% of babies). Asian flu and infectious mononucleosis appear to result in occasional cases. In addition, CMV (cytomegalovirus) contracted from the mother at the time of delivery may lead to hearing defects. The drugs that have been implicated range from the so-called ototoxic antibiotics (i.e., ones that can destroy otoliths or hair cells, such as streptomycins, neomycin, kanamycin) and thalidomide to those for which the evidence is not clear, such as quinine, aspirin, various aniline dyes, and carbon monoxide (Gluck, 1971). In addition, severe hyperbilirubinemia at birth (from whatever cause) may produce hearing loss, probably due to loss of neurons in the cochlear nuclei (Konigsmark, 1971).

WAYS TERATOGENS CAN AFFECT DEVELOPMENT

Many environmental factors can operate to affect the developing embryo or fetus. In this chapter they have been grouped according to the nature of the environmental agent (for example, drugs, diseases, stresses). It might be more logical, though less obvious to the layperson, to group the environmental agents that can affect viability and constitution in terms of the mechanisms that may mediate the effects or be the direct cause of the problems:

(1) Environmental agents may operate at a genetic level, causing damage to chromosomes or genes or the splicing mechanisms that affect the instructional map for development prior to embryogenesis.

(2) Environmental agents may operate at the level of causing destruction of or damage to organ systems at the time of their rapid growth and differentiation.

(3) Environmental agents may operate to slow down or stunt normal growth and development during fetal development.

The first two modes of operation may give rise to physically obvious problems (teratological effects) or affect internal structures and become obvious only after death or as a result of special examination procedures (e.g., X rays, EEGs, CAT scans). Other effects may be biochemical, analogous to the inborn errors of metabolism. The third class is visible when total growth is affected and is often indexed by low birth weight or head circumference.

The brain is an organ of special interest to this discussion. Damage to it can occur through any of the three mechanisms. Because only gross defects can be detected, even with special techniques, and because its gross characteristics are not closely related to its function, behavioral teratology tries to assess damage to function.

Much of the work reviewed in this chapter has concentrated on easily measured characteristics, such as proportions who die or who have low birth weights. Not only are these measures crude indices of the underlying problems, they are usually a result of many different influences. When the effects of a teratogen are startling, clear-cut, and distinctive, as is the case with thalidomide and rubella, it is possible to pinpoint the primary causative agent. When the effects are limited to low birth weight or slightly lowered behavioral functioning, it is difficult to assign primary responsibility to any one of the potential causes.

Summary

Teratogens, external agents that can cause abnormalities in the development of the embryo or fetus, include infectious agents, maternal diseases, drugs, radiation, and possibly maternal stress. Teratogens can cause obvious problems such as pregnancy wastage, malformations or growth retardation, and neurological, intellectual, or behavioral problems, which may be difficult to detect. The study of these is called behavioral teratology or developmental pharmacology.

MATERNAL DISEASES AND CHRONIC CONDITIONS

Maternal infectious diseases such as rubella may affect the embryo or fetus early in pregnancy, during embryogenesis, and do structural damage. Syphilis appears to attack the fetus only after 16 weeks. Herpes simplex (which can cause death or severe CNS disorders), group B streptococcus (which can cause meningitis and death), and gonorrhea (which can cause blindness) are transmitted during childbirth. We do not yet know when during gestation AIDS is most likely to be acquired or most dangerous. It can cause physical malformations and neurological problems due to brain infection.

Chronic hormonal disorders of the mother such as hypo- and hyperthyroidism and diabetes affect prenatal development. Adequate medication blocks effects for hypothyroidism and diabetes, but the medication for hyperthyroidism can itself do harm. Chronic maternal conditions such as high blood pressure and heart and kidney disease pose risks for mother and fetus. Discontinuation of the pregnancy or premature delivery is often indicated. Growth retardation is a likely outcome for the fetus.

Babies of older mothers are at higher risk for Down syndrome. Babies of very young mothers may be at risk for prematurity or SGA due to inadequate prenatal care and nutrition.

MALNUTRITION, OXYGEN DEPRIVATION, AND HYPERTHERMIA

The nutritional status of the mother affects her reproductive functions as well as the health of her baby. A proper balance of vitamins, minerals, and calories, especially protein calories, is essential both before and during pregnancy. Severe malnutrition can cause permanent growth retardation that will have effects in the following generation. Other infant malnutrition is usually due to poor fetal environment: implantation where the blood supply is inadequate, placental inadequacy, or multiple fetuses.

Oxygen deprivation as a result of certain maternal conditions or the mother's dwelling at very high altitudes may result in maternal changes that cause growth retardation. Although hyperthermia, especially in interaction with alcohol or other drugs, alters brain growth in animals, its effects on human pregnancies are not known. The heating produced by using saunas is not harmful. Other teratogens may affect nutrition or oxygen supply and thus have indirect effects.

NONPSYCHOTROPIC DRUGS

Thalidomide, the first drug identified as a human teratogen, proved that drugs pass the placental barrier. It also dramatized the necessity of conducting clinical trials with pregnant humans before licensing a drug for their use.

Some steroid hormones have teratogenic effects. Both natural and synthetic sex hormones can cause fetal loss, prematurity, low birth weight, or abnormalities in sexual differentiation. Evidence for behavioral differences is more complex and controversial. Adrenal hormones can affect growth and development.

Antiepileptic drugs, folic acid antagonists, inhalant anesthetics, certain vitamins in excessive doses, some antibiotics, and some antidepressants are teratogenic. Many substances are suspect (quinine, insulin, oral hypoglycemic drugs, drugs used in the treatment of tuberculosis, pesticides, and even aspirin), but the evidence is not clear, which means that their effects are not likely to be major.

LEGAL PSYCHOTROPIC DRUGS AND PROBLEMS IN THE STUDY OF DRUGS

Research on the direct effects of alcohol (and other drugs) is difficult. Such effects are apt to be confounded with those of other substances, including those of cigarettes. Effects such as intellectual and behavioral deficits, measured at later times, can be confounded with effects of inadequate environment. Questions about the amount, frequency, and timing of use during pregnancy, as well as both the mother's and the father's prepregnancy use need to be answered. Differential effects on male and female offspring need to be better understood.

Alcohol is an important drug, in terms of both frequency of use and severity of effects. Fetal alcohol syndrome, the direst outcome, includes growth deficiencies and dysmorphic characteristics, as well as mental retardation. The milder FAE is less definite. Outcomes are worse when alcohol is combined with smoking than when either is used alone. More data on the amount, time during pregnancy (or before), and frequency of consumption are badly needed.

Research on the impact of cigarette smoking is inconsistent and incomplete. Prematurity and low birth weight are common effects, especially for male children and those of older mothers. Increased fetal and neonatal death rates are still controversial, as are effects on later intellectual functioning. Whether effects are directly caused by nicotine (or tars), or whether insufficient oxygen, malnutrition, twinning, placental abnormalities, lead accumulation, or other drugs used are mediating causes, or interact with nicotine to cause the problems, is unknown. Postnatal exposure to smoking may add to differences in long-term outcomes such as increased morbidity.

The effects of caffeine are also difficult to separate from other life-style variables, including smoking and drinking, but they may relate to birth weight as well as parental fertility.

ILLEGAL PSYCHOTROPIC DRUGS

Illegal drugs such as heroin, methadone, and cocaine are behavioral teratogens that affect behavior and physiological functioning as well as fetal growth and development. Heroin causes neonatal addiction and problems in motor activity and sleep. Methadone, the legal treatment drug for heroin withdrawal, can itself cause addiction and CNS damage. Behaviors in children of addicts in later life may be affected by child-rearing variables as well as by prenatal exposure.

Marijuana effects have not been well studied in humans, but it has been shown to cause fetal loss in animals. Its active ingredient (THC) causes retardation in placental development, which could lead to other problems. Neurobehavioral effects have been found in sleep and vision neonatally, which may be lasting, but effects seem to depend on ethnic group and maternal nutrition as well as amount of usage.

Cocaine causes pregnancy loss, premature birth, and low birth weight, as well as urinary tract abnormalities. It also affects a wide variety of emotional, social, and cognitive behaviors. Postnatal treatments are only beginning to be tested. Other illegal drugs with teratogenic potential include LSD, PCP, and crystal methamphetamine.

RADIATION AND OTHER POSSIBLE EXTERNAL ENVIRONMENTAL AGENTS

Radiation, which can pass through the mother's body to affect the eggs, embryo, or fetus directly, is often called the "universal teratogen." It causes malformations, CNS damage, and increased susceptibility to cancer. Exposure of the embryo or fetus at any stage of conception can have an effect, but the effect will depend on when during development the exposure occurred. Among potential effects are brain malformations, Down syndrome, various other birth defects, and mental retardation. Effects can also occur from the mother's exposure before conception having affected her ova.

Hard blows to the fetus or unusual noise levels (e.g., proximity to airports) may have a direct effect on the fetus, although it is well protected in the amniotic fluid from the environment outside the mother's body. Apparent effects could be indirect ones mediated by changes in the mother produced by the stresses.

PHYSICAL AND PSYCHOLOGICAL STRESS DURING PREGNANCY

The mother's physical stress is believed to affect the embryo or fetus, although whether the effects are direct or indirect is not known. Hard physical labor, work that involves being on one's feet for long periods, or exposure to chemicals or extreme noise are possible stressors. The effects of such work in interaction with factors such as maternal malnutrition, poverty, and illness, as well as postnatal stresses, need to be determined. An optimal level of maternal activity for fetal development, be it in athletics or in work, needs to be determined.

Animal studies using cross-fostering techniques show more anxious behavior in offspring of psychologically stressed mothers as well as deficits in male sexual behavior. Human studies indicate that babies from stressed mothers exhibit greater irritability, lower infant test scores, and increased morbidity. Again, it must be considered that other life-style variables associated with stress may cause the differences found.

The mother's reactions to psychological stress are thought to affect the embryo or fetus through stress-produced hormones that cross the placental barrier. Techniques for measuring hormones are now available that would permit clarifying research.

References

ABEL, E. L. (1980a). Fetal alcohol syndrome. *Psychological Bulletin, 87,* 29-30.

ABEL, E. L. (1980b). *Marijuana: The first twelve thousand years.* New York: Plenum.

ABEL, E. L. (1981). Behavioral teratology of alcohol. *Psychological Bulletin, 90,* 564-581.

ABEL, E. L. (1984). Prenatal effects of alcohol. *Drug and Alcohol Dependence, 14,* 1-10.

ABEL, E. L. (1985). Fetal alcohol effects: Advice to the advisors. In Malnutrition and tissue injury in the chronic alcoholic [Special issue]. *Alcohol and Alcoholism, 20,* 189-193.

ALFORD, C. A., Reynolds, D. W., & Stagno, S. (1974). Current concepts of chronic perinatal infections. In L. Gluck (Ed.), *Modern perinatal medicine.* Chicago: Year Book Medical Publishers.

AMARO, H., Heeren, T., Morelock, S., Kayne, H., Hingson, R., Alpert, J., & Zuckerman, B. (1986, August). *Effect of maternal marijuana use on birth weight: Ethnic differences.* Paper presented at 93rd Annual Meeting of the American Psychological Association, Washington, DC.

ANDO, Y., & Hattori, H. (1970). Effects of intense noise during fetal life upon postnatal adaptability. *Journal of the Acoustical Society of America, 47,* 1128-1130.

ANDO, Y., & Hattori, H. (1973). Statistical studies on the effects of intense noise during human fetal life. *Journal of Sound Vibration, 27,* 101-111.

AVERY, N. E., & Taeusch, H. W. (1984). Maternal conditions and exogenous influences that affect the fetus/newborn. In M. E. Avery & H. W. Taeusch (Eds.), *Schaffer's diseases of the newborn* (5th ed.). Philadelphia: W. B. Saunders.

BADR, F. M., & Badr, R. S. (1975). Induction of dominant lethal mutation in mice by ethyl alcohol. *Nature, 253,* 134-136.

BARR, H. M., Streissguth, A. P., Darby, B. L., & Sampson, P. D. (1990). Prenatal exposure to alcohol, caffeine, tobacco, and aspirin: Effects on fine and gross motor performance in 4 year old children. *Developmental Psychology, 26,* 339-348.

BARR, H. M., Streissguth, A. P., Martin, D. C., & Herman, C. S. (1984). Infant size at 8 months of age: Relationship to maternal use of alcohol, nicotine, and caffeine during pregnancy. *Pediatrics, 74,* 336-341.

BAUCHNER, H., Zuckerman, B., McClain, M., Frank, D., Fried, L. E., & Kayne, H. (1988). Risk of sudden infant death syndrome in infants with in utero exposure to cocaine. *Journal of Pediatrics, 123,* 831-834.

BECK, F., Moffat, D. B., & Lloyd, J. B. (1973). *Human embryology.* Oxford: Basil Blackwell.

BECKWITH, L. (1988). Intervention with disadvantaged parents of sick preterm infants. *Psychiatry, 51,* 242-247.

BEDI, K. S. (1987). Lasting neuroanatomical changes following undernutrition during early life. In J. Dobbing (Ed.), *Early nutrition and later achievement* (pp. 1-49). London: Academic Press.

BERAL, V. (1990). Leukaemia and nuclear installations: Occupational exposure of fathers to radiation may be the explanation. *British Medical Journal, 300,* 411-412.

BERG, A. T. (1989). Indices of fetal growth: Retardation, perinatal hypoxia-related factors and childhood neurological morbidity. *Early Human Development, 19,* 271-283.

BERGER, A. (1988). Effects of caffeine consumption on pregnancy outcome: A review. *Journal of Reproductive Medicine, 33,* 946-956.

BERKOWITZ, G. S., Skovron, M. L., Lapinski, R. H., & Berkowitz, R. I. (1990). Delayed childbearing and the outcome of pregnancy. *New England Journal of Medicine, 322,* 659-664.

BINGOL, N., Fuchs, M., Diaz, V., Stone, R. K., & Gromish, D. S. (1987). Teratogenicity of cocaine in humans. *Journal of Pediatrics, 110,* 93-96.

BLAIR, V. W., Hollenbeck, A. R., Smith, R. F., & Scanlon, J. W. (1984). Neonatal preference for visual patterns: Modification by prenatal anesthetic exposure? *Developmental Medicine and Child Neurology, 26,* 476-483.

BLOT, W. J., & Miller, R. W. (1973). Mental retardation following in utero exposure to atomic bombs of Hiroshima and Nagasaki. *Radiology, 106,* 617-619.

BOWELL, P., Mayne, K., Puckett, A., Entwistle, C., & Selkon, J. (1989). Serological screening tests for syphilis in pregnancy: Results of a five year study (1983-87) in the Oxford region. *Journal of Clinical Pathology, 42,* 1281-1284.

BROMAN, S. H., & Nichols, P. L. (1981, August). *Predictors of superior cognitive ability in young children.* Paper presented at the meeting of the American Psychological Association, Los Angeles.

BROOKE, O. G., Anderson, H. R., Bland, J. M., Peacock, J. L., & Stewart, C. M. (1989). Effects on birth weight of smoking, alcohol, caffeine, socioeconomic factors, and psychosocial stress. *British Medical Journal, 298,* 795-801.

BROWN, N., Goulding, E., & Fabro, S. (1979). Ethanol embryotoxicity: Direct effects on mammalian embryo in vitro. *Science, 31,* 573-575.

BROWN, S. S. (1991). *Children and parental illicit drug use: Research, clinical, and policy issues* (Summary of a workshop). Washington, DC: National Academy Press.

BURROW, G. (1965). Neonatal goiter after maternal propylthiouracil therapy. *Journal of Clinical Endocrinology, 25,* 403-408.

BUTLER, N. R., & Alberman, E. D. (Eds.). (1969). *Perinatal mortality.* Edinburgh: E. & S. Livingston.

BUTLER, N. R., & Golding, J. (1986). *From birth to five: A study of the health and behavior of Britain's five year olds.* Oxford: Pergamon.

BYERS, J. (1989). AIDS in children: Effects on neurological development and implications for the future. *Journal of Special Education, 23,* 5-16.

CAHALAN, D., Cissin, I. H., & Crossley, H. M. (1969). *American drinking practices: A national study of drinking behavior and attitudes.* New Brunswick, NJ: Rutgers University Press.

CALABRI, G., Polvi, G., Nieri, R. M., et al. (1989). Expected risk of congenital toxoplasmosis in Florence and its province: Statistical research in 1984. *Minerva-Pediatria, 41,* 445-448.

California Department of Health Services. (1989, September 7). *State health director announces final results of study of HIV infection* (Press release).

CARLSON, D. E. (1988). Maternal diseases associated with intrauterine growth retardation. *Seminars in Perinatology, 12,* 17-22.

CARTER, M. P. (1965). A probable epidemic of congenital hydrocephaly in 1940-1941. *Developmental Medicine and Child Neurology, 7,* 61-64.

CEPICKY, P., & Mandys, F. (1989). Reproductive outcome in women who lost their husbands in the course of pregnancy. *European Journal of Obstetrics, Gynecology and Reproductive Biology, 30,* 137-140.

CHANDLER, D. L. (1990, November 5). How much is too much? *Boston Globe,* pp. 45, 47.

CHARLEBOIS, A. T., & Fried, P. A. (1980). The interactive effects of nutrition and cannabis upon rat perinatal development. *Developmental Psychobiology, 13,* 591-605.

CHASNOFF, I. J., Burns, K. A., & Burns, W. J. (1987). Cocaine use in pregnancy: Perinatal morbidity and mortality (Meeting of the Committee on Problems of Drug Dependence: Developmental Effects of Drug Dependence). *Neurotoxicology and Teratology, 9,* 291-293.

CHASNOFF, I. J., Burns, W. J., Schnoll, S. H., & Burns, K. A. (1985). Cocaine use in pregnancy. *New England Journal of Medicine, 313,* 666-669.

CHASNOFF, I. J., & Griffith, D. R. (1989). Cocaine: Clinical studies of pregnancy and the newborn. In D. E. Hutchings (Ed.), Prenatal abuse of licit and illicit drugs [Special issue]. *Annals of the New York Academy of Sciences, 562,* 260-266.

CHASNOFF, I. J., Griffith, D. R., MacGregor, S., Dirkes, K., & Burns, K. A. (1989). Temporal patterns of cocaine use in pregnancy: Perinatal outcome. *Journal of the American Medical Association, 261,* 1731-1744.

CHASNOFF, I. J., Hatcher, R., & Burns, W. (1980). Early growth patterns of methadone-addicted infants. *American Journal of Diseases of Children, 134,* 1040-1051.

CHAVEZ, G. F. O., Mulinare, J., & Cordero, J. F. (1989). Maternal cocaine use during early pregnancy as a risk factor for congenital urogenital anomalies. *Journal of the American Medical Association, 262,* 795-798.

CHRISTOFFEL, K. K., & Salofsky, I. (1975). Fetal alcohol syndrome in dizygotic twins. *Journal of Pediatrics, 87,* 963-967.

CLARREN, S. K., & Smith, D. W. (1978). The fetal alcohol syndrome. *New England Journal of Medicine, 298,* 1063-1067.

COHEN, B. H., & Lilienfeld, A. M. (1970). The epidemiological study of mongolism in Baltimore. *Annals of the New York Academy of Sciences, 171,* 320-327.

COHEN, E. N., Belleville, J. W., & Brown, B. W. (1971). Anesthesia, pregnancy, and miscarriage: A study of operating room nurses and anesthetists. *Anesthesiology, 35,* 343-347.

COHEN, L. (1981). *The effects of maternal psychological stress during pregnancy on subsequent postnatal behavior in 2 day old infants.* Unpublished senior honors thesis, Wheaton College, Norton, MA.

COLES, C. D., Platzman, M. J., & Herbert, S. (1990, April). *Prenatal phenothiazine exposure and neonatal behavior.* Paper presented at the International Conference on Infant Studies, Montreal.

COLLMAN, R., & Stoller, A. (1962). A survey of mongoloid births in Victoria, Australia. *American Journal of Public Health, 52,* 813-829.

Committee on Hearing, Bioacoustics, and Biomechanics, National Research Council. (1982). *Prenatal effects of exposure to high-level noise.* Washington, DC: National Academy Press.

COONEY, G. H., Bell, A., McBride, W., & Carter, C. (1989). Low-level exposures to lead: The Sydney Lead Study. *Developmental Medicine and Child Neurology, 31,* 640-649.

COUSTAN, D. R., Reece, E. A., Sherwin, R. S., Rudolf, M. C., Bates, S. E., Sockin, S. M., Halford, T., & Tamborlane, W. V. (1986). A randomized clinical trial on the insulin pump vs. intensive conventional therapy in diabetic pregnancies. *Journal of the American Medical Association, 255,* 631-636.

CRUMP, C. J., & Chevins, P. F. (1989). Prenatal stress reduces fertility of male offspring in mice without affecting their adult testosterone levels. *Hormones and Behavior, 23,* 333-343.

CURATOLO, P., Brinchi, V., Cusmai, R., Vignetti, P., & Benedetti, P. (1986). Increased chromosomal breakage in epileptic children after long-term treatment. *European Journal of Pediatrics, 145,* 439-442.

DALTON, K. (1968). Ante-natal progesterone and intelligence. *British Journal of Psychiatry, 114,* 1377-1383.

DALTON, K. (1976). Prenatal progesterone and educational attainments. *British Journal of Psychiatry, 129,* 438-442.

DAVIDS, A., & DeVault, S. (1962). Maternal anxiety during pregnancy and childbirth abnormalities. *Psychosomatic Medicine, 24,* 464-470.

DAVIDS, A., DeVault, S., & Talmadge, M. (1961). Anxiety, pregnancy, and childbirth abnormalities. *Journal of Consulting Psychology, 25,* 74-77.

DAVIDS, A., Holden, R. H., & Gray, G. B. (1963). Maternal anxiety during pregnancy and adequacy of mother and child adjustment eight months following childbirth. *Child Development, 34,* 993-1002.

DAVIE, R., Butler, N., & Goldstein, H. (1972). *From birth to seven: The second report of the child development study (1958 cohort).* London: Longman/National Children's Bureau.

DAVIS, J. M., & Svendsgaard, D. J. (1987). Lead and child development. *Nature, 329,* 297-300.

DICKINSON, J., & Gonik, B. (1990). Teratogenic viral infections. *Clinical Obstetrics and Gynecology, 33,* 242-252.

DISHOTSKY, N. I., Loughman, W. D., Mogar, R. E., & Lipscomb, W. R. (1971). LSD and genetic damage: Is LSD chromosome damaging, carcinogenic, mutagenic, or teratogenic? *Science, 172,* 431-440.

DIXON, S. D., & Bejar, R. (1989). Echoencephalographic findings in neonates associated with maternal cocaine and methamphetamine use: Incidence and clinical correlates. *Journal of Pediatrics, 115,* 770-778.

DORRIS, M. (1989). *The broken cord.* New York: Harper & Row.

DOW-EDWARDS, D. L., Freed, L. A., & Milhorat, T. H. (1988). Stimulation of brain metabolism by perinatal cocaine exposure. *Developmental Brain Research, 42,* 137-141.

DOWLER, J. K., & Jacobson, S. W. (1984, April). *Alternative measures of maternal smoking and caffeine consumption as predictors of neonatal outcome.* Paper presented at the International Conference on Infant Studies, New York.

DRILLIEN, C. M., Jameson, S., & Wilkinson, M. E. (1966). Studies in mental handicap: I. Prevalence and distribution by clinical type and severity of defect. *Archives of Diseases of Childhood, 41,* 528-538.

DUMONT, M. (1989). Grippe et grossesse [Influenza and pregnancy]. *Revue Française de Gynecologie et d'Obstetrique, 84,* 605-607.

DURAK, E. P., Jovanovic-Peterson, L., & Peterson, C. M. (1990). Comparative evaluation of uterine response to exercise on five aerobic machines. *American Journal of Obstetrics and Gynecology, 162,* 754-756.

DUTTON, G. N. (1989). Recent developments in the prevention and treatment of congenital toxoplasmosis. *International Ophthalmology, 13,* 407-413.

ECKHOFF, E., Gawsha, J., & Baldwin, A. L. (1961). Parental behavior towards boys and girls of preschool age. *Acta Psychologica, 18,* 85.

EHRHARDT, A. A., & Money, J. (1967). Progestin induced hermaphroditism: IQ and psychosexual identity in a study of 10 girls. *Journal of Sex Research, 3,* 83-100.

ELLERT, D., Carly, D., Delcroix, M., Vittu, G., Houze de l'Aulnoit, D., & Brabant, S. (1989). Les enfants des meres hyper et hypothyroidiennes [Children of hyper- and hypothyroid mothers]. *Revue Française de Gynecologie et d'Obstetrique, 84,* 923-927.

ELLIS, F. W., & Pick, J. R. (1980). An animal model of the fetal alcohol syndrome in beagles. *Alcoholism: Clinical and Experimental Research, 4,* 123-134.

ELLIS, L., Ames, M. A., Peckham, W., & Burke, D. (1988). Sexual orientation of human offspring may be altered by severe maternal stress during pregnancy. *Journal of Sex Research, 25,* 152-157.

EMOND, S. E. (1990). Baby aspirin. *Harvard Health Letter, 16*(2), 4-6.

ENKIN, M., Keirse, M. J. N. C., & Chalmers, I. (1989). *A guide to effective care in pregnancy and childbirth.* Oxford: Oxford University Press.

EPSTEIN, L. G., Sharer, L. R., Oleske, J. M., Connor, E. M., Goudsmit, J., Bagdon, L., Robert-Guroff, M., & Koenigsberger, M. R. (1986). Neurologic manifestations of human immunodeficiency virus infection in children. *Pediatrics, 78,* 678-687.

ERIKSSON, M., Billing, L., Steneroth, G., & Zetterstrom, R. (1989). Health and development of 8-year-old children whose mothers abused amphetamine during pregnancy. *Acta Paediatrica Scandinavica, 78,* 944-949.

ERNHART, C. B., Sokol, R. J., Martier, S., Moron, P., Nadler, D., Ager, J. W., & Wolf, A. W. (1987). Alcohol teratogenicity in the human: A detailed assessment of specificity, critical period, and threshold. *American Journal of Obstetrics and Gynecology, 156,* 33-39.

ERNHART, C. B., Wolf, A. W., Linn, P. L., Sokol, R. J., Kennard, M. J., & Filipovich, H. F. (1985). Alcohol-related birth defects: Syndromal anomalies, intrauterine growth retardation, and neonatal behavioral assessment. *Alcoholism: Clinical and Experimental Research, 9,* 447-453.

FECHTER, L. D. (1987). *Neurotoxicity of prenatal carbon monoxide exposure* (Research Report No. 12). Cambridge, MA: Health Effects Institute.

FEDRICK, J., & Alberman, E. D. (1972). Reported influenza in pregnancy and subsequent cancer in the child. *British Medical Journal, 2,* 485-488.

FEIN, G. G., Schwartz, P. M., Jacobson, W. S., & Jacobson, J. L. (1983). Environmental toxins and behavioral development. *American Psychologist, 38,* 1188-1197.

FINNEGAN, L. P., Reeser, P. S., & Connaughton, J. F. (1977). The effects of maternal drug dependence on neonatal mortality. *Drug and Alcohol Dependence, 3,* 131-140.

FLETCHER, J. L., & Gordon, R. C. (1990). Perinatal transmission of bacterial sexually transmitted diseases: Part I. Syphilis and gonorrhea. *Journal of Family Practice, 30,* 448-456.

FLYNN, A., Martier, S. S., Sokol, R. J., Miller, S. I., Golden, N. L., & Del Villano, B. C. (1981). Zinc status of pregnant alcoholic women: A determinant of fetal outcome. *Lancet, 2,* 572-574.

FOX, N. L., Sexton, M., & Hebel, J. R. (1990). Prenatal exposure to tobacco: I. Effects on physical growth at age three. *International Journal of Epidemiology, 19,* 66-71.

FRANK, D. A., Zuckerman, B. S., Amaro, H., Aboagye, K., Bauchner, H., Cabral, H., Fried, L., Hingson, R., Kayne, H., Levenson, S. M., Parker, S., Reece, H., & Vinci, R. (1988). Cocaine use during pregnancy: Prevalence and correlates. *Pediatrics, 82,* 888-895.

FRASER, F. C. (1984). Other congenital defects involving bones. In M. E. Avery & H. W. Taeusch (Eds.), *Schaffer's diseases of the newborn* (5th ed.). Philadelphia: W. B. Saunders.

FRAZIER, T. M., Davis, G. H., Goldstein, H., & Goldberg, I. E. (1961). Cigarette smoking and prematurity: A prospective study. *American Journal of Obstetrics and Gynecology, 81,* 988-996.

FRIDA, E., & Weinstock, M. (1988). Prenatal stress increases anxiety related behavior and alters cerebral lateralization of dopamine activity. *Life Science, 42,* 1059-1065.

FRIED, P. A. (1989a). Cigarettes and marijuana: Are there measurable long-term neurobehavioral teratogenic effects? *Neurotoxicology, 10,* 577-583.

FRIED, P. A. (1989b). Postnatal consequences of maternal marijuana use in humans. In D. E. Hutchings (Ed.), Prenatal abuse of licit and illicit drugs [Special issue]. *Annals of the New York Academy of Sciences, 562,* 123-132.

FRIED, P. A., & Makin, J. E. (1987). Neonatal behavioral correlates of prenatal exposure to marijuana, cigarettes and alcohol in a low risk population. *Neurotoxicology and Teratology, 9,* 1-7.

FRIED, P. A., & Oxorn, H. (1980). *Smoking for two: Cigarettes and pregnancy.* New York: Free Press.

FRIED, P. A., & Watkinson, M. A. (1990). 36- and 48-month neurobehavioral follow-up of children prenatally exposed to marijuana, cigarettes, and alcohol. *Developmental and Behavioral Pediatrics, 11,* 49-58.

FRIED, P. A., Watkinson, M. A., Dillon, R. F., & Dulberg, C. S. (1987). Neonatal neurological status in a low-risk population after prenatal exposure to cigarettes, marijuana, and alcohol. *Journal of Developmental and Behavioral Pediatrics, 8,* 318-326.

GALLER, J. R., Ramsey, F., Solimano, G., Kucharski, L. T., & Harrison, R. (1984). The influence of early malnutrition on subsequent behavioral development: IV. Soft neurological signs. *Pediatric Research, 18,* 826-832.

GARDNER, M. J., Snee, M. P., Hall, A. J., Powell, C. A., Downes, S., & Terrell, J. D. (1990). Results of case-control study of leukaemia and lymphoma among young people near Sellafield nuclear plant in West Cumbria. *British Medical Journal, 300,* 423-429.

GARLAND, S. M., & Kelly, V. N. (1989). Is antenatal screening for syphilis worthwhile? *Medical Journal of Australia, 151,* 368, 370, 372.

GENTRY, J. T., Parkhurst, E., & Bulin, G. V. (1959). An epidemiological study of congenital malformations in N.Y. state. *American Journal of Public Health, 49,* 1-22.

GEORGAS, J., Giakoumaki, E., Georgoulias, N., Koumandakis, E., & Kaskarelis, D. (1984). Psychosocial stress and its relation to obstetrical complications. *Psychotherapy and Psychosomatics, 41,* 200-206.

GLUCK, L. (1971). Neurosensory factors in newborn hearing. In *Conference on newborn hearing screening: Proceedings summary and recommendations.* Sacramento: California State Department of Public Health.

GOFMAN, J. W. (1990). *Radiation-induced cancer from low-dose exposure: An independent analysis.* San Francisco: Committee for Nuclear Responsibility.

GOLUB, M. S., Sassenrath, E. N., & Chapman, C. F. (1981). Regulation of visual attention in offspring of female monkeys treated chronically with delta-9-tetrahydrocannabinol. *Developmental Psychobiology, 14,* 507-512.

GORDON, N. (1968). Folic acid deficiency from anti-convulsant therapy. *Developmental Medicine and Child Neurology, 10,* 497-504.

GOTTESFELD, Z., & Silverman, P. B. (1990). Developmental delays associated with prenatal alcohol exposure are reversed by thyroid hormone treatment. *Neuroscience Letters, 109,* 42-47.

GOY, R. W., Bercovitch, F. B., & McBriar, M. C. (1988). Behavioral masculinization is independent of genital masculinization in prenatally androgenized female rhesus macaques.

Hormones and Behavior, 22, 552-571.

GOY, R. W., & McEwen, B. S. (1980). *Sexual differentiation of the brain.* Cambridge: MIT Press.

GRAHAM, J. M., Jr., Hanson, J. W., Darby, B. L., Barr, H. M., & Streissguth, A. P. (1988). Independent dysmorphology evaluations at birth and 4 years of age for children exposed to varying amounts of alcohol in utero. *Pediatrics, 81,* 772-778.

GRANTHAM-McGREGOR, S., Schofeld, W., & Powell, C. (1987). Development of severely maladjusted children who received psychosocial stimulation: Six-year follow-up. *Pediatrics, 79,* 247-254.

GREENE, M. F., Hare, J. W., Cloherty, J. P., Benacerraf, B. R., & Soeldner, J. S. (1989). First-trimester hemoglobin A1 and risk for major malformation and spontaneous abortion in diabetic pregnancy. *Teratology, 39,* 225-231.

GREENE, M. F., Hare, J. W., Krache, M., Phillippe, M., Barss, V. A., Saltzman, D. H., Nadel, A., Younger, M. D., Heffner, L., & Scherl, J. E. (1989). Prematurity among insulin-requiring diabetic gravid women. *American Journal of Obstetrics and Gynecology, 16,* 106-111.

GRIMM, V. E. (1987). Effect of teratogenic exposure on the developing brain: Research strategies and possible mechanisms. *Developmental Pharmacology and Therapy, 10,* 328-345.

GROSE, C., & Weiner, C. P. (1990). Prenatal diagnosis of congenital cytomegalovirus infection: Two decades later. *American Journal of Obstetrics and Gynecology, 163,* 447-450.

GUNDERSON, V., & Sackett, G. P. (1982). Paternal effects on reproductive outcome and developmental risk. In M. E. Lamb & A. L. Brown (Eds.), *Advances in developmental psychology* (pp. 85-123). Hillsdale, NJ: Lawrence Erlbaum.

HAAS, J. D. (1970). Prenatal and infant growth and development. In P. T. Baker & M. A. Little (Eds.), *Man in the Andes.* Stroudsburg, PA: Dowden, Hutchinson, & Ross.

HAAS, J. D. (1973, December). *Biocultural factors relating to infant growth and motor development in Peru.* Paper presented at the annual meeting of the American Anthropological Association, New Orleans.

HACKMAN, E., Emanuel, I., van Belle, G., & Daling, J. (1983). Maternal birthweight and subsequent pregnancy outcome. *Journal of the American Medical Association, 250,* 2016-2019.

HAGLUND, B., & Cnattingius, S. (1990). Cigarette smoking as a risk factor for sudden infant death syndrome: A population-based study. *American Journal of Public Health, 80,* 29-32.

HANS, S. L. (1989). Developmental consequences of prenatal exposure to methadone. In D. E. Hutchings (Ed.), Prenatal abuse of licit and illicit drugs [Special issue]. *Annals of the New York Academy of Sciences, 562,* 195-207.

HANSON, S. W., Streissguth, A. P., & Smith, D. W. (1978). The effects of moderate alcohol consumption during pregnancy on fetal growth and morphogenesis. *Journal of Pediatrics, 92,* 457-460.

HARDY, J. B., & Mellits, E. D. (1972). Does maternal smoking during pregnancy have a long-term effect on the child? *Lancet, 2,* 1332-1336.

HARLAP, S., & Shiono, P. H. (1980). Alcohol, smoking and incidence of spontaneous abortions in the first trimester. *Lancet, 1,* 173-176.

HATCH, E. E., & Bracken, M. B. (1986). Effect of marijuana use in pregnancy on fetal growth. *American Journal of Epidemiology, 124,* 986-993.

HEUYER, C., Mises, R., & Dereux, J. F. (1957). La descen-

dance des alcoholiques [The descendants of alcoholics]. *La Presse Medicale, 29,* 657-658.

HILL, R. M., Verniaud, W. M., Deter, R. L., Tennyson, L. M., Rettig, G. M., Zion, T. E., Vorderman, A. L., Helms, P. G., McCulley, L. B., & Hill, L. L. (1984). The effect of intrauterine malnutrition on the term infant: A 14-year progressive study. *Acta Paediatrica Scandinavica, 73,* 482-487.

HINES, M., Alsum, P., Roy, M., Gorski, R. A., & Goy, R. W. (1987). Estrogenic contributions to sexual differentiation in the female guinea pig: Influences of diethylstilbestrol and tamoxifen on neural, behavioral and ovarian development. *Hormones and Behavior, 21,* 402-417.

HIRAOKA, T. (1989). [Relationship between social factors and urinary catecholamine concentration in pregnant women] (in Japanese). *Nippon Sanka Fujinka Gakkai Zasshi, 41,* 20-26.

HOCKMAN, C. H. (1961). Prenatal maternal stress in the rat: Its effects on emotional behavior in the offspring. *Journal of Comparative and Physiological Psychology, 54,* 679-684.

HOHLFELD, P., Daffos, F., Thulliez, P., Aufrant, C., Couvreur, J., MacAleese, J., Descombey, D., & Forestier, F. (1989). Fetal toxoplasmosis: Outcome of pregnancy and infant follow-up after in utero treatment. *Journal of Pediatrics, 115,* 765-769.

HOLDINESS, M. R. (1987). Teratology of the antituberculosis drugs. *Early Human Development, 15,* 61-74.

HORNER, J. S. (1972). *The health of Hillington.* Uxbridge, Middlesex: Health Department.

HOWARD, J. (1989). Cocaine and its effects on the newborn. *Developmental Medicine and Child Neurology, 31,* 255-257.

HOWARD, J., Beckwith, L., Rodning, C., & Kropenske, V. (1989, June). The development of young children of substance-abusing parents: Insights from seven years of intervention and research. *Zero to Three: Bulletin of the National Center for Clinical Infant Programs, 9.*

HUME, R. F., Jr., O'Donnell, K. J., Stanger, C. L., Killam, A. P., & Gingras, J. L. (1989). In utero cocaine exposure: Observations of fetal behavior state may predict neonatal outcome. *American Journal of Obstetrics and Gynecology, 161,* 685-690.

HUSSEIN, L., el Shawarby, O., Elnaggar, B., & Abdelmegid, A. (1988). Serum vitamin A and carotene concentrations among Egyptian fullterm neonates in relation to maternal status. *International Journal for Vitamin and Nutrition Research, 58,* 139-145.

HUTCHINGS, D. E. (1978). Behavioral teratology: Embryopathic and behavioral effects of drugs during pregnancy. In G. Gottlieb (Ed.), *Various influences on the brain and behavioral development.* New York: Academic Press.

HUTCHINGS, D. E. (1982). Methadone and heroin during pregnancy: A review of behavioral effects in human and animal offspring. *Neurobehavioral Toxicology and Teratology, 4,* 429-434.

HUTCHINGS, D. E. (1987). Drug abuse during pregnancy: Embryopathic and neurobehavioral effects. In M. D. Braude & A. M. Zimmerman (Eds.), *Genetic and perinatal effects of abused substances* (pp. 131-151). New York: Academic Press.

HUTCHINGS, D. E. (Ed.). (1989). Prenatal abuse of licit and illicit drugs [Special issue]. *Annals of the New York Academy of Sciences, 562.*

HUTCHINGS, D. E., et al. (1985). Design considerations in screening for behavioral teratogens: Results of the collaborative behavioral teratology study (1985, Cincinnati, OH). *Neurobehavioral Toxicology and Teratology, 7,* 639-642.

IANNACCONE, P. M., Bossert, N. L., & Connelly, C. S. (1987). Disruption of embryonic and fetal development due to preimplantation chemical insults: A critical review. *American Journal of Obstetrics and Gynecology, 157,* 476-484.

IANNETTI, P., Falconieri, P., & Imperato, C. (1989). Acquired immune deficiency syndrome in childhood: Neurological aspects. *Child's Nervous System, 5,* 281-287.

Institute of Medicine. (1982). *Marijuana and health.* Washington, DC: National Academy of Sciences Press.

IOFFE, S., & Chernick, V. (1988). Development of the EEG between 30 and 40 weeks gestation in normal and alcohol-exposed infants. *Developmental Medicine and Child Neurology, 30,* 797-807.

JACOBSON, S. W., Fein, G. G., Jacobson, J. L., Schwartz, P. M., & Dowler, J. K. (1984). Neonatal correlates of prenatal exposure to smoking, caffeine, and alcohol. *Infant Behavior and Development, 7,* 253-265.

JACOBSON, J. L., Fein, G. G., Jacobson, S. W., Schwartz, P. M., & Dowler, J. K. (1984). The transfer of polychlorinated biphenyls (PCBs) and polybrominated biphenyls (PBBs) across the human placenta and into maternal milk. *American Journal of Public Health, 74,* 378-379.

JACOBSON, J. L., Jacobson, S. W., & Humphrey, H. E. (1990a). Effects of exposure to PCBs and related compounds on growth and activity in children. *Neurotoxicology and Teratology, 12,* 319-326.

JACOBSON, J. L., Jacobson, S. W., & Humphrey, H. E. (1990b). Effects of in utero exposure to polychlorinated biphenyls and related contaminants on cognitive functioning in young children. *Journal of Pediatrics, 116,* 38-45.

JAHAN, M. (1987a). Role of psychological factors in complications during first trimester of pregnancy. *Journal of Personality and Clinical Studies, 3,* 11-16.

JAHAN, M. (1987b). Stress and complications of pregnancy. *Journal of the Indian Academy of Applied Psychology, 13,* 7-11.

JOHNSON, H. L., Diano, A., & Rosen, T. S. (1984). 24-month neurobehavioral follow-up of children of methadone-maintained mothers. *Infant Behavior and Development, 7,* 115-123.

JONAS, M. M., Reddy, R. K., DeMedina, M., & Schiff, E. R. (1990). Hepatitis B infection in a large municipal obstetrical population: Characterization and prevention of perinatal transmission. *American Journal of Gastroenterology, 85,* 277-280.

JONES, F. N., & Tauscher, J. (1978). Residence under an airport landing pattern as a factor in teratism. *Archives of Environmental Health, 35,* 10-12.

JONES, K. L., Smith, P. W., Streissguth, A. P., & Myrianthopoulis, N. C. (1974). Outcome in offspring of chronic alcoholic women. *Lancet, 2,* 1076-1078.

JONES, W. S., & Man, E. B. (1969). Thyroid function in human pregnancy: VI. Premature deliveries and reproductive failures of pregnant women with low serum butanolextractable iodines. *American Journal of Obstetrics and Gynecology, 104,* 909-914.

KALLEN, B. (1987). Search for teratogenic risks with the aid of malformation registries. *Teratology, 35,* 47-52.

KALTENBACH, K., & Finnegan, L. P. (1984). Developmental outcome of children born to methadone maintained women: A review of longitudinal studies. *Neurobehavioral Toxicology and Teratology, 6,* 271-275.

KALTER, H. (1968). *Teratology of the central nervous system.* Chicago: University of Chicago Press.

KALTER, H., & Warkany, J. (1983). Congenital malformations: Etiologic factors and their role in prevention. *New England Journal of Medicine, 308,* 424-431.

KAMINSKI, M., Funeau, C., & Schwartz, D. (1978). Alcohol consumption in pregnant women and the outcome of pregnancy. *Alcoholism: Clinical and Experimental Research, 2,* 155-164.

KAPLAN, K. M., Cochi, S. L., Edmonds, L. D., Zell, E. R., & Preblud, S. R. (1990). A profile of mothers giving birth to infants with congenital rubella syndrome: An assessment of risk factors. *American Journal of Diseases of Children, 144,* 118-123.

KARMEL, B. Z., Gardner, J. M., & Magnano, C. L. (1990). Neurofunctional consequences of in utero cocaine exposure. In *Problems of drug dependence: Proceedings of the 52nd Annual Scientific Meeting (Richmond, VA)* (NIDA Research Monograph). Richmond, VA: Committee on Problems of Drug Dependence.

KATO, H., Yoshimoto, Y., & Schull, W. J. (1989). Risk of cancer among children exposed to atomic bomb radiation in utero: A review. *IARC Scientific Publications, 96,* 365-374.

KATZ, V. L., Miller, N. H., & Bowes, W. A., Jr. (1988). Pregnancy complications of physicians. *Western Journal of Medicine, 149,* 704-707.

KENDALL, S. R., Albin, S., Lowinson, J., Berle, B., Eidelman, A. J., & Gartner, L. M. (1976). Differential effects of maternal heroin and methadone use on birthweight. *Pediatrics, 58,* 681-685.

KENDELL, R. E., & Kemp, I. W. (1989). Maternal influenza in the etiology of schizophrenia. *Archives of General Psychiatry, 46,* 878-882.

KITZMILLER, J., Brown, E., Philippe, M., et al. (1981). Diabetic nephropathy in perinatal outcome. *American Journal of Obstetrics and Gynecology, 141,* 741-751.

KLEBANOFF, M. A., & Berendes, H. W. (1988). Aspirin exposure during the first 20 weeks of gestation and IQ at 4 years of age. *Teratology, 37,* 249-255.

KLEIN, P. S., Forbes, G. B., & Nader, P. R. (1976). Short term starvation in infancy regarding subsequent learning disabilities: A proven relationship? [Letter]. *Journal of Pediatrics, 88,* 702-703.

KLINE, J., Shrout, P., Stein, Z., Susser, M., & Warburton, D. (1980). Drinking during pregnancy and spontaneous abortion. *Lancet, 1,* 176-180.

KLINE, J., Stein, Z., & Hutzler, M. (1987). Cigarettes, alcohol, and marijuana: Varying associations with birthweight. *International Journal of Epidemiology, 16,* 44-51.

KONIGSMARK, B. W. (1971). *Hereditary and congenital factors affecting newborn sensorineural hearing* (Publication of the Conference on Newborn Hearing Screening, San Francisco). San Francisco: California State Department of Public Health.

KUHNERT, P. M., Erhard, P., & Kuhnert, B. R. (1977). Lead and delta-aminolevulinic acid dehydrastase in RBC's of urban mothers and fetuses. *Environmental Research, 14,* 73-80.

KUMAR, M. L., Gold, E., Jacobs, I. E., Ernhart, C. B., & Nankervis, G. A. (1984). Primary cytomegalovirus infection in adolescent pregnancy. *Pediatrics, 74,* 493-500.

KUMAR, R., & Chadhuri, B. N. (1989). Altered maternal thyroid function: Fetal and neonatal development of rats. *Indian Journal of Physiology and Pharmacology, 33,* 233-238.

LAMMER, E. J., Sever, L. E., & Oakley, G. P., Jr. (1987). Teratogen update: Valproic acid. *Teratology, 35*, 465-473.

LANDESMAN-DWYER, S., Keller, L. S., & Streissguth, A. P. (1978). Naturalistic observations of newborns: Effects of maternal alcohol intake. *Alcohol: Clinical and Experimental Research, 2*, 171-177.

LAURENCE, K. M. (1985). Prevention of neural tube defects by improvement in a maternal diet and preconceptional folic acid supplementation. In M. Marois (Ed.), *Prevention of physical and mental congenital defects: Part B. Epidemiology, early detection and therapy, and environmental factors* (pp. 383-388). New York: Allan R. Liss.

LEFKOWITZ, M. M. (1981). Smoking during pregnancy: Long-term effects on offspring. *Developmental Psychology, 17*, 192-194.

LEMOINE, P., Haronsseau, H., Borteryll, J. P., & Menuet, J. C. (1968). Les enfants de parents alcoholiques: Anomalies observees à propos de 127 cas [Infants of alcoholic parents: Anomalies observed in 127 cases]. *Quest Medical, 25*, 476-482.

LENZ, W. (1966). Malformations caused by drugs in pregnancy. *American Journal of Diseases in Children, 112*, 99-105.

LESTER, B. M., Corwin, M. J., Sepkoski, C., Feifer, R., Peucker, M., McLaughlin, S., & Golub, H. L. (1991). Neurobehavioral syndrome in cocaine-exposed newborn infants. *Child Development, 62*, 694-705.

LEVIN, J. S., & DeFrank, R. S. (1988). Maternal stress and pregnancy outcomes: A review of the psychosocial literature. *Journal of Psychosomatic Obstetrics and Gynaecology, 9*, 3-16.

LEWIS, K. L., Bennett, B., & Schmeder, N. (1989). The care of infants menaced by cocaine abuse. *American Journal of Maternal Child Nursing, 14*, 324-329.

LIS, S. (1989, July). *Psycho-social development of twins born with dissimilar birth weight.* Paper presented at the meeting of the International Society for the Study of Behavioural Development, Jyyväskyla, Finland.

LITTLE, B. B., Snell, L. M., Klein, V. R., & Gilstrap, L. C. (1989). Cocaine abuse during pregnancy: Maternal and fetal implications. *Obstetrics and Gynecology, 73*, 157-160.

LITTLE, R. E., Schultz, F. P., & Mandell, W. (1976). Drinking during pregnancy. *Journal of Studies of Alcohol, 37*, 375-379.

LITTLE, R. E., & Sing, C. F. (1987). Father's drinking and infant birth weight: A report of an association. *Teratology, 36*, 59-65.

LOUGHNAN, P. M., Gold, H., & Vance, J. C. (1973). Phenytoin teratogenicity in man. *Lancet, 2*, 70-72.

LUKE, B., Hawkins, M. M., & Petrie, R. H. (1981). Influence of smoking, weight gain, and pregravid weight for height on intrauterine growth. *American Journal of Clinical Nutrition, 34*, 1410-1417.

MacGREGOR, S. N., Keith, L. G., Chasnoff, I. J., Rosner, M. A., Chisum, G. M., Shaw, P., & Minogue, J. P. (1987). Cocaine use during pregnancy: Adverse perinatal outcome. *American Journal of Obstetrics and Gynecology, 157*, 686-690.

MAN, E. B., Holden, R. H., & Jones, W. S. (1971). Thyroid function in human pregnancy: VII. Development and retardation of 4-year-old progeny of euthyroid and of hypothyroxinemic women. *American Journal of Obstetrics and Gynecology, 109*, 12-19.

MAN, E. B., & Jones, W. S. (1969). Thyroid function in human pregnancy: V. Incidence of maternal low serum butanol-extractable iodines and of normal gestational TBG and TBPA capacities; retardation of 8-month-old infants. *American Journal of Obstetrics and Gynecology, 104*, 898-908.

MAN, E. B., Jones, W. S., Holden, R. H., & Mellits, E. D. (1971). Thyroid function in human pregnancy: VIII. Retardation of progeny aged 7 years; relationships to maternal age and maternal thyroid function. *American Journal of Obstetrics and Gynecology, 111*, 905-916.

MAN, E. B., & Serunian, S. A. (1976). Thyroid function in human pregnancy: IX. Development or retardation of 7-year-old progeny of hypothyroxinemic women. *American Journal of Obstetrics and Gynecology, 125*, 949-957.

MANSFIELD, P. K. (1988). Midlife childbearing: Strategies for informed decision making. In Women's health: Our minds, our bodies [Special issue]. *Psychology of Women Quarterly, 12*, 445-460.

MARCUS, J., Hans, S. L., & Jeremy, R. J. (1982). Differential motor and state functioning in newborns of women on methadone. *Neurobehavioral Toxicology and Teratology, 4*, 459-462.

MARTIN, J. C., Martin, D. C., Lund, C. A., & Streissguth, A. P. (1977). Maternal alcohol ingestion and cigarette smoking and their effects on newborn conditioning. *Alcoholism: Clinical and Experimental Research, 1*, 243-247.

MARTIN, J. C., Martin, D. C., Sigman, P., & Redow, B. (1978). Offspring survival, development and operant performance following maternal ethanol consumption. *Developmental Psychobiology, 10*, 435-446.

MASSA, G., Vanderschueren-Lodeweyckz, M., Van Vliet, G., Craen, M., de Zegher, F., & Eggermont, E. (1989). Hypothalamo-pituitary dysfunction in congenital toxoplasmosis. *European Journal of Pediatrics, 148*, 742-744.

MASTROGIANNIS, D. S., Decavalas, G. O., Verma, U., & Tejani, N. (1990). Perinatal outcome after recent cocaine usage. *Obstetrics and Gynecology, 76*, 8-11.

MATEJCEK, Z., Dytrych, Z., & Schuller, V. (1985). Follow-up study of children born to women denied abortion. In *Abortion: Medical progress and social implications* (CIBA Foundation Symposium 115). London: Pitman.

Maternally transmitted HIV infection. (1990, August). *Research Resources Reporter.*

MAU, G., & Netter, P. (1974). Kaffee und Alkoholkonsum: Riskfaktoren in der Schwangerschaft? [Are coffee and alcohol consumption risk factors in pregnancy?]. *Geburtshilfe und Frauenheilkunde, 34*, 1018-1022.

MAUSS, E. A. (1983). Health effects of ionizing radiation in the low-dose range. *Annals of the New York Academy of Sciences, 403*, 27-36.

McANARNEY, E. R., & Stevens-Simon, C. (1990). Maternal psychological stress/depression and low birth weight. *American Journal of Diseases of Children, 144*, 789-792.

McCARTER, R. J., Kessler, I. I., & Comstock, G. W. (1987). Is diabetes mellitus a teratogen or a coteratogen? *American Journal of Epidemiology, 125*, 195-205.

McDONALD, A. D., McDonald, J. C., Armstrong, B., Cherry, N., Cote, R., Lavoie, J., Nolin, A. D., & Robert, D. (1988). Fetal death and work in pregnancy. *British Journal of Industrial Medicine, 45*, 148-157.

McDONALD, A. D., McDonald, J. C., Armstrong, B., Cherry, N., Delorme, C., Nolin, A. D., & Robert, D. (1987). Occupation and pregnancy outcome. *British Journal of Industrial Medicine, 44*, 521-526.

McDONALD, J. C., Lavoie, J., Cote, R., & McDonald, A. D. (1987). Chemical exposures at work in early pregnancy and congenital defect: A case-referent study. *British Journal of Industrial Medicine, 44*, 527-533.

McFINN, J. H., & Robertson, J. (1973). Psychological-test results of children with thalidomide deformations. *Developmental Medicine and Child Neurology, 15,* 719-727.

McINTOSH, K. (1984). Viral infections of the fetus and newborn. In M. E. Avery & H. W. Taeusch, Jr. (Eds.), *Schaffer's diseases of the newborn* (5th ed.). Philadelphia: W. B. Saunders.

McLAREN, A. (1985). Early stages of development of mammalian embryos. In M. Marois (Ed.), *Prevention of physical and mental congenital defects: Part A. The scope of the problem.* New York: Allan R. Liss.

MEHES, K. (1987). *Informative morphogenetic variants in the newborn infant* (2nd ed.). Budapest: Akademia Kiado.

MEYER, L. S., & Riley, E. P. (1986). Behavioral teratology of alcohol. In E. P. Riley & C. V. Vorhees (Eds.), *Handbook of behavioral teratology.* New York: Plenum.

MEYER, M. B., Jones, B. S., & Tonascia, J. A. (1976). Perinatal events associated with maternal smoking during pregnancy. *American Journal of Epidemiology, 103,* 464-476.

MEYER-BAHLBURG, H. F. L., Feldman, J. R., Cohen, P., & Ehrhardt, A. A. (1988). Perinatal factors in the development of gender-related play behavior: Sex hormones versus pregnancy complications. *Psychiatry, 51,* 260-271.

MIDA, M., Verhoest, P., Boulanger, J. C., & Vitse, M. (1989). Role de la thyroide dans les fausse-couches du premier trimestre [Role of the thyroid in first trimester miscarriage]. *Revue Française de Gynecologie et d'Obstetrique, 84,* 901x.

MILUNSKY, A., Jick, H., Jick, S. S., Bruell, C. L., MacLaughlin, D. S., Rothman, K. J., & Willett, W. (1989). Multivitamin/folic acid supplementation in early pregnancy reduces the prevalence of neural tube defects. *Journal of the American Medical Association, 262,* 2847-2852.

MIODOVNIK, M., Mimouni, F., Siddiqi, T. A., Khoury, J., & Berk, M. A. (1990). Spontaneous abortions in repeat diabetic pregnancies: A relationship with glycemic control. *Obstetrics and Gynecology, 75,* 75-78.

MOORE, C. L., & Power, K. L. (1986). Prenatal stress affects mother-infant interaction in Norway rats. *Developmental Psychobiology, 19,* 236-245.

MORGAN, M. G. (1989). *Electric and magnetic fields from 60 Hertz electric power: What do we know about possible health risks?* Pittsburgh, PA: Carnegie-Mellon University, Department of Engineering and Public Policy.

MORISHIMA, H. O., Pedersen, H., & Finster, M. (1978). The influence of maternal psychological stress on the fetus. *American Journal of Obstetrics and Gynecology, 131,* 286-290.

MUKHERJEE, A., & Hodgen, G. (1982). Ethanol exposure induces transient impairment of umbilical circulation and severe fetal hypoxia in monkeys. *Science, 218,* 700-702.

MULDER, E. J., Visser, G. H., Bekedam, D. J., & Prechtl, H. F. (1987). Emergence of behavioral states in fetuses of type-1-diabetic women. *Early Human Development, 15,* 231-251.

MYERS, R. E., & Myers, S. E. (1979). Use of sedative analgesic and anaesthetic drugs during labor and delivery: Bane or boon? *American Journal of Obstetrics and Gynecology, 133,* 83-104.

NAEYE, R. L. (1978). Effects of maternal smoking on the fetus and placenta. *British Journal of Obstetrics and Gynaecology, 85,* 732-737.

NAEYE, R. L. (1979a). The duration of maternal cigarette smoking and fetal and placental disorders. *Early Human Development, 3,* 229-237.

NAEYE, R. L. (1979b). Relationship of cigarette smoking to congenital anomalies and perinatal death. *American Journal of Pathology, 90,* 289-293.

NAEYE, R. L., Blanc, W., & Paul, C. (1973). Effects of maternal nutrition on the human fetus. *Pediatrics, 52,* 494-503.

National Academy of Sciences. (1975). *Nutrition and fertility: Interrelationships. Implications for policy and action.* Washington, DC: National Academy of Sciences Press.

NEERHOF, M. G., MacGregor, S. N., Retzky, S. S., & Sullivan, T. P. (1989). Cocaine abuse during pregnancy: Peripartum prevalence and perinatal outcome. *American Journal of Obstetrics and Gynecology, 161,* 633-638.

NEWTON, R. W. (1985). The influence of psychosocial stress on low birth weight and preterm labour. In R. W. Beard & F. Sharp (Eds.), *Preterm labour and its consequences: Proceedings of the Thirteenth Study Group of the Royal College of Obstetricians and Gynaecologists.* Manchester: Richard Bates.

NEWTON, R. W. (1988). Psychosocial aspects of pregnancy: The scope for intervention. *Journal of Reproductive and Infant Psychology, 6,* 23-29

NICHOLS, P. I., & Chen, T. (1981). *Minimal brain dysfunction: A prospective study.* Hillsdale, NJ: Lawrence Erlbaum.

NOMURA, T. (1989). Role of radiation-induced mutations in multigeneration carcinogenesis. *IARC Scientific Publications, 96,* 375-387.

NORDBERG, L., Rydelius, P. A., Nylander, I., Aurelius, G., Zetterström, P. (1989). Psychomotor and mental development during infancy: Relation to psychosocial conditions and health: 4. Of a longitudinal study of children in a new Stockholm suburb. *Acta Paediatrica Scandinavica* (Suppl. 353), 3-35.

O'CONNOR, M. J., Sigman, M., & Brill, N. (1986). Alcohol use in primiparous women older than 30 years of age: Relation to infant development. *Pediatrics, 78,* 444-450.

OLSHAN, A. F., Baird, P. A., & Teschke, K. (1989). Paternal occupational exposures and the risk of Down syndrome. *American Journal of Human Genetics, 44,* 646-651.

ORO, A. S., & Dixon, S. D. (1987). Perinatal cocaine and methamphetamine exposure: Maternal and neonatal correlates. *Journal of Pediatrics, 111,* 571-578.

OSBORN, L. M., Harris, D. L., Reading, J. C., & Prather, M. B. (1988). Female residents not at increased risk for adverse pregnancy outcome. *Proceedings of the Annual Conference for Residents' Medical Education, 27,* 120-128.

OSTREA, E. M., Chavez, C. J., & Strauss, M. E. (1975). A study of factors that influence the severity of neonatal narcotic withdrawal. *Addictive Diseases, 2,* 187-199.

OTTINGER, D. R., & Simmons, J. E. (1964). Behavior of human neonates and prenatal maternal anxiety. *Psychological Reports, 14,* 391-394.

OULLETTE, E. M., Rosett, H. L., & Rosman, N. P. (1977). Adverse effects on offspring of maternal alcohol abuse during pregnancy. *New England Journal of Medicine, 297,* 528-530.

OVERPECK, M. D., & Moss, A. J. (1991, June 18). Children's exposure to environmental smoke before and after birth: Health of our nation's children, United States, 1988. *Advance Data From Vital and Health Statistics of the National Center for Health Statistics, 202.*

PALMER, R. H., Ouellette, E. M., Warner, L., & Leichtman, S. R. (1974). Congenital malformations in offspring of a chronic alcoholic mother. *Pediatrics, 53,* 490-494.

PARKER, C. R., Jr., & Wendel, G. D. (1988). The effects of syphilis on endocrine function of the fetoplacental unit. *American Journal of Obstetrics and Gynecology, 159,* 1327-

1331.

PEDERSON, L. M., Tygstrup, I., & Pederson, J. (1964). Congenital malformations in newborn infants of diabetic women. *Lancet, 1*, 1124-1126.

PERSSON, B., & Gentz, J. (1984). Follow-up children of insulin-dependent and gestational diabetic mothers: Neuropsychological outcome. *Acta Paediatrica Scandinavica, 73*, 349-358.

PETERS, D. A. (1982). Prenatal stress: Effects on brain biogenic amine and plasma corticosterone levels. *Pharmacology, Biochemistry and Behavior, 17*, 721-725.

PETRAKIS, P. L. (1987). *Alcohol and birth defects: The fetal alcohol syndrome and related disorders.* Washington, DC: U.S. Department of Health and Human Services.

PFEIFER, W. D., Mackinnon, J. R., & Seiser, R. L. (1977). *Adverse effects of paternal alcohol consumption on offspring in the rat.* Paper presented at the annual meeting of the Psychonomic Society, Washington, DC.

PHELAN, S. T. (1988). Pregnancy during residency: II. Obstetric complications. *Obstetrics and Gynecology, 72*, 431-436.

PICONE, T. A., Allen, L. H., Olsen, P. N., & Ferris, M. E. (1982). Pregnancy outcome in North American women: II. Effects of diet, cigarette smoking, stress, and weight gain on placentas and on neonatal physical and behavioral characteristics. *American Journal of Clinical Nutrition, 36*, 1214-1224.

PIERCE, D. R., & West, J. R. (1986a). Alcohol-induced microencephaly during the third trimester equivalent: Relationship to dose and blood alcohol concentration. *Alcohol, 3*, 185-191.

PIERCE, D. R., & West, J. R. (1986b). Blood alcohol concentration: A critical factor for producing fetal alcohol effects. *Alcohol, 3*, 269-272.

PITTS, K. S., & Weinstein, L. (1990). Cocaine and pregnancy—a lethal combination. *Journal of Perinatology, 10*, 180-182.

PORATH, A., McNutt, R. A., Smiley, L. M., & Weigle, K. A. (1990). Effectiveness and cost benefit of a proposed live cytomegalovirus vaccine in the prevention of congenital disease. *Reviews of Infectious Diseases, 12*, 31-40.

PREECE, P. M., Pearl, K. N., & Peckham, C. S. (1984). Congenital cytomegalovirus infection. *Archives of Diseases in Childhood, 59*, 1120-1126.

PRESTON, M. S. (1989). Epidemiological studies of perinatal carcinogenesis. *IARC Scientific Publications, 96*, 289-314.

PUESCHEL, S. M. (1983). The child with Down syndrome. In M. D. Levine, W. B. Carey, A. C. Crocker, & R. T. Gross (Eds.), *Developmental behavioral pediatrics.* Philadelphia: W. B. Saunders.

REINISCH, J. M. (1977). Prenatal exposure of human foetuses to synthetic progestin and estrogen affects personality. *Nature, 266*, 561-562.

REINISCH, J. M., & Karow, W. G. (1977). Prenatal exposure to synthetic progestins and estrogens: Effects on human development. *Archives of Sexual Behavior, 6*, 257-288.

REINISCH, J. M., Simon, N. G., Karow, W. G., & Gandelman, R. (1978). Prenatal prednisone exposure in humans and animals retards intrauterine growth. *Science, 202*, 436-438.

RICCI, J. M., Fojaco, R. M., & O'Sullivan, M. J. (1989). Congenital syphilis: The University of Miami/Jackson Memorial Medical Center experience, 1986-1988. *Obstetrics and Gynecology, 74*, 687-693.

RICHARDSON, G. A., & Day, N. L. (1986, April). *Alcohol use during pregnancy and neonatal outcome.* Paper presented at International Conference on Infant Studies, Los Angeles.

RIESE, S. L. (1989). Size for gestational age and neonatal temperament in full-term and preterm AGA-SGA twin pairs. *Journal of Pediatric Psychology, 13*, 521-530.

RILEY, J. B., Brodsky, N. L., & Porat, R. (1988). Risk for SIDS in infants with in utero cocaine exposure: A prospective study [Abstract]. *Pediatric Research, 23*, 454A.

ROBERTS, T., & Frenkel, J. K. (1990). Estimating income losses and other preventable costs caused by congenital toxoplasmosis in people in the United States. *Journal of American Veterinary Medicine Association, 196*, 249-256.

ROSENBLITH, J. F. (1979). The Graham/Rosenblith Behavioral Examination for Newborns: Prognostic value and procedural issues. In J. D. Osofsky (Ed.), *Handbook of infant development.* New York: John Wiley.

ROSENBLITH, J. F. (1990, April). *Relations between Graham/Rosenblith neonatal measures and seven year assessments.* Paper presented at the International Conference on Infant Studies, Montreal.

ROSETT, H. L. (1980). Guest editorial: A clinical perspective on the fetal alcohol syndrome. *Alcoholism: Clinical and Experimental Research, 4*, 119-122.

ROSETT, H. L., Ouellette, E. M., & Weiner, L. (1976). A pilot prospective study of the fetal alcohol syndrome at the Boston City Hospital: Part I. Maternal drinking. *Annals of the New York Academy of Science, 273*, 118-122.

ROSETT, H. L., Ouellette, E. M., Weiner, L., & Owens, E. (1978). Therapy of heavy drinking during pregnancy. *Obstetrics and Gynecology, 51*, 41-46.

ROSETT, H. L., & Sander, L. W. (1979). Effects of maternal drinking on neonatal morphology and state regulation. In J. D. Osofsky (Ed.), *Handbook of infant development.* New York: John Wiley.

ROSETT, H. L., Snyder, P., Sander, L. W., Lee, A., Cook, P., Weiner, L., & Gould, J. (1979). Effects of maternal drinking on neonate state regulations. *Developmental Medicine and Child Neurology, 21*, 464-473.

ROSETT, H. L., Weiner, L., Lee, A., Zuckerman, B., Dooling, E., & Oppenheimer, E. (1983). Patterns of alcohol consumption and fetal development. *Obstetrics and Gynecology, 61*, 539-546.

ROSSI, N. (1987). La ricerca psicologica di fronte alla vita fetale. Prospettive e metodi di indagne [Psychological research into fetal life]. *Eta-evolutive, 26*, 65-70.

ROTHENBERG, S. J., Schnaas, L., Cansino-Ortiz, S., Perroni-Hernandez, E., et al. (1989). Neurobehavioral deficits after low level lead exposure in neonates: The Mexico City pilot study. *Neurotoxicology and Teratology, 11*, 85-93.

RUBIN, D. H., Krasilnikoff, P. A., Leventhal, J. M., Weile, B., & Berget, A. (1986). Effect of passive smoking on birthweight. *Lancet, 2*, 415-417.

RUSH, D. (1973). A correction by author: Maternal smoking: A reassessment of the association with perinatal mortality. *American Journal of Epidemiology, 97*, 425.

RUSH, D. (1974). Examination of the relationship between birthweight, cigarette smoking during pregnancy and maternal weight gain. *Journal of Obstetrics and Gynecology of the British Commonwealth, 81*, 746-752.

SANDROCK, D. H., Hankoff, L. D., Broking, S., & Massoth, N. (1990, August). *Substance abuse during pregnancy.* Paper presented at the annual meeting of the American Psychological Association, Boston.

SASSENRATH, E. N., Chapman, L. F., & Goo, G. P. (1979). Reproduction in rhesus monkeys chronically exposed to moderate amounts of delta-9-tetrahydrocannabinol. In G. G. Nahas & W. D. Patton (Eds.), *Marijuana: Biological effects.* Elmsford, NY: Pergamon.

SAVITZ, D. A., Whelan, E. A., & Kleckner, R. C. (1989). Self-reported exposure to pesticides and radiation related to pregnancy outcome: Results from National Natality and Fetal Mortality Surveys. *Public Health Reports, 104,* 473-477.

SAXEN, L., Holmberg, P. C., Kurppa, K., Kuosma, E., & Pyhala, R. (1990). Influenza epidemics and anencephaly. *American Journal of Public Health, 80,* 473-475.

SCHER, M. S., Richardson, G. A., Coble, P. A., Day, N. L., & Stoffer, D. S. (1988). The effects of prenatal alcohol and marijuana exposure: Disturbances in neonatal sleep cycling and arousal. *Pediatric Research, 24,* 101-105.

SCHMAND, B., Neuvel, J., Smolders-de-Haas, H., Hoeks, J., Treffers, P. E., & Koppe, J. G. (1990). Psychological development of children who were treated antenatally with corticosteroids to prevent respiratory distress syndrome. *Pediatrics, 86,* 58-64.

SCHNORR, T. M., Grajewski, B. A., Hornung, R. W., Thun, M. J., Egeland, G. M., Murray, W. E., Conover, D. L., & Halperin, W. E. (1991). Video display terminals and the risk of spontaneous abortion. *New England Journal of Medicine, 324,* 727-733.

SEELIG, H. P., & Roemheld, R. (1969). Untersuchungen zur histochemischen lokalisation der leucin und cystinamino-pepidase (oxytocinase) in der placente [The search for hostochemical localization of leucin- and cystinamino-pepidase (ocytocinase) in the placenta]. *Histochemie, 18,* 30-39.

SEVER, J. L., Ellenberg, J. H., Ley, A., & Edmonds, D. (1985). In M. Marois (Ed.), *Prevention of physical and mental congenital defects: Part B. Epidemiology, early detection and therapy, and environmental factors* (pp. 317-326). New York: Alan R. Liss.

SEVER, J. L., Larsen, J. W., Jr., & Grossman, J. H., III. (1979). *Handbook of perinatal infections.* Boston: Little, Brown.

SEXTON, D. W. (1978). The behavior of infants whose mothers smoke in pregnancy. *Early Human Development, 2,* 363-369.

SEXTON, M., Fox, N. L., & Hebel, J. R. (1990). Prenatal exposure to tobacco: II. Effects on cognitive functioning at age three. *International Journal of Epidemiology, 19,* 72-77.

SHIOTA, K., & Kayamura, T. (1989). Effects of prenatal heat stress on postnatal growth, behavior and learning capacity in mice. *Biology of the Neonate, 56,* 6-14.

SHIOTA, K., Shionoya, Y., Ido, M., Uanobe, F., Kuwahara, O., & Fukui, Y. (1988). Teratogenic interaction of ethanol and hyperthermia in mice. *Proceedings of Society for Experimental Biology and Medicine, 187,* 142-148.

SILVERMAN, D. T. (1977). Maternal smoking and birth weight. *American Journal of Epidemiology, 105,* 513-521.

SINGLETON, E. G., Harrell, J. P., & Kelly, L. M. (1986). Racial differentials in the impact of maternal cigarette smoking during pregnancy on fetal development and mortality: Concerns for Black psychologists. *Journal of Black Psychology, 12,* 71-83.

SINISTERRA, L. (1987). Studies on poverty, human growth and development: The Cali experience. In J. Dobbing (Ed.), *Early nutrition and later development.* New York: Academic Press.

SMITH, M. S. R., Edwards, J. J., & Upfold, J. B. (1986). The effects of hyperthermia on the fetus. *Developmental Medicine and Child Neurology, 28,* 803-813.

SNOW, M. H. L. (1985). Restorative growth and its problems

for morphogenesis. In M. Marois (Ed.), *Prevention of physical and mental congenital defects: Part C. Basic and medical science, education, and future strategies* (pp. 295-299). New York: Allan R. Liss.

SOKOL, R. J., Miller, S. I., & Reed, G. (1980). Alcohol abuse during pregnancy: An epidemiological study. *Alcoholism: Clinical and Experimental Research, 4,* 135-145.

SONTAG, L. W. (1941). Significance of fetal environmental differences. *American Journal of Obstetrics and Gynecology, 42,* 996-1003.

SONTAG, L. W., Steele, W. G., & Lewis, M. (1969). The fetal and maternal cardiac response to environmental stress. *Human Development, 12,* 1-9.

SPOHR, H. L., & Steinhausen, H. C. (1987). Follow-up studies of children with fetal alcohol syndrome. *Neuropediatrics, 18,* 13-17.

STEIN, Z. A., & Susser, M. W. (1975a). The Dutch famine, 1944/45 and the reproductive process: I. Effects on six indices at birth. *Pediatrics Research, 9,* 70-76.

STEIN, Z. A., & Susser, M. W. (1975b). The Dutch famine, 1944/45 and the reproductive process: II. Interrelations of caloric rations and six indices at birth. *Pediatrics Research, 9,* 75-83.

STEIN, Z. A., Susser, M. W., Saenger, G., & Marolla, F. (1975). *Famine and human development: The Dutch hunger winter of 1944-1945.* New York: Oxford University Press.

STEPHENSON, J. B. P. (1978). Epilepsy: A neurological complication of thalidomide embryopathy. *Developmental Medicine and Child Neurology, 18,* 189-199.

STEVENS, R. J., Becker, B. S., Krumpos, G. L., Lanz, L. J., & Tolan, C. J. (1988). Postnatal sequelae of parental smoking during and after pregnancy. *Journal of Reproductive and Infant Psychology, 6,* 61-81.

STEWART, A. M. (1955). A note on the obstetric effects of work during pregnancy. *British Journal of Preventative and Social Medicine, 9,* 57-61.

STOCKARD, C. R. (1913). The effect on the offspring of intoxicating the male parent and the transmission of the defects of subsequent generations. *American Naturalist, 47,* 641-682.

STOCKARD, C. R., & Papanicolaou, G. (1916). A further analysis of the hereditary transmission of degeneracy and deformities by the descendants of alcoholized mammals. *American Naturalist, 50,* 65-88.

STOTT, D. H. (1972). The congenital background to behavior disturbance. In L. W. Robbins & M. Pollack (Eds.), *Life history research in psychopathology* (Vol. 2). Minneapolis: University of Minnesota Press.

STOTT, D. H. (1973). Follow-up study from birth of the effects of prenatal stresses. *Developmental Medicine and Child Neurology, 15,* 770-787.

STOTT, D. H., & Latchford, S. A. (1976). Prenatal antecedents of child health, development, and behavior. *Journal of the American Academy of Child Psychiatry, 15,* 161-190.

STRAUSS, M. E., Lessen-Firestone, J. K., Starr, R. H., Jr., & Ostrea, E. M. (1975). Behavior of narcotics addicted newborns. *Child Development, 46,* 887-893.

STRAUSS, M. E., Starr, R. H., Jr., Ostrea, E. M., Jr., Chavez, C. J., & Stryker, J. C. (1976). Behavioral concomitants of prenatal addiction to narcotics. *Journal of Pediatrics, 89,* 842-846.

STREISSGUTH, A. P. (1977). Maternal drinking and the outcome of pregnancy: Implications for child mental health.

American Journal of Orthopsychiatry, 47, 422-431.

STREISSGUTH, A. P., Barr, H. M., & Martin, D. C. (1983). Maternal alcohol use and neonatal habituation assessed with the Brazelton scale. *Child Development, 54*, 1109-1118.

STREISSGUTH, A. P., Barr, H. M., Sampson, P. D., Darby, B. L., & Martin, D. C. (1989). IQ at age 4 in relation to maternal alcohol use and smoking during pregnancy. *Developmental Psychology, 25*, 3-11.

STREISSGUTH, A. P., Herman, C. S., & Smith, D. W. (1978a). Intelligence, behavior, and dysmorphogenesis in the fetal alcohol syndrome: A report on 20 patients. *Journal of Pediatrics, 92*, 363-367.

STREISSGUTH, A. P., Herman, C. S., & Smith, D. W. (1978b). Stability of intelligence in the fetal alcohol syndrome: A preliminary report. *Alcoholism: Clinical and Experimental Research, 2*, 165-170.

STREISSGUTH, A. P., Martin, D. C., Barr, H. M., Sandman, B. M., Kirchner, G. L., & Darby, B. L. (1984). Intrauterine alcohol and nicotine exposure: Attention and reaction time in 4-year-old children. *Developmental Psychology, 20*, 533-541.

STREISSGUTH, A. P., Martin, D. C., Martin, J. C., & Barr, H. M. (1981). The Seattle longitudinal prospective study of alcohol and pregnancy. *Neurobehavioral Toxicology and Teratology, 3*, 223-233.

STREISSGUTH, A. P., Sampson, P. D., & Barr, H. M. (1989). Neurobehavioral dose-response effects of prenatal alcohol exposure in humans from infancy to adulthood. In D. E. Hutchings (Ed.), Prenatal abuse of licit and illicit drugs [Special issue]. *Annals of the New York Academy of Sciences, 562*.

STREISSGUTH, A. P., Treder, R. P., Barr, H. M., Shepard, T. H., Bleyer, W. A., Sampson, P. D., & Martin, D. C. (1987). Aspirin and acetaminophen use by pregnant women and subsequent child IQ and attention decrements. *Teratology, 35*, 211-219.

STYLIANOPOULOU, F. (1983). Effect of maternal adrenocorticotropin injections on the differentiation of sexual behavior of the offspring. *Hormones and Behavior, 17*, 324-331.

TAKAHASHI, L. K., Kalin, N. H., Barksdale, C. M., Vanden Burgh, J. A., & Brownfield, M. S. (1987). Stressor controllability during pregnancy influences pituitary-adrenal hormone concentrations and analgesic responsiveness in offspring. *Physiology and Behavior, 42*, 323-329.

TANAKA, H., Nakasawa, K., & Arima, M. (1987). Effects of maternal caffeine ingestion on the perinatal cerebrum. *Biology of the Neonate, 51*, 332-339.

TEITELMAN, A. M., Welch, L. S., Hellenbrand, K. G., & Bracken, M. B. (1990). Effect of maternal work activity on preterm birth and low birth weight. *American Journal of Epidemiology, 131*, 104-113.

THALER, I., Goodman, J. D. S., & Davies, G. S. (1980). Effects of maternal cigarette smoking on fetal breathing-fetal movements. *American Journal of Obstetrics and Gynecology, 138*, 282-287.

THOMPSON, W. R. (1957). Influence of prenatal maternal anxiety on emotionality in young rats. *Science, 125*, 698-699.

THOMPSON, W. R., Watson, J., & Charlesworth, W. R. (1962). The effects of prenatal maternal stress on offspring behavior in rats. *Psychological Monographs, 76*(Whole No. 38).

THOMSON, A. M., & Billewicz, W. Z. (1963). Nutritional status, maternal physique, and reproductive efficiency. *Proceedings of the Nutrition Society, 22*, 55.

U.S. Department of Health, Education and Welfare. (1979).

Smoking and health: A report of the surgeon general (CDHEW Publication No. PNS 79-50066). Washington, DC: Government Printing Office.

UHLIG, H. (1957). Missbildungen unerwunschler Kinder [Mishaps of unwanted children]. *Arztlische Wochenshrift, 12*, 61-66.

ULSTEIN, M., Jensen, T. S., Irgens, L. M., Lie, R. T., Sivertsen, E., & Skjeldestad, F. E. (1990). [Pregnancy outcome in some Norwegian counties before and after the Chernobyl accident] (in Norwegian). *Tidsskr Nor Leegeforen, 110*, 359-362.

ULTMAN, M. (1988). Developmental abnormalities in infants and children with acquired immune deficiency syndrome (AIDS) and AIDS-related complex. *Developmental Medicine and Child Neurology, 27*, 563-571.

UPFOLD, J. B., & Smith, M. S. (1988). Maternal hyperthermia as a cause of "ideopathic" mental retardation. *Medical Hypotheses, 27*, 89-92.

VAN-DEN-BERGH, B. R., Mulder, E. J., Visser, G. H., Poelmann-Weesjes, G., Bekedam, D. J., & Prechtl, H. F. (1989). The effect of (induced) maternal emotions on fetal behavior: A controlled study. *Early Human Development, 19*, 9-19.

VARDARIS, R. M., Weisz, D. J., Fazel, A., & Rawitch, A. B. (1976). Chronic administration of delta-9-tetrahydrocannabinol to pregnant rats: Studies of pup behavior and placental transfer. *Pharmacology and Biochemistry of Behavior, 4*, 249-254.

VERGEL, R. G., Sanchez, L. R., et al. (1990). Primary prevention of neural tube defects with folic acid supplementation: Cuban experience. *Prenatal Diagnosis, 10*, 149-152.

VIERCK, C., King, F. A., & Ferm, V. H. (1966). Effects of prenatal hypoxia upon activity and emotionality of the rat. *Psychonomic Science, 4*, 87-88.

VISSER, G. H., Mulder, E. J., Bekedam, D. J., van Ballegooie, E., & Prechtl, H. F. (1986). Fetal behaviour in type-1 diabetic women. *European Journal of Obstetrics, Gynecology and Reproductive Biology, 21*, 315-320.

VOORHEES, C. V., & Mollnow, E. (1987). Behavioral teratogenesis: Long-term influences on behavior from early exposure to environmental influences. In J. Osofsky (Ed.), *Handbook of infant development* (2nd ed.). New York: John Wiley.

VOS, O. (1989). Effects and consequences of prenatal irradiation. *Bolletino Societa Italiana Biologia Sperimentale, 65*, 481-500.

WACHSMAN, L., Schuetz, S., Chan, L. S., & Wingert, W. A. (1989). What happens to babies exposed to phencyclidine (PCP) in utero? *American Journal of Drug and Alcohol Abuse, 15*, 31-39.

WAHA, E. K., & Erkkola, R. (1988). The sauna and pregnancy. *Annals of Clinical Research, 20*, 279-282.

WAINWRIGHT, R. C. (1983). Changes in observed birth weight associated with change in maternal cigarette smoking. *American Journal of Epidemiology, 117*, 668-675.

WARD, I. L. (1984). The prenatal stress syndrome: Current status. *Psychoneuroendocrinology, 9*, 3-11.

WARKANY, J. (1986). Teratogen update: Hyperthermia. *Teratology, 33*, 365-371.

WARKANY, J., & Kalter, H. (1961). Congenital malformations. *New England Journal of Medicine, 265*, 993-1001, 1046-1052.

WEATHERSBEE, P. S., Olsen, L. K., & Lodge, J. R. (1977). Caffeine and pregnancy. *Postgraduate Medicine, 62*, 64-69.

WEINBERG, J. (1989). Prenatal ethanol exposure alters adrenocortical development of offspring. *Alcoholism, 13*, 73-83.

WEN, S. W., Goldenberg, R. L., Cutter, G. R., Hoffman, H. J., Cliver, S. P., Davis, R. O., & DuBard, M. B. (1990). Smoking, maternal age, fetal growth, and gestational age at delivery. *American Journal of Obstetrics and Gynecology, 162*, 53-58.

WERBOFF, J., & Gottlieb, J. S. (1963). Drugs in pregnancy: Behavioral teratology. *Obstetrical and Gynecological Survey, 18*, 420-423.

WERLER, M. M., Mitchell, A. A., & Shapiro, S. (1989). The relation of aspirin use during the first trimester of pregnancy to congenital cardiac defects. *New England Journal of Medicine, 321*, 1639-1642.

WERNER, E. E. (1979). *Cross cultural child development: A view from planet earth.* Monterey, CA: Brooks/Cole.

WERTELECKI, W., Hoff, C., & Zansky, S. (1987). Maternal smoking: Greater effect on males, fetal tobacco syndrome? *Teratology, 35*, 317-320.

WEST, J. R. (1986). Long-term effects of developmental exposure to alcohol. *Neurotoxicology, 7*, 245-256.

WHITLY, R. J., Nahmias, A. J., Visintine, A. M., Fleming, C. L., & Alford, C. A. (1980). The natural history of herpes simplex virus infection of mother and newborn. *Pediatrics, 66*, 489-494.

WILD, N. J., Sheppard, S., Smithells, R. W., Holzel, H., & Jones, G. (1989). Onset and severity of hearing loss due to congenital rubella infection. *Archives of Disease in Childhood, 64*, 1280-1283.

WILLARD, D. (1989). Les enfants de femmes ayant presente une affection maligne [Children born to mothers with malignant disease]. *Pediatrie, 44*, 621-625.

WILSON, G. S. (1989). Clinical studies of infants and children exposed prenatally to heroin. In D. E. Hutchings (Ed.), Prenatal abuse of licit and illicit drugs [Special issue]. *Annals of the New York Academy of Sciences, 562.*

WILSON, G. S. R., McCreary, J. K., & Baxter, J. C. (1979). The development of preschool children of heroin addicted mothers: A controlled study. *Pediatrics, 63*, 135-141.

WINICK, M. (1969). Malnutrition and brain development. *Journal of Pediatrics, 74*, 667-679.

WINICK, M. (1976). *Malnutrition and brain development.* New York: Oxford University Press.

WINICK, M., & Noble, A. (1966). Cellular response in rats during malnutrition at various ages. *Journal of Nutrition, 89*, 300-306.

WINICK, M., & Rosso, P. (1969). Head circumferences and cellular growth of the brain in normal and marasmic children. *Journal of Pediatrics, 74*, 774-778.

WITTER, F. R., & Niebyl, J. R. (1990). Marijuana use in pregnancy and pregnancy outcome. *American Journal of Perinatology, 7*, 36-38.

WOLFE, L. A., Hall, P., Webb, K. A., Goodman, L., Monga, M., & McGrath, M. J. (1989). Prescription of aerobic exercise during pregnancy. *Sports Medicine, 8*, 273-301.

WOODS, J. R., Jr., Plessinger, M. A., Scott, K., & Miller, R. K. (1989). [Article]. In D. E. Hutchings (Ed.), Prenatal abuse of licit and illicit drugs [Special issue]. *Annals of the New York Academy of Sciences, 562*, 267-279.

YERUSHALMY, J. (1964). Mother's cigarette smoking and survival of the infant. *Journal of Obstetrics and Gynecology, 88*, 505-518.

YERUSHALMY, J. (1971). The relationship of parents' cigarette smoking to outcome of pregnancy: Implications as to the problem of inferring causation from observed associations. *American Journal of Epidemiology, 93*, 443-456.

YERUSHALMY, J. (1972). Infants with low birth weight born before their mothers started to smoke cigarettes. *American Journal of Obstetrics and Gynecology, 112*, 277-284.

ZELSON, C., Sook, J. L., & Casalino, M. (1973). Neonatal narcotic addiction: Comparative effects of maternal intake of heroin and methadone. *New England Journal of Medicine, 289*, 1216-1220.

ZIERLER, S., & Rothman, K. (1985). Congenital heart disease in relation to maternal use of bendectin and other drugs in early pregnancy. *New England Journal of Medicine, 313*, 347-352.

ZIMMERBERG, B., & Reuter, J. M. (1989). Sexually dimorphic behavioral and brain asymmetries in neonatal rats: Effects of prenatal alcohol exposure. *Brain Research and Developmental Brain Research, 46*, 281-290.

ZUCKERMAN, B., Amaro, H., Bauchner, H., & Cabral, H. (1989). Depressive symptoms during pregnancy: Relationship to poor health behaviors. *American Journal of Obstetrics and Gynecology, 160*, 1107-1111.

ZUCKERMAN, B., Frank, D., Hingson, R., Amaro, H., Levenson, S., Kayne, H., Parker, S., Vinci, R., Aboagye, K., Fried, L., Cabral, H., Timperi, R., & Bauchner, H. (1989). Effects of maternal marijuana and cocaine use on fetal growth. *New England Journal of Medicine, 320*, 762-768.

Perinatal Events That Affect Constitution or Mother-Infant Interaction

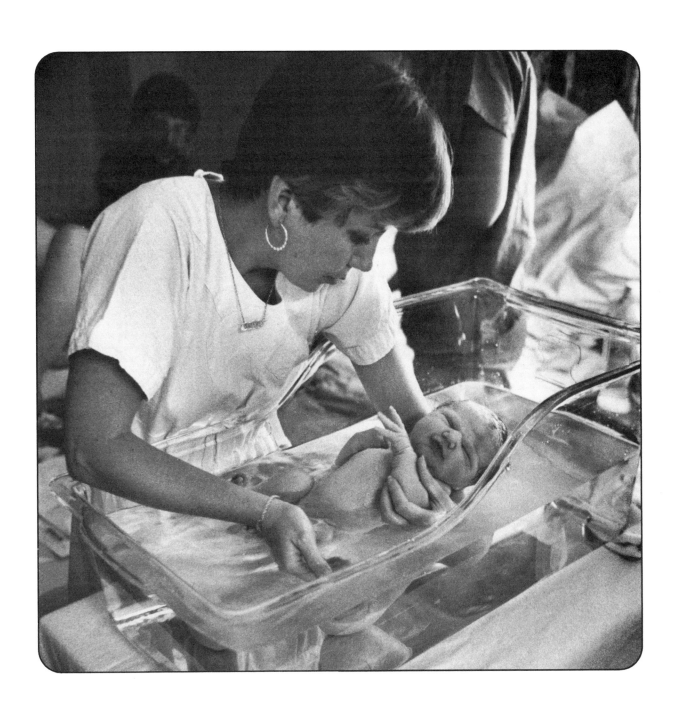

Chapters 2-4 discussed the development of the infant prior to birth and the genetic and environmental problems that may occur then. Another set of environmental determinants of the baby's constitution are associated with the birth process itself and with the immediate postnatal events in the baby's life.

A number of factors associated with the delivery process are clearly capable of harming the infant. Others are thought to be harmful or are considered less than optimal from the standpoint of the infant's current health or later development. Still others may hinder interactions of the infant with the mother or other family members. This chapter discusses the possible influences in the following categories: complications of delivery and ways to avoid or counteract them, drugs used during delivery, childbirth practices, and mother-infant bonding. Before the discussion of these topics, however, a brief overview of the process of labor and delivery is in order.

Labor is a very appropriate name for what goes on in childbirth; it is hard physical work. There are three stages. In the first, the cervix expands or dilates so that it will be large enough to allow the infant to pass through. At the beginning, the contractions are relatively mild and far apart, but they gradually increase in intensity and come more frequently. The woman normally goes to the hospital when they reach a frequency that her doctor has suggested as appropriate. It is during this stage that the controlled breathing of childbirth preparation classes can be used to manage discomfort. This normally takes 8 to 10 hours in first pregnancies.

In the second stage, the baby passes through the birth canal and is born (Beynon, 1975). This stage usually lasts 1 to 2 hours in first pregnancies. During this stage, when the mother uses her abdominal muscles to push the baby out, the presence of a supportive person can be most crucial. In the third stage the placenta, or "afterbirth," is expelled, a matter of great importance if serious hemorrhaging or later infection is to be avoided. This normally takes 15 or 20 minutes. For a more thorough, yet brief, review of the nature of childbirth, see Herzfeld (1985).

Complications of Delivery

SPEED OF DELIVERY

As is true of many things, both too much and too little speed in delivery are bad. Labors that are too long or too short are more likely to result in problems than are those of moderate length. The length of the second stage is most crucial. If the baby is squeezed through the birth canal very rapidly (in less than 10 minutes, according to most views), the delivery is called *precipitate*.

There are two dangers in precipitate delivery: First, contractions prevent the normal flow of blood to the fetus, and they may be too close together to provide adequate oxygen for the fetus; second, the head may be subjected to such pressure that blood vessels in the brain hemorrhage and cause injury to the brain. Babies whose heads have been squeezed often look rather peculiar. Normally the different bones of the skull meet smoothly, except for the **fontanelle** (the soft spot at the top of the skull). However, there are joints between all the skull bones that are still soft, and babies who have suffered a lot of pressure during delivery may be born with each bone at a very different level from that of its neighbor. Because the joints or **sutures** are flexible, the bones level out in a matter of days or weeks and the odd appearance goes away. However, this recovery does not indicate whether any minor damage has been done to the brain cells. It is thought that very small hemorrhages that are not severe enough to be detected in the newborn period may occur and cause the child problems in later life. Such problems may take the form of poor motor coordination, learning disabilities, mental retardation, or, in more severe cases, even cerebral palsy or epilepsy. The strength of contractions, or the amount of pressure on the baby when in the uterus, has some of the same potential for doing minor brain damage.

A long, drawn-out delivery is also considered undesirable. As in a precipitate delivery, a long delivery can lead to brain damage. In this case, it is usually caused by **anoxia** (lack of sufficient oxygen), rather than by hemorrhaging. Anoxia can be caused by long-term squeezing of the umbilical cord during delivery or by a decrease in maternal blood pressure.

PRESENTATION AT DELIVERY

The normal way for the baby to "present" (that is, the part of the baby that enters the birth canal first) is the crown of the head. Occasionally the face presents first, which is not desirable because there is a greater possibility of damage to the neck and spinal cord. About 4% of babies do not arrive head first at all. Some come buttocks first (breech deliveries), others feet first (footling breech), and still others have one or both hands coming first (see Figure 5.1). All the unusual presentations are more dangerous for the baby and more difficult for the mother. When it is known that it is not the baby's head but some other part that is engaged at the exit of the uterus, doctors may attempt to manipulate the fetus into proper position. If such attempts fail, a **cesarean section** (**CS**, or **C-section**) may be used. In this procedure the abdomen and uterus are opened surgically, and the baby and placenta are removed.

All of the unusual presentations make physical injury to both the baby and the mother more likely. In these positions, at some point, a surface that is both larger and softer than the head, and hence does not afford the proper pressure, must pass through the cervix. Umbilical circulation may be cut off, thus depriving the baby's brain of adequate oxygen. Babies who are born buttocks first usually have quite abnormal patterns of muscle tonus after birth. These tend to disappear in a matter of weeks to months. Nevertheless, lasting damage may be done. In a study reported by Ingemarsson et al. (1978), breech babies delivered vaginally were compared with those delivered by cesarean over a period of from 1 to 5 years. Not only was mortality lower for the CS group, but neurological and developmental outcomes were more optimal.

"ENTANGLING ALLIANCES"

Another variable is whether the umbilical cord has become wrapped around the baby's neck during intrauterine growth or the process of delivery. It may be wrapped around the neck one or more times, and the wrapping may be loose or quite tight. Some deaths in late fetal development (stillbirths) are caused by strangulation due to multiple, tight wrapping of the cord. Fetuses who do not die prior to birth are still at risk if the cord is sufficiently tightly wrapped to cause anoxia, or if it passes through the cervix before the baby does (technically a prolapsed cord). Other complications of delivery may be exacerbated in a baby who is also entangled.

PROBLEMS OF ANOXIA

The importance of the fetus receiving enough oxygen has been mentioned, but what do we know about the effects? Anoxia can occur as a result of complications of delivery, but also as a result of maternal conditions. It can also have occurred prenatally, but it is anoxia occurring at birth with which we are concerned here. Severe oxygen deficiency leads to asphyxiation and death, but what about brain damage from less severe anoxia?

Benaron et al. (1960) report that neonates with severe anoxia were eight times more likely than their siblings who had no anoxia to show intellectual retardation. However, only 20% of the anoxics became abnormal, and some had superior intelligence. Lowered average intelligence, compared with unrelated controls, has been found in children with chemically well-

Figure 5.1. Various deviations from the most optimal vertex presentation. The first drawing on the left shows a minor deviation in which the head is first but is turned to the side. The next shows a prolapsed cord. The more extreme presentations are shown in the three drawings on the right.

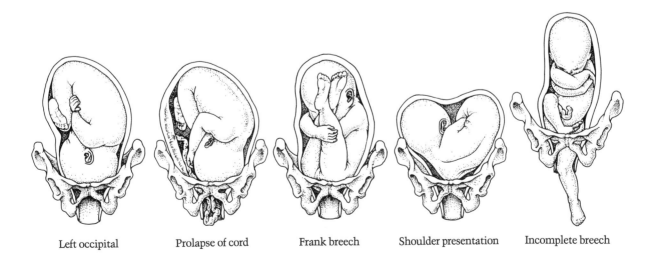

Left occipital   Prolapse of cord   Frank breech   Shoulder presentation   Incomplete breech

defined levels of anoxia, but in that study there was no evidence for improved intelligence (Ernhart et al., 1960). By 7 years of age the children who had been anoxic no longer differed in IQ from the controls, but did show impairment in abstract verbal ability, perceptual skills, and social competence (Corah et al., 1965).

Animal data are more clear-cut. According to Windle (1966), neurological symptoms of monkeys asphyxiated at birth tended to become less severe over time, although brain damage increased. Some animals were better able to compensate for their early deficits than others. Monkey babies that suffered anoxia at birth were more apt to die as a result of failure of the heart and circulatory system than to survive to exhibit later brain damage (R. E. Myers, 1972). Recent animal data suggest that the fetal or neonatal brain may be protected from the effects of anoxia by the release of endogenous opioids, which act to diminish the rate at which the brain metabolizes oxygen (Lou et al., 1989).

A large body of data indicates that anoxia leads to a greater risk for various problems, but it fails to tell us which infants will have problems. Data are unclear due to different definitions of anoxia, methodological flaws, limited choice of outcome measures, and the use of retrospective data. Certainly much greater knowledge of the mechanisms that produce individual differences in reactions are needed if we are to understand why oxygen deprivation has such different effects in different individuals, human or monkey.

Graham et al.'s (1957) call for more studies using accurate definitions of the degree, duration, and clinical features of asphyxia or anoxia has not been heeded. Now people are calling for the use of sophisticated techniques such as brain imaging, EEGs, and brain stem auditory responses to provide more knowledge of the location and degree of damage (e.g., Amiel-Tison & Ellison, 1986). These, rather than increased knowledge about oxygen deprivation, are hoped to lead to better individual prediction of outcomes.

However, there are data that suggest all of this research may be addressed to the wrong question, the question of the effects of acute anoxia at the time of birth. The data of the extensive CPRP indicate strongly that if social and demographic differences are taken into account, there is no effect of acute hypoxia on lowered IQ at age 7 (Naeye & Peters, 1987). In contrast, chronic hypoxia during pregnancy is negatively related to long-term cognitive performance. In addition to these data, new ways of imaging the premature brain through the fontanelle are providing data that cast doubt on the critical role of oxygen in brain damage ("Fetal Monitoring," 1981).

Ways to Avoid or Counteract Complications

Over the years various techniques have been developed to counteract birth complications. Most are addressed to trying to avoid anoxia or asphyxiation, but some are aimed at avoiding injuries.

FETAL MONITORING

There are a number of levels of fetal monitoring. The nurse, midwife, or doctor who listens to the fetal heartbeat is monitoring the fetus. Such monitoring can determine the fetal heart rate response to contractions by monitoring before, during, and after contractions. Currently the term *monitoring* is often used to refer to continuous external electronic monitoring. This does not require the mother to identify contractions and permits her to remove the abdominal belt with its electrodes and move around freely. (It does interfere with Lamaze techniques.) Monitoring is sometimes done much more invasively, using electrodes put through the vagina and cervix and attached to the baby, a technique that deprives the mother of most movement. The mother's contractions and the baby's blood gases and acid-base balance (or pH) may also be monitored using scalp needles. These supposedly give information about both the degree of anoxia and the physiological responses of the fetus to it. However, experts asked to interpret the records often disagree about the degree of distress, and they only agree half of the time about what should be done. It has been estimated that invasive monitoring was used in 60-80% of births in 1981 ("Fetal Monitoring," 1981).

Invasive electronic fetal monitoring (EFM) has problems. The mother's delivery is disturbed, which may result in her needing more drugs or in a slowing down of labor even if extra drugs are not used. The risks of infection to both mother and fetus are also increased (Gassner & Ledger, 1976). The question of whether either the psychological or monetary costs are worth the possible benefits to the baby has been reviewed by Banta and Thacker (1979). These authors estimate that EFM of 50% of births adds $411 million to the annual cost of childbirth. The effectiveness of fetal monitoring in lowering neonatal death rates has also been questioned (Anthony & Levene, 1990; Banta & Thacker, 1979; Freeman, 1990; Neutra et al., 1978; Shy et al., 1990). It is my conclusion that invasive monitoring should be used only in high-risk situations.[1] And I ask: Why, when researchers were pointing out at the end of the 1970s that EFM led to more C-sections, without improvement in perinatal mortality, do studies and reviews making this same point in 1990 appear as news?

It is quite possible to diagnose a normal heart rate pattern (by any of the methods of monitoring) and avoid an unnecessary intervention. However, it is more difficult to determine whether an abnormal heart rate pattern really indicates fetal distress. As noted earlier, agreement among experts is far from perfect. Untested rules of thumb are adopted, and even the interpretation of lowered pH may be difficult.

Very recently it has been suggested that determining whether a fetus responds to acoustic stimulation in early stages of labor can help determine its being at risk. Nonresponders were at greater risk for a number of unfavorable outcomes in a sample dominated by complicated pregnancies (Sarno et al., 1990).

AIDS FOR THE DELIVERY PROCESS

Normally babies are delivered by what is called *spontaneous vaginal delivery*. This means that little or no outside help is needed. When labor is very extended (more than 24 hours for a first delivery), or when the fetus shows signs of distress, additional help may be needed. Monitoring fetal heart rate helps to determine whether to use other aids. Despite reservations about the inevitability of bad outcomes for babies who were anoxic at birth, mothers and doctors would prefer to avoid this risk factor. If fetal distress appears, what can lessen its duration? Here I will discuss only what has traditionally been done. In the later section on types of childbirth, alternatives will emerge.

To speed up delivery, three major interventions can be used: administration of oxytocin or related drugs to speed up contractions, use of mechanical aids for speeding delivery (forceps and vacuum extraction), and doing a C-section to deliver the fetus surgically. Oxytocin will be discussed in the section on drugs; discussion of the others follows.

Forceps

In a forceps delivery, the doctor clamps the infant's head with a tonglike instrument much like that used to lift corn on the cob from boiling water. The forceps are applied while the infant is in the birth canal. There are three types of forceps: high, medium, and low. The type used depends on how far into the birth canal the infant is and how much and which parts of the infant's head can be grasped. High forceps are used when the baby is still high in the birth canal. Fortunately, these are rarely seen in today's world.[2] They can cause (a) enough pressure to cause brain hemorrhaging; (b) a

precipitate delivery, with accompanying problems; or (c) a sudden release of pressure when the baby comes out that can fracture, rupture, or tear the baby's spinal cord, resulting in death or severe handicap.

Medium forceps are used in intermediate placements, and low forceps are applied when the infant's head is almost through the birth canal. Neither is apt to cause problems other than superficial bruising, which passes rapidly. Nevertheless, the use of medium forceps seems to be declining markedly, mostly in favor of C-sections, which replaced high forceps earlier.[3] Long-term consequences of low forceps have been little studied. A study of 28 low-forceps babies whose mothers received regional anesthetics compared them to babies with normal, unmedicated deliveries (Murray et al., 1981). At birth the babies delivered with forceps and exposed to anesthetics were more disorganized in terms of their motoric, physiological, and state behaviors. At 1 month they were fed less often and seen by their mothers to be more bothersome and more poorly organized. Whether such differences would last, and what the relative roles of forceps and anesthesia are, is not clear.

Vacuum Extraction

In some places, doctors and hospitals have substituted vacuum extraction for forceps.[4] Properly used, vacuum extraction probably has less potential for harming the brain than either precipitate delivery or medium forceps, *if* the head is low enough and *if* there are no other risk factors. Distortion of the shape of the skull may occur, but this is often less unsightly than forceps bruises and passes relatively quickly.

There are sharp differences in the Western world about the value of vacuum extraction. Experience in Sweden and Germany in the 1960s indicated that it might be safer than forceps, except for preterm fetuses, and it was widely used. The technique did not become

---

1. The Banta and Thacker review covers 296 articles; the Anthony and Levene paper covers 34 more recent ones. It has a good description of the techniques and discussion of the hoped-for results.

2. Old-time obstetricians delight in telling of the "terrible old days" when doctors frequently used high forceps. Each seems to have a tale of at least seeing a doctor pull so hard that when the baby came out the doctor flew across the room as a result of the release of pressure.

3. It is interesting to note that in a university hospital in France between 1981 and 1986, the use of forceps decreased without an increase in cesareans and without affecting outcomes.

4. The technique is the same as that used in extracting menses or in abortions, but the scale is larger.

popular in Britain or the United States, but it is replacing medium forceps in some places (Broekhuizen et al., 1987). It has been considered ideal for the family physician who practices obstetrics (Epperly & Breitinger, 1988; for a review of its history, use, and findings, see Galvan & Broekhuizen, 1987).

Vacuum extraction is easier on the mother than either a cesarean delivery or the use of forceps. It produces fewer bad tears and requires fewer postdelivery bladder catheterizations (Meyer et al., 1987).

No long-term effects on the infants are found (Bjerre & Dahlin, 1974; Carmody et al., 1986; Ngan et al., 1990). Short-term effects seem to be related to the conditions that led to intervention, except for an increase in jaundice (Broekhuizen et al., 1987; Carmody et al., 1986; Gale et al., 1990; Meyer et al., 1987). Japanese data do not show differences between infants delivered after oxytocin-induced labors using vacuum extraction, with or without epidural block, and those with neither (Ochi et al., 1989). Hong Kong data on 295 10-year-olds who had been delivered by vacuum extraction and compared with well-matched controls showed no differences in neurological or cognitive functioning (Ngan et al., 1990). Present data do not permit distinguishing the problems caused by either medium forceps or medium vacuum extraction from those caused by the conditions that led to their use.

Cesarean Section

The other basic type of delivery that an infant may experience is surgical delivery by C-section, which has replaced high-forceps and even medium-forceps deliveries. The modern cesarean, with sterile surgical practices and anesthesia (originally done under general anesthesia, now often done with epidural anesthesia), represented a tremendous advance in obstetrics for mothers and infants. In the past, when the infant's head was too large to pass through the pelvic opening, death for both mother and baby resulted. With current techniques the mother can be awake and have her husband there.

When C-sections became relatively safe and pain free, but when still done with general anesthesia, some mothers and doctors found them convenient because they made it possible to plan the time of birth. Some women even found them attractive because they made childbirth less "animallike."

However, there are disadvantages to the use of C-sections, including a higher maternal death rate. Although the chances that the mother may die are very small, they are 3 to 30 times greater than the chances

of women vaginally delivered (Benaron & Tucker, 1971; Evrard & Gold, 1977; Nielsen & Hokegård, 1984a). Swedish data show that from 1973 to 1979 the maternal death rate for vaginal deliveries was 1/100,000, but for C-sections it was 12.7/100,000 (Nielsen & Hokegård, 1984a). Part of this difference in rate can be accounted for by the fact that women who are at high risk are more likely to have cesareans. Nevertheless, some of the higher maternal mortality stems from the method of delivery itself. Evrard and Gold (1977) found that four of the nine deaths in their sample could be attributed to the method.

Other disadvantages from the maternal point of view include the fact that surgery requires a longer recovery period (see, e.g., Robertson et al., 1990). This is accentuated by the greater frequency of complications in C-sections. Even in Sweden, with its excellent health care system, almost 12% of CS mothers in one study had some complication, and 2% had major complications (Nielsen & Hokegård, 1984a). Complications were primarily found among emergency and not elective cases (19% versus 4%). Uterine (and bladder) infections are more likely with C-sections than with vaginal deliveries (Gassner & Ledger, 1976), running as high as 38% in a major New York teaching hospital (Petrie, 1981).

Finally, it has long been accepted doctrine that "once a cesarean, always a cesarean." Some mothers were upset by the fact that they were told they could have no more than four children this way. As early as 1982 the American College of Obstetricians and Gynecologists issued guidelines that permitted trying a vaginal delivery after a CS. A national conference at which all concerned disciplines were represented supported an effort to increase this practice (National Institutes of Health, 1981). Despite (a) these official proddings, (b) the fact that no death from a ruptured uterus (the feared consequence of a vaginal delivery) had been reported in 20 years (as of 1985), and (c) data showing that vaginal delivery is successful in 50-82% of cases in which it is tried (Meehan, 1989; Meehan et al., 1989; Paul et al., 1985), hospitals and doctors have been slow to offer this alternative to mothers. Even the judicious use of oxytocin does not seem harmful in women trying vaginal delivery after a CS (Flamm et al., 1987), although if it is used together with epidural anesthesia it can lead to some scar ruptures (Molloy et al., 1987). The percentage of women who delivered vaginally after CS rose from about 4% in 1980 to almost 10% in 1987 (Taffel et al., 1989).

In spite of the disadvantages of cesareans and the diminution in those done for "convenience," the rates for this method of delivery rose sharply in the last two decades; they showed signs of leveling off only in 1987 (Taffel et al., 1989). Rates differ markedly in different countries, and low rates of infant mortality can be achieved in some populations despite very low rates of cesareans (Notzon, 1990). For the period 1981-1986, the United States had a CS rate of 23% of all births. This rate was exceeded by Brazil (32%) and Puerto Rico (29%), but is much greater than those of the Netherlands, Japan, and Czechoslovakia, which had rates of 10% or less (Althaus, 1990).

The medical data indicate that the rate of CS for first births has increased for the following major reasons: Cephalopelvic disproportion (baby's head too big for mother's pelvis) has doubled and fetal distress has increased 70-fold (Haddad & Lundy, 1978). The increase in fetal distress is probably related to increased fetal monitoring, but breech presentation and cephalopelvic disproportion are the major reasons for C-sections. Breech presentation accounted for 11% of C-sections in 1970-1973, but for 19% in 1978-1981. The proportion of breech presentations that were CS deliveries increased from 23% in the earlier period to 64% in 1978-1981 ("Avoiding Unnecessary Repeat Cesarean Deliveries," 1985). The latter is also the percentage found in a British study (Bingham et al., 1987); 40% were planned and 24% occurred after vaginal delivery was unsuccessful.

Repeat CS is said by some not to be a major reason for the increased rate, but National Center for Health Statistics data indicate that they account for 55% of the increase, and data from Ontario, Canada, indicate that repeats account for 68% of a rise from 16.5% in 1979 to 18.7% in 1982 (Anderson & Lomas, 1984).

The roles of finances and of doctors' motivations to be in control have been questioned by some. The latter charges seem neither testable nor fair. However, financial reasons need some scrutiny. First is the question of medical malpractice suits and the cost of medical insurance. While I have stated that it is believed that EFM is not a major reason for the increase in doing C-sections, it is a fact that it leaves a lasting record that can be used in a later lawsuit. Hence it is tempting to do a CS if a few squiggles from a monitor record look suspicious.

Data on the prevalence of CS in different economic groups lend some credence to financial motivations. The CS rate for private patients is higher than that for clinic patients, two to three times higher in Denver (Neuhoff et al., 1989; Porreco, 1985) and twice as high in an Australian study (Cary, 1990), with about equal perinatal mortality. First-time C-sections are linearly related to income; according to Gould et al. (1989), in Los Angeles County, among those whose annual income is $30,000, the rate is almost double that of the lowest income group. These researchers speculate that doctors are more afraid of being sued by affluent patients, but some assert that poor patients are more likely to sue. Data are lacking to support either view.

Many elements in our society, from the medical profession to parts of the women's movement and to various alternative childbirth advocates, have become concerned with the rise in cesareans. They argue that doctors are becoming more inclined to intervene, and to intervene more drastically, in the birth process when it may not be necessary. At least two hospitals (Mount Sinai in Chicago and Columbia Presbyterian in New York) have guidelines for doing a CS and require either a second opinion or a board review of all C-sections. In Chicago the rate dropped from 17% to 11% in just two years (and the hospital lost $2 million in fees), but there was a possible increase in fetal deaths of breech babies. In New York the rate went from 25% to 19% over four years (Brody, 1989).[5] Studies in Ireland and Great Britain have shown that what is called "active management of labor" (this includes more accurate definition of when labor has

Table 5.1
Percentage of C-Section Deliveries for Different Age Groups (United States) at Different Periods

Year	Overall	Teenagers	Ages 20-24	Ages 25+
1965	4.5			
1970	5.5	3.9	4.9	8.3
1980	16.5			
1983	20.3	15.0	19.0	25.4
1987[a]	24.4			

SOURCE: Data from "Avoiding Unnecessary Repeat Cesarean Deliveries" (1985).
a. Data for 1987 are from Taffel et al. (1989).

started and early diagnosis and treatment of failure to progress) can lead to a decrease in the number of first-time C-sections (O'Driscoll et al., 1984; Turner et al., 1988).

Because a CS is relatively safe, one could argue that the best medical practice is to do one if there is the slightest doubt about the infant's or mother's safety. But one can argue that doctors may overrespond when the risk is slight, and that they may be more worried about malpractice suits than about the quality of the birth experience for the woman and her family.[6] As more women become involved in planning their own deliveries and argue for vaginal deliveries, doctors may have to become less conservative. It has recently been suggested that even for deliveries involving medium forceps or vacuum extraction, the gains for the mother need to be weighed against increased problems for the fetus (Robertson et al., 1990), and that a trial of either with readiness to proceed to a CS if necessary is safe (Lowe, 1987). This issue is part of the more general one of hospital childbirth practices, which will be discussed later in this chapter.

An important question not yet addressed is whether babies so delivered are adversely affected. In studies of humans it is difficult to separate the effects of the CS from those of the problems that led to doing it or of the anesthetics used. In the immediate postnatal period, babies born by CS are more apt to develop acute respiratory distress (RDS). Swedish data show an incidence of 1.6% for vaginal, 6.4% for elective, and 10.1% for emergency C-section deliveries (Nielsen & Hokegård, 1984b). According to White et al. (1985), premature infants born after 30 weeks' gestation are 2.3 times as likely to develop RDS as those born vaginally, especially if the C-section was started prior to the onset of labor. These authors hypothesize that corticosteroids produced by the fetus in response to the stress of labor enhance lung maturity, thus reducing RDS for those for whom labor precedes the CS. Four times the amount of umbilical catecholamines (and other biochemical differences) have been found in vaginally delivered babies compared with elective CS

babies (Irestedt et al., 1989). Twin pairs in which one was delivered by CS after the first was born vaginally are not a clear-cut case of whether the second twin has been exposed to labor. In any event, the CS babies in these cases do not appear to be more compromised than their vaginally delivered twins (Riese, 1988).

Several studies reported at the 1980 International Conference on Infant Studies failed to agree on what, if any, effects cesareans have on babies' later development. Father-infant interactions were affected: Fathers of CS babies not only do more caretaking, but they feel better about themselves as fathers (Grossman, 1980; Pederson et al., 1980; Vietze et al., 1980). Some studies have found that children delivered by CS develop lower IQs and some have found higher IQs.

Monkey data enable assessment of the effects of C-sections done without any medical reason. In one study, CS babies had lower total activity, *less vocalization*, and later acquisition of learning than vaginally delivered monkeys (Meier, 1964). In a study reported by Field and Widmayer (1980), CS human newborns (lower-SES blacks) did not differ from vaginally delivered controls matched on variables other than obstetric complications. At 4 months they vocalized *more* and showed more contented facial expressions during feeding interactions, but were rated as less adaptable by testers. CS mothers interacted more positively with their babies, rated their temperaments more positively, and were more realistic about when to expect their first words or to be able to potty train them. Mothers still rated their babies more favorably at 8 months, although there were few differences on objective measures.

In sum, cesareans have a number of negative features for mothers and may lead to more cases of RDS and some other problems in neonates, but appear to have no consistent effects on later development. Mother-infant relations do not seem negatively affected (and are perhaps positively affected for lower-class black mothers), and father-infant relations may be improved.

If we think about all of the ways to avoid or counteract complications, we see that, together with other factors such as replacing opiate sedation by epidural anesthesia, they have led to dramatic reduction in perinatal death and in neonatal brain damage due to birth asphyxia and trauma (Cyr et al., 1984). Despite this, the frequency of severe birth asphyxia has not changed, and birth injuries actually increased in 1984. Furthermore, cerebral palsy has not declined, and has even increased for low birth weight infants, probably as a result of the fact that more of them are now kept alive (Pharoah et al., 1987).

---

5. Dr. Rosen of Columbia Presbyterian has recently written a paperback (with Thomas) titled *The Caesarean Myth* (1989).

6. A 1983 poll of Florida physicians showed that more than 20% of them had stopped doing deliveries and a similar percentage were considering doing so because of the risk of being sued for various errors of omission or commission that might have led to the brain damage of an infant they delivered. Minimal malpractice insurance now costs $27,000 per year, and the coverage a doctor might need to settle such a case would cost $54,000 per year.

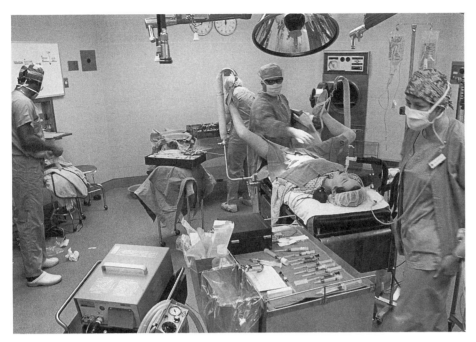

Figure 5.2. This is a picture of a standard delivery room scene as it was frequently seen in the past and not infrequently still today: bright lights, clutter, no friendly person, and an extreme of the lithotomy position in which the legs are up in the air instead of over supports at the knee level. (Photograph courtesy of J. W. Myers, Stock, Boston.)

Drugs Used During Delivery

During hospital delivery mothers are often, even usually, given drugs to reduce pain, to relieve anxiety, or both. As previously noted, drugs are sometimes given to speed up delivery. Although other drugs might be given for various reasons, this discussion will be concerned only with drugs given in connection with these two major purposes.

TYPES OF DRUGS

The most universally used drugs are those for pain or anxiety. In the earlier stages of labor three classes of drugs are often given: (a) tranquilizers, which do not reduce pain but reduce the woman's reaction to it; (b) sedative-hypnotics, which make the woman drowsy and reduce her reaction to pain; and (c) narcotic-analgesics, which reduce but do not eliminate pain. In later stages of labor, anesthetics (drugs designed to eliminate or greatly reduce pain) are often given.

Drugs may also be given to combat low blood pressure in the mother and thus protect the fetus from anoxia and resulting acidosis, which increases the difficulty of resuscitation. Both narcotic antagonists (drugs designed to reduce the bad effects of the narcotics)

and antihypotensive drugs may be given. Low blood pressure may be brought on by drugs used during delivery and may be exacerbated by the **lithotomy** position. This is the typical delivery position, in which the woman lies on her back, often on a hard surface, with her legs drawn up to the sides of her abdomen, and sometimes fastened over supports (see Figure 5.2).

Anesthetics are sometimes given to affect only part of the body. A whole family of drugs (drugs with some chemical similarity) are given by spinal injection (see Figure 5.3). The height of the spinal cord at which they are injected determines the area that has no pain and over which the patient has no voluntary control. In general this includes all points below the site of injection.

General anesthetics affect the entire body. These include the volatile anesthetics, which are inhaled, and barbiturates (and some nonbarbiturate agents), which are given by intravenous injection. The inhalants include nitrous oxide, cyclopropane, and ether compounds such as Penthrane and Fluorthane that have replaced the ether and chloroform used earlier. (A comprehensive review of anesthetics appears in Brackbill, 1979b.)

Before discussing possible effects of these drugs, I would like to enumerate some reasons for concern

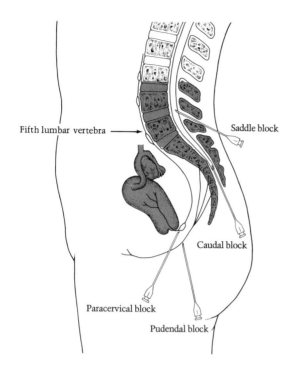

Figure 5.3. Diagram of the spine with needles inserted at various points to illustrate where drugs used to block pain are injected.

about their use. First, most drugs cross the placental barrier, hence the fetus is not protected from them. Second, they can cross the blood-brain barrier, which consists of the membranes between the circulating blood and the brain. Because they can cross this barrier, they can directly affect the brain of the fetus. Third, the amount of a drug given the mother is determined by her size or body weight. If placental exchange allows this concentration in the fetal system, it is an incredibly larger dose. Fourth, the liver and kidneys of the fetus or newborn are quite immature, so drugs will remain in the infant's system for a much longer time than they would stay in an adult's system.[7] The actual amount of a drug that will remain in the newborn's system depends not only on the amount given the mother, but on the time at which it was given in relation to when the umbilical cord was cut.

Drugs differ markedly in the time they take to cross the placental barrier and in how rapidly they are metabolized by the mother's system. A rapidly acting drug that is also rapidly metabolized by the mother's body may be effectively removed from mother and fetus if it is given substantially prior to birth. The same drug given shortly before the cord is cut will remain in the infant's system, since the baby can only metabolize and excrete substances very slowly.[8]

A fifth, and very different, reason for concern is the prevalence of the use of drugs in delivery. The degree to which their use has diminished is not clear. A 1974 poll of 18 American teaching hospitals (i.e., hospitals in which medical students and interns are taught) conducted by Brackbill (1979a) found that only 5% of their deliveries were accomplished without anesthesia. Comparable figures for the numbers in which no analgesics were used are not available, but one can guess that they would be even fewer in number. Brackbill did report that some drugs, such as barbiturates and scopolamine, might be used less than formerly. However, Field and Widmayer (1980) found that scopolamine was used in 12 of 20 CS deliveries.

DIFFICULTIES OF ESTABLISHING DRUG EFFECTS

Having established that there are reasons to want information about the effects of drugs, I must note also how difficult it is to achieve clear-cut answers. For ethical reasons, random assignment of subjects to receive particular drugs or drug combinations is not possible. Also, mothers are apt to reject random assignment to receive drugs or no drugs during delivery. Thus researchers are limited to correlational studies that explore the relation between drugs received during labor and delivery and behaviors of the offspring in the newborn period or later.

The large numbers of drugs, the different quantities administered, the different times in relation to birth they are given, and the fact that they may be given orally or by injection make adequately controlled studies very difficult. It is particularly hard to assess the effects of a single drug, because most women are given analgesics or sedative-hypnotics in combination with anesthetics. Inasmuch as few deliveries in the United States are undrugged, it is hard to arrive at a view of what the totally undrugged newborn is like. Adams (1989) combed 600 records to find 22 mothers who received no medication.

The outcomes of studies of drug effects are apt to be influenced by a variety of extraneous variables. Mothers who receive no anesthetic and no other drugs

---

7. This is because the liver is the principal agent for metabolizing drugs and the kidneys must excrete them and their metabolic products.

8. While it is not directly relevant to the effects of drugs used during delivery, the fact that drugs taken after delivery may be excreted in the breast milk and thus affect nursing infants should be noted.

(or only small quantities) are likely to be better educated, to have received better prenatal care, to be in better social economic circumstances, to have attended childbirth preparation classes, and to have different ideas about interacting with their babies than mothers who are more heavily drugged. Drug-free deliveries are more likely in easy labors, which often are not the first. The potential influence of all these variables should be controlled for by such techniques as matching or statistical techniques, available to correlational research. Alternatively, one can do studies in other societies where large numbers of women (hence less preselected or biased samples) do not have drugs—at least not anesthetics.

Measuring the dependent variable in studies of obstetric medication is also complex. Multiple effects are usually measured, and they may be measured at various ages. Physiological effects are often assessed neonatally, and psychological and psychophysiological effects may be assessed at birth, in infancy, or in childhood. If measures are made in childhood, there need to be controls for, or at least assessment of, the intervening environmental factors.

Effects of Drugs

Methodological problems have certainly not prevented researchers from doing studies, especially of the effects of drugs on some aspect of behavior in the neonatal period (Aleksandrowicz, 1974; Aleksandrowicz & Aleksandrowicz, 1974, 1976; Brackbill, 1979b; Brumitt & Dowler, 1984; Friedman et al., 1978; Moreau & Birch, 1974; Murray et al., 1981; for a critique, see Federman & Yang, 1976). Indeed, the number of studies and the complexities involved would require a chapter (or better, a book) to review adequately. Most of the above-cited studies were done when dosages tended to be higher than now, and hence should not be generalized to current usage. Most used small numbers of infants (20 to 30 per group) and were not able to control for agents other than the one or two under study. Medically oriented studies have used larger numbers of subjects, but more limited measures of effects. The fetal respiratory and circulatory systems are particularly vulnerable to injury during labor and delivery (see Chapter 2); hence much medical research has focused on neonatal depression (the slowing of physiological functions, especially of respiratory and heart functions).

PREANESTHETICS

Preanesthetics (drugs given during labor, prior to use of an anesthetic that might be given during delivery) include tranquilizers, narcotic-analgesics, and sedative-hypnotics. These are discussed in turn below.

Tranquilizers

Many different tranquilizers are used, such as (by trade name) Thorazine, Vistaril, Phenergan, and Largon. The effects of tranquilizers are particularly hard to assess because they are usually used in conjunction with other drugs. Clearly some of them potentiate (magnify) the effects of analgesics, making it possible to get good pain relief with smaller doses. Tranquilizers appear to have little or no depressant effect on the fetus, according to several studies (cited in Bowes et al., 1970). Groups that received Valium or Phenergan together with the narcotic-analgesic Demerol did not differ from those receiving Demerol alone in terms of their EEGs, but all differed from a group receiving no Demerol (Brower, 1974), thus indicating that the tranquilizers had no effect, but Demerol may have. However, one must note that it is said that the current dosage of Demerol is one-third to one-fourth of what it was at the time of the cited study.

In a well-controlled study of the tranquilizer Largon used together with the analgesic Demerol in women, most of whom had spinal anesthesia, no medical side effects could be attributed to Largon. Its short duration of action enabled dosing to be done as needed, thus reducing the risk of overdosing (Farley, 1961). Behavioral differences were assessed for a subsample of 47 babies by an examiner who did not know whether the mother had received Largon or water. There were no differences between the groups at 6 to 16 hours after birth. Babies whose mothers had received water were more variable in performance at 16 to 36 hours after birth, suggesting that Largon masks some individual differences otherwise present.

By far the largest study of the effects of drugs is that by Brackbill and Broman (n.d.). It drew on the data of the Collaborative Perinatal Research Project, a major study done under the auspices of the National Institutes of Health.[9] Data for the 3,528 full-term, singleton infants born to healthy, usually economically disadvantaged mothers, ages 16 to 40, with low-risk pregnancies and uneventful vertex, vaginal deliveries were examined. Sparine (given to one-fifth of sample) and Phenergan (given to one-seventh) were related to half of the 4-month pediatric-neurological items.

However, for Sparine half of the relations were to presumably better outcomes, compared with only one-fifth for those exposed to Phenergan. There were some statistically significant but small relations of both drugs to measures at 8 and 12 months. Again, Sparine, but not Phenergan, was related to positive as often as to negative outcomes. Overall, the pattern of findings in these studies does not suggest that the use of tranquilizers during labor is harmful, but Sparine and Largon would seem preferable to Phenergan.

Narcotic-Analgesics

The narcotic-analgesics include morphine, Demerol, and Nisintil. The most studied is Demerol. It has been found to be related to response decrement in newborns (Brackbill et al., 1974). In the CPRP data, it was related to pediatric items at 4 months and Bayley items at 8 months, but it was related to positive outcomes as often as to negative ones, and the strength of the relations was low. Labor analgesia (usually Demerol) has been shown not to relate to behaviors of first-time mothers or their infants in a sample of well-educated women (Muir, 1988).

Behavioral effects of Demerol in the neonatal period (assessed using the NBAS) depended on how it was administered (intravenously or intramuscularly) and on other drugs given with it (Brumitt & Dowler, 1984). Intramuscular Demerol had no effect, but intravenously it led to better muscle tone at 3 days of age. But when combined with the tranquilizer hydroxyzine hydrochloride (perhaps best known as Vistaril), Demerol was associated with poorer muscle tone. When oxytocin had been used, Demerol had the depressant effect found by Brackbill and colleagues. Here is another instance of the difficulties of determining the effects of one drug when so many other variables come into play. This study did not consider timing, which would almost certainly also have affected the results.

An unusually well-controlled study of babies exposed to only a single dose of Nisintil (a synthetic narcotic) compared them to those exposed to no drugs of any kind. Visual habituation and fixation times were compared. They did not differ significantly on the number of trials needed to habituate, but first and total fixation times were about twice as long for the no-drug as for the Nisintil group. The latter is not necessarily a good sign, as will be shown in Chapter 8. Further, three times as many of the no-drug babies

failed to complete testing (Adams, 1989). It is difficult to conclude anything of practical relevance from these data.

Sedative-Hypnotics

The sedative-hypnotics include various barbiturates (e.g., Nembutal, Seconal, Amytal) and nonbarbiturates (e.g., Valium, scopolamine). The most studied is scopolamine. In the original CPRP sample, it had been given to 36% of the mothers. Infant behaviors on the 8-month Bayley were affected, usually negatively. Scopolamine-exposed children had slightly lower scores on some cognitive tasks at both 4 and 7 years (Brackbill & Broman, n.d.; Broman, 1981, 1983). Among all the preanesthetic agents, scopolamine is the drug that appears most suspect. It is the drug that was a major ingredient of so-called twilight sleep, in which the mother would remember nothing of her delivery, used in the 1930s.

The effect of scopolamine on mothers, at least in the doses used earlier, is pronounced. They may not remember anything about the birth or even that they have given birth. More adequate data on its effects on both mothers and infants are certainly called for, with greater caution in its use until they are available.

Results for other drugs in this category are neither consistent enough nor strong enough to raise questions as to their safety with respect to the behavioral development of the infant. The evidence about their physiological or medical effects, which may not always be benign, has not been reviewed.

REGIONAL ANESTHETICS

There are actually two issues involved in studying the effects of regional anesthetics. One is the level of the spinal cord injected to obtain regional anesthesia and the other is the drug used. This discussion begins with evidence focused on the level at which the drug is administered.

Where Administered

Spinals not only numb pain, but also paralyze a woman from her waist down. They are used in second-stage labor when there is a medical reason to shorten it. Saddle blocks (see Figure 5.3 to see where they are administered) deaden the area that a saddle touches and to some extent the legs, and are currently not as much used (or studied) as epidurals. One study shows that sucking behaviors of infants whose mothers received saddle blocks (with either Xylocaine or Pon-

---

9. For a description of the project, see Niswander and Gordon (1972).

tocaine) were affected (Sanders-Phillips et al., 1988). Multiparous mothers who received anesthesia (either blocks or general) have been found to engage in significantly fewer face-to-face interaction behaviors at 2 months (Muir, 1988).

The most used form of pain relief today is the lumbar epidural block (described as anesthesia by some and analgesia by others). With it, women can feel pressure, but no pain. Although it is considered the most desirable form of regional anesthesia, contractions often slow and the urge to push is lost.[10] This may soon be a matter of the past, as it is now possible to administer it on a continuous basis, which permits stopping administration when the woman needs to push and resuming it as the baby emerges. With the single-injection method there is an increased possibility that oxytocin, forceps, vacuum extraction, or C-section will be used (Avard & Nimrod, 1985; Murray et al., 1981; Poore & Foster, 1985; Thorp et al., 1989) and that more postpartum bladder catheterizations will be needed (Poore & Foster, 1985). Like other regional anesthesias, epidurals can affect the mother's blood pressure; hence monitoring is used. However, babies whose mothers had received epidurals did not have lower 5-minute **Apgar** scores (an index of physiological status or depression at birth) or umbilical cord arterial and venous blood gases than those whose mothers received no analgesia or only narcotics (Thorp et al., 1989).

Effects of epidurals on the baby beyond this immediate postbirth period were judged unclear by Avard and Nimrod in a 1985 review because of contradictory findings. Subsequent data show that fewer infants exposed to epidurals either in vaginal or CS deliveries were optimal on the NBAS at 28 days, compared with those exposed to nitrous oxide. Optimal motor scores were 23% less frequent in the epidural CS group than in the epidural vaginal group, which itself had almost 20% fewer optimal scores than other medication groups (Muhlen et al., 1986). A smaller study that tested at 3 hours, day 1, day 2, and day 4 or 5 found better scores on alertness on all tests except at day 1 for epidural-exposed babies (Kangas et al., 1989). Still another study found poorer NBAS scores than for babies from unmedicated deliveries, both overall and on several subscales, but only the state control differences persisted to the fifth day, and there were no differences at 1 month. The epidural babies cried more in the neonatal period (which might go with the greater alertness noted in one study).

Epidural mothers have been found to differ both in their behaviors and in their perceptions of their ba-

bies. In one study, they saw their babies as less adaptable, more intense, having less good interactive capacities and poorer state control, and as being more "colicky" than did mothers with unmedicated deliveries (Murray et al., 1981). Given the absence of behavioral differences in the babies it is hard to know the source of these maternal perceptions. If the differences are real, did they result from differences in anesthesia or from different maternal behaviors? At 1 month they fed their babies less often, responded less promptly to their cries, spent more time stimulating them to suck, and gave them slightly less affectionate handling. Babies from unmedicated deliveries made more eye contact with their mothers, but their mothers were more likely to rate them as "at risk" (Murray et al., 1981). The research since 1985 has not led to more definitive conclusions about the potential for harm of epidurals, but it would appear that maternal reactions play a role in any effects on babies at 1 month, and demonstration of effects beyond that time are not available.

Caudal blocks cut off sensations and stop the urge to push, but trained women can be instructed to push. With proper doses they do not affect contractions. Some data on outcomes are reviewed in the section on the effects of the drugs used.

Pudendal and paracervical blocks (see Figure 5.3) are generally considered local anesthetics. The pudendal block numbs the vagina and **perineum** (the region from the vagina to the anus), and hence is useful for forceps deliveries. The woman loses the urge to push, but can do so when asked to. A paracervical block stops pain in the pelvis from the uterus and cervix. It can temporarily decrease intensity and frequency of contractions, but rarely slows labor. A study of paracervical blocks with low doses showed no risk for the 261 mothers, although the intensity of uterine contractions decreased (Freeman & Arnold, 1975). The risk to the infants appeared to be minimal inasmuch as their Apgar scores were not affected, although in 6% of the 104 monitored cases heart rate was affected. The doctors thus could not exclude the possibility of minor and/or subtle fetal damage resulting from hypoxia (too little oxygen) related to the heart rate changes. Nevertheless, they judged that the potential fetal risks from this type of anesthesia were acceptable given the ease of the procedure and the degree of pain relief obtained.

---

10. Anyone desiring a review of all its possible effects on the mother should consult Nicholson and Ridolfo (1989).

What Is Administered

Mepivicaine and lidocaine (Xylocaine), both of which are used in epidurals and caudals, cross the placenta rapidly and are relatively stable in the blood (Bowes et al., 1970; Morishima & Adamson, 1967). They have been shown to affect muscle strength and muscle tone in the newborns, but the effects wear off rapidly in the first day (Scanlon, 1976; Tronick et al., 1976). Mepivicaine was also shown to lead to physiological depression in about 20% of the 56 infants in another study (Morishima et al., 1966). Maximum effects of this agent occur if the infant is born 20 to 30 minutes after administration of the drug.

Bupivicaine, which is chemically similar to mepivicaine and lidocaine, is also used for caudal and epidural blocks. It has effects that persist for at least several days after birth (Lieberman et al., 1979; Murray et al., 1981). Evidence for negative effects of other regional anesthetics is even less convincing. Two drugs commonly used in spinal and saddle blocks, procaine (or Novocaine) and tetracaine (or Pontaine), are inactivated more rapidly than lidocaine and mepivicaine, and thereby may have less effect.

As part of a study assessing a new procedure for determining visual acuity in newborns, Dobson et al. (1987) tested for effects of anesthetics on results. Whether their mothers had spinals, epidurals, local anesthesia, or no anesthesia had no effect on the babies' visual acuity.

Where women are given choices, those choices are influenced by characteristics that can influence the results. A study that controlled for some of these characteristics (age, education, financial security, and orientation to the pregnancy) found that regional anesthetics had no influence on neonatal behaviors of babies whose mothers chose medicated births. Specifically, none of the items assessing motor maturity and irritability on the NBAS differed (Standley, 1974, 1976).

GENERAL ANESTHETICS

General anesthetics produce a lack of sensation throughout the entire body, as opposed to locally or only below a certain level of the body, and a loss of consciousness. General anesthesia can be produced by intravenous injection or by inhalation of anesthetic agents. It is indicated in cases where intrauterine manipulation of the fetus is required, or when the woman feels she cannot cope with being awake during delivery. These needs can also be met by regional anesthesia combined with sleep-inducing drugs. General anesthesia used to be common when a C-section was done.

Anesthetists tend to prefer intravenous anesthetics (primarily barbiturates) that act quickly and allow rapid recovery of consciousness. This is fortunate, because there is evidence that inhalants may be harmful. As a class the inhalants are more often related to the outcomes at each age studied, and the relations are predominantly negative (Brackbill & Broman, n.d.; Broman, 1981, 1983). In particular, the results suggest that "inhalants are associated with defects in psychomotor and neuromotor functioning in the first year" (Broman, 1981, p. 134). These results may underestimate their harm inasmuch as nitrous oxide was included with all other inhalants in the analysis, an inclusion that is frequent, but probably inappropriate (Cosmi & Marx, 1968; Horowitz et al., 1977; Moya & Thorndike, 1962).

Nitrous oxide ("laughing gas") is the most fre-

Table 5.2
Characteristics of Infants Whose Mothers Received Different or No Drugs

	No Drug (15 cases)	*Bupivicain* (20 cases)	*Oxytocin and Bupivicaine* (20 cases)
Length of second-stage labor (minutes)	100	84	48
Malposition of fetus (cases)	0	5	8
Use of low forceps (cases)	0	12	6
Mother-infant separation[a] (cases)	0	4	6
Phototherapy for jaundice (cases)	0	1	5[b]

SOURCE: Data from Murray et al. (1981).

a. Done for observation of the newborn
b. There were other cases of jaundice in this group, but they did not require therapy.

quently used inhalant in the United States. When administered together with oxygen, it is not considered to have a significant depressive effect (Horowitz et al., 1977; Moya & Thorndike, 1962), unlike other inhalant anesthetics that are known to produce medical depression in newborns. The use of nitrous oxide at delivery was not related to any maternal or infant behaviors in a well-educated sample (Muir, 1988), although its use has been questioned if there are other problems (Zelcer et al., 1989). A larger percentage of infants exposed only to nitrous oxide were optimal at 28 days on the NBAS state control and interaction subscales than for any other medication (including minimal). Fewer were optimal on the motoric processes subscale (Muhlen et al., 1986).

As long ago as 1961, Brazelton suggested that nitrous oxide might provide protection against the effects of other medications. This idea has never been seriously tested, to my knowledge. One study appears to offer some support for this hypothesis. Field and Widmayer (1980), in a study of cesarean deliveries, found much less effect of drugs on Brazelton scores than anticipated. They speculate that the lack of effects in babies whose mothers had high levels of narcotics and barbiturates and frequently had had oxytocin may have resulted from the ability of nitrous oxide to provide an antagonistic or protective effect.

OVERALL LEVEL OF MEDICATION

Although the thrust of most research has been to identify whether particular drugs are harmful, another valid question is whether a certain level of medication, regardless of the specific drugs used, is harmful.

Horowitz and her collaborators (1977) have attempted to answer the question of harmful levels of medication in three different studies. They had to go to different countries to find a wide range of medication levels. In the United States they found that among medicated mothers, higher levels of medication were correlated with negative outcomes in the neonatal period, but there were not enough unmedicated cases to allow comparison of drugged with nondrugged groups.

In Israel they compared a moderately medicated group (one that had no anesthetics) to a completely drug-free group. Israel was a particularly fortunate site for study, because drug choices of women there did not seem to be associated with extraneous variables such as education and social class, as they are in the United States. The infants were tested with the NBAS (Kansas version) for the first 4 days and at 1 month, and with the Bayley scales at 3 months. Only two items on the Brazelton scale differentiated the drug group from the nondrug group: (a) a measure of the lability of the infant's states (see Chapter 6 for a discussion of state) and (b) defensive responses to cloth being placed over the face. Horowitz's third study, in Uruguay, found the opposite difference between medicated and nonmedicated groups; there, drugged babies did better. In general the differences among the groups in the three different locales were much greater than the differences between the different levels of medication.

The three studies taken together suggest that low levels of medication are less likely to result in problems in the neonatal period than are higher levels. Whether drug-free labors and deliveries are safer for newborns than those with low levels of medication is not clear. It has been suggested that, because anxiety and pain may affect the mother's hormone secretions so as to reduce blood flow to the uterus, too little use of drugs to relieve the mother may increase the risk of anoxia in the fetus or newborn (Shnider, 1981). In an Australian sample, minimal anesthetics were not found to be optimal for NBAS functioning at 28 days (Muhlen et al., 1986). However, the authors suggest that this may have been due to the administration of local anesthetics used for perineal repairs, but whether they were used prior to clamping the cord is not recorded.

It is unfortunate that oxytocin, a drug used to induce or speed up delivery, has often been included in studies that assess the effects of overall levels of medication. Both its purpose and the nature of the drug are very different from those of the drugs used to reduce pain or change the mother's reaction to it.

Before turning to the effects of a non-pain-killing drug, I would like to say something about the dangers of anesthesia (both general and regional) for mothers. In a study of all maternal deaths in Massachusetts between 1954 and 1985, Sachs et al. (1989) found that 4.2% were related to anesthesia. In 1955-1964 the maternal death rate was 1.5 per 100,000, and the anesthetic-related deaths were primarily due to aspiration in the course of administering inhalant anesthetics using a mask over the face. For the period 1965-1974 the maternal death rate remained the same, and the primary cause of deaths was cardiovascular collapse associated with regional anesthesia. The death rate fell to .4 per 100,000 for 1975-1984, and all deaths were associated with general endotracheal anesthesia. The authors offer suggestions for even further improvements in the safety of anesthesia, but 1 death in 250,000 deliveries is already a startling contrast to the maternal death rates found 50 to 100 years ago.

EFFECTS OF OXYTOCIN

Oxytocin, also called Pitocin, is used to induce labor, to speed up labors that are not progressing, and to stimulate expulsion of the placenta. Labor induction is important when a relatively quick delivery is called for and a C-section is not desired. Maternal high blood pressure, kidney disease or diabetes, and fetal postmaturity are common reasons. Oxytocin is often combined with amniotomy (surgical breaking of the membranes) and sometimes with other drugs. Oxytocin as a single technique to induce labor has been shown not to have the best results (Bakos & Backstrom, 1987), but in a network of community hospitals it did not lead to more use of epidurals and episiotomy, as it has in other settings (Crump, 1989). Induction by amniotomy plus oxytocin and oxytocin alone have been shown to increase the risk of postpartum hemorrhage compared with oxytocin plus an ergot compound (Gilbert et al., 1987).

Oxytocin's use to speed up labor is more frequent and is my chief concern here. Because it acts to increase the intensity of contractions, it increases pain. Further, if it is not administered carefully, it can result in a precipitate delivery. The effects of oxytocin can be estimated by comparing women who had bupivicaine alone with those who had both bupivicaine and oxytocin (see Table 5.2). In this sample, low forceps were more often needed in those receiving regional anesthesia with bupivicaine. They were used less often if oxytocin was also used. They were not used with those who received no drugs (but drugs would normally be used if the doctor is going to use forceps). However, better muscle control, or having been allowed to remain in second-stage labor for a longer time, may have reduced the use of forceps. Variables related to delivery that could affect infant outcomes differed among the groups, which complicates interpretation.

Oxytocin's effects on the fetus have not been subject to sufficient scrutiny. Babies whose mothers had received oxytocin (and bupivicaine) had lower scores on the NBAS than either the bupivicaine-only or unmedicated groups (Murray et al., 1981). They were tense and hypertonic, which interfered with their motor activity. The state control differences persisted in the fifth day of life. Unlike the others, babies exposed to oxytocin rarely woke for feedings. At 1 month there were no longer any differences on the NBAS, but mothers who had had oxytocin spent more time stimulating their babies to feed. If the babies needed the stimulation this would not be optimal.

Phototherapy for jaundice was more frequent in the oxytocin group in the Murray et al. (1981) study (see Table 5.2). This is in agreement with the more recent finding of increased risk of jaundice in babies whose mothers' labors were induced with oxytocin (Maisels et al., 1988), but other research has found that oxytocin is not related to jaundice if other factors are controlled for (Johnson et al., 1989). Neurological disorders at age 2 have been shown not to be related to the use of oxytocin (Rosen et al., 1989).

Researchers working on the Collaborative Perinatal Research Project did not routinely collect data on oxytocin use, but the data they have show very small negative effects of oxytocin at ages beyond 1 month. Its use was related to some psychomotor deficit on the 4-month pediatric and neurological and 8-month psychological assessments. At school age it was associated with lower achievement test scores (Broman, 1981). None of the other studies separated the use of oxytocin to induce labor from its use to speed labor, a topic for which more research might be productive.

Recently, prostaglandins have been used both to replace oxytocin and to precede its usage. Many studies from many countries indicate that vaginal or cervical suppositories of prostaglandin are as effective as, or more effective than, intravenously administered oxytocin (see, e.g., Bernstein et al., 1987; Dommisse & Wild, 1987; el-Qarmalaw et al., 1990; Goeschen, 1989; Lyndrup et al., 1990; Nager et al., 1987; Silva-Cruz et al., 1988). They are also more acceptable to women and easier for hospital personnel. In one study, priming with oral prostaglandin followed by induction with oxytocin had the best results of the methods tested, resulting in 71% vaginal deliveries (Somell, 1987). Other work has found that after prostaglandin use oxytocin is often not needed (Nager et al., 1987). One study in Finland has reported complications from the use of prostaglandin (Ekblad & Erkkola, 1987).

Studies are more unanimous in finding negative effects of oxytocin than they are for most of the pain-reducing drugs. These data and others indicating that oxytocin may produce contractions that are severe enough to produce fetal anoxia indicate that considerably more caution might be exercised in elective use of oxytocin.

CONCLUSIONS

Conclusions about the effects of obstetric drugs are difficult to reach because of the methodological problems intrinsic to research in this field and the sparseness of and inconsistencies in the data. Nevertheless, I will attempt a summary.[11]

---

11. For a reasonably up-to-date review, see Sepkoski (1985).

First, not all drugs have the same effects. Most have no long-term negative consequences, and parents can compensate for short-term consequences, such as increased crying and decreased feeding. Tranquilizers, most sedative-hypnotics, analgesics, and most regional anesthetics do not have long-term or serious short-term consequences for babies. Oxytocin used to induce or augment labor, scopolamine, and inhalant anesthetics, other than nitrous oxide, are more suspect.

Second, the overall amount of medication may be an important variable. Though some studies have shown that large proportions of mothers currently receive some drug during delivery, there is reason to believe that dosing is more carefully done now than previously.

Third, we need more information on the effects of drugs that themselves appear harmless, but may be harmful when used in combination with other drugs. High total dosage or interaction effects among specific drugs might produce negative effects. The timing of administration of the drugs may be a major factor.

Fourth, the magnitude of drug effects is usually small. The effects of birth weight, parity (particularly the first versus subsequent deliveries), and SES, for example, are much larger.

Fifth, a given drug may affect some, but not other, outcomes. Not all effects are negative. Positive effects have been found for some drugs on some outcomes (a factor overlooked by would-be policymakers). Drugs may reduce stress during labor and delivery, thus reducing the probability of negative effects on the fetus. Alternatively, they may increase stress, which may help inoculate the baby against future stress. Research on animals has demonstrated the existence of such inoculation effects.

Sixth, the fact that a medicated group may be advantaged on some outcomes and disadvantaged on others may reflect the operation of chance factors. If a drug truly had no consistent effects but the investigators calculated many statistical tests, some results would be significant merely by chance. Half of those should favor the drug group and half the nondrug group. Some of the findings reported above were like this. In other studies more than a chance number of significant findings occurred or most of the significant findings were in one specific direction (that is, were good or bad).

Seventh, not all babies respond in the same way to a given drug at a given dosage. Individual differences in babies' abilities to metabolize a given drug undoubtedly contribute to the conflicting findings. Babies' capacities in this regard cannot be known before birth,

so a mother's decision to use or not use drugs during delivery cannot be influenced by this factor.

I cannot leave the topic without expressing regret that very little research seems to have been conducted on the topic in the last five years.[12] Given what we know, I would be hesitant to give up the advantages of many of these drugs out of fear of damaging my infant, although I would avoid certain drugs. Some of the alternative childbirth systems to be described in the next section are intended to obviate or reduce the need for drugs.

Childbirth Practices

Discussion has been presented on the known and potential impacts of various perinatal factors—obstetric medication and type of delivery—on the physical well-being of infants. Another set of potentially important variables revolves around the impact of labor and delivery upon the mother's feelings toward her infant and their possible effects upon the quality of her subsequent mothering.

STANDARD DELIVERY PRACTICES AT MID-CENTURY

For some time now there has been considerable controversy over hospital practices with respect to childbirth. This controversy stems from several sources: (a) the various movements for childbirth reform that have focused on the delivery itself (e.g., those of Dick-Read, Lamaze, and Leboyer), (b) those segments of the feminist movement that have been concerned with the impact of delivery practices on the woman or family unit (e.g., see Livingston, 1987), and (c) the doctors, nurses, and researchers concerned with the maternal bond to the infant.

Before these influences had any effect, the standard childbirth in the United States took place in a hospital with a doctor in charge of the delivery. The woman was admitted to the hospital, "prepped" or prepared for labor (this did not mean she was instructed or given counsel, but that she had her pubic hair shaved and was given an enema). When labor was well under way she was separated from the father and any relatives by being placed in a "labor room," often with several other women in labor, some of whom might be screaming or crying. Then, when she was about to

---

12. An annotated bibliography of studies that looked at effects of obstetric drugs on NBAS behaviors up until 1982 can be found in Larin (1982).

deliver, she was taken to the "delivery room," where she was placed on a hard table in the lithotomy position and the obstetrician delivered the baby with appropriate help from an anesthetist and a nurse or nurses. Once the baby was delivered, he or she was held up for the mother to see and then whisked away to be cleaned up, measured, and examined; drops were put in the baby's eyes and the baby was warmed and observed. The whole setting was like that of an operating room (see Figure 5.2). The following sections describe criticisms of these practices and other approaches to childbirth.

Criticisms of These Practices

There are three major criticisms of these earlier standard hospital practices: the exclusion of persons significant to the mother from the whole delivery process, the separation of the mother from her newborn baby in the first minutes and hours after birth, and the treatment of childbirth as surgery or disease and of women who are in labor as sick patients. To understand all these criticisms, it is important to put current American childbirth procedures into some anthropological and historical perspective. Unfortunately, the popular literature on these topics contains much romantic lore about the superiority of the methods used in other cultures or at other times or about what is "natural," so it is essential to know something about the origins of the "standard practices."

The procedures described above resulted from efforts to make childbirth as safe as possible for both mother and infant. Infant and maternal death rates dropped remarkably with the advent of modern hospital practices; that is, after the roles of germs and infection were understood. Few would want to return to practices that result in the higher mortality rates that were an aspect of the "good old days" or of doing what is "natural." At the same time, many hospitals were reluctant to accept newer techniques for avoiding infections and keeping infants well that would allow changes such as not shaving and the presence of others, including children. Instead, they maintained customs that by then were for the convenience of hospital staff rather than the safety of the mother and infant.

Excellent historical views of childbirth in our own culture can be found in several relatively recent books: *Lying-In: A History of Childbirth in America* (Wertz & Wertz, 1979), *Childbearing in American Society: 1650-1850* (Scholten, 1985), and *In the Family Way: Childbearing in the British Aristocracy, 1760-1860* (Lewis, 1986).

Exclusion of Significant Others. Most criticism about the exclusion of significant persons centers on the exclusion of the father from labor and delivery rooms. Some persons are also concerned about the exclusion of children, other relatives, and friends. Some proponents of alternative childbirth systems decry this as going against nature. An examination of practices in various cultures demonstrates that there is, in fact, no one norm. Although fathers are allowed at deliveries in some cultures, other cultures, both literate and preliterate, have throughout history excluded *all* men (including husbands, doctors, and medicine men). Some continue the exclusion for weeks or even months after birth because the mother is considered to be unclean during this time. Other cultures vary from one in which the father takes to a labor bed himself (a practice known as *couvade*) to one in which he may be chained in the sea so that the tide will drown him if his wife does not have a suitably rapid delivery. The impact of these customs on the woman must differ greatly and surely differ from the effects of the husband's mere exclusion. In our own culture the exclusion of fathers was common long before hospitals were invented. The father pacing outside the room where his child was being born is an old and widespread image, whether he was excluded by his wife, her mother, the midwife, or the doctor. All of these patterns are "natural"; that is, they occur (or occurred) in viable cultures—ones that survived for long periods of time without their children becoming so abnormal as to threaten this survival.

Whether fathers are excluded from labor and delivery thus depends largely on cultural traditions, although there are often practical realities underlying the cultural practices. For example, where population densities were low, fathers often had to help at their wives' deliveries, as they still do in remote places or when labor moves faster than the mother can get to the hospital. I know of one case in which the mother, a doctor, delivered herself in the backseat of a car while the father drove and the parents together provided commentary for a young sibling for whom there had been no available baby-sitter.

Exclusion of the father was challenged in connection with several alternative childbirth movements, most of which did not originally concern themselves with fathers being present, but with the presence of a supportive other, often a midwife. Today most hospitals allow fathers to be present throughout labor, delivery, and most of the immediate postdelivery period. Unlimited visiting is often allowed subsequent to birth. Not every hospital allows all of these, and they may be allowed only if the father fulfills certain conditions (e.g., attends childbirth classes).

Cultural norms concerning the exclusion of other people important to the mother also vary widely. Such others include siblings of the infant being born, male or female relatives, and friends. Some cultures allow children (siblings or others), some allow only one sex, some only those below a certain age, and some only those above a certain age. In some cultures birth takes place with all the relatives and friends present, but in others the mother is isolated from all but one or two special persons. In still another she is expected to deliver herself while working in the fields, with no one present.[13]

In Western European cultures, siblings usually have been cared for by relatives or friends for a period of time around birth. They were long banned from obstetric units even for visits to their mothers, who often were there for 10 days or more. Hospitals now vary widely in their practices in this regard. Children are often allowed to visit their mothers in the hospital (a safer practice now that vaccines have conquered many childhood diseases) and are sometimes allowed to touch and hold the newborn as well. In the mid-1980s a male sibling who attended childbirth classes was given court permission to attend his mother's hospital delivery.

In present-day Western cultures, one can find both mothers who would hate and mothers who would love to have the presence of their children, their friends, and/or their husbands during childbirth. In short, one can find cultural or historical evidence for almost any practice that happens to please one. There is no reason to think that any one approach has all the virtues.

Separation of Mother and Newborn. A second major focus of attack on the once-standard hospital procedures for deliveries and mother-child care involves the fact that mothers were routinely separated from their newborns for anywhere from hours to days. Those concerned with maternal bonding were especially vocal in their objections to early separation. In the past, all babies were removed to another room or a different part of the room as soon as the cord had been cut in order to allow some people in the delivery room to concentrate on the infant's well-being while the obstetrician concentrated on the mother's. When these procedures were completed, babies were taken to a nursery and mothers to a recovery room (or to their own rooms, depending on hospital practice and the characteristics of the delivery, such as use of anesthetics or C-sections). Indeed, in an earlier era, when mothers were often so deeply anesthetized that they

were unable to respond to their infants (a condition found with general anesthesia), separation was mandatory. However, it was not limited to those cases.

In addition to the separation of the mother from her infant right after birth, it was standard to allow the infant to be in the mother's room only during feeding time (or perhaps at normal feeding time if that occurred before the infant was due to receive a first feeding). From the 1940s to the 1960s, when very few American mothers were nursing their infants, feeding periods were quite short. Although strict scheduling no longer pervaded the culture by the 1960s, hospitals still adhered rather strictly to schedules (whether for the good of the infant or of the hospital staff may be debatable). These practices, which extended through the hospital stay of 10 to 14 days, were supposed to enable the mother to rest and recover, and to allow her to receive visitors without exposing her baby to their germs. Many would argue that the more important effects were to make the mother feel incapable of caring for her own infant, especially if she was having her first baby and had had little previous experience caring for infants (as is common in cultures in which small nuclear families are the norm). A capable nurse was needed for newborn care.

The perception of the appropriateness of having people other than the mother provide primary care for newborns varies greatly across cultures and history. In some cultures the mother is the primary caregiver from the moment her baby is born. In others she is thought to be able to care for her newborn only if other women take over all of her other responsibilities (from cooking and cleaning to having intercourse with her husband). In some cultures the mother is considered incapable of doing anything for her newborn, other than nursing it, for weeks and often for months. It is rare, however, to separate infants from their mothers to the extent that occurred in "standard" hospital practices, because until 75 years ago infants had to be breast-fed, and that requires frequent interactions; a baby nursed on demand will nurse every 2 to 3 hours.[14] The sooner and more frequently a baby nurses after birth, the sooner the mother's milk comes in. If the mother's breasts are not stimulated in the first few days after she gives birth, her milk production

---

13. Konner (1980) discusses a culture in which this was the cultural ideal, but where it was acknowledged that the ideal was reached only in higher parities (not for first or second children).

14. Among the upper classes in Western cultures, women called "wet nurses" often have been hired to nurse babies and thus relieve the mother of the (animal-like?) chore of nursing. For a discussion of the effect of this on the infants of the women hired, see Maria Piers's book, *Infanticide* (1978).

system will turn off, thus nursing mothers and their infants need more frequent access to each other in the newborn period than has been standard hospital practice. In fact, the desire to have mothers nurse was part of the impetus for the movement in the 1940s to have newborns "room-in" with their mothers in the hospital. Today the desire to encourage breast-feeding is one reason for the objection to hospital practices that separate mothers from infants.

A second basis for objection to the separation of mother and infant concerns the psychological well-being of the pair. Proponents of rooming-in argued that such contact promotes the development of the mother-infant relationship. Indeed, a study that randomly assigned low-income mothers to rooming-in or routine care found overwhelmingly more cases of parental inadequacy in the latter (O'Connor et al., 1980). To some extent the bonding hypothesis seems a modification of rooming-in. Bonding, in the strongest form of the hypothesis, is proposed to occur in a critical period in the first few hours after birth. It is suggested that separation from her baby during that time will interfere with the mother's development of maternal love (the evidence in support of this hypothesis will be discussed later in this chapter). It is quite possible that rooming-in has other benefits. Babies who had it had more quiet sleep and cried less than those in the nursery at nighttime in a small study (Keefe, 1987).

Pregnancy as Illness. The third major criticism of earlier standard practices is related to the perception of pregnancy as an illness. Since the development of modern medicine, doctors have managed pregnancy and birth, and usually have taken the medically safest route, arguing that if there is a potential danger it is best to avoid it. This has led them to require women to restrict their activities in substantial ways during pregnancy. Before modern childbirth movements and the women's movement began to challenge the concept of pregnancy as an illness, doctors commonly forbade many activities during the latter part of pregnancy, such as intercourse and exercise, ranging from driving an automobile to running. Many women objected to such restrictions, but were afraid to go against the doctor's advice because the doctor's word has often been considered law. Thus women have been made to feel dependent and helpless in the face of their doctors' demands (social psychologists have a subfield that deals with such "learned helplessness"). Alternatively, if a woman rebelled, she was apt to feel guilty, especially if anything went wrong.

Cultural and social class norms influence pregnancy

practices as they do other human endeavors, and doctors are not immune to such influence. In some cultures and classes pregnant women have been considered much more delicate than in others. Women in the upper classes were more likely to be treated as ill and to be pampered during pregnancy than those in the lower classes or in subsistence economies, where work throughout pregnancy is required for survival. This has reversed a lot with the emphasis on careers for middle- and upper-class women, whose jobs are more apt to be psychologically stressful than physically stressful.

Attitudes toward sexual intercourse during pregnancy provide a good example of cultural variation. Some cultures (usually polygamous) ban intercourse for much of pregnancy; ours tended to ban it for the last 6 weeks to 3 months; others permit it throughout. There is at least one culture in which frequent intercourse throughout pregnancy is urged because it is thought that the husband's ejaculate is necessary to nourish the growing child (this certainly gives the father a role in pregnancy). Western research shows that, for healthy women, intercourse almost up to the delivery date neither induces premature labor nor leads to greater infection rates.

Delivery as Surgical. The treatment of women during labor and delivery as if they were surgical patients contributes to the depersonalization and loss of control women often feel. Four practices related to such treatment that have fallen under attack include electronic fetal monitoring, delivery position, episiotomies, and length of hospital stay. These are discussed in turn below.

Electronic fetal monitoring, as noted earlier, involves placing electrodes on the scalp of the fetus or bands around the mother's abdomen, hence it interferes with her freedom of movement during labor. This can lead to discomfort and can interfere with the progress of labor. The invasiveness of the internal technique conveys an aura of medicine and surgery that may not be necessary. As noted above, it has been overused because of maternal demand as well as doctor's desires. Its widespread use has not decreased the incidence of cerebral palsy or improved the long-range outcomes of prematures compared with monitoring with a stethoscope, hence the high rate of usage (about 75% of births) clearly seems uncalled for (Shy et al., 1990).

The lithotomy position and episiotomies. The standard lithotomy position, on a hard table with legs up in stirrups in an operating room setting, is uncomfortable and makes the woman feel helpless. It stretches the perineum because the feet are apart, and thus the perineum has less elasticity and is more likely to tear. The doctor (more than 90% of the time in the United States) makes a surgical incision in the perineum; that is, does an **episiotomy**. Presumably this facilitates delivery, is easier to repair than a jagged tear, and prevents dangerous tearing (to the anus); therefore, doctors consider the procedure good preventive medicine (Banta, 1981; Thacker & Banta, 1980).

However, episiotomies have been attacked for a number of reasons. For one thing, an episiotomy is more uncomfortable while it is healing than are tears (Banta, 1981). Also, an episiotomy often interferes with sexual intercourse for many months after birth (as do spontaneous tears). Some object to the fact that episiotomies are done routinely rather than in response to danger of extensive tearing, and suggest that changes in delivery practices might eliminate the need for them in many instances. Recently, it has been asserted that episiotomies may lack medical efficacy.

Borgatta et al. (1989) found that deep perineal tears were much less frequent in women who had no episiotomy and who did not use stirrups in delivery (.9%) than in women who had episiotomies and used stirrups (27.9%). Use of either alone produced an intermediate rate. Green and Soohoo (1989) analyzed the risk of rectal injury for 2,700 spontaneous cephalic (head-first) deliveries and found that having a midline episiotomy increased the risk more than any other factor. The baby's having a large head increased the risk the same amount as being delivered by a physician rather than a midwife, and delivery in a delivery room rather than a labor bed increased it some. In another study of 24,000 deliveries Shiono et al. (1990) found that, even after statistical adjustment for other risk factors, a midline episiotomy resulted in a 4-fold increase in the risk of severe lacerations among first births and an almost 13-fold increase for later births. Mediolateral episiotomies were related to a 2.5-fold reduction in the risk of severe lacerations in first births.

In short, routine episiotomies do not seem to be called for, especially not midline ones, although mediolateral episiotomies may be useful. The lithotomy position is again challenged.

Length of hospital stay. A few decades ago women were routinely kept in the hospital for 10 to 14 days after childbirth, the length of time that would have been prescribed at that time for a surgical patient. Such a long period of recuperation encouraged women to see themselves as ill and in need of medical care. Today many women go home between 2 and 5 days after delivery, as do many surgical patients. Whether this resulted from changes in doctors' perceptions caused by women's objections to being

treated like surgical patients, from medical knowledge about the disadvantages of being bedridden after either delivery or surgery, or from rising hospital costs is unclear. In any case, women today certainly have less time to feel ill or pampered. Indeed, given that there is often no extended family to help out at home, mothers may now find that the fatigue of coping with everything alone when they go home seriously hampers their recovery, and their fatigue may hamper their relationships with their new babies.

It should be noted that today many hospitals offer birthing rooms and other alternative childbirth arrangements.

OTHER APPROACHES TO CHILDBIRTH

Now let us turn to some of the movements for alternative childbirth practices that are followed by substantial numbers of people in our culture. The several methods of prepared childbirth (also called educated or natural childbirth) were developed to allow women to deal with the pain and discomfort of labor and childbirth and therefore to reduce or eliminate obstetric medication. Vertical deliveries were developed in several contexts. Home and birthing center deliveries and use of midwives, monotrices, or doulas have generally centered on psychological support for the mother.

Childbirth Without Fear

British obstetrician Grantly Dick-Read began the first modern movement toward "natural" childbirth. He believed that such a natural process as childbirth should not be full of pain, and decided that women's fear of labor (instilled by other women and even by the Bible) and not labor itself was the source of pain. If this were true and one could eliminate fear, then the pain would be reduced or eliminated also. Dick-Read's classic book *Childbirth Without Fear* (1944/1972) was designed to convince women that childbirth could be a positive experience if only they were not fearful. Dick-Read did not provide any techniques for reducing pain other than positive thinking, and many other obstetricians who attempted this form of childbirth with their patients were much less successful than he had been. The role of hypnosis and self-hypnosis thus came to be questioned as a possible basis for his successes.

Lamaze Childbirth

Russian obstetricians, goaded by a lack of drugs

during World War II, applied the classical conditioning paradigm to labor and called it psychoprophylaxis (mind-prevention). The unconditioned stimulus, the labor contraction, leads to unconditioned responses of pain and tension. The "therapeutic" technique involves conditioning women (through breathing and muscular relaxation responses) to respond positively to the onset of contractions. The conditioned relaxation then competes with the tension associated with the pain of the contractions, and the relaxation responses of women who are well practiced win the battle and reduce the pain.

These techniques were adopted and developed in France in the 1950s by Dr. Ferdinand Lamaze and were introduced into the United States through the missionary work of Marjorie Karmel (1959) (see Lamaze, 1970). By 1983 a survey of 400 hospitals across the United States showed that almost all obstetricians associated with them recommended psychoprophylactic preparation (Wideman & Singer, 1983; cited in Wideman & Singer, 1984). Fathers were allowed in labor and delivery rooms in 99% of these hospitals. Although only 37% of the hospitals offered Lamaze preparation, more than 70% reported that more than half of the mothers delivering at them had had it. Lamaze training classes can be found in rural and city areas, in hospitals and churches; region, income level, and ethnic origin were unrelated to electing a Lamaze delivery in the Wideman and Singer study.

Unlike Dick-Read advocates, Lamaze parents are usually taught that medication may become desirable (to the mother) or required (by the physician) and that such eventualities should not be interpreted as failure. If a cesarean becomes advisable, Lamaze parents are encouraged to accept that as an unfortunate, but acceptable, outcome.

Lamaze classes usually involve six weekly sessions, in which (a) the childbirth process is described in detail so that mothers can estimate the time between contractions and the likely duration and intensity of the pain, (b) the relaxation and breathing exercises are introduced and practiced, (c) mothers are taught to focus cognitively on relaxing thoughts and told to bring objects or pictures that are relaxing to them on which they can focus during contractions, and (d) the father or other companion is taught to help. The goal is to enable the woman to deal with her pain. Taken together, these techniques can maximize the likelihood that mothers-to-be will be awake and alert and in a positive frame of mind to enjoy the birth of their babies.

The role of the father in Lamaze deliveries as practiced in the United States was originally filled by trained women called *monotrices* in France. Such assistants are not generally available in the United States, so fathers came to assume their function and became participants in the labor and delivery process. They learn the breathing techniques, and they help time contractions and massage the mothers as well as provide emotional support. This involvement of the father has come to be seen as one of the major desirable features of Lamaze childbirth, American style. A retrospective study of fathers indicates that being coaches was highly stressful for them, and that they spent much of the time trying to hide their feelings and worrying about their usefulness (Berry, 1988).

Does Lamaze really lead to the results that advocates expect? Evidence on this subject is lacking, and what there is, is conflicting. (See Wideman & Singer, 1984, for documentation of the low amount of research to that date and an interesting survey of the relevance of different aspects of the Lamaze technique.) Broome and Koehler (1986) report that of the women they studied, both prepared mothers and those whose husbands were present reported less pain and more positive feelings. Similarly, Leventhal et al. (1989) report that pain and negative moods in second-stage labor declined for Lamaze-trained women and for those who were told to monitor their contractions. It has also been reported that 10-20% of prepared-childbirth women, but only 3-14% of women in general, say they had no pain. One study has found that psychological pain-control techniques did not reduce the intensity of pain or reduce the frequency of using epidural anesthetics in first-time mothers unless they were consistently supported throughout labor and it was relatively short (Copstick et al., 1986). Lamaze-trained mothers were found not to differ from matched controls in use of analgesia and anesthesia, length of labor, type of delivery, fetal distress, or complications, but to be given oxytocin more frequently (Patton et al., 1985). Finally, Lamaze-trained mothers who had not only their partners with them during labor but also professional support persons have been shown to be less likely to have pain medication or episiotomies (Hodnett & Osborn, 1989).

Prepared-childbirth techniques may affect relations among mothers and fathers and their infants in a number of ways. If mother and infant do receive less medication, both are apt to be more alert in the immediate postbirth period. The mother is more able to respond to her baby and the baby to her, and the baby is more likely to nurse with sufficient vigor to stimulate the mother's milk production. All of this should lead to better maternal bonding according to proponents of that theory. Finally, Lamaze deliveries provide an explicit and necessary role for the father. He not only gets to watch his child aborning, in a context where his emotional bond to his spouse may well be strengthened, but his initial bonding to the baby may also be facilitated.

To evaluate the desirability of Lamaze childbirth, it is necessary to consider the effects on the family separately from those on the baby. It is one thing to engage in prepared childbirth for the sake of the parents' emotional experience. That decision is one that is properly up to each family. It is quite another thing to argue that prepared childbirth will lead to advantages for the offspring. The answer to this question is not known.

Leboyer: Birth Without Violence

Another set of alternative delivery practices is known as "birth without violence," from the title of Leboyer's (1975) book, or simply as Leboyer delivery. These practices assume an alert, awake mother at delivery and, in fact, they are most often paired with a Lamaze type of preparation and delivery. The focus, however, is on the infant's birth experience. The techniques are derived from the theories of Reich, Rank, and Janov, all of whom consider birth to be *the* prototypical emotional trauma that leads to emotional difficulties later in life. Leboyer developed techniques designed to minimize the infant's trauma. Bright, glaring operating room lights are replaced with dim, indirect lighting; the temperature of the room is kept close to that of the mother's body (rather than cool, like a delivery room, which is kept comfortable for working persons in surgical garb). After delivery and before the umbilical cord is cut, the naked baby is put on the mother's bare belly, thus providing skin-to-skin contact. People refrain from talking loudly or making noise, soft music may be played, and the baby is handled gently and slowly, which is presumably the way he or she was jostled in the womb. The cord is cut only after it stops pulsating, a practice around which there is considerable medical argument. The infant is then given a warm bath, presumably to re-create the experience of the womb.

Leboyer deliveries are controversial for many reasons. They are very intrusive on hospital staff, and nonbelievers are not likely to be amenable to such disruptions. More theoretically, some authorities argue that the shocks of bright lights and noise may help to establish regular breathing. The "proof of the pudding" is to be found in research on infant outcomes. Early reports were enormously positive. According to

Rappoport (1976), Leboyer-delivered babies walked sooner than average, were unusually adept with their hands, toilet trained easily, and learned to feed themselves early. Unfortunately, she made no direct comparisons with traditionally delivered infants of similar women. Women who are concerned with the delicate sensibilities of their newborns may be generally sensitive to their infants' emotional needs, and, as we shall see in Chapter 12, this apparently is a major variable in child rearing. And those who choose a new procedure may differ in important ways from those who stick with tradition. When subjects are not randomly assigned to the delivery techniques being compared, the effects of the technique are confounded by those of the type of parents who chose it.

One recent study attempted random assignment (Nelson et al., 1980). However, out of 153 women with low-risk pregnancies who were interested in the Leboyer approach, who intended to attend prenatal classes and would be available for 3-day and 8-month follow-ups, only 56 were willing to be randomly assigned. These were stratified according to whether it was a first or later pregnancy and according to social class. Within these groupings women were randomly assigned to the Leboyer group or to the control group. Control deliveries took place in a cool, well-lit delivery room, the cord was cut within 60 seconds, and the baby was wrapped in a blanket and returned to the mother. Leboyer deliveries took place in the mother's bed in a warm, dimly lit labor room. The baby was placed in skin-to-skin contact with the mother and massaged by her. The cord was cut only after it stopped pulsating and the infant was given a warm bath by the father.

Both groups were the same in that fathers participated actively, no "prepping" was done (i.e., no shaving or enemas), and no medication other than epidurals was used. Bulb suctioning of the nasopharynx was done as needed for both groups and no infants were weighed or given silver nitrate drops in the eyes in the first hour. The groups did not differ significantly in actual medications used, use of labor induction, spontaneous rupture of membranes, rooming-in (all had it at least part-time), or feeding practices (most breast-fed). All cesarean (5) and forceps (8) deliveries in both groups were excluded from the study.

The Leboyer group had significantly shorter first-stage labor (median 7.5 hours, compared with 14 hours for the control group). Although the authors did not report on it, it seems plausible that the absence of the lithotomy position and the more relaxed setting could have led to the shorter labors in the ex-

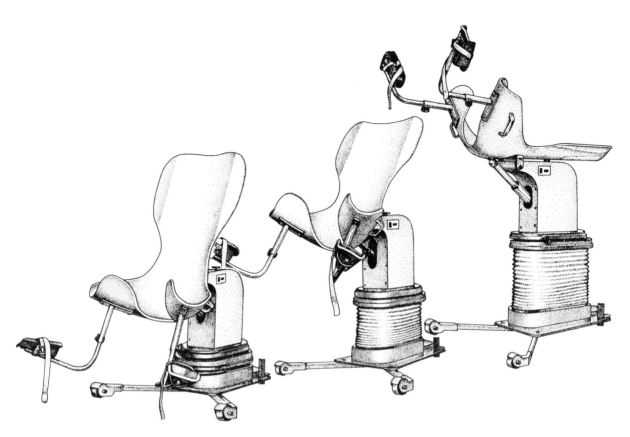

**Figure 5.4. An obstetrical chair that is currently available commercially in the
United States. While it was to be modified to be more adjustable, or more like that
used by Caldeyro-Barcia (or the sixteenth-century French), its fate seems to be that
it is primarily used as a urology chair.**

perimental group. The authors note that the Leboyer
mothers may have expected easier births, and the belief may have led to greater relaxation and easier labors
(Nelson et al., 1980). Mothers in the two groups did
not differ in their ratings of the birth experience, their
psychological adjustment, or their perceptions of their
babies as difficult (compared with the average baby).
Initially mothers did not differ in their perceptions of
the delivery's effect on their babies, but at 8 months
the Leboyer mothers were more likely to think the delivery had influenced their babies' behavior. Maternal
perceptions can, of course, be influenced by beliefs
about the effects of delivery practices.

Nelson and colleagues (1980) also measured infants' behaviors and did not find the advantages predicted by Leboyer proponents. Proponents have
reported that babies born in this fashion are quieter,
more alert, and cry less, but in this study the babies in
the two groups did not differ on any of these behaviors. The calming effect of the bath was also not obvious, since 9 of the 19 babies observed in it reacted

with irritable crying. Brazelton assessments done at 24
and 72 hours by examiners with no knowledge of the
baby's method of delivery showed no statistically significant differences in interactive or motor processes,
state control, or response to stress. Neither the Bayley
scales nor the Carey assessment of temperament at 8
months showed any differences. As I will describe in a
subsequent section, one of the ingredients of a
Leboyer delivery, early, tactile contact between mother
and infant, is thought by some to be important for
maternal bonding, a question that was not directly addressed in this research.

It thus appears that evidence for the claimed superiority of Leboyer-delivered babies does not seem to
exist in a controlled randomized study. However, all
mothers were given prenatal education, delivered with
a significant other present, received little anesthesia or
other drugs, and participated in several other features
of various systems that have challenged conventional
procedures, some of which are a part of the Leboyer
total package. What effect the fact that only one-third

of the mothers agreed to random assignment might have had on results is unknown. In any event, the lack of significant differences between the groups in morbidity or negative outcomes should be reassuring to doctors and patients when the latter desire Leboyer delivery.

Vertical Delivery Position

A movement to permit women a choice of a vertical or semivertical delivery position (in a birthing chair or propped against pillows or another person, or squatting on a floor or in a wading pool) has arisen in several contexts. There is much historical and cultural precedent for vertical delivery positions. In many preliterate societies, women give birth in a squatting position. Throughout history, women in various cultures have used semiupright positions. As a teenager, I discovered that an English obstetrician had invented a delivery chair.[15] It made good sense to me, and I wondered why it had gone out of favor. I later learned that this was a reinvention of the obstetrical chair. The Old Testament refers to the obstetrical chair, the walls of the tomb of Queen Hatshepshut of Egypt (who died in 1468 B.C.) show its use for the delivery of her son, and in some places it was part of a midwife's equipment until the nineteenth century.

More recently, Caldeyro-Barcia built his own obstetrical chair modeled after a sixteenth-century French one, all of the parts of which were adjustable. All of his mothers chose the chair in preference to the lithotomy position. Figure 5.4 shows a currently available obstetrical chair, but it is not as adjustable as Caldeyro-Barcia's.

Other forms of vertical delivery are becoming more common. In many places women may choose their birthing position, which may be squatting, squatting in a wading pool, sitting in a chair, or propped against pillows (see Figure 5.5). Most women offered a choice opt for a vertical position (see, for example, Odent, 1982, 1984). Subsequent to Odent's work a water birth movement has arisen (Daniels, 1989). Separately from it, soothing effects of a warm bath during labor as an alternative to epidural anesthesia has been assessed in terms of subjective reactions. Normal primiparas and multiparas with pathological pregnancies were found to be positive about the experience (Gillot-de-Vries et al., 1987).

There is growing medical evidence that lying down may not be the best position for either labor or delivery. Both a vertical position and movement strengthen contractions (Mendez-Bauer et al., 1975) and shorten labor. Caldeyro-Barcia (1981) found first-stage labor

to be 25% shorter for 40 patients who were primarily vertical (median 147 minutes compared with 225 minutes for 5 who were horizontal; all were having their first babies and had had normal pregnancies). Rates of assisted and cesarean deliveries are reportedly much lower. Caldeyro-Barcia reports that with mothers in a vertical position, even breech deliveries do not require maneuvers. Perhaps reclining and being quiescent to permit monitoring led to some of the great increase in breech presentation reported earlier. Odent reports a cesarean rate of only 8% among 1,800 deliveries in 1977 and 1978. A review of research points out the difficulties and concludes cautiously that ambulation, standing, and sitting in labor *may* shorten its length, and that there is no evidence for their being harmful (Lupe & Gross, 1986). Japanese data indicate that while sitting is advantageous for first deliveries, the supine position seems to better for subsequent deliveries (Mizuta, 1987).

The mother's circulatory system may be stressed by a horizontal delivery, because the lungs and the major blood vessels are compressed when one is lying down. This affects the amount of oxygen the mother and her infant receive. An index of anoxia (PCO^2 level) does not rise in sitting-up deliveries, even after 200 minutes, although it rises after only 50 minutes in horizontal deliveries. Oxygen levels are also better for mothers in a sitting position than for those in the lithotomy position (Wood et al., 1964-1965). Furthermore, in vertical deliveries the perineum is less stretched than in the lithotomy position, hence the likelihood of tears or need for episiotomies is much less frequent (Caldeyro-Barcia, 1981; Odent, personal communications, 1981, 1982).

Infants born in vertical deliveries appear to be either at no increased risk or at reduced risk compared with those born in horizontal deliveries. Odent found a perinatal death rate of only 9 per 1,000, compared with 20 per 1,000 for all French infants at that time. Only 1.7% of the babies had to be transferred to intensive care hospitals. Infections in babies and mothers were infrequent even though mothers wore their own clothes, used the wading pool (even during birth), and had fathers present.[16] Drs. Moyses and Claudio

---

15. I learned this from a book called *Devils, Drugs and Doctors* (Haggard, 1929/1959), the first two parts of which were devoted to surveying the history of practices surrounding childbirth historically. Although this volume was first published in 1929, I still recommend it to students. It is, of course, less up to date than the Wertz and Wertz book.

16. The wading pool referred to is the foot-high, inflatable, backyard type of pool.

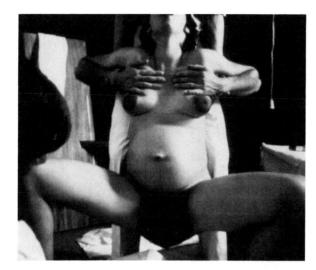

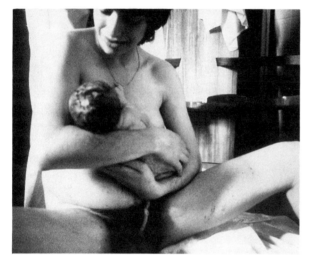

Figure 5.5. One kind of alternative birthing experience. (top) The mother in a squatting position. She is supported by the father and attended by a midwife, the back of whose head is visible. The midwife monitors the delivery and calls on the doctor only if necessary. The baby's head is crowning, as can be seen in the bulge at the vaginal opening. (bottom) A mother nursing her newborn. The umbilical cord is still attached and the placenta has not yet been delivered. This illustrates some of the bonding practices discussed in the next section: skin-to-skin contact, early suckling, no early separation. In fact, all mothers in this hospital have rooming-in, including those whose babies must be in incubators but do not require intensive care. (Photographs courtesy of Dr. Michael Odent.)

Paciornik (1976) found fewer neurological problems in Indian babies in Brazil whose mothers squatted during delivery than in their urban, "modern" counterparts delivered with the mothers lying on their backs.

(Their film is referenced in the manual.)

In sum, giving birth in a sitting or squatting position seems to be safer for both mothers and infants than delivering in the lithotomy position. If future research replicates these findings, these positions should become popular. However, resistance to change is strong. I know of a maternity hospital that was loaned a commercial birthing chair and had many mothers who asked for it, but the doctors ordered it returned at the end of the loan period.

Home Deliveries

The movement to give birth at home has gathered strength in the United States in the last few years. It is another way of objecting to treatment of childbirth as a semisurgical procedure and a response to the resistance of doctors and hospitals to modification of their practices. Home deliveries permit parents to control the process and thereby design a birth experience according to their own ideas. Indeed, most women who deliver at home, usually with prepared-childbirth techniques, report their deliveries as peak experiences.

Home deliveries are standard practice in some Western countries. Women who are at minimal risk (many social as well as medical factors are defined as risks) deliver at home in the Netherlands, assisted by professional midwives, an honored profession there, and in most of Scandinavia and many other countries. The midwife is also in attendance at the hospital deliveries of at-risk pregnancies, but will be joined by a doctor at any sign of a problem. The neonatal death rate for all deliveries in Holland is considerably lower than that for the United States.

Home deliveries are becoming more prevalent in the United States, both for couples concerned about the birth experience (usually educated) and probably for persons unable to afford hospital delivery (statistics are less reliable on this). Mothers in this group are also less likely to have had adequate, or even any, prenatal care, which would define them as at risk in Holland. Can we expect them to be as safe? Not necessarily.

In the United States, home deliveries are often not attended by medical professionals. This is true for several reasons: (a) Many doctors refuse to attend home deliveries, (b) trained midwives are in relatively short supply and are even illegal in some states, (c) some persons opting for home delivery (and a nonillness model) do not wish to have any medical personnel present, and (d) some mothers cannot afford any trained help. In Holland a trained midwife is routinely present. Even the lower-SES mothers who are considered at risk in Holland are considerably better off in social and economic terms than lower-SES mothers in the United States.

Although the overall question of the safety of home deliveries in the United States is not fully agreed upon, some conclusions can be drawn:

(1) *If* a careful assessment of risk is made, and *if* an adequately trained midwife or doctor is present, and *if* hospital facilities are not too far away should there be a need for them for mother or infant, there seems to be no reason home deliveries would not be as safe as in other countries.

(2) Home deliveries that do not have the above safeguards would seem to be unnecessarily risky.

Some data from Australia show that midwife-attended home deliveries (1983-1986) had the following results: Only 1% had cesareans and only 5% assisted births, and no labor was induced among the 84% who were not transferred to a hospital in advance. The only neonatal death was due to congenital anomalies (Howe, 1988). A study in the United States that closely matched every home-delivery case for risk factors with a hospital case and where 66% were delivered by family physicians and only 31% by lay midwives showed no maternal deaths in either group and infant deaths did not differ (were low in both). The hospital-delivered group had a large excess of many factors judged nonoptimal: 3 times as many cesareans, 20 times more frequent use of forceps, twice as frequent use of oxytocin, more use of analgesia and anesthesia, both more tears and more surgical cuts, 6 times as many infants showing distress in labor, 5 times as many cases of maternal high blood pressure, 3 times as many cases of maternal hemorrhaging, 4 times as many infections among newborns, 3 times as many babies who needed help to initiate breathing at birth, and more babies with breathing difficulties in the first days of life. In addition, there were 30 cases of physical injury to the newborn among the 1,064 hospital births, and none among the home deliveries.

Both the Australian and U.S. studies indicate that home deliveries are safer than those in hospitals. The precautions advocated above held for both of these studies. Unfortunately, most studies have been conducted by avowed advocates, which reduces the amount of reliable data available.

Birthing Centers

A compromise between hospital and home delivery is provided in a number of areas of the country by so-called freestanding birthing centers. *Freestanding* sim-

ply means that they are not directly associated with any hospital. There are also birthing centers within some hospitals. Most birthing centers are staffed by medically trained midwives who carefully screen their clients to be "low risk" and promptly refer them to traditional care if they develop any problems. Individual centers may follow some of the specific practices described above or others. A recent study reports the outcomes for almost 12,000 deliveries of low-risk mothers in 84 such centers (Rooks et al., 1989). Almost 16% were transferred to hospitals, most of them first-time deliveries. There were only 4.4% cesareans, no maternal deaths, and the combined neonatal deaths and deaths at delivery were 1.3 per 1,000 births. Hence for selected patients, and especially women not in their first pregnancies, these birthing centers provided safe alternatives. However, only half of the known birthing centers participated in this study; it is likely that nonparticipants were not a random selection of birthing centers. Even among participants, 5 centers were excluded from the data analyses because they did not conform to the standards set for patient enrollment or records; they had a much higher mortality rate. (See Lieberman & Ryan, 1989, for discussion of these issues.)

In a smaller study with a large number of comparisons, Feldman and Hurst (1987) also found maternity center births to be safe for low-risk pregnancies. These researchers' detailed comparisons indicate that although labors are longer in such centers, the proportion of fetal heart rate abnormalities is lower. They call attention to the "obstetrical cascade," in which one hospital intervention leads to another (oxytocin use to need for epidurals, for example), described by Mold and Stein (1986).

Midwives in the United States

Much of the above discussion has proceeded as if we do not have midwives in the United States. Although they were illegal in many states until relatively recently, this does not mean they did not exist.[17] The levels of training of midwives vary greatly. Certified nurse-midwives (CNMs) not only have R.N. degrees plus special training, they often work only in hospital settings with obstetricians as consultants, and they do no surgery or even use forceps. Currently CNMs have hospital privileges in only three of the nine hospitals

---

17. Midwives were outlawed in Massachusetts at the beginning of the century; they regained legal recognition there in 1977.

providing obstetrical services in Washington, D.C., and even there they cannot admit patients themselves (Langton & Kammerer, 1989). They sometimes operate birthing centers, using physicians only as consultants. In Florida, so-called empirical midwives constitute more than 90% of all midwives. Their training includes a two- to three-year apprenticeship to another empirical midwife and self-training, and they rarely have working relationships with physicians. With the current crisis in medical care for pregnancy and delivery, doctors are calling for a much larger role for trained midwives in inner cities as well as in rural areas. Incidentally, it is not only doctors who are being driven out of obstetrics by insurance costs; midwives working at birthing centers are also having their insurance rates raised markedly.

The family physician who practices obstetrics may offer many of the advantages of a midwife. A large-scale Canadian study shows that for women whose deliveries were categorized as low risk (even though from a population at higher social risk), the rates of interventions other than C-sections were much lower and the complications for mothers and infants did not differ when the birth was attended by a family physician as opposed to an obstetrician (Reid et al., 1989). Family physicians less often artificially ruptured the membranes, induced or augmented labor, used low forceps or vacuum extraction, did episiotomies, or used epidural anesthesia.

Female Support Persons

It is possible that the midwife serves not only a medical function but one of being a closely interacting supportive female. A number of people have called attention to the fact that historically and cross-culturally female support figures have played an important role in childbirth. In one locale where prepared childbirth was practiced and the father was present together with a midwife, if labor progressed too slowly the doctor would find an errand for the father to run, which often served to speed up labor (Odent, personal communication, 1982).

A woman experienced in childbirth who stays with the mother throughout labor but has no medical role is called a *doula* by Klaus and colleagues (1986). A trained monitrice was involved in the Leboyer deliveries on Odent's OB service. Twice as many women randomly assigned to have a monitrice had no medication, fewer used stirrups, and more had intact perineums (Hodnett & Osborn, 1989). There were no differences between those with or without a monitrice in the number of C-sections or in use of

forceps. Inasmuch as the use of medications differed between the groups, the role of the monitrice in reducing length of labor was significant.

DeLay et al. (1987) have described the activities of a doula: She stays close to the mother, talks to her, and has a great deal of tactile contact with her, which tends to become clutching in late stages. Compared with a control group that labored alone, the presence of a doula has been shown to lead to many fewer C-sections and fewer perinatal complications (Klaus et al., 1986). In addition, the length of labor was cut almost in half (8 versus 14 hours). In a study done in the United States with random assignment to having or not having a doula, labors conducted with a doula were 2 hours shorter than those of the control group; even the group that was just observed had a 1-hour shorter labor (Kennell et al., 1988; McGrath et al., 1991). Less than 8% of the doula group had epidural anesthesia, compared with 23% of the observed and 55% of the control groups. Forceps were used three times as often in the control group, and C-sections were done twice as often. Maternal fever was more than twice as frequent in the control group, as was a prolonged stay in hospital for the infant.

These studies have been of women's first deliveries, and Kennell (1990), in a discussion of his paper, points out that first-time fathers are apt to be worried and anxious too, and hence less able to reassure their wives. In addition, the mother may try to protect the father instead of just drawing support from him. The great individual differences in fathers' effectiveness as support figures have been documented (Nagashima et al., 1987). A study that looked at continuous one-on-one support of a nurse in Lamaze-trained deliveries where the father was present found that those with the nurse present were less likely to have pain medication or episiotomies (Hodnett & Osborn, 1989). One must of course remember that not all women want the same amount or kinds of support, a commonsense view supported by data (Mackey & Lock, 1989).

*Difficulty of Arriving at Conclusions
About Alternative Childbirth*

In evaluating the safety, effectiveness, and benefits of any of the alternative forms of childbirth, researchers are confronted by the problem that different types of people choose these alternatives. Only a few studies have randomly assigned mothers to a treatment group. In the absence of that, one needs to know the effects of the type of people compared with those of the childbirth format. In a study of drug knowledge and usage in hospital deliveries compared with birthing center and home deliveries, Brackbill et al. (1985) found the following differences, all of which could affect outcomes for the delivery type: Hospital mothers were (a) younger, (b) less educated, (c) less often white, (d) more often not living with the father, (e) less often worked during pregnancy, and (f) much more often recipients of some form of aid during pregnancy. Mothers attending birthing centers were more apt not to have any religious affiliation, and those having home births were more apt to belong to fundamentalist or nontraditional religious groups. In addition, hospital-delivered mothers drank more caffeine-containing beverages and were more apt to smoke during pregnancy. Clearly, many of these factors might be expected to affect outcomes for a baby regardless of the other delivery factors.

Conclusions

Despite the above cautions, it does seem possible to draw several conclusions. Home and birthing center deliveries are safe if appropriately supervised, and may lead to fewer complications than hospital deliveries. Support during delivery, whether by husbands, medical personnel, or relatively untrained persons (monotrices or doulas), helps reduce complications of childbirth. Many of the alternative childbirth strategies as well as the alternative settings for childbirth should operate to reduce stress. The possibility has been raised that these may operate through the action of endogenous analgesics. Research has not really started, but one study showed that multiparas who exercised throughout pregnancy had more endogenous hormones and fewer stress hormones, and reported less pain throughout labor (Varrassi et al., 1989).

Finally, it is important to remember that mothers are individuals with different needs. Few studies have looked at women's choices. Mackey's (1990) study of choices of childbirth settings emphasizes the importance of flexibility and choice in maternity care. For an excellent discussion of how to find the kind of care a woman or family wants, see Herzfeld (1985).

Mother-Infant Bonding

Many people believe that the emotional attachment of mothers to their infants is set in a profound way during the first hours or days after birth. They see circumstances related to delivery that prevent, or make more difficult, the establishment of a bond to the infant at that time as likely to result in suffering for the infant. Premature infants are more isolated from their

mothers than full-term infants, and hence are likely to be particularly at risk. But term infants also may be at risk, because most Western deliveries take place in hospitals where it is common practice to remove infants from their mothers for considerable periods of time right after birth and where a mother may have received enough drugs to lower her responsiveness to her baby and her baby's responsiveness to her.

Although most psychologists are delighted to see humanizing changes in hospital practices, many disagree with the notion that experiences during the immediate postnatal period are crucial to the mother's ability to mother her child. That is, they doubt that there is a critical or sensitive period for human maternal bonding to infants. In this section I will first provide some background and outline pros and cons of the issues, and then proceed to the detailed research evidence.

There are two bases for the recent thinking about the mother's attachment to her infant. One is the impact of **ethology** (a branch of zoology that studies animal behavior in its evolutionary and developmental context) on behavioral scientists and students of infancy in particular. Research inspired by ethological concepts has demonstrated that when mothers of some mammalian species are separated from their offspring for relatively short periods of time, it becomes difficult to get them to reaccept those offspring and provide normal mothering. This is true with cows, sheep, and goats (all of which are ungulates). In the case of goats, the data are particularly clear that the mother will not reaccept her kid and mother it even though rejection will lead to its death unless the experimenters intervene. The second basis stems from anecdotal evidence about infants who failed to thrive after being sent home from the hospital as presumably healthy. The pioneer work that is most often cited is that by Klaus and Kennell (1976), which will be discussed in detail shortly.

Before discussing the research evidence, I would like to cite a few important considerations that might lead to some skepticism about a critical period for human mothers to attach to their infants. First, ungulates are one branch of the mammalians; other nonhuman species of mammals do not show any strong rejection of their offspring if separated from them after delivery. Many species will accept and nurture not only their own separated offspring, but those of other mothers, and even of other species, although they may require a little extra time to accept them. Some primates will even provide compensatory care for experimentally damaged infants (Berkson, 1974; Rosenblum & Youngstein, 1974). The dangers of extrapolating from one species to another are compounded because we do not know what species might provide the most appropriate model.

Second, the original work in this field focused on premature infants and was extrapolated to term infants. Many factors other than the mother's lack of contact with her infant in the newborn period may operate to reduce the effectiveness of her bonding to (or forming a strong attachment for) her premature infant, if indeed she is less attached. The infant may be less physically attractive; the mother may regard her preemie as "made of egg shells," and may be afraid to handle or express love toward the baby; the infant's behavior may be more difficult than that of other infants, and hence less likely to trigger affectionate responses (and, in extreme cases, may trigger hostile ones). Even if the behavior is not difficult in some absolute sense, it may be so different from the mother's previous experience or from her expectations that she may react negatively. Physical as well as psychological reasons may play a role in failure to thrive. Thus many factors may explain failure of maternal bonding or be related to poor outcomes for infants. Nevertheless, it is possible that procedures to enhance bonding could help some mothers deal more adequately with any of these factors and thus lead to lower risk for their infants.

A third reason for skepticism about the criticality of early contact is the fact that for many centuries, the world over, there have been cases of successful adoption. These occur not only with "mothers" who have not given birth to a particular baby or child, but with "mothers" who have never given birth to any baby.

Methodological problems of research in this area are great, and the outcomes are not entirely clear. It is important to be alert to the danger that belief in the bonding hypothesis may arouse guilt in parents who may question the adequacy of their attachment to their offspring because they had no opportunity for immediate maternal bonding experiences. Mothers should not be made to feel that they must opt for and attain these procedures if they are not to deprive their children.

The following subsections will discuss whether the differences in childbirth practices affect the infant through the mechanism of maternal bonding. If the process of the mother attaching to her infant is disrupted by hospital practices, will this affect her ability to mother and hence the well-being of the infant? Although the hospital practices discussed earlier have dealt with the birth of full-term babies, the consideration of bonding here begins with studies of the premature infant. One reason for this is that the impetus for

the original studies came from clinicians' experiences with prematures. Any discussion of bonding with prematures must be separated from that with term infants because hospital practices differ so much for the two groups, and because prematures may be more vulnerable to any deficiencies in the quality of their mothers' bonds to them.

BONDING TO PREMATURE INFANTS

Pediatricians were aware of babies whose lives had been saved, often by heroic efforts, and who were developing very well when discharged, but who returned to the hospital after a period at home with what is known as "failure to thrive." They did not gain weight or develop appropriately, and there seemed to be no physical reason. Indeed, they often began to develop normally again after nothing more than routine hospital care. Also, according to some data, more premature or LBW babies were abused than would be expected by chance. Klaus and Kennell (1970), and others, hypothesized that the mothers of these infants might be inadequate because they had been separated from their infants in the immediate postbirth period. The standard hospital practices for such babies had been to isolate them in special nurseries, never take them to their mothers, and often not to allow the mother to touch or feed her infant until weeks or even months after birth.

Had hospital practice followed the advice given in the first textbook on neonatology (Budin, 1907), some of these problems might have been avoided. Budin reported that some mothers of prematures lost all interest in their babies and subsequently abandoned them. He advised that mothers of prematures should breast-feed their infants and be allowed to visit and look at (he invented the glass-walled incubator) and even care for them, even though that might have to be in the hospital for considerable periods of time.

Unfortunately, Budin's pupil and disciple, Cooney, who publicized the methods for care of prematures, left out the factors of maternal care and feeding. Indeed, his publicity techniques seem quite astounding and certainly dictated against involvement of the mothers. From 1896 through 1940, Cooney exhibited premature infants in glass incubators at major fairs and expositions in Berlin, London, and various parts of the United States, offering the mothers free passes to the fairs. At the Chicago World's Fair in 1932, the receipts from Cooney's exhibit were second only to those for Sally Rand, the famed fan dancer (Liebling, 1939; cited in Klaus & Kennell, 1976). At the New York World's Fair of 1940 he exhibited and successfully cared for 5,000 prematures!

In the 1920s, hospitals began to establish nurseries, and they were run in ways designed to avoid infections. Practices for nursery management, like those for maternal care, did not change as techniques for prevention and cure of infections improved. Nor did they change as a result of studies in England in the late 1940s and early 1950s that demonstrated that maternal care and even home maternal care (Miller, 1948; cited in Klaus & Kennell, 1976) did not increase infections or substantially raise mortality rates.[18] As Klaus and Kennell (1976) note, "Standard textbooks on the care of the newborn from 1945 to 1960 continued to reflect the traditions and fears of the early 1900s, recommending only the most essential handling of the infants and a policy of strict isolation (exclusion of visitors)" (p. 6). These recommendations were in part based on a desire to protect prematures from overstimulation, which was seen as overtaxing their limited resources, a viewpoint that is being returned to in part today.

Klaus was among the colleagues of C. R. Barnett who started the first study in the United States (in 1964 at the Stanford University Hospital) of the effects of permitting parents into the premature nursery. Not only was parent visitation safe, but nurses, who were originally quite skeptical, became enthusiasts when they found that their routines were not interfered with and that most mothers were a real help in caring for their infants. Nevertheless, nurseries in the United States were slow to change. In 1970 only a third of 1,400 premature nurseries answering a questionnaire allowed mothers to enter the premature nursery. Only 12% allowed them to touch their babies in the first few days (C. R. Barnett, R. Grobstein, & M. Seashore, personal communication with Klaus & Kennell, 1972; cited in Klaus & Kennell, 1976).

Research Supporting the Bonding Hypothesis

What were the actual effects of early contact on the mothers and their infants? First of all, 2 of the 13 mothers selected for the Stanford program refused to enter the nursery. They feared becoming more attached to their babies and then having to suffer more if they should die. Neither of these infants' families named their babies for a month, though the babies had been declared out of danger well before that.[19]

The 11 mothers who entered the nursery touched, explored, fed, diapered, and talked and cooed to their babies despite the plastic barrier between them. The investigators felt that the mothers were more committed to their babies, had more confidence in their mothering abilities, and showed greater skill in stimu-

lating and caring for their infants than the mothers who were not selected for visiting. Few objective data are provided, but the mothers touched and explored their babies' bodies differently. Although the investigators may have been biased, the outcomes seem highly reasonable.

Mothers of prematures began to behave more like those of term babies by their third visit, increasing their fingertip contacts, the number of times they touched the trunk as opposed to the extremities, and the proportion of time spent in the *en face* (face-to-face) position. But they still spent only about half as much time in contact, and about one-third as much contacting with the palm or contacting the baby's trunk, as mothers of full-term infants did on their first visit. Figure 2.12 may help those who are not familiar with small prematures understand why mothers were inhibited from touching the baby's trunk. Indeed, parents have reported that the most stressful aspect of their premature's being in the intensive care unit is the infant's appearance and behavior (Miles, 1989).

The first long-term studies of the effects of separation on mother-infant interaction and development of premature infants were done at Stanford University (Leifer et al., 1972) and at Case Western Reserve University (Klaus et al., 1972; Klaus & Kennell, 1970, 1976). At both places the early-contact mothers were allowed in the intensive care unit (ICU, also called NICU, or neonatal intensive care unit) in the first 5 days after birth; the comparison group had only visual contact for the first 21 days. In the Stanford study, an additional comparison group of mothers of full-term infants had the usual contacts at feeding time for the 3 days they were hospitalized. Both at Case and at Stanford the investigators found it impossible to study early- and routine-contact groups simultaneously, because the staff would not permit some mothers to be denied contact with their infants when others had it, so the groups were studied sequentially. Although participants were thus not randomly assigned, there is no reason to assume that the population was different in

---

18. It should be noted that current procedures for monitoring and controlling fluid levels and acid-base balance used with very small and/or sick prematures could not be instrumented at home.

19. It is interesting that in a number of cultures where infant mortality is high, customs do not call for naming infants for considerable periods of time. For example, in Egypt, I was told that it is difficult to get good infant mortality figures because parents do not register the birth of a baby for several weeks or until they feel the infant is sure to live for some months. They used to register births even later when neonatal mortality was higher.

one year than in another. The Stanford groups were all middle-class and the Case Western Reserve groups covered a range of social classes.

Let us look first at the Stanford study (Leifer et al., 1972). Early-contact mothers averaged visits only once every 6 days and had only 3 or 4 more visits than the low-contact group. Either the privilege was not seen as one or the practical difficulties of arranging visits to the hospital did not permit parents to take advantage of it. Both early- and low-contact mothers could spend as much time with their babies as they wanted for the last week to 10 days before discharge when the babies were out of intensive care. It is thus not surprising that there were few differences between early- and late-contact mothers of prematures, although the late-contact mothers, especially of firstborns, did feel less capable at 1 week, but not at 1 month, after discharge (Seashore et al., 1973). The contrast between mothers of preterm and of full-term infants was clear: Mothers of preterms had less physical and social contact with their infants. But by 21 months there were no differences in maternal behavior between groups, except that mothers of prematures touched and attended to their children *more* than did mothers of full-term infants.

One incidental difference between early- and late-contact mothers impressed the investigators. At the start of the study, all mothers were married and intended to keep their infants. Only 1 of 22 mothers in the early-contact group, but 5 of 22 mothers in the late-contact group, had divorced by the time the babies were 2 years old (Leifer et al., 1972). Although one cannot put much faith in uncontrolled, incidental findings, the role of the stress of coping with a premature baby might add to other marital stresses to increase divorce rate. Rosenfield's (1980) study of parental visiting found serious marital disturbances centered on conflicts related to infants in several families. Perhaps it is plausible that even such limited early contact helped the early-contact group cope with the stress.

The Stanford study suggests that having a premature baby is a greater problem than being separated from it. It is a weak test of the bonding hypothesis, since the early-contact mothers did not take maximal advantage of their opportunity. (For an overview of the study, see Leiderman, 1981.)

---

20. These are movies made in extremely slow motion so that frames are exposed after longer lapses of time than needed for natural movement. They require much less film to shoot and less time to watch and analyze.

The mother-infant pairs in the Case Western Reserve study were filmed in the process of feeding their infants, using time-lapse photography.[20] The films were made just before discharge from the hospital and 1 month later, when the babies were brought back. In addition, Bayley developmental examinations were given to the babies just before their discharge from the hospital and at 9, 15, and 21 months of age. A Stanford-Binet IQ test was given at 42 months of age.

Differences related to treatment groups were few, whether maternal or infant behaviors were examined. Mothers with early contact looked more at their babies during feeding. The babies did not differ in Bayley scores at any of the ages tested, but, of the 18 (out of 53 original infants) available for testing at 42 months, those whose mothers had early contact averaged 14 points higher (99 versus 84) in IQ. Whether those tested were representative of the total cannot be determined, hence it is impossible to interpret the finding. It is likely that the stablest mothers were the ones who brought their babies back at 42 months, hence better performance could be related to any number of variables other than early contact. At best it is very tentative evidence in favor of the hypothesis (as Klaus and Kennell themselves have pointed out).

A separate study at Case Western Reserve found that infrequent visiting was related to a number of the negative outcomes that had initially stimulated studies of the effects of contact with premature infants (Fanaroff et al., 1972; cited in Klaus & Kennell, 1976). Only 2% of mothers who visited their babies more than three times in two weeks battered, abandoned, or fostered their babies, but 25% of mothers who visited less than three times did so. This was in a nursery where mothers could telephone and visit as often as they wished. Although these differences are substantial (and similar differences have been found in at least three other retrospective studies), two contrasting interpretations are possible, because, as is the case with all correlational studies, extraneous variables may have influenced the findings. Specifically, the *reasons* some parents visited more than others, rather than the *number* of visits, may be what influenced the outcome. Put another way, the parent, not the number of visits, may determine the outcome.

Those who favor the bonding hypothesis need to assume that less frequent visiting was due to reasons that are not relevant to the outcomes, such as transportation difficulties. If this were so, the correlations of frequency of visiting with outcome variables could be reasonably attributed to better bonding among high-frequency visitors. Those skeptical of the bonding hypothesis would point out that high-frequency visitors might differ from low-frequency visitors in ways that influence outcomes. For example, mothers who are unstable prior to delivery would be likely to visit less and also be more likely to abuse, abandon, or foster their babies regardless of the frequency of visits to the hospital. Likewise, if the mother found her newborn baby unattractive or unrewarding, she would probably visit the baby less frequently and also be more likely to abuse it.[21] Data presented in Chapter 2 support the likelihood that stimulated babies became more appealing to their mothers, thus encouraging more frequent visits. Mothers of low birth weight babies in an extra stimulation program gradually increased their frequency of visiting to a greater degree than did mothers of control babies (Rosenfield, 1980). This indirectly supports the likely relation between attractiveness and visiting. A third important difference between high- and low-frequency visitors might be marital stress. The families in Rosenfield's study who experienced serious marital stress all exhibited unusual visiting patterns.

Thus the findings of both Fanaroff and colleagues (1972) and Rosenfield (1980) are consistent with the hypothesis that the characteristics of the mother that influence her behavior during the postpartum period, including her frequency of visits, also affect her child-rearing behaviors at later ages. If this interpretation is correct, researchers should look for continuing, long-term influences of mother and baby on each other rather than for strong effects of critical experiences in the first hours or days after birth.

Research Challenging the Bonding Hypothesis

The evidence in favor of the bonding hypothesis has been sporadic at best, and evidence that disconfirms or fails to support it has grown. I will separate these disconfirmatory studies into two kinds: (a) those that explored mothers' bonding responses themselves, and (b) those that explored the long-term consequences for the offspring of their mothers' hypothesized failure to bond properly.

Remember that the bonding hypothesis posits that mothers of preterm infants should have more difficulty bonding than mothers of term infants because preterm infants are separated from their mothers during the hypothesized critical period for bonding. A number of recent studies have suggested that babies at risk (for prematurity or other reasons) receive more, not fewer, favorable interactions. Compared with normal infants, they received more interaction, holding, and affection from their mothers (Campbell, 1977; Crawford, 1982; Field, 1977). Their cries elicited more tender re-

sponses and responses that were likely to be more effective from adults (Zeskind, 1980). Furthermore, among high-risk babies, those whose obstetrical and postnatal course was less optimal received more interactions from their mothers even though their behaviors could be described as less rewarding. They cried and fussed more, slept more, and made fewer nondistress vocalizations (Beckwith & Cohen, 1978; Beckwith et al., 1976). Good sample sizes and controls and the partial replications of these results (true for various of the studies cited) lend them considerable credence. In addition, all the results are in the same direction, so that although the relations between risk and maternal interaction are small, they strongly suggest that most mothers of nonoptimal babies provide compensatory care for them rather than neglecting or abusing them. This conclusion is, of course, hard to reconcile with the notion that mothers have more trouble loving their premature infants because they lack early contact with them.

The second set of studies challenging the bonding hypothesis deals with infant outcomes. Two studies had as their major finding that experience in the neonatal period was not related to infant behaviors at later times. The first was a longitudinal study of premature or ill babies who had been separated from their mothers at birth and for prolonged periods thereafter (Rode et al., 1981). According to the bonding hypothesis, such separation should mean that the babies' mothers could not bond properly, which might be expected to affect the infants' attachment to their mothers. In spite of their early separation, they were not more likely than other year-old babies to be insecurely attached to their mothers (security of attachment is discussed in Chapter 12). In addition, other neonatal factors—birth weight, gestational age, number of days spent in neonatal intensive care units, and parental visiting patterns—were unrelated to security of attachment. These data disconfirm the hypothesis that maternal bonding should affect infant attachment, and support the notion that preterm babies are resilient with respect to their neonatal experiences.

The babies in the study were from intact, middle-class families, where caring for a sick or premature infant is less stressful than it would be in families with greater economic and family stresses (Rode et al., 1981). Deficits in bonding might be expected to have their strongest effects when the mother-infant pair is

---

21. Nurses (both those experienced in caring for prematures and those not so experienced) are able to rate differential attractiveness of premature infants reliably.

under stress. The Stanford study found no differences in Bayley mental or motor scores that were related to the hospital experience.

Another study of infant outcomes examined the relation between mother-infant interactions and subsequent development in both preterm and term disadvantaged babies (Bakeman & Brown, 1980; Brown & Bakeman, 1980). The preterm babies in this study were all healthy enough to be out of intensive care by 24 hours of age. Standard hospital practices were followed, and thus the term babies had not been separated from their mothers as long as the preterm babies. Interactions during the neonatal period (assessed in three 30-minute sessions devoted primarily to feeding) differed profoundly between the two groups, but were not related to the Bayley Mental Development Index at 12 or 24 months, or to Stanford-Binet IQ at 3 years. Although knowing whether babies were preterm or term helped to predict later IQ, adding knowledge about the nature of their early feeding interactions with their mothers did not improve the predictions. These data actually suggest that the neonatal period might be a time in which infants are buffered against any long-term consequences of their early interactions with their mothers.

Conclusions

While some evidence suggests that early contact experiences influence mother-infant outcomes, more evidence suggests that they are not important determinants of either later maternal behaviors or infant outcomes. Finding apparently contradictory results often means that the research questions were inappropriate or asked in an inappropriate fashion. The original hypothesis was formulated as a critical period hypothesis, that is, that the necessity for bonding is biologically based and therefore crucial for all mother-infant pairs. The research described above renders that formulation very unlikely. Early contact might still be important in some contexts or for some women. It may be that mothers who avoid visiting their infants in the hospital, even though it would be feasible, have trouble dealing with having birthed an at-risk infant. The lack of early contact may intensify their difficulty in accepting their babies; early contact and other early support services may help them to overcome these difficulties.

Klaus and Kennell designed a new program to maximize attachment of both mothers and fathers to their premature infants. Unfortunately, they were not able to maintain the study (Kennell, personal communication, spring 1984). Indeed, in many settings it is now impossible to do studies of bonding because hospital

nursery practice dictates that all mothers must have such opportunities.

The changed practices of neonatal intensive care units in support of parental visits and encouragement of appropriate touching and other interaction with their premature (or sick) infants seem highly appropriate despite the lack of firm research evidence for their importance. One would certainly doubt that such practices could do harm, unless the pressures on mothers make them feel guilty if they are unable to engage in these practices.

BONDING TO TERM INFANTS

The evidence that immediate and continuing post-birth contact is important for maternal bonding is even more tenuous for term than for premature infants. Evidence from samples that are modest in size and not representative, and with few significant findings, is used as support for a sensitive period immediately after birth for the formation of the maternal bond to the infant. Although I personally would choose the type of contact that is advocated as a result of the sensitive period hypothesis, I would not feel guilty if for some reason this type of contact were not possible (as, indeed, it was not when my children were born). The evidence presented below demonstrates why I believe personal choice is appropriate.

The first study on bonding to term infants included 28 mothers and their babies (Klaus et al., 1972). The mother-infant pairs were randomly assigned to experimental and control groups and the groups were matched on parity (first), age (teens), marital status (about 65% unmarried), race (black), and SES (very low). Birth weights, sex distributions, amount of nursing care received, and length of time in the hospital (almost 4 days) did not differ for the two groups. In short, the study was a true experiment with random assignment of subjects, but the subjects were not representative of the population at large.

Control mothers received routine treatment for that hospital at that time: a glimpse of the baby at birth, another brief contact at 6 to 8 hours, and then every 4 hours for feeding. Experimental mothers had their nude babies in bed with them for 1 hour in the 12 hours after birth and had 5 extra hours of contact on each of the next three days. Many dependent variables were examined, a fact that poses problems of interpretation when only a few of them turn out to be significant.

Mothers brought their babies back for a checkup at 1 month and answered a questionnaire concerning their behaviors toward and feelings about their babies. Interactions during the examination and a feeding session were scored blind from videotapes. The extra-contact mothers spent more time during feeding either fondling their babies or in the *en face* position or a combination of the two (18% versus 5%). Six control but no experimental mothers had questionnaire scores indicating inadequate mothering. Higher scores for experimentals on items presumed to index attachment could be interpreted to mean that the mothers were "overprotective" and did not allow their babies an optimal degree of autonomy according to Brazelton (Klaus & Kennell, 1976).

At 1 year, during the infants' physical checkups, the extended-contact mothers spent more time near the examining table and soothing their infants (Kennell et al., 1974), but there were no differences in the other 23 behaviors measured. Follow-ups of small subsamples at later ages produced few and somewhat contradictory findings (Ringler et al., 1975, 1978). Klaus and Kennell note that the effects might have been stronger had the infants been placed with their mothers immediately after birth and left with them continuously, and had the mothers received no medication.

The experiment did not test the hypothesis of a critical period immediately after birth, but tested whether exposure to infants in the first 2 hours together with greater-than-average exposure throughout the hospital stay affected the dependent variables assessed. Even the few findings of effects might not occur in a less disadvantaged sample.

With Guatemalan colleagues, Klaus and Kennell (1976) tested the critical period hypothesis by varying only immediate contact for mothers in a social security hospital that cares for very low SES cases. Experimental mothers had their babies and privacy for 45 minutes on the delivery table (nude, under a heat panel) immediately after delivery. The control mothers' babies were taken away immediately after birth, but there were no other differences between groups in the rest of their two-day stay in the hospital, and all mothers were given a free supply of powdered milk at discharge. More infants from the experimental group were still breast-feeding at 6 months, they had gained 1.5 lb more, and had had fewer infections—differences that may simply reflect the advantages of breast- over bottle-feeding. Mother's milk provides better immunity, and the dangers of contaminating the formula are avoided. Separate data analyses for nursing and non-nursing mothers would be needed to know whether any effects of postbirth "bonding" would exist if nursing were held constant. All the differences found could have been due to early contact having facilitated breast-feeding. Other studies have shown that immediate contact helps to establish breast-feeding (Souza

et al., 1974; Winters, 1973; both cited in Klaus & Kennell, 1976). However, in the Souza et al. (1974) study, early contact was confounded with rooming-in and the aid of a special nurse to stimulate breast-feeding. The mechanism by which this early contact affects nursing may be hormonal rather than psychological.

A study in a Guatemalan hospital serving a higher-SES population failed to replicate (cited in Klaus & Kennell, 1976), suggesting that early contact operates more powerfully in groups at socioeconomic risk. Other laboratories have conducted similar studies to try to replicate Klaus and Kennell's results. The outcomes do not permit a clear-cut resolution of the controversy.

Two series of studies in Sweden, one at the University of Göteborg and one by de Chateau and colleagues, provide some confirmation for the bonding hypothesis (Carlsson et al., 1978, 1979; de Chateau, 1977a, 1977b, 1979; de Chateau & Wiberg, 1977a, 1977b, 1984; Schaller et al., 1979). Both groups found an increase in affective aspects of nursing behavior in the immediate postpartum period for mothers given extended body contact with their newborns in the first 2 hours (de Chateau & Wiberg, 1977a; Carlsson et al., 1978). One found no effects at 6 weeks of age (Carlsson et al., 1979), while the other found some differences among the many variables tested at 3 months, 1 year, and 3 years (de Chateau, 1979; de Chateau & Wiberg, 1977b, 1984).

The findings of all these studies are sporadic. Differences were found in only 2 of 25 observational categories (Kennell et al., 1974), and in only 3 out of 35 observational measures in the newborn period (only 1 of which had any connotation of affection) in the de Chateau and Wiberg (1977a) study. Differences were found in only a few of the 61 behavior categories at 3 months (de Chateau & Wiberg, 1977b), and none of those was found in both sexes. Another study that permitted separation of the effects of early contact from those of extended contact had the same finding of only a few differences among many variables tested (Vietze et al., 1978).

Furthermore, the actual behaviors that differed were rarely the same in different studies, and not even in the same direction from one age to another. For example, Klaus et al. (1972) found that *en face* contact was more frequent at 1 month, but Schaller and colleagues (1979) found no differences either in the first week of life or at 6 weeks, and Svedja et al. (1980) found differences at 36 hours of age, but only for males. Language findings at 2 years of age were often in the opposite direction from those at 1 year and not relevant to affection (Ringler et al., 1975, 1978).

Other studies provide even less support for either

the critical period or early-contact view of bonding. In a study with excellent methodological controls (random assignment of subjects to groups, use of a double-blind procedure, where neither the subjects nor the experimenters knew who was in what group, and response measures that were closely tied to the construct of attachment), significant differences were found only when the data were analyzed by sex (Svedja et al., 1980). Female babies received a higher number of touches and males higher numbers of *en face* interactions. A pooled group of behaviors considered affectionate did occur more often in the 10 minutes of free interaction for both sexes of experimental babies. Entwisle and Doering (1981) found that the amount of contact mothers had with their infants in the first 3 days did not predict nurturant behavior even 3 to 4 weeks later if preexisting differences among mothers were statistically controlled for.

Svedja and colleagues argue that the positive findings of other studies may have been due to the fulfillment of **experimenter expectations** (a variable that has been shown in social psychological research to affect outcomes). Those who favor the bonding or early-contact hypothesis argue that population differences, especially those related to social class, might account for the differences in results. It is easy to assume that such experimental manipulations could have effects in deprived but not nondeprived mothers, as was found in the Central American studies. Nevertheless, the one Swedish study with a few long-term effects had middle-class subjects. Thus we cannot simply conclude that bonding variables are more important in deprived populations.

A German study of middle-class, stable families manipulated bonding separately from more general early contact. There were four groups: Those in one had their nude babies with them for at least 30 minutes after birth (bonding), one had rooming-in for 5 hours on each of the 10 days in hospital (extended contact), one had both, and one had the standard hospital practice, which was neither. The primary dependent variable was the amount of cuddling and tender touching that occurred at times other than during caretaking (Grossmann et al., 1981).

The researchers found effects largely for mothers whose pregnancies were planned. Mothers with early contact were highest in tender touching and mothers

with extended contact were lowest. But about twice as many mothers in the extended-contact group had not planned their pregnancies. When planning was controlled for statistically, there was no longer any effect of extended contact. The effect of the early contact was highest for those who had planned their pregnancies or was most helpful for those who seemed least likely to need it. But these positive effects did not last through the 7 to 9 days the German mothers spent in the hospital. Attachment behaviors of the infants did not differ at 12 months as a result of either early postpartum contact (bonding) or extended contact. Bonding advocates could argue that the effects might have been stronger if only first-time mothers were considered (half of the Grossmann sample), because Klaus and Kennell's mothers had all been first-time mothers. One bonding advocate (Anderson, 1977) has suggested that a major weakness of studies of bonding is that contact is given according to an experimental protocol and not according to the mother's wishes or the baby's demands. More technically, contact is on a scheduled, not a self-regulatory, basis, and this would be expected to weaken effects.

A more recent study in this country was able to assign middle-class participants randomly to either 15 or 60 minutes of contact (none was not allowed) and either skin-to-skin contact or contact between a covered mother and a swaddled baby. None of these groups differed in infant or maternal behaviors, unless in interaction with feeding, which was a much more powerful determinant of behaviors (Gewirtz et al., 1989). The authors suggest that if their findings are accurate, then "parents and professionals should be more concerned with the behavioral factors that ensure a higher quality of parental-infant interactive life instead of concern about unique contact opportunities following birth" (p. 8).

SUMMARY OF BONDING RESEARCH

It is clear from the research on maternal bonding that strong conclusions are unwarranted. If hypotheses were validated by counting the number of findings for or against them, the bonding hypothesis would surely be found invalid. Many more similarities between extended-contact and control groups than differences characterize all studies. The number of differences is so small compared with the number of variables analyzed that we must suspect that many of the positive findings are likely to be chance events.[22]

Other reviewers have reached similar, or harsher, conclusions (Lamb, 1982; McCall, 1982; B. J. Myers, 1984a, 1984b, 1987). B. J. Myers's (1984a) review

---

22. If the criterion of significance is a *p* level of .05, then 5 of every 100 findings will be significant by chance. Therefore, if 50 differences were tested, as was typical in these studies, 2 or 3 of them would be significant by chance alone.

has been commented on by Kennell and Klaus (1984), who make the point that, given the life-sustaining nature of attachment, it is unlikely to be dependent on a single process, but to have many failsafe routes to it. Myers's (1984b) rejoinder to that commentary stresses the value of humanistic birthing practices regardless of the role of early contact in attachment. It is interesting to note the very modest claims made by de Chateau in 1987.

Science does not proceed entirely by tallying scores for and against hypotheses. Inconsistent findings may mean that the research question has not been properly asked. In the case of bonding, the strong form of the hypothesis—that there is a biologically based, universal critical period during which mothers *must* have contact with their babies in order to develop a strong emotional bond to them—is clearly *not* correct. Early, extended, or enriched contact may be important in some contexts. Restricted access to their babies may have deleterious effects on some mothers and not on others. Greater difficulties in bonding might be expected in mothers who feel a high degree of stress (who feel inadequate, who have at-risk babies, or who feel excessive need to be "perfect" mothers) and have limited resources to deal with their stress. Bonding practices may affect mother-infant pairs only for women who are at the extremes on one or more of these variables. Further research is necessary to determine whether there are particular kinds of mothers who could be helped by having special assistance in the postpartum period.

Bonding practices might influence only those maternal behaviors, or mother-infant relationships, or children's behaviors, that were not the ones chosen for study. Nursing may be positively affected by early contact. At least two studies have failed to find a relation between neonatal contact and later toddler attachment, the infant behavior most likely to be affected by bonding practices. Inasmuch as many other influences may have affected the mother-infant relationship between birth and the measurement of attachment (typically at about 1 year), and because the standard measures of attachment leave out important areas of infant love (see Chapter 12), the existence of a relation between bonding practices and a baby's love for mama is not ruled out.

I have not tried to cover the meager evidence for father-infant bonding, but it should be noted that a large number of men who have been surveyed believe in father-infant bonding, and in there being scientific evidence for it. A subsample questioned about the sources of their beliefs cited "general knowledge," mass media, classes, and popular readings, in that order, with only one having seen a scientific article (Palkovitz, 1988). Unfortunately, the media and the public jump on bandwagons, despite a lack of scientific evidence. In the case of bonding, the overall effect on childbirth practices has been good, but it is hard to know to what extent guilt has been engendered and had a bad effect.

I hope that the weakness of the findings for bonding will not be used as an excuse to keep mothers and their infants separated in the hospital. Although such separation may do no permanent harm for most mother-infant pairs, providing contact in a way that is acceptable to the mother surely does no harm and gives much pleasure to many. It is my belief that anything that may make the postpartum period more pleasurable surely is worthwhile, a conclusion similar to that reached by McCall (1982) and B. J. Myers (1984a).

Summary

A number of aspects of the birth process may affect the well-being of the newborn and the experience of birth for the mother. The duration of labor (especially of second-stage labor), atypical presentations at birth, and how the umbilical cord is entwined around the fetus all may influence the neonatal outcome. They may lead to oxygen deprivation, brain hemorrhages, damage to the spinal cord, and, in extreme cases, death.

WAYS TO AVOID OR COUNTERACT COMPLICATIONS

Fetal monitoring can reduce some of the risks of delivery. It may be external, using a stethoscope (which is just as efficacious as more intrusive methods, unless for high-risk deliveries) or electrodes on an abdominal belt, or internal, using electrodes attached to the fetus through the vagina and cervix. If fetal heart rate appears problematic, blood gases can be obtained using needles inserted in the scalp. Apparent fetal distress often leads to a cesarean delivery. Invasive monitoring poses some risks for both mother and fetus/baby, and may serve to lengthen labor due to inhibited motion for the mother.

Prevention of anoxia is a major goal of monitoring. If anoxia becomes so severe that asphyxia results, the baby may die. It was originally thought that preventing anoxia during delivery would greatly reduce the incidence of cerebral palsy, but this has not been borne out. Anoxia can lead to brain damage and to lowered intelligence, but individual differences in susceptibility are great and the reasons for them are not known.

Three major interventions to speed up delivery when that is considered desirable are (a) administration of oxytocin, (b) use of mechanical aids (forceps and vacuum extraction), and (c) cesarean section. Use of oxytocin is reviewed below. High forceps, which are very dangerous, and even medium forceps, which are not clearly dangerous, have been largely replaced by cesareans. Low forceps are frequently used, particularly when the mother has been anesthetized, to help pull the baby through the birth canal when it is already well into it. Vacuum extraction is used in some countries for the same purpose, and may be increasing in use here.

Cesarean sections can save the lives of mothers and infants in cases where normal deliveries are impossible. They are relatively safe for the mother and often safer for the fetus in complicated deliveries. However, the mother must recover from surgery, a longer process than recovery from childbirth, and has a greater risk of infections. There is little agreement on whether there are any long-term effects on the baby from the C-section as opposed to those from the condition that led to its being done.

DRUGS USED DURING DELIVERY AND THEIR EFFECTS

Drugs used in early stages of labor to reduce pain or anxiety, or both, include tranquilizers, narcotic-analgesics, and sedative-hypnotic agents. There are numerous drugs in each category, and the effects of each may vary. During delivery itself, anesthetics are often given. A different class of drugs is made up of those used to speed up delivery by increasing the strength of the contractions. All of these drugs, given at the mother's dosage level, cross the placental and blood-brain barriers to provide the fetus, whose liver and kidneys do not dispose of them well, a high dose.

Determining the effects of drugs is very complex due to the many combinations, the varied dosages, and the timing with respect to the separation of the infant from the mother. Using infants whose mothers had no drugs as controls is problematic in a culture in which that is not the norm, so that such women are likely to be atypical. When effects are measured after the neonatal period, environmental and social variables confound the drug effects. Hence statements made here about the effects of drugs must be considered tentative.

Negative effects are not found for tranquilizers, do not appear serious for most narcotic-analgesics, but

seem potentially serious for the sedative-hypnotic scopolamine. Regional anesthetics may interfere with contractions and the woman's ability to push, thus increasing the need for delivery aids. General anesthetics provided by injection are probably safer than inhalants (other than nitrous oxide, which may even be protective). The effects of oxytocin, which is frequently used to speed up labor, need to be studied more carefully, as it appears this drug may have negative effects on the fetus.

CHILDBIRTH PRACTICES

The standard delivery in the United States from the 1940s through the 1960s was in a medical context of illness and surgery. Infant and maternal mortality rates were reduced, but complaints arose: Electronic fetal monitoring, the lithotomy position, routine episiotomies, and a possible excess in cesareans all promote the medical model and depersonalize childbirth. The mother was separated from significant others during delivery, and from her newborn after delivery; routine practices induced feelings of helplessness in the mother with respect to her delivery and with respect to the care of her infant.

This type of delivery was challenged by doctors who proposed alternate systems, by feminists who challenged the doctor's role, and by women who wanted more psychologically meaningful birth experiences. Dick-Read, in England, wrote a book called *Childbirth Without Fear* (1944/1972) and Lamaze (1970), in France, developed techniques for controlling the pain of labor and delivery that have been widely accepted in the United States. Both stressed knowledge and preparation as well as techniques for minimizing pain. Leboyer's *Birth Without Violence* (1975) focused on the child's experience of childbirth and maternal bonding. Hard data on the benefits of these systems for mothers or infants are sparse, but they do not appear to be harmful and they are psychologically meaningful and satisfying to many couples.

These systems led to a number of changes: to many hospitals offering childbirth classes, to fathers being allowed to be present during labor and delivery, to mothers being allowed to hold their babies right after birth, to longer feeding times and more opportunities for both mothers and fathers to hold their infants, and to sibling visits. A number of doctors in various countries practice deliveries that do not use the standard lithotomy position. Birthing chairs, squatting deliveries, and deliveries while seated in wading pools or reclining on pillows or the father's lap fit this group. Research indicates that such labors go better, with less chance for fetal damage and less need to resort to medical interventions. The usefulness of a totally non-medical support person (doula) is also being explored, to avoid the excess demands placed on the father in Lamaze father-assisted deliveries.

In addition, there are challenges from alternative birthing arrangements such as home delivery, birthing centers, and the use of midwives instead of medical doctors to do normal deliveries in any of these settings. The specific questions addressed to the illness model of childbirth are centered on electronic fetal monitoring, the lithotomy position, routine episiotomies, and a possible excess in the number of cesareans.

MATERNAL BONDING

An early critical period for mother-infant bonding, during which close contact is essential, was proposed by pediatricians concerned with failure-to-thrive premature infants whose mothers had a long separation from them. The hypothesis was bolstered by reference to those animal species that will not accept or nurse their young if separated from them immediately after birth. Given the prevalence of adoption in other animal species, as well as in preliterate human cultures and our own, the importance of contact in the immediate postbirth period seems questionable. Thus it is hardly surprising that the research on the importance of such contact has failed to yield clear-cut results in its favor, other than that it promotes breast-feeding. The methodological problems of these studies have been considered at length in this chapter.

References

ADAMS, R. J. (1989). Obstetrical medication and the human newborn: The influence of alphaprodine hydrochloride on visual behavior. *Developmental Medicine and Child Neurology, 31,* 650-656.

ALEKSANDROWICZ, M. K. (1974). The effect of pain relieving drugs administered during labor and delivery on the behavior of the newborn: A review. *Merrill-Palmer Quarterly, 20,* 121-141.

ALEKSANDROWICZ, M. K., & Aleksandrowicz, D. R. (1974). Obstetrical pain relieving drugs as predictors of infant behavior variability. *Child Development, 45,* 935-945.

ALEKSANDROWICZ, M. K., & Aleksandrowicz, D. R. (1976). Obstetrical pain relieving drugs as predictors of infant behavior variability: A reply to Federman and Yang's critique. *Child Development, 47,* 297-298.

ALTHAUS, F. (1990). Higher income women are more likely to have a caesarean delivery. *Family Planning Perspectives Digest, 22,* 43-44.

AMIEL-TISON, C., & Ellison, P. (1986). Birth asphyxia in the fullterm newborn: Early assessment and outcome. *Develop-mental Medicine and Child Neurology, 28,* 671-682.

ANDERSON, G. C. (1977). The mother and her newborn: Mutual caregivers. *Journal of Gynecological Nursing, 6,* 50-57.

ANDERSON, G. M., & Lomas, J. (1984). Determinants of the increasing Cesarean birth rate: Ontario data 1979 to 1982. *New England Journal of Medicine, 311,* 887.

ANTHONY, M. Y., & Levene, M. I. (1990). An assessment of the benefits of intrapartum fetal monitoring. *Developmental Medicine and Child Neurology, 32,* 547-553.

AVARD, D. M., & Nimrod, C. M. (1985). Risks and benefits of obstetric epidural analgesia: A review. *Birth Issues in Perinatal Care and Education, 12,* 215-225.

Avoiding unnecessary repeat caesarean deliveries may help stem overall rise in C-section rates. *Family Planning Perspectives Digest, 17,* 125-127.

BAKEMAN, R., & Brown, J. V. (1980). Early interaction: Consequences for social and mental development at three years. *Child Development, 51,* 437-447.

BAKOS, O., & Backstrom, T. (1987). Induction of labor: A prospective, randomized study into amniotomy and oxytocin as induction methods in a total unselected population. *Acta Obstetricia et Gynecologica Scandinavica, 66,* 537-541.

BANTA, H. D. (1981, October). *The risks and benefits of episiotomy.* Paper presented at the conference, Obstetrical Management and Infant Outcome 1981: Implications for Future Mental and Physical Development, sponsored by the American Foundation for Maternal and Child Health, New York.

BANTA, H. D., & Thacker, S. B. (1979). *Costs and benefits of electronic fetal monitoring: A review of the literature* (NCHSR Research Report Series, DHEW Publication No. PHS 79-3245). Washington, DC: Government Printing Office.

BECKWITH, L., & Cohen, S. E. (1978). Preterm birth: Hazardous obstetrical and postnatal events as related to caregiver-infant behavior. *Infant Behavior and Development, 1,* 403-411.

BECKWITH, L., Cohen, S. E., Kopp, C. B., Parmelee, A. H., & Marcy, T. G. (1976). Caregiver-infant interaction and cognitive development in pre-term infants. *Child Development, 47,* 579-587.

BENARON, H. B. W., & Tucker, B. E. (1971). The effect of obstetric management and factors beyond clinical control on maternal mortality rates at the Chicago Maternity Center from 1959 to 1963. *American Journal of Obstetrics and Gynecology, 110,* 1113-1118.

BENARON, H. B. W., Tucker, B. E., Andrews, J. P., Boshes, B., Cohen, J., Fromm, E., & Yacorzynski, G. K. (1960). Effect of anoxia during labor and immediately after birth on the subsequent development of the child. *American Journal of Obstetrics and Gynecology, 80,* 1129-1142.

BERKSON, G. (1974). Social responses of animals and infants with defects. In M. Lewis & L. A. Rosenblum (Eds.), *The effect of the infant on its caregiver.* New York: Wiley-Interscience.

BERNSTEIN, P., Leyland, N., Gurland, P., & Gare, D. (1987). Cervical ripening and labor induction with prostaglandin E2 gel: A placebo-controlled study. *American Journal of Obstetrics and Gynecology, 156,* 336-340.

BERRY, L. M. (1988). Realistic expectation of the labor coach. *Journal of Obstetric, Gynecologic, and Neonatal Nursing, 17,* 354-355.

BEYNON, C. L. (1975). The normal second stage of labor. *Journal of Obstetrics and Gynecology, 64,* 815-820.

BINGHAM, P., Hird, V., & Lilford, R. J. (1987). Management

of the mature selected breech presentation: An analysis based on the intended method of delivery. *British Journal of Obstetrics and Gynaecology, 94,* 746-752.

BJERRE, J., & Dahlin, K. (1974). The long-term development of children delivered by vacuum extraction. *Journal of Developmental Medicine and Child Neurology, 16,* 378-381.

BORGATTA, L., Piening, S. L., & Cohen, W. R. (1989). Association of episiotomy and delivery position with deep perineal laceration during spontaneous delivery in nulliparous women. *American Journal of Obstetrics and Gynecology, 160,* 294-297.

BOWES, W. A., Jr., Brackbill, Y., Conway, E., & Steinschneider, A. (1970). The effects of obstetrical medication on fetus and infant. *Monographs of the Society for Research in Child Development, 35*(4, Serial No. 137).

BRACKBILL, Y. (1979a, November). *Effects of obstetric drugs on human development.* Paper presented at a symposium of the American Foundation for Maternal and Child Health, New York.

BRACKBILL, Y. (1979b). Obstetrical medication and infant behavior. In J. Osofsky (Ed.), *Handbook of infant development.* New York: John Wiley.

BRACKBILL, Y., & Broman, S. H. (n.d.). *Obstetrical medication and development in the first year of life.* Unpublished manuscript.

BRACKBILL, Y., Kane, J., Manniello, R. L., & Abramson, D. (1974). Obstetrical meperidine usage and assessment of neonatal status. *Anesthesiology, 40,* 116-120.

BRACKBILL, Y., McManus, K., & Woodward, L. (1985). *Medication in maternity: Infant exposure and maternal information.* Ann Arbor: University of Michigan Press.

BRAZELTON, T. B. (1961). Psychophysiologic reaction in the neonate: II. The effects of maternal medication on the neonate and his behavior. *Journal of Pediatrics, 58,* 513-518.

BRODY, J. E. (1989). Personal health: Research casts doubt on need for many Caesarean births as their rate soars. *New York Times,* p. B5.

BROEKHUIZEN, F. R., Washington, J. M., Johnson, F., & Hamilton, P. R. (1987). Vacuum extraction versus forceps delivery: Indications and complications, 1979-1984. *Obstetrics and Gynecology, 69,* 338-342.

BROMAN, S. H. (1981). Risk factors for deficits in early cognitive development. In G. G. Berg & H. D. Maillie (Eds.), *Measurement of risk.* New York: Plenum.

BROMAN, S. H. (1983). Obstetric medications. In C. C. Brown (Ed.), *Childhood learning disabilities and prenatal risk.* Skillman, NJ: Johnson & Johnson Baby Products.

BROOME, M. E., & Koehler, C. (1986). Childbirth education: A review of effect on the woman and her family. *Family and Community Health, 9,* 33-44.

BROWER, K. R. (1974). *Effects of intranatal drugs on the newborn EEG.* Unpublished master's thesis, University of Hawaii, Honolulu.

BROWN, J. V., & Bakeman, R. (1980). Relationships of human mothers with their infants during the first year of life. In R. W. Bell & W. P. Smotherman (Eds.), *Maternal influences and early behavior.* Jamaica, NY: Spectrum.

BRUMITT, G. H., & Dowler, J. K. (1984). *Behavioral effects of obstetrical medication on the newborn.* Paper presented at the Fourth Biennial International Conference on Infant Studies, New York.

BUDIN, P. (1907). *The nursling.* London: Caxton.

CALDEYRO-BARCIA, R. (1981, October). *The scientific basis for preserving the natural physiology of labor and birth through non-intervention.* Paper presented at the Conference on Obstetrical Management and Infant Outcome, New York.

CAMPBELL, B. K. (1977). An assessment of early mother-infant interaction and the subsequent development of the infant in the first two years of life. *Dissertation Abstracts International, 38,* 1856-1857.

CARLSSON, S. G., Fagerberg, H., Horneman, G., Hwang, P., Larsson, K., Rodholm, M., Schaller, J., Danielsson, B., & Gunoewall, C. (1978). Effects of amount of contact between mother and child on the mother's nursing behavior. *Developmental Psychology, 11,* 143-150.

CARLSSON, S. G., Fagerberg, H., Horneman, G., Hwang, P., Larsson, K., Rodholm, M., Schaller, J., Danielsson, B., & Gunoewall, C. (1979). Effects of various amounts of contact between mother and child on the mother's nursing behavior: A follow-up study. *Infant Behavior and Development, 2,* 209-214.

CARMODY, F., Grant, A., Mutch, L., Vacca, A., & Chalmers, I. (1986). Follow-up of babies delivered in a randomized controlled comparison of vacuum extraction and forceps delivery. *Acta Obstetricia et Gynecologica Scandinavica, 65,* 763-766.

CARY, A. J. (1990). Intervention rates in spontaneous term labour in low risk multiparous women. *Australian and New Zealand Journal of Obstetrics and Gynaecology, 30,* 46-51.

COPSTICK, S. M., Taylor, K. E., Hayes, R., & Morris, N. (1986). Partner support and the use of coping techniques in labour. *Journal of Psychosomatic Research, 30,* 497-503.

CORAH, N. L., Anthony, E. J., Painter, P., Stern, J. A., & Thurston, D. L. (1965). The effects of perinatal anoxia after seven years. *Psychological Monographs, 79*(Whole No. 596).

COSMI, E. V., & Marx, G. F. (1968). Acid-base status and clinical condition of mother and foetus following methoxythrane anesthesia for vaginal delivery. *British Journal of Anesthesia, 40,* 94-98.

CRAWFORD, J. W. (1982). Mother-infant interaction in premature and full-term infants. *Child Development, 53,* 957-962.

CRUMP, W. J. (1989). Oxytocin and the induction of labor: Use in a network of community hospitals. *Family Medicine, 21,* 110-113.

CYR, R. M., Usher, R. H., & McLean, F. H. (1984). Changing patterns of birth asphyxia and trauma over 20 years. *American Journal of Obstetrics and Gynecology, 148,* 490-498.

DANIELS, K. (1989). Water birth: The newest form of safe, gentle, joyous birth. *Journal of Nurse Midwifery, 34,* 198-205.

DE CHATEAU, P. (1977a). The importance of the neonatal period for the development of synchrony in the mother-infant dyad: A review. *Birth and the Family Journal, 4,* 10-23.

DE CHATEAU, P. (1977b). The influence of early contact on maternal and infant behavior in primiparae. *Birth and the Family Journal, 3,* 149-155.

DE CHATEAU, P. (1979). Effects of hospital practices on synchrony in the development of the infant-parent relationship. *Seminars in Perinatology, 3,* 45-60.

DE CHATEAU, P. (1987). Parent-Infant socialization in several Western European countries. In J. D. Osofsky (Ed.), *Handbook of infant development* (2nd ed., pp. 642-668). New York: John Wiley.

DE CHATEAU, P., & Wiburg, B. (1977a). Long-term effect on mother-infant behavior of extra contact during the first hour post-partum: I. First observation at 36 hours. *Acta Paediatrica Scandinavica, 66,* 137-144.

DE CHATEAU, P., & Wiburg, B. (1977b). Long-term effect on

mother-infant behavior of extra contact during the first hour post-partum: II. Follow-up at three months. *Acta Paediatrica Scandinavica, 66,* 145-151.

DE CHATEAU, P., & Wiberg, B. (1984). Long-term effect on mother-infant behavior of extra contact during the first hour post-partum: III. One year follow-up. *Scandinavian Journal of Social Medicine, 12,* 91-103.

DeLAY, T., Kennell, J., & Klaus, M. (1987, April). *Supportive companions of women in labor: A descriptive analysis.* Paper presented at the annual meeting of the Society for Research in Child Development, Baltimore.

DICK-READ, G. (1972). *Childbirth without fear: The principles and practices of natural childbirth* (H. Wessel & H. E. Ellis, Eds.; 2nd rev. ed.). New York: Harper. (Original work published 1944)

DOBSON, V., Schwartz, T. L., Sandstrom, D. J., & Michel, L. (1987). Binocular visual acuity of neonates: The acuity card procedure. *Developmental Medicine and Child Neurology, 29,* 199-206.

DOMMISSE, J., & Wild, J. M. (1987). Assessment of a new prostaglandin E2 gel in labour induction. *South African Medical Journal, 71,* 506-507.

EKBLAD, U., & Erkkola, R. (1987). Intracervical prostaglandin EZ gel for cervical ripening. *Annales Chirurgiae et Gynaecologiae-Supplementum, 202,* 23-25.

EL-QARMALAW, A. M., Elmardi, A. A., Saddik, M., el-Abdel-Hadi, F., & Shaker, S. M. (1990). A comparative randomized study of oral prostaglandin E2 (PGEZ) tablets and intravenous oxytocin in induction of labor in patients with premature rupture of membranes before 37 weeks of pregnancy. *International Journal of Gynaecology and Obstetrics, 33,* 115-119.

ENTWISLE, D. R., & Doering, S. G. (1981). *The first birth: A family turning point.* Baltimore: Johns Hopkins University Press.

EPPERLY, T. D., & Breitinger, E. R. (1988). Vacuum extraction. *American Family Physician, 38,* 205-210.

ERNHART, C. B., Graham, F. K., & Thurston, D. (1960). Relationship of neonatal apnea to development at three years. *Archives of Neurology, 2,* 504-510.

EVRARD, J. R., & Gold, E. M. (1977). Caesarean section and maternal mortality in Rhode Island. *Obstetrics and Gynecology, 50,* 594-597.

FANAROFF, A. A., Kennell, J. H., & Klaus, M. H. (1972). Follow-up of low birth-weight infants: The predictive value of maternal visiting patterns. *Pediatrics, 49,* 288-290.

FARLEY, J. E., Jr. (1961). [Unpublished data].

FEDERMAN, E. J., & Yang, R. K. (1976). A critique of obstetrical pain relieving drugs as predictors of infant behavior variability. *Child Development, 47,* 294-296.

FELDMAN, E., & Hurst, M. (1987). Outcomes and procedures in low risk birth: A comparison of hospital and birth center settings. *Birth, 14,* 18-24.

Fetal monitoring: For better or worse? (1981, December 10). *Harvard Medical Area Focus,* pp. 1-3, 8.

FIELD, T. M. (1977). Effects of early separation, interactive deficits, and experimental manipulation on mother-infant face-to-face interaction. *Child Development, 48,* 763-771.

FIELD, T. M., & Widmayer, S. M. (1980). Developmental follow up of infants delivered by Caesarean section and general anesthesia. *Infant Behavior and Development, 3,* 253-264.

FLAMM, B. L., Goings, J. R., Fuelhurst, N. J., Fischermann, E., Jones, C., & Hersh, E. (1987). Oxytocin during labor after previous cesarean section: results of a multicenter study. *Obstetrics and Gynecology, 70,* 709-712.

FREEMAN, D. W., & Arnold, N. I. (1975). Paracervical block with low doses of chloroprocaine. *Journal of the American Medical Association, 231,* 56-57.

FREEMAN, R. (1990). Intrapartum fetal monitoring: A disappointing story [Editorial]. *New England Journal of Medicine, 322,* 624-626.

FRIEDMAN, S. L., Brackbill, Y., Caron, A. J., & Caron, R. F. (1978). Obstetric medication and visual processing in 4- and 5-month-old infants. *Merrill-Palmer Quarterly, 24,* 11-128.

GALE, R., Seidman, D. S., Dollberg, S., & Stevenson, D. K. (1990). Epidemiology of neonatal jaundice in the Jerusalem population. *Journal of Pediatrics, Gastroenterology and Nutrition, 10,* 82-86.

GALVAN, B. J., & Broekhuizen, F. F. (1987). Obstetric vacuum extraction. *Journal of Obstetric, Gynecologic, and Neonatal Nursing, 16,* 242-248.

GASSNER, C. B., & Ledger, W. J. (1976). The relationship of hospital-acquired maternal infection to invasive intrapartum monitoring techniques. *American Journal of Obstetrics and Gynecology, 126,* 33-37.

GEWIRTZ, J. L., Hollenbeck, A. R., et al. (1989). *Maternal-infant behavior at 2-days and at 28-days post-partum following maternal-infant contact in the recovery room.* Unpublished manuscript, Florida International University, Department of Psychology.

GILBERT, L., Porter, W., & Brown, V. A. (1987). Postpartum haemorrhage: A continuing problem. *British Journal of Obstetrics and Gynaecology, 94,* 67-71.

GILLOT-DE-VRIES, F., Wesel, S., Busine, A., Adler, A., et al. (1987). Influence of a bath during labor on the experience of maternity. *Pre- and Peri-Natal Psychology Journal, 1,* 297-302.

GOESCHEN, K. (1989). Premature rupture of membranes near term: Induction of labor with endocervical prostaglandin E2 gel or intravenous oxytocin. *American Journal of Perinatology, 6,* 181-184.

GOULD, J. B., Davey, B., & Stafford, R. S. (1989). Socioeconomic differences in rates of cesarean section. *New England Journal of Medicine, 321,* 233-239.

GRAHAM, F. K., Caldwell, B. M., Ernhart, C. B., Pennoyer, M. M., & Hartmann, A. F., Sr. (1957). Anoxia as a significant perinatal experience: A critique. *Journal of Pediatrics, 50,* 556-569.

GREEN, J. R., & Soohoo, S. L. (1989). Factors associated with rectal injury in spontaneous deliveries. *Obstetrics and Gynecology, 73,* 732-738.

GROSSMAN, F. K. (1980, April). *Psychological sequelae of Caesarean delivery.* Paper presented at the International Conference on Infant Studies, New Haven, CT.

GROSSMANN, K., Thane, K., & Grossmann, K. E. (1981). Maternal tactual contact of the newborn after various postpartum conditions of mother-infant contact. *Developmental Psychology, 17,* 158-169.

HADDAD, H., & Lundy, L. (1978). Changing indications for Caesarean section. *Obstetrics and Gynecology, 51,* 133-137.

HAGGARD, H. W. (1959). *Devils, drugs, and doctors.* New York: Pocket Books. (Original work published 1929)

HERZFELD, J. (1985). *Sense and sensibility in childbirth.* New York: W. W. Norton.

HODNETT, E. D., & Osborn, R. W. (1989). A randomized trial of the effects of monotrice support during labor: Mothers' views two to four weeks postpartum. *Birth, 16,* 177-184.

HOROWITZ, F. D., Ashton, J., Culp, R., Gaddis, E., Levin, S., & Reichmann, B. (1977). The effects of obstetrical medication on the behavior of Israeli newborn infants and some comparisons with Uruguayan and American infants. *Child Development, 48,* 1607-1623.

HOWE, K. A. (1988). Home births in south-west Australia. *Medical Journal of Australia, 149,* 296-297, 300, 302.

INGEMARSSON, I., Westgren, M., & Svenningsen, N. W. (1978). Long-term follow-up of preterm infants in breech presentation delivered by Caesarean section: A prospective study. *Lancet, 2,* 172-175.

IRESTEDT, L., Dahlin, I., Hertzberg, T., Sollevi, A., & Lagercrantz, H. (1989). Adenosine concentration in umbilical cord blood of newborn infants after vaginal delivery and cesarean section. *Pediatric Research, 26,* 106-108.

JOHNSON, C. A., Giese, B. S., & Hassanein, R. E. (1989). Factors predictive of heightened third-day bilirubin levels: A multiple stepwise regression analysis. *Family Medicine, 21,* 283-287.

KANGAS, S. T., Jouppila, R., Alahuhta, S., Jouppila, P., & Hollmen, A. (1989). The effect of lumbar epidural analgesia on the neurobehavioral responses of newborn infants. *Acta Anaesthesiolog Scandinavica, 33,* 320-325.

KARMEL, M. (1959). *Thank you Dr. Lamaze.* Philadelphia: J. B. Lippincott.

KEEFE, M. R. (1987). Comparison of neonatal nighttime sleep-wake patterns in nursery versus rooming-in environments. *Nursing Research, 36,* 140-144.

KENNELL, J. H. (1990). Doula-mother and parent-infant contact. In N. Gunzenhauser (Ed.), *Advances in touch* (pp. 53-62). Skillman, NJ: Johnson & Johnson Consumer Products.

KENNELL, J. H., Jerauld, R., Wolfe, H., Chesler, D., Kreger, N. C., McAlpine, W., Steffa, M., & Klaus, M. H. (1974). Maternal behavior one year after early and extended post-partum contact. *Child Neurology, 16,* 172-179.

KENNELL, J. H., & Klaus, M. H. (1984). Mother-infant bonding: Weighing the evidence. *Developmental Review, 4,* 275-282.

KENNELL, J. H., Klaus, M., McGrath, S., Robertson, S., & Hinkley, C. (1988). Medical interventions: The effect of social support during labor. *Pediatric Research, 61,* 211.

KLAUS, M. H., Jerauld, R., Kreger, N. C., McAlpine, W., Steffa, M., & Kennell, J. H. (1972). Maternal attachment: Importance of the first post-partum days. *New England Journal of Medicine, 286,* 460-463.

KLAUS, M. H., & Kennell, J. H. (1970). Mothers separated from their newborn infants. *Pediatric Clinics of North America, 17,* 1015-1037.

KLAUS, M. H., & Kennell, J. H. (1976). *Maternal-infant bonding.* St. Louis, MO: Mosby.

KLAUS, M. H., Kennell, J. H., Robertson, S., & Sosa, R. (1986). Effects of social support during parturition on maternal and infant morbidity. *British Medical Journal, 293,* 585-587.

KONNER, M. J. (1980, April). *Functional consequences of nursing frequency among hunter-gatherers.* Paper presented at the International Conference on Infant Studies, New Haven, CT.

LAMAZE, F. (1970). *Painless childbirth: Psychoprophylactic method.* Chicago: Regnery.

LAMB, M. E. (1982). Early contact and maternal-infant bonding: One decade later. *Pediatrics, 70,* 763-768.

LANGTON, P. A., & Kammerer, D. A. (1989). Childbearing and women's choice of nurse-midwives in Washington D.C. hospitals. *Woman's Health, 15,* 49-65.

LARIN, H. M. (1982). Drug and obstetric medication effects on infant behavior as measured by the Brazelton Neonatal Behavioral Assessment Scale. *Physical and Occupational Therapy in Pediatrics, 2,* 75-84.

LEBOYER, F. (1975). *Birth without violence.* New York: Knopf.

LEIDERMAN, P. H. (1981). Human mother to infant social bonding: Is there a sensitive phase? In K. Immelmann, G. Barlow, et al. (Eds.). *Behavioral development.* New York: Cambridge University Press.

LEIFER, A. D., Leiderman, P. H., Barnett, C. R., & Williams, J. A. (1972). Effects of mother-infant separation on maternal attachment behavior. *Child Development, 43,* 1203-1218.

LEVENTHAL, E. A., Leventhal, H., & Shacham, S. (1989). Active coping reduces reports of pain from childbirth. *Journal of Consulting and Clinical Psychology, 57,* 365-371.

LEWIS, J. S. (1986). *In the family way: Childbearing in the British aristocracy, 1760-1860.* New Brunswick, NJ: Rutgers University Press.

LIEBERMAN, B. A., Rosenblatt, D. B., Belsey, E., Packer, M., Redshaw, M., Mills, M., Caldwell, J., Notarianni, L., Smith, R. L., Williams, M., & Beard, R. W. (1979). The effects of maternally administered pethidine or epidural bupivicaine on the fetus and newborn. *British Journal of Obstetrics and Gynaecology, 86,* 598-606.

LIEBERMAN, E., & Ryan, K. J. (1989). Birth-day choices [Comment]. *New England Journal of Medicine, 321,* 1824-1825.

LIEBLING, A. (1939, June 3). Profile: Patron of the preemies. *New Yorker,* pp. 20-24.

LIVINGSTON, M. (1987). Choice in childbirth: Power and the impact of the modern childbirth reform movement. *Women and Therapy, 6,* 239-261.

LOU, H. C., Tweed, W. A., & Davis, J. M. (1989). Endogenous opioids may protect the perinatal brain in hypoxia. *Developmental Pharmacology and Therapy, 13,* 129-133.

LOWE, B. (1987). Fear of failure: A place for the trial of instrumental delivery. *British Journal of Obstetrics and Gynaecology, 94,* 80-86.

LUPE, P. J., & Gross, T. L. (1986). Maternal upright posture and mobility in labor: A review. *Obstetrics and Gynecology, 67,* 727-734.

LYNDRUP, J., Legarth, J., Dahl, C., Philipsen, T., Eriksen, P. S., & Weber, T. (1990). Induction of labour: The effect of vaginal prostaglandin or I.V. oxytocin—a matter of time only? *European Journal of Obstetrics, Gynecology, and Reproductive Biology, 37,* 111-119.

MACKEY, M. C. (1990). Women's choice of childbirth setting. *Health Care for Women International, 11,* 175-189.

MACKEY, M. C., & Lock, S. E. (1989). Women's expectations of the labor and delivery nurse. *Journal of Obstetric, Gynecologic, and Neonatal Nursing, 18,* 505-512.

MAISELS, M. J., Gifford, K., Antle, C. E., & Leib, G. R. (1988). Jaundice in the healthy newborn infant: A new approach to an old problem. *Pediatrics, 81,* 505-511.

McCALL, R. B. (1982). A hard look at stimulating and predicting development: The cases of bonding and screening. *Pediatrics in Review, 3,* 205-212.

McGRATH, S., Kennell, J., Klaus, M., Robertson, S., & Hinckley, C. (1991). Continuous emotional support during labor in a U.S. hospital: A randomized control trial. *Journal of the American Medical Association, 265,* 2197-2201.

MEEHAN, F. F. (1989). Trial of scar with induction/oxytocin in delivery following prior section. *Clinical and Experimental Obstetrics and Gynecology, 15*, 117-123.

MEEHAN, F. F., Burke, G., & Kehoe, J. T. (1989). Update on delivery following prior cesarean section: A 15-year review 1972-1987. *International Journal of Gynaecology and Obstetrics, 30*, 205-212.

MEIER, G. W. (1964). Behavior of infant monkeys: Differences attributable to mode of birth. *Science, 143*, 968-970.

MENDEZ-BAUER, C., Arroyo, J., Garcia-Ramos, C., et al. (1975). Effects of standing position on spontaneous uterine contractility and other aspects of labor. *Journal of Perinatal Medicine, 3*, 89-100.

MEYER, L., Mailloux, J., Marcoux, S., Blanchet, P., & Meyer, F. (1987). Maternal and neonatal morbidity in instrumental deliveries with the Kobayashi vacuum extractor and low forceps. *Acta Obstetricia et Gynecologica Scandinavica, 66*, 643-647.

MILES, M. S. (1989). Parents of critically ill premature infants: Sources of stress. *Critical Care Nursing Quarterly, 12*, 69-74.

MILLER, F. J. W. (1948). Home nursing of premature babies in Newcastle-on-Tyne. *Lancet, 2*, 703-705.

MIZUTA, M. (1987). [Studies on the influence of maternal delivery position on fetal status] (in Japanese; abstract only). *Nippon Sanka Fujinka Gakkai Zasshi, 39*, 965-971.

MOLD, J. W., & Stein, H. F. (1986). The cascade effect in the clinical care of patients. *New England Journal of Medicine, 314*, 512-514.

MOLLOY, B. S., Sheil, O., & Duignan, N. M. (1987). Delivery after Caesarean section: Review of 2176 consecutive cases. *British Medical Journal of Clinical Research, 294*, 1645-1647.

MOREAU, T., & Birch, H. G. (1974). Relationship between obstetrical general anesthesia and rate of neonatal habituation to repeated stimulation. *Developmental Medicine and Child Neurology, 16*, 612-619.

MORISHIMA, H. O., & Adamson, K. (1967). Placental clearance of mepivicaine following administration to guinea pigs. *Anesthesiology, 28*, 147-154.

MORISHIMA, H. O., Daniel, S. S., Finster, M., Poppers, P. J., & James, L. S. (1966). Transmission of mepivicaine hydrochloride (Carbocaine) across the human placenta. *Anesthesiology, 27*, 147-154.

MOYA, F., & Thorndike, V. (1962). Passage of drugs across the placenta. *American Journal of Obstetrics and Gynecology, 84*, 1778-1798.

MUHLEN, L. Pryke, M., & Wade, K. (1986). Effects of type of birth and anaesthetic on neonatal behavioral assessment. *Australian Psychologist, 21*, 253-270.

MUIR, L. E. (April, 1988). *Effect of obstetric medication on maternal-infant interaction.* Paper presented at the International Conference on Infant Studies, Washington, DC. (Abstract from *Infant Behavior and Development, 11*, 230)

MURRAY, A. D., Dolby, R. M., Nation, R. L., & Thomas, D. B. (1981). Effects of epidural anesthesia on newborns and their mothers. *Child Development, 52*, 71-82.

MYERS, B. J. (1984a). Mother-infant bonding: The status of this critical-period hypothesis. *Developmental Review, 4*, 240-274.

MYERS, B. J. (1984b). Mother-infant bonding: Rejoinder to Kennell and Klaus. *Developmental Review, 4*, 283-288.

MYERS, B. J. (1987). Mother-infant bonding as a critical period. In M. H. Bornstein (Ed.), *Sensitive periods in development: Interdisciplinary perspectives.* Hillsdale, NJ: Lawrence Erlbaum.

MYERS, R. E. (1972). Two patterns of perinatal brain damage and their conditions of occurrence. *American Journal of Obstetrics and Gynecology, 112*, 246-276.

NAEYE, R. L., & Peters, E. C. (1987). Antenatal hypoxia and low IQ values. *American Journal of Diseases in Childhood, 141*, 50-54.

NAGASHIMA, L., Bertsch, T., Dykeman, S., McGrath, S., DeLay, T., & Kennell, J. (1987). Fathers during labor: Do we expect too much? *Pediatric Research, 21*, 62.

NAGER, C. W., Key, T., & Moore, T. R. (1987). Cervical ripening and labor outcome with preinduction intracervical prostaglandin EZ (Prepidil) gel. *Journal of Perinatology, 7*, 189-193.

National Institutes of Health. (1981). Consensus development statement on cesarean childbirth. *Obstetrics and Gynecology, 63*, 485.

NELSON, N. M., Enkin, M. W., Saigel, S., Bennett, K. J., Milner, R., & Sackett, D. L. (1980). A randomized clinical trial of the Leboyer approach to childbirth. *New England Journal of Medicine, 302*, 655-660.

NEUHOFF, D., Burke, M. S., & Porreco, R. P. (1989). Cesarean birth for failed progress in labor [Comment]. *Obstetrics and Gynecology, 73*, 915-920.

NEUTRA, R. R., Fienberg, S. E., Greenland, S., & Friedman, E. A. (1978). Effect of fetal monitoring on neonatal death rates. *New England Journal of Medicine, 299*, 324-326.

NGAN, H. Y., Miu, P., Ko, L., & Ma, H. K. (1990). Long term neurological sequelae following vacuum extraction delivery. *Australian and New Zealand Journal of Obstetrics and Gynaecology, 30*, 111-114.

NICHOLSON, C., & Ridolfo, E. (1989). Avoiding the pitfalls of epidural anesthesia in obstetrics. *Journal of the American Association of Nurse Anesthetists, 57*, 220-230.

NIELSEN, T. F., & Hokegård, K. H. (1984a). Cesarean section and intraoperative surgical complications. *Acta Obstetricia et Gynecologica Scandinavica, 63*, 103-108.

NIELSEN, T. F., & Hokegård, K. H. (1984b). The incidence of acute neonatal respiratory disorders in relation to mode of delivery. *Acta Obstetricia et Gynecologica Scandinavica, 63*, 109.

NISWANDER, K. R., & Gordon, M. (Eds.). (1972). *The women and their pregnancies.* Philadelphia: J. B. Saunders.

NOTZON, F. C. (1990). International differences in the use of obstetric interventions. *Journal of the American Medical Association, 263*, 3286-3291.

OCHI, M., Ishikawa, H., Morikawa, S., Chihara, H., Nagata, T., & Kometani, K. (1989). [The assessment of the safety of vacuum extraction deliveries under routine epidural block] (in Japanese). *Nippon Sanka Fujinka Gakkai Zasshi, 41*, 826-832.

O'CONNOR, S. O., Vietze, P. M., Sherrod, K. B., Sandler, H. M., & Altemeier, W. A., III. (1980). Reduced incidence of parenting inadequacy following rooming-in. *Pediatrics, 66*, 176-183.

ODENT, M. (1982). The milieu and obstetrical positions during labor: A new approach from France. In M. H. Klaus & M. O. Robertson (Eds.), *Birth, interaction, and attachment: Exploring the foundations for modern perinatal care* (pp. 23-28). Skillman, NJ: Johnson & Johnson Baby Products.

ODENT, M. (1984). *Birth reborn.* New York: Pantheon.

O'DRISCOLL, K., Foley, M., & MacDonald, D. (1984). Active management of labor as an alternative to cesarean section for dystocia. *Obstetrics and Gynecology, 63,* 485-490.

PACIORNIK, M., & Paciornik, C. (1976). Do not disturb the deliverance of Indians: The squatting deliverance confronting the dorsal decubitus deliverance. *Annals: III. Paraguayan Congress of Gynecology and Obstetrics.*

PALKOVITZ, R. (1988). Sources of father-infant bonding beliefs: Implications for childbirth educators. *Maternal and Child Nursing Journal, 17,* 101-113.

PATTON, L. L., English, E. C., & Hambleton, J. D. (1985). Childbirth preparation and outcomes of labor and delivery in primiparous women. *Journal of Family Practice, 20,* 375-378.

PAUL, R. H., Phelan, J. P., & Yeh, S. (1985). Trial of labor in a patient with a prior Cesarean birth. *American Journal of Obstetrics and Gynecology, 151,* 297-304.

PEDERSON, F., Zaslow, M., Cain, R., & Anderson, B. (1980, April). *Caesarean childbirth: The importance of a family perspective.* Paper presented at the International Conference on Infant Studies, New Haven, CT.

PETRIE, R. H. (1981, October). *The challenge of the 80's: Balancing medical education and humanistic obstetrics in a teaching hospital.* Paper presented at the Conference on Obstetrical Management and Infant Outcome, New York.

PHAROAH, P. O., Cooke, T., Rosenbloom, I., & Cooke, R. W. (1987). Trends in birth prevalence of cerebral palsy. *Archives of Diseases of Childhood, 62,* 379-384.

PIERS, M. (1978). *Infanticide: Past and present.* New York: W. W. Norton.

POORE, M., & Foster, J. C. (1985). Epidural and no epidural anesthesis: Difference between mothers and their experience of birth. *Birth Issues in Perinatal Care and Education, 12,* 205-212.

PORRECO, R. D. (1985). High cesarean section rate: A new perspective. *Obstetrics and Gynecology, 65,* 307.

RAPPOPORT, D. (1976). Pour une naissance sans violence: Resultats d'une première enquête [For a birth without violence: Results of a first investigation]. *Bulletin Psychologie, 29,* 552-560.

REID, A. J., Carroll, J. C., Ruderman, J., & Murray, M. A. (1989). Differences in intrapartum obstetric care provided to women at low risk by family physicians and obstetricians. *Canadian Medical Association Journal, 140,* 625-633.

RIESE, M. L. (1988). Temperament in full-term and preterm infants: Stability over ages 6 to 24 months. *Journal of Developmental and Behavioral Pediatrics, 9,* 6-11.

RINGLER, N. M., Kennell, J. H., Jarvella, R., Navojosky, B. J., & Klaus, M. H. (1975). Mother-to-child speech at 2 years: Effects of early postnatal contact. *Journal of Pediatrics, 86,* 141-144.

RINGLER, N. M., Trause, M. A., Klaus, M. H., & Kennell, J. H. (1978). The effects of extra postpartum contact and maternal speech patterns on children's IQs, speech, and language comprehension at five. *Child Development, 49,* 862-865.

ROBERTSON, P. A., Laros, R. K., Jr., & Zhao, R. L. (1990). Neonatal and maternal outcome in low-pelvic and midpelvic operative deliveries. *American Journal of Obstetrics and Gynecology, 162,* 1436-1442.

RODE, S. S., Chang, P., Fisch, R. O., & Sroufe, L. A. (1981). Attachment patterns of infants separated at birth. *Developmental Psychology, 17,* 188-191.

ROOKS, J. P., Weatherby, N. L., Ernst, E. K., Stapleton, S., Rosen, D., & Rosenfield, A. (1989). Outcomes of care in birth centers: The National Birth Center Study. *New England Journal of Medicine, 32,* 1804-1811.

ROSEN, M., & Thomas, L. (1989). *The Caesarean myth: Choosing the best way to have your baby.* New York: Penguin.

ROSEN, M. G., Debanne, S. M., & Thompson, K. (1989). Arrest disorders and infant brain damage. *Obstetrics and Gynecology, 74,* 321-324.

ROSENBLUM, L. A., & Youngstein, K. P. (1974). Developmental change in compensatory dyadic response in mother and infant monkeys. In M. Lewis & L. A. Rosenblum (Eds.), *The effect of the infant on its caregiver.* New York: Wiley-Interscience.

ROSENFIELD, A. B. (1980). Visiting in the intensive care nursery. *Child Development, 51,* 939-941.

SACHS, B. P., Oriol, N. E., Ostheimer, G. W., Weiss, J. B., Driscoll, S., Acker, D., Brown, D. A., & Jewett, J. F. (1989). Anesthetic-related maternal mortality, 1954 to 1985. *Journal of Clinical Anesthesiology, 1,* 333-338.

SANDERS-PHILLIPS, K., Strauss, M. E., & Gutberlet, R. L. (1988). The effect of obstetric medication on newborn infant feeding behavior. *Infant Behavior and Development, 11,* 251-263.

SARNO, A. P., Ahn, M. O., Phelan, J. P., & Paul, R. H. (1990). Fetal acoustic stimulation in the early intrapartum period as a predictor of subsequent fetal condition. *American Journal of Obstetrics and Gynecology, 162,* 762-767.

SCANLON, J. W. (1976). Effects of local anesthetics administered to parturient women on the neurological and behavioral performance of newborn children. *Bulletin of the New York Academy of Medicine, 52,* 231-240.

SCHALLER, J., Carlsson, S. G., & Larsson, K. (1979). Effects of extended post-partum mother-child contact on the mother's behavior during nursing. *Infant Behavior and Development, 2,* 319-324.

SCHOLTEN, C. M. (1985). *Childbearing in American society: 1650-1850.* New York: New York University Press.

SEASHORE, M. J., Leifer, A. D., Barnett, C. R., & Leiderman, P. H. (1973). The effects of denial of early mother-infant interaction on maternal self-confidence. *Journal of Personality and Social Psychology, 26,* 369-378.

SEPKOSKI, C. (1985). Maternal obstetric medication and newborn behavior. In J. W. Scanlon (Ed.), *Perinatal anesthesia.* London: Basil Blackwell.

SHIONO, P., Klebanoff, M. A., & Carey, J. C. (1990). Midline episiotomies: More harm than good? *Obstetrics and Gynecology, 75,* 765-770.

SHNIDER, S. (1981). Choice of anesthesia for labor and delivery. *Journal of Obstetrics and Gynecology, 58*(Suppl. 5), 24S-34S.

SHY, K. K., Luthy, D. A., Bennett, F. C., et al. (1990). Effects of electronic fetal-heart-rate monitoring, as compared with periodic auscultation, on the neurologic development of premature infants. *New England Journal of Medicine, 322,* 588-593.

SILVA-CRUZ, A., Godinho, F., Pinto, J. M., Andrade, L., & Sim, D. (1988). Prostaglandin E2 gel compared to oxytocin for medically-indicated labour induction at term: A controlled clinical trial. *Pharmatherapeutica, 5,* 228-232.

SOMELL, C. (1987). Induction of labor and cervical ripening with oral PGE2 in risk pregnancies: A placebo controlled study. *Acta Obstetricia et Gynecologica Scandinavica.*

SOUZA, P. L. R., Barros, F. C., Gazalle, R. V., Begeres, R. M., Pinheiro, G. N., Menezea, S. T., & Arruda, L. A. (1974, October). *Attachment and lactation.* Paper presented at the Fifteenth International Congress of Pediatrics, Buenos Aires.

STANDLEY, K. (1974, August). *Prenatal and perinatal correlates of neonatal behaviors.* Paper presented at the annual meeting of the American Psychological Association, New Orleans.

STANDLEY, K. (1976, April). *Sources of variation in the behavior of normal newborns: Consequences of obstetric medication.* Paper presented at the annual meeting of the Eastern Psychological Association, New York.

SVEDJA, M. J., Campos, J. J., & Emde, R. N. (1980). Mother-infant "bonding": Failure to generalize. *Child Development, 51,* 775-779.

TAFFEL, S. M., Placek, P. J., & Moien, M. (1989). Cesarean section rate levels off in 1987. *Family Planning Perspectives, 21,* 227-228.

THACKER, S. B., & Banta, H. D. (1980). Benefits and risks of episiotomy: An interpretive review of the English-language literature, 1860-1980. *Obstetrical and Gynecological Survey, 34,* 627-642.

THORP, J. A., Parisi, V. M., Boylan, P. C., & Johnston, D. A. (1989). The effect of continuous epidural analgesia on cesarean section for dystocia in nulliparous women. *American Journal of Obstetrics and Gynecology, 161,* 670-675.

TRONICK, E., Wise, S., Als, H., Adamson, L., Scanlon, J., & Brazelton, T. B. (1976). Regional obstetric anesthesia and newborn behavior: Effect over the first ten days of life. *Pediatrics, 58,* 94-100.

TURNER, M. J., Brassil, M., & Gordon, H. (1988). Active management of labor associated with a decrease in the cesarean section rate in nulliparas. *Obstetrics and Gynecology, 71,* 150-154.

VARRASSI, G., Bazzano, C., & Edwards, W. T. (1989). Effects of physical activity on maternal plasma beta-endorphin levels and perception of labor pain. *American Journal of Obstetrics and Gynecology, 160,* 707-712.

VIETZE, P. M., MacTurk, R. H., McCarthy, M. E., Klein, R. P., & Yarrow, L. J. (1980, April). *Impact of mode of delivery on father- and mother-infant interaction at 6 months.* Paper presented at the International Conference on Infant Studies, New Haven, CT.

VIETZE, P. M., O'Connor, S., Falsey, S., & Altemeier, W. A. (1978, August). *Effects of rooming-in on maternal behavior directed towards infants.* Paper presented at the annual meeting of the American Psychological Association, Toronto.

WERTZ, R. W., & Wertz, D. C. (1979). *Lying-in: A history of childbirth in America.* New York: Schocken.

WHITE, E., Shy, K. K., & Daling, J. R. (1985). An investigation of the relationship between Cesarean section birth and respiratory distress syndrome of the newborn. *American Journal of Epidemiology, 121,* 651.

WIDEMAN, M. V., & Singer, J. E. (1983). *Psychosocial trends in obstetrical practices in American hospitals.* Unpublished manuscript, Uniformed Services University of the Health Sciences, Bethesda, MD.

WIDEMAN, M. V., & Singer, J. E. (1984). The role of psychological mechanisms in preparation for childbirth. *American Psychologist, 39,* 1357-1371.

WINDLE, W. F. (1966). An experimental approach to prevention or reduction of brain damage of birth asphyxia. *Developmental Medicine and Child Neurology, 8,* 129-140.

WINTERS, M. (1973). *The relationship of time of initial feeding to success of breast feeding.* Unpublished master's thesis, University of Washington, Seattle.

WOOD, C., et al. (1964-1965, Winter). Effects of meperidine on the newborn infant. *Collaborative Project Reporter, 33,* 1-8.

ZELCER, J., Owers, H., & Paull, J. D. (1989). A controlled oximetric evaluation of inhalational, opioid and epidural analgesia in labour. *Anesthesia and Intensive Care, 17,* 418-421.

ZESKIND, P. S. (1980). Adult responses to cries of low and high risk infants. *Infant Behavior and Development, 3,* 167-177.

PART II

Early Characteristics and Development

The Development of Basic Characteristics of Infants

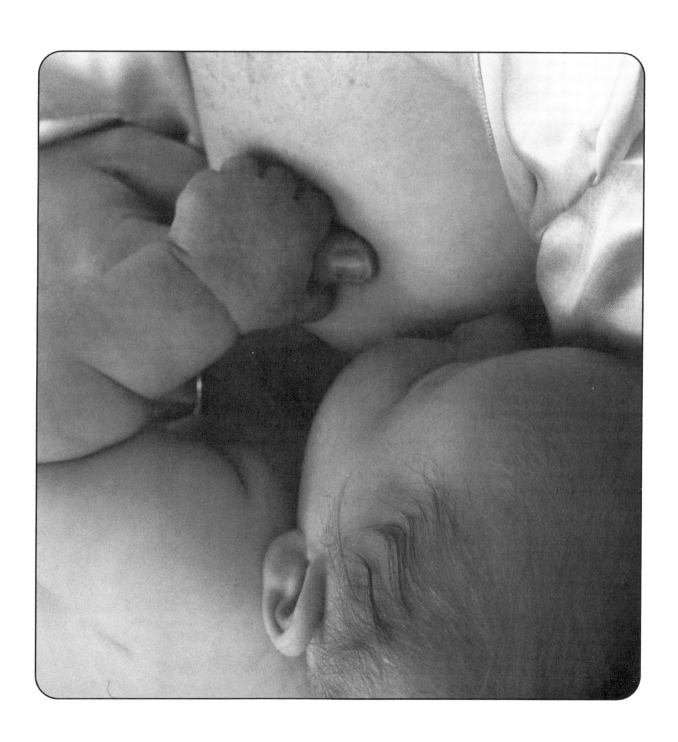

Newborns are often described as creatures who only eat, sleep, and cry. Although babies do spend much of their time in such activities, this description by no means fully represents their abilities. This chapter explores the basic response systems of young babies, beginning with a discussion of three aspects of their activities: sleep, activity, and attention. These, and crying, which will be considered later in the chapter, are all aspects of what is called **state**. Studies of learning, perception, and cognition, as well as the testing of infants, especially young ones, are all dependent on state.

Next, sucking is considered. As a behavior of primary importance to infant survival, sucking has been the focus of a major theoretical debate within the field of child development. Finally, the discussion turns to three affective behaviors of infants that also serve important communicative functions for both biological survival and social development: crying, smiling, and laughing.

The research relevant to these topics focuses on whether and how these response systems operate in newborns. This permeates the study of infants, inasmuch as one of the major purposes in studying infants is to discover when and how human characteristics get started. In addition, knowing the basic response of normal, full-term infants helps in the recognition or diagnosis of abnormality. Although development of the basic systems is discussed here when information is available (the best example is sucking), the information is sporadic at best. It is important to realize that all these systems undoubtedly change radically as infants grow.

How Babies Spend Their Time

SLEEP

The sleep of infants interests parents and researchers alike. It starts during fetal life and its patterns change throughout infancy. Researchers are interested in specific types of sleep, in sleep patterns, their variability, and such questions as the proportions of sleeping time in quiet versus active sleep (Dreyfus-Brissac, 1968; Thoman & Whitney, 1989). In quiet sleep the baby shows little or no motor activity, the eyes are firmly closed and motionless, and respiration is relatively slow and constant in depth. In active sleep a wide range of motor activity may be seen. The eyes are usually closed, but brief eye opening may accompany rapid eye movement (**REM**); respiration is more rapid and less regular in deep than in quiet sleep. There is also a

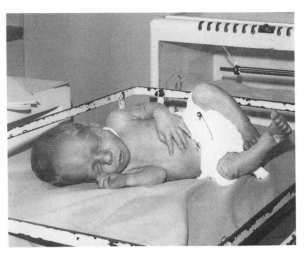

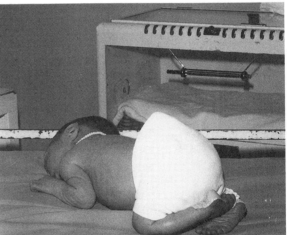

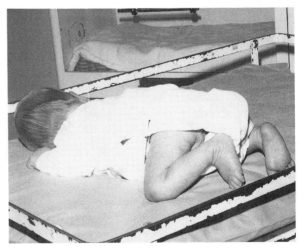

Figure 6.1. Some common postures of newborns during sleep. Most babies sleep better on their sides or on their tummies (prone). The baby on his back is in a more active stage of sleep—he has just kicked his foot. (Photograph courtesy of Judy F. Rosenblith.)

transitional stage that is a mixture of these two (see Figure 6.1).

Parents are interested in how much and when their baby will sleep. A good starting point for examining this question would seem to be to study naturally occurring sleep patterns in newborns. But most hospitals, and many families, awaken babies for feedings at regular intervals, so no accurate picture of spontaneous sleep patterns can be obtained. Given this limitation, one of the best studies of the neonatal period is that by Parmelee et al. (1961). They obtained a sample of 100 babies approximately evenly divided between breast- and bottle-fed and males and females. The 75 babies whose mothers made adequate records averaged 17, 16.5, and 16.2 hours in the first, second, and third days. They fed more frequently on Day 3, more than 6 times per day. Although total sleeping time averaged 16-17 hours, the babies differed greatly. Some slept twice as much as others, ranging from 10.5 to 23 hours on Day 2 and 11.4 to 21 hours on Day 3. Those who slept long on Day 2 tended to sleep long on Day 3. Hence trying to tell a parent how much his or her child will sleep would be rather futile.

Sleeping times of 19 infants studied over the first months of life showed that babies slept less than 15 hours on average from 3 through 15 weeks of age (Kleitman & Engelmann, 1953). A recent study by Bamford et al. (1990) confirms many of these older findings with a population of inner-city infants in Manchester, England, as do recent Finnish data (Michelsson et al., 1990). As can be seen in Table 6.1, the number of episodes of sleep declines steadily from 6 to 52 weeks, but with considerable individual differences. The decline in total amount of sleep is much more gradual, but individual differences are striking, with some infants sleeping more than twice as much as others at all ages. There were no significant sex differences. Babies tended to be similar from one age to another, but the correlations were not large (range .18 to .45).

Parmelee et al.'s (1961) data confirm something parents have often noted during their long walks in the middle of the night: Many babies (43%) do not have their longest period of sleep between 11 p.m. and 7 a.m., and many do not have any long periods of sleep. The lengths of the longest periods of sleep vary from 2 to 10 hours. More recent data give the average as 3.5 hours at 3 weeks and 6 hours at 6 months (Coons & Guilleminault, 1984). Finnish data showed 6 hours of continuous sleep for 35% of infants under 3 months, increasing to 72% by 9 to 12 months (Michelsson et al., 1990). These sleep patterns do not seem to be affected by the sex of the infant or the type of feeding. Although total sleep stays about constant, it tends to change from 3- to 4-hour periods evenly distributed throughout the day and night to two such periods **entrained** into a night diurnal cycle. (*Entrainment* refers to the ways in which the external environment affects basic biological rhythms.) Over the first 5 weeks of life the amount of wakefulness during the day increases, but the amount of wakefulness at night does not (Thoman & Whitney, 1989). There is already a definite tendency to sleep more at night by 6 weeks (Bamford et al., 1990). The longest waking period is still randomly distributed throughout the 24 hours at 3 months, but not at 4½ months (Coons & Guilleminault, 1984).

Scientists and pediatricians are interested in the amounts of time spent in quiet versus active sleep. Stern et al. (1969) have reported cyclic fluctuations between quiet and active sleep for newborns and for 3- and 8-month-olds. These researchers recorded eye and body movements, respirations, and **EEGs** (electroencephalograms, which are records of the electrical activity of the brain). Quiet-active cycles in the sleep of the term infants lasted only 47 minutes, compared with 90 minutes in adult sleep (46 minutes for prematures at 31-34 weeks according to Curzi-Dascalova et al., 1988). The length of these cycles increased very slowly, to 49 minutes at 3 months and 50 minutes at 8

Table 6.1

Number of Episodes of Sleep and Total Sleep Time According to Age

Postnatal Age in Weeks	Number of Infants	Median[a] Number of Sleep Episodes	Median Total Sleep Time
6	156	7 (3-14)[b]	950 (530-1310)
13	156	6 (2-17)	905 (105-1300)
26	145	5 (2-13)	843 (545-1190)
52	148	4 (2-7)	820 (475-1085)

SOURCE: Adapted from Bamford et al. (1990).
[a] Medians rather than averages are shown to reduce the effect of any few extreme cases.
[b] Range is shown in ( ).

months. There was also a change in the proportion of each cycle that was composed of quiet sleep. At birth, quiet sleep time equaled active sleep time, but at from 3 to 8 months it was twice as long as active sleep (compared with three times as long in adults).

Studies of sleep patterns in prematures shed light on the neurological organization of the premature and on the development of sleep. In extremely premature infants (24 to 27 weeks of conceptional age), the primitive sleep state that exists has no cyclic organization (Dreyfus-Brissac, 1968). Sleep cycles shorten with age after 32 weeks, and the amount of quiet sleep in a cycle increases (Dittrichova & Paul, 1984). Both preterm and SGA babies have been shown to have a greater rate of state change than term infants (Watt & Strongman, 1985). In a study by Curzi-Dascalova et al. (1988), indeterminate sleep (sleep that cannot be classified as either active or quiet) made up roughly 30% of the total sleep cycle at 31-34 weeks, but only 12% by 35-36 weeks. At this age the duration and percentage of active and quiet sleep has increased and remains stable up to 39-40 weeks.

When development of sleep patterns in prematures is compared with that of term babies, interesting features emerge. Prematures do not simply lag behind their term peers by a factor that reflects their age since conception, as one might expect. They show greater maturity than term infants of the same conceptional age for some aspects of sleep, and less maturity for others (see, for example, Booth et al., 1980; Yokochi et al., 1989), a fact that leads to intriguing research questions. What are the environmental or experiential factors that lead to these differences in state organization? Are there long-range consequences of such differences?

Sleep-wake state organization of prematures is related to performance on neonatal assessment batteries, and both are related to developmental quotients at 6 months and 1 year (Anders et al., 1985). Beckwith and Parmelee (1986) showed that prematures with less **trace alternant** EEG patterns (bursts or clusters of high-amplitude slow waves interspersed with periods of more attenuated activity) in their sleep records, especially in quiet sleep, had lower IQs from 4 months to 8 years of age. This did not hold true if they were reared in consistently attentive and responsive environments. In a study by Whitney et al. (1990), prematures with neurobehavioral problems had markedly different sleep patterns than normal prematures (shorter longest-sleep periods, awake more, lower state stability scores) over the first 5 weeks of life. Significant but small differences were found on other variables.

Recently, stable individual differences in sleep measures have been demonstrated for both premature (Davis & Thoman, 1988) and term babies (Thoman & Whitney, 1989). The new automated techniques developed by the researchers involved in this work make large-scale studies and studies over longer age spans more feasible.

Weissbluth (1983) has shown that total sleep duration, the variable of greatest interest to parents, is highly negatively correlated with four of five infant temperament characteristics used to define easy/difficult children. In that study's sample, difficult children slept 2 hours less at night and 1 hour less in the daytime than did easy children. Brief daytime sleep was associated with high persistence ratings or short attention spans, an odd dichotomy.

Recently it has been suggested that the developmental norms for sleep-wake cycles may be artifacts of the feeding practices (exclusive bottle-feeding) current in our society when the research establishing most of them was done (Elias et al., 1986). Breast- versus bottle-feeding affects newborn state (diPietro et al., 1987), as does varying the amino acid content of formula (Yogman & Zeisel, 1983). Increasing the amino acid content of formula can promote sleep, as can the introduction of solid food (Bamberg et al., 1990). Another cultural limitation is that all data are based on infants who sleep alone, not those who sleep with their mothers, a common practice in many non-Western cultures (McKenna, 1987). Data on British infants who sleep with their mothers and are breast-fed confirm the findings of Elias and colleagues (1986) that they tend to sleep in shorter periods with frequent wakings (Odent, 1990).

I cannot begin to do justice to the literature on sleep and its development in this short discussion, but hope I have demonstrated that (a) it is not a single phenomenon, (b) different aspects develop on different schedules, and (c) there are great individual differences in sleep behaviors.

ACTIVITY

Activity is an aspect of behavior that varies in the awake state as well as in sleep, and that can be studied prior to birth. The levels of activity displayed by different newborns and fetuses vary markedly. This has led some to wonder whether the activity level of an infant is indicative of a lifelong or enduring constitutional or temperamental trait. Babies differ not only in the amount of activity they show spontaneously, which is what is usually studied, but also in how their activity changes (or fails to change) in response to stimulus situations (see Figure 6.2).

Background Issues

Before focusing on current research on activity, it is appropriate to review the history of debates on the nature of newborn activity and the progress made in measuring it.

History of Debates on the Nature of Newborn Activity. Let us begin with a discussion of the history of the arguments about the nature of activity. Preyer (1880/1888) questioned the relation between early general activity and later adaptive behaviors. He even proposed a mechanism resembling what is now called reinforcement that operated to determine the aspects of activity that remained stable. His view can be seen as fitting either of the polar positions about the nature of activity that developed later. One of these positions is represented by Dennis (1932) and Watson (1937), who saw the infant's "stream of activity" as made up of unlearned responses (that is, of discrete activities) that quickly became conditioned. At the opposite extreme were those such as Coghill (1929a, 1929b), Irwin (1930), and Weiss (1929), who found that the infant's activity was better described by the phrase *mass activity* than as reflexes or discrete behaviors. Weiss, for example, found that 30-40% of newborns' movements were rapid, unorganized, and involved the entire body. Irwin (1930) and Coghill (1929a, 1929b) proposed that growth proceeded by the differentiation of specific movements out of this mass activity, rather than by the conditioning of specific responses. Subsequently, researchers have tended to ignore the theoretical issue and to use measures of activity to study other aspects of infant behavior.

Measurement of Activity. Many observational schemes have been used to measure activity. Some are directed toward assessing mass activity, others toward specific movements, and some toward both; there has been one attempt at a choreographic description of "rhythms of movement" (Kestenberg, 1965). As in all observational techniques, the problems of definition are great and always involve some judgment. What constitutes a specific movement? How much activity constitutes "mass activity"? How many different kinds of activity are there? Thus it is crucial that workers es-

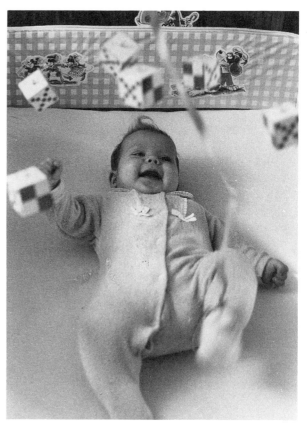

Figure 6.2. An active baby, responding to the stimulus of a mobile. (Photograph courtesy of Carolyn Rovee-Collier.)

tablish **reliability** in scoring.[1] This requires careful descriptions of categories, considerable training or experience, and avoidance of an excessive number of categories (which demand that overly fine distinctions be made). Given these conditions, which are demanding, the human observer can be a rather good instrument for measuring activity. Hence investigators searched for more objective and less demanding ways of recording activity. The result was the early development of various kinds of apparatuses to aid in measurement.

A number of devices called stabilimeters were developed for this purpose. They involve some system for measuring movements of the mattress on which the infant is lying, and they usually enable analyses of the directions of motions—that is, left-right or up-down (see Weiss, 1929). Photoelectric cells and spring suspensions of the infant have been used to provide information that can be fed directly into computers (e.g., Crowell et al., 1964). Such devices are best at recording mass activity, although some systems have allowed recording of a finite number of specific responses (see,

---

1. Reliability means that two (or more) persons' scoring behaviors agree most of the time. Agreement is measured by determining the correlation coefficients for the two persons' sets of scores (or ratings), or the percentage of all instances of the behavior on which they agree. A more complete discussion of reliability appears in the manual.

for example, Lipsitt & DeLucia, 1960). Changes in the amount of activity from before to after administration of a stimulus can be assessed by any of the systems. Unfortunately, differences among the stabilimeter systems used to study activity are so great that it is hard to compare results from a study using one with those from another.

Some researchers returned to using direct observations with various methods to increase their precision. For example, Gordon and Bell (1961) observed the movements of each body part and used these movements to arrive at activity levels only after the movements were scored in relation to the normal amount of movement for that body part. Film has long been used to measure activity of infants, and today videotape is frequently used. Observation of the films or tapes allows the checking and rechecking of observations as often as necessary. In the 1930s, Gesell and his colleagues developed objective methods for scoring filmed records (Gesell & Thompson, 1934; Gesell, 1948) and used them to study individual differences in activity (Ames, 1942, 1949), as did Bell (1960). Observers must still be able to score the behaviors in films or videotapes. Aids to accuracy are used such as projecting a film onto a screen with a superimposed grid to enable scoring the number of times a given body part crosses a grid line, or the number of grid lines it crosses. Because these features can be counted any number of times by any number of people, the observational scheme can be refined repeatedly until reliability is achieved. The tedium of this process can be reduced by having the camera take only one picture every few seconds. This time-lapse photography has been used with a wrist band on the baby to enable easy scoring of grid crossings (Robertson, 1982).

The relation between activity level and crying is a problem in activity measurement. Korner and her colleagues showed that all measures of total activity are badly contaminated by the amount of time spent crying (Korner, Kraemer, et al., 1974; Korner, Thoman, & Glick, 1974). A crying baby produces about 12,000 movements per hour, compared with about 2,000 for a noncrying baby. Because some babies practically never cry and others cry as much as 22% of the time, measures of overall activity levels that do not take crying into consideration can be grossly misleading. When noncrying activity alone is measured, babies still show strong individual differences. The range found by Korner et al. was 1,100 to 4,500 movements per hour. Activity in noncrying periods was fairly highly correlated with activity when crying ($r = .62$), which suggests that babies who are more active than most

when quiet are also likely to be more active when crying. Activity measures made in either quiet or crying periods may provide a valid index of activity level, but when measured in periods in which both occur, they may be confounded by the amount of crying.

Not all measures of activity are based on direct observation and quantification of number or location or vigor of movements. Data from various neonatal and infant tests are also used to arrive at activity measures or ratings (see Chapter 8). Prenatal activity is measured using polygraphic records and ultrasound pictures, as well as maternal observations.

Activity Level in Response to Stimulation

The preceding discussion has focused on spontaneous activity. We now turn to how activity is affected by all kinds of stimuli, both internal and external.

Internal Stimuli. The activity level of newborns clearly is responsive to internal stimuli, but in complicated ways. Hunger is the only generally occurring internal stimulus for which we have good operational definitions. In general, one can say that hunger increases activity level, but the pattern of changes differs in different babies. Five infants observed by Wolff (1966) showed a sharp increase in activity from the period just after feeding to the mid-feeding time and then dropped slightly just before the next feeding. In contrast, six infants showed a small increase between the postfeeding and midway periods, with a sharp rise in the period just before feeding. It would be interesting to know whether these two activity patterns are related to differences in total consumption (or total consumption in relation to weight) or to differences in metabolic rates. Clearly, individual differences in the relations between hunger and activity level are marked.

External Stimuli. Young babies become more active in response to external stimuli, and they again show large individual differences. Some examples of environmental events that stimulate changes in activity level are rubbing the forehead with a soft cloth, holding a nipple (without food) in the mouth, visual and auditory stimuli, and removing a nipple from the mouth (McGrade, 1968).

Cossette et al. (1991) studied motor activity in a variety of situations, with varying degrees of external stimulation, at 2½ and 5 months of age to determine whether there were any sex differences. They found virtually no significant sex differences, and the varied situations affected both sexes similarly.

Table 6.2

Correlations Between Fetal Activity and Gesell Scores

	Gesell Motor Score at			Gesell Total Score at		
Prenatal Month	*12 Weeks*	*24 Weeks*	*36 Weeks*	*12 Weeks*	*24 Weeks*	*36 Weeks*
Seventh	.29	.54	.53	.29	.44	.51
Eighth	.32	.33	.38	.35	.31	.23
Ninth	.26	.37	.51	.40	.40	.40
Average	.53	.44	.53	.40	.31	.31

SOURCE: Adapted from Walters (1965).

Activity Level as a Predictor of Later Development

Both pre- and postnatal activity have been shown to relate to later behaviors or development of the infant.

Prenatal Activity. In the 1930s, researchers asked whether prenatal activity level was related to later outcomes. Richards and Newberry (1938) studied 12 pregnant women for 5 to 6 hours every week or two. The number of minutes the mothers-to-be reported the fetus to be active in any way was determined and an activity rate (number of minutes of activity per 10 minutes of observation) was obtained. This rate in the last 2 months of pregnancy was correlated with the babies' total Gesell scores (see Chapter 8) at 6 months and to half of the items at 12 months. The correlations were positive (i.e., the higher the activity level, the better the Gesell scores) and highly significant. The authors thus concluded that 30-70% of the variance in developmental level at 6 months is accounted for by fetal activity level (percentage of variance is explained in the manual).

Walters (1965) replicated this study with a larger sample (35) of largely college-educated women. Seven babies exposed to pregnancy or delivery factors that might have affected prenatal activity level, postnatal development, or both were eliminated from the main sample used to test the hypothesis. Activity levels were recorded by mothers during the last 3 months of pregnancy (1.5 hours each week, averaged to provide a monthly score). Babies were tested on the Gesell Scales at 12, 24, and 36 weeks by persons with no knowledge of their fetal activity scores. Fetal activity scores for each month were correlated with total Gesell scores and those for each area of development. Even after taking account of birth weight, activity in each of the last 3 prenatal months was related to the total Gesell score (see Table 6.2), thus replicating the previous findings, even to finding similar strengths of relationships. Activity in each of these prenatal months was also related to motor development at all three postnatal ages. For reasons that are unclear, the 8-month prenatal measures were less related to later Gesell scores than those at 7 or 9 months (or than the average for the 3 months). Contrary to expectations, the strength of the relations did not decline as postnatal age increased. Fetal activity was as strongly related to development at 36 weeks as it had been at 12 or 24 weeks.

The activity levels of the seven babies eliminated because of prenatal or delivery problems were negatively (but not significantly) correlated with the total Gesell scores. Had these cases been kept in the main study, this negative relation would have weakened the total correlation, possibly making it appear that prenatal activity and postnatal development were not significantly related. Since subjects were from middle- or upper-middle-class families who had normal pregnancies and deliveries, the results can be generalized only to other such families and births. For these babies the data suggest that fetal activity would be positively correlated with development in the first 8 months of life. However, given the modest size of the correlations, this prediction would hold only for the group and could not be expected to hold for individual cases. In one study pregnant women scored different types of fetal activity (Ishikawa & Minamide, 1984). Kicking, rolling, and total fetal movement were negatively related to visual orientation to animate stimuli on the Brazelton Neonatal Behavioral Assessment Scales (see Chapter 8). These data are hard to reconcile with the earlier findings.

A recent study that has no follow-up on the infants has tried to establish that fetal activity as recorded by the mother has the characteristics of a temperamental trait (Eaton & Saudino, 1991). This study established that activity increases from 29 to 34 weeks, then declines to 39 weeks, and that individual differences are substantial and relatively stable.

Postnatal Activity. If activity level is a **trait** (that is, if there are stable individual differences in it), then spontaneous postnatal activity scores should have the measurement characteristics that are typical of traits, such as height, weight, and IQ. And they do. Measures of postnatal activity exhibit a wide range of scores, and they are approximately normally distributed. For example, in one study scores ranged from 34 to 134, with an average score of 80 and a standard deviation of 19, with no sex differences (Brownfield, 1956). Inasmuch as activity level has these measurement features, it is plausible to conceive of activity level as a trait; however, evidence for this is sporadic and inconsistent. The strongest evidence that activity over at least the first month of life predicts later activity is that from a study by Lancione et al. (1980). They found stability over the first month of life, using the activity measures of the Kansas version of the NBAS. In fact, of all the characteristics measured, activity was the one that showed the greatest evidence of stability over the first month of life. However, even this stability was modest despite being based on 106 infants assessed five times during the first month (three times in the first three days). Korner, Thoman, and Glick (1974) found very modest correlations of noncrying activity from one feeding interval to another (in the mid .30s range), which certainly does not suggest strong stability even in such short intervals. McGrade (1968), assessing spontaneous activity on two consecutive days from motion picture records, found no relation between newborn spontaneous activity level and performance at 8 months on the Bayley tests of infant development.

It is possible that measures of activity that include activity in response to stimulation might be stabler or better predictors. In the McGrade (1968) study, activity in response to external stimuli—the forehead being rubbed with a soft cloth, having a nipple without food held in the mouth, or having it removed from the mouth—were compared with baseline activity. Neonates who had responded with high activity to nipple withdrawal (a stressor) were significantly more active, happier, and less tense at 8 months of age (measures based on the Infant Behavior Profile of the Bayley test). McGrade concludes that it was the reaction to neonatal stress that was related to reactions to stress at 8 months. Her conclusion is consistent with Lancione et al.'s (1980) finding that defensive movements (high activity plus a focus) in response to a cloth over the face were as stable over the period from birth to 1 month as was activity itself.

Goldsmith and Gottesman (1981), using a different research strategy, also found evidence that activity level is a trait, if spontaneous and reactive activity were both included. They first demonstrated that a broad set of behaviors from the Bayley examination at 8 months clustered into an activity factor. The cluster included speed of response, active manipulation, re-

sponse duration, pursuit persistence, and activity level. Thus the cluster involved both spontaneous activity and activity in response to stimulation. They next demonstrated a genetic component to this activity factor by showing that identical twins were more similar than fraternal twins. Although this demonstrated a genetic contribution to activity level, this genetic factor accounted for less than 35% of the variance in the activity factor scores. Hence there are other important influences.

Stability in activity level from birth to age 2 was found, but the degree of stability was too low to give strong support to the idea of activity level as a stable genetic or constitutional trait Thomas et al. (1963). Let me hasten to add, however, that it is premature to conclude that activity level is *not* an important predictor of later development.

Conclusion

Activity shows strong individual differences from prenatal life throughout infancy, differences about which parents, caretakers, and scientists can agree. There is less agreement about whether activity is a stable trait. Data from twin studies indicate some genetic or biological basis for individual differences in activity, but the lack of evidence for long-term stability of individual differences makes the status of activity as a biological trait somewhat questionable. Whether or not postnatal activity is a stable trait, prenatal activity is related to general later developmental outcomes.

ATTENTION

Attention is another topic of importance in the study of infants. In the discussion of state that follows, each system of descriptions has one or two categories in which attention is most likely (or that describes an attentive state). Attentiveness is an important topic for our knowledge of infancy; it is while infants are awake and attentive that they can best perceive and process their world.

Attention, or attentiveness, has been relatively ignored in the study of infancy. In disguised form it is frequently found in the description of the numbers of infants who had to be excluded from a study because their states were inappropriate (that is, they were sleeping or crying or inflexibly focused) or because they failed to attend to the stimuli although they apparently were awake. Eliminating babies for these reasons can be a serious source of bias, because those eliminated may differ in important ways from those who completed the study.

Visual attention is a moderately stable characteristic of the infant from one week to another and is somewhat stable from 4 to 7 months, if it is measured across a number of situations (Colombo et al., 1988). Wider-ranging measures of attention at 1 year of age are related to similar measures at 2 and 3½ years of age (Ruff et al., 1990).

Attention Getting Versus Attention Holding

Attention is the focus of many studies of infants' responses to particular stimuli. Cohen (1972) distinguished between what he called attention getting and attention holding. *Attention getting* refers to how readily the infant will turn toward (orient to) a stimulus. *Attention holding* refers to how long the infant looks at a stimulus (Cohen was studying vision). Auditory stimuli can elicit attending even in sleeping or drowsy infants. Cohen originally hypothesized that attention getting is a reflexive response, but subsequent work (Cohen et al., 1975; DeLoache et al., 1978) has indicated that attention getting is a more active process in which orienting is partially a function of prior experience, at least in 16-week-old infants.

Attention holding is often used as a dependent variable in studies of infant perception and cognition. For example, if infants look longer at one of two geometric shapes presented side by side, we can conclude that the infants can perceive the difference between the two (see Chapter 7 for more examples). It is also used as a measure of individual differences in attentiveness, which have been related to such variables as prematurity, perinatal events (including obstetric medication and Apgar scores), and maternal caretaking behaviors. For example, term infants who are less attentive are likely to have more neurological problems than those who are more attentive (Sigman et al., 1973). Full-term infants who are more attentive to visual and auditory stimuli during neonatal testing are likely to have mothers who are later more attentive and sensitive to them (Osofsky, 1976; Osofsky & Danzger, 1974; Sigman & Beckwith, 1980), presumably because more attentive babies elicit more positive caretaking responses from their mothers.

Attention in Term Versus Preterm Babies

Visual attentiveness in preterm infants is quite different from that in full-term infants. To begin with, preterm infants tested at 40 weeks postconceptional age (i.e., when they should have been born) show much longer fixation times (attention spans) than full-term babies do at birth (Kopp et al., 1975; Sigman & Beckwith, 1980; Sigman et al., 1973). Furthermore, the relations between attentiveness and maternal caregiving behaviors are in general opposite to those found for full-term infants. Although these findings are complicated by sex differences (Sigman & Beckwith, 1980), it is generally fair to say that more attentive preterm babies receive less caregiving from their mothers. Since in their study high attentiveness in preterm babies was negatively related to later Bayley scores in girls, Sigman and Beckwith (1980) conclude that in preterm infants high attentiveness reflects an inability to turn off stimulation rather than a state in which the ability to process information is maximal.

Attention as a Predictor of Later Development

Researchers are beginning to attend more to attention, especially to its possible predictive value. Babies who are alert and process information efficiently as newborns may become children who are more intelligent and better thinkers.

Attention of preterm infants, measured by a composite of fixation measured by a visual checkerboard at term age, was negatively related to intelligence at age 5 (Cohen & Parmelee, 1983; Sigman, 1983) and at age 8 (Sigman et al., 1986) in one sample. Attention (measured somewhat differently) at 4 months of age was positively correlated with intelligence at 8 years for the English-speaking subsample of the same group of infants.

Attention at 4 months of age as measured by habituation rate or frequency (see Chapter 9) was related to Bayley test results and to the size of the babies' vocabularies at 12 months of age for a small sample ($N = 20$) of middle-class healthy babies (Ruddy & Bornstein, 1982). Sustained attention in 8-month-old male preterm infants is related to cognitive competence at 2 years of age as measured by both the Gesell and Bayley tests (Kopp & Vaughn, 1982).

Richards (1985, 1987, 1989) has pointed out that sustained visual attention at 14, 20, and 26 weeks is related to heart rate and to heart rate variability (as indexed by respiratory sinus arrhythmias). He posits that stability of attention responses over age may be mediated by the stability of the physiological systems and their relation to attention at the different ages.

As the reader may have noted, all of the above studies concern infants under 1 year of age. One of the few studies conducted with older infants found that the proportion of time spent in focused attention, during a play situation, doubled between ages 1 and 2 (Ruff & Lawson, 1990). It was found that 1-year-olds spent longer times in episodes of focused attention if only one toy was present rather than several. Because deficits in attentional behavior are found in learning disorders and other problems in the school years, this is an important area of research.

STATE

Clearly sleep and activity, which have already been discussed, are aspects of state; perhaps attention is also. These topics have been considered separately here because much research has done so and because it may be easier to look at states in general after having some concrete information.

Classification of State

Close observation of newborns reveals a number of gradations of sleep and waking beyond those already discussed that can be accurately identified by researchers or parents. These states reflect both the babies' needs and their availability for contact with the external environment. This last aspect is very important to many types of research, as well as to parents. For example, when an infant is brought in to the mother for a feeding, its state appears to be the main factor in whether or not the mother greets the baby (Levy, 1958). Of 19 mothers studied, all greeted their babies when they were brought to them in an awake, quiet state; one-third greeted them if they were crying or whimpering; and only one-sixth greeted them if they were asleep.

All studies of infants demand that the state of the infant be taken into account (e.g., Bell, 1963; Escalona, 1962; Hutt et al., 1969; Korner, 1972). Infants are differentially responsive to various stimuli, depending on their states. Thus all perceptual and cognitive studies of infants must take account of state. Numerous researchers have been interested in the question of unusual state patterns in infants (e.g., babies who cry a lot and sleep little) that might affect mother-infant interaction.

To study state and its patterns successfully, it is

Table 6.3
Four Systems for Classifying States

Brown	Wolff	Korner	Prechtl
(S₃) Deep sleep	(1) Regular sleep; comparable to Brown's S3, but low muscle tone is a descriptor and eye movements visible under lids is not	(1) Regular sleep	(I) Eyes closed; regular respiration
(S₂) Regular sleep	(2) Periodic sleep; respiration periodic, with bursts of rapid shallow and deep slow breathing		(II) Eyes closed
(S₁) Disturbed sleep	(3) Irregular sleep; some irregularities in respiration; better muscle tone than in state 1; frequent grimaces and occasional REMs	(2) Irregular sleep	
(A₁) Drowsy	(4) Drowsiness	(3) Drowsiness	(III) Eyes open; no gross movement
(A₂) Alert activity	(5) Waking activity; frequent spurts of diffuse motor activity; no auditory or visual pursuit	(4) Waking activity (diffuse), eyes open, not alert	(IV) Eyes open; gross movements; no crying
(A₃) Alert and focused	(6) Alert inactivity; eyes open, alert; has conjugate focus	(5) Alert inactivity	(V) Crying; eyes open or closed
(A₄) Inflexibly focused	(7) Crying; does not include sucking or inflexibility	(6) Crying; vigorous diffuse movements	
		(7) Indeterminate	

SOURCE: Systems are from Brown (1964), Prechtl (1965), Korner (1972), and Wolff (1966).

necessary to describe them in such a way that two observers working independently can judge the same infant to be in the same state. A variety of schemes for
classifying states have been proposed, and all of them
can be used reliably by researchers. I will describe
Brown's scheme here in greater detail; this scheme and
those of three other researchers are presented in Table
6.3 to illustrate the differences among the classifications used.

Brown (1964) used three stages of sleep and four of
wakefulness to describe the states that encompass the
range of observed behaviors. A brief description of her
seven states follows:

- S₃ (deep sleep): motionless, eyes closed, regular respiration (breathing), no vocalizations, unresponsive
  to external stimulation
- S₂ (regular sleep): hardly any movements except for
  periodic discharges (a topic we will return to); skin
  may be mottled or pale, breathing may be raspy or
  wheezing, and respirations may be regular or pass
  from regular to irregular
- S₁ (disturbed sleep): variable amounts of movement,
  eyelids closed but may flutter, breathing regular or
  irregular, squawks, sobs, and sighs
- A₁ (drowsy): eyes open or semiopen and glassy, little movement (startles or free movements may
  occur), breathing regular, skin mottled or pale,
  more regular vocalizations than in S1 and with transitional sounds
- A₂ (alert activity): the state commonly seen by the
  parent as awake—eyes open and bright, many free
  movements, possible fretting, skin reddening and irregular respirations as tension mounts
- A₃ (alert and focused): comparable to attention in
  an older child but quite uncommon in the newborn;
  eyes open and bright (The little motor activity that
  occurs is integrated around a specific activity. In
  Brown's study, this state occurs in listening or auditory focus and in looking or visual focus; see Figure
  6.3.)
- A₄ (inflexibly focused): awake, but nonreactive to
  external stimuli; found in concentrated sucking and
  wild crying; in sucking, all motor reactivity is integrated around it, eyes are closed or glassy; in crying,
  a lot of free activity (thrashing), eyes are often
  squeezed shut and the skin reddens as the baby
  screams

Recently Thoman (1990) has presented a classification consisting of 10 primary states: alert, nonalert
waking, fuss, cry, drowse, daze, sleep-wake transition,
active sleep, active-quiet transition, and quiet sleep.
She derives 6 states from these and demonstrates their
reliable measurement and stability over a week's time

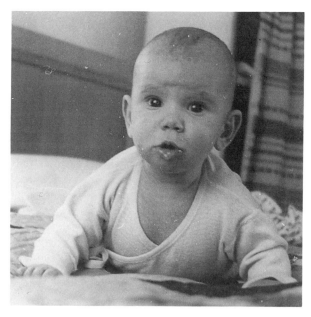

Figure 6.3. A 3-month-old infant in a quiet, alert
state, showing fixed visual regard. (Photograph by
Judy F. Rosenblith.)

for the given infant. The consistency of state patterning over successive time periods is used to characterize
infants, and those who are not stable over time appear
to be at higher risk than those who are stable. Thoman
also compares her system with those of Prechtl and
Wolff and discusses the implications they have for investigation of the functions of state.

The various states reflect different kinds of organization in the central nervous system. Crying might appear to be the least organized state to the lay observer,
but in fact irregular sleep is. Regular sleep demands
the strongest organization (or homeostatic control).
Infants with CNS damage seem unable to achieve it
(Hutt et al., 1969).

States and the Baby's Day

Using the classification schemes in Table 6.3, a large
number of researchers have mapped out how babies
spend their time. As already noted, they have found
that newborns spend most of their time asleep (about
17 hours a day, three-fourths of it in regular sleep).
Newborns are awake and quiet for 2 to 3 hours, awake
and active for 1 to 2 hours, and cry or fuss the remainder of the time. These figures do not tell the whole
story, however; individual differences among babies
are quite striking. For example, in an intensive observational study of six full-term babies, one infant at-

tained an alert receptive state only 4% of the time, but two infants spent 30% or more of the time in this state; one baby slept 56% of the time and cried only 17% of the time, but the baby with only 4% alert receptive periods slept 37% of the time and cried 39% (Brown, 1964). Brown found that some babies seemed to have better capacities than others to lower their own arousal (e.g., from crying to alert inactivity), a point featured in Brazelton's neonatal examination. These differences did not appear to be related to delivery factors, and they tended to be consistent from the first three to the second three days of life (i.e., over the hospital stay at that time). Environment also affects babies' states. For example, both temperature and relative humidity affect the length of time spent in regular sleep, a fact that was taken advantage of by Skinner's Air Crib.[2] In addition to the individual differences noted here, significant sex differences in the amount of time spent in the amounts of active and quiet sleep have been found in the first two days of life (Freudigman & Thoman, 1991) using the Thoman and Glazier (1987) Motility Monitoring System.

The tremendous variations among babies in the ways they spend their days can be expected to have profound effects upon parents. The amount and pattern of babies' sleep influences the amount of rest their parents get. The amount of time the baby spends crying determines how much of their parents' time is spent trying to soothe their bawling newborn. Parents who are unable to soothe their babies are likely to feel incompetent. Pleasant social interactions are most likely in alert, focused states, hence babies who spend much time in such states will be more engaging to parents than babies who rarely achieve them. The baby who sleeps for long, regular periods during the night, cries little, and spends a lot of time in an alert, focused state is a very easy baby. One who sleeps irregularly, and not at night, cries a lot, is not easily soothed, and spends little time in an alert, focused state is likely to have tired, irritable parents who feel incompetent and who get little pleasure or reward from their newborn.

Luckily, parents and other adults are not helpless and can often help infants to change states. The actions found to lower arousal are, in descending order of effectiveness, picking the baby up, auditory stimulation, restraint of limbs, and position changes. Two of these (auditory stimulation and position changes) may also serve to arouse the infants, but they are far less arousing than undressing. Individual differences are important. Different babies respond differently to soothing techniques, and the differences between babies have been found to be stable from one testing to another (Korner & Thoman, 1972). Thus parents

need to find the techniques that work best for their own babies. A pacifier at will (nonnutritive sucking) affects states, as most parents discover. It increases the amount of time spent in quiescent states and decreases the frequency of state transitions and overall motor activity in both term and preterm babies (Woodson et al., 1985). Other ways parents can soothe crying babies are discussed below, in the section on crying. States have also been shown to be related to such environmental variables as light (Grauer, 1989) and the constituents of formula (Yogman & Zeisel, 1983).

It is clear that the individual differences discussed above mean something to parents, but do they mean anything for the subsequent development of the infant? Individual differences in the stability of state profiles over repeated observations have been shown to be related to outcomes for low-risk term infants (Thoman et al., 1981). The stability index has been related to outcome for high-risk and low-risk prematures in NICUs (Tynan, 1986). In the latter study it was also related to neonatal behavioral deficits, as well as to underlying physiological dysfunction.

Other individual differences in states have been studied in relation to various outcomes. Moss and Robson (1970) hypothesized that infants who spent more time in an awake, alert, nonirritable state would be likely to have more advanced visual behaviors. The states of 42 infants (21 of each sex) were assessed during home observations at 1 and 3 months of age and from maternal reports. As expected, the babies were awake more and drowsy or crying less at 3 months than at 1 month. The amount of fussing stayed about the same (with boys fussing more than girls). The only relations between state and visual behaviors were for boys. Those who spent more time in an awake state at 1 month fixated on social stimuli longer at 3 months ($r = .59$, $p < .01$), and boys whose mothers viewed them as fussy or demanding spent less time looking at geometric designs. Boys who enjoyed or were quieted by visual stimuli (according to their mothers) tended to look more at both geometric and social stimuli. There were no significant relations between any of these variables for girls. In short, at least for some outcomes, it is important to analyze the relation between states and outcomes separately for the two sexes.

Research that measured state when neonates were undisturbed related it to performance on the Kansas adaptation of the Brazelton (NBAS-K) at 2 weeks of age (Colombo et al., 1989). Neonates grouped, on

2. See Skinner (1945) for a popularized description of this temperature- and humidity-controlled crib.

the basis of their state distributions, into sleep, alert-crying, and unstable groups differed at 2 weeks (but not neonatally). The sleep group scored higher on the NBAS-K cluster assessing regulation of state control, and the alert-crying group scored higher on a cluster of orientation items.

States and Responsiveness

The states of newborns clearly affect the kind and degree of responsiveness they will show. This is true of even the most basic spinal reflexes—those that are not transmitted to the brain and that involve only one **synapse** (nerve junction). Different groups of reflexes can be obtained in different states. Very simple one-synapse reflexes, such as the knee jerk and Moro, occur strongly during regular sleep and wakefulness (Prechtl's States I and III; see Table 6.2), but are absent or weak in irregular sleep (Prechtl's State II). Reflexes that involve many synapses, such as the grasp reflex, can be elicited in their strongest form only during wakefulness. Reflex responses to stimuli that cause pain or damage, such as a pin scratch, can be obtained in all states (Hutt et al., 1969; Lenard et al., 1968). These noxious stimuli are the only ones to which infants are responsive in all states, and even then they may not be equally responsive.

Responses that are less clearly reflexive and that have adaptive significance are produced in a wide vari-

ety of states by only a few stimuli. Visual evoked potentials (EEG responses to light stimuli) of term newborns are influenced by state (DeGuire et al., 1983), as are those of preterm neonates (Whyte et al., 1987). Fetal responses to sound near due date also depend on state, but this is partly because higher amounts of activity can mask a response (Schmidt et al., 1985). Prestimulus state is related to the intensity of response to sound and touch stimuli but not to cold applied to the thigh (Lamper & Eisdorfer, 1971). It appears that cold is such an intense stimulus that it overrides the effects of state. Responses to cotton (or cellophane) covering both nostrils do not appear to be influenced by state when tested in the context of an examination in which efforts are made to keep the baby's state optimal. They are attenuated, but not eliminated, in quiet sleep when no efforts are made to control their state (Rosenblith & Anderson-Huntington, 1975). Thus evidence from three different kinds of threatening stimuli (pain, cold, and those threatening the air supply) suggest that responses that are of special adaptive value may be obtained in wider ranges of state than responses to less threatening stimuli.

Brown (1964) examined infants' responsivity to nonreflex stimulation and found that infants are least responsive in deep sleep (S_3) and in the inflexibly focused state (A_4), are relatively unresponsive in regular sleep and alert inactivity (S_2 and A_2), are somewhat responsive in disturbed sleep and in the drowsy state (S_1

Figure 6.4. The relations among responsivity to stimulation, wakefulness, and arousal. The states represented by the letters A (awake) and S (sleeping) are found to be related to responsivity to external stimulation (Brown, 1964). The Roman numerals represent the corresponding states according to Prechtl's scheme, which ranges from I (low arousal) to V (high arousal). (Scheme developed by Judy F. Rosenblith.)

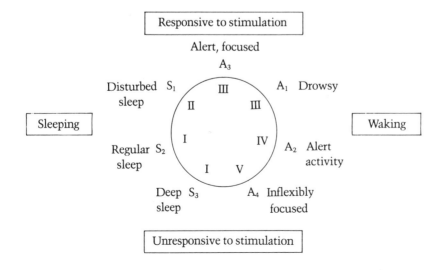

and A_1), and are most responsive in the alert focused state (A_3).

One conceptual and methodological issue raised by these findings is the necessity of clearly distinguishing responsivity to stimulation from arousal. Most of the schemes in Table 6.3 represent a continuum from low arousal (deep sleep) to high arousal (crying). But babies are not least responsive to external stimulation in State I and most responsive in State V. If there were such a continuum, we should expect reflexes to be more or less strongly elicited as an infant goes from sleeping to waking states or vice versa, and that, as we have seen, is not the case (Lenard et al., 1968).

Brown's characterization of responsivity to external stimuli also does not fit a model of a single continuum of arousal. Figure 6.4 shows her state categories arrayed around the outside of the circle with the Prechtl states on the inside. States on the left side of the circle are sleep states, while those on the right side are waking states. The state in which babies are most responsive, alert focused (A_3 or III), is at the top of the circle, and those in which they are least responsive, deep sleep and inflexibly focused (S_3 or I and A_4 or V), are at the bottom. The states of intermediate responsivity are appropriately arranged in between, so that the upper half of the circle represents relatively responsive states and the lower half relatively unresponsive states. Notice that the unresponsive states include all arousal levels. Responsivity does not correspond to a continuum from waking to sleeping. Except for the most responsive state (A_3 or III), all levels of responsivity are found in both sleeping and waking states, and three of the four levels of availability to external stimulation include both a waking and a sleeping state. Perhaps the complexities illustrated in Figure 6.4 will make it easier to conceive of states as qualitatively different systems or organizations rather than as a simple continuum of arousal, responsivity, and wakefulness.

As complex as this description of the relation of state to responsivity is, it is oversimplified. The relation between state and responsivity differs somewhat for different sensory modalities (Brown, 1964), and babies differ somewhat from each other in respect to the states in which they are most responsive. Furthermore, visual preferences are affected by the level of arousal (McKeever & Gardner, 1991). These are complexities that are beyond the scope of this discussion.

States: A Problem in the Study of Newborns

The amount of time spent in an awake, alert state is very small for most newborns, but this state is assumed by many to be optimal or even necessary for certain types of studies. Although infants may be responsive in light or active sleep, they will be unresponsive if too deeply asleep. If they are very active, it may be impossible for the experimenter to detect a response to a stimulus in the midst of all the other activity. Babies are also unresponsive when they are in the state Brown calls inflexibly focused, that is, when they are deeply involved in crying or sucking. Different states do not simply result in response or no response. Babies may respond in two different states, but the responses may be different. Thus responses obtained in different states can lead us to markedly different views of the functional capacities of young babies. The fact that researchers' findings often are not in agreement can be a result of their failure to use the same state criteria for examining babies or for excluding them.

Physicians have typically examined newborns in ways that lead to their rapid arousal and crying. This, combined with the fact that the physician rarely has time to calm the infant, means that during most of an examination the infant is inflexibly focused. When researchers began to devise tests that measured infants' abilities to respond to stimuli, they typically tried to use less aversive techniques or techniques that enabled them to observe the babies' responses when in different states (Brazelton, 1973; Graham et al., 1956; Korner et al., 1987; Rosenblith, 1961a, 1961b).

The problems of state definition and states present during testing arise in research contexts such as general level of functioning in the newborn as determined by a "test" (see Chapter 8), learning abilities (see Chapter 9), or perceptual abilities (see Chapter 7). The problem is compounded when the same infant is examined on several occasions. Particularly for newborns, the question of whether their responses are reproducible at different times of the day or on different days may be influenced more by fluctuations in state than by changes in the babies' behavioral capacities or qualities. To assess true developmental change in infants (or stable individual characteristics), we need first to make sure that results are not inadvertently produced by changes in state. (For an interesting discussion of the role of state in neonatal research, see Colombo & Horowitz, 1987.)

Before describing some solutions to the state problem, I wish to point out that state is an issue in the measurement of all dependent variables. Not only are reflexes and behavioral responses to sensory stimuli dependent on state, but so are more physiological responses, such as heart and respiration rates, EEGs, and the **galvanic skin response** (**GSR**, a measure of changes in the skin's conductivity to electrical stimulation that usually indicates emotional reactions or arousal). Thus the approaches described below must be applied to all types of measures.

One approach to solving the problem of state is for the researcher to wait for the infant to be in the desired state for the study, which may be very time-consuming. Another technique is to try to manipulate the state. An example of state manipulation is to produce a sleeplike state by swaddling babies and keeping them in an environment that is monotonous (e.g., constant temperature and light). Inasmuch as there are differences between "normal" quiet sleep and that induced by sound (Wolff, 1966), it would be important to see a study comparing the sleep induced by swaddling with normal sleep. Another way to manipulate state is by soothing and rousing manipulations designed to keep the baby in an appropriate state for the desired observation.

If researchers do not wish to manipulate state and do not have time to wait for optimal states, they can simply assess or measure state in addition to measuring the behaviors of central interest. Then they can relate the infants' behaviors to the state at the time of response. This can be done at the observational level by using any of the schemes shown in Table 6.3, or it can be done by using physiological measures of state. In general, physiological measures may appear simple and objective, but in practice they do not necessarily enable a simpler solution. EEG is often used in this connection, either to assess state in order to time the presentation of stimuli or to judge state at the time the stimulus was presented. In the former usage, it probably does not represent much improvement over behavioral observations. In the second usage it may. A second approach to the problem is to consider only those results obtained in the most appropriate states.

All of this leaves researchers with a lot of complexities to deal with. The technique used to control for state may influence the research outcomes (dependent variables). Furthermore, when researchers control by assessing state through observational or physiological techniques, they will find different results depending

on which observational scheme or which physiological index is used.[3] It is also the case that different dependent variables may be differently affected by the way the state problem is addressed.

States in Preterm Babies

States and state organization are very different in preterm compared with full-term babies. Indeed, prior to sometime between 34 and 38 weeks postconceptional age, preterms do not show clearly identifiable states (see Dittrichova & Paul, 1983; also see the review by Parmelee & Garbanati, 1986). Starting at 34 to 36 weeks, ultrasound scans can identify states (Fagioli & Salzarulo, 1987; Nijhuis et al., 1982; van Vliet et al., 1985b). This indicates the importance of maturation of physiological systems, including the CNS, for state organization. Using both ultrasound and heart rate, a group of Dutch researchers has found organized behavioral states (Prechtl's States I-IV) only at 38 to 40 weeks (Nijhuis et al., 1982). They appear somewhat later in the fetus of a first than of a later pregnancy (van Vliet et al., 1985a) and in growth-retarded than normal fetuses (van Vliet et al., 1985b).

Aylward (1981) has provided a very useful series of state observations showing state both before being disturbed and after various arousing manipulations (in the course of a modified Prechtl neurological assessment). In Aylward's study unstimulated infants of 29 to 30 weeks conceptional age were all in Prechtl's State II. As they approached normal term age they were increasingly in other states, especially State III. The youngest infants moved into State III after moderate amounts of manipulation, and 30% of the older ones showed moderate amounts of State IV. Stimulation, such as that provided by a pin prick, did not rouse the youngest to more than State III. Crying, which occurred 75% of the time in 40-week-olds, was present only 33-40% of the time at 34 to 38 weeks, and did not appear prior to 31 weeks. Prematures respond to gravitational changes (such as occur in raising to a sit, suspending in a prone position, or spinning) at younger ages and with greater arousal than they respond to other types of stimulation. Aylward's prematures, like those studied in a different manner by Prechtl et al. (1979), were all healthy, so his data, though based on only 58 babies, provide a basis for judging the typicality, or normality, of the state change responses of prematures from 31 to 38 weeks conceptional age.

The largest and most systematic study of state in prematures rated it 22 times in each weekly standardized neurobehavioral maturity assessment (Korner et

---

3. Individual physiological measures have their own special problems. For example, a range of heart rates cannot be used as an index of state across a group of infants being studied, because a given heart rate (e.g., 90-100) may be associated with different states in different infants—say, with awake and active in one, drowsiness in another, and quiet sleep in still another. Thus if you are reading studies of perception and you see initial heart rate being used to control for state, as is common, you should remember that the control is not fully adequate unless the relation of heart rate to state is determined separately for each infant.

al., 1987). Korner et al. (1988) did this for 175 preterm infants from 32 to 40 weeks postconceptional age (or discharge). The percentages of all ratings in which the babies were asleep, awake, and crying were stable from one day to the next, but not the percentage of quiet sleep. Sleep decreased markedly with age, while drowsiness and alert inactivity decreased only slightly. While the general tendency to be either asleep or awake was not stable over 3 weeks, being irritable, alert, or drowsy was. There was also some consistency in the number of state changes and the number of mixed states, which did not decrease over time as the authors had expected. There were sizable sex differences in the distributions of states. Girls slept less and were awake more, which may reflect earlier maturation. By the third testing differences had decreased, but girls were still higher on alert inactivity; boys were higher on alert activity. An earlier study also found decreased sleep, greatly increased crying, and increased awake state with increased age (Michaelis et al., 1973). The agreement in the findings of the two studies is remarkable in view of the fact that the methods of examining the infants as well as the ethnic makeup of the samples differed.

Rhythmic Activities

AN OVERVIEW

Several of the behavior systems to be discussed (e.g., sucking, crying, Piaget's circular reactions) show strong rhythmic characteristics. Certain rhythmic behaviors, such as rocking and head banging, have long attracted the attention of clinicians, but rhythmic behaviors in their totality have been little studied. Rhythmic motoric behaviors (such as stepping and kicking) have been studied by Thelen (1981), who made a natural history and an ethological catalog of all rhythmic stereotyped behavior bouts from 4 weeks to 1 year. More than 16,000 bouts were recorded, and there were great individual differences. Some infants spent only 5% of their time in such behaviors and others spent 40%. Most bouts were associated either with a change in stimuli or with being in a nonalert state.

There were developmental (or age) changes both in the amount of rhythmic behaviors and in the type of stimuli that elicited them. Rhythmic movements of given body systems appear to increase just before the infant achieves voluntary control of that system. Indeed, maturational level seems to be the primary determinant of these behaviors, inasmuch as there are no differences between normal-term infants and prematures who had respiratory distress or postmatures *if* gestational age is controlled (Field et al., 1979).

The CNS mechanisms governing rhythmicity in motor behaviors are little known. Robertson (1982) has found rhythmicity, in the form of periodic spontaneous wrist movements, in the awake infant similar to that of movements and startles during sleep. Robertson's studies of motility cycles in the fetus and newborn, and their relation to state, should ultimately help us integrate our understanding of rhythmic and cyclic activities (see, e.g., Robertson, 1986, 1989). More normative data on these activities might allow us to detect abnormal patterns or amounts of these behaviors, even if we have not understood the mechanisms.

It is to be hoped that more research in these areas will enable testing of some of the deductions made by Thelen (1981), who ties these behaviors to a wide range of other observations in developmental psychology (both human and animal).

SUCKING

Getting Started

Sucking is a rhythmic activity that is actually one of a group of feeding reflexes that include the rooting reflex, the lip and sucking reflexes, and the swallowing reflex. The rhythmicity of sucking bursts is not present in very young prematures, but usually appears at 31 to 33 weeks postmenstrual age (Hack et al., 1985).

The Sucking Reflexes. The rooting reflex is the name given to a reflexive response to touch stimulation of the area around the mouth (the perioral region). It has been described by Kussmaul (1859) and detailed by Prechtl (1958), who differentiated a side-to-side head-turning reflex from a directed head-turning response. In the former the head turns first one way, usually toward the stimulus (gentle tapping or stroking of some perioral area), and then the other. The swings become progressively smaller until the mouth is sufficiently oriented toward the stimulus to bring the lips into contact and allow sucking to follow. This reflex disappears or shades into the directed head-turning response by 3 weeks of age in normal newborns. The directed head-turning response involves a single well-aimed (or purposeful) head movement that brings the infant's mouth into contact with the stimulus. It can be elicited only from areas close to the mouth, but can include up, down, or rotational movements of the head in response to stimulation of the middle of either lip, or at an angle from the corners of the mouth. While the directed reflex is usually present at birth, it is more difficult to elicit and often found together with the more predominant side-to-side reflex.

In the normal course of feeding, the rooting reflexes lead to contact with the nipple, especially in breast-feeding babies, whose rooting response is said to be better developed than that of bottle-fed babies after the first 2 or 3 weeks (Ingram, 1962). Even though rooting is unnecessary for bottle-fed babies, unless they are left with propped bottles, they often root when nipples are inserted in their mouths.

Although the strength of the rooting reflex varies from time to time, we know of no systematic studies linking these changes to changes in hunger. In general, rooting seems to be more easily obtained when infants are hungry or drowsy and when they are in the normal feeding position (Ingram, 1962). Some parents feel that the ease of eliciting and strength of the rooting response can be used to determine whether their infant's fussing is related to hunger.

Rooting reflexes have not been found to be useful for neurological diagnosis, because of their relative invulnerability to neurological deficits and the wide range of individual differences in the ease of eliciting them (Ingram, 1962). They have been found in babies with severe cortical damage, and even, temporarily, in **anencephalics** (babies who lack a cortex). This invulnerability seems sensible from an evolutionary perspective. The reflexes necessary to ingest food would be expected to be among the most built-in, or most resistant to damage.

There is a lip reflex (sometimes called the cardinal point sign) that is similar to the head movement reflexes. It can be elicited by touching or stroking. This causes the lips to move toward the stimulus when the head does not (André-Thomas & Saint-Anne Dargassies, 1952; Thompson, 1903). In the newborn the mouth opens and the tongue protrudes and at the end of the motion the tongue retracts, the lips close, and swallowing and sucking movements follow. Occasionally there is an inverted response, similar to those found in the 3- to 4-month-fetus (Minkowski, 1922, 1928; Prechtl, 1958), in which the movements are away from the stimulus.

The behavior of sucking is triggered by an object (especially a nipplelike one) touching the lips, gums, hard palate, or front of the tongue. Repetitive sucking usually follows such a touch, often after an initial swallow. If it does not, gentle movements of the object within the mouth will usually produce sucking. This is, of course, the time-honored technique by which mothers encourage their babies to nurse or to suck their bottle nipples.

Thus far, the sucking part of this whole complex has been discussed as if it were a unitary process. However, within it there are two separate processes: One, called **expression**, is the squeezing of the nipple between tongue and palate; the other is the "suction" or negative pressure generated in the mouth cavity (Ardran et al., 1958; cited in Sameroff, 1968). Normally the two components are linked—in other words, when one occurs so does the other—but they can be separated under experimental conditions. There are stable individual differences in both the suction pressure and expression amplitudes, as well as in the number of responses (Sameroff, 1968).

Sucking and Feeding. Sucking, or the whole complex of feeding behaviors, is often described as a reflex or innate response, but many mothers know that these reflexes do not always work well. There are great individual differences in the efficiency with which normal-term newborns take to sucking or feeding. For efficient feeding, not only must all of these reflexes be present and coordinated, they must also be coordinated with another reflex in the complex of feeding reflexes—the swallowing reflex. This reflex is less studied than the others, probably because it is less visible and less likely to need any special stimulation. Indeed, reflex swallowing is produced by many stimuli that have no relation to feeding. In addition, the pattern of sucking and swallowing in the newborn makes it hard to differentiate swallowing from sucking.

Sucking and swallowing must also be coordinated with breathing or respiratory activity. Although each reflex can be tested separately, the coordinated presence of all them is necessary for successful feeding. In particular, the coordination of sucking and swallowing with breathing is necessary if the baby is to avoid getting food into the lungs instead of the stomach. Lack of this coordination, more often than the absence of reflexes, leads to the necessity of premature infants being fed by gavage, that is, with a tube inserted directly into the esophagus or stomach.

Although the individual reflexes are not useful for neurological diagnosis, spontaneous feeding behavior, which involves their integration, does help identify infants with physiological and motor problems and with retardation. For example, there is evidence showing that high bilirubin levels (severe jaundice) lead to a disintegration of the sucking pattern (Kazmeier, 1973; Kazmeier et al., 1977). This relation is dramatically evident in infants who receive exchange transfusions in which all of the blood in their bodies is replaced by new blood with normal bilirubin levels. The degree to which the sucking pattern is organized is directly related to the bilirubin levels. There is a gradual decrease in the level of organization as bilirubin levels build up, followed by a dramatic increase in the organization after the exchange, followed by a gradual decrease again, for as many times as the baby receives exchanges to stabilize its bilirubin at a normal level. (It should be noted that exchange transfusion has largely been displaced by treating jaundiced babies under lights, a treatment that is effective in reducing jaundice, but the implications of which for the infant are just starting to be studied.)

Changes in Sucking Pressure During the Perinatal Period. A variety of data suggest a very early readiness to suck in both premature and term infants (Anderson et al., 1982; Gaulin-Kremer et al., 1977; Koepke & Barnes, 1982). Sucking pressures do not increase gradually, but, in fact, decline by 6 to 8 hours of age. Note that this is before many hospitals provide feeding or nonnutritive sucking (the latter occurs in breast-fed babies). The maximal sucking pressures in the first hours of life may act to improve the establishment of the maternal milk supply (remember that long-range effects of "bonding" practices were found primarily in nursing variables). This illustrates that maternal-infant interaction in the immediate postbirth period results partly from infant behaviors, not just maternal behaviors.

Sucking and Experience. It has already been shown that sucking reflexes change rapidly, even before sucking experience can modify them. But early sucking responses are modified by experience. Sameroff (1968) systematically studied the influence of learning on the two components of the sucking response. He used the technique of operant conditioning, by which newborns were rewarded (given milk) if they sucked (one condition) or if they expressed (another condition). He found that the sucking component was governed largely by the reward—when sucking got them milk, they sucked more; when it did not get them milk, they sucked less. Expression movements were less responsive to reward. The expression pressure increased when that was necessary to get milk, but did not decrease when it was not rewarded. Thus sucking is in part governed by basic biological mechanisms and is in part a response to environmental events.

Because sucking develops so rapidly in the first 3 weeks of life, partly in response to the environment, the lack of opportunity to suck may be disadvantageous to infants. This reasoning has led several investigators to question common hospital practices for prematures. Although prematures at all stages of de-

velopment show some sucking behaviors, many nevertheless are fed by tubes down the esophagus in order to make certain that the liquid reaches their stomachs and is not breathed into the lungs, where it can cause pneumonia. Thus the infant does not have to coordinate sucking with swallowing and breathing movements and is denied the opportunity to establish sucking patterns during the immediate postpartum period.

In three studies reported in a symposium at the 1980 International Conference on Infant Studies, prematures were given sucking experience in the hospital. When allowed to keep pacifiers in their mouths, many prematures sucked for as much as an hour at a time. A variety of indices showed these prematures to be physiologically and neurologically in better condition and better organized than those who were not given pacifiers (Anderson, Burroughs, et al., 1980). Secondborn twins, who are usually more at risk, given nonnutritive sucking together with their tube feeding were ready to suck for food three days earlier, had fewer complications in general, and were discharged for home many days earlier than the firstborn who received routine procedures (Anderson, Fleming, & Vidyasagar, 1980).

A third set of studies compared a randomly assigned (stratified) experimental group of 16 prematures with 17 control prematures (Ignatoff, 1980; Ignatoff & Field, 1982). All weighed less than 1,800 g and were less than 35 weeks gestational age, with no genetic or physical abnormalities. Both groups received pacifiers, according to the normal practice of the unit, but the pacifiers were linked with food intake only for the experimentals. The experimentals were given the largest pacifiers they could tolerate with each tube feeding, a procedure that is possible because the tubes used to feed prematures are usually put down the nostril, not the mouth. The experimentals had better weight gain and were ready to be sent home earlier, thus leading to a shorter separation from their parents and lower hospital costs. The evidence with respect to long-term differences is not available, so we do not yet know whether there are any subsequent advantages or harmful side effects.

Overall, the evidence seems to indicate that both nonnutritive sucking in general and nonnutritive sucking that is linked to the delivery of food are good for prematures. In addition, it has been shown that both crying and stress responses of minimal-care NICU infants to heel sticks are reduced by giving a pacifier. Crying is reduced in the younger prematures, but not the stress responses (Field & Goldson, 1984).

The Socialization of Sucking

As mentioned above, individual reflexes in feeding behaviors can be elicited without actually feeding the infant. Even if sucking is not elicited, both newborns and older infants will suck things that do not lead to their obtaining nourishment or food. This is commonly described as **nonnutritive sucking** (**NNS**). Babies do nonnutritive sucking prior to birth, as has often been illustrated by photos showing a fetus in utero sucking its thumb. Some newborns even have damaged fingers or thumbs that appear to result from excessive sucking prior to birth. But massive numbers of ultrasound pictures of fetuses in utero show us that such sucking is not common, although raising the hand toward the mouth is. Again, NNS is another behavior that shows strong individual differences in utero and well beyond babyhood.

Nonnutritive Sucking: Good or Bad? NNS has aroused a great deal of interest throughout history, both in relation to practical questions of the managing of infants and with respect to theoretical questions. The infant management questions center on whether to allow thumb or finger sucking or to give pacifiers. Nutritive sucking is central only to the management problem of when to wean the infant (except for some newborns who need to be taught to suck). Attitudes toward NNS vary widely in different cultures and in our own culture at different points in history. So, too, have the attitudes toward the proper age at which to wean babies from nutritive sucking. Sucking, be it of fingers, fists, pacifiers, blankets, toys, or whatever, has been perceived as a tool by which the infant can achieve self-quieting, as a form of self-gratification or indulgence, and as a nasty habit that should not be allowed to develop or, if developed, that should be gotten rid of as soon as possible. When experts in the United States considered NNS to be a nasty habit, they advised the following steps (in this order) to prevent its continuation: (a) Paint the baby's hands with iodine or other unpleasant tasting substances; (b) fasten cuffs over the baby's arms so that he or she cannot get

hands to mouth; and (c) tie the sleeves of the baby's clothes to the sides of the crib.[4]

It is tempting to think that the view of nonnutritive sucking as bad reflects a puritan heritage that considers any pleasure as necessarily sinful. Superimposed on this view was the Watsonian behaviorist view that the more pleasure (reward) infants receive from undesirable behaviors, the harder it will be to "break" them of these "bad" habits. Thus parents should prevent the habit of NNS from getting started. Subsequently, Freudian theories began to have an impact on some parents and on the advice given them in women's magazines, government booklets, and newspapers. To oversimplify, Freud saw sucking as a normal need that could be dealt with satisfactorily only by gratifying it. That is, he considered sucking to be a psychological need, analogous to the physical need for food, which must be satisfied if growth is to proceed normally. If properly gratified, this need would be outgrown in a healthy way. If the need were gratified too little or too much, the baby would not outgrow the need and would develop emotional problems, such as oral addictions (liquor, pills, cigarettes, excessive talking).

The Clash of Theories About the Role of Sucking. The contrast between Freud's view and the "learned bad habit" view led to theoretical debates on the role of NNS. One debate was over the question of whether sucking was innately pleasurable or became so only after being associated with feeding (that is, as a result of learning). Indeed, a whole chapter of a book on the history of selected problems in psychology (McKee & Honzik, 1963) is devoted to the sucking of mammals as an illustration of the nature/nurture issue and that scientists as far back as Darwin had suggested that both learning (habit) and an "inherited or instinctive tendency" might be necessary for sucking. The authors comment on the preoccupation with the single behavior of sucking, especially thumb sucking or pleasure sucking, that characterized the period from the early 1920s to the early 1960s, when they wrote. They discuss the controversy between psychoanalytic and behavioristic views in greater detail than I can here, but I would like to illustrate the issue by describing several classic studies on both sides.

The first is a study by David Levy, an important child psychiatrist (1892-1977). Having interviewed mothers and found that thumb suckers had had less opportunity to suck in nursing, a finding that would be expected from Freudian theory, Levy (1928) designed a study to test the Freudian hypothesis. A litter of six puppies was separated into three pairs at 10 days of age. One pair continued to nurse from the mother,

---

4. Much of the advice to parents given earlier in this century treated both sucking and masturbation as nasty habits. The techniques described to cope with sucking were similar to those prescribed to prevent infants from "handling themselves." Boy babies who moved their thighs to produce genital stimulation were to have their legs tied to the bars of the crib. Babies who both sucked their fingers and masturbated might have both hands and legs tied to the bars of their cribs if parents followed the government's booklet of advice on infant care.

one pair was bottle-fed from very slowly flowing nipples, and the third was fed by tube for 3 days, when they were shifted to very fast-flowing nipples because they were losing weight. When all the pups were later tested for sucking on a nipple-covered finger (i.e., for NNS), the pair that had had least chance to suck (fed on rapidly flowing nipples) sucked most, appeared more restless, and required more formula to achieve normal weight gain. This study was replicated in 1957. These research efforts provide support for the Freudian idea that infants (here, puppies) need a certain amount of sucking or gratification from sucking, and that those denied it during nutritive sucking will do more nonnutritive sucking. Such research contributed to the change in strict limits on sucking time allowed during feeding.

The second study stemmed from learning theory, although at least one of its authors (Sears) was trained both in learning theory and in psychoanalytic theory. In this study by Davis et al. (1948), a group of infants were fed by cup from birth. Because they did not get nutritional sucking from which they could develop a learned drive to suck, learning theory would predict that they should show less NNS than the control groups fed normally. According to Freudian theory, the cup-fed infants should show more NNS because they had not experienced adequate oral (sucking) gratification. The sample included 20 cup-fed, 20 bottle-fed, and 20 breast-fed newborns. All the infants were observed in nonnutritive sucking test behaviors (as in Levy's study) for 10 days. The breast- and cup-fed groups behaved as learning theory would predict. Breast-fed infants showed larger amounts of nonnutritive sucking, and cup-fed infants showed low amounts. The bottle-fed group, predicted to be intermediate, were, on the contrary, like the cup-fed infants. The authors' post hoc explanation was that the nipples were so easy that bottle-feeding was like cup-feeding in the amount of oral gratification received. Indeed, bottle-fed babies, like cup-fed babies, consumed their food in half the time taken by breast-fed babies. If this explanation is true, then both cup- and bottle-fed babies fulfilled the learning expectations that they would engage in less NNS than the hard-sucking breast-fed babies. A replication study designed to test this interpretation both confirmed the earlier results and made the explanation more plausible (Brodbeck, 1950).

These two sets of studies support opposing theoretical positions, and other studies have yielded inconsistent results. The Freudian oral drive view that adequate sucking during feeding leads to little nonnutritive sucking has been supported by Fleischl (1957)

and Ross (1951). The learned-habit view has been supported by Blau and Blau (1955), Brodbeck (1950), and Sears and Wise (1950). A more recent study looked at the amount of NNS in 1- to 13-month-old infants who had never experienced nutritive sucking (due to continuous feeding for medical conditions) (Lepecq et al., 1985). They were compared with normally fed age-matched controls using behavioral and polygraphic observation for a 24-hour period. There were no differences between groups in the amount of NNS overall or during different sleep or waking states. These data suggest that nutritive reinforcement does not play a role in maintaining NNS activity.

Let us look at a well-designed study of infant monkeys to see what light it can shed on this controversy. In this study by Benjamin (1961), infants with no experience sucking for food (cup-fed) were compared with those who sucked for food from a bottle with the smallest nipple holes from which they would feed. During the first three months of life the two groups differed in oral activities. However, the direction of the effects on NNS were opposite to those for nonsucking oral activities. Bottle-fed infants did more NNS than cup-fed ones, thus supporting learning theory prediction that the sucking habit would be strengthened by reinforced sucking experience. However, NNS showed various changes over the course of the study that cannot be interpreted easily in terms of either theory. NNS increased in both groups over the first 70 days. It started to wane for the bottle-fed at that point, and somewhat later for the cup-fed group. The differences between the groups in NNS waxed and waned during the first three months, but became very small after 90 days. These data could be seen as supporting the Freudian view that once the need is adequately met, the behavior will wane, and this will be later for the cup-fed infants. Oral behaviors other than NNS were lower for bottle-fed than for cup-fed infants, which supports Freudian theory. Again the differences between the groups decreased after 90 days.

The fact that all infants engaged in nonnutritive oral behaviors during the first three months and then decreased in both sucking and other forms of oral activity suggests the existence of an underlying oral responsiveness (orality or oral drive) that waxes and wanes during infancy. This idea is in semiagreement with Freud's views. The finding that NNS was the preferred form for the bottle-fed group and that other nonnutritive oral behaviors were the preferred form for cup-fed infants suggests that the form that oral behaviors take depends on the kind of experience the baby has had. This finding is in semiagreement with a learning theory view. Benjamin's study also leads to the conclusion that Freud was wrong in his claim that early sucking experience has long-lasting effects. Even monkeys who experienced no nutritive sucking were no different in oral behaviors from those with adequate nutritive sucking experience after 90 days of age.[5]

Benjamin's study might resolve the discrepancies of the previous studies, given its good controls, the varied outcome measures assessed (NNS, weight gain, time taken in feeding, and degree of postfeeding disturbance—crouching and rocking), and its long time span (longitudinal over six months, equivalent to a much longer time in humans). However, it is limited by the facts that monkeys are not humans and that these monkeys were being raised on artificial mothers. (Artificial mothers enabled easier control of sucking experiences, but may limit the generalizability of the results, even for monkeys.)

All the human studies discussed thus far have focused on NNS during infancy, but the crucial Freudian hypothesis is that infant sucking experiences have permanent effects on personality. Unfortunately, adequate tests of long-term outcomes are rare. Most Freudian studies are **retrospective**; persons with behavior problems presumed to indicate high orality (e.g., pencil chewing or addiction to alcohol) are asked to recall their early experiences, an extremely problematic procedure, because everyone's memory of long past events is faulty.

I know of only one long-term prospective study of the development of oral behaviors in humans. Skard (1966) followed the development of children and their parents from the prenatal months to the children's ninth year using interviews with the parents and observations and tests of the children. She determined feeding practices, finger sucking, hand-mouth reactions, and other oral activity during free play when they were babies and during school class sessions and in sandbox play when they were older. Her sample was too small for statistical analyses to be helpful; therefore, I will describe the data for her strongest findings in terms of the individual children.

During infancy almost all babies sucked their fingers, hence there was no relation between feeding

practices and finger sucking. The onset of finger sucking was related to the age of weaning in a way that suggests that finger sucking was a compensation for the loss of nutritive sucking, which is consistent with Freudian theory and the conclusions that can be drawn from Benjamin's study of monkeys. Babies who were allowed to regulate their own food intake and sucking time were not likely to finger suck early (only 1 in 7 did). In contrast, babies whose food intake or sucking time, or both, were regulated by their mothers were likely to finger suck early (7 of 9 did). This agrees with an earlier finding based on a larger sample (Yarrow, 1954), and both are consistent with others discussed in this section: Babies who are allowed to suck enough to meet their needs have less need to suck their fingers.

The long-term outcomes in Skard's study generally support and extend Benjamin's conclusion that early sucking experiences (in monkeys) have no long-term

Figure 6.5. In some cultures, nursing is a casual affair. (Photograph courtesy of N. Konner/Anthro-Photo File.)

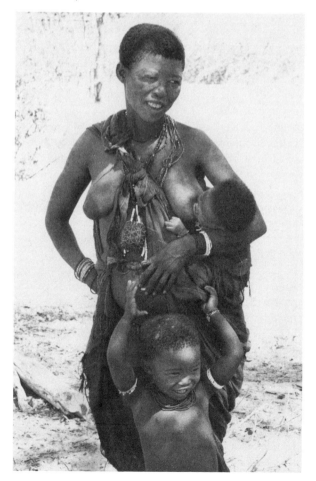

---

5. Benjamin also indicates that her data suggest that masturbation and thumb sucking enhance each other; that is, both are forms of sexual gratification, a Freudian notion. The only masturbators in the group studied were four males who were thumb suckers and who had rocking mothers. Equally this might suggest that rocking mothers may enhance both thumb sucking and masturbation. In other words, the pleasures of rhythmic activity, learned from a rocking mother, may produce a secondary drive for rhythmic activity in at least some monkey infants.

consequences. Amount of orality or mother's attitude toward need gratification in the first year, weaning age, and self-demand food intake, measures of oral activity, were not related to oral behaviors at 3½ years. The relations between early sucking experience and oral behaviors at 6, 7, 8, and 9 years were only slightly more impressive. The only apparent relation between an infant variable and later oral activity was between the duration of breast-feeding and oral activity at 7 years. This relation was curvilinear, but in the direction opposite to what would be predicted by Freud. Those with a short duration of breast-feeding (less than 1 month) or a long duration by current Western standards (more than 7 months) had less oral activity at 7 years than those breast-fed for from 2½ to 5 months. All 8 of the latter had high oral activity, compared with only 2 of the 7 from the extreme groups. The finding of long-term negative consequences for children in the middle range is compatible with Childers and Hamil's (1932) finding that children weaned between 1 and 5 months of age are overrepresented in behavior problem groups. However, Sewell and Mussen (1952) found no outcome differences for such children at ages 5 and 6. If children weaned between 1 and 5 months are at risk for later problems— and the data are by no means conclusive—this would support Freud's general claim that feeding practices in infancy have long-term consequences but disconfirm his hypothesis that moderate levels of oral gratification are optimal. A reasonable explanation of the findings results if we posit that the infants' sucking needs (or their needs for comfort provided by breast-feeding, that is, longer and more frequent intimate interaction) are highest during the 1- to 5-month period, so that denial of needs in that period has more impact than denial when the needs are less strong. In many cultures, nursing is much more prolonged (see Figure 6.5).

Skard's study provides additional evidence that Freud may have been correct in his hypothesis of long-term effects of early experience but wrong about those of oral gratification. Parents' attitudes and behaviors toward crying in the first year were related to oral behaviors at 3½ years. Of the 6 children usually picked up when they cried, only 1 showed much finger sucking at 3½ years, while 7 of the 10 usually left to cry showed a lot. It could be argued that both this finding and the relation between the length of breast-feeding and oral behaviors at 7 years show the long-term negative effects of lack of comfort during infancy. Skard notes that failure to provide comfort (for crying, at least) is likely to be a general parental characteristic that lasts beyond a child's infancy, and that the 7-year finding may be a cumulative effect, rather than the result of treatment in infancy.

To make matters more complicated, Skard's data provide indications of still other possible influences on orality. Children who came from very warm, accepting homes showed more orality, a result found also by McFarlane et al. (1954). Somewhat in contrast is Skard's finding that only 1 of 10 children from homes with low conflict between parents showed high orality, whereas 4 of the 5 children from homes with high conflict showed high orality.

Taken in their entirety, Skard's data show that the factors that determine later orality are complex. Freud may be correct that experiences in infancy affect later orality, but, if so, they are not the experiences he proposed. Some Freudians might still object because the outcome measures used in these studies are not the pathological adult behaviors with which Freud was concerned.

Skard's findings that parental warmth and responsivity and low conflict in the home are related to later behaviors are consistent with much research in the last 20 years. These variables have been found to be relatively more important in explaining development in several domains than are sucking and feeding experiences during infancy (see Chapters 12 and 13).

Because earlier research did not find profound effects of early sucking experiences on orality and because later work (to be discussed in Chapter 12) showed that nursing variables were not important determinants in the development of infants' attachment to their mothers, few researchers today are exploring the role of sucking in personality development. Instead, there is increased emphasis on using sucking as a tool to explore other aspects of the infant's behavior (see, e.g., Chapter 7). The role of NNS in the development of prematures is an active area of research, and sucking is used to indicate something about the medical status of newborns. The recording of sucking behavior has become automated and computerized so that objective records of the behavior are now relatively easy to obtain.

Practical Issues. As for the practical problems of nonnutritive sucking (of thumbs, fingers, pacifiers), the research suggests that it is unlikely that a parent's personal decision will have long-term consequences for the child's later personality. The issues to consider, then, are more immediate and practical. As noted by many, most babies suck their fingers at some time during infancy (Simsarian, 1947; Skard, 1966) and that seems to be because babies do have a basic need to suck.

Both nutritive and nonnutritive sucking will usually produce quieting (Fisher & Ames, 1989), a connection that is innate (Kessen et al., 1967). NNS for 5 minutes prior to feeding of prematures in NICUs alters their state in ways that are more optimal for feeding, thus saving time for the nurses (Gill et al., 1988). (For an interesting view of the calming effects of sucking in the first days of life, see Smith et al., 1990.) Allowing an upset baby to suck (fingers, blankets, or pacifiers) can be a boon to baby and parent alike.

Sucking shows a normal progression of waxing and waning, so parents do not condemn their children to a difficult habit by allowing sucking. Many parents worry about the difficulty of later "breaking the habit" if they allow their babies to suck. It is true that about 40% of children continue to suck their fingers even after they start school (Kessen et al., 1970). It is not clear what current figures, when a more tolerant attitude toward NNS has prevailed, would be. A strong late sucking need is at least as likely to be from constitutional individual differences as it is to be due to parental behaviors. One small study found great individual differences in the length of time and degree to which five babies breast-fed on demand sucked their fingers (Simsarian, 1947). It is not likely that differences in sucking experience produced these individual differences. If parental behaviors are important in preventing school-age finger suckers, it is not known what those behaviors are, unless perhaps they include parental warmth and responsiveness to crying, as identified by Skard.

Affective Behaviors

The three prominent emotionally expressive behaviors—smiling, laughing, and crying—have received a great deal of attention from infant researchers. The more general issues of whether infants exhibit other emotional expressions that can be recognized by adults and whether infants can recognize adults' emotional expressions have received only sporadic study until recently. This section first reviews research on the communicative nature of facial and vocal expressions in infancy,[6] and then describes the particular research on crying, smiling, and laughing that focuses on the development of these responses and the environmental stimuli that elicit them.

---

6. Another recent review pertinent to this topic can be found in Tronick (1989).

Most studies in this field have, like Darwin's, focused on facial expressions. A few have focused on vocal expressions of emotion.

Communication by Facial Expressions

Darwin (1872) made observational studies of the expression of emotion in animals and humans, including the facial grimaces associated with crying in children, and he included observations of these expressions in his infant diary (see Chapter 1). Recently, a spate of studies have appeared that demonstrate that it is possible for adults to identify facial expressions of babies accurately in the first year of life (Hiatt et al., 1979; Izard et al., 1980, 1983; Sternberg et al., 1983). The stimuli used to produce the expressions judged are those adults deem likely to lead to the emotions whose labels are used. The infants' expressions are judged as resembling those of adults we would judge to be expressing that emotion, and the labels given are those given to adult expressions. Experienced health professionals, college students, and trained and untrained judges have all reliably judged what they called facial expressions of interest, joy, surprise, anger, disgust, sadness, and fear. Training primarily improves observers' identification of negative emotions (although not positive ones) and improves the performance of those that were least accurate initially. Raters are as accurate using videotapes and slides as in actual observations. Facial expressions of sadness, anger, and physical distress of 15-month-old infants not only can be differentiated by mothers of young infants, but also they trigger different caregiving and socializing interventions (Huebner & Izard, 1988).

Facial expressions are related to physiological measures. Fox and Davidson (1988) have found that facial signs of emotion in 10-month-old infants are related to differences in EEG activation of left and right hemispheres, hence they propose that EEG may be useful in differentiating among emotional states associated with differences in facial and vocal expressivity. Facial expressions of interest and joy, as well as looking-away behaviors in the presence of an interacting stranger, have been related to heart rate variability in 5- but not in 10-month-old infants (Stifter et al., 1989).

It must be noted that a given stimulus produces different emotional responses as infants become older. For example, Izard and colleagues (1983) found that distress reactions to "shots" declined from 2 to 18 months, whereas anger responses increased dramatically after 6 months of age.

If adults can discriminate the affective expressions of infants, can infants make such discriminations about the expressions of adults or peers? Newborns' responses to various facial expressions made by a single model have been explored (Field et al., 1982). The adult model would first elicit the newborns' attention and then make a happy, sad, or surprised face. Newborns did discriminate among the various expressions. This was detected by an experimental technique known as the habituation-dishabituation paradigm (see Chapters 7 and 9). A similar study included a condition that exposed infants to a similar expression, such as happy, in four different faces and then determined whether the infants detected the difference between a new expression, such as surprise, and the first expression (Caron et al., 1982). The researchers found that 18- or 24-week-olds were unable to differentiate between happy and surprised expressions, but 30-week-olds could. A second task determined whether the infants could discriminate between two faces with the same expression. Babies from 18 weeks on were able to do this, with girls doing better than boys. It is reasonable that this simpler task develops earlier.

The studies by Caron and colleagues, taken together with those of Nelson and colleagues (Ludemann & Nelson, 1988; Nelson, 1985; Nelson & Dolgin, 1985) indicate that between 4 and 7 months infants become able to classify some pictured emotional expressions. This is true even when the examples vary on several dimensions, including the intensity of the expression. (This work is well reviewed by Nelson, 1987.) However, subsequent work by Caron et al. (1985) has cast doubt on this interpretation, and makes it appear that 7-month-olds may have detected such invariant features as toothiness or wide-eyedness, not specific emotions. The ecological validity of static pictures as stimuli for judging infants' abilities to judge emotion is raised by these authors. A recent study used videotapes with happy, angry, and neutral expressions, silent or with sound tracks that either matched or did not, to study 7-month-olds. In the silent condition they looked longest at the happy expression, then the angry, and least at the neutral. With sound they looked longer if it matched, even when happy was not included (a first-ever finding). Dynamic visual input is thus enough to enable infants to distinguish affective expressions (Soken et al., 1991).

None of the above-cited studies addressed the question of what such expressions mean to infants. Behavioral responses that might indicate something about the meaning have been little studied. There are observational data in naturalistic settings that shed some light on this question for older infants. In one study,

10- to 29-month-olds (most under 2 years) responded with distress to high-intensity anger expressed by a parent to someone other than themselves in 69% of episodes that involved hitting—usually of a sibling—and in 41% of episodes of anger without hitting (Cummings et al., 1981). Exposure to such angry behaviors did not lead to angry responses on the part of the infants. However, the more fights between parents that infants had been exposed to, the more likely they were to respond emotionally, with affectional/prosocial behaviors or with anger or distress. Positive emotional expressions of affection of parents toward someone other than the infant elicited affectional/prosocial behaviors from the infant in 61% of instances, but jealous affection and anger were also relatively frequent responses. In specially staged incidents of expression of affect, negative responses were much less frequent, suggesting that the infants could discriminate between these dramas and the real thing.

Another approach to looking for meaning in infants' responses to pictures that convey emotion to adults comes from so-called metaphorical studies. Information is presented in another sense modality (auditory) that is supposed to share an abstract dimension with the pictured emotion—for example, a rising tone with joy. One then determines whether the infant shows differential looking to the visual stimulus that supposedly matches the auditory one. Phillips et al. (1990) found that 7-month-olds who did not categorize distinct facial expressions of joy or anger when they also varied on some other salient feature did respond differentially in the presence of the auditory pattern. They looked longer at joy and surprise faces when in the presence of ascending, pulsing tones, and longer at sad ones in the presence of descending, continuous tones.

Termine and Izard (1988) found that 9-month-old infants exposed to their mothers expressing joy or sadness, both facially and vocally, watched them longer, played more, and expressed more joy than when the mother expressed joy only facially. They showed more sadness, anger, and gaze aversion in the sadness condition.

After this glimpse at infants' discrimination of and response to affective visual displays (sometimes accompanied by sound), we turn to the adult's and child's ability to judge emotional state from vocal expressions.

Communication by Vocal Expressions

Nearly all research addressing responses to infant vocal productions as signals of emotional state has been on crying. Work on sounds indicating pleasure, contentment, or joy is extremely rare. M. Papoušek (1989) provides a notable exception. She studied responses to tapes of single voiced sounds of 2-month-olds made in states of varying degrees of discomfort and comfort, cry, and joy. Judges were persons with different levels of experience with infants (mothers and fathers of young infants, multiparous and primiparous mothers of newborns, speech therapists, and 8-year-old children). These extremely brief (all less than 2 sec), isolated sounds communicated about emotional state to all groups studied, but not equally. All identified cry sounds, but only parents of young infants were good at decoding sounds of joy. Children judged joy sounds higher on discomfort than any discomfort sounds other than cries, presumably as a response to such negative aspects as shrillness in the joy sounds.

The milder comfort and discomfort sounds were correctly categorized (as on the comfort or discomfort side) 72% and 83% of the time, respectively. Accuracy was higher for those with more experience or who were older, but was not affected by parental status or gender. Having a same-age infant (currently or previously) or having professional experience with children and sounds improved performance equally. It is to be hoped that more work will be done in this field. The Infant State Barometer used by Papoušek (1989) would seem a valuable tool for further studies in these areas.

We now turn to the most studied infant expression of affect, one that has always had powerful effects on parents: crying.

CRYING

The most important mechanism newborns have for communicating with their world is crying. This is true from the first cry, which tells the mother and doctor that the baby's lungs have filled with air. Cries may also tell a doctor or scientist something about the state of the baby's central nervous system. Cry patterns are intimately related to respiration, hence are also thought to be partially controlled by the **autonomic nervous system** (the nervous system that governs actions that are relatively automatic). Hence cries may tell us something about its function, and knowledge of it may tell us something about cries.

Characteristics of Cries

People have long tried to describe cries in some systematic way. In the early 1800s different types of cries were described in terms of musical notations (Gardiner, 1838). By 1906 it was possible to use recording

discs to study the **acoustical** (or sound) properties of cries. Even then, researchers noticed that the pitch of the cries of an infant with breathing problems was about an octave higher than that of normal infants. With the development of the sound spectrograph, which allows visual presentation of acoustic characteristics of sounds, it became possible to analyze cries in more detail.

The cry of the newborn is described by Lind (1965) as "a vivid manifestation." It is a complex motor act in response to some stimulus, starting with that provided by the birth experience, and a vocalization containing acoustic information. Taken in its entirety, including actions of pharynx, soft palate, tongue, larynx, and even the trunk as it participates in respirations, the performance pattern of the cry may be the infant's most distinctive motor activity. Indeed, just as infants are footprinted for identification, the concept of a "cryprint" was introduced in 1960 (Truby, 1959, 1960; cited in Lind, 1965). Thus it is not surprising that mothers sometimes correctly identify the cries of their own unseen baby.

Researchers differ in the number of types of cry they describe: four types (birth, hunger, pain, and pleasure) by Wasz-Hockert et al. (1968) or three types (basic, anger, and pain) by Wolff (1969). The basic cry is a rhythmic pattern that typically consists of the basic cry, followed by a briefer silence, then a shorter inspiratory whistle that is of somewhat higher pitch than the cry proper, and another brief rest period before the next cry. Wolff believes the hunger cry is really an instance of the basic cry and not specifically caused by hunger, but most researchers still talk about a hunger cry. The anger cry, so called because most mothers infer exasperation or rage from it, is a variation of the basic cry, differing in that excess air is forced through the vocal cords. The pain cry, which is elicited by high-intensity stimuli, differs from the others in that there is a sudden onset of loud crying without preliminary moaning and a long initial cry followed by an extended period of breath holding. Even this cry gradually subsides into the basic cry. The actual sound characteristics used to identify cries and the ways they are measured are well described by Lester and Zeskind (1982).

Wolff (1969) found that crying before feeding differs from that after feeding based on his observations of three infants for 16 to 18 hours a day. Before feeding, crying was rhythmic, had a braying quality, and was accompanied by kicking that seemed governed by the same rhythm. Crying after meals tended to be less rhythmic, more shrill, and not synchronized with kicking. Wolff found few individual differences in the amount of time spent crying before meals, but after meals one infant cried only 4 minutes, one 89 minutes, and the third 361 minutes.

The infant has a remarkable capacity to produce varied sounds. The pitches in a single infant's hunger cries may span a range of from two octaves below middle C (a note sustained by bassos) to three octaves above middle C (higher than the top notes of a coloratura; Fairbanks, 1942). Pitch is largely determined by tension in the vocal folds as determined by the laryngeal muscles. Pitch varies in relation to both the infant's neurological status and the cause of crying. The pitches that make up hunger cries differ from those of attention-getting cries (Lynip, 1951). Distress cries are louder, less varied, and longer lasting than hunger cries and tend to be more irregular. The cries of medically at-risk infants tend to be higher in pitch and shorter in duration than those of normals. Cries in response to the most invasive aspects of circumcision are at the high pitches and short durations characteristic of damaged infants (Porter et al., 1988).

Both diary studies (Brazelton, 1962) and actual tapes of infant vocalizations (Rebelsky & Black, 1972) have been used to follow the developmental course of crying. Both show that crying increases over the first 6 weeks of life, then decreases; that the timing of maximum crying is in the evening in the first weeks of life, then shifts toward feeding times; and that there are marked differences among babies. Recently St. James-Roberts (1989) has confirmed a crying peak in late afternoon and evening, as well as an increase in daily crying that peaks at 6 to 8 weeks. There are differences, of course, in the same baby from day to day or week to week. I trust that readers will remember this when they are faced with crying newborns.

Diagnostic Value of Cries

What about the neurological or medical information to be found in the cry? Can an infant's cry help a doctor diagnose a neurological abnormality? Infants diagnosed at birth as normal but noted by nurses or others to have unusual cries are often later found to have CNS abnormalities, even to the extent of lacking a cerebral cortex. Differences in pitch, duration, or patterns of cries could be examined to determine the role they play in producing these different-sounding cries.

Prechtl et al. (1969) note that there are marked and stable individual differences in the duration of the cry over the first 8 days of life (.4 to .9 sec). They found the duration of spontaneous crying to rise over the first 3 days, stay high until day 5, and then decline until day 8, but not to decline for infants with neurological problems. The duration of such babies' cries in

response to pinching is also markedly longer than that of normals, with practically no overlap between the two groups. Furthermore, cries in the neonatal period have been shown to be related to mental and motor development at 4, 8, 12, 18, and 24 months of age (Huntington et al., 1990), and at 5 years (Lester et al., 1989).

A different approach to diagnostic usefulness of cries is related to the autonomic nervous system. Parasympathetic or **vagal tone** (an inhibitory mechanism that helps control tension of the laryngeal muscles) is related to pitch of cry. Low vagal tone leads to high pitch. High-pitched cries are characteristic of infants with CNS damage, but they also occur in normal babies who are acutely stressed, such as by the most invasive aspects of circumcision (Porter et al., 1986). Prestress or resting vagal tone predicts the level of response to circumcision. Infants with high vagal tone respond more dramatically to the surgery, hence might be considered in need of analgesia, anesthesia, or soothing of some type (Porter et al., 1988). Those with low resting vagal tone might be considered suspect for neurological problems and hence deserving of special examination.

Computers have recently been added to the array of devices used to study cry patterns. Golub and Corwin (1982, 1985) extracted 88 characteristics of the cries produced by heel sticking (used to get routine blood samples) and used them to provide a "cry model." From the model, the researchers selected 8 abnormal cry patterns based on differing characteristics. They then compared the cry patterns of 55 normal, term infants with those of 17 infants with multiple or severe abnormalities and those of 12 infants who had moderately elevated bilirubin levels (moderately to severely jaundiced). Tapes (not necessarily neonatal) of 3 other infants who later died of **sudden infant death syndrome (SIDS)** were also analyzed. Of the 55 normal, term infants, only 10 had any of the 8 abnormal patterns and none had more than 1. In contrast, all of the 17 abnormal infants had at least 1 abnormal pattern, and 14 of them had 2 or more.

The cry model also predicted specific patterns for specific problems. Infants with respiratory distress were predicted to have the pattern called *abnormal respiratory efforts*. Of the 12 infants with respiratory distress, 10 had this pattern, compared with 4 of the 77 infants without respiratory distress. Of the 12 jaundiced babies, 11 had the pattern called *glottal instability*, but no other abnormal pattern. Muscle tonus and states, which affect this pattern, are both affected by jaundice, hence patterns for all jaundiced babies, including those in the group with multiple abnormalities, were examined. Glottal instability was found in 22 out of 24, but only in 8 out of 63 without jaundice. The 3 infants who died of SIDS all had cry patterns associated with constriction of the vocal tract. Further support for this association is found in Lester et al. (1989).

This computerized analysis was modified by Lester (1987) and used to look at a number of risk factors and outcomes. Both alcohol consumption (more than five drinks per week) and marijuana smoking were related to cry characteristics. For both term and premature infants, cry characteristics were related to Bayley scores at 18 months and to the General Cognitive Index of the McCarthy Scales at 5 years (Lester, 1987; Lester et al., 1989).

Effects of Cries on Adults

Much of the evidence on adult reactions to crying is anecdotal or derived by inference from naturalistic observations of mothers and infants. Let us examine the research evidence relevant to both theoretical and practical questions:

(1) Do adults (especially parents) react differently to cries than to other expressions of affect, and do they react differently to different types of cries?

Frodi and colleagues investigated parents' physiological responses to smiles and cries and obtained their answers to a mood adjective checklist (Frodi, 1985; Frodi, Lamb, Leavitt, & Donovan, 1978; Frodi, Lamb, Leavitt, Wilberta, et al., 1978). The 48 couples who watched 6-minute videotapes of a baby who either cried or smiled in the middle 2 minutes had different physiological responses (diastolic blood pressure and skin conductance) and indicated different moods in response to the crying and smiling tapes. Parents also respond more to audiotapes of cries compared with tapes of pure tones (Wiesenfeld et al., 1981). In one study, 16 mothers and fathers also listened to audiotapes of anger and pain cries. Physiological indices of stress (skin conductance and EKG) differed for the two types of cry, as did parents' ratings of their tension while listening and the pleasantness and unusualness of the tapes. Dependent measures did not all show the same relationships, and some of the differences depended on the type of cry (see Question 4).

Berry (1975) showed that children as young as 7 years of age could distinguish cry types. Thus it seems that babies' cries do serve the purpose of communicating to others, even to young others.

(2) Do parents distinguish the different cries of their own baby better than those of a strange baby?

The answer to this question also appears to be positive. Wiesenfeld et al. (1981) showed that both parents were good at identifying cries taped from their own baby, but when tapes were of cries from another baby they were less accurate. In the Frodi studies both parents found the pain cries of their own child to be the most unpleasant and most tension provoking.

(3) Do parents distinguish cries better or respond to them differently than do people who are not parents?

Zeskind and colleagues (1984; Zeskind & Lester, 1978) have shown that both inexperienced and experienced adults can distinguish different cry sounds. The latter study showed that even for very brief segments of cry tapes, pain cries were more aversive and arousing and seemed more urgent than hunger cries. Zeskind (1980) had parents and nonparents choose from a list of six caretaking behaviors (feed, cuddle, pick up, clean, give pacifier, wait and see) which one they would use in response to the cry they had just heard. They later were asked to rate each of the caretaking behaviors as to "how tender and caring the response is" and "how immediately effective it would be in terminating the crying." Parents and nonparents did not differ in responses to low-risk infants, but parents were more responsive to the cries of infants at greater risk. There is reason to believe that the amount of experience with infants is a more meaningful distinction than parental status (Boukydis & Burgess, 1982; Lounsbury & Bates, 1982). However, in the study by Gustafson and Harris described below, parity did not affect the results.

Actual, not predicted, behavior is the real concern. Gustafson and Harris (1990) tried to approach its study by determining caregiving behaviors to an extremely lifelike mannequin programmed to cry in different ways. It weighed 6.5 lb and it had a soft spot on its head, flexible joints, and a head that fell back if not supported; it could drink and wet. Participants were asked to "baby-sit" this "1-month-old infant" in an equipped nursery and were told it needed a nap. After 5 minutes in its crib, the "baby" cried. The tapes were of cries of either hunger or distress (taped during circumcision).

The behaviors of mothers and nonmothers were extremely similar. All picked up the mannequin, and more than 90% talked to it and attempted to feed it, and 62% checked its diaper. The crying was terminated if it was a hunger cry and the sitter fed it, or if it was a distress cry and she pulled the diaper pin out of its skin. Both mothers and nonmothers took more than three times as long to solve the pain cry as the hunger cry. At least four nonspecific comforting behaviors (such as picking up, talking to, holding to shoulder, providing tactile and vestibular stimulation) were performed by 87% of the sitters before feeding or diapering. Both mothers and nonmothers tried to feed the baby sooner in response to the pain cry. Mothers held the baby to their shoulder more and provided more vestibular stimulation, both effective techniques (see the section below on how to soothe). More nonmothers attempted to demonstrate a toy in response to the pain cry, a technique that is unlikely to be effective.

Both mothers and nonmothers were equally good at judging intensity, and both were less good at scoring a specific cause for the cries in other tapes played without a doll.

(4) Do fathers or other men respond differently than mothers or other women?

This question is derived from the hypothesis that women are biologically preprogrammed by evolution to respond to the cries of babies in ways that men are not (see, for example, Klaus et al., 1975; Money & Tucker, 1975). The answer to this question is not clear-cut. In the Frodi studies already described, mothers and fathers did not differ in their physiological responses (Frodi, Lamb, Leavitt, & Donovan, 1978; Frodi, Lamb, Leavitt, Wilberta, et al., 1978). However, mothers had somewhat more extreme mood ratings. Nevertheless, the same pattern of effects in relation to the nature of the stimulus held for both mothers and fathers. In the pain study by Craig and colleagues (1988), mothers rated babies after heel stick as experiencing it as less intense than did fathers. A study using college students did not show any sex differences in the responses (Freudenberg et al., 1978).

Zeskind (1980) does not report separate analyses for the sexes, but differences seem unlikely in view of the strength of the results. Zeskind and colleagues (1984) found very minimal sex differences, and Boukydis and Burgess (1982) found no sex differences in skin potential responses to different types of cries, but fathers were more likely than mothers to judge that cries indicated the infant was spoiled and to react with irritation rather than caregiving.

The one study that showed quite a few differences between mothers and fathers had the greatest number of complexities in its design (Wiesenfeld et al., 1981).

Cries were of anger or pain, of the parents' own or another baby, and there were pure tones. The dependent measures were of both physiological responses (skin conductance and EKG) and self-ratings. Each parent listened to six tape segments (two of which were pure tones) and judged whether the cry segments were of his or her own or of another baby and whether it was a pain or an anger cry.

There were a number of differences between mothers and fathers. Fathers and mothers were alike in showing heart rate responses that indicated orienting (or that the stimulus was heard and attended to) to the cries of other infants. Both parents found pain cries more unpleasant and tension evoking than anger cries. The next most unpleasant and tension provoking for mothers were their own infants' anger cries, but for fathers they were the pain cries of the other baby. Fathers had orienting responses to the cries of both their own and the other infant, but mothers responded with defensive-type heart rate changes to their own babies' cries of anger or pain. The mothers' GSRs were strongest to their own babies' pain cries.

Mothers were better than fathers (and correct from 63% to 81% of the time) at identifying cries as not coming from their own babies, as being anger cries, and as being anger cries of their own babies. Pain cries were less well recognized by either parent, but better recognized for own baby than for another, especially by mothers (50% compared to 38% for fathers) versus 25% and 31% for another baby, with the fathers having the edge.

Thus mothers were somewhat better than fathers on several of the measures. Although the differences were small, these findings could be taken as support for the view that women, but not men, are biologically preprogrammed to respond to stimuli that are relevant to infant survival. However, the fact that pain cries were less well recognized than anger cries, by either parent, would seem directly counter to an evolutionary hypothesis, inasmuch as response to pain is important in guaranteeing the survival of babies.

In sum, there is little consistent evidence to support the hypothesis that females, but not males, are innately programmed or predisposed to respond nurturantly to infant signals. Whatever differences exist could be easily interpreted as a result of greater encouragement for women to give expression to emotions, greater experience of women with babies, or more socialization to caretake, and hence to heed signals for the need to caretake. The findings provide little support for the ethological view.

(5) Do the cries of abnormal infants affect adults dif-

ferently than those of normal babies?

The fifth question may have some relevance to evolutionary thinking, but quite opposite reasonings are possible. One could argue that the species should be preprogrammed to respond more to the cries of abnormal or at-risk infants. However, over most of history societies have not had enough resources to allow spending them on abnormal or difficult infants. Indeed, many cultures have had practices to ensure against such waste of resources: abandoning sickly infants (and even adults), abandoning one member of any twin pair, or testing the strength of infants so that only the strong survived to be raised. Hence, no matter what the research findings are, they will not be conclusive with respect to evolutionary theory.

Answers to Question 5 are complicated by the great variety of stimuli used to study the question. Stimuli compared include the following: pain cries of high-risk and low-risk term infants (Zeskind, 1980); cries of Down syndrome babies and those of normals (Freudenberg et al., 1978); cries of prematures and those of term infants (Frodi, Lamb, Leavitt, & Donovan, 1978; Frodi, Lamb, Leavitt, Wilberta, et al., 1978); labels of normal, difficult, or premature applied to the cries of normal babies (Frodi, Lamb, Leavitt, & Donovan, 1978; Frodi, Lamb, Leavitt, Wilberta, et al., 1978); ratings of cries of difficult, average, or easy babies (Boukydis & Burgess, 1982; Lounsbury & Bates, 1982); responses of adults to pain cries of normal, Down syndrome, asphyxiated, and cri du chat infants (Frodi & Senchak, 1990). In some studies the cries were considered to be hunger cries, while in others they were pain induced. In only a few of these studies were the actual acoustic properties of the cries analyzed.

The difficulties of noncomparable stimuli are compounded by the use of different measures of the adults' responses, or the use of more than one measure, with different results for each. The most frequently used measures are (a) various physiological responses, especially heart rate and GSR; (b) statements of what the subject would do in response to the cries; and (c) ratings of mood when listening to the cries. In one study, whether the mother judging cries of "difficult" infants had a difficult infant herself was a variable (see, e.g., Bates et al., 1982), and whether respondents are nonparents, first-time parents, or multiparous parents is often varied. Small wonder that different and even opposite conclusions have been reached from these studies, and that the data are hard to integrate to provide answers to our questions.

To answer Question 5 adequately, it seems impera-tive to use acoustic analyses of pitch, intensity, and rhythmic pattern (especially the pattern of pauses) and to use cries from babies with a wide range of abnormalities. At present there is some evidence to support almost any answer to questions of whether problem babies elicit more TLC (tender, loving care) responses, or are aversive to caretakers and elicit avoidance, abuse, or both. It is clear that inexperienced adults have different heart rate responses to the pain cries of normal and at-risk babies. Cries of high-risk babies elicit greater changes (either acceleration or deceleration, depending on the person), while those of normal infants elicit smaller accelerations (Zeskind, 1987). Factor analyses of the acoustic properties of cries have identified a factor (composed of energy, duration, and number of short utterances) that is related to the later likelihood of mothers' seeking support from family and friends (Boukydis & Lester, 1990).

One study that partially supports the idea that unusually high-pitched cries of high-risk infants may trigger less optimal responses from parents and college students was conducted by Frodi and Senchak (1990). In it, subjects filling out questionnaires "overheard" cries from the infant research waiting room next door. Actually, they heard one cry tape from a collection that included two normal newborns, one Down and one cri du chat syndrome infant, and two asphyxiated infants (one with and one without brain damage). The asphyxiated infants had pitches that were two to three times as high as any of the others. The subjects were videotaped during the cry. After they finished their questionnaires, they were asked whether they had heard something; if they had, they were asked to fill out the Perceptions of Infant Cry Inventory. The asphyxiated infant without brain damage had the highest-pitched cries and elicited from its listeners the least positive affect, significantly less than to one normal, the Down, or the brain-damaged asphyxiated infant. The second-highest pitch was that of the asphyxiated infant with brain damage, and it was most often ignored. Listeners to both asphyxiated infants were more apt to perceive the cries as being due to the infant entertaining itself. These data not only seem contrary to the theory that cries of high-risk infants elicit most concern and care, but to contradict the synchrony between pitch and responsivity found by Zeskind and Marshall (1988), a finding that might hold over a less extreme range of pitches.

Little work has been done on analyzing responses to cries as a function of their intensity. However, the general ideas about crying that prevail would indicate that responses should be faster to more intense stimuli. On the contrary, DeConti and Gustafson (1990) have shown that mothers take almost twice as long to respond to their infants' cries of medium intensity as to those of low intensity.

There is one study that analyzed pitch of cries of older children in a child-care setting and showed that higher-pitched cry sounds, which are characteristic of abnormal infants, elicited more urgent and comforting responses from the caretakers (Zeskind & Collins, 1987). However, none of these cries would be at the extremely high pitches shown by the asphyxiated infants.

(6) Do child abusers respond differently to cries than nonabusers?

Various persons have speculated that child abusers may abuse those whose emotional expressions are abnormal. It has also been hypothesized that child abusers may react differently than nonabusers to the communicative signals their infants provide. However, few controlled data exist on this subject. Frodi and Lamb (1980) used the techniques already described to study responses of child abusers (recruited from Parents Anonymous) in comparison with those of a control group (recruited from a YWCA and a well baby group). Responses of the abusers to both the smile and cry stimuli were markedly different from those of the controls or from the participants in the earlier Frodi studies. The abusers (compared with controls) showed greater arousal as indexed by both cardiac and skin conduction responses, but less blood pressure increase. They reported less sympathy toward and were more annoyed by the crying baby than were control parents. But abusers also rated a smiling baby as less pleasant than did the control group and reported themselves as less attentive and less willing to interact with the smiling baby than did nonabusers. They also were more indifferent toward the smiling baby, though their blood pressure and skin conduction responses were greater than those of nonabusers. In short, their responses to the smiling baby were very like those to the crying baby.

Frodi and Lamb (1980) theorize that this response pattern, in which any social solicitation on the part of an infant (i.e., crying or smiling) is seen as aversive by abusers, had developed through the abusers' transactions with children who, "because of their temperament or their parents' incompetence, are difficult to care for" (p. 243). They point out the need for studies that would directly link behavior patterns of abusive and nonabusive mothers (or fathers) to their physiological responses.

Lamb (1978) has argued, as has Bowlby (1969),

that responses to smiling and crying should be sharply differentiated, but that both have evolutionary survival value. The data seem to support this position, but there is a very real question as to whether the aversive nature of the cry that leads to attention and care might be, or become, so aversive that it hinders care or leads to avoidance or abuse. Clearly, much more work is necessary before we can say with any certainty what features of cries adults respond to and how they respond to them. An excellent and very brief overview of much of this research can be found in M. Papoušek (1989).

How to Soothe Crying Babies

What most concerns parents about crying is how to soothe their babies. A fair amount of work has explored the relative effectiveness of various soothing responses. Study after study has found that picking up a baby is the most effective method of getting the baby to stop crying (Bell & Ainsworth, 1972; Brown, 1964; Wolff, 1969). A high, front-to-front position, such that the baby looks over the adult's shoulder, is the most effective holding position (Korner & Thoman, 1972). Bell and Ainsworth (1972) found this technique effective in stopping 85% of crying episodes in both the first and last quarters of the first year.

Other techniques that were effective more than half of the times tried were sucking (Bell & Ainsworth, 1972; Wolff, 1969), rocking (Gordon & Foss, 1966; Kopp, 1971), and auditory stimulation (Bell & Ainsworth, 1972; Brown, 1964; Kopp, 1971; Wolff, 1969). The kind of auditory stimulation that is effective depends in part on the infant's age. For newborns, nonsocial auditory stimuli seem most effective. For example, white noise soothed 1-month-old babies 56% of the time, compared with 6% for their mothers' voices (Kopp, 1971). The most effective nonsocial auditory stimuli are low-pitched continuous or rhythmic sounds (Brackbill, 1970). Continuous stimulation of other senses (light, warmth, swaddling) also has soothing effects and often leads to quiet sleep (Brackbill, 1971). It is no wonder, then, that for generations mothers have sworn by such soothing techniques as turning on music and putting babies on top of or next to vibrating, humming machinery, such as clothes washers or dryers and vacuum cleaners. Recent fads include a machine that reproduces the human heartbeat for the purpose of soothing babies and a record that reproduces the intrauterine sounds to which the baby was exposed before birth.

The most effective stimuli change rapidly, and by 3 months of age the mother's voice is more effective than white noise (Kopp, 1971). Visual stimulation, initially rather ineffective, becomes an increasingly effective soother, and by 3 to 4 months it works about half the time (Kopp, 1971; Wolff, 1969). Giving a toy to babies of this age, who do not yet reach, is actually presenting visual and sometimes auditory stimulation. It is no surprise, then, that it is an effective soother (Ainsworth, 1972). By 4 months of age the combination of visual and auditory stimulation is more effective than either is alone.

Tactile (touching) and movement and balance control (besides rocking and holding) are often effective infant soothers—sometimes by decreasing and sometimes by increasing stimulation. Swaddling or restraining the limbs of very young infants often quiets them (Wolff, 1969; Brown, 1964). Touching successfully soothes 50% of the time, according to Bell and Ainsworth (1972). Rhythmic patting is effective 15-20% of the time (Kopp, 1971), and changing the baby's position sometimes reduces arousal (Brown, 1964). In none of the studies cited is the reason for the baby's crying considered independently. Babies who are crying because they are hungry can be quieted only temporarily by these techniques. However, NNS can reduce responses to such painful stimuli as heel sticks and circumcision (see the section on pain in Chapter 7).

Virtually all of this information deals with infants in the first 3 to 4 months of life and would have to be modified considerably for older infants. Bell and Ainsworth (1972) demonstrated that in the first 3 months crying was less frequent when the mother was in close, physical contact and was most frequent when the mother was out of sight or earshot. In the last 3 months of the first year, crying of the same infants was more frequent when the mother was close physically. This supports the view that crying has become a true communication; that is, it is under the infant's control and not just a response to stimulation. However, recent data contradict those of Bell and Ainsworth. DeConti and Gustafson (1990) found that infants observed and videotaped with their mothers from just after a nap until they fell asleep again (about 2 hours per day for 2 days) initiated half of all cry bouts when in the mothers' arms, and only 18% when beyond arm's reach. These authors hypothesize that, since most cry bouts were of low or medium intensity and took place close to the mother, cry primarily serves a social communication purpose as early as 3 months. Indeed, in their data crying led only to social interaction with the caregiver in 65% of crying bouts, and social interaction was the first response in all mother-infant dyads. Earlier findings that caretakers usually engage in several social

behaviors before doing such caretaking as feeding or diapering lends additional credence to this hypothesis (Gustafson & Harris, 1990).

All this information can help caregivers to deal with infants in several ways. It provides alternative soothing techniques and a knowledge of which ones are most likely to work. A parent can run through the different techniques with a baby, realizing that none will work all the time. It also focuses attention on the fact that babies change rapidly; hence techniques that were maximally effective for newborns become minimally effective with older infants, changing even within the first 3 months of life. There is much truth in mothers' complaints that as soon as they figure out how to handle their babies, the babies change and the mothers have to figure them out all over again.

There are great individual differences in what soothes babies. For example, babies who are less active in the first quarter of life are more soothed by visual or tactile-kinesthetic techniques (Kopp, 1971). Even more important, babies differ greatly in how soothable they are by any technique, a feature that is related to the concept of the "difficult" baby mentioned earlier. Parents of babies who cry a lot or who have very unpleasant cries may wear themselves out trying to soothe their infants. Trying many different techniques may yield one that successfully quiets a particular child, but it may also be that such crying is physiologically produced and cannot be controlled by parental soothing techniques. Parents must then find their ways of coping, be it with ear plugs, loud stereo or TV, putting the baby at the far end of the house and closing all doors, drugging the baby (or themselves), or beating the baby (not recommended!). We know very little about what happens in these circumstances. One study has suggested that mothers whose babies cry frequently and for long periods of time have decreased affectionate contact with their babies at later ages, although there was no relation between the babies' crying and their mothers' affectionate contact at that same age (Dunn, 1975). This suggests that regardless of mothers' immediate responses to high levels of infant crying, they eventually lead to decreased contact.

To Soothe or Not to Soothe

The idea that prompt, efficient response to babies' crying is optimal has been implicit, if not explicit, in the discussion of adult responses to cries. Whether such prompt responsiveness is a good idea has been the center of intense theoretical debate. According to the Freudian-influenced ethological school of Ainsworth and others (Bell & Ainsworth, 1972; Ainsworth &

Bell, 1977), prompt response to crying makes infants feel secure and promotes their sense of efficacy and their attachment (see Chapter 12). Bell and Ainsworth (1972) report that the babies of mothers who responded promptly to their babies' cries in the first 3 months cried less later in their first year. These babies were also more likely to exhibit more clear and varied noncrying modes of communication later in their first year of life.

Learning theorists from Watson to the present day would counsel that if parents reinforce crying by attending to it, either positively or negatively, it will increase in frequency. Gewirtz (1977; Gewirtz & Boyd, 1977a, 1977b) critiqued Ainsworth's methodology, leading to a rejoinder from Ainsworth and Bell (1977) that admitted their thesis was unproven. Etzel and Gewirtz (1967) had previously shown that crying (as well as fussing) can be decreased through procedures in which it is ignored (not reinforced) and a competing response (smiling) is reinforced.

Several studies have supported the learning theory view. For example, Moss (1967) found that prompt response to crying (or fussing) in the first 3 weeks of life led to higher rates of fussing at 3 months; Bedouin infants, who are not allowed to fuss, being fed as soon as they begin to fuss, were found by Landau (1982) to be fussier than three other Israeli groups and to show the highest rates of fussing when their mothers attempted to elicit smiling behavior from them.

Hubbard and van IJzendoorn (1988, 1990) have attempted to meet the criticisms of the Ainsworth and Bell study by Gewirtz and to meet Ainsworth and Bell's call for an intensive naturalistic replication of their study. They found a high correlation (.81 to .90) between current maternal unresponsiveness and infant crying in each quarter, a relation not analyzed by Bell and Ainsworth. A more modest correlation was found between maternal unresponsiveness in one quarter and infant crying in the next quarter, the correlation that led to the original hypothesis that one could not spoil a baby by attending to its crying. Statistical analyses showed that mothers who ignored more crying had babies who cried less frequently in the next quarter. Hubbard and Van IJzendoorn point out that they have no alternate slogan to offer and opine that in the absence of scientifically justified advice, caretakers should rely on their intuition ("intuitive parenting"; Papoušek & Papoušek, 1987).

Another aspect of infant learning is that by 1 month infants start to soothe before they are picked up, which could represent classical conditioning or a cognitive expectation (Lamb & Malkin, 1986). If the adult inhibits the picking up after approaching the cry-

ing baby, it leads to protest by 3 or 4 months, especially to the mother. The older the infant, the less the expectation is generalized to a stranger. These findings are judged to agree with Piagetian predictions.

A resolution of the controversy is likely to require a more complex formulation. Prompt response to crying may reinforce it, but it is apt to reinforce only mild crying. In contrast, when a mother is slow to respond to her infant's cries they are likely to become stronger and more noxious. If she responds only when they have become too unpleasant for her to bear, she would be reinforcing noxious crying. That is the sort of crying Etzel and Gewirtz (1967) successfully reduced through learning procedures. More sophisticated and more naturalistic studies are needed. DeConti and Gustafson (1990) found that nearly a third of cry bouts began as protests of the mother's caretaking, another indication that we may need to rethink our conceptualization of the communicative nature of crying.

Aside from this contemporary argument, different cultures (and the same culture at different times) have had very different attitudes about appropriate responses to a crying infant. It has often been held that crying is good for the infant. Even those who are not oriented toward learning theory, such as Brazelton (1962) and Emde et al. (1976), have noted that a certain amount of crying is necessary for infants' organization. The questions then become, How much? At what ages? In what circumstances? I have no answers to these questions.

Figure 6.6. A sleep or reflexive smile. Only the mouth is smiling; the eyes are not. To see this fully, cover the lower half of the picture. (Photograph courtesy of Judith E. Sims-Knight.)

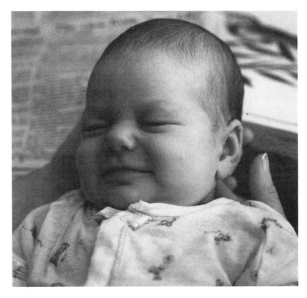

Table 6.4
The Development of Smiling and Laughter

Age	Response	Stimulation	Latency	Remarks
		SMILING		
Neonate	Corners of mouth	No external stimulation		Due to CNS fluctuations
Week 1	Corners of mouth	Low-level, modulated sound	6-8 sec	During sleep, boosting of tension
Week 2	Mouth pulled back	Low-level, modulated voices		When drowsy, satiated
Week 3	Grin, includes eyes	Moderate-level voices	4-5 sec	When alert, attentive (nodding head with voices)
Week 4	Grin, active smile	Moderate or moderately intense sounds	Reduced	Vigorous tactile stimulation effective
Weeks 5-8	Grin, active smile, cooing	Dynamic stimulation, first visual stimulation	Less than 3 sec	Nodding head, flicking lights, stimulation that must be followed
Weeks 9-12	Grin, active smile, cooing	Static visual stimulation, moderately intense	Short	Trial-by-trial effects, effortful assimilation, recognition; static at times more effective than dynamic
		LAUGHTER		
Month 4	Laughter	Multimodal, vigorous stimulation	1-2 sec	Tactile, auditory
Months 5-6	Laughter	Intense auditory stimulation and tactile	Immediate	Items that may previously have caused crying
Months 7-9	Laughter	Social, visual stimulation, primarily dynamic	Immediate	Tactile, auditory decline
Months 10-12	Laughter	Visual, social	Immediate or anticipatory	Visual incongruities, active participation

SOURCE: From "The Ontogenesis of Smiling and Laughter: A Perspective on the Organization of Development in Infancy," by A. Sroufe & E. Waters. *Psychological Review*, 1976, *83*, 173-187. Copyright 1976 by the American Psychological Association. Reprinted by permission.

SMILING

Smiling is perhaps the earliest clearly social and positive behavior. Like crying, it is a behavior that communicates affect, or is perceived to do so. All baby books give ages at which parents can expect their infants to smile. Parents who think they see their infant smiling earlier than this are usually politely told that what they saw was a grimace due to gas pains. This condescending response does not, however, jibe with what we now know of smiling. There is a form of smiling during the neonatal period, called reflex smiling to differentiate it from the later-developing "real" or "social" smiling. The characteristics of this early reflex smile have been explored by Wolff (1959, 1963, 1966) and Korner (1969), who agree on the characteristics of this smile, but found very different amounts of it in their observations, perhaps because Wolff observed babies in incubators and Korner observed them in bassinets.

Reflex smiling involves only the muscles of the lower face, but later smiling involves the eye muscles as well. Early smiling occurs when the baby is in different states than does later smiling, and often occurs without outside stimulation. Reflex smiles occur most often in irregular sleep, occasionally in a drowsy state, and never in deep sleep or in alert states (see Figure 6.6). Those of you who have cared for or observed very young babies will probably recall having seen them "smile" as they were falling asleep. They are often described as looking as if they are having a pleasant dream. The smiles occur spontaneously and are considered discharge behaviors, "released" or triggered by the sudden absence of inputs into the CNS. They occur in bursts and do not come soon after a startle, but are similar to the muscle jerks or startles that sometimes reawaken adults as they are falling asleep. There is a marked difference between sexes in the number of spontaneous smiles per hour. Girls have twice as many smiles as boys, but only half as many smiles as startles.

Although these reflex or spontaneous smiles can also be elicited by gentle stimulation or by high-pitched sounds in 30-40% of tries, after one or two responses the infant habituates and no longer responds. It is easy to understand how a mother, cooing or talking gently to her baby as she puts it to sleep and seeing these smiles "in response" might consider them to be social. Whether these smiles can be considered social or not depends on what one means by *social*. They are generally not considered social because (a) they occur spontaneously (without external stimulation); (b) they can be elicited by nonhuman auditory stimuli, especially high-pitched sounds, as well as by a human voice; and (c) they contrast markedly with later smiling, in which alert babies selectively smile in response to purely social stimuli, such as the reappearance of a familiar person. Despite all this, early smiles can be considered social in that they serve as social stimuli to mothers.

Smiling rapidly changes into a more responsive form (see Table 6.4). In the second week it is not unusual to see smiling movements when the eyes are partially open. These usually occur at the end of a feeding, when the baby is drowsy and the mother is making soft sounds. At this age, visual stimuli are not effective in producing smiles. After the second week smiling gradually shifts to periods when the infant is awake and in a state of alert inactivity. Smiles are still triggered best by sounds, and a high-pitched voice is more effective than a low-pitched one (whether live or taped). This may be why some studies have shown fathers to be less effective in eliciting smiles than mothers.

Toward the end of the fourth week the combination of visual and auditory stimuli is more effective than an auditory stimulus alone. Silent nodding of the head is sometimes effective, and pat-a-caking is also, even if the infant has no previous experience with it. Indeed, pat-a-caking can get 20 to 30 smiles, whereas other stimuli elicit only 8 to 10. By 1 month visual stimuli tend to become more effective than auditory ones. Vocalizations now tend to elicit gurgling (inexact imitation) rather than smiling. Human faces are effective, but a change in a rhythmic visual stimulus also evokes a smile. Masks or glasses evoke smiles, but mirror glasses tend to evoke a crying type of face.

After the first month smiling appears to become almost an obligatory response. A crying infant will stop crying to smile at an effective stimulus and resume crying when the smile is completed. By another month the response becomes selective. This selectivity of the smile is part of what people mean when they consider these later smiles to be truly social (see Figure 6.7). Babies by this age respond clearly to humans and do so differentially. This selectivity continues to develop and change during infancy. For example, Hetzer and

Tudor-Hart (1927) found that at 6-8 weeks babies smiled to humans regardless of the person's expression or voice tone, but by 5 to 7 months the baby would adopt the adult's facial expression, angry or friendly, and cry at a scolding voice with an angry face. Nonsocial stimuli continue to be effective elicitors of smiles from older babies (see Figure 6.2), especially when the baby successfully manipulates them in some way (as in the experimental situation in which the photo in Figure 6.2 was taken).

Smiling has been studied from a wide variety of perspectives:

(1) as an innate indicator of emotion or pleasure, as Darwin approached it (e.g., Sroufe & Waters, 1976)

(2) as related to arousal as indexed by heart rate deceleration (Brock et al., 1986)

(3) as a stimulus for adult responses (Frodi, Lamb, Leavitt, & Donovan, 1978; Frodi, Lamb, Leavitt, Wilberta, et al., 1978)

(4) as a response that can be learned—that is, can be enhanced and diminished in accordance with learning principles (e.g., Brackbill, 1958; Gewirtz, 1965; Rheingold, 1961; see also even Bühler, 1930, 1931; Preyer, 1880/1888)

(5) as an indicator of cognitive processing (e.g., Kagan, 1971; McCall, 1972; Schultz & Zigler, 1970; Sroufe & Wunsch, 1972; Zelazo & Komer, 1971)

Figure 6.7. A social smile. This baby is responding to a stimulus from his (off-camera) father. Notice that his whole face is smiling. (Photograph courtesy of Judith E. Sims-Knight.)

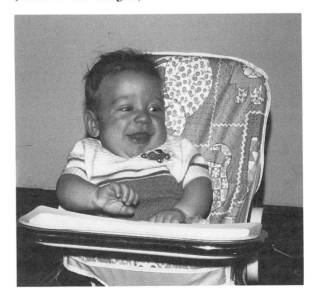

(6) as related to the broader theories of nonverbal communication (e.g., Zivin, 1982)

Despite all of this interest, a coherent view of smiling's developmental aspects does not currently exist.

Recent studies have looked at smiling in later infancy (at 17 months). Jones and Raag (1989) found that an inattentive mother did not reduce the level of nonsocial smiling (to toys) and that social smiles were directed to a friendly stranger when the mother was inattentive. A subsequent study found that the nature of the smile (closed lips, bared teeth, or open mouth) varied as a function of whether it was directed toward toys or the mother (Jones et al., 1990). Bared-teeth smiles, started when the infant was looking at or playing with toys, were directed toward the mother when she was being attentive. Although mothers were equally likely to smile in response to all three types of smiles, they were more likely to nod or vocalize to bared-teeth smiles. Hence different smiles at this age appear to function as different social cues for mothers. (See Table 6.4 for summary information on smiling and laughing; also see Sroufe & Waters, 1976, on which the table is based, for a more comprehensive account of these behaviors.)

LAUGHING

Laughter is not present in the newborn and usually follows smiling by at least 1 month (Rothbart, 1973). In home situations some infants appear to laugh as early as 5 to 9 weeks (see such baby biographers as Church, 1966; Darwin, 1872; Major, 1906). Parents and other adults call these early responses laughter, but researchers are more hesitant to do so (Wolff, 1963). In a laboratory situation Washburn (1929) obtained clear instances of laughter only at 12 to 16 weeks, and even then not in all babies. While four babies laughed at one or more stimulus situations as early as 12 weeks, one did not laugh until 52 weeks.

When Washburn asked parents to make their babies laugh, the most frequent parental behavior was tickling, which parents found effective for infants between the ages of 24 and 52 weeks of age. Washburn herself was successful in eliciting laughter by tickling only once; after that, the babies either responded negatively or smiled. Wilson (1931) had 14 mothers keep records of what made their babies laugh when they were between 1 and 29 months of age. The effective stimuli reported were boisterous play, tickling, surprising sounds, sights, and movements, and such motor accomplishments as rolling over or standing up.

Sroufe and Wunsch (1972) studied laughter and its

eliciting stimuli systematically in a series of one longitudinal and two cross-sectional studies. The infants were 4 to 12 months old. Strong patterns emerged: Tactile and kinesthetic stimuli were most potent in producing laughter; 7- to 9-month-olds laughed more and in response to more things than did 4- to 6-month-olds. When the younger babies laughed, it was more likely to be in response to items with tactile or auditory components. Visual stimuli (such as mother covers face, makes object disappear, sucks baby bottle) and social stimuli (such as mother plays tag, "gonna get you," or peekaboo) elicited increasing responses with increasing age. The social items peaked in effectiveness earlier than the visual ones.

There are a number of similar theories concerning what produces laughter (Ambrose, 1963; Berlyne, 1960; Rothbart, 1973; for a review, see Sroufe & Waters, 1976). Following is a discussion of Rothbart's arousal theory.

Sudden, intense, or discrepant stimulation arouses individuals. They then attend to and evaluate the stimulus. If they perceive it to be dangerous, they become fearful, and, if babies, they often cry. If it is not dangerous but is difficult to understand, they attempt to figure it out. Once they understand it (either with or without problem solving at the time), their arousal decreases and they either smile or laugh. Rothbart hypothesizes that the more arousing the nondangerous stimulus, the more likely it is that it will evoke laughter rather than smiling.

If this arousal theory is correct, we should expect to see fear and laugh responses in similar situations. Several studies with infants have supported this relation between fear and laughter. Further, the sounds of laughs are difficult (require more experience with infants) to distinguish from discomfort sounds (Papoušek, 1989). Sroufe and Wunsch (1972) found that an object coming straight toward the infant (looming), which is an arousing stimulus, leads to both laughter and fear. One of their stimulus situations produced laughter, while a very similar situation in another study (Scarr & Salapatek, 1970) produced fear. In Sroufe and Wunsch's laughter-producing situation, masks were put on by the infants' mothers while the infants were watching. In the fear reaction study, the experimenter put on a mask out of the infants' sight and then appeared before them. Lewis and Brookes-Gunn (cited in Rothbart, 1973), in a study of responses to strangers, mothers, and selves in a mirror, found both positive (smiling and laughing) and negative (crying) reactions were most likely when the stimulus person was close to the child and least likely when he or she was across the room. In addition, the direction of the affect depended on the stimulus. The mother and mirror self generally elicited positive reactions, while adult strangers elicited negative reactions. Parents and other caretakers are aware of the fact that laughter can shift quickly to crying, possibly in ways that are compatible with this theory.

The arousal theory involves cognitive processes in several ways. First, laughter should occur only in response to stimuli that are understood. This appears to be supported by the fact that more cognitively complex stimuli evoked laughter in older infants but not in younger ones, and younger infants laughed only after the stimulus, while older infants often laughed before the stimulus ended (Sroufe & Wunsch, 1972). It takes more cognitive capacity to understand an event well enough to anticipate its end, a capacity only the older infants had, and so they could laugh before the stimulus ended. Second, the theory proposes that achieving understanding of something initially not understood should produce laughter. For example, babies laugh when they achieve mastery (Rothbart, 1973; Wilson, 1931). Stimuli that are moderately difficult to figure out should be more likely to elicit laughter, according to the theory; stimuli that are too easy to process may not be arousing enough; and stimuli that are too difficult will be either ignored or responded to with fear. This is also in keeping with White's (1959) effectance concept and his conclusion that "children enjoy most that which lies at the growing edge of their capacities" (p. 335). It is also possible that laughter may be evoked by a violation of an expectation, perhaps because such a situation is arousing.

The arousal model of laughter explains a large body of research in both infants and other organisms, but it is not the whole story. Rothbart (1973) points out that laughter serves a very useful role in giving infants control over their environment. When a baby laughs, the caregiver tends to repeat whatever he or she has just done; the baby's laugh is reinforcing to the caregiver (and to other humans, such as big brothers and sisters). Thus through their laughter babies learn that they can affect other people, an important aspect of White's concept of effectance motivation. They also learn about their world. Consider the contingencies in a laughter "game." If the baby laughs, the person repeats; if the baby does not laugh, the person does not repeat. Therefore, the stimulus is repeated only if it is at an appropriate cognitive level for the infant. The repetition may be important, because babies often need long or repeated presentations of a stimulus to process it. The "power" of the rewarding properties of their laughter helps to keep the stimulus around. Similar learning occurs with crying. When babies cry, their caregivers respond to them. If they continue to cry, their caregivers change behaviors, over and over again until the baby stops crying or the caregiver gives up.

Traits or Temperament

At several points in the book I have mentioned the relation of some pre-, peri-, or postnatal characteristic to later aspects of behavior. Sometimes the characteristic is considered to be the precursor of personality or is labeled a temperamental characteristic, or **trait**. Activity level and possibly attentiveness, discussed earlier in this chapter, are such characteristics. The findings of presumably stable temperamental characteristics, or traits, by the New York Longitudinal Study (Thomas et al., 1963) generated renewed interest in questions about temperamental characteristics: What are they? How stable are they? How can they be measured? To what degree do they have genetic or constitutional determinants?

Research in the area of temperament is extremely difficult to summarize due to the diverse definitions of temperament used by different researchers and the different behaviors used to index it. Some include the criterion that it be inherited (Buss & Plomin, 1984; Plomin, 1987; Plomin & Dunn, 1986) or primarily biologically based (see Rothbart's comments in Goldsmith et al., 1987), or exclude cognitive factors (Goldsmith & Campos, 1982). Others focus on behaviors without regard to their presumed biological or genetic bases (Chess & Thomas, 1959; Goldsmith & Campos, 1986; Thomas & Chess, 1977). Still others focus their research on single aspects of behavior, such as activity level (Eaton et al., 1989; Saudino & Eaton, 1989, in press), behavioral inhibition (Kagan, 1989; Kagan et al., 1984, 1988; Kagan & Snidman, 1991), or "difficultness," a concept derived from the work of Thomas, Chess, and colleagues (Bates, 1980, 1987). All agree that (a) they are interested in behavioral tendencies, not in specific behavioral acts; (b) continuity over time is important to the construct; (c) it has some biological underpinnings; and (d) it, or its expression, is modifiable. Another important theoretical question is whether a temperamental characteristic should be conceived as belonging to a continuous dimension or as a qualitative characteristic (see Kagan, 1989; Kagan et al., 1989), a strategy adopted by Gandour (1989). I tend to adhere to the former view, but agree that labels on a characteristic should be applied only to the extremes, and that study of the extremes may be a good research strategy.

Interest in modifiability has led to a focus on studies

of infants where fewer environmental influences have acted. How much continuity over time is needed to assume support for any temperamental trait is a question that is answered in different ways by different researchers.

DEFINITIONS OF TEMPERAMENT

Buss and Plomin (1984) specify three traits of temperament: (a) emotionality or distress, together with difficulty of being soothed; (b) activity, with tempo and vigor as its components; and (c) sociability. All of these they find to be among the more heritable traits (Buss & Plomin, 1975, 1984). Rothbart's Infant Behavior Questionnaire (IBQ) has scales for smiling and laughter, fear, distress to limitations (frustration), soothability, activity level, and duration of orienting (attention). Rothbart (1984) has proposed that individual differences in negative reactivity are present at birth, those in positive affect by 2-3 months, and cortically regulated approach and avoidance as well as behavioral inhibition by 4-6 months. A potential fourth dimension, the ability to focus and shift attention, develops toward the end of the first year. Matheny et al. (1984) constructed a temperament profile from laboratory behavior ratings that formed three factors or aspects of temperament: positive emotional tone, sustained attention, and receptiveness to staff and strangers. Let us begin by examining some research evidence relevant to activity as a trait.

TEMPERAMENTAL TRAITS STUDIED

Activity Level

Postnatal activity scores have the measurement characteristics typical of such traits as height, weight, and IQ. Measures of postnatal activity exhibit a wide range of scores, and they are approximately normally distributed, with no sex differences (Brownfield, 1956). If activity level (AL) is a temperamental trait there should be stable individual differences in it. Evidence for this is not entirely consistent. Sex (and ethnic) differences in data from the CPRP indicate a need for more consideration of these variables in studies of AL (Eaton et al., 1989).

Stability of noncrying activity from one feeding interval to another has been found, but correlations were only in the mid .30s (explained only 9-13% of the variance), which certainly does not suggest strong stability (Korner, Thoman, & Glick, 1974). The strongest evidence that activity over the first month of life predicts later AL is that of Lancione et al. (1980).

They found stability over the first month of life using the more global assessment of activity from the Kansas version of the NBAS. Activity was the stablest of all characteristics measured, though its stability was modest.

Evidence for an AL factor with a genetic component exists in later behavior. Goldsmith and Gottesman (1981) clustered a broad set of behaviors from the Bayley examination at 8 months into an activity factor. The items include speed of response, active manipulation, response duration, pursuit persistence, and activity level, hence the cluster includes both spontaneous activity and activity in response to stimulation. These authors found that identical twins were more similar to each other than were fraternals, indicating a genetic component. However, it accounted for less than 35% of the variance in the activity factor scores. Hence there are other important influences. ALs of 31-week-old twins assessed by mechanical recorders, called actometers, showed correlations for MZ and DZ twins that fit the classic twin model with $r = .88$ for MZ and $r = .54$ for DZ twins (Saudino & Eaton, 1989). Whether the larger correlations in this study result from the better measuring device is not clear.

Moderate stability in AL has been shown between 3 months and 2 years (Thomas et al., 1963); between 2 weeks and 2 months and between 2 months and 1 year, but not from 2 weeks to 1 year (Worobey & Blajda, 1989); and between 3 and 6 months, 6 and 9 months, and even 3 and 9 months (Rothbart, 1986). In the last study parental responses on the IBQ were stabler than measures based on home observations, suggesting that stability may sometimes be in the eye of the parent, not in the baby. Neonatal activity when awake is also related to the variability of activity at 2 years (Riese, 1987).

Parental ratings on the Toddler Temperament Scale (see Fullard et al., 1984) were used by Gandour (1989) to classify 5-month-old infants as high or low active (more than one standard deviation from the mean). AL interacted with the stimulation level provided by the mother in determining the level of exploratory behavior of the infants. High-AL toddlers were more exploratory if they had low-stimulating mothers and low-AL toddlers tended to be higher in exploratory behavior if they received high levels of stimulation. This kind of interaction between infant characteristics and maternal treatment or other environmental events is what temperamental traits have been posited to mediate.

In conclusion, AL shows strong individual differences from prenatal life throughout infancy and beyond, differences about which parents, caretakers, and scientists can agree. The interpretation of the modest evidence for its stability over time is less agreed upon. Data from twin studies seem to show some genetic or biological basis for individual differences in activity. AL's apparent stability or instability may depend on the ways and times in which it is measured.

Attention or Duration of Orientation

Attention is considered a component of temperament by several researchers in the field. It was discussed briefly in an earlier section, and in a later chapter its ability to predict future cognitive behaviors is addressed. Persistence is a related trait that has been found to have some connection to social and adaptive competence at 8 years of age (Bathurst et al., 1988).

Emotionality/Distress and Soothability

A variety of studies from the Louisville twin study are relevant here. Emotional tone at 9 months is well predicted by that in the neonatal period (Matheny et al., 1985). Neonatal irritability is negatively related to emotional tone at 2 years, as well as to attentiveness and social orientation toward staff, and positively related to variability of activity. Neonatal activity in sleep is related to variability of emotional tone at age 2. Neonatal measures are not related to those at 12 or 18 months, but 9-14% of the variance in behaviors at 2 years is accounted for by them (Riese, 1987).

Negative reactivity was not found by Rothbart (1986) to be as stable as positive reactivity, but Worobey and Blajda (1989) found a similar factor (called Irritability) based on the IBQ was strongly correlated over time: between 2 weeks and 2 months (.64), between 2 months and 1 year (.50), and between 2 weeks and 1 year (.46). In addition, Worobey and Lewis (1989) have found reactivity to stress to have continuity. Infants who react strongly to heel pricks for blood samples at 2 days also react strongly to immunization shots at 2 months (86% of high reactors remained high). Time to dampen the reaction did not correlate at the two times, but analysis of the extremes again showed continuity, with 95% of those with short duration of reaction at 2 days being short at 2 months.

In concluding this section there are two things I would like to stress: First, these variables appear to yield more meaningful results than some others, hence they justify a renewed interest in temperament research; second, research that looks for correlations between two points in time within extreme cases seems to produce more meaningful results.

Finally, a note of caution about sex differences, which have been reported in only a few studies (not all have looked for them). Riese (1986) has found sex differences in irritability in opposite-sex twins, with girls being more irritable and more difficult to soothe. Rothbart (1986) has found no sex differences in her measures, but great sex differences in their stability over time. Reactivity is correlated .62 from 6 to 9 months for boys, but .00 for girls. Clearly, some understanding of these kinds of results is necessary if we are to arrive at any satisfactory understanding of temperament.[7]

Inhibited-Uninhibited (Shy-Sociable)

In line with his belief that temperament should be conceived of as a qualitative trait, Kagan and colleagues followed infants and toddlers who were at the extremes on these characteristics to age 7½ years (Kagan, 1989; Kagan et al., 1988, 1989). They used a variety of both physiological and behavioral measures in varied settings, with a number in realistic social settings. The infant sample (21 months initially) showed more continuity over time ($r = .67$, 45% of variance accounted for, compared with $r = .39$, 15% of variance accounted for in the toddler sample). The inhibited children differed from the uninhibited in a variety of physiological measures, which Kagan and colleagues take to mean lower thresholds of reaction in certain areas of the brain and to support a genetic basis for the traits. Support is found in the findings (a) for a relation between measures of heart period variability and reactivity (Bell et al., 1988) and (b) that sociability at 18 months is related to socialization and the adaptive behavior composite of the Vineland Adaptive Behavior Scales at 8 years, accounting for about 25% of the variance (Bathurst et al., 1988). Sociability has also been shown to add significantly to the variance associated with SES in predicting performance on intellectual tests at 3, 4, and 7 years (Larson et al., 1989).

Kagan and Snidman are currently looking at younger infants to find behaviors that would predict inhibited and uninhibited behavior in the second year. Their preliminary data reveal a subsample of infants (about 14%) who show very high motor arousal, high irritability, and high heart rate at 2 and 4 months, all of whom were fearful in response to unexpected events in the laboratory at 9 and 14 months (Kagan & Snidman, 1991). Of the 14 (28%) who had been low

---

7. A more thorough summary of the field of temperament up to 1986 can be found in Bates (1987).

on all three, all but one were smiling and sociable with the examiner and showed little fear at the later ages.

CLINICAL CONCERN WITH TEMPERAMENT

The work of Thomas et al. (1968) was more clinically oriented than that discussed above. Their work led to the development of questionnaires (Carey & McDevitt, 1978; Fullard et al., 1984) and also gave rise to the concept of the "difficult child" (for a multifaceted discussion of this concept, see Kagan, 1982; Plomin, 1982; Rothbart, 1982; Thomas et al., 1982; see Thomas, 1982, for a reply to Kagan, Plomin, and Rothbart). Bates (1980, 1987, 1990; Bates et al., 1982) focused on this research area, as did others. Several studies have questioned the concept as more than a very weak constitutional trait (e.g., St. James-Roberts & Wolke, 1988; see also Sanson et al., 1990). But both difficultness and adaptability, measured by maternal questionnaire at 18 months, were related to preschool behavior problems (as seen by the mothers, not the teachers) and accounted for as much as 15-25% of the variance (Guerin & Gottfried, 1986).

These findings suggest a clinical aspect of the work of Kagan and his colleagues on inhibition. Three-fourths of the inhibited, but only one-fourth of the uninhibited, had unusual fears at 7½.

Bates et al. (1982) report that the role of mothers in the development of difficultness reveals a significant but modest (.30) correlation between a mother's perception of her 6-month-old infant as difficult and the infant's actual fussy behaviors as seen in home observations. The infant's "difficultness" was not related to negative aspects of maternal behaviors. The authors conclude that if the difficult infant becomes the difficult child as a result of negative interactions with the mother, the crucial interactions must occur later than infancy. Social class, which is related to child-rearing practices, has been found to be related to some aspects of temperament, including the easy/difficult dimension (Prior et al., 1987).

The question of whether premature infants would differ in temperament from term infants has been studied by several without a clear pattern of results. The largest study found no differences at corrected ages of 4 and 8 months, *if* high-risk cases with medical complications and prolonged intensive care were excluded (Oberklaid et al., 1986).

Clinical interest in this concept continues, but the lack of stability prior to 3 or 4 years, and the danger of creating a self-fulfilling prophecy by labeling infants with "difficult" temperaments as "at risk" (Rothbart,

1982; Rothbart & Derryberry, 1981) may be related to the current lower emphasis on this aspect of temperament research.

ASSESSMENT OF TEMPERAMENT

There are a number of tests used to assess temperament, most of which leave a great deal to be desired. In a review of the instruments designed to assess temperament from infancy into the school-age period, Hubert et al. (1982) found 26 such instruments, at least 16 of which were designed for use in some portion of infancy. While most of these showed good interjudge reliability and moderate to good test-retest reliability, the stability data were inconsistent. When validity data were available they were inconsistent and not similar from one instrument to another. Another critical review is found in Bornstein et al. (1986). The categories assessed lack internal consistency in at least some tests (Huitt & Ashton, 1982). Theories of temperament are rather controversial, hence only operational definitions of the construct of temperament are possible (Hubert et al., 1982). This makes it imperative to pay attention to the measuring instruments used.

Most measures are based on questionnaires filled out by the mother. If studies using such measures find continuity (ergo support for some trait), the similarity over time may be in the parent rather than in the infant. This issue is addressed in some of the papers cited, but I would like to discuss two relevant studies.

More of the scales on Carey's Infant Temperament Questionnaire (ITQ; Carey & McDevitt, 1978) were related to maternal characteristics than to child variables (six versus four) in two samples. In addition, four of the six ITQ scales that were related to maternal characteristics were still related after all effects of the children's behaviors were removed (partialed out statistically). Only one ITQ scale, adaptability, was still related to children's characteristics after maternal characteristics were partialed out. Thus we see that maternal characteristics have more effect on mothers' ratings of their infants' temperaments than do the infants' behaviors. (See also Vaughn et al., 1987, for a similar point based on several studies.)

A different kind of study, which bears on the issue of the source of stability, examined the degree to which different persons (and persons in different settings) rated infants and older preschoolers similarly (Field & Greenberg, 1982). They found that ITQ scores for mothers and fathers correlated significantly for four traits: activity, rhythmicity, approach, and the summary rating. However, parent and teacher ratings did not agree, although the two teachers making ratings each had more than four months' experience with the infant. Mothers' scores were not related to teachers' on a single ITQ scale, and fathers and teachers were related only for mood. (The correlations obtained ranged from .54 to .59.) Thus there seems to be no stability of perceptions of temperamental traits across settings. Significant teacher-teacher correlations were found for both adaptability and mood. But if the various adults were asked how many behavior problems an infant had, correlations ranged from .50 to .80, and the setting in which children were observed was no longer a large influence.

Taken together, these studies suggest that much that is measured by infant temperament questionnaires is in the eye of the beholder or in the setting in which the child is observed. Both of these are contrary to the idea that stable characteristics of the child are being assessed by temperament questionnaires. In contrast, children's behavior problems seem to be stable across settings and are seen similarly by parents and teachers.

Overall, with respect to all research on temperament, Bornstein et al. (1986) conclude: "At this juncture, with so little known about temperament as a developmental phenomenon, child clinicians can neither evaluate nor predict what temperamental differences will mean in the family or in other social contexts." We might take as an example of this the contradictory findings of two studies. Wachs and Gandour (1983) found negative effects of a "difficult" temperament on cognitive functioning at 6 months of age, while Maziade et al. (1987) found that the "difficult" infants in their study had higher IQs at 4½ years. The latter were in good homes, the former from a wider range, and the ages of assessment of cognitive functioning were different, but this does illustrate that drawing conclusions concerning outcomes is likely to be premature.

Summary

Learning about infant response systems helps us understand how humans develop. The systems reviewed here include sleep, activity, attention, and other states; rhythmic behaviors (especially sucking); and affective behaviors (crying, smiling, and laughing). The question of temperamental characteristics in infancy was also discussed. There are large individual differences in all of the behaviors discussed.

SLEEP, ACTIVITY, ATTENTION, AND OTHER STATES

Sleep is the activity in which most young babies

spend the greatest proportion of their time. Sleep patterns change throughout infancy. The number of sleep episodes and total sleeping time decline, and the infant gradually sleeps longer at night and is more wakeful during the day. Sleep is not a unitary state, but can be divided into quiet and active (or REM) sleep. The relative proportion of each changes with age. Premature babies show unusual sleep patterns, developing more slowly in some ways and faster in others.

Activity level varies in both sleep and waking states. It is affected by both internal and external stimuli. Theoretical arguments about the nature of newborn activity were once an active focus of research. The methods for measuring activity have become more sophisticated over time, and they provide good examples of measurement problems in infant studies. One must be careful in comparing results of different studies to see that measures are comparable as well as that each is reliable.

Fetal activity levels, in healthy babies, have been found to be related to later motor development and even to general development. More active babies have higher scores. Postnatal activity is only moderately stable from one time to another and is only moderately correlated with later development. Some genetic component is indicated by identical twins being more alike than fraternals. Activity in response to external stress may be a stabler characteristic, but thus far it has been little explored.

One of the most dramatic changes in behavior from birth to 2 years is the increasing ability of infants to be attentive to things in their environment. What catches the infant's attention is not necessarily what keeps it. The baby whose attention is most easily caught is not necessarily the one who will pay sustained attention to stimuli, a behavior necessary for certain kinds of cognitive processing. Attention is affected by other variables, such as prematurity, perinatal events, and maternal caretaking. Hence it is used as a dependent measure, and it appears to affect the behavior of the mother. Research into the long-range meaning of early differences in attentive behaviors is under way.

Sleep, activity, and attention (alertness) are all aspects of state, as is crying. States differ qualitatively from one another on the dimensions of arousal and availability to external stimuli. Infant studies usually require that babies be in an awake, alert state, and they can be soothed or roused to the desired state, or the researcher can record state and relate it to the behaviors measured, or use only the results from the appropriate states. There are several reliable systems for classifying state, and either observational or electrophysiological techniques may be used to determine states. Only intense noxious stimuli are partially exempt from the rule that state determines responsivity.

Very premature infants have no state variations, but gradually develop them as the CNS develops. Females differ from males, probably as a result of earlier maturation of the CNS. A baby's day can be described in terms of the amount of time spent in each state. The variations in state patterns may have profound effects on parents, and instability of states is related to behavioral deficits and physiological dysfunction.

RHYTHMIC ACTIVITIES

The amount of time babies spend in rhythmic activities varies greatly. These behaviors include sucking, crying, kicking, arm waving, head banging, rocking, and all of Piaget's circular reactions. The first two are most studied and are what we have been concerned with in this chapter. Which rhythmic behaviors are most frequently found changes with age, as do the stimuli that evoke them.

Sucking is a primary behavior system on which life normally depends. It is not a single reflex, and it involves the coordination of a whole group of reflexes, including those of swallowing and breathing, for feeding to be assured. Prematures often lack this coordination, and hence are tube-fed, and may need NNS to help them organize behavior patterns. Sucking develops rapidly after birth because of both experience and maturation. Serious deficiencies in feeding behaviors may help professionals to diagnose major problems.

The attitudes prevalent in the culture about oral gratification and nonnutritive sucking change over time and differ from one culture to another. The Freudian-ethological view that adequate sucking satisfies innate oral needs and the learning view that sucking reinforces the sucking habit have both been supported by animal research. Oral needs appear to fluctuate in infancy. There is no good evidence for long-term differences as a result of different patterns of early feeding and oral behaviors, but there is evidence for effects on later oral behaviors of early experience variables, such as familial warmth, that are probably continuous over time.

CRYING, SMILING, AND LAUGHING

Affective behaviors have been studied from several points of view. Starting with Darwin, both the built-in nature of certain expressions and the abilities of persons to judge the meanings of expressions have interested people. The expression of emotion as judged by facial and vocal expressions can be accurately judged by parents and by trained and untrained judges. As infants mature, their emotional responses to stimuli change. Newborns can discriminate among changing facial expressions in a single adult, and older infants can discriminate on several dimensions. Older infants respond with emotion when their parents direct anger or affection toward another.

The very first affective behavior is crying. Cries communicate to adults: to doctors or researchers about the neurological status of the infant, and to parents and others about the distress of the infant. Cry sounds vary greatly in frequency (or pitch), intensity, and pause patterns, all of which can be analyzed using objective techniques. Computers have been used to analyze cry patterns and to identify specific problems associated with specific patterns. The nature of the stimulus and the physiological and neurological status of the baby determine the variation. Very young prematures do not cry at first; when they start to cry it is at a higher pitch than a term infant's cry, and hence may be more unpleasant. Normal full-term newborns vary tremendously in the amount they cry.

Most adults show stress reactions to cries more than to smiles, and they respond differently to various types of cries. Parents are both able to distinguish their own babies' cries from those of other babies and somewhat better at distinguishing different cry meanings of their own babies' cries. On the whole, fathers/males appear to respond to cries similarly to mothers/females. Research on adult responses to abnormal cries is not conclusive, but it appears that the nature of the abnormality (or cry pattern) may be crucial. Whether such cries make it less likely that parents (especially stressed parents) can attend adequately is not well answered. One study indicated that the physiological responses of child abusers to both cries and smiles may differ from those of others. This study should be replicated and behavioral responses studied.

As with sucking, the theoretical and value-laden arguments over whether to soothe crying babies (or under what circumstances to do so) are vigorous. Prompt soothing promotes security according to the Freudian-ethological viewpoint, but leads to increased crying according to learning theory. I do not feel that the two positions are as antithetical as they are presented by their proponents. The ways in which babies can be soothed are many, vary from one baby to another and from one time to another, and change as babies develop.

Smiles are present in reflex form from birth, and depend primarily on state. They rapidly become responsive to auditory and later to visual stimuli and are said to become social inasmuch as humans usually provide these stimuli. Smiling has been studied in a variety of contexts, and there is currently no comprehensive theory.

Laughter appears somewhat later. It is elicited primarily by tactile or auditory stimuli, or roughhousing at 4-6 months, but by visual events and more subtle social interactions later. It is difficult to elicit laughter reliably in laboratory settings until long after its home occurrence. Arousal theory has been used to account for laughter. Sudden, intense, or discrepant stimuli arouse the infant and, if judged not threatening, result in laughter. This calls for considerable cognitive ability.

TEMPERAMENT OR TEMPERAMENTAL TRAITS

If an infant characteristic such as activity level is stable across time, it is considered to be a temperamental trait. How much stability is needed to qualify it is not agreed upon, nor is the degree to which it should be influenced by heredity. Hence the rather large body of research in this field has not yielded very many satisfactory answers about the degree to which temperamental characteristics can be found in infancy. There are promising new leads, however.

Activity level shows some stability, and identical twins are more similar than fraternals. It interacts with environment, in that high-activity toddlers explore more if they receive low levels of home stimulation, and vice versa. Emotional tone, ease of arousal, and soothability show some stability over time, especially for extreme groups, as do inhibition and its lack. Because of the instability of the traits identified to date, it may be important to avoid labeling an infant to the parents as X or Y, lest unnecessary worry or a self-fulfilling prophecy is created.

Much of the work on infant temperament has relied on questionnaires filled out by parents or others. Mothers, fathers, and teachers often disagree in their answers on such questionnaires. Respondents bring their own biases into their perceptions of a given infant, a factor that can be lessened only if questions address very specific behaviors.

References

AINSWORTH, M. D. S. (1972). Attachment and dependency: A comparison. In J. L. Gewirtz (Ed.), *Attachment and dependency*. Washington, DC: Winston & Sons.

AINSWORTH, M. D. S., & Bell, S. M. (1977). Infant crying and maternal responsiveness: A rejoinder to Gewirtz and Boyd. *Child Development, 48*, 1208-1216.

AMBROSE, J. A. (1963). The concept of a critical period for the development of social responsiveness in early infancy. In B. M. Foss (Ed.), *Determinants of infant behaviour* (Vol. 2, pp. 201-225). London: Methuen.

AMES, L. B. (1942). Supine leg and foot postures in the human infant in the first year of life. *Journal of Genetic Psychology, 61*, 87-107.

AMES, L. B. (1949). Bilaterality. *Journal of Genetic Psychology, 75*, 45-50.

ANDERS, T. F., Keener, M. A., & Kraemer, H. (1985). Sleep-wake state organization, neonatal assessment and development in premature infants during the first year of life. *Sleep, 8*, 193-206.

ANDERSON, G., Burroughs, A., Measel, C., Afone, U., & Vidyasagar, D. (1980, April). *Non-nutritive sucking opportunities: A safe and effective treatment for premature infants.* Paper presented at the International Conference on Infant Studies, New Haven, CT.

ANDERSON, G. C., Fleming, S., & Vidyasagar, D. (1980, April). *Effect of position on infant behavior and physiologic stabilization during the first four hours postbirth.* Paper presented at the International Conference on Infant Studies, New Haven, CT.

ANDERSON, G. C., McBride, M. R., Dahm, J., Ellis, M. K., & Vidyasagar, D. (1982). Development of sucking in term infants from birth to four hours postbirth. *Research in Nursing and Health, 5*, 21-27.

ANDRÉ-THOMAS, & Saint-Anne Dargassies, S. (1952). *Études neurologiques sur le nouveau-ne* [Neurological studies of the newborn]. Paris: Masson.

ARDRAN, G. M., Kemp, F. H., & Lind, J. (1958). A cineradiographic study of bottle feeding. *British Journal of Radiology, 31*, 11-22.

AYLWARD, G. P. (1981). The developmental course of behavioral states in pre-term infants: A descriptive study. *Child Development, 52*, 564-568.

BAMFORD, F. N., Bannister, R. P., Benjamin, C. M., Hillier, V. F., Ward, B. S., & Moore, W. M. O. (1990). Sleep in the first year of life. *Developmental Medicine and Child Neurology, 32*, 718-724.

BATES, J. E. (1980). The concept of difficult temperament. *Merrill-Palmer Quarterly, 26*, 299-319.

BATES, J. E. (1987). Temperament in infancy. In J. D. Osofsky (Ed.), *Handbook of infancy* (2nd ed., pp. 1101-1149). New York: John Wiley.

BATES, J. E. (1990). Conceptual and empirical linkages between temperament and behavior problems: A commentary on Sanson, Prior, and Kyrios. *Merrill-Palmer Quarterly, 36*, 193-199.

BATES, J. E., Olson, S. L., Pettit, G. S., & Bayles, K. (1982). Dimensions of individuality in the mother-infant relationship at six months of age. *Child Development, 53*, 446-461.

BATHURST, K., Gottfried, & Guerin, D. (1988, April). *Infant temperament as a predictor of adaptive behavior at six and eight years of age.* Paper presented at the International Conference on Infant Studies, Washington, DC.

BECKWITH, L., & Parmelee, A. H. (1986). EEG patterns of preterm infants, home environment, and later IQ. *Child Development, 57*, 777-789.

BELL, M. A., Sutton, D. B., Luebering, A., & Aaron, N. A. (1988, March). *Relationships among maternal-report of temperament, lab measures of reactivity, and heart period variability at 5 and 14 months.* Paper presented at the Conference on Human Development, Charleston, SC.

BELL, R. Q. (1960). Relations between behavior manifestations in the human neonate. *Child Development, 31*, 463-477.

BELL, R. Q. (1963). Some factors to be controlled in studies of the behavior of newborns. *Biologia Neonatorum, 5*, 200-214.

BELL, S. M., & Ainsworth, M. D. S. (1972). Infant crying and maternal responsiveness. *Child Development, 43*, 1171-1190.

BENJAMIN, L. S. (1961). The effect of frustration on the non-nutritive sucking of the infant rhesus monkey. *Journal of Comparative and Physiological Psychology, 54*, 700-703.

BERLYNE, D. (1960). *Conflict, arousal, and curiosity.* New York: McGraw-Hill.

BERRY, K. K. (1975). Developmental study of recognition of antecedents of infant vocalization. *Perceptual and Motor Skills, 41*, 400-402.

BLAU, T. J., & Blau, L. R. (1955). The sucking reflex: The effects of long feeding vs. short feeding on the behavior of a human infant. *Journal of Abnormal and Social Psychology, 51*, 123-125.

BOOTH, C. L., Leonard, H. L., & Thoman, E. B. (1980). Sleep states and behavior patterns in preterm and full term infants. *Neuropédiatrie, 11*, 354.

BORNSTEIN, M. H., Gaughran, J., & Homel, P. (1986). Infant temperament: Theory, tradition, critique, and new assessments. In C. E. Izard & P. B. Read (Eds.), *Measurement of emotions: Vol. 2. Studies in social and emotional development* (pp. 172-199). New York: Cambridge University Press.

BOUKYDIS, C. F. Z., & Burgess, R. L. (1982). Adult physiological response to infant cries: Effects of temperament of infant, parental status, and gender. *Child Development, 53*, 1291-1298.

BOUKYDIS, C. F. Z., & Lester, B. M. (1990, April). *Cry characteristics and social support in preterm infants.* Paper presented at the International Conference on Infant Studies, Montreal.

BOWLBY, J. (1969). *Attachment and loss: Vol. 1. Attachment.* London: Hogarth.

BRACKBILL, Y. (1958). Extinction of the smiling response in infants as a function of reinforcement schedule. *Child Development, 29*, 115-124.

BRACKBILL, Y. (1970). Acoustic variation and arousal level in infants. *Psychophysiology, 6*, 517-526.

BRACKBILL, Y. (1971). Cumulative effects of continuous stimulation on arousal level in infants. *Child Development, 42*, 17-26.

BRAZELTON, T. B. (1962). Crying in infancy. *Pediatrics, 29*, 579-588.

BRAZELTON, T. B. (1973). *Neonatal Behavioral Assessment Scale* (Clinics in Developmental Medicine No. 50). Philadelphia: J. B. Lippincott.

BROCK, S. E., Rothbart, M. K., & Derryberry, D. (1986). Heart-rate deceleration and smiling in 3-month-old infants. *Infant Behavior and Development, 9*, 403-414.

BRODBECK, A. J. (1950). The effect of three feeding variables on the non-nutritive sucking of newborn infants. *American Psychologist, 5*, 292-293.

BROWN, J. L. (1964). States in newborn infants. *Merrill-Palmer Quarterly, 10*, 313-327.

BROWNFIELD, E. D. (1956). An investigation of the activity and sensory responses of healthy newborn infants. *Dissertation Abstracts, 16*, 1288-1289.

BÜHLER, C. (1930). *The first year of life* (P. Greenberg & R. Ripin, Trans.). New York: Day. (Original works published 1927, 1928, 1930)

BÜHLER, C. (1931). The social behavior of the child. In C. Murchison (Ed.), *A handbook of child psychology.* Worcester, MA: Clark University Press.

BUSS, A. H., & Plomin, R. (1975). *A temperament theory of personality development.* New York: Wiley-Interscience.

BUSS, A. H., & Plomin, R. (1984). *Temperament: Early developing personality traits.* Hillsdale, NJ: Lawrence Erlbaum.

CAREY, W. B., & McDevitt, S. C. (1978). Revision of the Infant Temperament Questionnaire. *Pediatrics, 61*, 735-739.

CARON, R. F., Caron, A. J., & Myers, R. S. (1982). Abstraction of invariant face expressions in infancy. *Child Development, 53*, 1008-1015.

CARON, R. F., Caron, A. J., & Myers, R. S. (1985). Do infants see emotional expressions in static faces? *Child Development, 56*, 1552-1560.

CHESS, S., & Thomas, A. (1959). Characteristics of the individual child's behavioral responses to the environment. *American Journal of Orthopsychiatry, 24*, 798-802.

CHILDERS, A. T., & Hamil, B. M. (1932). Emotional problems in children as related to duration of breastfeeding in infancy. *American Journal of Orthopsychiatry, 2*, 134-142.

CHURCH, J. (1966). *Three babies: Biographies of cognitive development.* New York: Random House.

COGHILL, G. E. (1929a). *Anatomy and the problem of behavior.* Cambridge: Cambridge University Press.

COGHILL, G. E. (1929b). The early development of behavior in amblystoma and in man. *Archives of Neurology and Psychiatry, 21*, 989-1009.

COHEN, L. B. (1972). Attention-getting and attention-holding processes of infant visual preferences. *Child Development, 43*, 869-879.

COHEN, L. B., DeLoache, J. S., & Rissman, M. W. (1975). The effect of stimulus complexity on infant visual attention and habituation. *Child Development, 46*, 611-617.

COHEN, S. E., & Parmelee, A. H. (1983). Prediction of five-year Stanford-Binet scores in preterm infants. *Child Development, 54*, 1242-1253.

COLOMBO, J., & Horowitz, F. D. (1987). Behavioral state as a lead variable in neonatal research. *Merrill-Palmer Quarterly, 33*, 423-437.

COLOMBO, J., Mitchell, D. W., & Horowitz, F. D. (1988). Infant visual attention in the paired-comparison paradigm: Test-retest and attention-performance relations. *Child Development, 59*, 1198-1210.

COLOMBO, J., Moss, M., & Horowitz, F. D. (1989). Neonatal state profiles: Reliability and short-term prediction of neurobehavioral status. *Child Development, 60*, 1102-1110.

COONS, S., & Guilleminault, C. (1984). Development of consolidated sleep and wakeful periods in relation to the day/night cycle in infancy. *Developmental Medicine and Child Neurology, 26*, 169-176.

COSSETTE, L., Malcuit, G., & Pomerleau, A. (1991). Sex differences in motor activity during early infancy. *Infant Behavior and Development, 14*, 175-186.

CRAIG, K. D., Grunau, R. V., & Aquan-Asee, J. (1988). Judgment of pain in newborns: Facial activity and cry as determinants. *Canadian Journal of Behavioral Science, 20*, 442-451.

CROWELL, D. H., Yasaka, E. K., & Crowell, D. C. (1964). Infant stabilimeter. *Child Development, 35*, 525-532.

CUMMINGS, E. M., Zahn-Waxler, C., & Radke-Yarrow, M. (1981). Children's responses to expressions of anger and affection by others in the family. *Child Development, 52*, 1274-1282.

CURZI-DASCALOVA, L., Peirano, P., & Morel-Kahn, F. (1988). Development of sleep states in normal premature and full-term newborns. *Developmental Psychobiology, 21,* 431-444.

DARWIN, C. (1872). *Expressions of the emotions in man and animals.* London: John Murray.

DAVIS, D. H., & Thoman, E. B. (1988). The early social environment of premature and fullterm infants. *Early Human Development, 17,* 221-232.

DAVIS, H. V., Sears, R. R., Miller, H. C., & Brodbeck, N. J. (1948). Effects of cup, bottle and breast feeding. *Pediatrics, 2,* 549-558.

DeCONTI, K. A., & Gustafson, G. E. (1990, April). *On some reasonable assumptions about cry-initiated interactions.* Paper presented at the International Conference on Infant Studies, Montreal.

DeGUIRE, A., Glaze, D. G., & Frost, J. D. (1983). Visual evoked potentials in the newborn: Awake and asleep. *American Journal of EEG Technology, 23,* 15-23.

DeLOACHE, J. S., Rissman, M. D., & Cohen, L. B. (1978). An investigation of the attention-getting process in infants. *Infant Behavior and Development, 1,* 11-25.

DENNIS, W. (1932). Discussion: The role of mass activity in the development of infant behavior. *Psychological Review, 39,* 593-595.

diPIETRO, J. A., Larson, S. K., & Porges, S. W. (1987). Behavioral and heart rate pattern differences between breast-fed and bottle-fed neonates. *Developmental Psychology, 23,* 467-474.

DITTRICHOVA, J., & Paul, K. (1983). Development of behavioral states in very premature infants. *Activitas Nervosa Superior, 25,* 186-188.

DITTRICHOVA, J., & Paul, K. (1984). Development of sleep cycles in premature infants. *Activitas Nervosa Superior, 26,* 167-168.

DREYFUS-BRISSAC, C. (1968). Sleep ontogenesis in early human prematurity from 24 to 27 weeks conceptional age. *Developmental Psychobiology, 1,* 162-169.

DUNN, J. F. (1975). Consistency and change in styles of mothering. In *Parent-infant interaction* (CIBA Foundation Symposium 33, New Series). Amsterdam: Elsevier.

EATON, W. O., Chipperfield, J. G., & Singbiel, C. E. (1989). Birth order and activity level in children. *Developmental Psychology, 25,* 668-672.

EATON, W. O., & Saudino, K. J. (1991). Prenatal activity level as a temperament dimension? Individual differences and developmental functions in fetal movement. *Infant Behavior and Development.*

ELIAS, M. F., Nicolson, N. A., Bora, C., & Johnston, J. (1986). Sleep/wake patterns of breast-fed infants in the first 2 years of life. *Pediatrics, 77,* 322-329.

EMDE, R. N., Gaensbauer, T. G., & Harmon, R. J. (1976). Emotional expression in infancy: A biobehavioral study. *Psychological Issues Monograph Series, 10*(37).

ESCALONA, S. (1962). The study of individual differences and the problem of state. *Journal of the American Academy of Child Psychiatry, 1,* 11-37.

ETZEL, B. C., & Gewirtz, J. L. (1967). Experimenter modification of caretaker maintained high-rate operant crying in a 6- and a 20-week old infant (infants tyrannotearus): Extinction of crying with reinforcement of eye-contact and smiling. *Journal of Experimental Child Psychology, 5,* 303-317.

FAGIOLI, I., & Salzarulo, P. (1987). Behavioral states and brain activity during the earliest developmental stages. *Eta-evolutiva, 26,* 78-82.

FAIRBANKS, G. (1942). An acoustical study of the pitch of infant hunger wails. *Child Development, 13,* 227-232.

FIELD, T., & Goldson, E. (1984). Pacifying effects of nonnutritive sucking on term and preterm neonates during heelstick procedures. *Pediatrics, 74,* 1012-1015.

FIELD, T. M., & Greenberg, R. (1982). Temperament ratings by parents and teachers of infants, toddlers, and preschool children. *Child Development, 53,* 160-163.

FIELD, T. M., Ting, G., & Shuman, H. H. (1979). The onset of rhythmic activities in normal and high-risk infants. *Developmental Psychobiology, 12,* 97-100.

FIELD, T. M., Woodson, R., Greenberg, R., & Cohen, D. (1982). Discrimination and imitation of facial expressions by neonates. *Science, 218,* 179-181.

FISHER, K., & Ames, E. W. (1989, April). *The relationship between non-nutritive sucking and respiration in 6- to 8-week-old infants.* Paper presented at the annual meeting of the Society for Research in Child Development, Kansas City, MO.

FLEISCHL, M. F. (1957). The problem of sucking. *American Journal of Psychotherapy, 1,* 86-87.

FOX, N. A., & Davidson, R. J. (1988). Patterns of brain electrical activity during facial signs of emotion in 10-month-old infants. *Developmental Psychology, 24,* 230-236.

FREUDENBERG, R. P., Driscoll, J. W., & Stern, G. S. (1978). Reactions of adult humans to crises of normal and abnormal infants. *Infant Behavior and Development, 1,* 224-227.

FREUDIGMAN, K. A., & Thoman, E. G. (1991, April). *Newborn sleep: Effects of age, sex, and mode of delivery.* Paper presented at the meeting of the Society for Research in Child Development, Seattle.

FRODI, A. M. (1985). When empathy fails: Aversive infant crying and child abuse. In B. M. Lester & C. F. Z. Boukydis (Eds.), *Infant crying: Theoretical and research perspectives* (pp. 241-261). New York: Plenum.

FRODI, A. M., & Lamb, M. E. (1980). Child abusers' responses to infant smiles and cries. *Child Development, 51,* 238-241.

FRODI, A. M., Lamb, M. E., Leavitt, L. A., & Donovan, W. L. (1978). Fathers' and mothers' responses to infant smiles and cries. *Infant Behavior and Development, 1,* 187-198.

FRODI, A. M., Lamb, M. E., Leavitt, L. A., Wilberta, L., Donovan, C. M., & Sherry, D. (1978). Fathers' and mothers' responses to the faces and cries of normal and premature infants. *Developmental Psychology, 14,* 490-498.

FRODI, A. M., & Senchak, M. (1990). Verbal and behavioral responsiveness to the cries of atypical infants. *Child Development, 61,* 76-84.

FULLARD, W., McDevitt, S. C., & Carey, W. B. (1984). Assessing temperament in one- to three-year-old children. *Journal of Pediatric Psychology, 9,* 205-217.

GANDOUR, M. J. (1989). Activity levels as a dimension of temperament in toddlers: Its relevance for the organismic specificity hypothesis. *Child Development, 60,* 1092-1098.

GARDINER, W. (1838). *The music of nature.* Boston: Wilkins & Carter.

GAULIN-KREMER, E., Shaw, J. L., & Thoman, E. B. (1977). *Temporal course of sucking responsiveness in the earliest hours of life.* Paper presented at the biennial meeting of the Society for Research in Child Development, New Orleans.

GESELL, A. (1948). *Studies in child development.* New York:

Harper & Brothers.

GESELL, A., & Thompson, H. (1934). *Infant behavior: Its genesis and growth.* New York: McGraw-Hill.

GEWIRTZ, J. L. (1965). The course of infant smiling in four child-rearing environments in Israel. In B. M. Foss (Ed.), *Determinants of infant behaviour* (Vol. 3). London: Methuen.

GEWIRTZ, J. L. (1977). Maternal responding and the conditioning of infant crying: Directions of influence within the attachment-acquisition process. In B. C. Etzel, J. M. LeBlanc, & D. M. Baer (Ed.), *New developments in behavioral research: Theory, method, and application.* Hillsdale, NJ: Lawrence Erlbaum.

GEWIRTZ, J. L., & Boyd, E. F. (1977a). Does maternal responding imply reduced infant crying? A critique of the 1972 Bell and Ainsworth report. *Child Development, 48,* 1200-1207.

GEWIRTZ, J. L., & Boyd, E. F. (1977b). In reply to the rejoinder to our critique of the 1972 Bell and Ainsworth report. *Child Development, 48,* 1217-1218.

GILL, N. E., Behnke, M., Conlon, M., McNeely, J. B., et al. (1988). Effect of nonnutritive sucking on behavioral state in preterm infants before feeding. *Nursing Research, 37,* 347-350.

GOLDSMITH, H. H., Buss, A. H., Plomin, R., Rothbart, M. K., Thomas, A., Chess, S., Hinde, R. A., & McCall, R. B. (1987). Roundtable: What is temperament? Four approaches. *Child Development, 58,* 505-529.

GOLDSMITH, H. H., & Campos, J. J. (1982). Toward a theory of infant temperament. In R. N. Emde & R. J. Harmon (Eds.), *The development of attachment and affiliative systems* (pp. 161-193). New York: Plenum.

GOLDSMITH, H. H., & Campos, J. J. (1986). Fundamental issues in the study of early temperament: The Denver Twin Temperament Study. In M. E. Lamb & A. Brown (Eds.), *Advances in developmental psychology* (pp. 231-283). Hillsdale, NJ: Lawrence Erlbaum.

GOLDSMITH, H. H., & Gottesman, I. I. (1981). Origins of variation in behavioral style: A longitudinal study of temperament in young twins. *Child Development, 52,* 91-103.

GOLUB, H. L., & Corwin, M. J. (1982). Infant cry: A clue to diagnosis. *Pediatrics, 69,* 197-201.

GOLUB, H. L., & Corwin, M. J. (1985). A physio-acoustic model of the infant cry. In B. M. Lester & C. F. Z. Boukydis (Eds.), *Infant crying: Theoretical and research perspectives* (pp. 59-82). New York: Plenum.

GORDON, N. S., & Bell, R. Q. (1961). Activity in the human newborn. *Psychological Reports, 9,* 103-106.

GORDON, T., & Foss, B. M. (1966). The role of stimulation in the delay of onset of crying in the newborn infant. *Quarterly Journal of Experimental Psychology, 18,* 79-81.

GRAHAM, F. K., Matarazzo, R. G., & Caldwell, B. M. (1956). Behavioral differences between normal and traumatized newborns: I. The test procedures. *Psychological Monographs, 70*(20, Whole No. 427).

GRAUER, T. T. (1989). Environmental lighting, behavioral state, and hormonal response in the newborn. *Scholarly Inquiry for Nursing Practice, 3,* 53-66.

GUERIN, D., & Gottfried, A. W. (1986, April). *Infant temperament as a predictor of preschool behavior problems.* Paper presented at the International Conference on Infant Studies, Los Angeles.

GUSTAFSON, G. E., & Harris, K. L. (1990). Women's responses to young infants' cries. *Developmental Psychology, 26,*

144-152.

HACK, M., Estabrook, M. M., & Robertson, S. S. (1985). Development of sucking rhythm in preterm infants. *Early Human Development, 11,* 133-140.

HETZER, H., & Tudor-Hart, B. H. (1927). Die Fruhesten reactionen auf die menschliche stimme. [The earliest reactions to the human voice.] *Quellen und Studien, 5,* 103-124.

HIATT, S., Campos, J., & Emde, R. (1979). Facial patterning and infant emotional expression: Happiness, surprise, and fear. *Child Development, 50,* 1020-1035.

HUBBARD, F. O. A., & van IJzendoorn, M. H. (1988, April). *Does maternal unresponsiveness increase infant crying?* Paper presented at the International Conference on Infant Studies, Washington, DC.

HUBBARD, F. O. A., & van IJzendoorn, M. H. (1990). Responsiveness to infant crying: Spoiling or comforting the baby? A descriptive longitudinal study in normal Dutch sample. In W. Koops, H. J. G. Soppe, J. L. van der Linden, P. C. M. Moelnaar, & J. J. F. Schroots (Eds.), *Developmental psychology behind the dikes.* Delft, Netherlands: Uitgeverij Eburon.

HUBERT, N. C., Wachs, T. D., & Peters-Martin, P. (1982). The study of early temperament: Measurement and conceptual issues. *Child Development, 49,* 571-600.

HUEBNER, R. R., & Izard, C. E. (1988). Mothers' responses to infants' facial expressions of sadness, anger, and physical distress. *Motivation and Emotion, 12,* 185-196.

HUITT, W. G., & Ashton, P. T. (1982). Parents' perception of infant temperament: A psychometric study. *Merrill-Palmer Quarterly, 28,* 95-109.

HUNTINGTON, L., Hans, S. L., & Zeskind, P. S. (1990). The relations among cry characteristics, demographic variables, and developmental test scores in infants prenatally exposed to methadone. *Infant Behavior and Development, 13,* 533-538.

HUTT, S. J., Lenard, H. G., & Prechtl, H. G. R. (1969). Psychophysiological studies in newborn infants. In L. P. Lipsitt & H. W. Reese (Eds.), *Advances in child development and behavior* (Vol. 4, pp. 128-172). New York: Academic Press.

IGNATOFF, E. (1980, April). *Effects of nonnutritive sucking on clinical course and Brazelton performance of ICU neonates.* Paper presented at the International Conference on Infant Studies, New Haven, CT.

IGNATOFF, E., & Field, T. (1982). Effects of non-nutritive sucking during tube feedings on the behavior and clinical course of ICU preterm neonates. In L. P. Lipsitt & T. Field (Eds.), *Infant behavior and development: Perinatal risk and newborn behavior.* Norwood, NJ: Ablex.

INGRAM, T. T. S. (1962). Clinical significance of the infantile feeding reflexes. *Developmental Medicine and Child Neurology, 4,* 159-169.

IRWIN, O. C. (1930). The amount and nature of activities of newborn infants under constant external stimulating conditions during the first ten days of life. *Genetic Psychology Monographs, 8,* 1-92.

ISHIKAWA, A., & Minamide, E. (1984). Correlation between fetal activity and the neonatal behavioral assessment scale. *Early Child Development and Care, 17,* 155-165.

IZARD, C. E., Hembree, E. A., Dougherty, L. M., & Spizzirri, C. C. (1983). Changes in facial expressions of 2- to 19-month-old infants following acute pain. *Developmental Psychology, 19,* 418-426.

IZARD, C. E., Huebner, R. R., Risser, D., McGinnes, G. C., & Dougherty, L. M. (1980). The young infant's ability to pro-

The Development of Basic Characteristics of Infants

243

duce discrete emotion expressions. Developmental Psychology, 16, 132-140.
JONES, S. S., & Raag, T. (1989). Smile production in older infants: The importance of a social recipient for the facial signal. Child Development, 60, 811-818.
JONES, S. S., Raag, T., & Collins, K. L. (1990). Smiling in older infants: Form and maternal response. Infant Behavior and Development, 13, 147-165.
KAGAN, J. (1971). Change and continuity in infancy. New York: John Wiley.
KAGAN, J. (1982). The construct of difficult temperament: A reply to Thomas, Chess, and Korn. Merrill-Palmer Quarterly, 28, 21-24.
KAGAN, J. (1989). Temperamental contribution to social behavior. American Psychologist, 44, 668-674.
KAGAN, J., Reznick, J. S., Clarke, C., Snidman, N., & Garcia-Coll, C. (1984). Behavioral inhibition to the unfamiliar. Child Development, 55, 2212-2225.
KAGAN, J., Reznick, J. S., & Snidman, N. (1988). Biological bases of childhood shyness. Science, 240, 167-171.
KAGAN, J., Reznick, J. S., & Snidman, N. (1989). Issues in the study of temperament. In G. A. Kohnstamm, J. E. Bates, & M. K. Rothbart (Eds.), Temperament in childhood. New York: John Wiley.
KAGAN, J., & Snidman, N. (1991). Infant predictors of inhibited and uninhibited profiles. Psychological Science, 2, 40-44.
KAZMEIER, K. J. (1973, March). Non-nutritive sucking patterns of jaundiced infants. Paper presented at the Sixth Annual Meeting of the Gatlinburg Conference on Research and Theory in Mental Retardation, Gatlinburg, TN.
KAZMEIER, K. J., Keenan, W. J., & Sutherland, J. M. (1977). Effects of elevated bilirubin and phototherapy on infant behavior. Pediatric Research, 11, 563.
KESSEN, W., Haith, M. M., & Salapatek, P. H. (1970). Infancy. In P. H. Mussen (Ed.), Carmichaels' manual of child psychology (Vol. 1, 3rd ed., pp. 287-445). New York: John Wiley.
KESSEN, W., Leutzendorff, A., & Stoutsenberger, K. (1967). Age, food deprivation, non-nutritive sucking and movement in the human newborn. Journal of Comparative Physiology and Psychology, 63, 82-86.
KESTENBERG, J. S. (1965). The role of movement patterns in development: I. Rhythms of movement. Psychoanalytic Quarterly, 34, 1-36.
KLAUS, M. H., Trause, M. A., & Kennell, J. H. (1975). Does human maternal behaviour after delivery show a characteristic pattern? In Parent-infant interaction (CIBA Foundation Symposium 33, New Series). Amsterdam: Elsevier.
KLEITMAN, N., & Engelmann, T. G. (1953). Sleep characteristics of infants. Journal of Applied Physiology, 6, 269-282.
KOEPKE, J. E., & Barnes, P. (1982). Amount of sucking when a sucking object is readily available to human newborns. Child Development, 53, 978-983.
KOPP, C. B. (1971, April). Inhibition of crying: A comparison of stimuli. Paper presented at the biennial meeting of the Society for Research in Child Development.
KOPP, C. B., Sigman, M., Parmelee, A. H., & Jeffrey, W. E. (1975). Neurological organization and visual fixation in infants at 40 weeks conceptional age. Developmental Psychology, 8, 165-170.
KOPP, C. B., & Vaughn, B. E. (1982). Sustained attention during exploratory manipulation as a predictor of cognitive development in preterm infants. Child Development, 53, 174-182.

KORNER, A. F. (1969). Neonatal startles, smiles, erections and reflex sucks as related to state, sex, and individuality. Child Development, 40, 1039-1053.
KORNER, A. F. (1972). State as variable, as obstacle, and as mediator of stimulation in infant research. Merrill-Palmer Quarterly, 18, 77-94.
KORNER, A. F., Brown, B. W., Reade, E. P., Stevenson, D. K., et al. (1988). State behavior of preterm infants as a function of development, individual and sex differences. Infant Behavior and Development, 11, 111-124.
KORNER, A. F., Kraemer, H. C., Haffner, M. E., & Thoman, E. B. (1974). Characteristics of crying and noncrying activity of full-term infants. Child Development, 45, 953-958.
KORNER, A. F., Kraemer, H. C., Reade, E. P., Forrest, T., Dimiceli, S., & Thom, V. (1987). A methodological approach to developing an assessment procedure for testing the neurobehavioral maturity of preterm infants. Child Development, 58, 1479-1487.
KORNER, A. F., & Thoman, E. B. (1972). Relative efficacy of contact and vestibular stimulation in soothing neonates. Child Development, 43, 443-453.
KORNER, A. F., Thoman, E. B., & Glick, J. H. (1974). A system for monitoring crying and noncrying, large medium, and small neonatal movements. Child Development, 45, 946-952.
KUSSMAUL, A. (1859). Unterschungen über das seelenleben des neugeborenen Menschen [Inquiries into the mental life of newborn humans]. Tübingen: Moser & C. F. Winter.
LAMB, M. E. (1978). Qualitative aspects of mother- and father-infant attachments. Infant Behavior and Development, 1, 51-59.
LAMB, M. E., & Malkin, C. M. (1986). The development of social expectations in distress-relief sequences: A longitudinal study. International Journal of Behavioral Development, 9, 235-249.
LAMPER, C., & Eisdorfer, C. (1971). Prestimulus activity level and responsivity in the neonate. Child Development, 42, 465-473.
LANCIONE, G. E., Horowitz, F. D., & Sullivan, J. W. (1980). The NBAS-K: I. A study of its stability and structure over the first month of life. Infant Behavior and Development, 3, 341-359.
LANDAU, R. (1982). Infant crying and fussing: Findings from a cross-cultural study. Journal of Cross-Cultural Psychology, 13, 427-444.
LARSON, S. K., Pizzo, S. L., & Gottfried, A. W. (1989, April). Infant temperament and developmental status from infancy through the early school years. Paper presented at the annual meeting of the Society for Research in Child Development, Kansas City, MO.
LENARD, H. G., Von Bernuth, H., & Prechtl, H. F. R. (1968). Reflexes and their relationships to behavioral state in the newborn. Acta Paediatrica Scandinavica, 55, 177-185.
LEPECQ, J. C., Rigoard, M. T., & Salzarulo, P. (1985). Spontaneous non-nutritive sucking in continuously fed infants. Early Human Development, 12, 279-284.
LESTER, B. M. (1987). Developmental outcome prediction from acoustic cry analysis in term and preterm infants. Pediatrics, 80, 529-534.
LESTER, B. M., Anderson, L. T., Boukydis, C. F. Z., Garcia-Coll, C. T., Vohr, B., & Peucker, M. (1989). Early detection of infants at risk for later handicap through acoustic cry analysis. Research in Infant Assessment, 25, 99-118.
LESTER, B. M., & Zeskind, P. S. (1982). Biobehavioral per-

spective on crying in early infancy. In H. E. Fitzgerald, B. M. Lester, & M. Yogman (Eds.), *Theory and research in behavioral pediatrics* (Vol. 1). New York: Plenum.

LEVY, D. M. (1928). Finger sucking and accessory movements in early infancy: An ethological study. *American Journal of Psychiatry, 7*, 881-918.

LEVY, D. M. (1958). *Behavioral analysis.* Springfield, IL: Charles C Thomas.

LEWIS, M., Bartels, B., & Goldberg, S. (1967). State as a determinant of infant's heart rate response to stimulation. *Science, 155*, 486-488.

LIND, J. (Ed.). (1965). Newborn infant cry [Special supplement]. *Acta Paediatrica Scandinavica* (Suppl. No. 163).

LIPSITT, L. P., & DeLucia, C. (1960). An apparatus for the measurement of specific responses and general activity of the human neonate. *American Journal of Psychology, 73*, 630-632.

LOUNSBURY, M. L., & Bates, J. E. (1982). The cries of infants of differing levels of perceived temperamental difficulties: Acoustic properties and effects on listeners. *Child Development, 53*, 677-686.

LUDEMANN, P. M., & Nelson, C. A. (1988). Categorical representation of facial expressions by 7-month-old infants. *Child Development, 24*, 492-501.

LYNIP, A. (1951). The use of magnetic devices in the collection and analysis of the preverbal utterances of an infant. *Genetic Psychology Monographs, 44*, 221-262.

MAJOR, D. R. (1906). *First steps in mental growth.* New York: Macmillan.

MATHENY, A. P., Riese, M. L., & Wilson, R. S. (1985). Rudiments of infant temperament: Newborn to 9 months. *Developmental Psychology, 21*, 486-494.

MATHENY, A. P., Wilson, R. S., & Nuss, S. M. (1984). Toddler temperament: Stability across settings and over ages. *Child Development, 55*, 1200-1211.

MAZIADE, M., Cote, R., Boutin, P., Bernier, H., & Thivierge, J. (1987). Temperament and intellectual development: A longitudinal study from infancy to four years. *American Journal of Psychiatry, 144*, 144-150.

McCALL, R. (1972). Smiling and vocalization in infants as indices of perceptual cognitive processes. *Merrill-Palmer Quarterly, 18*, 341-347.

McFARLANE, J. W., Allen, L., & Honzik, M. P. (1954). A developmental study of the behavior problems of normal children between 21 months and 14 years. *University of California Publications in Child Development, 2*, 1-122.

McGRADE, B. J. (1968). Newborn activity and emotional response at eight months. *Child Development, 39*, 1247-1252.

McKEE, J. P., & Honzik, M. P. (1963). The sucking behavior of mammals: An illustration of the nature-nurture question. In L. Postman (Ed.), *Psychology in the making: Histories of selected research problems.* New York: Knopf.

McKEEVER, N., & Gardner, J. M. (1991, April). *Shifts in neonatal visual pattern preference as a function of arousal.* Paper presented at the Society for Research in Child Development, Seattle.

McKENNA, J. J. (1987). An anthropological perspective on the sudden infant death syndrome: A testable hypothesis on the possible role of parental breathing cues in promoting infant breathing stability: I. *Pre- and Peri-Natal Psychology Journal, 2*, 93-135.

MICHAELIS, R., Parmelee, A. H., Stern, E., et al. (1973). Activity states in premature and term infants. *Developmental Psychobiology, 6*, 209-215.

MICHELSSON, K., Rinne, A., & Paajanen, S. (1990). Crying, feeding and sleeping patterns in 1- to 12-month-old infants. *Child Care, Health and Development, 16*, 99-111.

MINKOWSKI, M. (1922). Über frühzeitige bewegungen Reflexe und Muskulare reaktionen beim menschlichen Fötus und ihre Heiziehungen zum totalen Nerven- und Muskelsystem. [About the early movement reflexes and muscle reactions of the human fetus and their incorporation in the total nerve and muscle systems.] *Schweizer Medizinische Wochenschrift, 52*, 721-751.

MINKOWSKI, M. (1928). Neurobiologische Studien am menschlichen Fötus. [Neurobiological studies of the human fetus.] *Abderhalden's Handbuch der Biologishe Arbeitsmethoden, 5.*

MONEY, J., & Tucker, P. (1975). *Sexual signatures.* Boston: Little, Brown.

MOSS, H. A. (1967). Sex, age and state as determinants of mother-infant interaction. *Merrill-Palmer Quarterly, 13*, 19-36.

MOSS, H. A., & Robson, S. (1970). The relation between the amount of time infants spend at various states and the development of visual behavior. *Child Development, 41*, 509-517.

NELSON, C. A. (1985). The perception and recognition of facial expressions in infancy. In T. M. Field & N. A. Fox (Eds.), *Social perception in infants* (pp. 101-125). Norwood, NJ: Ablex.

NELSON, C. A. (1987). The recognition of facial expressions in the first two years of life: Mechanisms of development. *Child Development, 58*, 888-909.

NELSON, C. A., & Dolgin, K. (1985). The generalized discrimination of facial expressions by 7-month-old infants. *Child Development, 56*, 58-61.

NIJHUIS, J. G., Prechtl, H. F., Martin, C. B., & Bots, R. S. (1982). Are there behavioural states in the human fetus? *Early Human Development, 6*, 177-195.

OBERKLAID, F., Prior, M., & Sanson, A. (1986). Temperament of preterm versus full-term infants. *Journal of Developmental and Behavioral Pediatrics, 7*, 159-162.

ODENT, M. (1990). The unknown human infant. *Journal of Human Lactation, 6*, 6-8.

OSOFSKY, J. D. (1976). Neonatal characteristics and mother-infant interaction in two observational situations. *Child Development, 47*, 1138-1147.

OSOFSKY, J. D., & Danzger, B. (1974). Relationships between neonatal characteristics and mother-infant interaction. *Developmental Psychology, 10*, 124-130.

PAPOUŠEK, H., & PAPOUŠEK, M. (1987). Intuitive parenting: A dialectic counterpart to the infant's integrative competence. In J. D. Osofsky (Ed.), *Handbook of infant development* (2nd ed., pp. 669-720). New York: John Wiley.

PAPOUŠEK, M. (1989). Determinants of responsiveness to infant vocal expression of emotional state. *Infant Behavior and Development, 12*, 507-524.

PARMELEE, A. H., & Garbanati, J. (1986, July). *Clinical neurobehavioral aspects of state organization in newborn infants.* Paper presented at the Fifth International Symposium on Developmental Disabilities, Osaka, Japan.

PARMELEE, A. H., Jr., Schulz, H. R., & Disbrow, M. A. (1961). Sleep patterns of the new-born. *Journal of Pediatrics, 58*, 241-250.

PHILLIPS, R. D., Wagner, S. H., Fells, C. A., & Lynch, M. (1990). Do infants recognize emotion in facial expressions?

Categorical and "metaphorical" evidence. *Infant Behavior and Development, 13,* 71-84.

PLOMIN, R. (1982). The difficult concept of temperament: A response to Thomas, Chess, and Korn. *Merrill-Palmer Quarterly, 28,* 25-33.

PLOMIN, R. (1987). Developmental behavioral genetics and infancy. In J. D. Osofsky (Ed.), *Handbook of infant development* (2nd ed., pp. 363-414). New York: John Wiley.

PLOMIN, R., & Dunn, J. (1986). *The study of temperament: Changes, continuities and challenges.* Hillsdale, NJ: Lawrence Erlbaum.

PORTER, F. L., Miller, R. H., & Marshall, R. E. (1986). Neonatal pain cries: Effect of circumcision on acoustic features and perceived urgency. *Child Development, 57,* 790-802.

PORTER, F. L., Porges, S. W., & Marshall, R. E. (1988). Newborn pain cries and vagal tone: Parallel changes in response to circumcision. *Child Development, 59,* 495-505.

PRECHTL, H. F. R. (1958). The directed head turning response and allied movements of the human baby. *Behavior, 13,* 212-242.

PRECHTL, H. F. R. (1965). Problems of behavioral studies in the newborn infant. In D. S. Lehrman, R. A. Hinde, & E. Shaw (Eds.), *Advances in the study of behavior* (pp. 75-96). New York: Academic Press.

PRECHTL, H. F. R, Fargel, J. W., Weinman, H. M., & Bakker, H. H. (1979). Postures, motility and respiration of low-risk pre-term infants. *Developmental Medicine and Child Neurology, 21,* 3-27.

PRECHTL, H. F. R., Theorell, K., Gramsbergen, A., & Lind, J. (1969). A statistical analysis of cry patterns in normal and abnormal newborn infants. *Developmental Medicine and Child Neurology, 11,* 142-152.

PREYER, W. (1888). *The mind of the child: Part I. The senses and the will* (N. W. Brown, Trans.). New York: Appleton. (Original work published 1880)

PRIOR, M., Sanson, A., Oberklaid, F., & Northam, E. (1987). Measurement of temperament in one to three year old children. *International Journal of Behavioral Development, 10,* 121-132.

REBELSKY, F., & Black, R. (1972). Crying in infancy. *Journal of Genetic Psychology, 121,* 49-57.

RHEINGOLD, H. (1961). The effect of environmental stimulation upon the social and exploratory behaviour in the human infant. In B. M. Foss (Ed.), *Determinants of infant behaviour* (pp. 143-172). London: Methuen.

RICHARDS, J. E. (1985). The development of sustained visual attention in infants from 14 to 26 weeks of age. *Psychophysiology, 22,* 409-416.

RICHARDS, J. E. (1987). Infant visual sustained attention and respiratory sinus arrhythmia. *Child Development, 58,* 488-496.

RICHARDS, J. E. (1989). Development and stability in visual sustained attention in 14, 20, and 26 weeks old infants. *Psychophysiology, 26,* 422-430.

RICHARDS, T. W., & Newberry, H. (1938). Studies in fetal behavior: III. Can performance on test items at 6 months postnatally be predicted on the basis of fetal activity? *Child Development, 9,* 79-86.

RIESE, M. L. (1986). Implications of sex differences in neonatal temperament for early risk and developmental/environmental interactions. *Journal of Genetic Psychology, 147,* 507-513.

RIESE, M. L. (1987). Temperament stability between the neonatal period and 24 months. *Developmental Psychology, 23,* 216-222.

ROBERTSON, S. S. (1982). Intrinsic temporal patterning in the spontaneous movement of awake neonates. *Child Development, 53,* 1016-1021.

ROBERTSON, S. S. (1986). Human cyclic motility: Fetal-newborn continuities and newborn state differences. *Developmental Psychobiology, 20,* 425-442.

ROBERTSON, S. S. (1989, April). *The dynamics of newborn cyclic motor activity.* Paper presented at the biennial meeting of the Society for Research in Child Development.

ROSENBLITH, J. F. (1961a). *Manual for behavioral examination of the neonate as modified by Rosenblith from Graham.* Unpublished manuscript, Brown University Institute for Health Sciences.

ROSENBLITH, J. F. (1961b). The modified Graham behavior test for neonates: Test-retest reliability, normative data, and hypotheses for future work. *Biologia Neonatorum, 3,* 174-192.

ROSENBLITH, J. F., & Anderson-Huntington, R. B. (1975). Defensive reactions to stimulation of the nasal and oral region in newborns: Relations to state. In J. Bosma & J. Showacre (Eds.), *Development of upper respiratory anatomy and function: Implications for sudden infant death syndrome* (pp. 250-263). Washington, DC: Government Printing Office.

ROSS, S. (1951). Sucking behavior in neonate dogs. *Journal of Abnormal and Social Psychology, 46,* 142-149.

ROTHBART, M. K. (1973). Laughter in young children. *Psychological Bulletin, 80,* 247-256.

ROTHBART, M. K. (1982). The concept of difficult temperament: A critical analysis of Thomas, Chess, and Korn. *Merrill-Palmer Quarterly, 28,* 35-40.

ROTHBART, M. K. (1984, April). Temperament and the development of behavioral inhibition. In M. K. Rothbart (Chair), *Developmental perspectives on infant temperament.* Symposium conducted at the International Conference on Infant Studies, New York.

ROTHBART, M. K. (1986). Longitudinal observation of infant temperament. *Developmental Psychology, 22,* 356-365.

ROTHBART, M. K., & Derryberry, D. (1981). Development of individual differences in temperament. In M. Lamb & A. Brown (Eds.), *Advances in developmental psychology.* Hillsdale, NJ: Lawrence Erlbaum.

RUDDY, M. G., & Bornstein, M. H. (1982). Cognitive correlates of infant attention and maternal stimulation over the first year of life. *Child Development, 53,* 183-188.

RUFF, H. A., & Lawson, K. R. (1990). Development of sustained focused attention in young children during free play. *Developmental Psychology, 26,* 83-93.

RUFF, H. A., Lawson, K. R., Parrinello, R., & Weissberg, R. (1990). Long-term stability of individual differences in sustained attention in the early years. *Child Development, 61,* 60-75.

ST. JAMES-ROBERTS, I. (1989). Persistent crying in infancy. *Journal of Child Psychology and Psychiatry and Allied Disciplines, 30,* 189-195.

ST. JAMES-ROBERTS, I., & Wolke, D. (1988). Convergences and discrepancies among mothers' and professionals' assessments of difficult neonatal behavior. *Journal of Child Psychology and Psychiatry, 29,* 21-42.

SAMEROFF, A. J. (1968). The components of sucking in the human newborn. *Journal of Experimental Psychology, 6,* 607-

623.

SANSON, A., Prior, M., & Kyrios, M. (1990). Further exploration of the link between temperament and behavior problems: A reply to Bates. *Merrill-Palmer Quarterly, 36,* 573-576.

SAUDINO, K. J., & Eaton, W. O. (1989, July). *Heredity and infant activity level: An objective twin study.* Paper presented at the meeting of the International Society for the Study of Behavioral Development, Jyvaskyla, Finland.

SAUDINO, K. J., & Eaton, W. O. (in press). Infant temperament and genetics: An objective twin study of motor activity level. *Child Development.*

SCARR, S., & Salapatek, P. (1970). Patterns of fear development during infancy. *Merrill-Palmer Quarterly, 16,* 53-90.

SCHMIDT, W., Boos, R., Gnirs, A., Auer, L., & Schulze, S. (1985). Fetal behavioral states and controlled sound stimulation. In Ultrasound studies of human fetal behavior [Special issue]. *Early Human Development, 12,* 145-153.

SCHULTZ, T. R., & Zigler, E. (1970). Emotional concomitants of visual mastery in infants: The effects of stimulus movement on vocalizing. *Journal of Experimental Child Psychology, 10,* 390-402.

SEARS, R. R., & Wise, G. (1950). Relation of cup feeding in infancy to thumb sucking and the oral drive. *American Journal of Orthopsychiatry, 20,* 123-138.

SEWELL, W. H., & Mussen, P. H. (1952). The effects of feeding, weaning and scheduling procedures on childhood adjustment and the formation of oral symptoms. *Child Development, 23,* 185-191.

SIGMAN, M. (1983). Individual differences in infant attention: Relations to birth status and intelligence at five years. In T. Field & A. Sostek (Eds.), *Infants born at risk: Physiological, perceptual and cognitive processes* (pp. 271-293). New York: Grune & Stratton.

SIGMAN, M., & Beckwith, L. (1980). Infant visual attentiveness in relation to caregiver infant interaction and developmental outcome. *Infant Behavior and Development, 3,* 141-154.

SIGMAN, M., Cohen, S. E., Beckwith, L., & Parmelee, A. H. (1986). Infant attention in relation to intellectual abilities in childhood. *Developmental Psychology, 22,* 788-792.

SIGMAN, M., Kopp, C. V., Parmelee, A. H., & Jeffrey, W. E. (1973). Visual attention and neurological organization in neonates. *Child Development, 44,* 461-466.

SIMSARIAN, F. P. (1947). Case histories of five thumbsucking children breast fed on unscheduled regimes, without limitation of nursing time. *Child Development, 18,* 180-184.

SKARD, A. G. (1966). Orality in the first nine years of life. *Nordisk Psykologi Monografiserien, 20.*

SKINNER, B. F. (1945). Baby in a box. *Ladies' Home Journal, 62,* 30-31.

SMITH, B. A., Fillion, T. J., & Blass, E. M. (1990). Orally mediated sources of calming in 1- to 3-day-old infants. *Developmental Psychology, 26,* 731-737.

SOKEN, N., Pick, A., Bigbee, M., Melendez, P., & Hansen, A. (1991, April). *The perception of happy, angry, and neutral expressions by 7-month-olds: The role of visual and vocal information.* Paper presented at the meetings of the International Society for the Study of Behavioral Development, Minneapolis.

SROUFE, L. A., & Waters, E. (1976). The ontogenesis of smiling and laughter: A perspective on the organization of development in infancy. *Psychological Review, 83,* 173-189.

SROUFE, L. A., & Wunsch, J. P. (1972). The development of laughter in the first year of life. *Child Development, 43,* 1326-1344.

STERN, E., Parmelee, A. H., Akiyama, Y., Shultz, M. A., & Wenner, W. H. (1969). Sleep cycle characteristics in infants. *Pediatrics, 43,* 65-70.

STERNBERG, C. R., Campos, J. J., & Emde, R. N. (1983). The facial expressions of anger in seven-month-old infants. *Child Development, 54,* 178-184.

STIFTER, C. A., Fox, N. A., & Porges, S. W. (1989). Facial expressivity and vagal tone in 5- and 10-month-old infants. *Infant Behavior and Development, 12,* 127-137.

TERMINE, N. T., & Izard, C. E. (1988). Infants' responses to their mothers' expressions of joy and sadness. *Developmental Psychology, 24,* 223-229.

THELEN, E. (1981). Rhythmical behavior in infancy: An ethological perspective. *Developmental Psychology, 17,* 237-257.

THOMAN, E. B. (1990). Sleeping and waking states in infants: A functional perspective. *Neuroscience and Biobehavioral Reviews, 14,* 93-107.

THOMAN, E. B., Denenberg, V. H., Sievel, J., Zeidner, L. P., & Becker, P. T. (1981). State organization in neonates: Developmental inconsistency indicates risk for developmental dysfunction. *Neuropediatrics, 12,* 45-54.

THOMAN, E. B., & Glazier, R. C. (1987). Computer scoring of motility patterns for states of sleep and wakefulness: Human infants. *Sleep, 10,* 122-129.

THOMAN, E. B., & Whitney, M. P. (1989). Sleep states of infants monitored in the home: Individual differences, developmental trends, and origins of diurnal cyclicity. *Infant Behavior and Development, 12,* 59-75.

THOMAS, A. (1982). The study of difficult temperament: A reply to Kagan, Rothbart, and Plomin. *Merrill-Palmer Quarterly, 28,* 313-315.

THOMAS, A., & Chess, S. (1977). *Temperament and development.* New York: Brunner/Mazel.

THOMAS, A., Chess, S., & Birch, H. G. (1968). *Temperament and behavior disorders in children.* New York: New York University Press.

THOMAS, A., Chess, S., Birch, H. G., Hertzig, M. E., & Korn, S. (1963). *Behavioral individuality in early childhood.* New York: New York University Press.

THOMAS, A., Chess, S., & Korn, S. J. (1982). The reality of difficult temperament. *Merrill-Palmer Quarterly, 28,* 1-20.

THOMPSON, J. (1903). On the lip-reflex (mouth phenomenon) of newborn children. *Revue of Neurological Psychiatry, 1,* 145.

TRONICK, E. Z. (1989). Emotions and emotional communication in infants. *American Psychologist, 44,* 112-119.

TRUBY, H. M. (1959). Acoustico-cineradiographic analysis considerations. *Acta Radiologica, Supplements, 182*(69).

TRUBY, H. M. (1960). *Some aspects of acoustical and cineradiographical analysis of newborn infant and adult phonation and associated vocal-tract activity.* Paper presented at the annual meeting of the Acoustical Society of America.

TYNAN, W. D. (1986). Behavioral stability predicts morbidity and mortality in infants from a neonatal intensive care unit. *Infant Behavior and Development, 9,* 71-79.

VAN VLIET, M. A., Martin, C. B., Jr., Nijhuis, J. G., & Prechtl, H. F. (1985a). Ultrasound studies of human fetal behaviour: The relationship between fetal activity and behavioral states and fetal breathing movements in normal and growth-retarded fetuses. *American Journal of Obstetrics and Gynecology,*

153, 582-588.

VAN VLIET, M. A., Martin, C. B., Jr., Nijhuis, J. G., & Prechtl, H. F. (1985b). Behavioral states in the fetuses of nulliparous women. *Early Human Development, 12*, 121-135.

VAUGHN, B. E., Bradley, C. F., Joffe, L. S., Seifer, R., & Barglow, P. (1987). Maternal characteristics measured prenatally are predictive of ratings of temperamental "difficulty" on the Carey Infant Temperament Questionnaire. *Developmental Psychology, 23*, 152-161.

WACHS, T. D., & Gandour, M. J. (1983). Temperament, environment, and six-month cognitive-intellectual development: A test of the organismic specificity hypothesis. *International Journal of Behavioral Development, 6*, 135-152.

WALTERS, C. E. (1965). Prediction of postnatal development from fetal activity. *Child Development, 36*, 801-801.

WASHBURN, R. W. (1929). A study of the smiling and laughing of infants in the first year of life. *Genetic Psychology Monographs, 6*, 397-535.

WASZ-HOCKERT, O., Lind, J., Vuorenkoski, V., Partanen, T., & Valanne, E. (1968). *The infant cry.* London: Spastics International Medical Publications.

WATSON, J. B. (1937). *Behaviorism.* Chicago: University of Chicago Press.

WATT, J. E., & Strongman, K. T. (1985). The organization and stability of sleep states in fullterm, preterm, and small-for-gestational-age infants: A comparative study. *Developmental Psychobiology, 18*, 151-162.

WEISS, A. P. (1929). The measurement of infant behavior. *Psychological Review, 36*, 453-471.

WEISSBLUTH, M. (1983). Sleep duration and infant temperament. In S. Chess & A. Thomas (Eds.), *Annual progress in child psychiatry and child development* (pp. 383-387). New York: Brunner/Mazel.

WHITE, R. (1959). Motivation reconsidered: The concept of competence. *Psychological Review, 66*, 297-333.

WHITNEY, M. P., Acebo, C., & Thoman, E. B. (1990, April). *Early state characteristics: Relationships between neonatal state patterns and later developmental dysfunction.* Paper presented at International Conference on Infant Studies, Montreal.

WHYTE, H. E., Pearce, J. M., & Taylor, M. J. (1987). Changes in the VEP in preterm neonates with arousal states, as assessed by EEG monitoring. *Electroencephalography and Clinical Neurophysiology, 68*, 223-225.

WIESENFELD, A. R., Malatesta, C. Z., & DeLoache, L. L. (1981). Differential parental response to familiar and unfamiliar infant distress signals. *Infant Behavior and Development, 4*, 281-295.

WILSON, C. D. (1931). *A study of laughter situations among young children.* Unpublished doctoral dissertation, University of Nebraska.

WOLFF, P. H. (1959). Observations on newborn infants. *Psychosomatic Medicine, 21*, 110-118.

WOLFF, P. H. (1963). Observations on the early development of smiling. In B. Foss (Ed.), *Determinants of infant behaviour* (Vol. 2, pp. 113-138). London: Methuen.

WOLFF, P. H. (1966). The causes, controls, and organization of behavior in the neonate. *Psychological Issues, 5*(Whole No. 7).

WOLFF, P. H. (1969). The natural history of crying and other vocalizations in early infancy. In B. M. Foss (Ed.), *Determinants of infant behaviour* (Vol. 4, pp. 81-109). London: Methuen.

WOODSON, R., Drinkwin, J., & Hamilton, C. (1985). Effects of nonnutritive sucking on state and activity: Term-preterm comparisons. *Infant Behavior and Development, 8*, 435-444.

WOROBEY, J., & Blajda, V. M. (1989). Temperament ratings at 2 weeks, 2 months, and 1 year: Differential stability of activity and emotionality. *Developmental Psychology, 25*, 257-263.

WOROBEY, J., & Lewis, M. (1989). Individual differences in the reactivity of young infants. *Developmental Psychology, 25*, 663-667.

YARROW, L. J. (1954). The relationship between nutritive sucking experiences in infancy and non-nutritive sucking in childhood. *Journal of Genetic Psychology, 84*, 149-162.

YOGMAN, M. W., & Zeisel, S. A. (1983). Diet and sleep patterns in new-born infants. *New England Journal of Medicine, 309*, 1147-1149.

YOKOCHI, K., Shiroiwa, Y., Inukai, K., Kito, H., et al. (1989). Behavioral state distribution throughout 24-hr video recordings in preterm infants at term with good prognosis. *Early Human Development, 19*, 183-190.

ZELAZO, P. R., & Komer, M. J. (1971). Infant smiling to nonsocial stimuli and the recognition hypothesis. *Child Development, 42*, 1327-1339.

ZESKIND, P. S. (1980). Adult responses to cries of low-risk and high-risk infants. *Infant Behavior and Development, 3*, 167-177.

ZESKIND, P. S. (1987). Adult heart-rate responses to infant cry sounds. *British Journal of Developmental Psychology, 5*, 73-79.

ZESKIND, P. S., & Collins, V. (1987). Pitch of infant crying and caregiver responses in a natural setting. *Infant Behavior and Development, 10*, 501-504.

ZESKIND, P. S., & Lester, B. M. (1978). Acoustic features and auditory perception of the cries of newborns with prenatal and perinatal complications. *Child Development, 49*, 580-589.

ZESKIND, P. S., & Marshall, T. R. (1988). The relation between variations in pitch and maternal perceptions of infant crying. *Child Development, 59*, 193-196.

ZESKIND, P. S., Sale, J., Maio, M. L., Huntington, L., & Weiseman, J. R. (1984, April). *Adult perceptions of pain and hunger cries: A synchrony of arousal.* Paper presented at the International Conference on Infant Studies, New York.

ZIVIN, G. (1982). Watching the sands shift: Conceptualizing development of nonverbal mastery. In R. S. Feldman (Ed.), *Development of nonverbal behavior in children.* New York: Springer-Verlag.

Chapter 7

Sensory and Perceptual Abilities

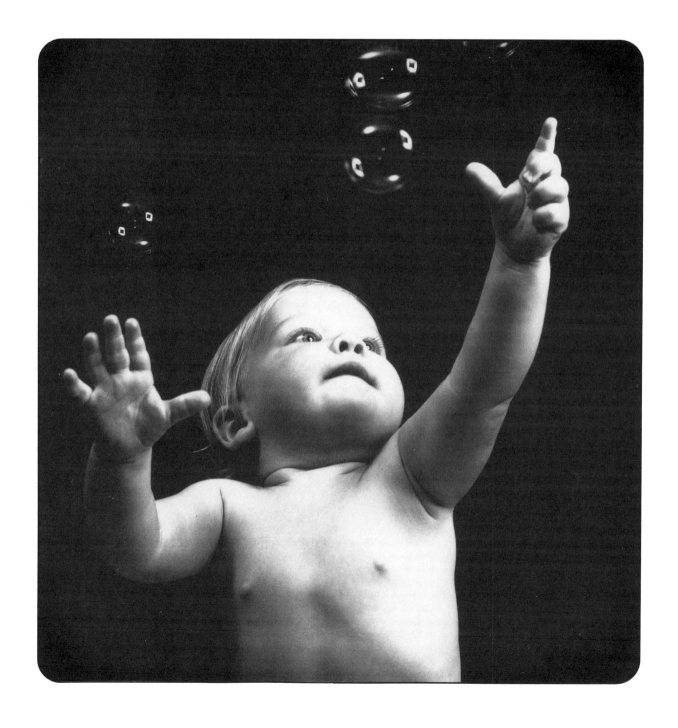

This chapter explores the abilities to touch, taste, smell, hear, and see. Three major questions have been asked in the research. First: What is the state of these sensory systems at birth? All of them function, and in many ways they are remarkably mature. Each system will be considered in turn.

Given that the sensory systems function, the second question is: What do infants perceive from the information their senses provide? It is possible that infants may see, hear, touch, and so forth, in a purely reflexive fashion. Alternatively, they may be able to attach some meaning to the information their senses process, and it is even possible that babies at birth are biologically preprogrammed to attach meaning to some stimuli. For example, if babies reach for something they see, does this imply that they know the object is at some point distant from themselves? Do they know that the thing that makes soft, appealing noises (the female voice) is part of the same object that has a peculiar configuration of what adults would call eyes, nose, and mouth? If they recognize the configuration of the human face, do they recognize it as belonging to one of their own kind?

The third major question is: What is the course of development of these sensory and perceptual systems over the first months and years of life? Although all five senses function at birth, none is totally mature; all undergo subsequent development. For example, if newborns are not able to recognize their mothers, when do they develop this ability and what do they need to learn in order to accomplish this goal?

Importance of Studying Sensory and Perceptual Development

Scientists explore the three questions outlined above for four important reasons. One is that the information is of practical use in medicine. Data about normative development, and about the amount and kind of perceptual development typical of infants of a given age, are needed if we are to be able to assess when development goes awry. Knowing the normal status of perceptual development at birth allows medical researchers to assess the influences of various prenatal factors and provides a way to predict later developmental outcome on the basis of the status at birth. Because the perceptual capacities are so highly developed at birth, they may be a good measure of general level of maturation and may become even better measures as new and better techniques by which to assess them are developed. Perception tests are also used to predict later cognitive development, as will be discussed in Chapter 8.

A second reason to study perceptual development is its relevance to traditional issues in psychology and philosophy concerning the basic nature of knowledge. For example, research on perception has been used to test empirically whether the basic ways humans structure the world (e.g., as objects that exist in a three-dimensional world) is innate or learned. **Empiricists** believe that everything humans know has to be learned, including depth perception and the understanding of what an object is. They argue that newborn babies are not able to perceive depth, nor would they know that a red, round ball they see is an object. They therefore do not know that what they see can be grasped and what they grasp can be seen, or that what they hear can be seen. In contrast, **nativists** believe that experience is not necessary for humans to have knowledge of spatial relations and objects. They believe that humans directly perceive depth and that, without having to learn, they know that objects have both visual and tactile aspects. Much research on perception in newborns is designed to see whether newborns act as if they already organize the world into objects in a three-dimensional space.

A third reason to do research in perceptual development is to assess the influences of environment on development. One of the most popular beliefs in all of developmental psychology is that the period of infancy is particularly important for the development of later functions. Some investigators focus on whether inadequate stimulation results in deficiencies in psychological development, while others are more interested in whether enriched environments improve it. Regardless of the focus, it is important to identify appropriate kinds of stimulation. To do this we need to know the nature of perceptual development. We now know that newborns look longer at patterned than at plain stimuli and at objects with a lot of contour (e.g., many sides) than at objects with little contour. Only when the basic perceptual capacities of infants are understood can we design stimuli to test adequately the role of environmental stimulation on development.

The fourth reason to do research on perceptual development is to understand more about other aspects of development, namely, affective, linguistic, and cognitive development. The so-called older senses (ones that are highly represented in the older parts of the brain) of smell, tactile sensitivity, and taste play an important role in our emotional lives. Despite the current increase in research interest in affective behaviors, few links to perceptual data have been forged. It is our hope that the current research in affective development will stimulate more work on the older senses (see Porter et al., 1988, for a similar plea for olfaction).

The auditory system is important for emotional development because it is a primary in much social interaction, but little research to date has focused on this. It is the means by which language is usually learned. The development of auditory capacities to process language begins at birth, or even before, and continues throughout infancy, even though infants do not start producing words before the end of their first year (see Chapter 11). Audition is also important for cognitive development, although research on its influence has focused on language and has relatively rarely explored the role of nonlinguistic auditory stimuli. All perceptual development is important for cognitive development, because all of infants' knowledge of the world must be obtained through their senses. Vision, the most widely studied sense, is crucial to the conception of the Piagetian stages of infancy (see Chapter 10).

Before turning to the research techniques used in these studies, we would like to call attention to the fact that an entire two-volume handbook has been devoted to infant perception (Salapatek & Cohen, 1987a, 1987b), and another entire book to measurement of vision and audition in the first year (Gottlieb & Krasnegor, 1985).

Research Techniques

To understand the research that explores infants' sensations and perceptions, it is necessary to know how researchers study and learn about infants' abilities, particularly those of newborns. They cannot talk or answer questions, they cannot locomote, and they have poor motor coordination. How, then, do researchers find out what infants can detect in the different sense modalities? Historically, the standard technique was naturalistic observation of the limited responses infants can make. Babies can move their eyes, blink, startle, cry, suck, turn their heads, pull their feet back, and so on. If babies make these responses immediately after some event in the environment, people infer that they are responding to that event and therefore perceiving it. Such simple techniques are limited in three ways. The first two limitations were discussed in Chapter 6: First, the observations may be unreliable; that is, observers may not always agree that the response in question has occurred. Second, the responses are not easily quantified. The third limitation is that it is impossible to tell what the infants have responded to. They may have responded only to the change from no stimulation to stimulation or to aspects of the stimulus that differ from those noted by the adults. That leaves unan-

swered such questions as, Do infants perceive color? Can they discriminate sweet from sour?

In the 1930s it became possible to study unseen responses such as heart rate, and the 1960s brought new advances, especially those related to computer processing of heart rate or EEG responses. Infrared photography, developed in the Vietnam era, enables study of what infants' eyes are focused on and how well. Thus it is now possible to study many aspects of physiological responses to sensory stimuli that could not be studied before.

Psychologists commonly use three basic techniques—preference, habituation, and conditioning (in different forms)—to study babies' sensory and perceptual abilities. Each will be discussed here in turn and compared with the others.

The simplest of the three is the **preference technique**, used primarily in the study of visual stimuli. Two stimuli are presented side by side. Infants, even newborns, look from one to the other of these stimuli. Both the number of times and the length of time they look at each stimulus can be measured. Basically this involves a sophisticated use of observational techniques combined with an experimental design for stimulus presentation. Photographic techniques can be used to determine when infants are actually looking at a stimulus by measuring the reflection of the stimulus on the infant's eye and timing its presence there very accurately (see Maurer's 1975 review of techniques, or Gottlieb & Krasnegor, 1985). If infants look at one stimulus longer (or more times) than they look at the other, one can conclude that they can discriminate between those two stimuli and that for some reason they find one more intriguing. If infants fail to show a visual preference, no clear interpretation can be made. Either they are unable to discriminate between the stimuli or they find them equally interesting.

Because this technique requires simultaneous presentation of two stimuli, it is most appropriate for visual stimuli. Preference techniques can be adapted for use with other senses. For example, in taste discrimination infants can be offered two fluids in alternation (with a pause between) and the amount they consume of each can be used as a measure of their preference for it. In such studies, half the sample of infants should have one substance offered first and the other half should have the second substance first, to control for satiation effects. Preference techniques can also be used to study responses to smell and sounds, although measuring infants' tendencies to turn toward or away from the stimulus would be cruder than the response measures for visual and taste stimuli.

The second technique is the **habituation-dishabit-**

uation paradigm, which will be discussed in greater detail in Chapter 9. It can be used to test infants' abilities to discriminate between two similar stimuli by habituating the infants to one (that is, presenting it until their responses are greatly diminished) and then presenting the other. If they perceive the second stimulus as different, they will dishabituate or again respond. If they do not perceive the new stimulus as different, they will continue to exhibit little or no response. Since the two stimuli are presented successively, the habituation-dishabituation paradigm is a good choice for studies of hearing and smelling. There has been some argument over whether habituation might not represent fatigue of relevant aspects of the sensory or motor apparatus. If so, the dishabituation stimulus might be responded to not because the infant discriminates, but because a different part of the sensory apparatus responds. Dishabituation to a lower level of stimulation would not occur if the sensory system were fatigued; indeed, stronger stimulation would be needed to produce a response. Thus the fact that even newborns dishabituate to a softer sounding of the same stimulus argues strongly against fatigue as an explanation (Tarquinio et al., 1990).

The third technique involves operant conditioning (see Chapter 9). In **discriminative learning**, operant conditioning is used to train infants to discriminate between two or more stimuli. In one type, infants are trained to respond when one stimulus is present and not to respond when it is absent. In another form, they are trained to make one response in the presence of one stimulus and a different response in the presence of a second stimulus. If an infant can be trained to respond differentially to the presence or absence of a stimulus or to two different stimuli, then we can conclude that the infant can discriminate between them.

Training infants to make discriminative responses is a time-consuming task. Luckily, conditioning also provides another, easier technique for testing infants' discriminative abilities. It uses the aspect of the conditioning paradigm called **generalization**. Once infants are conditioned to respond to a particular stimulus, they will also respond to stimuli that are similar to the original. If, for example, they are trained to turn their heads when they see a square, they are also likely to turn their heads when they see a rectangle. The tendency to generalize in this way is so strong that subjects' responses form a generalization gradient, such that the more similar a stimulus is to the training stimulus, the stronger the subjects' responses, and the more dissimilar it is, the weaker the response until it becomes so dissimilar that there is no response. Thus

generalization provides two kinds of information. First, it tells us whether infants perceive two stimuli to be similar or different, just as the preference and habituation-dishabituation paradigms do. Second, it can provide comparative responses; that is, it can tell which among several stimuli are perceived by infants to be most similar to the training stimulus.

Classical conditioning is probably the least popular measurement technique, because establishing the basic conditioned response is time-consuming with young infants. It is, however, the best technique to use when one wants to establish the degree to which stimuli are perceived to be similar or to be different. Operant conditioning is intermediate in difficulty and depends on the response being conditioned. (See Chapter 9 for a discussion.)

Tactile Sensitivity (The Skin Senses)

We start with tactile sensitivity, or the skin senses. A variety of sensory nerve endings located just below the surface of the skin convert mechanical energy into electrical signals that travel to the brain. Their greatest concentrations are in the tongue, lips, palms, fingertips, nipples, clitoris, and tip of the penis.

One reason to discuss skin senses first is the fact that they are first to appear during fetal development (Gottlieb, 1971), especially in the region around the mouth (perioral region), where responsiveness is present by the eighth week of intrauterine development. Aversive reactions to being touched in other areas by an amniocentesis needle are present in the third trimester (Birnholz, 1988). Primacy of the tactile sense is demonstrated by the fact that older infants can judge tactile stimulation for self, other, and in reality a year younger than they can make these discriminations in the visual modality (Flavell et al., 1989). The presence or absence of any differences between the sexes in sensitivity to stimuli in this domain will also be considered here, because many people believe that there are such differences, and some people have built them into their theories of sex differences. We will also return to these senses in the discussion of maternal interaction and attachment in Chapter 12.

Cutaneous senses are also old, inasmuch as they have been studied since early in the scientific study of infancy. Renewed interest in them occurred as part of the wave of neonatal and infancy studies that started in the 1920s (Dockeray & Rice, 1934; Pratt, cited in Kessen et al., 1970; Sherman & Sherman, 1925; Sherman et al., 1936).

Much of the early research explored responses designated as pain responses. One of the major motivations was to determine whether newborns experience pain. Many doctors and nurses have been indoctrinated with the idea that newborns do not feel pain. One result of this is that they have assured mothers that various medical procedures (including circumcision) do not hurt infants. Some have expostulated on the wonderful design of nature, which makes the fetus/newborn insensitive to pain, hence not responsive to the pain of being born (or circumcised, or operated on). Others remain unconvinced. If babies do not feel pain, why do baby boys scream so violently when they are circumcised? Why are they so hard to rouse from sleep afterward? And why are they so irritable when roused that one gives up on trying to get them into a state suitable for neonatal testing? The denial that neonates feel pain goes so far that the medical profession does major surgery using only muscle relaxants and perhaps a little nitrous oxide. To be sure, originally this was done to protect the baby from the dangers of anesthetics, but the belief became so strong that the practice persisted after anesthesia became safe. An editorial in the November 1987 issue of the *New England Journal of Medicine* said the evidence was "so overwhelming that physicians can no longer act as if all infants were indifferent to pain."

In part, the erroneous belief that babies do not feel pain stemmed from labeling responses to relatively mild aversive stimuli as studies of pain. Often the stimuli were slight pinpricks that were not sufficiently strong to elicit crying, other signs of bodily discomfort, or even pulling away. Recent studies have examined responses to the painful stimuli of heel sticks, immunization shots, and circumcision. These studies have often addressed questions of the type of reaction shown, how that changed over time, and whether there was individual stability in reactivity over time (as discussed in Chapter 6) rather than whether the babies felt pain.

Indeed, it is now considered a fact that while babies may not experience pain the same way older organisms do, they feel pain. Indeed, boys respond with sharp rises in plasma cortisol levels (a stress response) to being circumcised (Gunnar et al., 1985). However, these levels subside quite rapidly, hence cannot ac-

count for the more lasting effects on behavior that are found.

A longitudinal study of facial expressions in response to immunization shots at 2, 4, 6, and 19 months (discussed in Chapter 6) showed that expressions of pain and anger predominated at all ages and accounted for 75% of all codable responses (Izard et al., 1987). Infants who took long to soothe showed more anger responses than those who were quickly soothed. The effects of circumcision on the behaviors assessed on the NBAS have been evaluated according to whether anesthesia was used or not (Dixon et al., 1984). Those who received local anesthetics were more attentive to animate and inanimate stimuli and better able to quiet themselves when disturbed, both on the day of circumcision and the next. Both swaddling and pacifiers reduce the heart rate and crying responses to heel sticks at 2 days and inoculations at 2 months, but their effects differ (Campos, 1989). It is possible that sucrose may serve as a way to reduce pain responses without administering drugs (this is discussed below, in the section on taste).

Let us now survey some of the earlier research that may indicate tactile responsiveness rather than pain responses. Early studies used pinpricks in different regions of the body and counted the number of pricks necessary to obtain withdrawal or avoidance. Different studies found opposite effects. Sensitivity was found to increase with age by Sherman and colleagues (Sherman & Sherman, 1925; Sherman et al., 1936), but not to change by Dockeray and Rice (1934). The head area was most sensitive and all extremities were less sensitive, according to Sherman and colleagues, which makes theoretical sense in terms of cephalocaudal development. Dockeray and Rice found an inverse cephalocaudal sensitivity, with legs more sensitive than arms or head.

More recent work on pain thresholds has used mild electric shock, which, in principle, can be much better controlled than pinpricks.[1] Sensitivity (in an area just below the kneecap) increased with age over the first 5 days of life (Graham et al., 1956; Lipsitt & Levy, 1959). Lipsitt and Levy did another study using different babies on different days to eliminate possible confounding from repeat testing of the same infants. Experience in the testing situation could result either in sensitization or conditioning, either of which (rather than age or maturation) might account for increased sensitivity. Results were equivocal, inasmuch as babies tested on day 3 were more sensitive than those tested on day 2, but also more than those tested on day 4.

Skin conductance (the mechanism by which the

---

1. In fact, the precision may be more apparent than real because of different amounts of fat under the electrode, different degrees of closeness to nerve endings, or imperfect contact.

electric current is transmitted) is directly related to sweat gland function, which in turn is affected by a wide variety of factors, including activity level and state of wakefulness. Since both increase in the first few days of life, they could lead to changes in sweat gland activity, which would be related to an apparent increased sensitivity. Early work in this area left many problems unresolved, but stimulated Kaye (1964; Kaye & Lipsitt, 1964) to use a variety of electrode placements in areas with different amounts of fat pad and sweat glands. An apparent increase in sensitivity with age (with marked individual differences) was found whether one group was studied longitudinally or different groups were tested on each day. The developmental change in sensitivity to aversive stimulation appeared to be produced by a developmental change in skin conductance resulting from an increase in general arousal level. Anoxia and drugs used during delivery, both of which affect sweat gland functioning, affected the developmental course of sensitivity. The data were not analyzed according to the infants' sex or state of arousal at the time the measurements were made, which might also have influenced the findings.

A different kind of aversive stimulation has been used in two of the neonatal assessment batteries, the Brazelton (NBAS) and the Graham/Rosenblith (G/R) test. In the NBAS, movements that appear to be directed toward getting rid of a cloth over the face are assessed. In the G/R, defensive responses elicited by two stimuli (cotton, which is held over the nostrils and reaches just to the top of the lip, and cellophane, which is held across the baby's face from just above the nostrils, but not touching eyes, to just below the mouth) are assessed. Newborns usually respond vigorously with various movements (including withdrawal responses analogous to those resulting from mild electrical stimulation) that would normally get rid of the stimulus (Rosenblith & DeLucia, 1963). Although the G/R scale was called Tactile-Adaptive (TA), the stimuli combine tactile stimulation with partial blocking of air supply, and so do not provide "pure" measures of tactile sensitivity. Evaluation of responses in the naso-oral region to purely tactile stimuli has not been carried out.

Evidence for sex differences has been inconclusive. On the G/R Rosenblith and DeLucia (1963) found no sex differences on the TA scale in normal babies examined at from 2 to 96 hours of age. Girls were more sensitive than boys in one of the Lipsitt and Levy (1959) studies. Even these weak sex differences might be an artifact, because male babies are, on average, heavier than females, hence may have more subcutaneous fat, which would interfere with the electric cur-

rent and make them appear less sensitive. On the other hand, the only sex difference in response to immunization shots, where fat pads are no protection, was that males showed twice as many pain as anger responses, whereas girls had the opposite pattern (Izard et al., 1987). These are older infants, and the stimuli are different. One could argue that girls show more anger responses because anger has a larger cognitive component and girls are cognitively more advanced.

In summary, a number of increasingly sophisticated studies have failed to find strong evidence that sensitivity to aversive tactile stimulation increases during the first several days of life. Studies definitely do not support an inability to experience pain around the time of birth. And evidence for sex differences is equivocal at best.

RESPONSIVITY TO
NONAVERSIVE STIMULI

Finding appropriate stimuli for testing tactile sensitivity is not simple. Bell and Costello (1964) tried three different stimuli: removal of a covering blanket, an air puff, and an aesthesiometer. Removing the blanket was unsatisfactory in two ways. It failed to give test-retest stability, and as a stimulus it involves temperature reduction and friction as well as tactile stimulation. Air puffs to the abdomen and various parts of the face were presented when the newborn was in quiet sleep, and the flow was gradually increased until the baby showed a response. Although the observations were not highly reliable, they suggested that newborns responded to the stimulation of an air puff to these areas. Girls were more responsive to removal of the blanket and to air puffs to the abdomen (but not to the face).

Bell and Costello's third stimulus was composed of 13 filaments, with carefully measured bending force (an aesthesiometer). It yielded high observer agreement on response to tactile stimulation to the foot. On retest, but not on initial test, greater sensitivity was shown by older babies and there were no sex differences. Bell and Costello conclude that the aesthesiometer is the most reliable way to assess tactile sensitivity. They note that complex research designs and controls for large numbers of variables are needed in this type of research (see also Bell, 1963).

Clear demonstrations of tactile sensitivity have been obtained using stimulation of the tongue. Weiffenbach (1972a, 1972b) discovered a stereotyped reflex response to tactile stimulation of the tongue, in which the tongue moves toward the side on which it is stimulated. The response is easily identified, reliably observed, consistent from test to test, and can be elicited by several different types of stimulation of the tongue near its tip. All newborns responded to the same filament aesthesiometer used by Bell and exhibited an orderly increase in responses as a function of the stimulus intensity (Thach & Weiffenbach, 1976). The sensitivity of the babies' tongues was about equal to that found for adults on the upper arm (Ghent, 1961). Both gestational age and postnatal age affected responsiveness. Recently, attention has been paid to young infants' use of the mouth and oral activity as a tactile tool for exploration (Rochat, 1984). Changes in shape and tactile qualities of nipples are actively explored by mouthing behaviors by 1 month of age, and even neonates respond to changes in the tactile qualities. The rigidity of objects presented for oral and manual action affects the behaviors, with soft objects eliciting more sucking-type behaviors, especially at birth (Rochat, 1984). Such exploration increases over the first 3 to 4 months of life. (Tactile habituation and discrimination have been compared with vision by Stréri & Pêcheux, 1986.)

To summarize, newborns respond to a wide variety of tactile stimuli, including some that are purely tactile (i.e., that do not include temperature changes or other sorts of stimulation). Apparent changes in sensitivity in the first few days of life may not be due to other factors. Presumed developmental changes often differ in unanticipated ways for different kinds of stimuli. Tactile responses vary as a function of characteristics such as activity level and kind of feeding, but research is not sufficient to allow general conclusions. Sex differences are not consistent, particularly if birth weight is controlled for. Newborns can discriminate between tactile stimuli on two different places on their bodies, and between a tactile and an auditory stimulus. Finally, I would like to note that there is a deplorable lack of current research in this area.

CLINICAL WORK WITH TACTILE AND KINESTHETIC STIMULATION

This chapter does not discuss kinesthetic or vestibular senses, but a brief look at clinical work that combines tactile and kinesthetic stimulation is in order. Current work addresses the role of a combination of tactile and kinesthetic stimulation in promoting optimal growth and behavioral development of premature infants. Its rationale lies in a long history of animal research on physiological effects of deprivation of tactile stimulation normally provided by mothers (Schanberg & Field, 1987). The combined stimulation program,

which is applied with prematures after they leave the NICU for the "growing" nursery, has been found to promote weight gain, amount of time spent awake and active, and performance on several aspects of the NBAS, as well as to lead to earlier hospital discharge (Field et al., 1986; Scafidi et al., 1986, 1990).

Taste

Like touch, taste has a long history of investigation, but is currently studied much less than vision or audition. Two important nineteenth-century researchers concluded that the sense of taste is well developed at birth. Kussmaul (1859) observed facial expressions and sucking movements to various solutions. Acid, salt, and quinine evoked grimaces, but sugar led to sucking movements (except in a few infants). Indeed, quinine was rejected and sugar accepted by prematures as much as 2 months before the normal time of birth. Preyer (1880/1888) similarly found that infants' facial expressions differed for bitter and sour, and both differed from those to sweet (a result much the same as one obtained recently using sophisticated coding of taped facial expressions; Rosenstein & Oster, 1988). Preyer also found individual differences and rapid development of sensitivity over the first few days of life and concluded that the gustatory (taste) sense was one of the most highly developed in the newborn. Early in this century workers cautioned against confusing responses to smell, temperature, and intensity of stimulation with those to taste, a problem that is still pertinent today.

At the turn of the century, researchers began to measure responses other than observed facial expressions and sucking reactions (see Figure 7.1). Canestrini (1913) found different pulse and respiration responses to different stimuli (controlled for temperature). Salt disrupted respirations and disrupted and increased pulse rate, as did sour and bitter even more profoundly, whereas sweet solutions lowered pulse and respiration rates, producing a calming effect. Canestrini was not able to show differences in response to cow's milk versus that of the mother.

Pratt et al. (1930), in their classic monograph on infant behavior, added bodily movements, recorded from stabilimeters, to sucking reactions and facial movements. Over the first 15 days of life, infants made some response to all stimuli except water on 85% of trials and engaged in sucking on 30%. They responded differently to the sugar, salt, bitter, and acid stimuli (the classic taste categories). Sucking to sugar and water increased over this period, while that to quinine

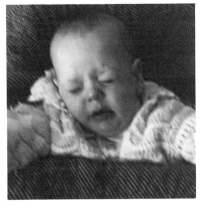 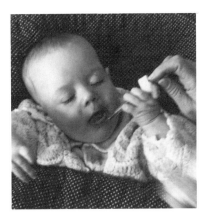 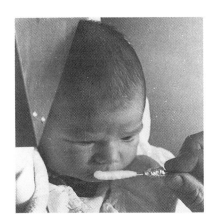

Figure 7.1. Babies responding to taste and smell stimuli: (left) lemon juice; (center) a sweetened medicine; (right) an odorant on a cotton swab. (Photographs left and center courtesy of Judith E. Sims-Knight; photograph on right courtesy of T. Engen, 1982. Used by permission.)

and acid decreased. Shortly after this work, Jensen (1932) recorded sucking responses to various solutions using an early automated nipple. Markedly different sucking responses were not always accompanied by differences in facial expressions, but if facial expressions changed, they were always accompanied by changes in sucking. Thus sucking was the more sensitive measure. Individual differences between infants were marked and stable. Inasmuch as Jensen tested infants both 15 minutes before and 15 minutes after feeding, he was able to note that moderately satiated infants were better discriminators of taste than were very hungry infants. For a more thorough review of the history of research in this area, see Lipsitt and Behl (1990).

Steiner (1977) returned to facial expressions as a way to study the affective dimension of food-related stimuli using an improved methodology in which videotapes, movies, or still photos are made of the facial expressions and these records are judged by persons who do not know what substance is being used to stimulate the baby. Observers of these records can reliably classify the expressions even when the taste stimuli were presented before the newborn had any experience of taste from feeding. Steiner thus concludes that discriminative taste sensitivity cannot depend on life experience. However, it should be noted that the taste of amniotic fluid, which has been swallowed for long periods prior to birth, may well provide an adaptation level against which new stimuli are judged. Inasmuch as infants without a cerebral cortex show facial responses, Steiner concluded that the gustofacial response is a reflexlike response that does not involve cortical structures. He interprets the fact that adults could interpret these responses to mean

that they are part of the infant's nonverbal communication equipment. However, recent research has indicated that there is no distinct facial pattern in response to salt, and adults are accurate only about the faces babies make in response to sweet stimuli (Rosenstein & Oster, 1988).

The genesis of preference for sweet tastes has intrigued a number of researchers. Desor et al. (1977) measured infants' preference for sweet over other tastes. Newborns 1 to 3 days old were tested midway between feedings with different sugars and at different concentrations. Preference was assessed by the amounts consumed. All sugars were preferred to water, but glucose least so, and a sucrose solution was preferred to milk. Older infants with varied amounts of experience with milk and other foods had the same preferences both at 5-11 and at 20-28 weeks, although they now consumed larger quantities. Desor et al. conclude that preference for sweet is characteristic of the human species, despite large individual differences in the degree of sweetness preferred. Studies of older twins indicate that preference for degree of sweetness or saltiness is based neither on inheritance nor on living in the same households. Preference for sweetness appears to be a unique sensory quality, inasmuch as similar universal preferences do not exist in other sensory domains.

It has recently been suggested, initially on the basis of animal data, that sugars, especially sucrose, trigger the release of endogenous opioids that reduce the reaction to pain. Consistent with that view is the fact that 1- to 2-day-old humans are immediately calmed by amounts of sucrose much too small to affect hunger or digestive processes (Blass et al., 1989). The calming lasts for some period thereafter, in contrast to that produced by a pacifier, which lasts only while it is being sucked (Smith et al., 1990). Indeed, sucrose is an effective analgesic, greatly reducing the amount of crying produced by heel lancing done to obtain blood for PKU testing (Blass, 1990) and even by circumcision (Blass & Hoffmeyer, in press).

Another current approach to the study of sweet preferences utilizes simultaneous and highly sophisticated recording of respiration and heart rate, as well as sucking. The measures are directly fed to computers, which give sucking response rates for each condition of testing for each child. The number of sucks per minute and the average interval between sucks are available (see Lipsitt, 1977; Lipsitt & Behl, 1990). Lipsitt and his collaborators have found that human newborns respond differently to sweet solutions than to water or to nonnutritive sucking; they suck more slowly, but more continuously, and their heart rates increase (Ashmead et al., 1980; Crook & Lipsitt, 1976; Lipsitt et al., 1976). These researchers interpret these reactions as reflecting pleasure.

Newborns also show evidence of adaptation to taste stimuli (Kobre & Lipsitt, 1972). The mean rates of sucking for very small drops of water or sucrose are stable over a 20-minute period and are about the same for both (about 55 per minute). But if water is alternated with sucrose, the rates for sucrose increase slightly (to about 60 per minute). Kobre and Lipsitt call this the "negative contrast effect," and say that it may represent an early and rudimentary learning phenomenon (see also Lipsitt & Behl, 1990).

Other researchers have studied responses to saltiness (for a review, see Weiffenbach et al., 1980). Studies using facial movements, tongue movements, modification of sucking pattern, physiological responses, and intake measures have all shown that newborns, and even preterms, respond to saltiness, usually negatively. However, whereas sucking will usually be inhibited to bad-tasting solutions, the amount of a salty solution consumed is not affected. Inhibition of sucking to salty solutions appears to be a different mechanism from merely reacting negatively to it, one that develops later. Thus newborns and young babies have been poisoned in some cases where salt has accidentally been substituted for sugar in their formula (Finberg et al., 1963). Babies who will vomit from the salt will not stop sucking salty solutions until they are very ill.

Unlike the innate preference for sweet tastes, that for salty tastes arises later, and it is not clear whether it results from dietary exposure or from the maturation of sensory or cortical mechanisms. From 2 to 4 months of age babies have no preference between water and a weak saline solution, but from 4 to 6 months of age

they prefer the weak saline (Beauchamp et al., 1986). However, these comparisons have all been made with water, and water may be an aversive rather than neutral stimulus for newborns (Desor et al., 1977).

Preferences for salty liquids and for salty foods are not parallel; indeed, as the latter develops the former declines. Most studies of preference for salt in food have been conducted with older infants, but one studied breast-fed babies, who have very little exposure to salt prior to starting solid foods. Preference for a lightly salted compared to an unsalted cereal for their first solids had a complicated relation to the age at which solids were introduced (Harris et al., 1990). It appears that a response mechanism for saltiness develops after the newborn period.

In summary, newborns do discriminate among tastes, as shown by several kinds of responses. Some, such as facial expressions, are obvious to the observer; others, such as sucking rates, need more than simple observation to be adequately quantified; still others, such as heart rate, are not directly observable. Sucking and heart rate appear to be more sensitive measures than simple observation of facial expressions. Our knowledge is still inadequate to allow us to tackle the practical health problems of preventing too great a preference for sweet or salt.

Smell

Another sense that is closely related to taste as we experience it is smell. In the evolutionary sense, smell is one of the oldest, and one of the most important, senses for many adaptations of other mammals. Eating behaviors, avoidance of predators, and sexual and maternal behaviors are all strongly influenced by the sense of smell (see Blass, 1990).

The portions of the brain devoted to smell appear to be much smaller in humans than in most other mammals, leading some to the conclusion that smell is not important in humans. Nevertheless, it is surprising that so little work has dealt with the infant's capacities in this sensory domain. The fact that many newborns do not seem to indicate displeasure when lying near the sour milk smells of their own regurgitation or the smells of their own diapers may have led parents (who sometimes are also scientists) to think that smell is not very important to the newborn. The difficulty of controlling the presentation of the stimuli, problems of rapid adaptation, and interactions among stimuli probably play a major role in the neglect of smell, or olfaction.

To be sure, early scientific researchers did look at

newborns' reactions to different odors. They found that the infants not only reacted to odors, but differentiated among some of the same odors that adults discriminate. Responses indicative of displeasure and/or avoidance were found to odors such as asafetida (which adults find nauseatingly bad), and responses indicative of pleasure were found to odors that adults find pleasant. A few studies conducted in the 1960s and 1970s reconfirmed what the early workers found: that newborns smell and discriminate between different smells, and that they improve somewhat over the first few days of life (Engen & Bosack, 1969; Engen & Lipsitt, 1965; Engen et al., 1963; Lipsitt et al., 1963; Self et al., 1972; see reviews in Engen, 1982; Porter et al., 1988).

Steiner (1977) suggested, on the basis of responses prior to their first feeding, that newborns have an inborn "hedonic monitor" that enables them to discriminate valuable foods from ones that should be rejected (e.g., rotten eggs). However, the idea of innate **hedonic tone** (pleasantness-unpleasantness) has been challenged by both animal and human data. If innate preferences and dislikes governed infant animal food intake, they might starve if the mother's diet contained an unusual substance that affected the odor and taste of her milk (see Blass, 1990, for a review of animal data and reasons this would be very maladaptive). Human work supporting the hypothesis that hedonic responses to odors are learned is surveyed by Engen (1986).

Inasmuch as preference can be taken to indicate hedonic tone, we can take data from several studies of naturalistic stimuli as supporting Engen's hypothesis. These studies strove for **ecological validity**; that is, they attempted to study the psychological phenomena of smell in a real-life context. MacFarlane (1975) explored newborns' responses to breast pads their mothers had been wearing, most of which were dry. At 6 days of age, but not at 2 days, babies turned toward their own mothers' breast pads significantly more than toward another mother's pads. Similar results are reported by Russell (1976) and Schaal et al. (1980). By about 2 weeks, breast-fed, but not bottle-fed, babies preferred their mothers' underarm odor to that of a nonnursing woman or of a strange nursing mother, but did not discriminate that of their fathers from that of an unfamiliar man (Cernoch & Porter, 1985). The role of familiarity was investigated by studying reactions of neonates to arbitrary odors to which they had been familiarized in their cribs. Girls showed a clearcut preference for the familiar odor (Balogh & Porter, 1986). This sex difference in sensitivity is found over the life span.

Recently it has been shown that 2-week-old bottle-fed girls (boys were not tested) preferred the odor of a breast pad from a lactating woman to that of a nonlactating woman, or to the armpit odors of the lactating woman, or to a clean pad (Makin & Porter, 1989).

Taken as a whole, these data indicate that learning or prior exposure is an important determinant of reaction to smells, a conclusion that is congruent with the role of previous exposure in determining initial suckling behavior in animals, as discussed by Blass. These data also indicate that smell may be more important in mediating social behaviors with familiar others than had been supposed (see Porter et al., 1988, for a further exploration of this theme), and would fit the Engen/Blass view that hedonic or affective reactions to smells are learned.

Development of odor preferences over the course of infancy has not been much studied. It has been accepted wisdom that children do not show adult preferences for odors before about 6 years of age. Schmidt and Beauchamp (1988) found that 3-year-olds in their sample had preferences very similar to those of adults, although fewer of them than adults judged the smell of spoiled milk to be unpleasant. These authors felt that the spoiled milk smell was close to that of infant vomit, which, as noted above, is not reacted to by most newborns. The 3-year-olds did not differ from adults on reactions to an odorant judged to represent strong cheese or vomit.

It is clear that experience governs both the ability to discriminate odors and the hedonic tone associated with many of them. The question of whether odors have any innate hedonic stimulus effect is not settled. Odors that are strong irritants and that activate the trigeminal nerve are responded to innately.

Audition

For hearing, as for the other senses, the first questions are, Can newborns respond to sound? Can they respond before the normal time of birth (prematurely delivered or in utero)? If not, how soon are they able to do so? If they can respond, to which aspects of the sound stimuli are they able to respond? To answer these questions, it is necessary to consider the various aspects of sounds. Sounds are characterized by loudness (intensity), measured in decibels (dB), a measure of sound pressure level; by pitch (determined by the frequency of the sound waves), measured in hertz (Hz); and by localization, or where in space they originate. In addition, there are differences in complexity. There are pure tones (sounds at a single frequency), combinations of pure tones, combinations of tones with a wide or narrow band of frequencies, noises, noises with various frequency components, and speech sounds (these last will be discussed in Chapter 11).

As in all studies of sensory and perceptual abilities in preverbal organisms, the behaviors of the organism used to judge the presence of responses have a profound influence on the answer obtained. The behaviors most often used by the earliest researchers were startles, eye blinks, turns toward the sound (which means that the infant not only heard the sound, but also detected something about where it came from), and quieting. All of these responses, plus internal responses, such as changes in heart rate or in the electrical activity of parts of the brain relevant to processing

Figure 7.2. Graphs showing how information can become clear as a result of using computer averaging, and showing the form that an auditory evoked potential takes. The numbers on the left show the number of responses that were averaged. The amount of amplification was increased fourfold between the top and the second graph. (This figure is modified from Figure 1 in "Average Responses to Clicks Recorded From the Human Scalp," by C. D. Geisler & W. A. Rosenblith. *Journal of the Acoustical Society of America*, 1962, 34, 125-127. These researchers were the first to use this technique.)

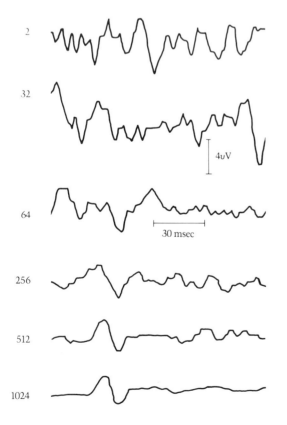

auditory stimuli (**auditory evoked potentials** or responses; see Figure 7.2), are studied. The interruption of sucking (often an orienting response) has also been used as an indication of hearing. Measurement of both the internal and some of the externally observable responses, such as activity and blink reflexes, has been automated, so researchers can depend less on human judgment to determine whether or not a response has occurred.

In a psychophysically sophisticated study, Spetner and Olsho (1990) showed that 3- and 6-month-olds have equally poor thresholds for 4,000-cycle tones. For 500- and 1,000-cycle tones 6-month-olds are better than 3-month-olds. At all of these frequencies adults have thresholds that are 10 to 30 dB lower than those of the infants.

In addition to the general question of understanding the functioning of infants, there is a clinical question involving the normalcy of any sensory system. In the case of hearing, this question has a particular relevance to infancy, since a large proportion of those in special education programs for the hearing impaired (a larger percentage now than in the past, since antibiotics that caused deafness are no longer used) were deaf at birth. Hearing loss is not discovered in more than a third of these children until after they are 3 years old. If they are in hearing families, this means that they are not exposed to language up to that time. If speech training is desired, 3 is a very late age to start. To detect deafness early, we must know the hearing capacities of normal infants in order to have a standard for comparison. We will return to this topic at the end of the section.

DO BABIES HEAR FROM BIRTH? BEFORE BIRTH?

Researchers in the nineteenth and early twentieth centuries did not agree on whether babies could hear from birth. Tiedemann (1897/1927) and Preyer (1880/1888) agreed that their sons heard after a few days. Kussmaul (1859), in contrast, was convinced that newborns did not hear. Genzmer (1882), however, repeated Kussmaul's experiments and concluded that infants heard on the first or at least the second day of life. In the early 1900s it was shown that newborns respond to a rattle within 10 to 360 minutes after birth (Peterson & Rainey, 1910). In 1960, Fröding established that 96% of infants responded with an eye blink to a gong that produced sounds of 126 to 132 dB (loud thunder is about 120 dB).

All of these workers used complex sounds (bells, rattles, human voices, hand claps) to obtain responses.

The responses noted were attentive or quieting responses (related to what would be called orienting responses now), reflex startles, eye blinks, and various bodily movements, especially of the face and eyes. As early as 1881 it was noted that the infants' states affected responses.

It would be strange if responses to sound did not occur in the newborn period, inasmuch as they occur prior to birth. Fetal movement or startle responses to a variety of stimuli were found by early researchers (Bernard, 1946; Bernard & Sontag, 1947; Forbes & Forbes, 1927; Peiper, 1924). With the advent of ultrasound to visualize the fetus, it was determined that sudden noises (above the background noise level of 50 to 80 dB that exists in utero) elicit startle responses in 50% of fetuses by 24 weeks and in 100% by 28 weeks (Birnholz & Benaceraff, 1983). After 28 weeks repeated presentations lead to a decrement in response, a primitive form of habituation that is apparently subcortically mediated, given that it occurs in infants lacking a cerebral cortex. The full-term infant has a well-myelinated auditory nerve and lower brain stem, while the myelination of midbrain structures continues for months and that of the auditory cortex for years (Eggermont, 1985; cited in Clarkson et al., 1989). We would therefore expect some responses to be quite mature at birth, but for a great deal of development to occur later.

Indeed, the fetus has a large variety of auditory experiences, which may play a role in neural as well as emotional and cognitive development (Fifer & Moon, 1988). A number of studies that show learning from these experiences will be reviewed below.

Starting in the 1920s, after Pavlov's work, classically conditioned responses were used to study infants' ability to respond to sound. Marquis (1931) established that seven out of eight neonates responded by sucking to the sound of a buzzer that had been paired with food during the first 10 days of life. While much argument exists as to whether this was conditioning, it clearly demonstrates that the infants responded to sound.

In short, it is hard to imagine why we needed so many proofs that newborns hear.

LOUDNESS (INTENSITY)

We shall start with perhaps the most fundamental characteristic of a stimulus, its loudness or intensity. How intense does a sound have to be to elicit a response from the infant? Can the infant detect differences in intensity (that is, respond differently to one intensity than to another)? If so, how large do the differences have to be?

Achieving answers to these questions is not simple, because responsivity to sounds of a given intensity depends on both the nature of the sound and the response measure used. For example, infants respond differently to sounds depending on their pitch, on the suddenness with which they begin (technically, speed of onset), and on their complexity. They respond more to noises that are complex than to pure tones.

Several studies have attempted to measure infants' absolute threshold for sound (the softest sound they can hear). Estimates vary depending on the response used. Increasing sound levels are required to produce responses as one goes from auditory evoked potentials to heart rate responses and to blink or startle responses. The estimate for the threshold also depends on the stringency of criteria used. Most studies yield estimates of around 40 dB (sound of a quiet office) to 60 dB (the level of a conversation). Wedenberg (1956) has shown that infants are awakened from deep sleep by 70-75 dB sounds (the noise of a busy street) and from light sleep by 55 dB sounds (a quiet car). In contrast, he found that it took sounds above 105 dB (the sound of a boiler shop) to elicit the eye blink response.

Newborns have been shown to respond differentially to different intensities of sounds. Both the number of startles and the latency of motor responses are related to intensity, as are heart rate accelerations. Both early and more recent studies have shown this (Bartoshuk, 1964; Bridger, 1961; Canestrini, 1913; Eichorn, 1951; Steinschneider et al., 1966). The size of auditory evoked responses to clicks in sleeping infants varies in a linear fashion with the intensity of the clicks (Barnet & Goodwin, 1965).

Thus neonates do respond to sounds, though not to sounds at intensities as low as those to which adults (who can hear approximately 0 dB) respond. They improve rapidly (by about 16 dB) over the first few days of life (Taguchi et al., 1969). This is apparently *not* due to loss of extra tissue in the middle ear, as had often been supposed, but may be partly due to loss of fluid in ear structures. Sharp decreases in the threshold have also been shown between 3 and 8 months (Hoversten & Moncur, 1969). Infants are able to respond to sounds over a wide range of intensities and frequencies (as shown in Figure 7.1), including to that stimulus of great interest, the human voice.

LOCALIZATION

Head turning and eye movements toward a sound were taken by the early baby biographers as signs of responding to sound. They found these occurrences occasionally in the first few weeks.

In light of all the early research, it is somewhat amazing to note that when Wertheimer (1961) reported that his newborn (delivered without drugs) responded by turning its head toward sound, this was considered controversial. Since then some researchers have found that newborns fairly consistently turn toward sounds (e.g., Field et al., 1980; Muir & Field, 1979; Turkewitz et al., 1966). Others have found no neonatal responsiveness (e.g., Butterworth & Castillo, 1976; Chun et al., 1960; McGurk et al., 1977; Zelazo et al., 1987). These discrepancies are apparently produced by differences in the kinds of sound stimuli used by various researchers. A good review of infant localization is found in Muir and Clifton (1985).

Soft sounds of more than 1 second's duration are more likely to produce head and eye movements toward the stimulus (Muir & Field, 1979; Turkewitz et al., 1966) than are loud or brief sounds. Pulsed continuous sounds may be even more effective, perhaps because newborns' responses are quite slow (Muir & Field, 1979). With the most effective stimuli, Muir and Field (1979) found that 11 of 12 infants (who had optimal characteristics at birth and who could be maintained in an alert state for the necessary 10 to 15 minutes) showed consistent orientation responses (on three-fourths of all trials). The importance of the duration of stimulation is shown by the following data from a series of methodologically sophisticated studies. Using a pulsed rattle sound, Clarkson et al. (1989) found that (a) an exposure longer than 1 second (but not one of .5 second) produced reliable orienting; (b) a .1-second exposure to the rattle sound at 69-71 dB produced reliable orienting, but a .014-second exposure at 89-91 dB (approximately equal energy) did not; and (c) the rate of repetition affects response. If the very brief stimulus is repeated several times at 2 times per second, it results in orientation, but not if it is repeated at the slightly lower rate of 1.3 times per second. Other researchers have found rather similar time constraints for evoking eye blinks.

A taped presentation of a word at 90° to left or right produced head turns in the direction of the sound in almost 90% of trials with newborns (Swain et al., 1989). Although infants tend to make only one head turn on a trial, if the stimulus was moved to the other side during the trial they made a second head turn toward it two-thirds of the time.

Studies using older infants found that responsivity decreased at around 2 months of age, a decline that was reversed by 3 to 4 months (Field et al., 1980; Muir et al., 1979) or by 4 to 5 months (Morrongiello & Clifton, 1984). By 5 to 6 months, the **latency** (the

amount of time before a response starts) of the response is less than half what it was in the newborn period (3 versus 7 seconds). At this age it will habituate unless reinforced (Clifton et al., 1984). By 3 to 6 months this response is so robust that head turning in the direction of a sound from an invisible source is used as a crude test of hearing on infant tests (Bayley, 1969; Cattell, 1940).

Recently a very different technique for determining infant responses has been adopted in a number of research areas. In it, an observer who is blind to the stimulus condition judges responses based on the totality of cues provided by the infant (Olsho et al., 1987). Morrongiello et al. (1990) have used this technique to study the minimum change in the angle of a sound that babies can discriminate. It allows for the fact that different babies may respond in different ways. The researchers found that babies discriminated a 27° shift at 8 weeks, and that age was linearly related to ability, with an 18° shift being detected at 24 weeks. Morrongiello (1988) previously showed a linear relation of threshold to age from 28 to 80 weeks, by which time it approximated the adult threshold.

Turning in the direction of a sound is a primitive form of localization, different from looking precisely toward the source of sounds coming from various places around them. Animal literature suggests that the latter requires cortical control, whereas a simple head turn in the direction of sound does not (Clifton et al., 1981). Most newborn research has looked at simple head turns, not at localizing more precise positions in space. Some of the large numbers of newborns tested on the G/R repeatedly localized correctly by head and/or eye turning to a rattle or bell, but they were a minority of all newborns tested (the sound stimuli were approximately 80 dB, sounded at the four cardinal points, and the infants' mothers had been relatively highly medicated). Recently, good evidence of newborns' abilities to turn toward a sound has been reported by Fenwick et al. (1991). Using an arch of eight loudspeakers (four on each side of the midline at from 36° to 90°), they found that the farther from the midline a sound was, the farther to that side infants turned. However, they turned less than half the distance to the speaker that was sounding.

The developmental course of localization has been followed by Morrongiello and Rocca (1987), who tested 6-, 9-, 12-, 15-, and 18-month-old babies using an array of 10 speakers and interspersed auditory and audiovisual trials. The average auditory error declined quite steadily from 16° at 9 months to 6° at 18 months. At that point auditory accuracy was about equal to that when both auditory and visual cues were presented (four clicks from the speaker followed by a light display and four more clicks). The audiovisual stimuli led to only 4° or 5° of error at all of these ages.

In older infants, auditory localization can be assessed using the reaching response to indicate the infants' appreciation of sounding objects in a three-dimensional space. To eliminate visual cues, one can test for reaching to auditory stimuli in the dark, a procedure difficult to use with young infants. Recently, Perris and Clifton (1988) developed an extremely ingenious method to test 7-month-olds in the dark. Reaching occurred on 77% of trials, and on trials with no reaching the infants oriented their heads toward the stimulus 80% of the time. Reaching occurred on 100% of trials in the light and more reaches produced contact with the sounding object, but even in the dark infants contacted the object on three-fourths of the trials. In further work on reaching in the dark with infants about 7 months of age, reaching occurred more often when the sounding object was within reach than when it was not (Clifton et al., 1991). If infants reached to the out-of-reach target their reach was less likely to be to the target area. Some of the data were consistent with the authors' hypothesis that head movements may be used to help locate the object. Hewett and Cornelisse (1991) have shown that 6- and 12-month-old infants can discriminate receding from approaching sounds, as shown by their conditioned head turning.

Sounds can be, and frequently are, used to help alert infants to attend visually. Sound has been used to get infants' eyes to midline in newborns (in the G/R test; Mendelson & Haith, 1976) and in 2-month-old infants (e.g., Culp, 1971; Self, 1971), and in numerous studies of vision at various ages. Sound can be used to elicit visual following or to make sure that a visual stimulus will be in the infant's field.

Among the major reasons for researchers' interest in auditory localization are the potential epistemological implications (that is, implications concerning the nature of human knowledge). Adults not only consistently turn their heads toward sounds, but they expect to see an object making the sound. In other words, for an adult a sound emanates from an object. The epistemological question is whether newborns also know that sounds emanate from objects. Some people argue that turning toward a sound demonstrates that newborns have that knowledge, even though they are probably unaware of it. Other researchers argue that the simple localization phenomenon found in newborns may not require the knowledge that an object has visual and auditory characteristics. Rather, they say, it appears to be a primitive, reflexlike mechanism that

drops out and is replaced by a more mature, cortically mediated, mechanism. Only then do infants understand that objects have both visual and auditory characteristics.

There is evidence that 3- to 4-month-olds understand that objects have different modalities—visual, auditory, tactile, and others (Broerse et al., 1983; Goldenberg et al., 1984; Spelke, 1976; Spelke & Owsley, 1979). The evidence that younger infants do so is inconclusive. Aronson and Rosenbloom (1971) found evidence that they do, but Condry et al. (1977) and McGurk and Lewis (1974) failed to replicate these findings. Earlier research found that it was not until 9 to 12 months that infants could use sound to search for a hidden object (Freedman et al., 1969). However, the data on reaching in the dark by 7-month-olds (Perris & Clifton, 1988) suggests that expecting a sound to emanate from an unseen object occurs earlier. Again, the cleverness of experimenters in asking research questions often determines the answers they get.

PITCH (FREQUENCY) AND COMPLEXITY

Sounds vary in pitch (high versus low tones) and in complexity (pure tones versus multitoned sounds). These characteristics affect responsivity to sound, as noted earlier. This section examines infants' responses to these specific characteristics. As noted earlier, the physical dimension underlying pitch is measured by the frequency of sound waves, given in units called hertz (Hz). For example, the range of a tuba is 45 to 350 Hz, of a baritone voice about 96 to 320 Hz; of a violin, 190 to 3,000 Hz. Adults generally can hear sounds anywhere from 20 to 20,000 Hz. *Complexity* refers to how many frequencies a given sound has. The flute makes an almost pure tone; it sounds almost exclusively at a single frequency. Most other sounds, including music from other instruments, voices, and noises, are complex; they include several frequencies. **White noise** is a particularly interesting complex sound that sounds like a waterfall. While the term is often used loosely to describe sounds with a wide spectrum of frequencies, technically it refers to a sound in which all audible frequencies are present and at equal intensities. Figure 7.3 illustrates the differences between simple and complex sounds.

Early studies used complex sounds (clicks, rattles, hand claps) and found that young infants were responsive to stimuli at a variety of pitches. As laboratory equipment and methods became more sophisticated, researchers confirmed that newborn infants do respond to sounds at a number of frequencies, but often depending on the circumstances. The complexity of

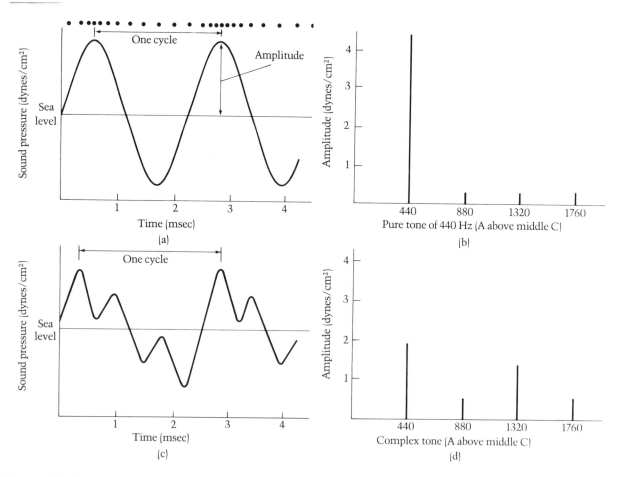

Figure 7.3. Sound waves are disturbances in air molecules caused by vibrating objects. The vibrations alternately push the air molecules together (compression, or increasing sound pressure) and allow the air molecules to spread out (expansion, or decreasing sound pressure). The number of such waves in a second (the frequency) determines the pitch of the tone. (a) The waves of compression and expansion of a pure tone such as that of a tuning fork or a flute. The dots above the tone represent the air molecules. The wave form is called a sine wave. This tone is the first A above middle C. The figure represents two waves; there will be 440 such waves in 1 second in a tone of this pitch. (b) A pure tone with just one frequency. This figure, which represents the same tone as in part a, shows that its fundamental frequency is 440 Hz. (c) A complex tone, typical of most sounds. Voices, bird songs, and most musical instruments produce complex tones. The fundamental frequency of this tone is also 440 Hz, which means that the same pitch will be heard as in part a. (d) Unlike pure tones, complex tones exhibit frequencies in addition to the fundamental frequencies. The fundamental frequency of complex tones is always their lowest frequency. The number of additional frequencies may vary from a few, as in this figure, to 20 to 30. (Adapted from *Psychology: Its Principles and Meanings*, 4th ed., by Lyle E. Bourne, Jr., and Bruce R. Ekstrand. Copyright © 1982 by CBS College Publishing. Reprinted by permission of CBS College Publishing.)

the sound is an important variable. White noise is a particularly effective stimulus (Lenard et al., 1969; Turkewitz et al., 1972a, 1972b), as are square-wave tones (selected fundamental tones with superimposed high frequencies), which have a broader band of frequencies than a pure tone sine wave (Bench, 1973; Hutt et al., 1968; Lenard et al., 1969; Leventhal & Lipsitt, 1964). Infants are much less likely to respond consistently to sustained pure tones (such as a flute note or a tone produced by a pure tone generator) than to other stimuli (Clarkson & Berg, 1978; Hutt et al., 1968; Lenard et al., 1969; Turkewitz et al., 1972b).

Studies seeking to determine the quietest sound to which newborns will respond (absolute threshold) at different frequencies yield inconsistent results. Some find different thresholds at different frequencies and others do not (Clarkson & Berg, 1978; Crowell et al., 1971; Werner & Gillenwater, 1990; see also the review by Eisenberg, 1976). If differences were found, they generally indicated greater sensitivity (response at lower dB levels) to moderately low tones (100-1,000 Hz) than to higher or very low frequencies. However, Werner and Gillenwater (1990) found that the threshold for 2- to 5-week-old infants was about the same at 4,000 as at 500 Hz (both were 55 to 60 dB) but that for 1,000 Hz was only about 25 dB (Werner & Gillenwater, 1990). In order to obtain a threshold for 100 Hz, they had to reduce the range of stimulus intensities from the 25-70 dB they had used at 500 and 4,000 Hz to 5-35 dB. This is one of many indications that in perceptual work the range of stimuli used (be it the highest and lowest of the tones, the loudest and softest of the sounds, the variety of colors, the intensities of the lights, or whatever) often influences the results.[2]

Other research exploring newborns' responsivity to pitch has examined responsiveness to stimuli that have more meaning than isolated tones. Two such avenues are the study of responsivity to human voices and of differential emotional responses to various sounds. Newborns have generally been found to be especially responsive to sounds in the 200 to 500 Hz range that parallels the frequencies of the human voice (Eisenberg, 1970a, 1970b; Hutt et al., 1968), a finding that is challenged by Werner and Gillenwater's data showing that the threshold at 500 was as poor as at 4,000 Hz.

In addition to what infants respond to, there is the question of what they prefer to listen to. Colombo and Bundy (1981) found that they prefer a human voice to silence or white noise. Butterfield and Siperstein (1974) report that they prefer music with voices ac-

companying it. Newborns will alter their sucking to listen to their own mothers' voices, but not strange women's voices, according to research by DeCasper and Fifer (1980). They do not prefer their fathers' voices to those of other males (DeCasper & Prescott, 1984), and they prefer the sound of an intrauterine heartbeat to that of a male voice (Panneton & DeCasper, 1984). They also prefer a melody sung during pregnancy to one not sung then (Panneton, 1985) and a prose passage read aloud by the mother during pregnancy to one not read at that time (DeCasper & Spence, 1986). They even prefer a tape of a female speaking their own language (be it Spanish or English) to one speaking the other (Moon et al., 1991).

In addition to studies using preference methods, newborns (16 out of 20) will learn (in the course of 12 minutes) to suck in response to a syllable that signals receiving maternal adult-directed speech as a reinforcer over one that signals quiet (Moon & Fifer, 1990). This tells us about their ability to detect differences in syllables as well as about the effectiveness of maternal speech as a reinforcer. When tapes of a mother's voice are filtered to sound more like they would have sounded in utero, newborns are equally reinforced by both, but when the voices are unfamiliar the unfiltered or "natural" extrauterine-sounding one is preferred (Spence & DeCasper, 1987). This finding is difficult to interpret in our current frame of thinking, as reflected in the following.

While much more research is needed on these topics, Aslin (1987), in his review of visual and auditory development in infancy, states, "These results strongly suggest that prenatal auditory exposure is sufficient to induce an auditory preference during the immediate postnatal period" (p. 67). It seems to me that a study should be undertaken that would compare the infant's preference for these songs and poems as they sound to the infant in utero against how they sound in "open-air" singing or reading. It has been determined that during labor intrauterine noises are predominantly low frequency, with maternal vocalization audible well above the background noise level (Benzaquen et al., 1990).

A preference that is probably not based directly on prenatal sound exposures is that for "motherese," a form of spoken language characterized by high pitch and exaggerated pitch contours compared with adult-

---

2. It would be surprising if newborns did not respond differently to pitches than adults, inasmuch as data on cats indicate that early responses to pitches are quite different from those in adults and appear to depend on anatomic changes in the cochlea during development (Walsh & McGee, 1990).

directed speech. This type of speech is characteristic of mothers' speech to infants and young children. The preference for infant-directed speech is present in newborns, though it is more pronounced at 2 months (Cooper & Aslin, 1990) and 4 months (Fernald, 1985). Computer simulations can remove actual speech but mimic various physical aspects of the sounds in motherese and adult-directed speech, to enable study of the physical features that might be responsible for the preference. Pitch- or frequency-mimicking computer samples have yielded a preference for the motherese pattern, while other aspects (amplitude and duration) did not affect preference (Fernald & Kuhl, 1987).

Several researchers are studying the perception of melody and rhythmic form by infants. This is one aspect of the more general question of the development of auditory pattern perception. This research goes beyond what can be encompassed here. The general question of auditory pattern perception is reviewed in Morrongiello (1988) and that of melodic perception in Trehub (1987) and Trehub et al. (1990).

Nonhuman sounds also can affect babies emotionally. They can soothe, alert, or distress infants. Both very high (above 4,000 Hz) and very low (70 Hz) frequencies appear to distress newborns (Haller, 1932; Hutt et al., 1968). In contrast, complex sounds in the low-frequency range appear to be soothing (Bench, 1969; Birch et al., 1965). These differential responses, which are similar to those of adults (Eisenberg, 1970a, 1970b), are of course clear evidence that newborns can distinguish between high- and low-pitched sounds.

An operant learning technique that is effective with infants 6 months old and older shows that they are more sensitive to higher frequencies of broad-band sounds than to low frequencies (Schneider et al., 1980; Trehub et al., 1980). At 24 months, infants were just as sensitive as adults at 19,000 Hz, and 6- to 18-month-olds were only 5 to 10 dB less sensitive. At 10,000 Hz, still a high tone, all 6- to 24-month-olds were slightly (12-16 dB) less sensitive than adults. Unlike what one would expect if the earlier data indicating special sensitivity to sound in the speech range were correct, response to low-pitched sounds (200 to 400 Hz) developed more slowly: 6-month-old babies have been found to be 5-8 dB less sensitive than 12-month-olds and 20-30 dB less sensitive than adults. New testing techniques have found a threshold of about 25 dB at 4,000 Hz for 6-month-olds (Trehub

et al., 1986), but the observer-based and conditioned head turns have both shown thresholds of about 10 dB at that age (Olsho et al., 1987).

Olsho (1984) found similar results in a study of sensitivity to differences between two tones (technically a difference threshold). Infants discriminated between high-frequency tones (4,000 and 8,000 Hz) as well as adults did, but were inferior at lower frequencies (250 and 2,000 Hz). However, Berg and Smith (1983) failed to find better high-frequency sensitivity in 6- to 18-month-old infants. The reasons for this inconsistency are not yet clear. Differential development of and deterioration of ear structures or differential development of or myelination of the auditory portions of the CNS could account for such differences.

Clarkson and Clifton (1985), using a visually reinforced head-turning response, taught 7-month-old infants to discriminate pitches that were only 20% apart in Hz. The infants subsequently showed evidence of perceptual constancy for the pitch of harmonic complexes, even when the fundamental frequency was removed.[3] This is a rather sophisticated ability for pitch perception, and is similar to that in adults.

CONTINUITY OR REPETITIVENESS OF STIMULATION

The research interest in rhythmic auditory stimulation probably started when Dr. Lee Salk (1962), a pediatrician who writes for parents, reported that recordings of a mother's heartbeat played in a newborn's nursery led to less crying and faster weight gain. Consistent with popular ideas at that time, he considered the possibility that infants were biologically set to respond to their mothers' heartbeats. He also speculated on the significance of mothers' usually holding their infants on the left side, where the heartbeat is best heard, and even on artists' depictions of mothers and infants in this position. However, it is possible that mothers hold their infants on the left side to free their right (usually preferred) hands for other uses.

To test Salk's hypothesis, Tulloch et al. (1964) compared the responses of newborns to heartbeats with their responses to other sounds—of a metronome's beating, a lullaby being sung, and silence. All three sounds led to quieting (less crying, less activity, less variable respirations, and a lower and less variable heart rate) compared with the condition of silence. The sounds were equally effective, hence no innate special responsivity to mother's heartbeat was evidenced. Detterman (1978) later attacked the heartbeat hypothesis on methodological grounds, and Salk (1978) defended his position.

---

3. I will not attempt to explain the intricacies of this phenomenon here.

CLINICAL ISSUES

The need to diagnose hearing loss within the first 6 months in order to start corrective measures is one reason for interest in the hearing capacities of normal infants. Corrective measures can range from instructing parents to provide loud sounds in the home (voices, TV) to providing a hearing aid. Where the loss is profound, training in American Sign Language can be started at the time that language acquisition is occurring in hearing infants.

This emphasis on early detection has led to a number of neonatal screening programs of dubious success. For example, of 6,184 newborns tested for behavioral responses to complex tones at 80, 90, and 100 dB, 17 failed on repeated testing to respond (see Rosenblith, 1970). These 17 were then tested for heart rate and respiratory responses to pure tone stimuli. Only 4 were judged not to hear using these techniques. By 12 to 14 months only 1 of the 4 was clearly deaf, 1 was not tested, and 2 appeared to have hearing within normal limits. Among the 13 behaviorally suspect infants who had been cleared on the physiological responses as neonates, 2 appeared to have hearing problems and a large number had behavioral peculiarities during testing at the later age. In a study she conducted in the early 1970s, Downs concluded on the basis of her own and other screening programs that a high-risk register would be an equally effective screening device (only 1 of 9 deaf infants in her study was not on such a register).

Subsequently, more sophisticated neurophysiological techniques, bolstered by the abilities of computers to average responses to large numbers of stimuli, have shown promise of being useful for screening at-risk populations. Galambos et al. (1984) obtained **auditory brain stem responses** (**ABRs**), responses that do not involve the cerebral cortex, for 1,613 infants leaving NICUs. Of these, 16% failed to meet the criteria for normal hearing. Nearly 60% of those who returned for testing at a later age still had hearing problems, and 35 were fitted with hearing aids. About two-thirds of the 40% whose hearing had become normal probably represented the clearing up of middle ear infections. A report by the National Research Council's Committee on Hearing, Bioacoustics, and Biomechanics (1987) concludes: "The consensus . . . is that the auditory brainstem evoked response . . . is the most objective measure currently available with which to assess the functional integrity of the peripheral auditory system in neonates." That report also contains qualifiers and detailed recommendations for future research.

In the meanwhile, psychophysical methods for measuring sound thresholds in infants as young as 6 months have improved (Trehub et al., 1986). Recently, adult observers have been successful in detecting infants' responses, with the result that function appears improved in relation both to age and to the intensity of stimulation needed (Trehub et al., 1991). The use of the human brain as a data processor to judge responses yields a lower threshold than other methods and holds promise as a potential screening tool for determining auditory handicaps.

The ABR is also correlated with both pre- and postnatal risk factors and with measures of concurrent functioning (Murray, 1988a). The ABR is associated with later deficits (delays in reaching gross motor milestones, fine motor skills, and perhaps speech motor skills up to 9 months of age), but not at a level that is useful for individual prediction (Murray, 1988b). However, aspects of the ABR predict gross motor delays and abnormal neurological findings at 1 year in a clinically significant fashion (Majnemer et al., 1988).

Vision

People have long been interested to know whether babies see when they are first born, or how soon they see. As noted in Chapter 1, both early baby biographers and the early scientists studying newborns concluded that they do see, a conclusion that later became unfashionable. Early researchers relied primarily on two responses to infer that babies see: (a) whether they turned toward light or objects, and (b) whether they followed the course of a moving object with their eyes.

The current cycle of interest in visual perception in infancy was stimulated by Fantz's (1961) development of the visual preference technique, described at the beginning of this chapter. It and other new techniques have permitted researchers to ask much more sophisticated questions concerning the nature of what infants might see—whether they discriminate colors, brightness, patterns, depth, and so forth. This research has also raised questions about the way infants explore visually: the nature and meaning of eye movements, how they scan stimuli, and how these abilities develop.

We shall begin with a discussion of the research on visual exploration, which has focused on development in early infancy. Then, research on various aspects of visual stimuli are considered. The standard questions are asked, concerning the age of onset of various aspects of vision and their subsequent development to a mature form.

VISUAL EXPLORATION

To process visual information, any organism needs to look at something. Even newborns have some capacity to find and look toward stimuli, although they are much more limited in such abilities than are older infants. This section will discuss infants' abilities to find visual stimuli and keep them before their eyes and in focus.

Eye Movements That Maintain Fixation on Large Moving Targets

The first eye movement to be discussed is **optokinetic nystagmus (OKN)**. OKN occurs when a large target with a repetitive pattern on it moves past a stationary observer (for example, vertical black and white stripes) or when an observer moves past a large pattern (for example, a person in a moving car watching telephone poles). In either case the person's eyes typically fixate on some part of the pattern (e.g., a particular telephone pole), follow that part with a smooth movement in the direction of the motion, then make a quick, jerky movement (a saccade) back toward the center of the visual field in the direction opposite to that of the motion. OKN seems to a certain extent to be involuntary, although a similar nystagmus can be started voluntarily. OKN is easily found in newborns, and its absence may be a sign of neurological pathology. Although OKN includes both smooth pursuit and the jerky saccadic movements discussed next, the total complex of OKN is apparently more mature at birth than are the saccadic movements by themselves, and is more easily elicited.

Saccades: Looking at Stimuli in the Corner of the Eye

When a stimulus appears in peripheral vision (anywhere outside the field of focus), a saccadic movement may occur. A **saccade** is a very rapid, usually accurate, movement that is ballistic (that is, it goes in a single motion from its origin to a predetermined end point). The eliciting stimulus may be small and nonrepetitive (unlike the kind that elicits OKN). Saccades bring peripheral stimuli into central focus, where adult vision is most acute. Motion is best detected in peripheral vision, and thus saccadic eye movements play an important role in the detection of potentially dangerous missiles. Consider, for example, a driver who sees another car out of the corner of her or his eye. Automatically, and very rapidly, the eyes (and even head, if the car is far to the side) turn toward the car so that it

comes into central vision. The same happens if a rock or ball is detected in peripheral vision.

Saccades not only help people process danger signals, and even save lives, they also help process visual materials, both pictures and print. Perusal of visual information takes place by a series of fixations and saccades. In reading, for example, saccades occur approximately every 250 msec and each one takes 25-40 msec.

The most striking thing about newborn saccades is that they exist. Infants evidently do not have to learn or practice for their eyes to move toward a peripheral target. Young infants look toward stimuli in the periphery even when they are already looking at something in their central vision, although saccades are less likely then. Infants are much more likely to make saccades to relatively near targets than to far objects and are more likely to make horizontal than vertical saccades. The form of the saccade is different from that in adults in ways that make it less efficient and perhaps less accurate. It also is slower to start, at least compared with the most rapid responses of adults, but it is still rapid—usually within 2 seconds of the onset of the peripheral target. The mature form does not develop until after 7 weeks of age, but the immature form may not pose any handicap to early vision (see a review by Aslin, 1987).

The saccadic movements of newborns show that they can detect the presence of peripheral stimuli, but do not tell whether they perceive their nature. Actually, the cells in the periphery of the retina appear more adultlike than those in the fovea (Yuodelis & Hendrickson, 1986). The binocular field has a shape similar to that of adults, but prior to 2 months it is only two-thirds the adult size (Mohn & van Hof-van Duin, 1986; Schwartz et al., 1987). By 10 months it is nearly the same size as an adult's. Adults apparently can process information in the periphery better than young children can (see Rayner, 1978, for a discussion). To find out how this ability develops in infants, researchers can study their discrimination of stimuli presented in the periphery. Maurer and Lewis (1979) found that infants as young as 3-4 months can discriminate stimuli in the periphery. Binocular recognition of peripheral targets at 10° from the midline increases over the first 4 months, then is stable for the next 8 (Sireteanu et al., 1984). At 20° from midline, acuity was twice as good at 3 months as at 1 to 2 months, but only one-sixteenth as good as that of adults (Courage & Adams, 1990).[4]

In summary, the research on saccadic eye movements shows that the basic physiological mechanisms for detecting and responding to stimuli in the periphery are present in newborns and develop rapidly in the early months of life. Thus newborns are well equipped to locate visual events in this world.

Do Newborns Search for Visual Stimuli?

The research on saccadic movements has established the existence of captured attention in the neonatal period. Nevertheless, there is disagreement over whether saccadic movements also are part of active visual exploration. Tronick and Clanton (1971) interpret the fact that very young infants often make saccades when no peripheral stimulus is present as their searching for a stimulus. But Salapatek (1975) has suggested that very peripheral stimuli, unnoticed by Tronick and Clanton, may have triggered the saccades.

Haith and his colleagues attacked this question in a quite different fashion (Haith, 1978, 1980; Haith & Goodman, 1982; Mendelson & Haith, 1976). They had observers judge whether infants' eye movements were controlled or were broad, uncontrolled jerks. The observers were able to make these judgments very reliably. In darkness newborns exhibited frequent and controlled eye movements that were not dependent on visual feedback. Haith believes that they did this to search for visual contours. In patterned light visual exploration was also controlled, as would be expected. Surprisingly, however, in light without patterns (a homogeneous field), the eye movements of newborns were uncontrolled, which suggests that they were not searching for visual information. Taking all three situations together, Haith concludes that newborns are active visual explorers and that lack of control will be found only when there is no contour to explore or if the visual information is uninteresting or unattended.

Tracking Moving Stimuli

From birth, infants attend to and track moving stimuli. As has already been described, optokinetic nystagmus has been found in newborns in response to moving vertically striped patterns. Newborns also track single moving objects for up to 90 degrees of arc, but in a quite immature fashion (Gregg et al., 1976; White, 1971). Kremenitzer et al. (1979) found that a sustained, smooth pursuit was found in less than 15% of the exposure time, with jerky pursuit in the remainder. Saccades occurred in the direction of moving objects with considerable latency, and the infants responded at their maximum to much more slowly moving targets than do adults (14 deg/sec and 40 deg/sec, respectively), which is consistent with many other findings that newborns require longer exposure times than older infants. Pursuit is often far less frequent when the

stimulus is a single target than when it is vertical stripes (OKN stimuli) (Kremenitzer et al., 1979).

Smooth pursuit develops by 6 to 8 weeks of age, at least for some speeds of stimulus movement (Aslin, 1981; Dayton et al., 1964; White, 1971). The infant now anticipates the movement of the object and with a smooth, continuous head and eye movement keeps the target in central vision. The ability to track stimuli moving at various speeds continues to develop in the first half year of life (Ames & Silfen, 1965; Aslin, 1981; Bertenthal et al., 1989).

Thus the research suggests that infants respond to movement of visual stimuli from birth and become more responsive as they develop. The shortness of this section may give the impression that perception of moving objects is not very important in early infancy, but such is certainly not my intent. Movement seems to play a very important role in the development of early social responsiveness (Moltz, 1960; Rheingold, 1961; Stern, 1977). It also appears to be of fundamental importance in infants' learning about objects. The role of movement in perceiving objects will be discussed later in this chapter.

Scanning Stationary Patterns

In addition to studying how infants get and keep visual events in their center of vision, researchers can study how they look at an object once they have focused on it. Newborns generally look at a single feature or contour of an object; for example, one corner of a triangle. By 2 months of age infants are beginning to scan more broadly, for example, along the sides and outer corners of a triangle (see Figure 7.4). Salapatek, in his 1975 review of this literature, points out that 2 months is also when infants become able to remember patterns and to make complex visual discriminations.

Another developmental trend in scanning in this age range is a shift from looking at external contours to examination of internal contours. Salapatek and Moscovich (in an unpublished study reported in Salapatek, 1975) presented squares embedded within squares to 1- and 2-month-old infants. The 1-month-olds looked at a corner of the big square, while the 2-month-olds typically selected the internal features. Similar results have been obtained with other geometric patterns (Bushnell et al., 1983) and with faces as stimuli. Infants younger than 2 months look at the ex-

---

4. There is a one-octave increase from 1 to 3 months, when it is still four octaves below the adult value. An octave is a halving or doubling of the spatial frequency (e.g., from 1.5 to 3 cycles/deg.).

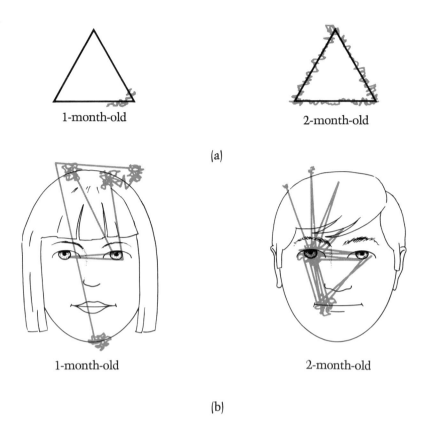

Figure 7.4. Schematic plots of visual scanning by representative 1- and 2-month-old babies. Infrared lights are placed behind the stimulus and reflect off the babies' eyes when they look at a picture. When their eyes change position to look at a new place, the infrared reflection changes position too. The tracings are drawn by observers who watch the videotape (but do not see the stimulus and thus cannot be biased by it). The tracings consist of zigzag lines because of the infants' saccades: their eyes jerk from one location to another. (a) Triangles. The 1-month-old fixates primarily on one corner of the triangle, while the 2-month-old scans all three corners. (b) Faces—pictures with internal contour. The younger infant scans mostly those external contours that have high contrast (the chin and hairline) and the older infant scans primarily internal contours. (Adapted from "Pattern Perception in Early Infancy," by P. Salapatek. In L. B. Cohen & P. Salapatek (Eds.), *Infant perception from sensation to cognition: Vol. 1. Basic visual processes.* Copyright 1975 by Academic Press. Used by permission.)

ternal contours (the hairline and chin, or ear), while 2-month-olds look at the eyes (see the section below on face perception).

Independent evidence that the scanning of patterns reflects infant processing has been presented by Milewski (1976), who habituated 1- and 4-month-old infants to a compound figure similar to that used by Salapatek and Moscovich. Older infants dishabituated in response to changes in shape of either the external or the internal contour, but younger infants dishabituated only to changes that involved the external contour. This suggests that 1-month-old infants not only ignore the internal contours in scanning, but also fail to remember anything about them.

DETECTING VISUAL INFORMATION

Having briefly addressed how babies explore their visual world, let us now examine what they see. Some of the information visual stimuli provide comes from their brightness and color, but most is carried by the pattern. Pattern includes external contour (shape) and internal features, but it also includes the more subtle and complex information that tells us what the object is and where it is located in space.

The most basic question asked about pattern perception was whether newborns detect patterns at all. Fantz's seminal work demonstrates that they do (e.g., see Fantz, 1961, 1963); they consistently look longer at patterns than at homogeneous fields. The next steps were to ask how well they see (acuity) and what kinds of patterns they see. Researchers have been particularly interested in infants' ability to perceive the visual patterns that signify human faces.

Visual patterns give one crucial kind of information about an object, but other kinds of information are just as important. Visual information provides the cues that tell us that an object is three-dimensional and how far away it is. Infant researchers are interested in the questions of when such object perception develops and how. What is known about infant perception of brightness and color is presented in the next section, followed by the various issues of pattern perception.

Brightness (Intensity) of Light

It seems clear that young infants are very good at discriminating among lights that vary in brightness. Hershenson (1964) found that 2- to 4-day-old babies looked longer at lights of medium intensity than they did at bright or dim lights. Peeples and Teller (1975) determined that 2-month-old babies could distinguish a bar of light from its background when the brightness of the two stimuli differed by only 5%, which is almost as good as adults, who can discriminate 1% difference. In both of these studies the two lights were presented at the same time. When lights are presented one after the other, infants as old as 4 months are very poor at discriminating differences in brightness (Kessen & Bornstein, 1978). This may be because of memory limitations.

Babies' ability to discriminate among lights of different brightness or intensity is clear, but what about the question of sensitivity to light in a more absolute sense? Gross observational methods suggest that newborns are more sensitive to light than older infants or children (or adults). They blink, close or squint their eyes, and turn away from lights of lower intensity than would cause this reaction in older children. Still greater hypersensitivity in newborns is a very rare occurrence and is associated with neurological damage (Anderson & Rosenblith, 1964). In a study of color preference, newborns preferred the less bright of two stimuli regardless of hue (Adams, 1987). However, we know of no studies in which early responses to intensity have been examined in a systematic way that explored responses to a number of intensities and controlled for light adaptation at the time of the study.

Color Vision

The physical stimulus for color is the wavelength of the light. Wavelengths vary continuously from infrared (too long for humans to see) through red, yellow, green, and blue to ultraviolet (wavelengths too short for humans to see) (see Figure 7.5).

It might seem a simple matter to determine whether infants can discriminate among colors, but in fact it is not. Because some colors are brighter than others, infants who discriminate between colors may be doing so on the basis of their brightness, not their hue or color. Equalizing the brightness of pairs of colors can only be done using adult data, and the interaction between color and brightness differs for adults and babies (for discussion of these and related problems, see Cohen et al., 1979; Teller & Bornstein, 1987).

Several researchers purposely varied brightness across color discriminations rather than trying to equalize it (Bornstein, 1976; Oster, 1975; Peeples & Teller, 1975; Schaller, 1975). Infants were presented the same pairs of colors (e.g., yellow and red) many times, but sometimes one and sometimes the other was brighter. Then if consistent preference was found for any one color it was assumed to be based on hue, not brightness. In this situation 8- to 12-week-old infants show a color preference. Babies younger than 3 months of age are not capable of discriminating all colors (see review by Banks & Salapatek, 1983) and, indeed, probably lack the physiological underpinnings for trichromatic color vision until about then (Teller & Bornstein, 1987). Recently, Adams (1987) has shown that 3-month-olds discriminate colors and prefer red and yellow (long-wave colors) over blue and green (short-wave colors), the reverse of adult preference. Even newborns preferred colored stimuli over gray ones.

Although people can discriminate among stimuli that differ by only a few wavelengths, they tend to give a single name to stimuli of many different, but similar, wavelengths. These naming practices reflect what is often called **categorical** or **discontinuous** perception. Similar wavelengths are grouped together and perceived as a single color, but those slightly longer or shorter are excluded from the category. For example, lights that differ in wavelength by only 10 nm may appear the same or different depending on where on the spectrum they are located (see Figure 7.5). For example, to adults 570 nm and 580 nm lights both appear yellow, but 560 nm, also a 10 nm difference from 570,

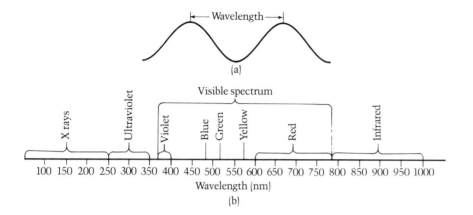

Figure 7.5. Light waves. (a) Like pure tones, the wave forms of light waves are sine waves, but they are measured by the distance between two crests rather than by time. The unit of measurement is a nanometer (nm), which is one billionth of a meter (1 m = 39.37 in.). (b) Wavelengths for the visible spectrum and those near the visible spectrum. Only wavelengths from about 380 to 780 nm are visible to humans. From 380 nm and up, humans see colors change from violet to blue to green and so forth through the colors of the rainbow, ending with red. The range of wavelengths both longer and shorter than those of visible light is much greater. This figure shows ultraviolet light (~300 nm), X rays (~10 nm), and infrared waves (≡1,000 nm). There are even shorter and longer wavelengths: gamma rays (~0.001 nm) and cosmic rays (~0.00001 nm) are much shorter, and microwaves (~0.001 ft), TV waves (~10 ft), and radio waves (~100 ft) are much longer.

appears green. Categorical perception of colors appears to be based in the physiology of our visual system and not to be a product of learning, since humans of other cultures and animals with similar color vision systems have the same sort of categorical perception.[5]

In studies conducted by Bornstein and colleagues, 3- and 4-month-old infants exhibited categorical color perception, but not to red; the investigators hypothesized that this was due to their strong preference for red (Bornstein, 1976; Bornstein et al., 1976). Others have questioned these conclusions (Banks & Salapatek, 1983; Werner & Wooten, 1979; but see also Bornstein's reply, 1981). Recent data would seem to confirm the categorical perception of hue in 20-week-old infants after ruling out many alternative causes for the results (Catherwood et al., 1989).

There is substantial development of the mechanisms involved in color vision in the first few months. Color preference appears almost immediately, hence it does not appear to depend on experience (see, e.g., Teller

& Bornstein, 1987). However, the colors preferred differ later in life. In sum, like other aspects of visual perception, color appears to be actively processed early in life.

PATTERN VISION

Does the visual input to the infant resolve into perceived patterns? Or is it all a buzzing, blooming confusion (as William James said)?

Acuity of Pattern Vision

The first question about infants' abilities to see patterns is, How accurately can they see? This is equivalent to asking what their visual acuity is. The most familiar test of visual acuity is the Snellen chart, which has a big E at the top with lines of successively smaller letters below. Patients read down the chart until the print is too small for them to make out. The results are reported in terms of what a person with unimpaired vision can see at 20 feet. Thus 20/20 is considered to be the norm. People's vision can vary in either direction from this. A person with 40/20 vision can see at 40 feet what the normal person can see only at 20 feet, but an individual with 20/400 vision can see at 20

---

5. Categorical perception is also found for speech sounds. Some researchers believe that the term *categorical perception* should be limited to situations in which subjects cannot discriminate among stimuli within a category (see Werner & Wooten, 1979). By this definition categorical perception would be characteristic of speech perception, but not color naming.

feet what the normal person can see at 400 feet (the big E on Snellen charts). I will use these equivalents in the discussion of infants' acuity, although the literature uses more technical measures.

Preference tests are the most widely used measures of infants' visual acuity, though OKN and **visual evoked potentials (VEPs)** or brain wave responses to visual stimuli are also used. Even newborn infants will look longer at a striped than at a plain gray stimulus. A striped pattern (called a grating) can be made with thinner and thinner stripes until the stripes appear to blend with each other and do not seem to the viewer to be different from the homogeneous gray field. Infants will cease to show a preference for the striped pattern when it looks like a gray blur. This technique has shown that the visual acuity of infants under 2 months of age is somewhere between 20/300 and 20/800. The same results are obtained when stripes are moved across the infants' visual field and acuity is measured by the width of stripe required to elicit OKN (see Banks & Dannemiller, 1987, for a review). Studies using the preferential looking technique may underestimate acuity inasmuch as infants actually prefer the plain gray when stripes are close to threshold separation (Held et al., 1979).

Acuity estimates are quite variable, ranging from 6/69 to 6/400 in a series of studies summarized in Dobson et al. (1987). The results differ somewhat depending on both the method and the stimuli used. VEPs tend to give slightly lower estimates. The most acute vision found in young infants has been about 20/150 when the stimulus used was a single line (Lewis & Maurer, 1977). In their review, Aslin and Dumais (1980) conclude 20/500 is the best estimate for newborns.

A relatively new technique in perceptual (and other) studies is to use the subjective judgment of an adult. An adult who does not know what stimulus the infant is being exposed to is asked to judge whether the infant has responded (or, in some studies of imitation, what the infant has responded to). When used to ascertain whether the infant is fixating a target (Morante et al., 1982), the results are very similar to those found using more elaborate techniques. Combined with fixed stimulus cards this enables practical clinical assessment of acuity in infants, even in newborns (Dobson et al., 1987; Teller et al., 1986).

Acuity develops rapidly during the first 6 months of life (see the review by Banks & Salapatek, 1983), reaching 20/200 by 6 months (see also Dobson & Teller, 1978). Acuity continues to improve to 20/50 at 12 months but does not reach 20/20 until 4 or 5 years, when both operant and preferential looking

methods yield this result (Birch et al., 1983). The reasons acuity increases during the first year of life and beyond are not fully known.[6] The early improvement is probably due to changes in cells of the retina (see Banks & Bennett, 1988). There is direct evidence that development in the first 12 weeks depends on maturation rather than experience (Dobson et al., 1980; Miranda, 1970). When full-term infants were compared with prematures matched on conceptional rather than postbirth age, the acuities of the two were similar, even though the preterm infants often had 4 weeks more experience than the full-term infants.

These studies assessed binocular acuity, but for purposes of clinical assessment it is important to know the visual acuity of each eye. Lewis and Maurer (1986) have compared different methods of doing this and found that preferential looking combined with their shortened method of testing appeared to be clinically useful. The monocular resolution of infants who had no visual problems improved from 6 to 36 months.

Another argument for the crucial role of neural maturation in visual performance can be found in the sudden development or improvement between 3 and 4 months of a number of visual functions. Vernier acuity, which depends on processing at higher levels of the visual system, is more acute than grating acuity in adults, but is poorer in infants under 3 months of age (Shimojo & Held, 1987). It rises sharply so that it exceeds grating acuity by 4 or 5 months (Shimojo et al., 1984). There are intriguing sex differences from the third through fifth months in vernier, but not in grating, acuity with girls being better than boys (see Gwiazda et al., 1989a, 1989b). Speculation as to the cause centers on the role of an early surge of testosterone affecting nerve growth (Held, 1991).

Acuity depends in part on contrast between the brightness of a target and that of its background. Infants' sensitivity to contrast is not mature at birth. Indeed, it shows a twofold increase between 1 and 3 months of age (Atkinson et al., 1977; Banks & Salapatek, 1978; Gwiazda et al., 1978).

Acuity may also depend on the distance from the baby's eyes to the stimulus. Special interocular eye muscles (as distinguished from extraocular muscles, which move the eyeball) automatically change the shape of the lens to bring an object into focus when an

---

6. It may be appropriate to note briefly here that acuity is also affected by astigmatism and young infants tend to have more astigmatism than older ones. While 55% of 11–20-week-old infants have significant degrees of astigmatism, by 50 weeks most of them have little or no astigmatism. Correction for astigmatism does result in increased acuity as measured by preference tests.

adult looks at targets at different distances. This is called **visual accommodation**. A procedure called dynamic retinoscopy allows measurement of the effects of lens changes by observing the focus of objects on the retina without cooperation from the testee other than keeping the eyes open. Haynes et al. (1965) used this technique to demonstrate that infants show no accommodation in the first month. According to these researchers, infants' eyes are fixed at one distance (like a fixed-focus camera), the average being 19 cm (7.5 in.), but by the fourth month, their accommodative ability nearly reaches adult levels.

This distance limitation was taken very seriously by infant researchers, and almost all subsequent studies of visual perception have presented stimuli at around 19 cm from the infants' eyes. Furthermore, researchers studying infant-mother interaction emphasized the fact that the mother's and infant's heads are approximately that distance apart in the normal nursing position, and argued that this provides an ideal situation for the infant to recognize the mother.

Such use of Haynes et al.'s data may have been premature. Reexamination of their procedure suggests that the targets may have been too small for infants to see beyond a certain distance. If so, the failure to discriminate at greater distances might be due to loss of acuity and not lack of accommodation. Two studies using different measurement techniques found accommodation nearly as good as that of adults at 2 months and partial accommodation as early as 1 month (Banks, 1980; Braddick et al., 1979).

The second reason for questioning Haynes et al.'s findings involves their implications. In adults, failure to accommodate produces an out-of-focus image, and thereby loss of acuity. It was naturally assumed that the same is true of infants, but this need not be so. Two studies, one done before (Fantz et al., 1962) and one done after the Haynes et al. study (Salapatek et al., 1976) found that visual acuity does not vary at distances from 12.7 cm (5 in.) to 150 cm (59 in.) for young babies even though it would in adults. This is presumably because small errors in accommodative focus will produce a greater loss of acuity in adults' more finely tuned systems. Thus young babies may be able to see at their maximal acuity across a substantial range of distances, which would mean that the nursing position is no more ideal for learning to recognize mother than many others.

Is There Foveal Vision at Birth?

Adults' vision is most acute in the **fovea**, that part of the **retina** (the part of the eye with the nerve cells

that transform light patterns into nerve impulses) that is most densely packed with sense receptors. The measures of acuity used with infants do not require that the subjects use foveal vision, since their heads are free to move, and thereby the stimulus may fall on areas outside the fovea. Indeed, in the OKN measure, peripheral vision must be involved. The sense receptors in the periphery of the retina are almost mature at birth, while those of the fovea are very immature. This has led some researchers to suggest that newborns lack foveal vision altogether. However, Lewis and Maurer (1980) found evidence to support the idea that the infant is maintaining fixation in the fovea, and hence can perceive foveally.

What Patterns Do Newborns Detect?

It has been noted that newborns prefer to look at patterned rather than plain stimuli. That preference is the basis for many studies of acuity. It has given rise to a large and complex literature exploring the kinds of patterns young infants discriminate, whether these early discrimination abilities mean that infants are prewired to perceive certain meaningful patterns, and whether changing preferences among visual stimuli mean that young infants are rapidly learning to extract information from their world.

This research enterprise is extremely difficult. There are an incredible number of two-dimensional patterns, both those in the natural world and those that can be created. Consider how difficult it is to select a few to present in the paired preference technique. Because of the complexities involved, I will not attempt to present the research in this area in a historical context, but will summarize the most widely accepted findings. Note that this will leave out many possibly important findings that have not yet been replicated or corroborated by other kinds of research.

It is quite clear that newborn infants look longer at figures with a high **contour density** (the total length of edges or contours in a given area). For example, a square with its four edges (sides) has higher contour density than a line, which has only one edge. Checkerboards with small squares have higher contour density than those with large squares. Contour density can account for infants' differentiating among a large number of patterns that were at one time thought to test more advanced abilities, such as the ability to perceive meaningful form or the ability to process large amounts of information (see Fantz et al., 1975; Karmel & Maisel, 1975; Salapatek, 1975). Detecting differences in contour density does not suggest advanced abilities, because our visual systems are physiologically structured to detect them, as we shall see shortly.

Newborns also respond to the sharpness of contours. Prior to 2 months infants look longer at stimuli that have (a) high contrast (are black and white rather than muted, such as gray on white or yellow on orange), (b) sharp rather than blurred edges, and (c) bright, flat surfaces rather than softer, textured ones (Fantz et al., 1975). This preference for sharp contrast, unlike that for contour density, disappears after 2 months of age.

Young infants, including newborns, prefer patterns with circular elements to those with straight elements (Fantz et al., 1975). This is true whether the circular elements are incorporated into a configuration (such as a bullseye or face) or are randomly placed.

There are a few other dimensions to which infants respond, but investigators disagree on whether the infant is cued by the dimension studied or by other dimensions that covary, such as contour density (or the contrast sensitivity function, as proposed by Banks & Salapatek, 1981). Newborns prefer large to small patterns (2 in. squares versus 1 in.). Fantz et al. (1975) found that 2-month-old infants are less sensitive to size, and are more sensitive to differences in number: They look longer at stimuli with many elements. There may also be a basic preference for irregular over regular figures, but, if so, it disappears for certain stimuli, such as those with circular elements, and at certain ages (Fantz et al., 1975). Throughout their first year infants prefer vertical and horizontal gratings to oblique ones, especially at spacings that are close to their acuity threshold (Leehey et al., 1975). At 2 months, infants seem to look longer at vertical than at horizontal lines (Salapatek, 1975). They discriminate oblique orientations by 5-6 weeks of age, but not when the gratings are static and the comparisons are made sequentially rather than simultaneously (Atkinson et al., 1988).[7] At approximately 6 weeks VEP responses can be found (Atkinson et al., 1988). By 4 months infants discriminate a 10° change in the orientation of a vertically symmetrical polygon and if habituated to multiple angles of it will not dishabituate to another similar angle, but will to a new stimulus, thus indicating they have formed some kind of concept of the stimulus (Bornstein et al., 1986). Earlier, Bornstein and Krinsky (1985) showed that 4-month-old infants did not prefer vertically symmetrical to vertically repeated or obliquely symmetrical patterns, but they processed them more efficiently.

Mechanisms to Explain These Phenomena

These pattern preferences and the developmental changes they undergo can be explained better by physiological maturation than by learning for several reasons. First, the visual system seems wired to respond to such aspects of visual stimuli as straight and curved edges, which are those involved in contours. Research on physiological responses in visual systems in other species can be helpful in explaining this. In such research, the firing of individual nerve cells is recorded by means of a very small needlelike instrument called a microelectrode. These electrodes are so small that their tips are usually less than one micron (one-thousandth of a millimeter) in diameter. They can record the firing of single cells in the **optic nerve** (the bundle of nerve fibers on their way to the higher centers of the brain) and the **visual cortex** (the part of the cortex devoted to perception of complex visual events). This discussion will concentrate on research with cats because (a) it is the most extensive, (b) cats' visual systems are similar to our own, and (c) research with humans (using both microelectrodes and other techniques) is limited, but what there is tends to be consistent with that on cats.

Two questions are addressed: Is pattern perception wired into the structure of the visual system?[8] If so, is this wiring innate? If a single nerve cell fires only in response to specific complex stimuli, the conclusion is that the visual system is anatomically structured to detect that pattern. If this single cell fires in newborn animals, it is possible to conclude that the anatomical wiring is innate. Briefly, the answers are that perception of some patterns is structurally wired and at least partly innate.

Many different kind of detectors have been found in cats and, directly or indirectly, in humans. In the visual cortex there are cells that fire in response to a border or edge (light on one side, dark on the other), others that respond to straight lines (dark line with light on either side) and still others to slits (lines of light, with dark on either side). Two levels of edge, line, and slit detectors have been found: simple cells and complex

---

7. However, the dishabituation stimuli were mirror images of the habituated ones, and much older children make errors in perceptual judgments that involve mirror images (Rosenblith, 1965).

8. Workers in this field talk about the nervous system in terms of a telephone or computer network. They use the expression *hard wired* to refer to established nervous system connections that are not easily subject to change. *Soft wiring* refers to connections that are plastic or learned.

cells. Simple cells respond to edges, lines, and slits only in a particular orientation in a particular place in the visual field. For example, one detector might fire for horizontal lines in the lower right of a cat's visual field, but not to vertical lines there or to horizontal lines anywhere. Complex cells fire for all stimuli of the particular pattern and orientation to which they are responsive, regardless of where in the visual field they are located. Cells can be further divided into those that respond optimally to bars or edges of one particular length and those that respond to a wider range of lengths. Some cells are sensitive to stimulus angles. This combination of types of detector cells allows cats to be sensitive to shape, size, and position of stimuli, and presumably to learn to respond appropriately to any of them.

The existence of these various kinds of receptors is firmly established in cats. While additional kinds of detectors are likely to be found, it is unlikely that the ones already found will be brought into disrepute by later research. Furthermore, both direct and indirect research with adult humans suggest that they exist in similar fashion in humans (for reviews of this research, see Leibowitz & Harvey, 1973; Sekuler, 1974). Thus we can say that the visual system is physiologically structured to detect the kinds of patterns described above. Many of the single-cell detectors in cats seem to be present in primitive form at birth or shortly thereafter (e.g., Hubel & Wiesel, 1963), although we will see later that these cells must receive visual stimulation to stay alive.

Let us now return to our thesis, that many of the early visual responses in human infants are due to neural functioning. These single-cell detectors respond to edges (contours), bars, angles, and slits, all of which involve light-dark patterning and are exactly the kind of stimuli to which newborn infants respond. Hence their responses may reflect firing of such detectors, and, indeed, newborns do not seem to respond to dimensions other than those to which single cells respond. A good example of a specific visual discrimination that is consistent with this hypothesis is from a study by Cohen and Younger (1984) in which they habituated young infants to an angle and tested dishabituation to various transformations of the habituated angle. Their results indicate that 6-week-olds process specific line segments in specific orientations, whereas 3-month-olds respond to the angle as a unit. Because single cells respond to individual lines in specific orientations, it is likely that the responses of younger infants were on that basis, whereas those of older infants evidently involved additional kinds of processing.

Infants' brain wave responses (EEGs) to visual pat-

terns support the conclusion that newborns' ability to distinguish contours is based on the early firing of these contour-receptive cells and that stimulation must occur if these cells are to continue to respond (Karmel & Maisel, 1975).

Studies that pit conceptional age against experience also support the role of physiological maturation. Fantz et al. (1975) found that the number of weeks of experience the infants had in the visual world was not an important determinant of their changing patterns of preference, but the number of weeks since they had been conceived was. Similarly, the blink response to a looming stimulus in postmature compared with term infants is determined by conceptional age, not by the amount of postnatal experience (Pettersen et al., 1980).

These data do not indicate whether infants perceive meaningful patterns. The ability to discriminate among stimuli varying in brightness, color, or contour density does not mean that they are perceived as meaningful. Young infants seem to perceive stimuli piecemeal, rather than as integrated figures. They scan only external contours (before 2 months) or internal features (from 2 to 3 months), but not both. Their preference for circularity does not require a complete configuration, and even early face recognition, as we shall see shortly, seems to be on the basis of a few pertinent features.

Preference for form or shape itself (except for curves)—for example, preference for X over O, or triangles over squares—has not yet been addressed. To claim that young infants can detect meaningful figures, it is necessary first to demonstrate that they perceive either shapes or configurations of groups of elements (such as dots). The early research on infant pattern perception was interpreted as a positive indication of such ability, but we know now that those early findings were due to differences in contour density, brightness, and so on. Salapatek (1975) found that 2-month-olds do not show preferences based on shape alone, and do not even necessarily look preferentially at central rather than at background figures (a very basic characteristic of visual perception). A compound figure, such as a cross within a circle, is not perceived as a single figure rather than as a cross and a circle until around 5 months of age (see Cohen et al., 1979). These findings strengthen the notion that perception in young infants is (a) of a piecemeal nature, (b) largely governed by the firing of single neurons in the visual system, and (c) controlled by the physiological maturation that naturally occurs in babies exposed to normal visual experiences.

Evidence has been found for greater perceptual or-

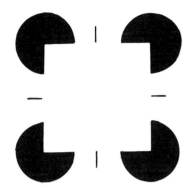

Figure 7.6. One of the stimuli used in Ghim's study. The perception of a square is clear, despite its not being physically outlined.

ganization as early as 2 to 4 months of age (e.g., Ghim & Eimas, 1988), but it has not been consistent (see Dodwell et al., 1987, for a review of the negative evidence). A recent series of well-controlled studies of perception of subjective contours (those perceived in the absence of physical stimuli for them) would indicate that infants as young as 3 months are able to perceive subjective contours (Ghim, 1990). Further, infants were able to use the percept of the subjective pattern as the basis for discrimination among forms with real contours, thus strengthening the idea that they saw them as equivalent (see Figure 7.6). These data lower the age of a fairly advanced percept, but not so much as to make visual experience irrelevant.

DEVELOPMENT OF FACE PERCEPTION

Research using abstract patterns as stimuli has failed to find clear evidence that newborns can perceive meaningful patterns. It does not rule out the possibility that infants innately perceive certain biologically important patterns, such as the face. If so, these configurations might provide the basis from which infants learn the meaning of other visual stimuli. Being able to recognize the configuration of a face early in infancy and to know (or rapidly learn) that it is associated with food, warmth, safety, and so on would be extremely adaptive in an evolutionary sense. Thus ethologists as well as psychologists are interested in early face perception, primarily to explore it as a basis for early attachment to the mother. Psychologists are interested in whether face perception is similar to or a precursor of perception of meaningful forms in general. This discussion will focus on the relevance of face perception to the general issue of what infants can perceive and

will examine research relevant to the questions of whether perception of the human face is innate and, if not, when and how it develops.

Researchers studying face perception have usually used one of two kinds of stimuli. One kind tests infants' ability to discriminate line drawings or other schematic representation of faces from other configurations of similar complexity, often schematic faces with the features scrambled (see Figure 7.7). The other kind compares two different faces, say, the mother's and a stranger's. Success on the latter sorts of discriminations obviously requires memory as well as perceptual ability.

Perception of Schematic Faces

It is clear that newborns prefer drawings of faces to less complex stimuli such as plain ovals, bullseyes, and newsprint (Fantz, 1963, 1966). The problem is that these results may be due to stimulus differences unrelated to the picture's representing a face, such as differences in contour density or brightness. Studies in the 1960s and 1970s that controlled for these confounding variables did not find consistent discrimination of faces prior to 4 months (Haaf, 1974; Haaf & Bell, 1967; Haaf & Brown, 1975; Kagan et al., 1966; Koopman & Ames, 1968). At that same age babies could discriminate their mothers' faces from those of strangers (Ambrose, 1961, 1963).

Subsequently, researchers have demonstrated face perception in younger infants using procedures in which the stimulus presentation is not controlled by the experimenter, but by the infant's own looking behaviors (Horowitz et al., 1972; described in Chapter 9). This results in a higher proportion of infants completing the experiment and in their spending longer times fixating the stimuli than when stimuli were presented for set, arbitrary times (usually no longer than 30 seconds). For example, the 2-month-old babies in Maurer and Barrera's (1981) study usually fixated for longer than 40 seconds per trial. Research using these techniques has established that face perception develops earlier than 4 months of age.

Maurer and Barrera (1981) reasoned that 2-month-olds should be capable of discriminating faces, but, because their scanning is still fairly primitive, they would need more time. Using infant-paced procedures that allow infants to look until they cease to fixate, the 2-month-olds did discriminate faces from scrambled faces (see Figure 7.7). The conclusion is especially strong since both the visual preference and the habituation-dishabituation paradigms achieved the same results. The researchers' interpretation that the devel-

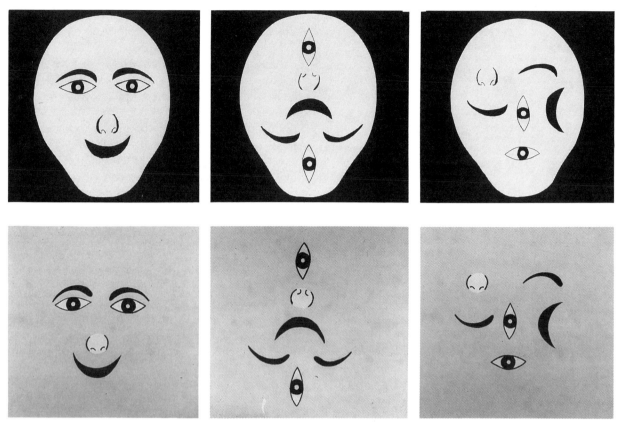

Figure 7.7. Diagrams of faces—scrambled and unscrambled, without external contours and with contours—used by Maurer and Barrera. (Photographs courtesy of Daphne Maurer.)

opment of scanning is the basis for the development of facial discrimination was enhanced by their earlier finding that 1-month-olds could not discriminate facial features from scrambled features when both lacked the external contours of a surrounding oval, but could distinguish them when they had borders (Maurer & Barrera, 1978). These results suggest that the reason very young babies do not discriminate between regular and scrambled faces is that they look primarily at the external contour (the boundary between face and hair), which does not provide enough information to enable them to make such discriminations.

A reanalysis of facial preference studies up to 1985 showed very high correlations ($r \geq .90$) between infants' ability to detect the pattern information associated with the stimuli and their preferences among them (Banks & Ginsburg, 1985). Infants prefer what is most visible.

Preference for schematic over scrambled faces is not necessarily driven by their similarity to natural faces in the infant's environment. Dannemiller and Stephens (1988) found that rearrangements usually alter many stimulus features besides face likeness. Using a facial and an abstract pattern that were equated for contrast, brightness, and size, and then reversing the contrast for both, they found that at 6 weeks babies had no preference for any of the patterns, but at 12 weeks the normal-contrast "face" was preferred to both the reverse-contrast face and the reverse-contrast pattern.

On the basis of data derived from exposing neonates to stimuli with elaborately controlled characteristics, Kleiner (1987) concludes that their preferences for facelike patterns are primarily governed by stimulus energy, not social significance. Her conclusions are disputed by Morton et al. (1990), who tend to argue for an innate template with which stimulus configurations are compared; Kleiner (1990) has defended her conclusions.

I find it difficult to generalize from the various studies using abstract (and often very different) representations of faces to perception of real faces, with their much more infinite variation.

Perception of Real and Photographic Faces

Several studies of infants' scanning of mirror reflections of real faces have found development comparable to that of scanning geometric figures (Haith et al., 1977; Maurer & Salapatek, 1976). It has been shown that 1-month-olds do not attend much to the faces at all, and when they do, they primarily scan borders that have high contrast, such as the hairline. Consistent with this, they look longer at Caucasian faces with dark hair (higher contrast) than they do at Caucasian faces with light hair (Melhuish, 1982). By 2 months infants attend much more to the faces (almost 90% of their time in the apparatus) and primarily scan internal features, such as the eyes.

Using actual faces as stimuli, newborns have been shown to prefer their mothers' faces to those of strangers (Bushnell et al., 1989; Field et al., 1984). Field et al. (1984) ruled out olfactory cues and found the preference when both faces were present simultaneously until the newborn had looked at one or both for a period of 20 seconds. Whether it was the first or second trial and whether the infant was breast- or bottle-fed, there was a significant preference for the mother, with infant looking for 57-69% of the 20 seconds at her rather than at the stranger whose coloring was similar (Bushnell et al., 1989). Bushnell (in an unpublished study cited in Bushnell et al., 1989) found that when both the mother and the other woman wore the same wig there was no preference (recognition).

It has been demonstrated that 3-month-old babies can discriminate between (a) photographed faces of their own mothers and fathers and those of strangers (Barrera & Maurer, 1981b; Maurer & Heroux, 1980), and (b) photographs of two same-sex strangers (Barrera & Maurer, 1981a; Maurer & Heroux, 1980). But the earliest age at which infants have been found to identify the equivalence between a photograph of a strange person and the actual person is at 5 months (Dirks & Gibson, 1977), although their ability to recognize photographs of their mothers earlier implies the recognition of some equivalence between mother and her picture. Even at 5 months infants' abilities to discriminate faces is still based on rather gross features. In Dirks and Gibson's (1977) study, photographs of both a person the infants had seen and a person with similar hair and features were recognized as similar to the live person by the 5-month-olds. Other studies show that 7-month-olds are able to make subtler identifications: They recognize the same person from different perspectives, such as full face versus profile (Cohen & Strauss, 1979; Fagan, 1976); they can iden-

tify as similar the same facial expression on different faces (Caron et al., 1982); and they can discriminate male from female faces (Cornell, 1974; Fagan, 1976). All of these require the perception of faces as integrated configurations of internal and external contours, an ability that develops with the ability to perceive compound patterns at 5 months.

In summary, babies' ability to perceive photographic or real faces apparently is a function of their general perceptual development and not innately given. We know a number of things relevant to this. For instance, 1-month-old babies attend primarily to regions of high contrast and do not process the internal features of a stimulus, thus they will fail to identify the features of a face (eyes, nose, mouth) or any rearrangement of these features. By 2 months they attend to internal features and thus can discriminate scrambled from regularly arranged features. By 3 months they process those internal features well enough to identify their mothers and to discriminate between some facial expressions. Subsequent development of face perception also seems consistent with general perceptual development (see Fagan, 1979, for a good review).

Studies claiming to have found face perception in even younger infants have not held up when replicated using stricter methodology (Maurer & Young, 1983; Melhuish, 1982). However, Haaf and Arehart (1988) have shown that exposure to photos of faces, as opposed to component elements of schematic faces, greatly increases the number of elements in a schematic face that 10-week-olds prefer. Infants in that study preferred a schematic face with complexity more at the level of the photos (7 or 13 elements), but preferred only 2 elements in the oval of a scrambled face.

As noted above, facial perception appears to be part of perceptual development and not a specifically prewired phenomenon. Infants' ability to perceive faces appears to develop gradually. You can be sure, however, that this issue has not been put to rest. Psychologists will continue to look for evidence of an innate ability to identify faces that is present in the neonatal period.

ABSTRACTION OF PERCEPTUAL INVARIANTS

Among the major influences on the field of perception have been the related theories of E. J. Gibson (1969) and J. J. Gibson (1966, 1979). Both these researchers believe that we learn to perceive objects by abstracting what is unchanging or **invariant** in a stimulus. For example, a face always has a particular configuration of eyes, nose, mouth, and so on. A set of in-variants uniquely specifies an object; for example, all closed-plane figures with three angles are triangles. That object may be a class (as in all men) or a particular object (my daddy). In either case it has a set of invariant features that differentiate it from all other stimuli.

The developmental question for infancy that Gibsonian theory raises is when and how the perception of invariants develops. Based on pattern perception data, a reasonable guess is that infants younger than 2 months probably do not abstract invariants, although they can make many of the discriminations that form the basis of distinctive features. By 2 to 3 months babies do recognize unchanging configurations in stimuli that vary in other ways. Milewski (1979) demonstrated this by habituating 3-month-olds to three-dot patterns in either a triangular configuration or a straight line. The crucial test of perception of invariance is whether the infants dishabituate to stimuli that have the same configuration as the habituation stimuli, but differ in other attributes (e.g., a longer straight line, or larger triangle). They did not, which indicates that they detected the invariant pattern. Inasmuch as they dishabituated to stimuli with the familiar size and position but in a new configuration, the interpretation that they abstracted the perceptual invariant is further strengthened.

It has been argued by J. J. Gibson and others that a caricature of a face accentuates the relevant features of a specific face and eliminates features that are not distinctive. Novelty preference has been shown by 24- to 36-week-old infants when they were familiarized with caricatures and tested on photos, but not in the reverse condition (Tyrrell et al., 1987). These data argue for better encoding of invariants when they are accentuated, as in the caricatures, or are gross features, as in Dirks and Gibson (1977).

If the development of face perception is analyzed in terms of perceptual invariants, the research is consistent with Milewski's findings. By 3 months of age babies recognize photographs of their mothers' faces. This means that they have abstracted some invariant characteristics of their mothers' faces (but not the same set an older baby would abstract, as shown by Dirks & Gibson's 1977 data already discussed). Only at 7 months did infants abstract the perceptual invariants of a strange face in a way we would expect of an older child or adult.

In a more complicated paradigm, which is related to the next topic as well, 3-month-old infants were exposed to films and sound tracks that were matched to each other or not and synchronous in time or not. Only those exposed to matched and synchronous stimuli showed evidence of intermodal learning (Bahrick, 1988). This technique could be used to explore further which kinds of invariant relations are detected earliest.

EXPECTANCY OF
DYNAMIC VISUAL EVENTS

Habituation studies could be said to involve the infant's forming an expectation about the stimuli. However, this can be seen as a relatively passive form of expectation. It has no overt result until it is violated. Haith and his colleagues have been asking the question of whether future-oriented expectancies exist in early infancy, expectancies that would lead the infant to behave in a given way prior to receiving a stimulus. This is another topic at the boundary of perception and cognition.

Short-term perceptual expectancies, involving dynamic visual stimulation over which the infant has no control, have been shown for 3½-month-olds (Haith et al., 1988). Slides were shown to the left (L) or right (R) of the infant's visual field, either in a simple alternating series (L-R-L-R-L-R) or in a series that appeared on either the L or R in a random fashion. The reflections of the stimuli on the infants' eyes were video recorded to enable measurement of reaction time (latency). Reaction times were shorter for the regularly alternating series, and there were more anticipatory movements of the eyes to where the next slide would be. While this indexes some kind of learning, it fits neither classical nor operant conditioning paradigms, as stimuli are not paired and responses are not reinforced.

When more complicated sequences were used (L-L-R or R-R-L and L-L-L-R or R-R-R-L), 3-month-olds showed anticipations and lower reaction times in the 2/1 condition, as well as in simple alternations, but they reacted faster to or anticipated the shift to the side of only the single presentation, not to the three side (Canfield & Haith, 1991). The 2-month-olds showed some evidence of being able to form some expectation in the simple alternating sequence. Incidentally, these expectancy measures are stable from one day to another in 3-month-olds (Haith & McCarty, 1990).[9]

In another study, the rule by which stimuli were presented was changed to see whether this would disrupt the infants' behavior, thus indicating a violation of expectations (Arehart & Haith, 1991). Infants saw either 40 pictures in a R-L-R-L pattern followed by 48 in a L-L-R sequence or the reverse. The rule change resulted in fewer anticipations, more anticipation errors, and slower reaction times. The second rule was harder to learn than the first, and the negative effect of a rule change was more lasting if it went from simple to complex.

Heart rate responses to predictable events have also been shown in 7-month-old infants in a study by Donohue and Berg (1991). When a white noise was followed by an interesting event, anticipatory heart rate decelerations occurred after about 12 trials, and they reached their peak just before the interesting event was to occur. The patterns of response were the same as for adults.

OBJECTS IN SPACE

Most of the research on pattern perception just discussed used two-dimensional stimuli, either line drawings or photographs. Our world, in contrast, is made up of three-dimensional objects situated in three-dimensional space. That we perceive visual patterns as objects at all is one of the great mysteries to be unraveled. Our eyes work similarly to a camera in that the image that is recorded on the retina (analogous to the film of the camera) is essentially two-dimensional. Yet on the basis of these two-dimensional images we perceive three-dimensional objects in space. How we come to perceive three dimensions is one of the major foci of the empiricist-nativist argument: Are we pre-wired to perceive three dimensions, or do we learn to do so?

I have selected three specific topics for discussion from the larger topic of perception of objects in space because these have been the focus of concentrated interest in infancy. They are (a) the role of movement in perceiving objects, (b) the implications for object knowledge in the two forms of reaching (see Chapter 8 also), and (c) development of depth perception.

The Role of Movement in Perception of Objects

The study of visual perception has been focused primarily on static (nonmoving) displays. Outside the laboratory, however, objects move a lot. The Gibsons have been instrumental in analyzing the role of kinetic information and in providing a basis for exploration of the development of sensitivity to such information. They argue that continuous motion of both target objects and of the viewer with respect to stationary ob-

jects provide the most fundamental mechanism for the extraction of information about objects. The simplest case is when a rigid object moves across a field (an action called **translation**). During such a movement the texture elements on the object remain in the same (invariant) relation because they move together. At the same time, the relation of the object to texture elements of the background changes. Thus movement helps to separate the expanse of the object from the background and from other objects and thereby to specify the nature of the object. Theoretically, similar patterns of invariance and change specify objects regardless of the kinds of motions they undergo. In addition, analogous patterns specify the nature of particular motions regardless of the particular object that is moving.

Even newborns are potentially capable of detecting such kinetic information. In fact, among the most salient visual cues for newborns are (a) contours that mark the boundaries between objects and backgrounds and (b) movement. Newborns can also track moving stimuli, although the kind of information picked up by the jerky, immature eye movements may be different from that resulting from continuous, smooth tracking.

Three distinct theoretical questions about kinetic information have been addressed in the infant research:

(1) Does movement provide a better basis for object recognition than static displays of the same object?
(2) What kinds of movements provide the best information for object recognition?
(3) Can babies detect different kinds of kinetic cues that carry various kinds of information?

Each of these questions will be discussed in turn.

The first question is perhaps most basic. When objects move, their parts move together. If we look at this phenomenon in reverse, we can see that perceptual configurations (e.g., eyes and nose) that move together provide a cue that they are parts of the same object. A number of recent studies demonstrate that movement often provides the information necessary for babies to recognize an object where a stationary pattern does not. These are discussed below in the order of the ages of the subjects.

Two-month-olds do not perceive two stationary surfaces as one, even if they are connected and have the same surface coloring, alignment, and so on (Kellman et al., 1987). Kellman and Spelke (1983) found that 4-month-old babies perceived a partly hidden object as a single, continuous object rather than two discontinuous objects only when the object moved behind an occluding object. When all was stationary, the babies acted as if they did not know whether the hidden pattern was one or two objects. When two surfaces moved together, either laterally or in depth, the infants perceived them as a unitary object (Kellman et al., 1986, 1987), but patterns of dishabituation indicated that they did not perceive them as connected if the surfaces were stationary. Owsley (1980) explored the relative effectiveness of continuous movement (as in a movie) versus a series of static displays of the same movement (as in a selection of individual frames of the movie). Continuous motion is hypothetically more effective, because it provides overlapping information that specifies the invariance. Owsley demonstrated that a moving object, but not a set of still views of the object in different orientations, was effective in producing recognition in 4-month-olds. Hofsten and Spelke (1985) presented 5½-month-old infants with two objects that were separated in depth and were either stationary or moved together. When they were stationary the infants reached for the nearer one, but when they moved together, they reached for the two objects as a single unit. The next step was to see what happened when the two objects were separated by a gap (Spelke et al., 1989). Since infants presented with two separate objects reach for only one, reaching can tell us whether they perceive one or two objects. When the separation was fully visible, the kinetic and spatial information interacted to determine the infant's response. The infants perceived adjacent objects as separate if they moved independently, but continued to react to visibly separated objects as a single unit if they moved together.

Ruff (1982a) presented complex objects moving in various ways (see Figure 7.8) to 6-month-old infants. After familiarizing them with one object, she presented a novel one and determined which they looked at longer. Infants exposed to moving objects exhibited recognition, but infants exposed to objects that were primarily stationary (they moved a little) did not. (See also Ruff, 1987.)

These studies demonstrate that movement is an effective cue to object recognition. In addition, movement appears to be necessary for object perception for young infants in some circumstances, although stationary cues are sufficient with older babies and adults. Unlike Owsley's 4-months-olds, 7-month-olds do abstract invariance from different discrete views (Cohen & Strauss, 1979; Fagan, 1976; McGurk, 1972). Thus there appears to be a developmental progression from reliance only on movement prior to 5 months to reliance on visual characteristics, as Spelke and her col-

leagues have shown. Movement cues provided by touch (not vision) may have the same effect on infants' treatment of objects as being one or two (Stréri &

Figure 7.8. Two distinct kinds of continuous movement used by Ruff in her study of 6-month-old infants (Ruff, 1982a). Arrows show the direction of movement. (a) A simple translation movement. The object stays facing the same way and is moved up, down, left, right, forward, and back. Watching these movements helped infants to recognize the object, whereas watching the same object when it moved just slightly (2.54 cm) in these directions (the control condition) did not. (b) Two of the three movements in a simple rotation condition. In the top drawing the object rotates in a frontal plane. In the bottom drawing the object rotates on its vertical axis and is in translational motion. This simple rotation condition moderately facilitated recognition, but only when infants were given more trials than was necessary for the translation condition to work. A more complex rotation condition (not illustrated) did not facilitate recognition. (From "Effects of Object Movement on Infant's Detection of Object Structure" by H. A. Ruff. In *Developmental Psychology, 18*, pp. 463-472. Copyright 1982 by the American Psychological Association. Reprinted by permission.)

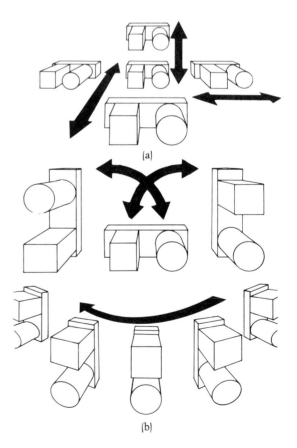

(a)

(b)

Spelke, 1989). The mechanisms that might account for these behaviors are not clear, but the data challenge some conventional conceptions of the infant's perception of the world.

Ruff (1982a) also explored the second question, that of the effect of different kinds of movements in promoting recognition. Simple translations (moving stimuli across the field) were more effective in promoting recognition than were more complex rotations (see Figure 7.8). Ruff further demonstrated that a simple rotation condition moderately facilitated recognition if infants were given more familiarization time than they needed for translation. One would expect this pattern of results, because in translation movements the object undergoes less change and hence the changing relation of object to background is clearly highlighted, whereas in rotation there is more internal change in the object and the relation of object to background is changing less.

The third question, identifying the sorts of kinetic cues babies respond to, is vast and largely uncharted territory. Several studies that have begun to map this territory will be discussed in this section. The most widely studied kinetic stimuli, looming objects (objects that look as if they are going to hit the observer), will be discussed in the section on depth perception, since it has most often been studied in that connection.

There are three other areas of visual perception that have been explored by infant researchers. First is whether babies can tell the difference between a rigid object and one that is elastic (changes shape when deformed). The cues that differentiate these two classes of objects are given only by differences in the ways the objects change when moved in particular ways (e.g., rotating a rigid object versus squeezing a sponge). Gibson et al. (1978) found that 5-month-olds discriminate between these two movements.

Second is Ruff's (1982b) work on infants' ability to detect different motions regardless of the object. She demonstrated that 5-month-olds differentiated between translation and rotation movements and between full rotations (repeated 360-degree turns in one direction—a spinning motion) and oscillating rotations (180-degree rotations—half turns back and forth). Ruff also explored in more depth exactly which changes in the stimulus the babies were responding to; readers interested in Gibsonian theory will want to read her study in its entirety.

The research described in this section usually used infants 4 to 6 months of age, by which time they are quite sensitive to kinetic information. An important aspect of 4 months as a dividing line in some percep-

tual abilities was shown by Yonas et al. (1987). By 4 months some infants can detect binocular disparity, which is related to depth perception (to be discussed later). Yonas and colleagues tested 4-month-olds to determine whether they could perceive binocular disparity (perception of disparity does not prove there is depth perception). They then related this ability to that of perceiving three-dimensional object shape from kinetic depth information. Those who could and those who could not detect disparity were tested (using the habituation-dishabituation paradigm) for their ability to perceive object shape from binocular information after having been exposed to kinetic displays of the shape. Those who showed disparity could, and those who did not yet show disparity could not. It appears that something—in the maturation of the visual system, in the amount of experience the system has had, or a combination of the two factors—is specifying the period around 4 months as one of new perceptual abilities.

The Role of Visually Guided Reaching in Perception of Objects

The development of visually guided reaching, much of which has been done to discover what infants know about objects and space, will be discussed in Chapter 8. That description is of what is generally accepted by experts in the field, but it masks some controversy about what the research tells us about what infants know about their world.

The existence and nature of visually guided reaching can elucidate three related epistemological issues. One is the infants' appreciation of three-dimensional space (depth). If they reach for objects they see, they in some sense must have an expectation (presumably unconscious) that there is an object out there (in three-dimensional space). Second, they must have an expectation that the object is graspable, that is, that it has three-dimensional mass. And third, they must expect that the stimulus with visual attributes also has tactile attributes. This is part of the issue of intercoordination of senses. Knowing that sensations in separate modalities come from the same object is an important part of knowing what an object is.

When infants develop visually guided reaching at 4 months of age, they presumably have all three of these sorts of knowledge. That conclusion is generally accepted. What is controversial is whether the earlier form, visually initiated prereaching behavior, also requires that knowledge. The subtleties of the reaching response can potentially resolve the controversy. If neonates have this underlying knowledge of objects, their reaching behaviors should reflect that knowledge through (a) success in grasping the object, and (b) different behavior for a graspable object than for no object or an object that is not graspable. They do not have success in grasping. The graspable object elicits more arm waving (prereaching?). If neonates lack this underlying knowledge, they should exhibit a variety of behaviors (looking, mouth opening and closing, hand movements, arm pumping, and leg kicking) in response to stimuli and spontaneously (that is, when adults cannot detect a specific stimulus). By chance just the right combination of stimuli and responses might occur so that the neonate grasps the object (see Figure 8.7 for an illustration of this).

We now turn to descriptions of the research studies designed to test these alternative hypotheses about what newborns know. First, there is disagreement over how frequently these responses occur. Discredited research found successful grasp on 40% of neonatal reaches, whereas Ruff and Halton (1978) found only 7%. Admittedly, discrepancies in research results can be due to differences in the criteria for reach (Rader, Opaluch, & Johnson; cited in Rader & Stern, 1982), and choice of criteria is a matter of the researchers' judgment and may reflect their biases.

Second, studies comparing neonatal arm movements when a stimulus object is present to when no stimulus is present have yielded somewhat conflicting results (Hofsten, 1982, 1984; Rader & Stern, 1982; Ruff & Halton, 1978), but all report some reaching type of behavior when there is *no* object. Thus the *most* we can say is that a pattern in the baby's visual field is more likely to elicit a reach than is a patternless field, and even that may be overstating the knowledge.

Third, there are conflicting results in studies that compare graspable to nongraspable stimuli. Reaching for three-dimensional objects more than for two-dimensional objects (pictures) should occur if the babies perceive that objects have mass and pictures do not. Two studies have failed to find this (Dodwell et al., 1976; Rader & Stern, 1982).

Fourth, slightly older infants have been found to reach differentially to a graspable object than to a nongraspable object or to the absence of an object (Brazelton et al., 1974; Bruner & Koslowski, 1972; Trevarthen et al., 1975). These findings may, however, reflect development since birth rather than innate knowledge of objects in space.

After examination of the methodologically more sophisticated studies and the findings that have been replicated, it seems reasonable to conclude that newborns do not know that there are three-dimensional objects in a three-dimensional space—they do not

know the difference between a picture and an object, they reach when there is no object, and in the majority of instances they do not reach even when there is an object. Newborns come equipped with the rudiments with which to acquire that knowledge—they respond to visual patterns with increased activity of their hands and arms that sometimes results in successful grasps.

Depth Perception

Depth perception has been one of the favorite topics of epistemology since long before scientists ever studied infants. Bishop Berkeley, an eighteenth-century British associationist, argued that we do not perceive depth directly. Rather, we must learn to perceive depth through associating varying sizes of objects with their varying distances. You know that if you are very far away from objects you are looking at (say, from the top of a tall building or in an airplane looking at objects on the ground) large objects look the size of toys. Berkeley believed that we have to learn that human beings that look like mere specks can nevertheless be real, full-sized human beings who are far away. He argued that we discover that very small images are really very far away because images get larger and larger as they get closer and closer, and we associate the changing visual image with the movements of our eye muscles as they converge to focus on the images. Other philosophers, such as Immanuel Kant, argue that knowledge of space is *innately given*. Sense impressions are not the bases by which we detect depth, but serve only as the grist for the organizing principles. Philosophers often argue that it was given to us by God or by an abstraction of the notion of God. Psychologists who are nativists tend to see it as given to us by our biological inheritance; in other words, our biological optical system is so organized that we see depth. The obvious way to resolve the nature/nurture argument is to study the development of depth perception in infants. The nativist position would be supported if newborns perceive depth when first exposed to patterned light. If the ability to perceive depth develops, then the situation is more complex. Such development may proceed as a function of experience or it may be governed primarily by a biological timetable in much the same way motoric skills are.

We can conclude that 4-month-olds act as if they perceive depth, but not that younger babies do (more evidence will be found in Chapter 8). This section will examine four additional areas of research in the order of the age at which they demonstrate evidence for depth perception, from earliest to latest. Such an ordering will facilitate the comparison of the various

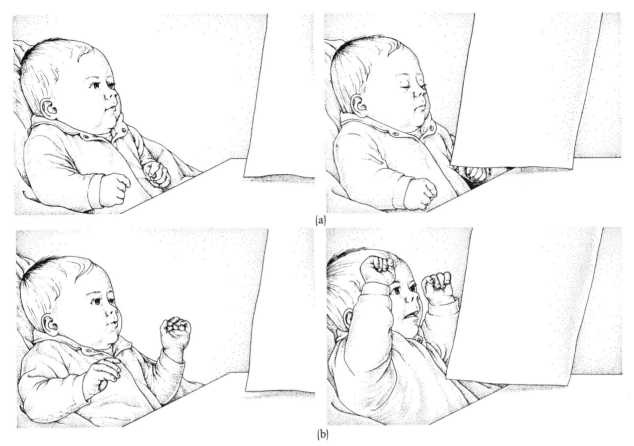

Figure 7.9. Responses to a looming stimulus. Whether researchers believe that young babies react defensively to impending collision depends in part on the dependent measures (infants' responses) they use. (a) Blinking: the response first used to explore response to a looming stimulus. It is a reliable measure, and studies using it show a developmental progression in the first 3 to 4 months of life. (b) An integrated avoidance response: eyes opening wide, head going back, both hands coming up between the object and the face. This response has been found in newborns in two studies, but not until 8 months in another. (Drawing in part b adapted from *Development in Infancy* (2nd ed.), by T. G. R. Bower. W. H. Freeman and Company. Copyright © 1982. Used by permission.)

methods and help our speculations both about what each technique is measuring and about when various components of depth perception develop.

Looming. First is the research on **looming**. A looming object is something that comes closer and closer as if it is going to hit the observer, such as a ball thrown at one's face (see Figure 7.9). It is easy to make a pictorial image of this by making a movie of a ball that gets larger and larger. The physical cue to depth is the apparent size of the ball. The ball seems small (subtends a smaller area on the retina) when far away and large when close up, and the change is marked by magnification of the contours corresponding to the edges of the object. The magnification increases as the object

approaches at a constant rate. The rate of magnification becomes explosive just before contact, and it is this accelerated expansion and the associated filling of the visual field until the ball becomes all we can see that specifies imminent collision (J. J. Gibson, 1958).

A looming stimulus obviously carries depth information, thus charting the development of responses to it can tell us something about the development of depth perception. There is a long history of research on blink responses to looming stimuli (Preyer, 1880/1888; Raehlman, 1891; for summaries of other German researchers at the beginning of this century, see Peiper, 1961/1963). The topic attracted the attention of Gesell (1925) and some of his contemporaries. The results of these early studies were quite consistent.

Babies under 2 months of age were found to stare at an approaching object, but not to blink. Blink responses arose at about 2 months of age and were virtually universal by 4 months.

Interest in looming then subsided until the explosion of infant perception work in the 1960s and 1970s. It reappeared with the publication of results showing defensive reactions (integrated avoidance responses involving the eyes opening wide, the head going back, and both hands coming up between the object and the face) in infants younger than 2 months (Ball & Tronick, 1971). In this context, a failure to blink is interpreted as part of an avoidance response, rather than as a failure to respond.

Yonas et al.'s (1977) replication of this work with additional controls did not find an integrated avoidance response, but did find that 1-2-month-olds made more backward head movements to looming than to nonlooming stimuli. The researchers note that a viable alternative interpretation to depth perception as an explanation for the response is that the infants may have been following the upper contour of the object as it moved upward in the process of getting larger. Young babies, who lack good motoric control of their heads, would be likely to jerk their heads backward as they tried to follow the upper contour. In several different manipulations, Yonas and his collaborators (1977, 1979) found that backward head movements occurred only when an upper contour moved upward and did not occur when the stimulus loomed but had no upward-moving contours. They did not find the integrated avoidance response until 8 months of age.

Blinking responses, in contrast, were elicited by the visual information of impending collision regardless of whether there was an upward-moving contour. In addition, Yonas et al. (1980) have shown that 3-month-old babies consistently blink (66% of the trials) only when the conditions specified by Gibson were met: explosive magnification and filling of the visual field (100 degrees of arc, which is 56% of the total visual field). Younger babies (1 month of age) responded both to the impending collision stimulus and to one in which the object appeared (to adults) to be slowing. Thus the response of younger babies can be said to be more general, less exact, and more rare. The frequency of response to approaching objects is about 16% at 6 weeks and increases with age, reaching 75% by 10 weeks (Yonas, 1981). Such development may, of course, reflect either maturation or experience.

One research technique that can help to distinguish between maturationally based and experientially based development is to compare babies with different gestational histories, as discussed earlier. In Pettersen et al.'s

(1980) study, the full-term 6-week-olds blinked to the approaching stimulus only 16% of the time, whereas the postmature 6-week-old babies (born at least 3 weeks after their expected delivery date) blinked on 37% of the trials. This supports the hypothesis that maturation underlies at least part of the increase in responsiveness.

Binocular Perception. The second area of depth perception research to be addressed here is that of **binocular perception** (the cues to depth given to us by the joint functioning of our two eyes). Because our eyes are separated but are both directed ahead, we see slightly different views of our visual field with our two eyes. You have undoubtedly experienced this at times. To see what I mean, look at something close up, and close first one eye and then the other. You will see two different views with the two eyes. The differences in these views provide the strongest cues to depth for objects that are relatively close to the viewer (beyond 30 ft the two images do not differ). The development of two binocular phenomena, convergence and stereopsis, have been demonstrated and replicated.

When a visual target is moved from a far to a near distance from the eyes, the eyes maintain fixation by moving inward toward the nose. If you watch someone else following a moving target coming toward his or her eyes, you will see the two eyes move inward, or converge. When objects move farther from the eyes, the eyes move to a straight-ahead position—they diverge. Convergence and divergence together are called **vergence**. It appears that even newborns under some conditions exhibit convergence: They show binocular fixation to stationary targets at certain distances from the target (Hershenson, 1964; Slater & Findlay, 1975), but they do not consistently exhibit appropriate vergence movements to moving stimuli. By 2 to 3 months of age, babies make reliable vergence movements (Aslin, 1977; Ling, 1942). Even newborns and 1-month-olds change their vergence in relation to target distance, but only at intermediate viewing distances, and they may be quite inaccurate on any given trial (Aslin, 1987).

The second binocular phenomenon is **stereopsis**, which is the perception of depth based solely on the information provided by the two different images of the two eyes. The difference in the two images is called **retinal disparity**. Stereopsis is difficult to study in infants because the perception of depth is a subjective experience. Nevertheless, it is possible to discover whether young infants detect the underlying cues given by changes in the degree of overlap between the two images (i.e., by the difference in retinal disparity).

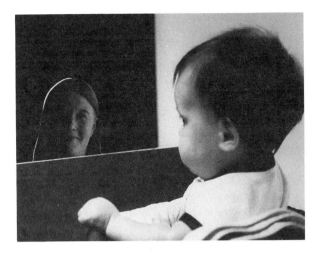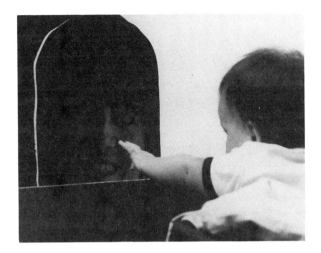

Figure 7.10. An example of the procedure used by Yonas to explore sensitivity to pictorial cues. The baby reaches for the larger face. (Photographs courtesy of Dr. Albert Yonas.)

This is done by presenting stimuli stereoptically, the same procedure used to make the 3D movies that require goggles for proper viewing. Two overlapping images are presented, one to each eye. The goggles are actually filters that allow one image to reach one eye and the other image to reach the other eye. Experimental procedures necessary to produce a convincing demonstration of this phenomenon have developed in the last two decades (see Aslin & Dumais, 1980, for a review). Three studies using these highly developed procedures have demonstrated that babies under 10 weeks of age do not detect the difference in retinal disparity and therefore do not experience stereopsis, our strongest single cue for depth. This ability develops during the period between 3½ and 6 months and by the end of that period is close to mature (Fox et al., 1980; Held et al., 1980; Petrig et al., 1981). Further, those 4-month-old infants who can detect binocular disparity can also perceive three-dimensional object shape from binocular depth information (Yonas et al., 1987). However, the procedure used does not allow separation of binocular disparity from vergence as an explanation of the results.

The ability to detect differences in retinal disparity is a prerequisite for binocular depth perception, but it is not sufficient to demonstrate that perceptual ability. Infants may be able to detect disparity cues but not perceive them as depth cues; that is, they may not perceive the stereoptic image as nearer to them than the background. Additional evidence to bolster the interpretation that older infants were really perceiving depth was obtained by presenting infants with a series of stereograms that adults did or did not find effective

in producing a fused image of an object in depth (Fox et al., 1980). Infants 3 to 5 months old detected the depth cues only with the stimuli that were the most effective producers of depth for adults. An indication of fusional vergence was also obtained by Aslin (1977) using displacing prisms (prisms that make an object appear to be at a different place than it is). Displacements of 2.5° or 5° did not induce fusional vergence eye movements until the fifth month (1-2° does so in adults). These studies suggests that infants of this age are truly perceiving depth binocularly.

Pictorial Cues. Also important in depth perception is a set of depth cues known as **pictorial cues**, because they produce a sense of depth in two-dimensional arrays. For example, if two cars known to be of comparable size are drawn different sizes and placed side by side in a picture, the smaller one is perceived to be farther away. The same cues also provide information concerning depth in our three-dimensional world. In fact, persons looking at a three-dimensional scene under conditions that eliminate other cues (they look through one eye only and do not move their heads or eyes, and the stimuli do not move) would still perceive depth because of the pictorial cues.

While there have been numerous sporadic attempts to explore the development of infants' knowledge of pictorial cues, systematic research to explore this problem is relatively recent (for reviews, see Yonas & Owsley, 1987; Yonas et al., 1987). This research, taken together, suggests that sensitivity to pictorial cues develops between 5 and 7 months. Yonas et al. (1982) presented infants with cutouts of photographs that were either larger or smaller than life-size. The 7-month-old infants, when looking with one eye only, were more likely to reach to the larger face than they were to the smaller face (see Figure 7.10). This is what one would expect them to do if they were responding to the size of the face. They knew what size faces normally are, and so responded to the larger face as if it were nearer (it actually was out of reach) and to the smaller face as if it were too far away to be reached, although it was not. To make certain that the infants were responding to the perceived distance, the researchers did two things: First, they presented the faces to infants who had both eyes uncovered, which destroys the illusion of depth for adults because of the availability of binocular cues; second, they created an analogous condition with checkerboard patterns, which should not produce an illusion of depth, because there is no standard size of checkerboards, hence a larger checkerboard will simply be perceived as larger rather than as closer. There were no differences in reaching in either control condition; that is, the infants, like adults, did not perceive the size differences as cues to depth.

Shading is another possible pictorial cue to depth. It and other pictorial depth cues that could be used to perceive shape are not effective for 5-month-olds (Granrud et al., 1985; Yonas et al., 1986). Linear perspective and texture gradients are not effective for 5-month-olds, but are for 7-month-olds (Yonas et al., 1986). This difference between 5- and 7-month-olds was replicated by Arterberry et al. (1989) using a more sensitive methodology. Furthermore, they found that the responses of 7-month-olds were not dependent on the degree of self-controlled locomotion they have experienced, an issue that will be raised below in relation to the responses to the visual cliff. In contrast, kinetic cues appear to be effective earlier (Yonas et al., 1987).

In sum, by 7 months of age infants respond to pictorial cues, which are the only source of depth information in pictures and a major source of depth information in our three-dimensional world, particularly at distances greater than 10 ft (when binocular cues become less effective). We do not know what maturational and experiential factors play a role in the major change in this ability that takes place between 5 and 7 months. It does seem that the knowledge 7-month-old infants have gathered in their brief lives influences their depth perception.

The Visual Cliff. The third area of depth perception research is that with an apparatus called the **visual cliff** developed by E. J. Gibson and Walk (1960; Walk &

Gibson, 1961). As Figure 7.11 shows, it is essentially a table divided into two halves and entirely covered by glass. One half of the table has an opaque surface immediately underneath the glass, and the other half has a drop of several feet before there is an opaque textured surface like the other. Down the center of the table dividing the two halves is a board raised slightly above the surface of the glass. The infant is put on the board and the mother stands across the table and tries to coax her baby to cross either the shallow or the deep side. If the infant refuses to cross to the mother on the deep side but crosses to the mother on the shallow side, this is taken to demonstrate that the baby perceives depth. Gibson and Walk found that when babies first crawl, at 6-9 months of age, most avoid the deep side as long as the depth cues are made obvious by making the floor of the visual cliff patterned. This is hardly clear support for innate depth perception, because a lot of development has occurred in the first 6 months of life. While babies do not have the experience of moving themselves through space prior to the time they start crawling, they clearly have the experience of being moved through space and of correlating this sensory experience with their reaching movements.

A series of studies by Campos and his collaborators has modified the visual cliff procedure for use with younger infants (Campos & Langer, 1971; Campos et al., 1970; Schwartz et al., 1973). These researchers placed infants on the visual cliff so that they looked at either the deep or the shallow side, and then measured responses such as heart rate, looking, and motor quieting. Babies between 1½ and 3 months of age oriented more to the deep side than to the shallow side, thus proving they could discriminate between the two sides. However, they could simply be discriminating between two visual patterns without knowing that one of those patterns is farther away than the other.

Another measure of response to the visual cliff used by Campos and his collaborators is fear. It can be assumed that babies who exhibit fear to deep places perceive the visual patterns of the deep side as deep. Thus if we see fear responses we can conclude with some confidence that the babies interpret the depth cues as depth. Babies 1½ to 5 months of age did not show fear (measured by acceleration of heart rate) of the deep side, but 9-month-olds did. In subsequent studies these researchers have demonstrated that experience in locomoting underlies wariness (Campos et al., 1978, 1981). They first showed this by correlating crawling experience with performance on the visual cliff and found that babies who had already started crawling exhibited fear to the deep side, whereas non-

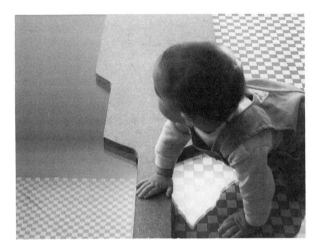

Figure 7.11. A baby on the visual cliff apparatus. The baby is intently exploring the glass surface above the deep side. (Photograph courtesy of R. D. Walk.)

crawling babies did not. Next, they tested their interpretation experimentally by exposing one group of noncrawling infants to a "walker" (a chair on wheels that infants can push). This experience accelerated the development of fear responses.

The evidence from fear responses may give us an upward boundary concerning depth perception—by 9 months of age babies perceive depth. It is possible that younger babies perceive depth (i.e., know that the deep side is farther away), but have no basis for fear of deep fall-offs. In fact, babies may need to perceive depth before they can learn which places result in their falling and hurting themselves, from which they learn to fear such places.[10]

The fear response may represent a separate developmental function that may possibly come after the development of depth perception; thus we cannot conclude that evidence that a role for experience in the development of fear to high places means that it is the same as the experience in the development of perception of deep places. Avoidance is the most convincing measure of depth perception on the visual cliff because (a) it implies both discrimination between the patterns on the two sides and perception of the deep side as farther away, and (b) it does not require the possibly extraneous variable of fear. There are two avenues of evidence using avoidance as a measure that suggest that avoidance of the cliff has a biological base. First, Walk and Gibson (1961) studied animals that could locomote at birth—chickens, rats, goats, sheep, cats, dogs, and monkeys. These studies indicated that newborns of those species avoid the deep side of the visual cliff when tested at birth or as soon as their eyes were

open. Second is evidence that the amount of experience in crawling did *not* predict avoidance of the visual cliff in human babies (Rader et al., 1980; Richards & Rader, 1981). Instead, age at onset of crawling predicted avoidance responses, and the babies who crawled early were more likely to cross the deep side. The authors of these studies hypothesize that if crawling develops before the maturation program that coordinates visual feedback with motoric development, then the infants will rely more on tactile than on visual feedback.

Even if Rader's explanation is correct, the demonstration that maturation plays a role in the development of avoidance of the deep side of the cliff does not mean experience is irrelevant. Babies less than 300 days of age avoid the deep side only if the surface has a visible texture (such as the checkerboard surface shown in the Figure 7.11), while older babies are more likely to avoid it even when it is an untextured gray (Walk, 1966). Walk attributes such improvement to maturation of acuity, but it may also be due to understanding that certain changes in the visual array indicate depth.

The research on the visual cliff reveals for us once more the complexity of the issues surrounding seemingly simple questions. We have learned that, methodologically speaking, there is a progression of criteria for responding to the visual cliff: (a) Babies discriminate differences between a shallow and a deep floor, but that does not imply that they perceive those differences as differences in depth; (b) babies make a response (e.g., avoidance) that implies depth perception; and (c) babies learn a fear response to the depth cues. We have seen that babies reach these different criteria at increasingly advanced ages. The research has shown that the developmental progression matches the order of complexity (from a to c). This is not trivial: Although we would expect a developmental progression to go from less to more complex, we would not necessarily predict that the steps in the progression should develop at different times. Indeed, a strong nativist would predict that the first two (detection of pattern differences and avoidance) should be present at birth. This research provides fertile ground for an exploration of the roles of maturation and experience. In its present state, it suggests that some components are governed by maturation and others by experience.

---

10. I am reminded of a 12-month-old infant being exposed for the first time to a porch with three steps down to the ground. He walked off the top step, thus falling to the ground, three times before changing his approach, but without showing fear.

In a cognitive task that does not involve fear, Benson and Uzgiris (1985) have shown that 10- to 11-month-old infants are more effective in searching for a hidden object if they have self-locomoted around a hiding box than if they were carried around it by a parent. They conclude that this supports Piaget's hypothesis that action-based knowledge during infancy is important for the development of spatial understanding. Ultimately, more knowledge of the role of locomotion and self-locomotion for acquisition of knowledge about the visual environment is needed.

The study of the development of depth perception is such a dynamic and rapidly changing field that it is difficult to draw any firm conclusions. This discussion has been confined, for the most part, to phenomena that have been replicated at least once. Also, the position taken here with respect to early development has been a conservative one, which allows me to suggest a consistent developmental progression.

Newborns show, at most, only very rudimentary abilities in depth perception. On rare occasions they reach for and grasp objects in space, in ways that do not indicate a knowledge of how far away in space the seen objects exist. They change the relative position of their eyes when they look at stimuli at 10 in. compared with those at 20 in., but make no further change when they look at those still closer (Slater & Findlay, 1975), thus showing rudimentary binocular skills.

After 1 month, the mechanisms for depth perception develop rapidly. By 2-3 months of age infants exhibit vergence and accommodation (accommodation was discussed above, in the section on acuity). They blink in response to the visual information of impending collision, and detect the differences between deep and shallow sides of the visual cliff, although more evidence is needed to determine that this is a discrimination between objects differing in depth.

By 4-6 months, sophisticated depth perception develops. The mature forms of visually guided reaching and binocular perception are developing. In the sixth and seventh months of life sensitivity to pictorial depth cues develops.

Thus we see that depth perception is a skill with many components that develop at different ages. The nature/nurture question has not been resolved, although the parameters of the problem are more clearly drawn. There is no real evidence that newborn babies perceive depth, although they have precursor responses from which responses to depth cues develop. Subsequent development of true depth responses is partly based on maturation and partly reflects experience, but the exact mechanisms require further exploration, as do the relations between maturation and experience.

Responses to Visual Stimuli in Relation to Other Senses

A number of studies have investigated presentation of stimuli to auditory and visual senses simultaneously. Many of these deal with determining which sense dominates; others address the effect of concordance, or a lack of it, between the two sources of information. Some studies, which will not be surveyed here, deal with visual and tactile stimuli not presented simultaneously; one example will be presented. Finally, it is proposed that visual preferences may depend in part on preceding stimuli in other sense modalities.

SENSORY DOMINANCE

In a lengthy series of studies, Lewkowicz (1985a, 1985b, 1988a, 1988b) examined the question of what changes 4-, 6-, and 10-month-old infants discriminate when presented with simultaneous auditory and visual stimuli. The visual stimulus used was a flashing checkerboard; the auditory stimulus was a sound that pulsed at the same rate as the flashing. After infants habituated to the compound stimulus, the pulsing rate of the audio, visual, or both was changed, and dishabituation was noted. At 6 months, infants discriminated the change in the audio component, but not that in the visual component, even when the intensity of the visual stimulus was greatly increased (Lewkowicz, 1988a). This is a task they have no difficulty with when there is only a visual stimulus. It was found that 10-month-olds discriminated the change both when only the audio changed and when both the audio and visual conditions changed together (1988b). When both stimuli varied in their rates and durations, the 10-month-olds discriminated the temporal change in the visual component. In short, where auditory and visual information competed for the infants' attention, the auditory modality was dominant at both ages, although the visual had some influence at 10 months. This is in sharp contrast to adults, for whom the visual information is dominant. The early prepotency of the auditory modality seems congruent with the fact that auditory stimuli are more effective in eliciting smiles in early infancy, but visual stimuli become more effective later.

Lewkowicz (1990) next studied the relative contribution of each stimulus modality using a different paradigm. The visual stimulus moved down a screen and a complex sound occurred when it reached the bottom, creating the impression of a bouncing object. The velocity of the visual stimulus, the repetition rate of the sound, or both were changed after habituation. The 4-month-olds in the study showed dishabituation to all three changes, as did the 6-month-olds, but for them and the 8-month-olds the change was significantly greater for the visual than for the auditory change. The salience of kinetic visual information thus appears much earlier than that of static visual information.

RESPONSE TO COHERENCE BETWEEN AUDIO AND VISUAL INFORMATION

This topic can be seen as cognitive rather than perceptual, inasmuch as it involves coordinating knowledge in two perceptual domains. However, I would like to present some examples of this type of research here. Kuhl and Meltzoff (1982) found that 4-month-olds hearing a sound track repeating *a* or *i* preferred to look at a video of a face that is saying the same thing. Spelke et al. (1983) showed babies two films in which an object moved up and down in a rhythmic sequence with an abrupt change in direction; the babies preferred to look at the one in which the abrupt change in direction corresponded with the playing of an abrupt noise. In a study by Schiff et al. (1989), 5-month-olds presented with a film of a talking person or of a car with its motor running, both of which either approached or receded, took longer to habituate to the sound when it did not agree with the visual input. They also took longer to habituate to a speaking person than to a running car. Walker-Andrews (1988) found that infants prefer looking at a face expressing the same emotion they are hearing expressed. In that study, 5-month-olds did not prefer a happy to an angry face (regardless of sound track) when the mouth was blocked out. This suggests that preference for happy expressions may rest on toothy smiles. If given a relatively large number of trials, 7-month-olds can exhibit a preference for the face matching the sound track, even if the sound is 5 seconds behind the visual presentation (Walker-Andrews, 1988).

At 10 months, 75% of infants who could see two videos of musicians playing instruments looked slightly longer at that of the instrument being played on the audiotape (Heinrichs et al., 1989). The cello, viola, and trombone were most effective in eliciting "correct" looking—that is, in infants preferring the coherent stimulus. Thus the size of the gross motor movements associated with the playing appears to be the cue used to judge coherence.

In a different type of study of coherence, 5- and 7-month-olds were shown filmed expressions of angry or happy faces that did or did not agree with a sound track. The lower part of the face was blocked out so that the synchrony of mouth movements and sound track could not be detected. The 7-, but not the 5-month-olds, increased their fixation to the face that agreed with the sound, hence they detected invariants across expression of a given emotion in different sensory modalities (Walker-Andrews, 1986). Work that involves expressive behaviors is reviewed in Walker-Andrews (1988).

Much of this research fits with a relatively new emphasis on dynamic as opposed to static stimuli in perceptual studies. These studies tend to make the infant look more competent, and that fits with the concept of **affordances** as propounded by J. J. Gibson (1979). The concept of affordances plays a major role in visual studies, but is a general concept of what activities the object shown or felt offers to a person's vision, touch, sucking, and so on. Can it be squeezed, banged, sucked, or what?

Gibson and Walker (1984) have shown that 1-year-olds familiarized with hard or spongy substances either in the dark or in the light prefer to look at a movie depicting an object being handled in the fashion appropriate to the familiarization stimulus; 1-month-olds familiarized orally with the affordances of hard and soft cylinders preferred to look at the novel one being manipulated. Gibson and Walker argue that the latter shows some intermodal knowledge of affordances at that early age. A review of infants' perception of the affordances of expressive behaviors can be found in Walker-Andrews (1988).

A different kind of relation between information in different sense modalities is provided by data showing that newborns' preference for the rate at which lights are flashing depends on their prior stimulation, whether internal or external. High prior levels of stimulation are related to preferences for lower rates of stimulation (Gardner et al., 1986). This can be conceived as part of their ability to self-regulate or to shut off excess stimulation, an aspect of neonatal behavior of great interest to Brazelton and some of his coworkers (see Chapter 8).

Summary

Researchers are interested in the development and function of the five sensory systems included in this chapter. Their state of functioning at birth, what it is babies perceive through them, and their course of development are of primary interest. Such information helps us to understand human maturation, sheds light on basic philosophical questions, and helps us determine which infants have sensory handicaps. Knowing the role that experience plays in the development of perception is crucial to several of these questions. In addition, we would like to know how perception is related to affective, linguistic, and cognitive development.

Naturalistic observation was long the method used to study infant perception. Movements of eyes, head, hands, and feet, and crying are all observable. Electronic devices now enable more accurate assessment of these responses and allow the study of heart rate and evoked responses from portions of the brain. In addition, the use of the habituation-dishabituation and conditioning paradigms permits early assessment of infant responses. Using an adult to judge whether an infant has made a response appears to be a highly sensitive instrument.

TACTILE SENSITIVITY

The skin senses develop early in fetal life. Early research claimed to show that newborns do not experience pain. This belief was based on using weak aversive stimuli, such as pinpricks, which did not elicit pain reactions. Newborns do react to more painful stimuli, such as heel sticks and circumcision, and older infants to immunization shots. They also react to such tactile stimuli as air puffs and slight pressure, but their reactions often depend on their state when tested. Some parts of the body are much more sensitive than others.

TASTE

At birth, the infant can differentiate among a number of substances. Early and current work shows this using facial expressions and mouth movements. More recent research has often made use of videotape, which can be scored more than once or by more than one person, for direct observation. Automated recordings of pulse and respiration rates, bodily movements, and sucking have been added. The preference for sweet taste appears to be innate; it has a calming and soothing effect that is not related to its relief of hunger. Preference for saltiness differs for liquids and solids. Facial expressions that would normally be interpreted as expressing a strong dislike do not affect the amount consumed in sucking studies.

---

11. Progress in electronics may have set back our research by making it so easy to use pure tones, which are not effective, as stimuli. It is also easy now to generate complex sounds with known characteristics, but even these may lack the complexity to be maximally effective.

SMELL

Smell is difficult to study because of difficulties in controlling the stimuli and because infants, like adults, adapt rapidly. The fact that babies appear to be insensitive to odors such as those of their own spitting up has led some to conclude that smell is not an important sense for the newborn. Reactions to both pleasant and unpleasant odors were found in early work, but the unpleasant odors were often strong enough to irritate nerves, not just to trigger the sense of smell. Babies do discriminate a number of smells at birth according to current research. They rapidly learn to discriminate odors from their mothers (breast pads or underarm odors) from those of others, and odors that they have been exposed to in their cribs from those they have not been exposed to. It appears that learning, not innate preferences, accounts for odors that are liked. Children as young as 3 years have preferences similar to those of adults.

AUDITION

Hearing is quite well developed prior to birth. Sound has a number of characteristics: pitch, loudness, complexity, and duration or continuity. Responses depend on all of these. Early research focused on observable responses such as startles, blinks, other movements, and quieting or orienting responses. Electronic techniques allowed more accurate control of stimuli and the recording of unseen responses such as heart rate and evoked brain stem responses.

The intensity of a sound required for a response depends on what response is measured and the nature of the stimulus (pure tone versus complex, onset time, pitch), as well as the age of the infant. The lowest response thresholds are found for averaged auditory evoked potentials, followed by increased heart rate, with blinks and startles requiring much stronger stimuli. The thresholds decrease rapidly in the first months of life.

Prior to 2 months, babies orient their eyes or heads toward the location of a sound, especially if it is soft, pulsing, and continuous. Between 2 and 4 months response decreases, then it increases again to remain highly predictable. Early orientation is not exact but becomes more so, and older infants can even reach quite accurately toward a sound in the dark.

Different pitches (frequencies of sound waves) are differentially effective in obtaining responses from babies. While early research indicated that infants were particularly sensitive in the pitch ranges of the human voice, newer research is less clear on this. Newborns respond more readily to complex sounds than to pure tones.[11] Development of structures of both the ear and the CNS may account for changing effectiveness of different pitches.

Babies' emotional reactions to sounds are similar to those of adults: Very high and very low sounds are alarming, whereas complex middle-range sounds and continuous and rhythmic sounds are soothing. Preferences appear to be affected by experiences in utero.

Understanding of normal hearing and developing ways to test hearing early in infancy are important for the diagnosis of hearing problems. Early detection is important to enable appropriate interventions to minimize the effects of the hearing loss.

VISION

Researchers are concerned with when infants can see what. What are their responses to moving stimuli? When and how well do they discriminate colors, brightness, patterns, or objects? When do they develop binocular vision and become able to discriminate three-dimensional objects in space?

Newborns respond to moving stimuli with OKN (nystagmus). They can follow a moving stimulus, although crudely, and can make saccades to find an object in the periphery even when focusing on a figure in central vision. Although babies will look toward a preferred stimulus in the periphery, suggesting that they process information there, the extent of the processing is not known. Infants explore their visual field, and show controlled eye movements in doing so, except when the field is empty or boring.

Newborns generally focus on a single feature of an object; scanning begins by 2 months. During this time, they shift from focusing on external to internal contours. They look longer at patterns than at homogeneous fields, and at lights of medium intensity rather than very bright or dim lights. They are more sensitive to light than adults or older children. Those who are hypersensitive compared to other newborns appear to have neurological damage, a finding that needs further study.

Newborns prefer colored stimuli to gray ones, and by 3 months they can discriminate colors. The mechanisms involved develop rapidly in the first few months.

Visual acuity, often measured by preferential looking, develops rapidly in the first year and reaches adult levels by 4 or 5 years. Both visual acuity and binocular vision appear to develop more rapidly in females. The ability to accommodate the eye to look at stimuli at different distances develops in the first few months. Although the receptor mechanisms for peripheral vi-

sion appear more mature than the fovea, newborns apparently have foveal vision, since they can focus on a small dot in central vision.

Pattern perception has focused on whether newborns perceive meaningful stimuli or have innate knowledge of the world, an old and still controversial topic in philosophy as well as psychology. It appears that much pattern perception in the first month is governed by single-cell detectors in the CNS. Faces and facial expressions are among the first meaningful patterns to be discriminated, but detection of subtle differences comes later. Moving objects are better perceived than are static ones. The question of how early depth perception is shown is important to the philosophical debate. It appears that while components may be present early, it develops over the first half year. The various cues used include binocular and pictorial.

RESPONSES TO VISUAL STIMULI
IN RELATION TO OTHER SENSES

Studies that use both auditory and visual stimuli are used to determine which sense dominates and whether or not infants perceive concordance between them. Auditory stimuli dominate initially, but later the visual do, as they do for adults. When auditory and visual stimuli match, infants habituate more rapidly than when they are not in agreement. The processes involved in the infant's perception of matching are not clear.

References

ADAMS, R. J. (1987). An evaluation of color preference in early infancy. *Infant Behavior and Development, 10,* 143-150.

AMBROSE, J. A. (1961). The development of the smiling response in early infancy. In B. M. Foss (Ed.), *Determinants of infant behaviour* (pp. 179-196). London: Methuen.

AMBROSE, J. A. (1963). The concept of a critical period for the development of social responsiveness. In B. M. Foss (Ed.), *Determinants of infant behaviour* (Vol. 2, pp. 201-225). London: Methuen.

AMES, E., & Silfen, C. (1965). *Methodological issues in the study of age differences in infant's attention to stimuli varying in movement and complexity.* Paper presented at the biennial meeting of the Society for Research in Child Development, Minneapolis.

ANDERSON, R. B., & Rosenblith, J. F. (1964). Light sensitivity in the neonate: A preliminary report. *Biologia Neonatorum, 7,* 83-94.

AREHART, D. M., & Haith, M. M. (1991, April). *Evidence for visual expectation violations in 13-week-old infants.* Paper presented at the meetings of the Society for Research in Child Development.

ARONSON, E., & Rosenbloom, S. (1971). Space perception in

early infancy: Perception within a common auditory-visual space. *Science, 172,* 1161-1163.

ARTERBERRY, M. A., Yonas, A., & Bensen, A. S. (1989). Self-produced locomotion and the development of responsiveness to linear perspective and texture gradients. *Developmental Psychology, 25,* 976-982.

ASHMEAD, D. A., Reilly, B. M., & Lipsitt, L. P. (1980). Neonates' heart rate, sucking rhythm, and sucking amplitude as a function of the sweet taste. *Journal of Experimental Child Psychology, 29,* 264-281.

ASLIN, R. N. (1977). Development of binocular fixation in human infants. *Journal of Experimental Child Psychology, 23,* 133-150.

ASLIN, R. N. (1981). Development of smooth pursuit in human infants. In D. F. Risher, R. A. Monty, & J. W. Senders (Eds.), *Eye movements: Cognition and visual perception.* Hillsdale, NJ: Lawrence Erlbaum.

ASLIN, R. N. (1987). Visual and auditory development in infancy. In J. D. Osofsky (Ed.), *Handbook of infancy* (2nd ed). New York: John Wiley.

ASLIN, R. N., & Dumais, S. T. (1980). Binocular vision in infants. In H. W. Reese & L. P. Lipsitt (Eds.), *Advances in child development and behavior* (Vol. 15). New York: Academic Press.

ATKINSON, J., Braddick, O., & Moar, K. (1977). Development of contrast sensitivity over the first 3 months of life in the human infant. *Vision Research, 17,* 1037-1044.

ATKINSON, J., Hood, B., Wattam-Bell, J., Anker, S., & Tricklebank, J. (1988). Development of orientation discrimination in infancy. *Perception, 17,* 587-595.

BAHRICK, L. E. (1988). Intermodal learning in infancy: Learning on the basis of two kinds of invariant relations in audible and visible events. *Child Development, 59,* 197-209.

BALL, W., & Tronick, E. (1971). Infant responses to impending collision: Optical and real. *Science, 171,* 818-820.

BALOGH, R. D., & Porter, R. H. (1986). Olfactory preferences resulting from mere exposure in human neonates. *Infant Behavior and Development, 9,* 395-401.

BANKS, M. S. (1980). The development of early infancy. *Child Development, 51,* 646-666.

BANKS, M. S., & Bennett, P. J. (1988). Optical and photoreceptor immaturities limit the spatial and chromatic vision of human neonates. *Journal of the Optical Society of America, 5,* 2059-2079.

BANKS, M. S., & Dannemiller, J. (1987). Infant visual psychophysics. In R. Aslin, J. Alberts, & M. Petersen (Eds.), *The development of perception.* New York: Academic Press.

BANKS, M. S., & Ginsburg, A. P. (1985). Early visual preferences: A review and a new theoretical treatment. In H. W. Reese (Ed.), *Advances in child development and behavior* (pp. 207-246). New York: Academic Press.

BANKS, M. S., & Salapatek, P. (1978). Acuity and contrast sensitivity in 1, 2, and 3-month-old human infants. *Investigative Ophthalmology, 17,* 361-365.

BANKS, M. S., & Salapatek, P. (1981). Infant pattern vision: A new approach based on the contrast sensitivity function. *Journal of Experimental Child Psychology, 31,* 1-45.

BANKS, M. S., & Salapatek, P. (1983). Infant visual perception. In P. H. Mussen (Ed.), *Handbook of child psychology: Vol. 2. Infancy and developmental psychobiology* (4th ed., pp. 435-571). New York: John Wiley.

BARNET, A. B., & Goodwin, R. S. (1965). Average evoked electroencephalographic responses to clicks in the human newborn. *Electroencephalography and Clinical Neurophysiology, 18,* 441-450.

BARRERA, M. E., & Maurer, D. (1981a). Discrimination of strangers by the three-month-old. *Child Development, 52,* 558-563.

BARRERA, M. E., & Maurer, D. (1981b). Recognition of mother's photographed face by the three-month-old infant. *Child Development, 52,* 714-716.

BARTOSHUK, A. K. (1964). Human neonatal cardiac responses to sound: A power function. *Psychonomic Science, 1,* 151-152.

BAYLEY, N. (1969). *Bayley scales of infant development: Birth to two years.* New York: Psychological Corporation.

BEAUCHAMP, G. K., Cowart, B., & Moran, M. (1986). Developmental changes in salt acceptability in human infants. *Developmental Psychobiology, 19,* 17-25.

BELL, R. Q. (1963). Some factors to be controlled in studies of the behavior of newborns. *Biologia Neonatorum, 5,* 200-214.

BELL, R. Q., & Costello, N. S. (1964). Three tests for sex differences in tactile sensitivity in the newborn. *Biologia Neonatorum, 7,* 335-347.

BENCH, J. (1969). In discussion of: Heron, T. G., Jacobs, R. Respiratory responses of the neonate to auditory stimulation. *International Audiology, 8,* 77.

BENCH, J. (1973). Square-wave stimuli and neonatal auditory behavior: Some comments on Ashton (1971), Hutt et al. (1968) and Lenard et al. (1969). *Journal of Experimental Child Psychology, 16,* 521-527.

BENSON, J. B., & Uzgiris, I. C. (1985). Effect of self-initiated locomotion on infant search activity. *Developmental Psychology, 21,* 923-931.

BENZAQUEN, S., Gagnon, R., Hunse, C., & Foreman, J. (1990). The intrauterine sound environment of the human fetus during labor. *American Journal of Obstetrics and Gynecology, 163,* 484-490.

BERG, W. K., & Smith, M. C. (1983). Behavioral thresholds for tones during infancy. *Journal of Experimental Child Psychology, 35,* 409-425.

BERNARD, J. (1946). Human fetal reactivity to tonal stimulation. *American Psychologist, 1,* 256.

BERNARD, J., & Sontag, L. W. (1947). Fetal reactivity to tonal stimulation: A preliminary report. *Journal of Genetic Psychology, 70,* 205-210.

BERTENTHAL, B. I., Bradbury, A., & Kramer, S. J. (1989, April). *Velocity thresholds in 5-month-old infants.* Paper presented at the meeting of the Society for Research in Child Development, Kansas City, MO.

BIRCH, E. E., Gwiazda, J., Bauer, J. A., Jr., Naegele, J., & Held, R. (1983). Visual acuity and its meridional variations in children aged 7-60 months. *Vision Research, 23,* 1019-1024.

BIRCH, H. G., Belmont, I., & Karp, E. (1965). Social differences in auditory perception. *Perceptual and Motor Skills, 20,* 861-870.

BIRNHOLZ, J. C. (1988). On observing the human fetus. In W. P. Smotherman & S. R. Robinson (Eds.), *Behavior of the fetus* (pp. 47-60). Caldwell, NJ: Telford.

BIRNHOLZ, J. C., & Benaceraff, B. R. (1983). The development of human fetal hearing. *Science, 222,* 516-518.

BLASS, E. M. (1990). Suckling: Determinants, changes, mechanism, and lasting impressions. *Developmental Psychology, 26,* 520-533.

BLASS, E. M., Fillion, T. J., Rochat, P., Hoffmeyer, L. B., & Metzger, M. A. (1989). Sensorimotor and motivational determinants of hand-mouth coordination in 1-3-day-old human infants. *Developmental Psychology, 25,* 963-975.

BLASS, E. M., & Hoffmeyer, L. B. (1991). Sucrose as an analgesic in newborn humans. *Pediatrics., 87,* 215-218

BORNSTEIN, M. H. (1976). Infants are trichromats. *Journal of Experimental Child Psychology, 21,* 425-445.

BORNSTEIN, M. H. (1981). "Human infant color vision and color perception" reviewed and reassessed: A critique of Werner and Wooten (1979a). *Infant Behavior and Development, 4,* 119-150.

BORNSTEIN, M. H., Kessen, W., & Weiskopf, S. (1976). The categories of hue in infancy. *Science, 21,* 425-445.

BORNSTEIN, M. H., & Krinsky, S. J. (1985). Perception of symmetry in infancy: The salience of vertical symmetry and the perception of pattern wholes. *Journal of Experimental Child Psychology, 39,* 1-19.

BORNSTEIN, M. H., Krinsky, S. J., & Benasich, A. A. (1986). Fine orientation discrimination and shape constancy in young infants. *Journal of Experimental Child Psychology, 41,* 49-60.

BOURNE, L. E., Jr., & Ekstrand, B. R. (1982). *Psychology: Its principles and meanings* (4th ed.). New York: Holt, Rinehart & Winston.

BOWER, T. G. R. (1982). *Development in infancy* (2nd ed.). San Francisco: Freeman.

BRADDICK, O., Atkinson, J., French, J., & Howland, H. C. (1979). A photorefractive study of infant accommodation. *Vision Research, 19,* 1319-1330.

BRAZELTON, T. B., Koslowski, B., & Main, M. (1974). The origin of reciprocity in the mother-infant interaction. In M. Lewis & L. Rosenblum (Eds.), *The effect of the infant on its caregiver.* New York: John Wiley.

BRIDGER, W. H. (1961). Sensory habituation and discrimination in the human neonate. *American Journal of Psychiatry, 117,* 991-997.

BROERSE, J., Peltolta, C., & Crassini, B. (1983). Infants' reactions to perceptual paradox during mother-infant interaction. *Developmental Psychology, 19,* 310-316.

BRUNER, J. S., & Koslowski, B. (1972). Visually preadapted constituents of manipulatory action. *Perception, 1,* 3-14.

BUSHNELL, I. W. R., Gerry, G., & Burt, K. (1983). The externality effect in neonates. *Infant Behavior and Development, 6,* 151-156.

BUSHNELL, I. W. R., Sai, F., & Mullin, J. T. (1989). Neonatal recognition of the mother's face. *British Journal of Developmental Psychology, 7,* 3-15.

BUTTERFIELD, E. C., & Siperstein, G. N. (1974). Influence of contingent auditory stimulation upon non-nutritional suckle. In J. F. Bosma (Ed.), *Proceedings of Third Symposium on Oral Sensation and Perception: The mouth of the infant.* Springfield, IL: Charles C Thomas.

BUTTERWORTH, G., & Castillo, M. (1976). Coordination of auditory and visual space in newborn human infants. *Perception, 5,* 155-160.

CAMPOS, J. J., Hiatt, S., Ramsay, D., Henderson, C., & Svedja, M. (1978). The emergence of fear on the visual cliff. In M. Lewis & L. Rosenblum (Eds.), *The origins of affect.* New York: Plenum.

CAMPOS, J. J., & Langer, A. (1971). The visual cliff: Discriminative cardiac orienting responses with retinal size held constant. *Psychophysiology, 8,* 264-265.

CAMPOS, J. J., Langer, A., & Krowitz, A. (1970). Cardiac responses on the visual cliff in prelocomotor human infants. *Science, 170,* 196-197.

CAMPOS, J. J., Svedja, M., Bertenthal, B., Benson, N., & Schmid, D. (1981, April). *Self-produced locomotion and wariness of heights: New evidence from training studies.* Paper presented at the biennial meeting of the Society for Research in Child Development, Boston.

CAMPOS, R. G. (1989). Soothing pain-elicited distress in infants with swaddling and pacifiers. *Child Development, 60,* 781-792.

CANESTRINI, S. (1913). Über das Sinnesleben des Neugeborenen [About the sensory life of the newborn]. *Monographien aus dem Gesamtgebiete du Neurologie und Psychiatrie, 5,* 104.

CANFIELD, R. L., & Haith, M. M. (1991). Young infants' visual expectations for symmetric and asymmetric stimulus sequences. *Developmental Psychology, 27,* 198-208.

CARON, R. F., Caron, A. J., & Myers, R. S. (1982). Abstraction of invariant face expressions in infancy. *Child Development, 53,* 1008-1018.

CATHERWOOD, D., Crassini, B., & Freiberg, K. (1989). Infant response to stimuli of similar hue and dissimilar shape: Tracing the origins of the categorization of objects by hue. *Child Development, 60,* 752-762.

CATTELL, P. (1940). *The measurement of intelligence in young children.* New York: Psychological Corporation.

CERNOCH, J. M., & Porter, R. H. (1985). Recognition of maternal axillary odors by infants. *Child Development, 56,* 1593-1598.

CHUN, R. W. N., Pawsat, R., & Forster, F. M. (1960). Sound localization in infancy. *Journal of Nervous and Mental Diseases, 130,* 472-476.

CLARKSON, M. G., & Berg, W. K. (1978). Cardiac deceleration in neonates is influenced by temporal pattern and spectral complexity of auditory stimuli [Abstract]. *Psychophysiology, 5,* 284.

CLARKSON, M. G., & Clifton, R. K. (1985). Infant pitch perception: Evidence for responding to pitch categories and the missing fundamental. *Journal of the Acoustical Society of America, 77,* 1521-1528.

CLARKSON, M. G., Clifton, R. K., Swain, I. U., & Perris, E. E. (1989). Stimulus duration and repetition rate influence newborns' head orientation toward sound. *Developmental Psychobiology, 22,* 683-705.

CLIFTON, R. K., Morrongiello, B. A., & Dowd, J. M. (1984). A developmental look at an auditory illusion: The precedence effect. *Developmental Psychobiology, 17,* 519-536.

CLIFTON, R. K., Morrongiello, B. A., Kulig, J. W., & Dowd, J. M. (1981). Newborns' orientation toward sound: Possible implications for cortical development. *Child Development, 52,* 833-838.

CLIFTON, R., Perris, E., & Bullinger, A. (1991). Infants' perception of auditory space. *Developmental Psychology, 27,* 187-197.

COHEN, L. B., DeLoache, J. S., & Strauss, M. S. (1979). Infant visual perception. In J. D. Osofsky (Ed.), *Handbook of infant development* (pp. 393-438). New York: John Wiley.

COHEN, L. B., & Strauss, M. S. (1979). Concept acquisition in the human infant. *Child Development, 50,* 419-424.

COHEN, L. B., & Younger, B. A. (1984). Infant perception of angular relations. *Infant Behavior and Development, 7,* 37-47.

COLOMBO, J., & Bundy, R. S. (1981). A method for the measurement of infant auditory selectivity. *Infant Behavior and Development, 4,* 219-233.

CONDRY, S. M., Haltom, M., & Neisser, U. (1977). Infant sensitivity to audio-visual discrepancy: A failure to replicate. *Bulletin of the Psychonomic Society, 9*, 431-432.

COOPER, R. P., & Aslin, R. (1990). Preference for infant-directed speech in the first month after birth. *Child Development, 61*, 1584-1595.

CORNELL, E. (1974). Infants' discrimination of photographs of faces following redundant presentations. *Journal of Experimental Child Psychology, 18*, 98-106.

COURAGE, M. L., & Adams, R. J. (1990). The early development of visual acuity in the binocular and monocular peripheral fields. *Infant Behavior and Development, 13*, 123-128.

CROOK, C. K., & Lipsitt, L. P. (1976). Neonatal nutritive sucking: Effects of taste stimulation upon sucking rhythm and heart rate. *Child Development, 47*, 518-522.

CROWELL, D. H., Jones, R. H., Nakagawa, J. K., & Kapuniai, L. E. (1971). Heart rate responses of human newborns to modulated pure tones. *Proceedings of the Royal Society of Medicine, 64*, 8-10.

CULP, R. (1971). *Looking response, decrement, and recovery of eight- to fourteen-week-old infants in relation to presentation of the infant's mother's voice.* Unpublished master's thesis, University of Kansas, Lawrence.

DANNEMILLER, J. L., & Stephens, B. R. (1988). A critical test of infant pattern preference models. *Child Development, 59*, 210-216.

DAYTON, G., Jones, M., Aiu, P., Rawson, R., Steele, B., & Rose, M. (1964). Developmental study of coordinated eye movements in the human infant: I. Visual acuity in the newborn human: A study based on induced optokinetic nystagmus recorded by electrooculography. *Archives of Ophthalmology, 71*, 865-870.

DeCASPER, A. J., & Fifer, W. P. (1980). Of human bonding: Newborns prefer their mothers' voices. *Science, 208*, 1174-1176.

DeCASPER, A. J., & Prescott, P. (1984). Human newborns' perception of male voices: Preference, discrimination, and reinforcing value. *Developmental Psychobiology, 17*, 481-491.

DeCASPER, A. J., & Spence, M. J. (1986). Prenatal maternal speech influences newborns' perception of speech sounds. *Infant Behavior and Development, 9*, 133-150.

DESOR, J. A., Maller, O., & Greene, L. S. (1977). Preference for sweet in humans: Infants, children and adults. In J. M. Weiffenbach (Ed.), *Taste and development: The genesis of sweet preference* (DHEW Publication No. NIH 77-1068). Bethesda, MD: National Institute of Dental Research.

DETTERMAN, D. K. (1978). The effect of heartbeat sound on neonatal crying. *Infant Behavior and Development, 1*, 36-48.

DIRKS, J., & Gibson, E. J. (1977). Infants' perception of similarity between live people and their photographs. *Child Development, 48*, 124-130.

DIXON, S., Snyder, J., Holve, R., & Bromberger, P. (1984). Behavioral effects of circumcision with and without anesthesia. *Journal of Developmental and Behavioral Pediatrics, 5*, 246-250.

DOBSON, V., Mayer, D. L., & Lee, C. P. (1980). Visual acuity screening of preterm infants. *Investigative Ophthalmology and Visual Science, 19*, 1498-1505.

DOBSON, V., Schwartz, T. L., Sandstrom, D. J., & Michel, L. (1987). Binocular visual acuity of neonates: The acuity card procedure. *Developmental Medicine and Child Neurology, 29*, 199-206.

DOBSON, V., & Teller, D. Y. (1978). Visual acuity in human infants: A review and comparison of behavioral and electrophysiological studies. *Vision Research, 18*, 1469-1483.

DOCKERAY, F. C., & Rice, C. (1934). Responses of newborn infants to pain stimulation. *Ohio State University Studies, Contributions to Psychology, 12*, 82-93.

DODWELL, P. C., Humphrey, G. K., & Muir, D. W. (1987). Shape and pattern perception. In L. Cohen & P. Salapatek (Eds.), *Handbook of infant perception* (Vol. 2, pp. 1-77). New York: Academic Press.

DODWELL, P. C., Muir, D. W., & DiFranco, D. (1976). Responses of infants to visually presented objects. *Science, 194*, 209-211.

DONOHUE, R. L., & Berg, W. K. (1991). Infant heart-rate responses to temporally predictable and unpredictable events. *Developmental Psychology, 27*, 59-66.

EGGERMONT, J. J. (1985). Evoked potentials as indicators of auditory maturation. *Acta Oto-laryngologica Supplementum, 421*, 41-47.

EICHORN, D. (1951). *Electrocortical and autonomic response in infants to visual and auditory stimuli.* Unpublished doctoral dissertation, Northwestern University.

EISENBERG, R. B. (1970a). The development of hearing in man: An assessment of current status. *Journal of the American Speech and Hearing Association, 12*, 119-121.

EISENBERG, R. B. (1970b). The organization of auditory behavior. *Journal of Speech and Hearing Research, 13*, 453-471.

EISENBERG, R. B. (1976). *Auditory competence in early life.* Baltimore: University Park Press.

ENGEN, T. (1982). *The perception of odors.* New York: Academic Press.

ENGEN, T. (1986). The acquisition of odour hedonics. In S. V. Toller & G. H. Dodd (Eds.), *Perfumery: The psychology and biology of fragrance* (pp. 79-93). London: Chapman & Hall.

ENGEN, T., & Bosack, T. N. (1969). Facilitation in olfactory detection. *Journal of Comparative and Physiological Psychology, 68*, 320-326.

ENGEN, T., & Lipsitt, L. P. (1965). Decrement and recovery of responses to olfactory stimuli. *Journal of Comparative Physiology and Psychology, 59*, 312-318.

ENGEN, T., Lipsitt, L. P., & Kaye, H. (1963). Olfactory responses and adaptation in the human neonate. *Journal of Physiology and Psychology, 56*, 73-77.

FAGAN, J. F., III. (1976). Infants' recognition of invariant features of faces. *Child Development, 47*, 627-638.

FAGAN, J. F., III. (1979). The origin of facial pattern perception. In M. H. Bornstein & W. Kessen (Eds.), *Psychological development from infancy: Image to intention* (pp. 83-113). Hillsdale, NJ: Lawrence Erlbaum.

FANTZ, R. L. (1961). A method for studying depth perception in infants under six months of age. *Psychological Record, 11*, 27-32.

FANTZ, R. L. (1963). Pattern vision in newborn infants. *Science, 140*, 296-297.

FANTZ, R. L. (1966). Pattern discrimination and selective attention as determinants of perceptual development from birth. In A. H. Kidd & J. L. Rivoire (Eds.), *Perceptual development in children.* New York: International University Press.

FANTZ, R. L., Fagan, J. F., III, & Miranda, S. B. (1975). Early visual selectivity as a function of pattern variables, previous exposure, age from birth and conception, and expected cognitive deficit. In L. B. Cohen & P. Salapatek (Eds.), *Infant perception from sensation to cognition: Vol. 1. Basic visual processes.* New York: Academic Press.

FANTZ, R. L., Ordy, J. M., & Udelf, M. S. (1962). Maturation of pattern vision in infants during the first six months. *Journal of Comparative and Physiological Psychology, 55,* 907-917.

FENWICK, K., Hillier, L., Morrongiello, B. A., & Chance, G. (1991, April). *Newborns' head orientation toward sound within hemifields.* Paper presented at the meeting of the Society for Research in Child Development, Seattle.

FERNALD, A. (1985). Four-month-old infants prefer to listen to motherese. *Infant Behavior and Development, 8,* 181-195.

FERNALD, A., & Kuhl, P. (1987). Acoustic determinants of infant preference for motherese speech. *Infant Behavior and Development, 10,* 279-293.

FIELD, J., Muir, D., Pilon, R., Sinclair, M., & Dodwell, P. (1980). Infants' orientation to lateral sounds from birth to three months. *Child Development, 51,* 295-298.

FIELD, T. M., Cohen, D., Garcia, R., & Greenberg, R. (1984). Mother-stranger face discrimination by the newborn. *Infant Behavior and Development, 7,* 19-25.

FIELD, T. M., Schanberg, S. M., Scafidi, F., Bauer, C. R., Vega-Lahr, N., Garcia, R., Nystrom, J., & Kuhn, C. M. (1986). Tactile/kinesthetic stimulation effects on preterm neonates. *Pediatrics, 77,* 654-658.

FIFER, W. P., & Moon, C. (1988). Auditory experience in the fetus. In W. P. Smotherman & S. R. Robinson (Eds.), *Behavior of the fetus* (pp. 175-190). Caldwell, NJ: Telford.

FINBERG, L., Kiley, J., & Luttrell, C. M. (1963). Mass accidental salt poisoning in infancy. *Journal of the American Medical Association, 184,* 121-124.

FLAVELL, J. H., Green, F. L., & Flavell, E. R. (1989). Young children's ability to differentiate appearance-reality and level 2 perspectives in the tactile modality. *Child Development, 60,* 201-213.

FORBES, H., & Forbes, H. (1927). Fetal sense reaction: Hearing. *Journal of Comparative Psychology, 7,* 353-355.

FOX, R., Aslin, R. N., Shea, S. L., & Dumais, S. T. (1980). Stereopsis in human infants. *Science, 207,* 323-324.

FREEDMAN, D. A., Fox-Kolenda, B., Margileth, D. A., & Miller, D. H. (1969). The development of the use of sound as a guide to affective and cognitive behavior. *Child Development, 40,* 1099-1105.

FRÖDING, C. A. (1960). Acoustic investigation of newborn infants. *Acta Oto-laryngolica, 52,* 31-40.

GALAMBOS, R., Hicks, G. E., & Wilson, M. J. (1984). The auditory brain stem response reliably predicts hearing loss in graduates of a tertiary intensive care nursery. *Ear and Hearing, 5,* 254-260.

GARDNER, J. M., Lewkowicz, D. J., Rose, S. A., & Karmel, B. Z. (1986). Effects of visual and auditory stimulation on subsequent visual preferences in neonates. *International Journal of Behavioral Development, 9,* 251-263.

GEISLER, C. D., & Rosenblith, W. A. (1962). Average responses to clicks recorded from the human scalp. *Journal of the Acoustical Society of America, 34,* 125-127.

GENZMER, A. (1882). Untersuchungen über die Sinneswahrnehmungen des neugeborenen Menschen [Investigation of the sensory perception of newborn men] (National Institute of Health, Trans., for J. F. Bosma, NIH 74-230c). Halle: Max Niemeyer.

GESELL, A. (1925). *Mental growth of the preschool child.* New York: Macmillan.

GHENT, L. (1961). Developmental changes in tactual thresholds on dominant and nondominant sides. *Journal of Comparative and Physiological Psychology, 54,* 670-673.

GHIM, H. (1990). Evidence for perceptual organization in infants: Perception of subjective contours by young infants. *Infant Behavior and Development, 13,* 221-248.

GHIM, H., & Eimas, P. D. (1988). Global and local processing by 3- and 4-month-old infants. *Perception and Psychophysics, 43,* 165-171.

GIBSON, E. J. (1969). *Principles of perceptual learning and development.* New York: Appleton-Century-Crofts.

GIBSON, E. J., Owsley, C. J., & Johnston, J. (1978). Perception of invariants by five-month-old infants: Differentiation of two types of motion. *Developmental Psychology, 14,* 407-415.

GIBSON, E. J., & Walk, R. (1960). The "visual cliff." *Scientific American, 202,* 64-71.

GIBSON, E. J., & Walker, A. S. (1984). Development of knowledge of visual-tactual affordances of substance. *Child Development, 55,* 453-460.

GIBSON, J. J. (1958). Visually controlled locomotion and visual orientation in animals. *British Journal of Psychology, 49,* 182-194.

GIBSON, J. J. (1966). *The senses considered as perceptual systems.* Boston: Houghton Mifflin.

GIBSON, J. J. (1979). *An ecological approach to visual perception.* Boston: Houghton Mifflin.

GOLDENBERG, I., Starkey, D., & Morant, R. B. (1984). *Auditory-visual integration: Face-voice mismatch.* Manuscript submitted for publication.

GOTTLIEB, G. (1971). Ontogenesis of sensory function in birds and mammals. In E. Tobach, L. R. Aronson, & E. Shaw (Eds.), *The biopsychology of development.* New York: Academic Press.

GOTTLIEB, G., & Krasnegor, N. A. (Eds.). (1985). *Measurement of audition and vision in the first year of postnatal life: A methodological overview.* Norwood, NJ: Ablex.

GRAHAM, F. K., Matarazzo, R. G., & Caldwell, B. M. (1956). Behavioral differences between normals and traumatized newborns: II. Standardization, reliability, and validity. *Psychological Monographs, 70*(20, Whole No. 28).

GRANRUD, C. E., Yonas, A., & Opland, E. A. (1985). Infants' sensitivity to the depth cue of shading. *Perception and Psychophysics, 37,* 415-419.

GREGG, C., Clifton, R. K., & Haith, M. (1976). A possible explanation for the frequent failure to find cardiac orienting in the newborn infant. *Developmental Psychology, 12,* 75-76.

GUNNAR, M. R., Malone, S., Vance, G., & Fisch, R. O. (1985). Coping with aversive stimulation in the neonatal period: Quiet sleep and plasma cortisol levels during recovery from circumcision. *Child Development, 56,* 824-834.

GWIAZDA, J., Bauer, J., & Held, R. (1989a). From visual acuity to hyperacuity: A 10-year update. *Canadian Journal of Psychology, 43,* 109-120.

GWIAZDA, J., Bauer, J., & Held, R. (1989b). Binocular function in human infants: Correlation of stereoptic and fusion-rivalry discriminations. *Journal of Pediatric Ophthalmology and Strabismus, 26,* 128-132.

GWIAZDA, J., Brill, S., Mohindra, I., & Held, R. (1978). Infant visual acuity and its meridional variation. *Vision Research, 18,* 1557-1564.

HAAF, R. A. (1974). Complexity and facial resemblance as determinants of response to facelike stimuli by 5 and 10 week old infants. *Journal of Experimental Child Psychology, 18,* 480-487.

HAAF, R. A., & Arehart, D. M. (1988, March). *Context and at-*

tention: Top-down processing by 10-week-olds? Paper presented at the Conference on Human Development, Charleston, SC.

HAAF, R. A., & Bell, R. Q. (1967). A facial dimension in visual discrimination by human infants. *Child Development, 38,* 893-899.

HAAF, R. A., & Brown, C. J. (1975). *Developmental changes in infants' response to complex facelike patterns.* Paper presented at the biennial meeting of the Society for Research in Child Development, Denver.

HAITH, M. M. (1978). Visual competence in early infancy. In R. Held, H. W. Leibowitz, & H. L. Teuber (Eds.), *Handbook of sensory physiology* (Vol. 8, pp. 311-356). New York: Springer.

HAITH, M. M. (1980). *Rules that infants look by.* Hillsdale, NJ: Lawrence Erlbaum.

HAITH, M. M. (1991). Gratuity, perception-action integration, and future orientation in infant vision. In F. Kessel, M. Bornstein, & A. Sameroff (Eds.), *The past as prologue in developmental psychology: Essays in honor of William Kessen.* Hillsdale, NJ: Lawrence Erlbaum.

HAITH, M. M., Bergman, T., & Moore, M. J. (1977). Eye contact and face scanning in early infancy. *Science, 198,* 853-855.

HAITH, M. M., & Goodman, G. S. (1982). Eye movement control in newborns in darkness and in unstructured light. *Child Development, 53,* 974-977.

HAITH, M. M., Hazen, C., & Goodman, G. S. (1988). Expectation and anticipation of dynamic visual events by 3.5-month-old babies. *Child Development, 59,* 467-479.

HAITH, M. M., & McCarty, M. E. (1990). Stability of visual expectations at 3.0 months of age. *Developmental Psychology, 26,* 68-74.

HALLER, M. (1932). The reactions of infants to changes in the intensity and pitch of pure tones. *Journal of Genetic Psychology, 40,* 162-180.

HARRIS, G., Thomas, A., & Booth, D. A. (1990). Development of salt taste in infancy. *Developmental Psychology, 26,* 534-538.

HAYNES, H., White, B. L., & Held, R. (1965). Visual accommodation in human infants. *Science, 148,* 528-530.

HEINRICHS, M., Gross, D., Miller, M., Melendez, P., & Pick, A. D. (1989, April). *Infants' perception of the unity of musical events.* Paper presented at the meeting of the Society for Research in Child Development, Kansas City, MO.

HELD, R. (1991). Development of binocular vision and stereopsis. In J. Cronly-Dillon (Ed.), *Binocular vision and psychophysics: Vol. 9. Vision and visual dysfunction.* London: Macmillan.

HELD, R., Birch, E., & Gwiazda, J. (1980). Stereoacuity of human infants. *Proceedings of the National Academy of Sciences USA, 77,* 5572-5574.

HELD, R., Gwiazda, J., Brill, S., Mohindra, I., & Wolfe, J. (1979). Infant visual acuity is underestimated because near threshold gratings are not preferentially fixated. *Vision Research, 19,* 1377-1379.

HERSHENSON, M. (1964). Visual discrimination in the human newborn. *Journal of Comparative and Physiological Psychology, 58,* 270-276.

HEWETT, K., & Cornelisse, L. (1991, April). *Infants' and adults' discrimination of sound distance.* Paper presented at the meeting of the Society for Research in Child Development, Seattle.

HOFSTEN, C. von. (1982). Eye-hand coordination in the newborn. *Developmental Psychology, 18,* 450-461.

HOFSTEN, C. von. (1984). Developmental changes in the organization of prereaching movements. *Developmental Psychology, 20,* 378-388.

HOFSTEN, C. von, & Spelke, E. S. (1985). Object perception and object-directed reaching in infancy. *Journal of Experimental Psychology: General, 114,* 198-212.

HOROWITZ, F. D., Paden, L. Y., Bhana, K., & Self, P. (1972). An infant control procedure for studying infant visual fixations. *Developmental Psychology, 7,* 90.

HOVERSTEN, G. H., & Moncur, J. P. (1969). Stimuli and intensity factors in testing infants. *Journal of Speech and Hearing Research, 12,* 687-702.

HUBEL, D. H., & Wiesel, T. N. (1963). Receptive fields of cells in striate cortex of very young, visually inexperienced kittens. *Journal of Neurophysiology, 26,* 994-1002.

HUTT, S. J., Hutt, C., Lenard, H. G., Bernuth, H. V., & Muntejewerff, W. J. (1968). Auditory responsivity in the human neonate. *Nature, 218,* 888-890.

IZARD, C. E., Hembree, E. A., & Huebner, R. R. (1987). Infants' emotion expressions to acute pain: Developmental change and stability of individual differences. *Developmental Psychology, 23,* 105-113.

JENSEN, K. (1932). Differential reactions to taste and temperature stimuli in newborn infants. *Genetic Psychology Monographs, 12,* 363-479.

KAGAN, J., Henker, B. A., Hen-Tov, A., Levine, J., & Lewis, M. (1966). Infants' differential reactions to familiar and distorted faces. *Child Development, 37,* 519-532.

KARMEL, B. Z., & Maisel, E. B. (1975). A neuronal activity model for infant visual attention. In L. B. Cohen & P. Salapatek (Eds.), *Infant perception from sensation to cognition: Vol. 1. Basic visual processes.* New York: Academic Press.

KAYE, H. (1964). Skin conductance in the human neonate. *Child Development, 35,* 1297-1305.

KAYE, H., & Lipsitt, L. P. (1964). Relation of electrotactual threshold to basal skin conductance. *Child Development, 35,* 1307-1312.

KELLMAN, P. J., Gleitman, H., & Spelke, E. S. (1987). Object and observer motion in the perception of objects by infants. *Journal of Experimental Psychology: Human Perception and Performance, 13,* 586-593.

KELLMAN, P. J., & Spelke, E. S. (1983). Perception of partly occluded objects in infancy. *Cognitive Psychology, 15,* 483-524.

KELLMAN, P. J., Spelke, E. S., & Short, K. (1986). Infant perception of object unity from translatory motion in depth and vertical translation. *Child Development, 57,* 72-86.

KESSEN, W., & Bornstein, M. H. (1978). Discriminability of brightness change for infant. *Journal of Experimental Child Psychology, 25,* 526-530.

KESSEN, W., Haith, M. M., & Salapatek, P. H. (1970). Human infancy: A bibliography and guide. In P. H. Mussen (Ed.), *Carmichael's manual of child psychology* (Vol. 1, 3rd ed., pp. 287-445). New York: John Wiley.

KLEINER, K. A. (1987). Amplitude and phase spectra as indices of infants' pattern preferences. *Infant Behavior and Development, 10,* 49-59.

KLEINER, K. A. (1990). Models of neonates' preferences for facelike patterns: A response to Morton, Johnson, and Maurer. *Infant Behavior and Development, 13,* 105-108.

KOBRE, K. R., & Lipsitt, L. P. (1972). A negative contrast effect in newborns. *Journal of Experimental Child Psychology, 14,* 81-91.

KOOPMAN, P., & Ames, E. (1968). Infants' preferences for facial arrangements: Failure to replicate. *Child Development, 39,* 481-487.

KREMENITZER, J. P., Vaughan, H. G., Jr., Kurtzberg, D., & Dowling, K. (1979). Smooth-pursuit eye movements in the newborn infant. *Child Development, 50,* 442-448.

KUHL, P. K., & Meltzoff, A. N. (1982). The bimodal perception of speech in infancy. *Science, 218,* 1138-1141

KUSSMAUL, A. (1859). *Untersuchungen über das Seelenleben des neugenobrenen Menschen* [Inquiries into the inner life of the newborn man]. Tübingen: Moser.

LEEHEY, S. C., Moskowitz-Cook, A., Brill, S., & Held, R. (1975). Orientational anisotropy in infant vision. *Science, 190,* 900-902.

LEIBOWITZ, H. W., & Harvey, L. O., Jr. (1973). Perception. *Annual Review of Psychology, 24,* 207-240.

LENARD, H. G., Bernuth, H. V., & Hutt, S. J. (1969). Acoustic evoked responses in newborn infants: The influence of pitch and complexity of the stimulus. *Electroencephalography and Clinical Neurophysiology, 27,* 121-127.

LEVENTHAL, A. S., & Lipsitt, L. P. (1964). Adaptation, pitch discrimination, and sound localization in the neonate. *Child Development, 35,* 759-767.

LEWIS, T. L., & Maurer, D. (1977, March). *Newborns' central vision: Whole or hole?* Paper presented at the meeting of the Society for Research in Child Development, New Orleans.

LEWIS, T. L., & Maurer, D. (1980). Central vision in the newborn. *Journal of Experimental Child Psychology, 29,* 475-480.

LEWIS, T. L., & Maurer, D. (1986). Preferential looking as a measure of visual resolution in infants and toddlers: A comparison of psychophysical methods. *Child Development, 57,* 1062-1075.

LEWKOWICZ, D. J. (1985a). Bisensory response to temporal frequency in 4-month-old infants. *Developmental Psychology, 21,* 306-317.

LEWKOWICZ, D. J. (1985b). Developmental changes in infants' visual response to temporal frequency. *Developmental Psychology, 21,* 858-865.

LEWKOWICZ, D. J. (1988a). Sensory dominance in infants 1: Six-month-old infants' response to auditory-visual compounds. *Developmental Psychology, 24,* 155-171.

LEWKOWICZ, D. J. (1988b). Sensory dominance in infants 2: Ten-month-old infants' response to auditory-visual compounds. *Developmental Psychology, 24,* 172-182.

LEWKOWICZ, D. J. (1990, April). *Developmental differences in infants' responses to auditory/visual compounds.* Paper presented at the International Conference on Infant Studies, Montreal.

LING, B. C. (1942). A genetic study of sustained visual fixation and associated behavior in the human infant from birth to six months. *Journal of Genetic Psychology, 61,* 227-277.

LIPSITT, L. P. (1977). Taste in human neonates: Its effects on sucking and heart rate. In J. M. Weiffenbach (Ed.), *Taste and development: The genesis of sweet preference* (DHEW Publication No. NIH 77-1068). Bethesda, MD: National Institute of Dental Research.

LIPSITT, L. P., & Behl, G. (1990). Taste-mediated differences in the sucking behavior of human newborns. In E. D. Capaldi & T. L. Powley (Eds.), *Taste, experience, and feeding* (pp. 75-93). Washington, DC: American Psychological Association.

LIPSITT, L. P., Engen, T., & Kaye, H. (1963). Developmental changes in the olfactory threshold of the neonate. *Child Development, 34,* 371-376.

LIPSITT, L. P., & Levy, N. (1959). Electrotactual threshold in the neonate. *Child Development, 30,* 547-552.

LIPSITT, L. P., Reilly, B. M., Butcher, M. J., & Greenwood, M. M. (1976). The stability and interrelationships of newborn sucking and heart rate. *Developmental Psychobiology, 9,* 305-310.

MacFARLANE, J. A. (1975). *Olfaction in the development of social preferences in the human neonate.* Amsterdam: Elsevier.

MAJNEMER, A., Rosenblatt, B., & Riley, P. (1988). Prognostic significance of the auditory brainstem evoked response in high-risk neonates. *Developmental Medicine & Child Neurology, 30,* 43-52.

MAKIN, J. W., & Porter, R. H. (1989). Attractiveness of lactating females' breast odors to neonates. *Child Development, 60,* 803-810.

MARQUIS, D. (1931). Can conditioned responses be established in the newborn infant? *Journal of Genetic Psychology, 39,* 479-490.

MAURER, D. (1975). Infant visual perception: Methods of study. In L. B. Cohen & P. Salapatek (Eds.), *Infant perception from sensation to cognition: Vol. 1. Basic visual processes* (pp. 1-76). New York: Academic Press.

MAURER, D., & Barrera, M. (1978). *Infants' perception of the natural and distorted arrangements of the human face.* Paper presented at the International Conference on Infant Studies, New Haven, CT.

MAURER, D., & Barrera, M. (1981). Infants' perception of natural and distorted arrangements of a schematic face. *Child Development, 52,* 196-202.

MAURER, D., & Heroux, L. (1980). *The perception of faces by three-month-old infants.* Paper presented at the International Conference on Infant Studies, New Haven, CT.

MAURER, D., & Lewis, T. L. (1979). Peripheral discrimination by three-month-old infants. *Child Development, 50,* 276-279.

MAURER, D., & Salapatek, P. (1976). Developmental changes in the scanning of faces by young infants. *Child Development, 47,* 523-527.

MAURER, D., & Young, R. E. (1983). Newborn's following of natural and distorted arrangements of facial features. *Infant Behavior and Development, 6,* 127-131.

McGURK, H. (1972). Infant discrimination of orientation. *Journal of Experimental Child Psychology, 14,* 151-164.

McGURK, H., & Lewis, M. (1974). Space perception in early infancy: Perception within a common auditory-visual space? *Science, 186,* 649-650.

McGURK, H., Turnure, C., & Creighton, S. J. (1977). Auditory-visual coordination in neonates. *Child Development, 48,* 138-143.

MELHUISH, E. C. (1982). Visual attention to mother's and stranger's faces and facial contrast in 1-month-old infants. *Developmental Psychology, 18,* 229-231.

MENDELSON, M. J., & Haith, M. M. (1976). The relation between audition and vision in the human newborn. *Monographs of the Society for Research in Child Development, 41*(4, Serial No. 167).

MILEWSKI, A. E. (1976). Infants' discrimination of internal and external pattern elements. *Journal of Experimental Child Psychology, 22,* 229-246.

MILEWSKI, A. E. (1979). Visual discrimination and detection of configural invariance in 3-month infants. *Developmental Psychology, 15,* 357-363.

MIRANDA, S. B. (1970). Visual abilities and pattern preferences of premature infants and full-term neonates. *Journal of Experimental Child Psychology, 10,* 189-205.

MOHN, G., & van Hof-van Duin, J. (1986). Development of the binocular and monocular visual fields of human infants during the first year of life. *Clinical Vision Science, 1,* 51-64.

MOLTZ, H. (1960). Imprinting: Empirical basis and theoretical significance. *Psychological Bulletin, 57,* 291-316.

MOON, C., Cooper, R. P., & Fifer, W. P. (1991, April). *Two-day-olds prefer the maternal language.* Paper presented at the meetings of the Society for Research in Child Development, Seattle.

MOON, C., & Fifer, W. P. (1990). Syllables as signals for 2-day-old infants. *Infant Behavior and Development, 13,* 377-390.

MORANTE, A., Dubowitz, L. M., Levene, M., & Dubowitz, V. (1982). The development of visual function in normal and neurologically abnormal preterm and fullterm infants. *Developmental Medicine and Child Neurology, 24,* 771-784.

MORRONGIELLO, B. A. (1988). Infants' localization of sounds in the horizontal plane: Estimates of minimum audible angle. *Developmental Psychology, 24,* 8-13.

MORRONGIELLO, B. A., & Clifton, R. K. (1984). Effects of sound frequency on behavioral and cardiac orienting in newborn and five-month-old infants. *Journal of Experimental Child Psychology, 38,* 429-446.

MORRONGIELLO, B. A., Fenwick, K. D., & Chance, G. (1990). Sound localization acuity in very young infants: An observer-based testing procedure. *Developmental Psychology, 26,* 75-84.

MORRONGIELLO, B. A., & Rocca, P. T. (1987). Infants' localization of sounds in the horizontal plane: Effects of auditory and visual cues. *Child Development, 58,* 918-927.

MORTON, J., Johnson, M. H., & Maurer, D. (1990). On the reasons for newborns' responses to faces. *Infant Behavior and Development, 13,* 99-104.

MUIR, D., Abraham, W., Forbes, B., & Harris, L. (1979). The ontogenesis of an auditory localization response from birth to four months of age. *Canadian Journal of Psychology, 33,* 320-333.

MUIR, D., & Clifton, R. K. (1985). Infants' orientation to the location of sound sources. In G. Gottlieb & N. A. Krasnegor (Eds.), *Measurement of audition and vision in the first year of postnatal life: A methodological overview* (pp. 171-194). Norwood, NJ: Ablex.

MUIR, D., & Field, J. (1979). Newborn infants orient to sounds. *Child Development, 50,* 431-436.

MURRAY, A. D. (1988a). Newborn auditory brainstem evoked responses (ABRs): Prenatal and contemporary correlates. *Child Development, 59,* 571-588.

MURRAY, A. D. (1988b). Newborn auditory brainstem evoked responses (ABRs): Longitudinal correlates in the first year. *Child Development, 59,* 1542-1554.

National Research Council. (1987). Report of Committee on Hearing, Bioacoustics, and Biomechanics. *Journal of American Speech and Hearing Association, 29,* 45-55.

OLSHO, L. W. (1984). Infant frequency discrimination. *Infant Behavior and Development, 7,* 27-35.

OLSHO, L. W., Koch, E. G., Halpin, C. F., & Carter, E. A. (1987). An observer-based psychoacoustic procedure for use with young infants. *Developmental Psychology, 23,* 627-640.

OSTER, H. S. (1975). *Color perception in ten-week-old infants.* Paper presented at the biennial meeting of the Society for Research in Child Development, Denver.

OWSLEY, C. J. (1980). *Perceiving solid shape in early infancy.*

Paper presented at the International Conference on Infant Studies, New Haven, CT.

PANNETON, R. K. (1985). *Prenatal auditory experience with melodies: Effects on postnatal auditory preferences in human newborns.* Unpublished doctoral dissertation, University of North Carolina, Greensboro.

PANNETON, R. K., & DeCasper, A. J. (1984, April). *Newborns prefer intrauterine heartbeat sounds to male voices.* Paper presented at the International Conference on Infant Studies, New York.

PEEPLES, D. R., & Teller, D. Y. (1975). Color vision and brightness discrimination in two month old human infants. *Science, 189,* 1102-1103.

PEIPER, A. (1924). Sinnesempfindungen des Kindes vor seiner Geburt [Sensory impressions of children prior to birth]. *Monatsschrift Kinderheilkunde, 29,* 236-241.

PEIPER, A. (1963). *Cerebral function in infancy and childhood* (3rd ed., B. Nagler & H. Nagler, Trans.). New York: Consultants Bureau. (Original work published 1961)

PERRIS, E. E., & Clifton, R. K. (1988). Reaching in the dark toward sound as a measure of auditory localization in infants. *Infant Behavior and Development, 11,* 473-491.

PETERSON, F., & Rainey, L. (1910). The beginnings of mind in the newborn. *Bulletin of Lying-In Hospital, City of New York, 7,* 99-122.

PETRIG, B., Julesz, B., Kropfl, W., Baumgartner, G., & Anliker, M. (1981). Development of stereopsis and cortical binocularity in human infants: Electrophysiological evidence. *Science, 213,* 1402-1405.

PETTERSEN, L., Yonas, A., & Fisch, R. O. (1980). The development of blinking in response to impending collision in preterm, full-term, and postterm infants. *Infant Behavior and Development, 3,* 155-165.

PORTER, R. H., Balogh, R. D., & Makin, J. W. (1988). Olfactory influences on mother-infant interaction. In C. K. Rovee-Collier & L. P. Lipsitt (Eds.), *Advances in infancy research* (Vol. 5). Norwood, NJ: Ablex.

PRATT, K. C., Nelson, A. K., & Sun, K. H. (1930). The behavior of the newborn infant. *Ohio State University Studies, Contributions to Psychology, 10.*

PREYER, W. (1888). *The mind of the child: Part I. The senses and the will* (N. W. Brown, Trans.). New York: Appleton. (Original work published 1880)

RADER, N., Bausano, M., & Richards, J. E. (1980). On the nature of the visual cliff avoidance response in human infants. *Child Development, 51,* 61-68.

RADER, N., & Stern, J. D. (1982). Visually elicited reaching in neonates. *Child Development, 53,* 1004-1007.

RAEHLMANN, E. (1891). Physiologisch-psychologische Studien über die Entwickelung der Gesichtswahrnehmungen bei Kindern und bei operierten Blindegeborenen [Physiological and psychological studies of the development of facial perception in children and children born blind and operated on (to restore sight)]. *Zeitschrift für Psychologie und Physiologie der Sinnesorgane, 2,* 53-96.

RAYNER, K. (1978). Eye movements in reading and information processing. *Psychological Bulletin, 85,* 618-660.

RHEINGOLD, H. L. (1961). The effect of environmental stimulation upon social and exploratory behavior in the human infant. In B. M. Foss (Ed.), *Determinants of infant behaviour* (pp. 143-177). London: Methuen.

RICHARDS, J. E., & Rader, N. (1981). Crawling-onset age predicts visual cliff avoidance in infants. *Journal of Experi-*

mental Psychology: Human Perception and Performance, 7, 382-387.

ROCHAT, P. (1984, April). *Oral activity by young infants: Development of two differentiated patterns of response.* Paper presented at the International Conference on Infant Studies, New York.

ROSENBLITH, J. F. (1965). Judgments of simple geometric figures by children. *Perceptual and Motor Skills, 21*(Monograph Suppl.), 2-V21.

ROSENBLITH, J. F. (1970). Are newborn auditory responses prognostic of deafness? *Transactions of the American Academy of Ophthalmology and Otolaryngology, 74,* 1215-1228.

ROSENBLITH, J. F., & DeLucia, L. A. (1963). Tactile sensitivity and muscular strength in the neonate. *Biologia Neonatorum, 5,* 266-282.

ROSENSTEIN, D., & Oster, H. (1988). Differential facial responses to four basic tastes in newborns. *Child Development, 59,* 1555-1568.

RUFF, H. A. (1982a). Effect of object movement on infants' detection of object structure. *Developmental Psychology, 18,* 462-472.

RUFF, H. A. (1982b). *Infants' detection of information specifying the motion of objects.* Paper presented at the International Conference on Infant Studies, Austin, TX.

RUFF, H. A. (1987). Preference for rotating objects in 5-month-old infants. *Infant Behavior and Development, 10,* 365-369.

RUFF, H. A., & Halton, A. (1978). Is there directed reaching in the human neonate? *Developmental Psychology, 14,* 425-426.

RUSSELL, M. J. (1976). Human olfactory communication. *Nature, 260,* 520-522.

SALAPATEK, P. (1975). Pattern perception in early infancy. In L. B. Cohen & P. Salapatek (Eds.), *Infant perception from sensation to cognition: Vol. 1. Basic visual processes.* New York: Academic Press.

SALAPATEK, P., Bechtold, A. G., & Bushnell, E. W. (1976). Infant visual acuity as a function of viewing distance. *Child Development, 47,* 860-863.

SALAPATEK, P., & Cohen, L. B. (Eds.). (1987a). *Handbook of infant perception: Vol. 1. From sensation to perception.* New York: Academic Press.

SALAPATEK, P., & Cohen, L. B. (Eds.). (1987b). *Handbook of infant perception: Vol. 2. From perception to cognition.* New York: Academic Press.

SALK, L. (1962). Mother's heartbeat as an imprinting stimulus. *Transactions of the New York Academy of Science, 24,* 753-763.

SALK, L. (1978). Response to Douglas K. Detterman (The effect of heartbeat sound on neonatal crying). *Infant Behavior and Development, 1,* 49-50.

SCAFIDI, F. A., Field, T. M., Schanberg, S. M., Bauer, C. R., Tucci, K., Roberts, J., Morrow, C., & Kuhn, C. M. (1990). Massage stimulates growth in preterm infants: A replication. *Infant Behavior and Development, 13,* 167-188.

SCAFIDI, F. A., Field, T. M., Schanberg, S. M., Bauer, C. R., Vega-Lahr, N., Garcia, R., Poirier, J., Nystrom, G., & Kuhn, C. M. (1986). Effects of tactile/kinesthetic stimulation on the clinical course and sleep/wake behavior of preterm neonates. *Infant Behavior and Development, 9,* 91-105.

SCHAAL, B., Montagner, H., Hertling, E., Bolzoni, D., Moyse, A., & Quichon, R. (1980). Les stimulations olfactives dans les relations entre l'enfant et la mere [Olfactory stimulation in the relationship between mother and infant]. *Reproduction, Nutrition et Développement, 20,* 843-858.

SCHALLER, M. J. (1975, April). *Chromatic vision in human infants: Conditioned fixation to "hues" of varying intensity.* Paper presented at the biennial meeting of the Society for Research in Child Development, Denver.

SCHANBERG, S. M., & Field, T. M. (1987). Sensory deprivation stress and supplemental stimulation in the rat pup and preterm human neonate. *Child Development, 58,* 1431-1447.

SCHIFF, W., Benasich, A. A., & Bornstein, M. H. (1989). Infant sensitivity to audiovisually coherent events. *Psychological Research, 51,* 102-106.

SCHMIDT, H. J., & Beauchamp, G. K. (1988). Adult-like odor preferences and aversions in three-year-old children. *Child Development, 59,* 1136-1143.

SCHNEIDER, B., Trehub, S. E., & Bull, D. (1980). High frequency sensitivity in infants. *Science, 207,* 1003-1004.

SCHWARTZ, A. N., Campos, J. J., & Baisel, E. J., Jr. (1973). The visual cliff: Cardiac and behavioral responses on the deep and shallow sides at five and nine months of age. *Journal of Experimental Child Psychology, 15,* 86-99.

SCHWARTZ, T., Dobson, V., Sandstrom, D., & van Hof-van Duin, J. (1987). Kinetic perimetry assessment of binocular visual field shape and size in the young infant. *Vision Research, 27,* 2163-2175.

SEKULER, R. (1974). Spatial vision. *Annual Review of Psychology, 25,* 195-232.

SELF, P. A. (1971). *Individual differences in auditory and visual responsiveness in infants from three days to six weeks of age.* Unpublished doctoral dissertation, University of Kansas, Lawrence.

SELF, P. A., Horowitz, F. D., & Paden, L. Y. (1972). Olfaction in newborn infants. *Developmental Psychology, 7,* 349-363.

SHERMAN, M. C., & Sherman, I. C. (1925). Sensory motor responses in infants. *Journal of Comparative Psychology, 5,* 53-68.

SHERMAN, M. C., Sherman, I. C., & Flory, C. D. (1936). Infant behavior. *Comparative Psychology Monographs, 12*(4).

SHIMOJO, S., Birch, E. E., Gwiazda, J., & Held, R. (1984). Development of vernier acuity in infants. *Vision Research, 24,* 721-728.

SHIMOJO, S., & Held, R. (1987). Vernier acuity is less than grating acuity in 2- and 3-month-olds. *Vision Research, 27,* 77-86.

SIRETEANU, R., Kellerer, R., & Boergen, K. (1984). The development of acuity in human infants: A preliminary study. *Human Neurobiology, 3,* 81-85.

SLATER, A. M., & Findlay, J. M. (1975). Binocular fixation in the newborn baby. *Journal of Experimental Child Psychology, 20,* 248-273.

SMITH, B. A., Fillion, T. J., & Blass, E. M. (1990). Orally mediated sources of calming in 1-3-day-old human infants. *Developmental Psychology, 26,* 731-737.

SPELKE, E. S. (1976). Infants' intermodal perception of events. *Cognitive Psychology, 8,* 553-560.

SPELKE, E. S., Born, W. S., & Chu, F. (1983). Perception of moving, sounding objects by four month old infants. *Perception, 12,* 719-732.

SPELKE, E. S., Hofsten, C. von, & Kestenbaum, R. (1989). Object perception in infancy: Interaction of spatial and kinetic information for object boundaries. *Developmental Psychology, 25,* 185-196.

SPELKE, E. S., & Owsley, C. J. (1979). Intermodal exploration and knowledge in infancy. *Infant Behavior and Development, 2,* 13-27.

SPENCE, M. J., & DeCasper, A. J. (1987). Prenatal experience with low-frequency maternal-voice sound influence neonatal perception of maternal voice samples. *Infant Behavior and Development, 10,* 133-142.

SPETNER, N. B., & Olsho, L. W. (1990). Auditory frequency resolution in human infancy. *Child Development, 61,* 632-652.

STEINER, J. E. (1977). Facial expressions of the neonate infant indicating the hedonics of food-related chemical stimuli. In J. M. Weiffenbach (Ed.), *Taste and development: The genesis of sweet preference* (DHEW Publication No. NIH 77-1068). Bethesda, MD: National Institute of Dental Research.

STEINSCHNEIDER, A., Lipton, E. L., & Richmond, J. B. (1966). Auditory sensitivity in the infant: Effect of intensity on cardiac and motor responsivity. *Child Development, 37,* 233-252.

STERN, D. (1977). *The first relationship.* Cambridge, MA: Harvard University Press.

STRÉRI, A., & Pêcheux, M. G. (1986). Tactual habituation and discrimination of form in infancy: A comparison with vision. *Child Development, 57,* 100-104.

STRÉRI, A., & Spelke, E. S. (1989). Effects of motion and figural goodness on haptic object perception in infancy. *Child Development, 60,* 1111-11254.

SWAIN, I. U., Clifton, R. K., & Clarkson, M. G. (1989, April). *Change in stimulus location influences newborns' head orientation to sound.* Paper presented at the Society for Research in Child Development, Kansas City, MO.

TAGUCHI, K., Picton, T. W., Orpin, J. A., & Goodman, W. S. (1969). Evoked response audiometry in newborn infants. *Acta Oto-laryngologica Supplementum, 252,* 5-17.

TARQUINIO, N., Zelazo, P. R., & Weiss, M. J. (1990). Recovery of neonatal head turning to decreased sound pressure level. *Developmental Psychology, 26,* 752-758.

TELLER, D. Y., & Bornstein, M. H. (1987). Infant color vision and color perception. In P. Salapatek & L. B. Cohen (Eds.), *Handbook of infant perception.* New York: Academic Press.

TELLER, D. Y., McDonald, M. A., Preston, K., Sebris, S. L., & Dobson, V. (1986). Assessment of visual acuity in infants and children: The Acuity Card procedure. *Developmental Medicine and Child Neurology, 28,* 779-789.

THACH, B. T., & Weiffenbach, J. M. (1976). Quantitative assessment of oral tactile sensitivity in premature and term neonates, and comparison with adults. *Developmental Medicine and Child Neurology, 18,* 204-212.

TIEDEMANN, D. (1927). Tiedemann's observations in the development of the mental faculties of children (S. Langer & C. Murchison, Trans.). *Pedagogical Seminary and Journal of Genetic Psychology, 34,* 205-230. (Original work published 1897)

TREHUB, S. E. (1987). Infants' perception of musical patterns. In The understanding of melody and rhythm [Special issue]. *Perception and Psychophysics, 41,* 635-641.

TREHUB, S. E., Bull, D., Schneider, B. A., & Morrongiello, B. A. (1986). PESTI: A procedure for estimating individual thresholds in infant listeners. *Infant Behavior and Development, 9,* 107-118.

TREHUB, S. E., Schneider, B. A., & Endman, M. (1980). Developmental changes in infants' sensitivity to octave-band noises. *Journal of Experimental Child Psychology, 29,* 282-293.

TREHUB, S. E., Schneider, B. A., Thorpe, L. A., & Judge, P. (1991). Observational measures of auditory sensitivity in early infancy. *Developmental Psychology, 27,* 40-49.

TREHUB, S. E., Thorpe, L. A., & Trainor, L. J. (1990). Infants' perception of good and bad melodies. In Music and child development [Special issue]. *Psychomusicology, 9,* 5-19.

TREVARTHEN, C., Hubley, P., & Sheeran, L. (1975). Les activités innée du nourrison [The inner activities of the newborn]. *La Recherche, 6,* 447-458.

TRONICK, E., & Clanton, C. (1971). Infant looking patterns. *Vision Research, 11,* 1479-1486.

TULLOCH, J. D., Brown, B. S., Jacobs, H. L., Prugh, D. G., & Greene, W. A. (1964). Normal heartbeat sounds and the behavior of human infants: A replication study. *Psychosomatic Medicine, 26,* 661-670.

TURKEWITZ, G., Birch, H. G., & Cooper, K. K. (1972a). Patterns of response to different auditory stimuli in the human newborn. *Developmental Medicine and Child Neurology, 14,* 487-491.

TURKEWITZ, G., Birch, H. G., & Cooper, K. K. (1972b). Responsiveness to simple and complex auditory stimuli in the human newborn. *Developmental Psychobiology, 5,* 7-19.

TURKEWITZ, G., Birch, H. B., Moreau, T., Levy, L., & Cornwell, A. C. (1966). Effect of intensity of auditory stimulation on directional eye movements in the human neonate. *Animal Behavior, 14,* 93-104.

TYRRELL, D. J., Anderson, J. T., Clubb, M., & Bradbury, A. (1987). Infant recognition of the correspondence between photographs and caricatures of human faces. *Bulletin of the Psychonomic Society, 25,* 41-43.

WALK, R. D. (1966). The development of depth perception in animals and human infants. *Monographs of the Society for Research in Child Development, 31,* 82-108.

WALK, R. D., & Gibson, E. J. (1961). A comparative and analytic study of visual depth perception. *Psychological Monographs, 75*(Whole No. 519).

WALKER-ANDREWS, A. S. (1986). Intermodal perception of expressive behaviors: Relation of eye and voice? *Developmental Psychology, 22,* 373-377.

WALKER-ANDREWS, A. S. (1988). Infants' perception of the affordances of expressive behaviors. In C. K. Rovee-Collier & L. P. Lipsitt (Eds.), *Advances in infancy research* (Vol. 5). Norwood, NJ: Ablex.

WALSH, E. J., & McGee, J. (1990). Frequency selectivity in the auditory periphery: Similarities between damaged and developing ears. *American Journal of Otolaryngology, 11,* 23-32.

WEDENBERG, E. (1956). Auditory tests on newborn infants. *Acta Oto-laryngologica, 46,* 446-461.

WEIFFENBACH, J. M. (1972a). Discrete elicited motion of the newborn's tongue. In J. F. Bosma (Ed.), *Third symposium on oral sensation and perception* (pp. 347-361). Springfield, IL: Charles C Thomas.

WEIFFENBACH, J. M. (1972b). Infants with clefts of lip and palate: Observations of touch elicited oral behavior. In J. F. Bosma (Ed.), *Third symposium on oral sensation and perception* (pp. 391-399). Springfield: Charles C Thomas.

WEIFFENBACH, J. M., Daniel, P. A., & Cowart, B. J. (1980). Saltiness in developmental perspective. In J. J. Fregly, R. A. Bernard, & M. R. Kare (Eds.), *Biological and behavioral aspects of salt intake.* New York: Academic Press.

WERNER, J. S., & Wooten, B. R. (1979). Human infant color vision and color perception. *Infant Behavior and Development, 2,* 241-274.

WERNER, L. A., & Gillenwater, J. M. (1990). Pure-tone sensitivity of 2- to 5-week-old infants. *Infant Behavior and Development, 13,* 355-375.

WERTHEIMER, M. (1961). Psychomotor coordination of auditory and visual space at birth. *Science, 134,* 1962.

WHITE, B. L. (1971). *Human infants: Experience and psychological development.* Englewood Cliffs, NJ: Prentice-Hall.

YONAS, A. (1981). Infants' responses to optical information for collision. In R. N. Aslin, J. Alberts, & M. Petersen (Eds.), *The development of perception: Psychobiological perspectives: Vol. 2. The visual system* (pp. 313-334). New York: Academic Press.

YONAS, A., Arterberry, M. E., & Granrud, C. E. (1987). Four-month-old infants' sensitivity to binocular and kinetic information for three-dimensional-object shape. *Child Development, 58,* 910-917.

YONAS, A., Bechtold, A. G., Frankel, D., Gordon, F. R., McRoberts, G., Norcia, A., & Sternfels, S. (1977). Development of sensitivity to information for impending collision. *Perception and Psychophysics, 21,* 97-104.

YONAS, A., Granrud, C. E., Arterberry, M. E., & Hanson, B. L. (1986). Infants' distance perception from linear perspective and texture gradients. *Infant Behavior and Development, 9,* 247-256.

YONAS, A., & Owsley, C. (1987). Development of visual space perception. In P. Salapatek & L. B. Cohen (Eds.), *Handbook of infant perception.* New York: Academic Press.

YONAS, A., Pettersen, L., & Granrud, C. E. (1982). Infants' sensitivity to familiar size as information for distance. *Child Development, 53,* 1285-1290.

YONAS, A., Pettersen, L., & Lockman, J. J. (1979). Sensitivity in 3- and 4-week-old infants to optical information for collision. *Canadian Journal of Psychology, 33,* 268-276.

YONAS, A., Pettersen, L., Lockman, J. J., & Eisenberg, P. (1980, April). *The perception of impending collision in 3-month-old infants.* Paper presented at the International Conference on Infant Studies, New Haven, CT.

YUODELIS, C., & Hendrickson, A. (1986). A qualitative and quantitative analysis of the human fovea during development. *Vision Research, 26,* 847-855.

ZELAZO, P., Weiss, M., Randolph, M., Swain, I., & Moore, D. (1987). The effects of delay on neonatal retention of habituated headturning. *Infant Behavior and Development, 10,* 417-434.

Developmental Milestones

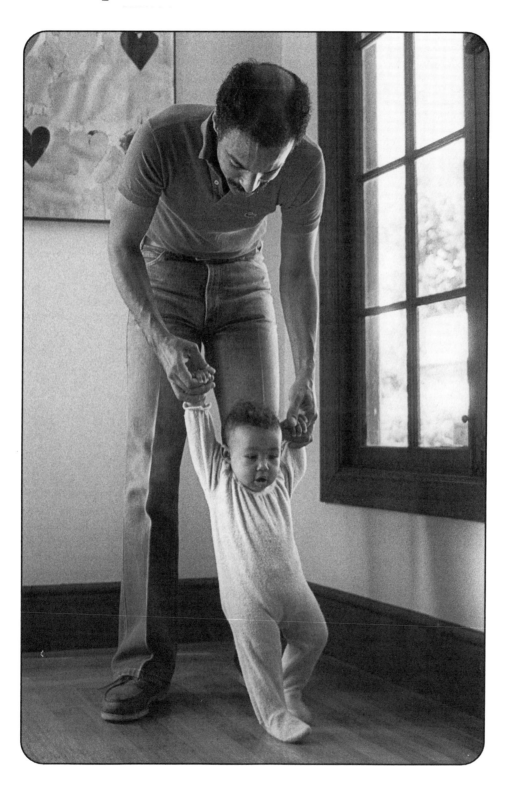

This chapter takes up some conventional topics of growth and development throughout the period of infancy. The discussion starts with physical growth, followed by aspects of motor development and developmental milestones. Finally, the neurological and psychological assessment of newborns and infants is addressed.

Physical Development

The most rapid growth of all life occurs prior to birth (see Chapter 2), but this growth is not seen and so must be admired in the abstract. Infancy is the next most rapid period of physical growth, particularly the first year, when birth weight triples and length increases 9 to 10 inches. This rate of growth is higher than that of any subsequent period, including the so-called adolescent growth spurt.

Parents and those who work with children are interested in the physical growth and development of infants. Health professionals are also interested, because physical growth often indexes problems in development. James M. Tanner, professor of child health and growth at the Institute of Child Health of the University of London and one of the world's experts in this field, elaborates this thesis at the end of his book *Foetus Into Man* (1978):

> Provided always that parental size is known, growth emerges as the prime measure of a child's physical and mental health. The study of growth emerges also as a powerful tool for monitoring the health and nutrition of populations, especially in ecological and economic circumstances that are sub-optimal. It is equally powerful for studying the effect of political organization upon the relative welfare of the various social, cultural, and ethnic groups which make up a modern state. Thus the study of growth has a very direct bearing upon human welfare. At the same time it gives us valuable lessons on the way in which our biological heritage and our technological culture interact. It warns us that all too soon we shall be technically capable of creating monstrously specialized, monstrously similar children. It points to our need to be reconciled with our origins, to see ourselves once again as a part of the natural order; not

foetus into angel, nor foetus into monster, but foetus into Man. (p. 219)

To give a concrete example, in rural Guatemala length and weight are the indices most strongly correlated with behavioral development over the first two years (Lasky, Klein, Yarbrough, Engle, et al., 1981). These relations are not accounted for by gestational age, food intake, prevalence of disease, or characteristics of the family.

The timetables of growth are largely genetically determined, and the ultimate height, body type, and, to a lesser degree, weight are largely influenced by an infant's genetic makeup. In interaction with genetic factors, living standards, nutrition, general health, and emotional health, all have a lot to do with optimal growth, as Tanner implies. Considerable attention will be devoted here to final or adult height, because differences in it represent the joint action of genetic and environmental factors in development.

Several important longitudinal studies that involved physical growth were started in the United States a century after the pioneer studies of Quetelet (1835). These include the Berkeley Growth Studies and those at the Fels Institute. These and other studies, usually cross-sectional, were used to provide norms by which pediatricians and parents could judge the development of a given child. They were usually based on samples from limited geographic areas and from only a narrow portion of the socioeconomic range, primarily middle or upper-middle class. Normative data based on representative samples of the population of the United States recently became available for older children.[1] These led to an assessment of existing norms and the combining of data from the Preschool Nutrition Survey (Owen et al., 1974) and the Fels longitudinal study to provide norms for the period from birth to 36 months of age. These data are referred to later in the chapter.

It is important to have up-to-date norms for physical development because of the so-called **secular trends** in growth. These are changes over time in heights and weights of given populations thought to be related to environmental influences. Upward secular trends are thought to reflect improved diet and health care that enable more infants to more nearly reach their genetic potential. Secular trends are especially obvious in countries where good diet and health care are prevalent. Height increased markedly in this century, especially after World War II, in such countries as the United States, Sweden, Japan, and Holland. In the United States today young adults are, on average, 1 inch taller than their parents. But in Japan

1. The Health Examination Survey and the Health and Nutrition Examination Survey of the National Center for Health Statistics are the studies. They were done to assess the health and nutritional status of noninstitutionalized people in the United States, not to provide growth norms.

after World War II, children could not use the school desks that their parents had used. Within each country the sex, or ethnic, or other grouping that had previously been most prevented from reaching their genetic potential had the greatest increases in height.

The secular trend toward increased average heights and weights appears to have nearly ceased, at least in the United States (National Center for Health Statistics, 1976). Increases ceased some time ago for advantaged Harvard students (Damon, 1968), and by now have ceased for the fairly representative sample of the National Center for Health Statistics (1976), which reports:

Whatever complex factors had been producing the secular trend to increasing body size of children (and adults) from the prenatal period onward had ceased to be of sufficient magnitude by 1955 or 1956 to affect these rather sensitive data across most socioeconomic levels of the American [U.S.] population. When the stragglers will finally achieve their genetic potential to full stature can probably be *better predicted by economic and social factors than by biologic ones.* (p. 19; emphasis added)

Secular trends are also found for birth weights and heights. Both have increased over the time spans discussed. Their change is less regular, due in part to changing fashions about the appropriate amount of weight for a pregnant woman to gain during pregnancy. A more detailed discussion of secular trends and issues associated with assessing them is available in Roche's (1979) monograph.

METHODOLOGICAL ISSUES IN
THE STUDY OF PHYSICAL
DEVELOPMENT

Any given set of figures on birth weight or birth height requires cautious interpretation because standardized measurements of these physical characteristics are not easy to make. For example, was the baby weighed with a wet or dry diaper, or with a blanket or not? Was the baby quiet for the weighing (a problem some modern digital scales can solve)? When in relation to feeding and elimination did the weighing take place? To use birth weights for comparative or diagnostic purposes, it is important to know not only whether similar measurement techniques were used, but also how soon after birth the weighing was done, the conceptional age of the baby, birth order, whether it was a multiple birth, and the heights and weights of the parents.

For height, the problems are greater. Measurement must be made on the horizontal, because newborns cannot stand. The head must be at the correct angle with respect to the head board; this is made harder by the fact that the head may be out of shape due to delivery. It is also difficult to extend a newborn's legs fully.

Thus in comparing any figures it is important to know that the same techniques were used to make the measurements. People often think that psychological data are peculiarly messy because of the problems of standardization of measurement techniques. It is important also to understand that measurement problems are not limited to psychological variables; they can exist in areas of physical measurement as well.

Another important methodological issue concerns assessment of the contribution of heredity to a characteristic. It is assessed by examining the degree to which characteristics are associated in persons with different biological relationships. The degree of association between any two groups on some trait (such as height, weight, or IQ) is assessed by the statistical technique of correlation (see Chapter 1). In general, the more closely the two groups are related, the higher the correlation coefficient (where 1.00 is a perfect correlation). Comparing groups who have the same genotype (that is, identical twins, with one in each group) yields the highest correlations in characteristics such as height and weight. Correlations between children and their siblings or parents are substantial for height and moderate even for weight.

A high correlation between groups does not preclude a substantial difference in their actual heights. Even if the correlations were perfect there could be marked differences in actual heights as long as the ordering of the heights remained the same in both groups. To take a hypothetical example, suppose we correlate the heights of a group of fathers born in a period of famine that extended from their prenatal pe-

Table 8.1
Father-Son Pairs Whose Heights Are Perfectly Correlated, but Differ

	Father's Height	*Son's Height*
Pair 1	5 ft, 6 in.	5 ft, 8 in.
Pair 2	5 ft, 7 in.	5 ft, 9 in.
Pair 3	5 ft, 8 in.	5 ft, 10 in.
Pair 4	5 ft, 9 in.	5 ft, 11 in.
Pair 5	5 ft, 10 in.	6 ft, 1 in.
Pair 6	5 ft, 11 in.	6 ft, 2 in.
Pair 7	6 ft, 0 in.	6 ft, 3 in.

riod through their infancy with the heights of their sons. The growth of the fathers would be stunted, but, if their sons were born in a period of prosperity, we might find data such as that in Table 8.1. The ordering of the heights is the same for fathers and sons, thus there is a perfect correlation, even though all the sons are taller than their own fathers, and hence the average heights of the two groups differs markedly. These data would also illustrate an extreme secular change.

NATURE OF PHYSICAL GROWTH

This section examines growth in height, weight, head circumference, and the brain. Several examples are presented to show how one system in the body would develop if it were to grow at the same rate as other systems. Such comparisons dramatically illustrate the uneven rates of growth of different body parts, organs, or tissues.

Height

At birth, full-term babies average 19 to 21 inches in length; boys are slightly longer than girls, and later-borns are slightly longer than firstborns. The growth curves for length published by the National Center for Health Statistics (1976) are shown in Figure 8.1 (a and b). Length at birth has little relation to adult height, but by the end of the first year there is a moderate correlation (.50 for boys and .60 for girls in the Berkeley Growth Study data). By the second year these correlations rise to the mid or high .70s (Tanner, 1978).

One way of looking at growth in this period is in terms of the proportion of adult height that infants have reached at a given age. By 2 years boys have reached 50% of their mature height and girls 53% (Harvard data, cited by Bayley, 1954). Another way of looking at it is in terms of the proportion of their birth length that infants grow over a given time period. By 1 year infants have grown by 50% of their birth height, and by 2 years by 75% of it (Stuart & Meredith, 1946).

Weight

Weight has to be considered separately for full-term and premature infants. We will start with term infants.

Term Infants. At birth, boys in the United States average 3.3 kg (7 lb, 4 oz) and girls 3.2 kg (National

Center for Health Statistics, 1976); British babies are about 0.1 kg heavier (Tanner, 1970). The curves of weight increase (Figure 8.1, c and d) are more varied than those for height (Figure 8.1, a and b). Birth weight is actually slightly more related to adult weight than length is to adult height, although weight is more affected by health and environmental factors, including even the seasons. For boys there is an r of .51 (Tanner et al., 1956, 1975). Girls, however, are 6 years old before their weight is significantly correlated with that of their mothers (Bayley, 1954). Birth weight does not predict weight at age 2 any better than it predicts adult weight.

Birth weight normally doubles in the first 5 months, triples in the first year, and quadruples by 22 years. If height did the same, 1-year-olds would be 5 feet tall. Children increase more in weight during their first year of life then between 2 and 5 years. At birth the body weighs only 5% of an adult's and does not reach 50% of adult weight until 10 years.

Premature Infants. It is important to distinguish between premature babies and those who are small for their gestational age, because the weight of the premature is particularly important in assessing the infant's risk status. Tanner and Thomson (1970) provided weight norms for babies born between 32 and 42 weeks of gestational age that show the average weights and those at different percentiles for boys and girls. Figures are given separately for first- and later-borns, and a correction factor based on the mother's height and weight is given. All of these factors need to be taken into account when the status of the infant is being interpreted.

Head Circumference

Another physical measurement of great interest to physicians, and one that has potential meaning for the psychologist, is head circumference. Infants who are outside the normal range (as determined by carefully standardized measurements) on either the large or the small side are at risk. Those with unusually large heads are likely to have **hydrocephaly**, a condition in which the cerebrospinal fluid that normally bathes the brain does not drain out of the skull properly. This results in pressure on both brain and skull, which leads to brain damage and a large head. If hydrocephaly is identified, the excess fluid in the head can often be drained or

Figure 8.1. Charts (produced by the National Center for Health Statistics) showing percentiles for length and weight development by age from birth to 36 months. (a) Girls' length, (b) boys' length, (c) girls' weight, (d) boys' weight.

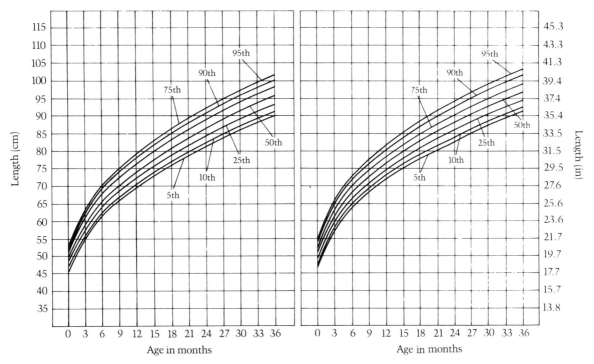

(a) Girls' length by age percentiles: Birth—36 months

(b) Boys' length by age percentiles: Birth—36 months

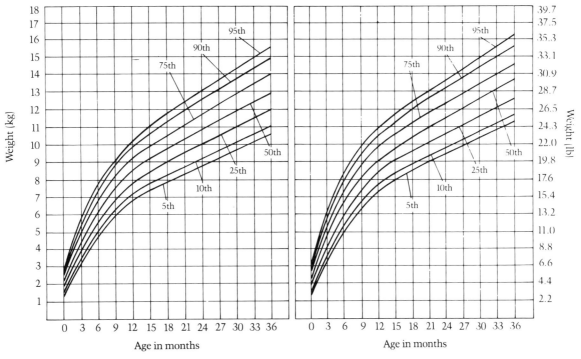

(c) Girls' weight by age percentiles: Birth—36 months

(d) Boys' weight by age percentiles: Birth—36 months

shunted to other parts of the body. This can even be done in utero. The degree of the problem and the rapidity of its correction both affect the outcome. Sometimes a large head may be the result of enlargement of the brain.

Babies whose heads are abnormally small may have **microcephaly**, in which the small size of the skull reflects a small brain, or **craniostenosis**, a condition that results from premature closure of one or more of the sutures between the bones of the skull. In the past the two were not clearly distinguished, which led to confusion about the success of surgery to separate the sutures (Menkes, 1984). Microcephaly is the result either of anomalous development in the first 7 months of gestation or of an insult in the last 2 months or perinatally. Anomalous development is sometimes a result of chromosomal or inherited problems (see Chapter 3) or of intrauterine causes such as rubella, CMV, toxoplasmosis, maternal PKU, irradiation, or drugs (see Chapter 4). Perinatal insults and those of the last 2 months of gestation include infections, trauma, and metabolic and anoxic destruction of brain tissues.

When microcephaly is part of general growth retardation, it appears to be less serious than when only the head is affected. In general, intellectual development in microcephalics is poor. Even if an infant's head circumference is smaller than normal, but above the microcephalic range, intellectual development is more likely to be handicapped (Broman, 1981).

Brain Growth

The brain, the largest part of the central nervous system, develops earlier than most other organs. From early fetal life its weight is closer to its adult level than that of any other organ except perhaps the eye (Tanner, 1978). The brain's weight at birth is 25% of its adult weight. By 6 months it weighs 50% as much as that of an adult, and at 2 years 75% as much. If the rates of growth for height and weight were as slow after birth as that for the brain, babies would grow only to be about 4 feet, 3 inches tall, and to weigh about 40 pounds.

The cortical portion of the brain is very poorly developed at birth, which suggests that little cortical function is possible. By 1 month cells appear in the primary motor area of the brain, which controls the upper limbs and trunk, suggesting that these may begin to be cortically controlled. By 3 months all primary cortical areas are relatively mature, with the motor areas most advanced, especially those controlling the hands, arms, and upper trunk. Their development earlier than the areas controlling the lower trunk and legs emphasizes the cephalocaudal principle of development.

Development of the primary sensory areas lags behind that of the primary motor areas, but by 2 years they have caught up. The association areas develop more slowly than either, and some of these areas are still immature at 2 years.

The maturation of these areas of the cortex does not mean that brain development is complete. Other aspects of development, such as myelination and the development of the neural processes (outgrowths)—the axons and dendrites—and of the synapses continues after cell division has ceased (see Chapter 2). Precise control of voluntary movement depends on fibers linking the cerebellum to the cortex, which are not fully myelinated until 4 years of age. Auditory system fibers begin to myelinate in the sixth fetal month and continue until the fourth year; visual system fibers start to myelinate just before birth, but complete the process rapidly; and still other structures continue to myelinate until puberty or beyond.

UNEVENNESS OF GROWTH

Although growth measured by height, weight, or head circumference is important and of interest to parents and pediatricians, one of the most striking features about growth is that different body parts grow or change at such different rates. As already noted, height, weight, head circumference, and brain do not grow at the same rates. One of the most striking results of differential growth is seen in the relative proportion of length that is accounted for by the length of the head compared to that of the legs (Figure 8.2). On the average, the head accounts for one-fourth of a baby's length at birth, compared with one-eighth of adult height. In contrast, the legs are only a third of the total length at birth, but half of adult length. The head doubles in length between birth and adulthood, whereas the trunk triples, the arms quadruple, and the legs quintuple.

Another, less obvious, aspect of growth is the fact that weight is made up of varied proportions of the different types of tissue that make up the body. For example, at birth 25% of weight is accounted for by muscle, 16% by vital organs, and 15% by the central nervous system. In the adult, 43% of weight is accounted for by muscle, 11% by vital organs, and 3% by the central nervous system. From this point of view, "growing up" physically seems to be disproportionately a matter of developing more muscle. The proportion of body weight that is accounted for by water changes from 75-80% at birth to only 59% by 1 year (Tanner, 1962).

Despite the separate weight norms shown for boys and girls, the differences are slight in the first year. Differences increase after age 1, when girls lose fat more rapidly than boys. At 6 this reverses. However, large individual differences in the amount of fat in relation to bone and muscle occur in both sexes and overwhelm the average differences between the sexes.

Motor Development

In addition to watching and charting physical growth and development, parents, pediatricians, and grandparents look for the milestones of motor development. When does the baby hold its head up steadily? Sit up? Stand up? Walk? Run? These motor accomplishments are aspects of gross motor development and are among the developmental milestones parents record in "baby books." Parents read books on development and discuss with their parents, friends, and pediatricians when to expect these milestones. They may also compare notes with friends and, usually inappropriately, feel good or bad because their baby is early or late to achieve a given skill.

Psychologists, pediatricians, and parents are also sometimes attentive to behaviors that are aspects of fine motor development. The abilities to grasp objects with the hands with ever greater smoothness and precision of movement and to grasp very small objects with neat pincer movements of thumb and one finger are aspects of fine motor development. These are probably less often carefully observed or charted by parents, but are often of greater importance for development.

BACKGROUND OF THE STUDY OF MOTOR DEVELOPMENT

Many of the early data describing the course of motor development came from Arnold Gesell and his colleagues and from Myrtle McGraw and M. M. Shirley. Their focus on motor behavior was not primarily diagnostic or on the provision of norms, but on processes of development. However, norms rather than processes were often what were picked up and accentuated by pediatricians, parents, and even other researchers. Motor development needs to be discussed separately from infant tests (from which much of the normative data came), because of the interest in process and because motor behaviors are a crucial element in Piaget's theory of sensorimotor stages of development (see Chapter 10). There is currently a resurgence of interest in motor development that is focused on process in contexts different from those found in the early work.

Let us begin with a discussion of Gesell, one of the pioneers of the detailed study of infants. In his original infant tests, he used seven categories of behaviors to cover the total development of the infant (Gesell, 1925). Three of them—postural, locomotive, and prehensive (grasping) behaviors—were relevant to motor development. The first two are gross motor behaviors,

Figure 8.2. The very different proportions of body length accounted for by the head, trunk, and legs at different ages or stages of development. The disproportion is greatest in fetal life: The head decreases from 50% of total body length at 2 months postconception to only 25% at birth and 12% in adulthood.

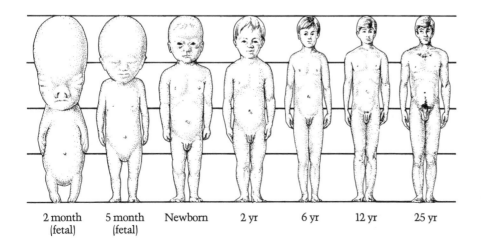

| 2 month (fetal) | 5 month (fetal) | Newborn | 2 yr | 6 yr | 12 yr | 25 yr |

while the third is fine motor behavior. It may seem strange to see posture listed as behavior; here is what Gesell et al. (1934) say about this:

> Posture is behavior. Postural patterns are behavior patterns. To be sure, these patterns are influenced by bodily size and proportions, by joints and ligaments, and even by abdominal viscera. But primarily they are determined by the maturity and organization of the infant's central neural equipment. The positions, the stances, the motor attitudes which he assumes are net resultants of a complicated system of reflexes and reaction trends which vary from age to age. Posture is not the manifestation of a discrete set of abilities which increase as the child grows stronger. (p. 44)

Locomotion, or the ability to move from one place to another by crawling or walking, is clearly important in infant development. In the very first known normative study, Feldman (1833) gave average ages of walking (and talking) for his French sample.

Prehension, or the ability to grasp things with the hands, is a fine motor behavior, often said to be one of the important features that differentiates humans from other animals, as it enables the precise use of tools. It is also crucial to the achievement of the developmental stages described by Piaget. We shall return to it later.

Although Gesell created one of the most used infant tests, he was also interested in process. He and other early pioneer students of motor development (including McGraw, 1935; Shirley, 1931) used observational techniques to study such motor behaviors as grasping, crawling or creeping, swimming, and walking. Gesell also pioneered the use of motion pictures that allow frame-by-frame analysis of the movement sequences. By comparing films made at different ages, a view of the process of development of motor skills is possible. The sequences of these developments are pictured in detail in Gesell's *An Atlas of Infant Behavior* (1934). This two-volume work contains 3,200 action photographs of infant behaviors.[2]

After the early research, psychologists concentrated for a long time on the average age and normal range of ages for the appearance of various motor skills. Gesell's work was often inappropriately cited as providing norms for the age of achievement of various skills, even though his observations were often made using relatively small numbers of infants in samples that were not representative of the population at large.

Now the age of these data makes them an inappropriate source of norms because of secular trends in the ages at which given skills normally develop, changes that are probably related to those for physical growth and development.

A number of factors affect the age at which motor skills are achieved. For example, appropriate motor development appears to depend not only on physical characteristics and growth factors, but also on the appropriate functioning of other systems, especially the perceptual systems. For example, infants who are congenitally blind are hypotonic, have slow motor development, do not tactilely (haptically) explore stimuli as much as normal infants—let alone more, as one might expect—and tend to walk before they crawl (Fraiberg, 1971, 1977). There is some suggestion from head shape that these infants may be left too much in the supine position and that this, rather than blindness, may be a partial cause of their differences from sighted infants (Fraiberg, 1971). The role of sensory deprivation (congenital blindness and deafness) in development will be addressed further in Chapter 12.

Neurologists interested in diagnostic problems have complained about the lack of detailed knowledge of normal motor performance that would enable them to be better judges of departures from it. Neuhauser (1975) called for getting away from task achievement (or motor ages) to an assessment of the quality of motor behavior. This has been heeded by some, as has his call for more detailed and specific analyses. Techniques that do not require verbal communication, developed earlier for sensory and perceptual development, are now beginning to be available for some motor behaviors.

Patterns of motor behavior are currently being studied in Holland. They have been found to distinguish fetuses that suffer intrauterine growth retardation from those growing normally (Bekedam et al., 1985). They distinguish anencephalic fetuses as early as the first half of pregnancy (Visser et al., 1985). Patterns of movement show stability from day 1 to day 4 in normal neonates (Cioni et al., 1989). A description of some work on fetal movements is found in McNay (1988).

McGraw, a pioneer student of motor development, noted in her 1977 address to the Society for Research in Child Development that researchers (herself in her earlier work included) have not paid enough attention to differences in the quality of motor performance. For example, three toddlers who can walk on a raised board may do so very differently. One may do it with what might be described as finesse, another with competence, and the third clumsily, often appearing to be

---

2. If your library has a copy, it is well worth looking at.

Table 8.2

Motor Milestones

Behavior	Average Age (Approximate)	Range of Ages
(A) Head control when held to shoulder		
Lifts head	Neonatal period	
Makes postural adjustment	Neonatal period	
Head erect—vertical	3 weeks	9 days-3 months
Head erect—steady	7 weeks	3 weeks-4 months
Holds head steady	2½ months	1 month-5 months
Head balanced	4 months, 1 week	2 months-6 months
(B) Motor behaviors in prone position		
Lateral head movements	Neonatal period	
Crawling movements	By 2 weeks	Neonatal period-3 months
Elevates self by arms	Just after 2 months	3 weeks-5 months
Able to progress (move) in some fashion	Just after 7 months	5 months-11 months
(C) Motor behaviors in supine position or on side		
Thrusts arms in play	3½ weeks	9 days-2 months
Thrusts legs in play	3½ weeks	9 days-2 months
Holds on to large plastic ring	3½ weeks	9 days-3 months
Lifts head (dorsal suspension)	1 month, 3 weeks	3 weeks-4 months
Turns from side to side	By 2 months	3 weeks-5 months
Turns from back to side	2½ months	2 months-7 months

SOURCE: Tables 8.2-8.5 are adapted from the Collaborative Perinatal Research Project form of the Bayley tests.

about to fall off. They would all pass the item, but they are not all functioning at the same level. The psychological consequences of such qualitative differences are just beginning to be studied.

DEVELOPMENTAL NORMS FOR GROSS MOTOR BEHAVIORS

The Bayley Motor Scale (Psychomotor Development Index or PDI, as used in the CPRP) has been chosen for this presentation of developmental norms for two reasons: First, the standardization sample on which it is based is closer to being representative of babies in the United States than that of any other test.[3] Second, the data for the PDI show not only the usual age at which the behaviors are achieved, but also the youngest and oldest ages at which any baby in the standardization sample demonstrated the behavior. These illustrate the extreme nature of individual differences. It is possible that babies who achieve a skill at the latest ages may have suffered damage. The rest of the variability is accounted for by an inextricable mixture of genetic and experiential factors.

These motor milestones were reached earlier in 1969 (Bayley, 1969) than in the earlier studies (Bayley, 1935; Gesell & Amatruda, 1947; Gesell et al., 1934). This seems to indicate secular trends similar to those found for height and weight. They are found despite

the fact that both Gesell's and Bayley's earlier samples represented a more privileged social group than the 1969 standardization sample. Better general health care and nutrition and changed ways of caring for children probably contributed to the observed changes over time, but unknown factors, including sampling differences, may have also played a role.

In presenting the normative data from the Bayley test, I have reorganized them at the earlier ages according to the postural position or stimulus situation in which the behaviors are found and, at later ages, by the type of motor behavior. (On the test, items are ordered according to the age at which they are normally passed.) Two developmental principles are illustrated in Tables 8.2-8.4. The first is that, as discussed in other contexts, development tends to proceed cephalocaudally. Head control is achieved before trunk control (sitting), which is achieved before leg control (walking). The second is the **proximodistal** (from the center out) character of development. It is illustrated in motor development by the fact that head control is achieved before arm control, which is achieved before hand control, which in turn precedes finger control.

I will not try to describe everything in the tables, but will comment on one or two highlights from each.

---

3. The publishers are starting a new standardization currently.

First, let us look at the behaviors that index head control and postural adjustment when the infant is held to the shoulder. Table 8.2A shows that the final stage of holding the head balanced is achieved after 4 months, on average, but by some babies at 2 months and by others only at 6 months. Table 8.2B shows behaviors exhibited when the baby is in the prone position (lying on the stomach). Both crawling and head control are involved here. The ability to move is achieved on the average at just over 7 months, but the range is from 5 to 11 months. Table 8.2C shows the motor behaviors that take place when the baby is supine (on the back) or on a side. In this position the baby is free to move the arms, to move the legs in a different fashion than when prone, and can turn over (see Figure 8.3). Actually, turning over is achieved earlier in the prone position. Once babies can use their arms to raise their heads and shoulders well above the rest of the body, their center of gravity and momentum can result in their turning over as a result of accidental movements. This is usually followed in a relatively short time by the baby appearing to carry out the sequence intentionally. Turning over was not included in prone-position behaviors, but in supine behaviors, perhaps because intentionality is more clearly demanded in the supine. Turning over is the capstone achievement of this sequence.

Sitting behaviors when the baby is placed in the sitting position by an adult are shown in Table 8.3A. Those that involve the baby's own efforts, but with some adult help, are shown in Table 8.3B. Table 8.3C

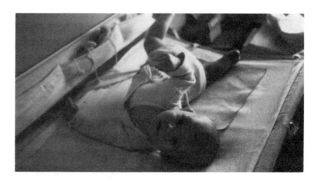

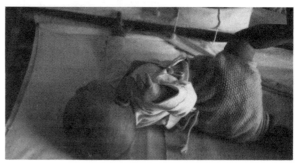

Figure 8.3. An infant just learning to turn from her back to her stomach. (Photographs by Judy F. Rosenblith.)

deals with efforts to gain a vertical position without the help of others, but using furniture as an aid, and with independent efforts to stand up.

Many different levels of a given behavior are charted in the tables. It is impossible to say at what age a baby

Table 8.3
Sitting Behaviors and Efforts to Achieve a Vertical Position

Behavior	Average Age (Approximate)	Range of Ages
(A) Placed by adult		
Sits with support	2 months, 1 week	1 month-5 months
Sits with slight support	3 months, 3 weeks	2 months-6 months
Sits alone, momentarily	5 months, 1 week	4 months-8 months
Sits alone, 30 seconds or more	6 months	5 months-8 months
Sits alone, steadily	6½ months	5 months-9 months
Sits alone, good coordination	7 months	5 months-10 months
(B) Helped by adult		
Makes effort to sit	4 months, 3 weeks	3 months-8 months
Pulls to sitting	5 months, 3 weeks	4 months-8 months
Pulls to standing	8 months	5 months-12 months
(C) Helped by furniture		
Raises self to sitting	8 months, 1 week	6 months-11 months
Stands up alone	8½ months	6 months-12 months
Stands up, level I	12½ months	9 months-18 months
Stands up, level II	By 22 months	11 months-30+ months
Stands up, level III	30+ months	22 months-30+ months

sits alone without specifying for how long and in what situation. Note that the differences between the earliest and latest ages for achieving the various sitting behaviors range from 3 to 5 months. For the different standing behaviors they range from 6 to over 19 months.

The behaviors relevant to the development of grasp and manipulation will not be presented here. They are related to fine motor development, which will be considered in the next section.

The last table in this sequence based on the Bayley Motor Scale covers walking, balance, and stair climbing (Table 8.4). Achievement of balance seems to be extremely variable. I know of no studies that explain the factors in this variability. The role of the mechanisms of balance relative to other physiological factors or relative to experience is interesting but largely unexplored terrain.

The tables, as presented here, omit a few behaviors that may occur by the end of the second year, but not many. The Bayley scales themselves extend beyond 2 years with a considerable number of items that are achieved, on the average, at over 30 months of age.

NATURE VERSUS NURTURE IN GROSS MOTOR DEVELOPMENT

Gesell assumed that postural, locomotive, and prehensive skills were biologically determined and depended primarily on the passage of time to unfold. Others working in the 1930s agreed (see Dennis, 1938, 1940, 1943; McGraw, 1935). A number of studies in that era attempted to assess the relative contributions of nature and nurture to motor skills, from the developmental milestones to such specialized skills as climbing, swimming, and roller-skating.

The age of walking was compared for Hopi infants reared on the traditional cradle board, Hopi infants with "Western" rearing, and non-Indian children (Dennis & Dennis, 1940). The age of walking was not affected by experience or by the opportunity for practice, a view W. Dennis later changed, as we will see in Chapter 13. The postural experience of being upright, which may be important for walking, was much more prevalent for the Hopi on cradle boards than for those with Western rearing. McGraw (1935) studied the role of practice. She gave one twin, but not the other, early practice on some motor skill such as roller-skating. The twin without the early training, given practice

Table 8.4
Walking,[a] Standing Balance, and Stair-Climbing Behaviors

Behavior	Average Age (Approximate)	Range of Ages
(A) Walking		
Early stepping movements	7 months, 2 weeks	5 months-11 months
Stepping movements	8 months, 3 weeks	6 months-12 months
Walks with help	9½+ months	7 months-12 months
Sits down	9½+ months	7 months-14 months
Stands alone	11 months	9 months-16 months
Walks alone	11 months, 3 weeks	9 months-17 months
(B) Balance		
Stands on right foot with help	16 months	12 months-21 months
Stands on left foot with help	16+ months	12 months-23 months
Stands on left foot alone	22 months, 3 weeks	15 months-30+ months
Stands on right foot alone	23½ months	16 months-30+ months
Jumps off floor, both feet	By 23½ months	17 months-30+ months
(C) Stair climbing		
Walks up stairs with help	16+ months	12 months-23 months
Walks down stairs with help	By 16½ months	13 months-23 months
Walks up stairs alone, both feet on each step	25+ months	18 months-30+ months
Walks down stairs alone, both feet on each step	25 months, 3 weeks	19 months-30+ months
Walks up stairs alternating forward foot	30+ months	23 months-30+ months

a. Includes motor control in standing position.

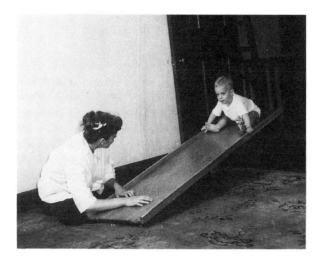

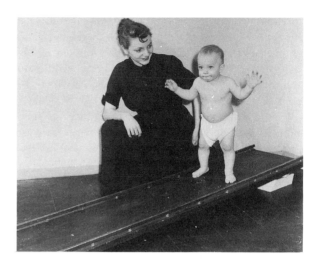

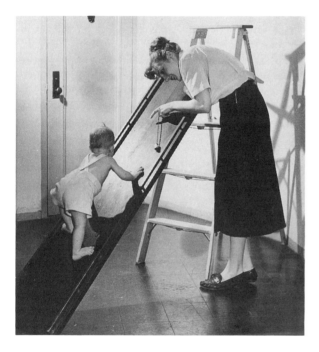

Figure 8.4. McGraw's early work, showing that babies need to be encouraged to learn unusual skills such as going up or down inclined boards. The first two pictures (top) show that as the baby's other motoric skills increase, the locomotor methods used to get down become more advanced. With encouragement the slightly older infant can make it up a much steeper incline (bottom), a highly unusual performance for infants of this age. Although much older children may master similar feats on their own, a certain fearlessness may be acquired, in addition to the motor accomplishment itself, by those who learn young. (Photographs courtesy of Dr. Myrtle McGraw.)

after the first was proficient, caught up rapidly. In short, biological readiness was most important. Unfortunately, the twins in McGraw's study turned out not to be identical. This spoiled its being a **co-twin control** study, a method initiated by Gesell in which one twin is treated differently from the other, enabling determination of the effect of the environmental variables, since genetics is constant.

Many ideas in the United States about waiting to teach a skill until a child is ready to learn it came from these studies. The idea applies to gross motor skills such as swimming and skating, but also to reading, which requires a great deal of fine motor skill. Even after learning theory dominated developmental psychology in the United States, motor skills were still thought of as primarily maturational, or as the result of genetic and constitutional factors in development. Special coaching did not greatly affect the time at which those skills that are universally acquired by the human species developed. When Piagetian ideas came to dominate developmental psychology, they fit well with this view of motor skills.

The pendulum of opinion is swinging back now, and psychologists are again exploring the role of experience as it interacts with maturation in motor development. McGraw (1977), who returned to developmental psychology after a considerable hiatus, had second thoughts about her earlier conclusions that maturation was all-important for motor development. She noted that the twins did differ in the quality of their motor performance, even as adolescents and young adults. Furthermore, as she now reflects on the total body of her work, she is convinced that if a function can be detected just as it is ready to emerge, and if it is then continuously challenged, its performance can be expanded (McGraw, 1977, personal communication, 1983). When she had placed a baby who was just starting to crawl on a slightly inclined surface and made it a little bit steeper every time the baby mastered the task, the result was a 6-month-old baby with the ability to crawl up a 70° incline (see Figure 8.4).

Cross-cultural psychology has provided new insights into the role of genetic and experiential factors in motor development. When Geber (1958; Geber & Dean, 1957) reported that African infants learned motor skills well in advance of children in the United States or France, the debate about the causes for the differences became a lively one. Many psychologists accepted the differences without much question, others speculated about possible environmental differences, and still others built the differences into their theoretical structures for the genetic inferiority of some racial groups. Precocious attainment of motor skills was seen as genetically determined and as providing a limit to intellectual growth (Jensen, 1973).

More careful analysis of the data on African precocity questions any genetic basis for it. Geber's own data had shown that Westernized Africans from the same genetic stock were not motorically precocious. Warren (1972) even concluded from his review of 30 articles that the methodological flaws in the studies made it impossible to be sure there was such a thing as African locomotor or postural precocity. However, in a survey of 50 cross-cultural studies of psychomotor development in infants from five continents, Werner (1972) concluded that African infants showed the greatest motor acceleration and Caucasians the least. Asian and Latin American infants were intermediate. In all of these groups traditionally reared rural infants showed more acceleration in the first year than Westernized urban infants. Thus the role of experience is important. But in all ethnic groups and in both traditional and Westernized samples, infants with higher birth weights were more accelerated. Thus the role of biological factors is also important.[4] It would be important to know the relation of different degrees of motor acceleration to the typical postures for babies in the different groups. Descriptions of postural manipulations of babies in other cultures will help us to understand some of the differences between them and Western cultures in their training or exercising of infants (see Brill & Sabatier, 1986; Hopkins & Westra, 1989).

Super (1976) tried to get around some of the problems of comparing apples and oranges—that is, the groups that had been compared differed not only genetically, but also in nutritional status, health, altitudes at which they lived, and amount of sun received, as well as in the child-rearing practices to which they were exposed. He did this by studying both the motor

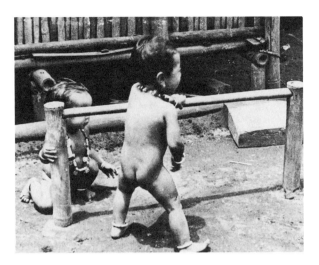

Figure 8.5. Encouragement for walking in Bali. This Balinese baby uses a rail built specially to help walking. In Western cultures aids take the form of furniture; special rails are not needed. (Photograph by Gregory Bateson, from the Library of Congress.)

behaviors of infants and the child-rearing practices of mothers across 14 African groups and 1 U.S. group. His data are compatible with an environmental explanation for the differences found. All infants born between 1972 and 1975 (in Kokwet, a prosperous community with good nutrition that is high enough in altitude to escape many tropical diseases) were tested on several Bayley test items once each month and observed at random times of day once a week to get a view of their everyday lives. Mothers were interviewed about their babies' motor development. These babies of the Kipsigis tribe were in fact able to sit, stand, and walk well in advance of their counterparts in the United States—about 1 month earlier, as judged by Bayley norms. But they were not advanced in all motor behaviors. Those involving motor control in the prone position, head control, and crawling were behind the U.S. norms. These differences in infant skills directly paralleled differences in maternal teaching practices. The Kipsigis consider it important to teach sitting and walking, and even have special words for the teaching of these skills. (See Figure 8.5 for an example of another culture's aid to walking.)

The proportion of mothers who said they taught their babies to crawl in each of six samples analyzed by Super (1976) was related to the age at which their

---

4. For a fuller picture of similarities and differences among infants from a wide variety of cultures, we recommend Werner's (1972) survey.

babies crawled ($r = .77$). Some 93% of the agricultural Teso mothers said they taught their babies to crawl, which they did at about 5½ months of age. The correlation of the combination of teaching and opportunity to practice (amount of time awake and lying down) with the age of crawling was .97. Only 13% of the desert Boran mothers thought it was important to teach their babies to crawl, and their babies did not crawl until they were 8 months old. Super (1976) writes: "Viewed in a cultural context, . . . these skills (which have so long been accepted by Western psychologists as genetically determined) look much more like other species-specific behaviors in the human." The basic structures may be in the genes, "but the environment contributes to how and how fast they develop" (p. 565).

A related theoretical issue concerns the relation between early reflexes and later similar voluntary behaviors. In Western cultures, many reflexes, including crawling, swimming, and stepping, drop out long before infants learn to do these things voluntarily. In cultures such as Kokwet there is little or no discontinuity between the reflexes and voluntary behaviors; that is, the standing, stepping, and placing reflexes do not disappear at around 2 months as they do in Western babies. Super found that other motor skills (such as sitting) were advanced in cultures that taught them, although the relation to reflexes was not specifically addressed.

Jamaican mothers living in England expect their infants to sit and walk alone earlier than do English mothers in the same neighborhoods, and they do. This is related to special handling routines they use relevant to these behaviors (Hopkins & Westra, 1989). The babies do not differ on crawling, for which Jamaicans have no special handling routine.

Returning to North America, Zelazo et al. (1972; Zelazo, 1983, 1984) found that when special exercise was given in stepping, it stayed in infants' behavior repertoires longer and walking occurred earlier. These researchers conclude that stepping drops out of the behavioral repertoire because of disuse. It is of some interest to note that the use of walkers, which is prevalent in Great Britain, delays crawling and does not serve to enhance walking (Crouchman, 1986).

Thelen and her colleagues have proposed that stepping drops out because the legs become too heavy, a view supported by their findings (Thelen, 1984; Thelen et al., 1984; see also Thelen, 1985). If weights are attached to the ankles of 4-week-olds, they reduce their rate of stepping, but if they are held upright in a tank of water so that the effects of gravity are decreased, they increase their rate of stepping (Thelen &

Fisher, 1982). Similar findings occur with kicking behaviors in 6-week-old infants (Thelen, Skala, & Kelso, 1987). In line with these researchers' biomechanical approach, both practice and maternal training operate to strengthen the muscles so that babies can lift the heavier legs. Thelen et al. (1982) have also explored both body build and arousal in relation to stepping.

In elaborate recordings of the biomechanical movements and muscular contractions of stepping at ages 1 and 2 months and at 1 and 2 months prior to independent walking, both similarities and differences were found (Thelen & Cooke, 1987). These suggest that there is not a discontinuity between the two behaviors, but an evolution from one to the other (see also Cooke & Thelen, 1987). This fits with Thelen's (1986) earlier findings that 7-month-olds placed on a small motorized treadmill exhibited well-coordinated stepping movements once it was turned on, but not before. They are even capable of adjusting their movements when each leg is on a different treadmill belt going at a different speed (Thelen, Ulrich, & Niles, 1987).

There is no known advantage in modern Western culture to having infants walk early. Indeed, there is a great disadvantage associated with their being able to get into things before they can learn what to avoid. However, there may be a practical question of interest. Could training techniques of Kokwet and other mothers be used with infants whose early motor development is at risk for neurological or other reasons? For example, would they serve any purpose with congenitally blind infants?

I find it interesting that there is no body of research on the relation of neonatal crawling to later crawling. However, one recent study has looked at the details of the development of crawling after 6 months. Goldfield (1989) looks at it not as a separate neuromuscular mechanism (à la Gesell and McGraw), but from the dynamic systems approach of Thelen and her colleagues. He examines the independent functions that lead to the development of crawling. First the infant supports its weight primarily on the hands and arms, and kicks without planting the feet on the support surface. Later the infant turns the head away from midline, uses the hands for reaching or support, and pushes the body forward by pressing the feet against the surface. Finally the baby crawls by raising the head and kicking first one leg and then the other while reaching forward with alternate hands to maintain balance or catch the fall with the hands.

Postures and postural control are currently being investigated in relation to their effects on other motor behaviors: on their relations to whether one- or two-

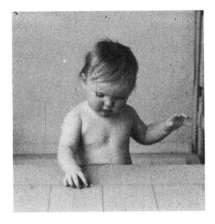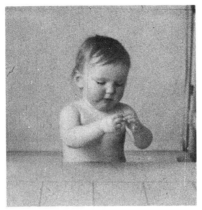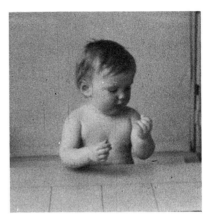

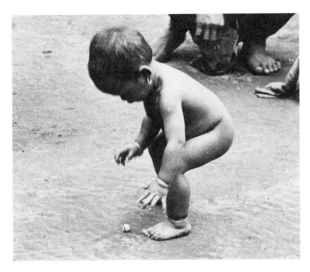

Figure 8.6. Three photographs from one of Gesell's sequences (top) showing fine motor coordination, in which a baby is picking up a pellet, and one of a Balinese baby (bottom) picking up something small. Although the babies both show mature grasping with complete thumb opposition, they do it in different ways. The Balinese infant exhibits the hand splaying characteristic of that culture, a demonstration that cultural experience can influence the nature of motoric behaviors. (Top photograph courtesy of Louise Bates Ames; bottom photograph by Gregory Bateson, from the Library of Congress.)

handed grasp is used (Rochat & Stacy, 1989), on the relation of the ability to control the body in a sitting position to reaching (Rochat & Senders, 1990), and on the relation of the ability to shift from a sitting to a quadrupedal position to reaching (Kamm & Thelen, 1989). Postural control in the face of conflicting cues from vision and proprioception is also being studied in infancy (Bertenthal & Bai, 1989; Stoffregen et al., 1987).

FINE MOTOR DEVELOPMENT

Infants have relatively little control over fine motor acts at birth, yet they have surprisingly many components of what later become finely coordinated arm, hand, and finger movements. At birth the infant has a grasp reflex. Any small rodlike object (including a finger) that is placed against the palm of the hand will be grasped. This reflex can be used to measure the strength of pull, as was shown by early workers who demonstrated that some babies (28% of 97 infants tested at less than 24 weeks of age, but fewer of those tested later, when the reflex has usually dropped out) could support their full weight by hanging from a rod by two hands. More recently, neonatal tests use this reflex to measure the strength of pull of the supine newborn. In the normal course of events this reflexive response is replaced by intentional object manipulation.

Halverson published seven studies between 1931 and 1937 of grasping responses and prehension using systematic movie records. He also pointed out that both maturation and learning are involved in these developments (see Halverson, 1931). An example of one of Gesell's grasping sequences is given in Figure 8.6.

In his 1931 study, Halverson describes this development:

The development of reaching and grasping affords excellent examples of the progress of maturation from the coarser to the finer muscles. The early approach patterns consist largely of crude shoulder and elbow movements . . . while the later approach patterns employ better directed shoulder and elbow action, in addition to wrist movements and hand-rotation, under the dominating influence of the forefinger and thumb. The early approach reveals a crudely functioning hand at the end of a poorly di-

Table 8.5

Grasping or Hand Usage in Sitting Position, and Fine Hand Control

Behavior	Average Age (Approximate)	Range of Ages
(A) Grasping		
Grasps cube with ulnar-palm prehension (1-inch cube)	3 months, 3 weeks	2 months-7 months
Grasps cube with partial thumb opposition	By 5 months	4 months-8 months
Grasps cube with complete thumb opposition (radial-digital)	By 7 months	5 months-9 months
(B) Manipulative capacity		
Reaches for object, one hand only	By 5½ months	4 months-8 months
Rotates wrist	5 months 3 weeks	4 months-8 months
Combines objects at midline (spoons or cubes)	8½ months	6 months-10 months
Plays pat-a-cake with midline skill	9 months, 3 weeks	7 months-15 months
(C) Small pellet skills		
Attempts to secure	5½ months	4 months-8 months
Scoops	6 months, 3 weeks	5 months-9 months
Grasps, partial finger prehension (inferior pincer)	7 months, 2 weeks	6 months-10 months
Grasps, fine prehension (neat pincer)	By 9 months	7 months-10 months

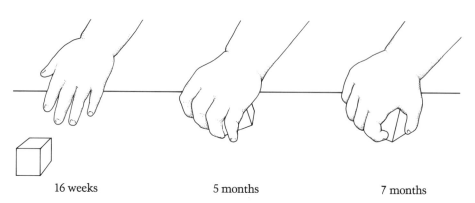

16 weeks   5 months   7 months

Figure 8.7. Grasping behaviors listed in Table 8.5A.

rected arm . . . while the later approach reveals a well coordinated arm under the directing influence of a pretty well developed prehensile organ. (p. 279)

This developmental sequence is also included in the Bayley Motor Scale, and the average age for achieving each item is shown in Table 8.5. Figure 8.7 illustrates the development of the grasping behaviors listed in Table 8.5A. Some of these behaviors are beginning to be studied with detailed measures of velocity and hand opening, similar to those Thelen and colleagues have used to analyze kicking, stepping, and walking. Beaudreau and Salmoni (1990), for example, document de-

tails of the greater proficiency of 9- to 10-month-olds than of 6- to 7-month-olds in reaching and grasping. Both ages had anticipatory hand preparations, and the maximum opening of the hand was highly correlated with the deceleration in the velocity of the reach, a relation that is found in adult grasping.

In addition to the direct effects of the infant's postural control (discussed earlier), the effect of the surface from which something is to be grasped has been studied. This too is affected by the internal stability of the upper extremities. When grasping a Cheerio from unstable surfaces, 7- to 8-month-old infants revert to less mature grasping patterns, but 13- to 14-months-olds use mature pincer grasp consistently (Hirschel et al., 1990).

A recent longitudinal study by Connolly and Dalgleish (1989) of the development of the skill required to use a spoon demonstrates the incredible complexity of the behaviors that are necessary to achieve smooth use of this tool.

Fine motor development generally seems to be handicapped by extremely premature birth, whereas gross motor behaviors appear to depend primarily on conceptional age (Piper et al., 1989).

Visually Guided Reaching

There has been little research done to explore the relation between the grasp reflex and more voluntary reaching and grasping. Much research has explored the nature of grasping in response to something seen, which in its mature form is called visually guided reaching, and the effects of experience on the development of this behavioral sequence.

A brief introduction to what is known about the development of visually guided reaching will be helpful here. Newborns not only grasp, they also make reaching motions (they extend their arms forward in space), and grasping sometimes follows reaching (Trevarthen, 1974). When the newborn's eyes are fixated on an object, the reaching movement is generally aimed in the direction of the object (Hofsten, 1982), but these primitive responses are not highly coordinated. Newborns rarely succeed in grasping the object (Dodwell et al., 1976; Ruff & Halton, 1978; Trevarthen, 1974), and they are unlikely to reach unless their trunks are supported in such a way that their arms are free of postural constraints. The extent to which the object itself plays a role in neonatal reaching is unclear. Some research cited in Chapter 7 has suggested that it does not matter whether there is an object or not. Reaching is apparently not guided by feedback. Newborns make one straight-line (ballistic) reach/grasp. If they happen to touch an object and if their hands happen to close at the right time, their grasp will be successful. They appear to be unable to make corrections during reaching (Dunkeld & Bower, 1981; McDonnell, 1975), and they immediately withdraw their hands after reaching rather than making adjustments (Trevarthen, 1974). Because of these characteristics, newborn reaching has been called by various names to distinguish it from visually *guided* reaching, the form that appears at 4 months of age. I will use the term visually *initiated* reaching (see Figure 8.8).

Visually initiated reaching is considered to be automatic and biologically organized and therefore to require little experience to develop. It disappears by 4 to 6 weeks of age (for reviews, see Bushnell, 1985; Hay, 1986). Bruner (1973) considers it a released action pattern (in the ethological sense) that needs only to be exposed to the appropriate environmental stimulus in order to emerge full blown. This position is supported by research on a similar visually triggered response (called placing) in kittens. Kittens need only to be exposed to unpatterned light to develop placing. If the kittens have been raised in the dark, only a very little experience in diffuse light will begin to trigger placing (Ganz, 1975).

In visually guided reaching, the object is usually grasped successfully. Both the reach and the grasp are more modulated; that is, the infant is more likely to take the characteristics of the object (for example, whether it is graspable, its size, its distance) into account. The reach undergoes corrections en route to the target and appears clearly intentional.

One type of research on reaching and grasping has focused on the roles of maturation and experience in such development. Hofsten (1984) has traced the development of reaching and grasping movements longitudinally, seeing 23 infants every 3 weeks from their first week of life to 16 weeks of age. The pattern of reaching changed at around 7 weeks of age. The number of reaches decreased from the first to the seventh week and then increased substantially at 10 weeks and at each subsequent test period. Hand movements during reaches changed at about the same age. At 7 weeks the percentage of reaches during which fists were clenched increased dramatically and did not depend on whether the infant was looking at the stimulus object. Clenched-fist reaches decreased at the later ages. After 7 weeks of age the percentage of reaches where the hand opened increased if the infant was looking at the stimulus. Hofsten argued on the basis of these and other findings that reaching in the first 2 months is reflexive and that, after that time, through maturation, it becomes reorganized and governed by cortical mechanisms. This reorganization produces more adaptive reaching, that is, reaching that is more responsive to the stimulus.

Early visually guided reaching and grasping are mainly **ipsilateral** (reaching for an object with the hand that is on the same side as the object). Provine and Westerman (1979) charted the development from 9 to 20 weeks of visually directed reaching that resulted in grasping or touching. At 9 weeks all infants touched objects on the ipsilateral side, one-third reached for objects at the midline, but none reached for objects on the **contralateral** side (the side opposite the hand that is reaching). This limits infants' ability to explore, particularly of objects on their left because

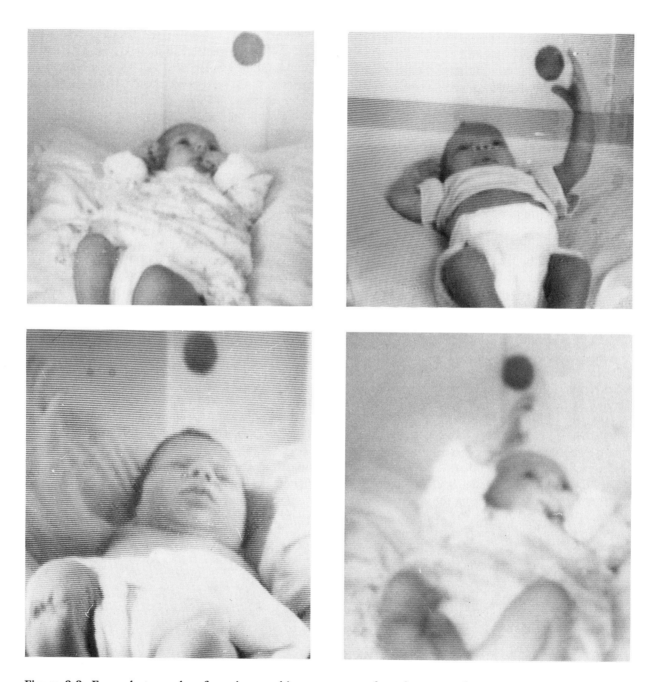

Figure 8.8. Four photographs of varying reaching responses of newborns, made from Ruff's videotaped records (hence their lack of sharpness). (Top, left) The infant gazes at the object, but makes no attempt to reach. (Top, right) The infant successfully reaches and grasps the object. (Bottom, left) and (Bottom, right) These infants are making arm and hand movements similar to those of the infant at the top, right, but the ball is in the background and out of the infant's sight. This is a control condition. It demonstrates that movements that might be interpreted as reaching and grasping are part of the repertoire of spontaneous activities in newborns. (Photographs courtesy of Holly Ruff.)

they are less likely to reach with their left hands (Hofsten, 1982). Contralateral and midline reaching develop gradually, so that by 20 weeks of age all infants contacted objects in all three positions (Provine & Westerman, 1979).

At about the same time that infants reach to all positions, they change their preferred reaching mode from a one-handed to a two-handed reach in the midline (White et al., 1964). This opens the door to the explosion of exploration that occurs at about 4 months. A further development takes place in more complex situations, such as when the infant holds an object in one hand and another object is presented to the same side. In this situation, 4- to 5-month-olds will not reach for the second object with the contralateral hand. Crossing the midline in this situation occurs several months later (Bruner, 1969, 1971). This achievement further increases the exploratory capacity of infants. The development of midline coordination and contralateral reaching apparently reflects important brain developments. Older handicapped children and adults with brain damage often show ipsilateral preference. Thus the development of laterality in reaching might be an index of normal versus abnormal development.

The role of experience in the development of visually guided reaching is clear. Visual enrichment provided to orphanage babies who were moderately deprived of social and visual stimulation affected the age at which they developed visually guided reaching (White, 1971; White & Held, 1966). The most effective form of enrichment was two pacifiers ringed by two disks (one was patterned) attached to the side of the crib. These enrichments allowed the infant to reach and touch the stimuli (accidentally or otherwise) and to see the stimuli and their hands simultaneously. Comparable research with animals indicates that experiencing visual feedback from reaching is necessary for the development of visually guided reaching (Hein & Diamond, 1971; Hein & Held, 1967; Walk & Bond, 1971).

This simple enrichment condition was more effective than a massive enrichment condition that included tactile stimulation from extra handling, improved mattresses that enabled easier movements, and a variety of visual stimuli that included a large, complex stabile, patterned crib sheets and bumpers, and removal of crib bumpers three times a day to enable babies to see the rest of the ward. Although less effective in advancing visually guided reaching, this program did increase visual attentiveness. I do not wish to give the impression that visually guided reaching must be laboriously taught or that parents must worry about providing the

appropriate environmental stimulation. First, virtually all homes provide sufficiently stimulating environments; in fact, many may be more like the massive enrichment condition. Second, the animal data indicate that recovery from even the most restrictive deprivation occurs after very short periods of normal visual experience, without any special enrichment or therapy (Hein, 1972). The human data are congruent, because, when compared with home-reared infants, White's (1971) visually deprived orphanage infants developed visually guided reaching within a reasonable time even if they received no enrichment. The importance of these studies is that they show the interrelation between experience and development.

Another line of research is represented by an ingenious series of studies conducted by Rochat and his colleagues, who have been exploring reaching, grasping, exploration of novel objects, and the relation of posture to reaching. This research becomes involved with another topic (that of tactile exploration or palpating, fingering, and so on). As such, it might have been covered in Chapter 6 with the tactile modality, but the actual research is closely linked to the studies that belong here, hence it is included here.[5] It is not possible to go into the details of all these studies, but the findings that are pertinent to motor development, visually guided reaching, and certain aspects of tactile manipulation can be summarized as follows:

(1) Whether 6- or 8-month-old infants grasp objects presented to them with one or both hands depends on the infants' posture—seated upright, seated reclined, lying supine, or lying prone on a board that is tilted to 75° (Rochat & Stacy, 1989). This agrees with observations of Piaget (1952).

(2) Bimanual coordination appears initially to be linked to the oral system, but is reorganized in relation to vision at around 4 months (Rochat & Senders, in press).

(3) Haptic exploration changes from mainly grasping movements (Rochat, 1987) to fingering or palpating of objects at around 4 months (Rochat, 1989). At that time the hands rapidly transfer objects from the mouth and its oral exploration to a position where visual exploration occurs, thus providing a basis for cross-modal comparisons.

(4) In fingering, one hand supports the object while the most sensitive portion of the other (the finger tips) explores it (Rochat, 1989). The fingering is

_____

5. For a review of haptic perception in infancy, see Bushnell and Boudreau (in press).

accompanied by visual exploration and decreases if there is no visual feedback (infant in the dark). Exploration by mouthing is not increased, suggesting the functional separateness of the systems.

(5) From 3 months on, the ways in which infants manipulate and explore objects are related to their physical properties or affordances (Rochat, 1989). Concretely, 3- and 4-month-olds given a large red ball with a sandy-textured surface wrapped in plastic and mounted on a wooden rod for grasping and with a small, soft object with many protuberances explore the two differently. They scratch the ball, which makes an interesting noise, but never attempt to scratch the soft toy.

Research related to the final point has explored the type of action or exploration that a variety of objects elicit in 6-, 9-, and 12-month-old infants (Palmer, 1989). Actions depend on both the age of the infant and the nature of the object. Further, they depend on the nature of the surface on which they are located. Mouthing and looking times and the amount of two-handed contact time decrease with age. Picking up, releasing, switching (from 6 to 9 months), and squeezing (from 9 to 12 months) increase with age. When objects were on a foam-covered table they were mouthed more and one-handed manipulations were used more, but fewer other actions were applied to the objects. After all, banging would have yielded little of interest and scooting of the toy car would have been difficult.

Palmer (1989) used pairs that differed on a particular dimension in one of her studies. Lighter objects led to more waving and mouthing and less scooting. Smaller objects led to more switching, picking up, releasing, and one-handed manipulation, and larger ones to more two-handed usage. Furry objects led to more picking up, releasing, squeezing, and scooting, and plastic ones to more mouthing. Squishy objects led to more mouthing and squeezing. A sounding bell led to more waving and a silent one to more mouthing. These results may sound obvious to us, but how do infants know to act in accordance with what are called the affordances of the objects?

These data indicate that infants utilize the affordances of two objects, the toy and the support surface. But when two or more detached objects are studied, an understanding of the affordances of both does not appear until after 2 years. Palmer points out that infants have had so much experience with support surfaces that they are in a relatively good position to know their affordances. The strength of the visual system in relation to a motor activity is dramatically illustrated by research examining the effects of lack of

visual feedback discussed in point 4 above. Hatwell (1987) found that when 5- or 6-month-olds were prevented by a horizontal screen from seeing their hands or lower body they often refused to grasp objects placed in their hands. When there were visual stimuli in the environment but no view of the hands, infants seemed more upset than in the absence of all visual stimulation. Older infants try to remove the screen, and fuss and cry when they do not succeed. A total of 60% of 7- to 15-month-olds failed to complete a haptic task in this situation, compared with only 20% of infants younger than 4 months, for whom vision is not yet so dominant. By 20 months 80% accepted the screen, but exploration was reduced to passive grasp for some.

One has to remember that reaching in the dark can be guided by auditory stimuli (Clifton et al., 1991). Both head and reaching movements are different from those elicited by the same object in the light. Infants only 26 to 32 weeks old will reach for a sounding object that they have previously seen and that now is within reach in the dark. This poses an interesting question with respect to Piaget's idea that infants lack object permanence at this age (see Chapter 10).

The strength of the visual system in relation to posture has also been explored recently (Bertenthal & Bai, 1989; Stoffregen et al., 1987). When 12- to 15-month-old infants are placed standing in a room with moving walls, they show a very adultlike response to such motion. They react as if *they* are in motion and attempt to compensate for their sway, with the result that they may fall (Bertenthal & Bai, 1989). When 5-, 7-, and 9-month-olds are tested in a seat that enables measures of their postural adjustment, 9- but not 5-month-olds show significant postural responses; 7-month-olds respond only under the strongest stimulus conditions.

You will have noted that the research findings cited here are largely devoid of descriptions of the experimental methodologies. This is because they are much too complicated to go into here. Thelen (1989) puts it this way: "The new ideas are not so simply told, but they are much more exciting"—a view I can only agree with.

Visually guided reaching as described here becomes less important toward the end of the first year (Hofsten, 1979; Lockman et al., 1984). Bushnell (1985) cites a variety of evidence to support this decrease and looks to overlearning of the skill as a factor in its decline. At this stage intermediate adjustments to reach the target are no longer necessary and the reach again becomes more ballistic, as it was in the first weeks of life. Bushnell also looks at the fit of these behaviors to

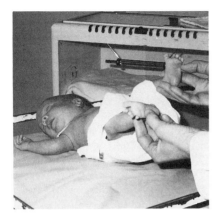
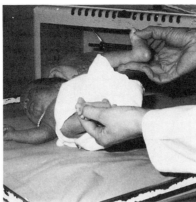
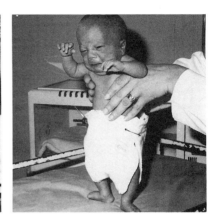
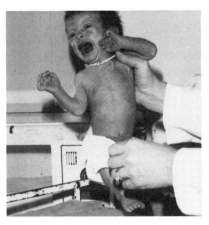
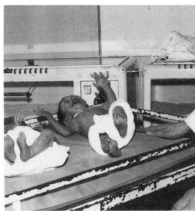
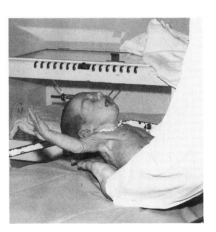

Figure 8.9. Some of the neonatal reflexes. (Top, left) Babinski, (top, center) plantar, (top, right) weight support, (bottom, left) stepping, (bottom, center) Moro reflex elicited by banging on the surface the baby is on (note that the other twin either received less stimulation or was less responsive), (bottom, right) Moro reflex elicited by removing support from head. (Photographs courtesy of Judy F. Rosenblith.)

various theories and calls attention to the fact that this new automatic stage means that much of the infant's attention becomes free for other tasks, including cognitive processing.

More research on fine motor development would be desirable, because it is more related to later developmental outcomes than is gross motor development. There are fewer items on the Bayley scales to assess fine motor development than gross motor development. Nevertheless, 8-month performance on the fine motor items is more related to IQ at 4 years of age than are the gross motor items or the entire Bayley Mental Scale (Kangas et al., 1966). Kopp's (1974) findings may provide a possible explanation for this. She studied infants who demonstrated the same level of development of grasp pattern and assigned them to coordinated or clumsy groups on the basis of five characteristics of their approach to objects, five characteris-

tics of the grasp itself, and two aspects of extraneous motor activity. Coordinated babies explored more frequently, for longer periods of time, and in different ways. Clumsy infants spent about half their time in some type of visual exploration, whereas coordinated infants spent only one-third of their time this way but more than half of their time in manipulation. Mouthing, an important form of exploration, was shown by 85% of coordinated infants at 8 months, but by only 40% of clumsy ones. Unfortunately, the clumsiness variable may have been confounded by the fact that 7 of the 12 clumsy infants were premature, although both groups of infants showed age-appropriate grasp patterns. The findings are very provocative. They suggest that the reason fine motor development is related to later IQ is that it influences the quantity and quality of cognitive exploration.

The study of motor development, and especially fine

motor development, has undergone a revolution in the last 5 to 10 years. For a brief and readable historical overview of the study of motor development, see Pick (1989).

Developmental Testing

Neonatal testing, which is done quite soon after birth, will be discussed here in some detail, followed by an examination of tests for use with prematures, which were developed later, and then tests used during infancy.

NEONATAL TESTING

Neurological Tests

Pediatric neurologists, especially in Europe, have devised standard examination schedules for neurological functioning in the neonatal period of both term and preterm infants. These batteries include tests of a variety of reflexes as well as of some behaviors not clearly reflexive (e.g., muscle tonus). Some examples of reflexes are shown in Figure 8.9. The ages of the onset and decay vary. Pediatric neurologists have made careful catalogs of which reflexes should be present at which times in development (see, e.g., Capute et al., 1984). Presence or absence of reflexes must take into account the baby's state at the time of testing, a fact that has made pediatric neurologists very concerned with state and its assessment (as noted in Chapter 6).

The Moro reflex and elicited nystagmus have long histories of use in assessing infant neurological status (articles appeared in 1910, 1921, 1927, 1941, 1953, and 1961). The **Moro reflex** is an infantile startle response in which an infant's arms spread wide in a curve and then slowly come together, while the legs are brought up in a similar fashion. It is typically elicited by a loud noise, by dropping the infant's head for a short distance, or by banging the side of the baby's bassinet or crib. Nystagmus, discussed in Chapter 7, is obtained by rotating the infant, and occurs after rotation ceases.

Prechtl and his colleagues developed a battery that meets the criteria for good test development: (a) detailed, exact procedures for eliciting responses; (b) quantification of responses; (c) consideration of state

of the infant (their definitions of state were given in Chapter 6); (d) reliability of administration; and (e) standardization on 1,500 infants (Prechtl, 1977; Prechtl & Beintema, 1964; Prechtl & Dijkstra, 1960). Both Prechtl (1977) himself and others (e.g., Aylward et al., 1985) have developed brief examinations based on Prechtl's.

Other neurological examinations popular in Europe include (a) those of the French workers André-Thomas and Saint-Anne Dargassies (André-Thomas et al., 1960; Saint-Anne Dargassies, 1972, 1977a, 1974/1977b, 1983); (b) that of Amiel-Tison (1976, 1982; Amiel-Tison & Grenier, 1986), a student of André-Thomas and Saint-Anne Dargassies;[6] (c) that of German researcher Peiper (1963); and (d) that of British workers Dubowitz and Dubowitz (1981). For a review of these European examinations, see Parmelee (1962) and Prechtl (1982). Parmelee (1974) developed a neurological examination based on his and his colleagues' extensive work with premature, term, and at-risk babies.

In some sense one needs to consider the modern imaging techniques as a type of neurological assessment or test, or adjunct to tests. While providing precise diagnosis of current damage, they do not suc-cessfully diagnose long-range problems, except for extreme cases.

Research Using Neurological Tests. Have these tests succeeded in identifying neurological problems that might presage difficulties in later development? Prechtl identified three patterns or syndromes in newborns: (a) apathy, found frequently in infants with a history of prenatal or perinatal complications; (b) hyperexcitability, characterized by tremor, but associated with only moderate complications; and (c) hemisyndrome, in which there are multiple lacks of symmetry between the left and right sides and an association with obstetric complications, including forceps deliveries. Both hyperexcitability and the hemisyndrome are found more often in boys. Prechtl also found that the strength of the stimuli needed to elicit the Moro and nystagmus reflexes was related to neurological status.

Performance on his test by high-risk infants was related to outcomes at 2, 4, and 8 years (Prechtl, 1965), but was not predictive for individuals. Other studies failed to replicate the long-term findings (H. F. R. Prechtl, personal communication, 1972). Data from Prechtl's laboratory show a sevenfold increase in the rate of mildly abnormal later development for those abnormal at birth, but with many who are normal (Hadders-Algra et al., 1986). And even after 13 years, neonatal neurological suboptimality was related to dif-

---

6. Students not wishing to read an entire book on neurological testing might find the 1988 review of the book by Bagnato published in *Developmental Medicine and Child Neurology* informative.

ferences in reaction time and neurophysiologically as reflected in evoked potential recordings (deSonneville et al., 1989). Prechtl (1990) has pointed out that brain imaging techniques plus repeated neurological examinations of brain-damaged infants only identify those more likely eventually to show a particular impairment.

Saint-Anne Dargassies (1983) found that infants whose normal developmental function had resumed by 15 days of age very gradually became normal. Among prematures the degree of prematurity was more important to their later intellectual development (to age 10 years) than the amount of neonatal abnormality. In addition, prematures were more likely than full-term babies with neurological problems as newborns to suffer long-term intellectual impairment.

Scores on Parmelee's neurological examination were related to concurrent behavior (visual fixation) in term infants (Kopp et al., 1975), but not in premature infants tested at 40 weeks of gestational age (Sigman et al., 1973, 1975).

The chances of finding long-term predictability are greater if the infant has appeared suspect or abnormal at several ages. For example, Rubin and Balow (1980) related IQ at 4 and 7 years and neurological abnormalities at age 7 to the number of earlier tests on which the children had been classified as abnormal or suspect neurologically. As Table 8.6 shows, those who were classified as abnormal or suspect only once were no more likely to have low IQs at 4 or 7 years than those always diagnosed as normal. In sharp contrast, the 22 children who had been classified as neurologically abnormal or suspect on two or three of the infant testings were 14 times as likely to have low IQs at age 7 as would be expected by chance. Nevertheless, less than one-third scored in the retarded IQ range. Similarly, while about 64% were either neurologically abnormal or suspect at age 7, at least 35% showed no neurological problems. A sample from a less optimal environment (pre- and postnatally) might produce a higher proportion of infants who continued to show deficits into middle childhood or later.

In short, neurological tests in infancy do not provide a diagnosis of which infants will later be handicapped, a point to be remembered when considering the efficacy of behavioral tests. The importance of repeated tests is stressed by most researchers. Even then, prediction is likely to be statistical and not accurate for a given individual. (For reviews of neurological tests from a psychological perspective, see Francis et al., 1987; Worobey, 1990. From a pediatric perspective, see Gorski et al., 1987. These reviews also cover behavioral assessments of neonates, which will be dis-

Table 8.6

Percentage of Infants With Negative Outcomes as a Function of Their Infant Neurological Functioning

	Number of Tests on Which Abnormal or Suspect		
	0	1	2 or 3
Number of cases	1,066	156	22
Outcomes			
IQ below 70 at 4 years	1.0	1.9	31.8
IQ below 70 at 7 years	0.7	1.3	21.1
Neurologically abnormal at 7 years	1.1	9.3	50.0[a]

a. Another 13.6% were neurologically suspect.

cussed next.)

In this context it is interesting to note that Prechtl (1990) is currently interested in the contribution to prediction that might be made by a study of the qualitative aspects of spontaneous general movements. He calls for a Gestalt judgment of a filmed sample of spontaneous movements, harking back to Konrad Lorenz's (1971) paper, "Gestalt Perception as a Source of Scientific Knowledge." Note that this is the technique (not so labeled) referred to previously several times in discussions of studies of perception and imitation where an adult judges whether the infant has responded or what the infant is responding to. Prechtl describes Gestalt perception as "an instrument that cannot be replaced by automatic quantification." (See his article for a fuller discussion, and Prechtl & Nolte, 1984, for more on the use of motor behavior as a neurological indicator.)

Behavioral Tests

Several of the neurological examinations of newborns long in existence were formalized in the period subsequent to the 1950s, when the current wave of research interest in newborns and young infants began. Behaviorally oriented examinations for newborns and young infants also were developed and standardized at that time. They owe more of a debt to the infant examinations developed earlier by Gesell and Bayley than to those developed by pediatric neurologists.

Graham Behavioral Test for Neonates. Graham and her collaborators adapted items from the earlier Gesell and Bayley scales, quantified them, and organized them into a battery (Graham, 1956; Graham et al., 1956). This provided a general maturation score,

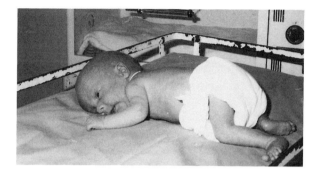

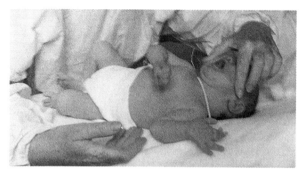

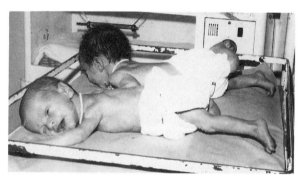

Figure 8.10. Items from the Graham/Rosenblith neonatal assessment. (top) Freeing nose after being placed flat on face, (center) responding to stimuli used to assess tactile-adaptive reactions, (bottom) muscle tonus assessment. In the bottom photo, twins are shown; the one on the right tends slightly toward hypertonicity. Photos coutesy of Judy F. Rosenblith

a visual following score, and an electrotactual threshold (the weakest amount of electrical stimulation to the skin just below the knee that the baby responded to). It also provided ratings of irritability and muscle tonus. Graham's test helped spawn two other neonatal batteries, the Graham/Rosenblith Behavioral Test for Neonates (G/R) and the Brazelton or Newborn

Behavior Assessment Scale (NBAS).

Graham/Rosenblith Behavioral Test. After a two-year study of the Graham tests in the early 1960s, Rosenblith undertook a revision of them. Based on her feelings, after many examinations of newborns, of what went with what in the babies' behaviors, she separated Graham's General Maturation Score into scores for (a) muscle strength and coordination (the Motor score), (b) adaptive (or defensive) responses to stimulation of the nose and mouth areas (the Tactile-Adaptive or TA score), and (c) reactions to sounds (rattle and bicycle bell). The first two, but not the third, were summed to obtain a General Maturation Score for a better comparison to Graham's Maturation Score. The individual items constituting both Motor and TA scores had been scored on 4-point scales (0 to 3). The G/R kept the 10-point scale for visual following. The techniques and specific responses of newborns to some items are illustrated in Figure 8.10. Ratings of muscle tonus were quantified differently than in the Graham. The G/R has ratings of actual irritable behavior as well as the examiner's judgment of irritability (that is, of whether the baby is irritable without good reason—is not sleepy, hungry, gassy). Rosenblith (1961a, 1961b) excluded the pain or electrotactual threshold, which required more elaborate instrumentation than was appropriate for a screening test.

Brazelton or Newborn Behavior Assessment Scales. This examination borrowed from Prechtl (1974, 1977) as well as from Graham in that it has a section devoted to reflexes and is very concerned with the states of the infant. Its purpose is less neurological, however, in that it is oriented toward detecting behaviors that affect mother-infant interaction. It was designed for use with the normal newborn. This test was used in several forms prior to its publication in a standardized form in 1973. The current version is found in Brazelton (1984).[7]

The NBAS considers state the single most important element, and attempts to track "the pattern of state change over the course of the examination, its lability and its direction in response to external and internal stimuli" (Brazelton, 1973, p. 2). Variability in state is seen as indicative of infants' abilities for self-organization and hence as important for behavior. The ability to self-quiet after experiencing aversive stimuli (as contrasted to needing external help to quiet) is another aspect of self-organization measured by the NBAS. External procedures are used to calm infants only after a 15-second period during which the infants' self-calming is noted. Calming procedures are

---

7. For an overview of the NBAS from the viewpoint of Brazelton and his colleagues, see Brazelton et al. (1987).

done in a set order: talking, hand on belly, restraint, holding, and rocking.

Responses to human stimuli (face, voice, cuddling) are compared with responses to inanimate auditory (rattle and bell) and visual (red ball and white light) stimuli and to what is described as temperature change associated with uncovering, which always has tactile as well as temperature components.[8] Habituation is assessed for three modalities: auditory, visual, and "pain" (light pinprick to heel of foot).

Some Comparisons of the G/R and NBAS. The G/R scores hand-to-mouth activity, trembling, startles, and general activity across the entire examination, but Rosenblith did not analyze these scores in relation to outcomes. Some of the information from these scores was used in scoring muscle tonus. On the NBAS these items have the same status as any other scored item. The NBAS scores reflexes from 0 to 3 (not elicited, low, medium, high responses). All other items are scored on 9-point scales, with behavioral definitions provided for each point. The differences between behaviors are very small for some items. The cuddliness scale provides a useful example, because it is also important to a discussion of the NBAS in relation to neonatal-maternal interactions in Chapter 12. In assessing cuddliness, the infant is held against the chest and shoulder of the examiner, who judges the extent to which the infant cuddles in response to the examiner's cuddle. The NBAS assumes that this response is a linear (straight-line) dimension, ranging in 9 equal steps from "very resistant to being held" to "extremely cuddly and clinging." The 9 steps of the scale are

Table 8.7
Cuddliness

Score	Behavior
1	Resists being held: continuously pushes away, thrashes, or stiffens
2	Resists being held most of time
3	Doesn't resist, doesn't participate (passive: rag doll)
4	Eventually molds into arms after lots of nestling and cuddling efforts by examiner
5	Usually molds and relaxes when first held, nestling into examiner's neck or crook of elbow; turns toward body when held horizontally; seems to lean forward when held on examiner's shoulder
6	Always molds initially, as above
7	Always molds initially with nestling, and turns toward body and leans forward
8	Molds and relaxes; nestles and turns head, leans forward on shoulder, fits feet into cavity of other arm; all of body participates
9	All of 8, plus baby grasps examiner and clings

listed in Table 8.7. Notice that the differences between scale points 5 and 6 and between 6 and 7 are rather small. The decision to score all behaviors in the finalized NBAS on a 9-point scale made such small distinctions necessary.

The different approaches to scoring taken by Rosenblith and Brazelton can be seen in a comparison of the scoring for defensive movements on the NBAS and that for responses on the tactile-adaptive responses on the G/R. Table 8.8 describes the specific stimuli used in both scales and the methods of scoring (Figure 8.10b shows the stimulus situation for the G/R and Figure 8.11 shows that for the NBAS). Note that the G/R has fewer categories, and that they are less specific but more clearly ordered along the single dimension of effectiveness in getting rid of the stimulus.

Although the NBAS was not originally structured to yield a small number of scores, Brazelton and his colleagues have devised an a priori group of clusters based on their conceptualizations of the nature of the infant. They assign the 26 9-point scales and the whole group of reflex items to one of four dimensions—physiological, motoric, state, or interaction (Adamson et al., 1975; Als, 1978; Als et al., 1977)—and describe the baby as "worrisome," "normal," or "superior" on each. Despite their conceptual ideas about the importance of these clusters, they accept the probability that

Figure 8.11. The stimulus situation for the defensive movement item on the NBAS. This can be contrasted with the similar Tactile-Adaptive item on the G/R shown in Figure 8.10b. (Photograph courtesy of T. B. Brazelton.)

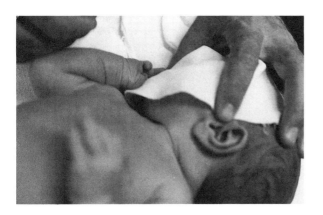

---

8. This is the reverse of my argument in Chapter 7 that when uncovering was used as a tactile stimulus, the temperature change was being ignored.

Table 8.8

Defensive Response Items of the NBAS Compared With the Tactile-Adaptive Scale of the G/R

	NBAS Defensive Movements	G/R Tactile-Adaptive Responses
Stimulus	Cloth over entire face	Cotton over nostrils, cellophane over nose and mouth
How held	Light pressure on upper part of face toward side of head in front of ears with one finger but other fingers touching head	Firm pressure against nostrils and upper lip Firm pressure against side of face or head in front of ears, one finger each side only
Length of application	1 minute or until a series of responses	20 seconds
Scoring categories	1 No response 2 General quieting 3 Nonspecific activity increase, long latency 4 Same as 3, but short latency 5 Rooting and lateral head turning 6 Neck stretching 7 Nondirected swipes of arms 8 Directed swipes of arms 9 Successful removal of cloth with swipes	0 No response 1 Any movement within 2 seconds 2 Specific movements of head or mouth, including rooting, neck stretching, head turning, back arching 3 Specific movements more than half of time (10 sec) 4 Responses of head and mouth and coordinated arm movements all present, and one or more for more than 10 of the 20 seconds (An additional one-half point was given if the infant responded persistently across trials for all but 4 seconds of each stimulus period on one-half of the 6 trials; a full point was given if persistent response occurred on at least two-thirds of the stimulus presentations.)[a]
Number of trials	Not specified	Three with each stimulus
Scoring	Best score	Best score based on sum for each stimulus Worst score based on sum for each stimulus

a. In Rosenblith's revision (in progress) this is 2 points or 1 point, thus eliminating half-point scores.

different studies with different specific goals may find different clusters useful.

Other workers using the NBAS have applied factor-analytic techniques to arrive at factors. These analyses have yielded 5 to 10 factors, with considerable similarity across various different studies and with several factors being similar to those of Brazelton (see, for example, Kaye, 1978; Lasky et al., 1983; Mitchell et al., 1977; Strauss & Rourke, 1978). However, a recent analysis of factor data from preterm infants indicates that the factors found are not statistically independent, an important criterion for the usefulness of factor-analytic techniques (Azuma et al., 1991). The use of only orientation and arousal factors provided the optimal model for describing the babies' behaviors. Azuma et al. (1991) conclude that a clearer "understanding of the underlying structure of the NBAS" is necessary if we are to "determine how well the instrument assesses infant behavior" (p. 223).

Reliability of Neonatal Tests

All of these tests attempt to describe a neonate's or young infant's developmental status or behaviors using a few scores or ratings, and all have resisted the temp-

tation to try to describe that status with a single score such as the IQ or developmental quotient (DQ). All have been shown to demonstrate satisfactory test characteristics. The interscorer agreement of two testers on the Graham and G/R has been shown to be satisfactory (Bench & Parker, 1970; Graham et al., 1956; Rosenblith & Lipsitt, 1959). The NBAS has been shown to be scored reliably by trained examiners (Brazelton & Tryphonopoulou, n.d.; cited in Brazelton, 1973; Brazelton et al., 1987; Horowitz & Brazelton, 1973). Nevertheless, some work has shown that despite good interscorer reliability there are large effects due to different examiners (Mitchell et al., 1977; Richardson et al., 1989; A. P. Streissguth, personal communication, 1982; Streissguth & Barr, 1977). Equivalent data do not exist for the Graham or G/R. These findings pose serious questions as to whether any neonatal examination should be considered as a standardized test in the way in which tests given to older children or adults are.

Another characteristic necessary in a good test is **test-retest reliability**. That is, a person (here, a newborn) tested on two occasions should, in general, have similar scores. All testers of newborns know that the newborn is making profound adaptations to extrauterine life and hence is in an unstable condition. They have therefore sought to determine stability of scores over short time spans (days or weeks). While the stabilities found for the Graham and G/R have been only modest to moderate, they have been considered acceptable for newborns (Bench & Parker, 1970; Graham et al., 1956; Rosenblith, 1961b). The NBAS has reasonable test-retest reliability (Brazelton et al., 1987; Horowitz et al., 1971, 1973; Lancione et al., 1980). Reliabilities were higher in an Israeli sample of babies whose mothers had received little or no medication (Horowitz et al., 1977). However, Worobey (1986) found that only autonomic stability was stable over a 1-month period.

Kaye (1978) repeatedly tested newborns with the NBAS, and his data accent the instability of behavior in newborns. But the point has been made that those critical of the reliability of the individual items on the NBAS from day to day (e.g., Horowitz et al., 1978; Sameroff et al., 1978) tend to ignore the stability over the entire item set for at least some individual infants (Linn & Horowitz, 1983). This stability of overall assessment despite instability of individual items occurs in the testing of older infants as well. They "accidentally" pass items and fail others they have previously succeeded at in ways that balance out their total scores.

Currently some researchers are looking at stability (or its lack) as another possibly important characteristic of the infant deserving to be assessed in its own right (Linn & Horowitz, 1983; Worobey, 1986, 1990). Instability has been posited by some (e.g., Emde, 1978) to be an indication of adaptability, potentially making mother-infant adjustment smoother. Linn and Horowitz found that babies whose scores were stable from one NBAS-K testing to another tended to elicit less responsiveness from the mother than those who were more variable, a finding compatible with such a hypothesis.

Worobey (1990) found evidence for a curvilinear relation between variability and outcome. Both the most variable and the most stable showed the least adaptive behaviors at 1 month. Inspection of the data revealed that the most stable group had also been higher in optimal performance at birth, hence subgroups were located who were matched on original performance. Alertness, looking at mother, and vocalizing were grouped into an attentiveness factor (see Worobey & Blajda, 1989). Babies who were most variable on this factor and on movement and crying were higher than stable babies on attentiveness and movement and lower on crying during mother-infant observations at 1 month. Similar relations were found using mothers'

ratings of their children on the IBQ at 2 months as the criterion. Hence it seems necessary to explore stability/variability further as itself an individual difference of importance.

Validity of Neonatal Tests

Once it has been established that a test consistently measures a domain by one or more reliability measures, the next question is whether the test measures something important or stable (or both) about infant functioning. If it does, the test is said to have **validity**. The two classic types of validity are concurrent and predictive validity.[9] To have **concurrent validity**, a test measure must be significantly related to some other aspect of behavior (or medical status) measured at the same point in time. To have **predictive validity**, a test should predict the same or related characteristics in the future. The lines between the two are not always sharp, because what is considered to be either the same point in time or in the future varies for different researchers and in relation to different research goals.

Relation of Neonatal Test Performance to Infant Variables: Concurrent Validity or Short-Term Prognostic Validity. The Graham tests, developed to study newborns with anoxia, differentiated those who had had anoxia from those who had not (Graham et al., 1956). Different degrees of anoxia, assessed biochemically and medically, were related to different levels of performance on these scales. This means there was concurrent validity. Scores for babies with problems other than anoxia also differed from those of normal term babies. These tests can thus be seen as indicative of the functional integrity of the CNS. Rosenblith assumed that Graham has established concurrent validity, and hence did not focus on relations of G/R measures to other neonatal measures.

The NBAS was designed to assess neonatal characteristics that might be related to mother-infant interaction. Both concurrent relations and those to short-term outcome measures of infant and maternal behaviors and their interactions are appropriate to examine here. Summary scores on the Kansas version of the NBAS (NBAS-K) and ratings of behaviors during mother-newborn feeding interactions were significantly related to infant state on the NBAS (Linn & Horowitz, 1983). It would appear that the two are simply different measures of the same type of behavior. However,

---

9. There is also something referred to as face validity. It simply means that on the face of it the scale appears to measure what it says it does.

the fact that there are similarities in the behaviors assessed on the NBAS to those in an interaction situation does not always lead to their being related. Cuddliness on the NBAS-K was not related to cuddling during the mother-baby interaction. Some relations found (in this and other studies) are difficult to understand or make no intuitive sense. For example, babies' orientation scores were negatively related to mothers' failures to interact and to keeping the baby's bassinet more than 3 feet away. Why should good orientation be associated with failures to interact? In addition, the NBAS-K examiners' ratings of how reinforcing the baby was to the examiner during the exam were negatively related to maternal interaction and bassinet positioning, but positively related to the baby being in a positive alert state and looking at the mother during the interaction. Such relations that appear counterintuitive and in disagreement with each other pose serious questions as to the meaning of the examination.

Osofsky and Danzger (1974) studied mothers interacting with their 51 newborn infants during feeding. Like the subjects in the Linn and Horowitz study, all were lower SES and black, and all mothers had fed their babies at least four times before the observation. The parts of the NBAS related to the largest number of infant behaviors during the mother-infant interactions were: babies' state at the start of the NBAS, cuddliness, self-quieting, and hand-to-mouth activity during the NBAS. For example, they were related to predominant state, to amount of eye contact, and to auditory responsiveness during the feeding. Again, these are characteristics that are quite similar to those assessed by the NBAS itself.

Mother-infant interactions and the relation of NBAS scores to the infants' behaviors in both a feeding and a semistructured situation designed to approximate NBAS assessments were subsequently studied in a larger, but similar, sample (Osofsky, 1976). There were relations between infant behaviors on the NBAS and those during the feeding interaction and the maternal stimulation situations. They were less strong, but similar in pattern to those in the first study. The lesser strength is surprising in view of the fact that the greater similarity between the NBAS test and maternal stimulation based on it leads to an expectation of higher correlations. A maternal variable (sensitivity) was related to infant responsiveness for four of the five stimuli presented by the mother.

Variables assessed during mother-infant interactions at 3 and 6 months of age were studied in relation to both the four Als cluster scores and scores on five factors derived by factor analysis of the NBAS items

(Vaughn et al., 1980). Three factors were derived from 33 ratings of the feeding interactions at 3 and at 6 months. Two of the feeding interaction factors reflected maternal behaviors, and one reflected the babies' sociable behaviors. Two of the Als a priori clusters, motoric processes and muscle tonus, distinguished babies who were at the extremes in terms of social behavior during feeding and play. Three of the five factor analytically derived NBAS scores (arousal, tonus, and quieting) discriminated the extreme group on the 6-month feeding factors. Hence for this population of 243 low-SES mothers and their firstborn babies, the aspects of the babies' behaviors assessed by the NBAS were related (significantly, but weakly) to the babies' later behaviors. However, they did not seem related to later maternal behaviors assessed during interaction with their babies during feeding or play.

NBAS Scores. Ploof (1976) examined mothers' perceptions of their infants in relation to the infants' performance on the NBAS. Newborn NBAS characteristics did not relate to their mothers' concurrent perceptions of them, except for alertness. They were related to the mothers' assessment of their babies' temperaments at 4 months of age, however. Inasmuch as mothers lacked much contact with their infants in the newborn period, the lack of relation then seems reasonable. Although the size of the relations was generally not great, several correlations were substantial (r about .50, or 25% of the variance in common). Activity, alertness, ease of arousal, difficulty of habituation, and self-quieting were related to similar characteristics at 4 months, but they were related more to the mothers' perceptions of their 4-month-olds than to the latter's actual behaviors. These data could be taken as providing some support for the idea that the NBAS taps temperamental or personality characteristics of infants, at least as they are seen by their mothers.

It would be nice to draw some neat set of conclusions with respect to the question of whether NBAS scores help to improve predictions of mother-infant interactions. Because the studies cited here have used different measures and measured different things at different times, and sometimes in different sorts of samples, this is not possible. In general it appears that state, alertness, and orientation variables are related to each other, whether they are assessed during the NBAS or during mother-infant interactions. Relations for variables such as cuddliness to maternal responsiveness are contradictory. Many more data and longitudinal data are needed to be able to determine an answer to this question.

There is one methodological question that affects both the above-cited work on the NBAS and much of that to follow. There is evidence that there are curvilinear relations between some NBAS items and outcome, where the highest score is not necessarily the best (Jacobson et al., 1984). This makes data analysis using Pearson correlation coefficients that are based on the assumption of linearity (that is, the higher the score on one variable, the higher the score on the other) suspect. Such analysis has, however, usually been used to determine the relations to later outcomes. Only the G/R did not, because Rosenblith assumed that we could not know in advance what was an optimal score, and hence did not know whether or not a linear model was appropriate.

Long-Term Predictive Value. To test long-term or predictive validity, Graham and her colleagues (1962) administered a battery of tests to the infants they had studied as newborns when they were 3½ years old. In general, there were no relations between their newborn measures and various measures of intellectual, perceptual, and emotional functioning at 3½. However, their analyses were all made within specific medical groups (normal, anoxic, other problems) and used Pearson correlation coefficients, which obscure any nonlinear relations.

Findings on the relation of the TA score on the G/R will illustrate this point. The TA score has been related to outcomes at 8 months and at 4 and 7 years (Rosenblith, 1973, 1974, 1979a), but for a number of outcomes a medium score was optimal, with a high score being better than a low one.

Other findings with respect to the predictive value of the G/R include the fact that the TA score has been related to more outcomes at 7 years than at 4 (Rosenblith, 1979b). This TA score is based on the best of three responses to each stimulus, as discussed in the description of the tests. A low Tactile-Adaptive (LTA) score based on the poorest performances has been related to the occurrence of sudden infant death syndrome (Anderson-Huntington & Rosenblith, 1971, 1976). The Motor score has been related to all outcomes at 8 months and to a few at 7 years, usually in a linear fashion.

The muscle tonus rating has been found to be the most powerful predictor of development at 7 years (Rosenblith, 1979a, 1979b; Rosenblith & Anderson, 1968). It is strongly related to a number of intellectual, perceptual, and behavioral outcomes for term infants. In addition, it accounts for 20% of the variance in reading achievement test scores at 7 years for premature babies. Pediatric neurologists have long been interested in muscle tonus (see Figure 8.12), but have not (to my knowledge) identified the specific pattern of tonus that has the poorest outcomes. It is a pattern in which the arms are relatively flaccid or hypotonic and the legs are relatively hypertonic or tense. The

Figure 8.12. Muscle tone as it affects being pulled to a sitting position. The infant at left shows excellent neck and shoulder tonus, enabling the baby to keep its head from drooping. The photo at right shows one twin who maintained control after reaching a sitting posture.

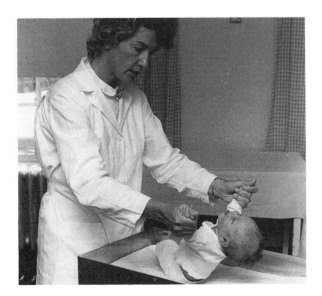
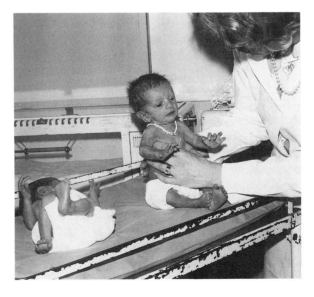

usual neonatal pattern is the reverse, and the difference in tonicity between arms and legs is smaller than in this at-risk pattern.

Scores obtained on examinations done in the first 2 days of life tend to be more related to later outcomes than those obtained on days 3 or 4. This is contrary to what one would expect if behaviors in the immediate postbirth period reflect only the rapid adaptations being made. A possible interpretation is that responses during a period of stress can reflect problems in adaptation, and these may be related to problems during later stressful adaptations (as, for example, the stresses of adapting to the academic demands of school at 7-8 years of age).

A surprising finding in the follow-up studies with the G/R is that although irritable behavior and ratings of irritability were generally not related to developmental outcomes at the earlier ages (8 months or 4 years), irritability was related to outcomes at 7 years for premature infants.

As is true for neurological tests, the G/R scores and ratings cannot be used to predict the outcome for an individual baby. However, in the course of studying more than 1,500 newborns, it was found that one behavior that was incidental to the examination and that was observed in only a small number of babies did predict the outcome for every one. All newborns are more sensitive to light than older infants, children, or adults. However, every newborn who was abnormally sensitive compared with other newborns showed later neurological abnormalities and intellectual retardation (Anderson & Rosenblith, 1964; Anderson-Huntington & Rosenblith, 1972; Rosenblith et al., 1970).

It is hard to know how to assess the long-term predictive value of the NBAS. It was not designed to predict later cognitive outcomes; nevertheless, it has been used this way. For example, Tronick and Brazelton (1975) compared the predictive value of the NBAS to that of a standard neurological examination in a sample of infants medically diagnosed as neurologically suspect or abnormal. They found that the NBAS diagnoses appeared to have greater long-range validity than the neurological tests. Babies identified by neurologists as suspect or abnormal and who later were found to be normal were less likely to have been called abnormal on the NBAS. These results utilized overall diagnoses based on two or more administrations of the NBAS.

There are also studies showing that the NBAS was related to performance on the Bayley scales (described later in this chapter) at 6 weeks (Sostek & Anders, 1977) and at 8 months (Field et al., 1978). One summary type score (motoric process) derived from either the NBAS or an adaptation of it for mothers (the MABI) was significantly related to the 8-month Bayley physical development scores in both normal and postmature babies. The NBAS done in the home on days 7 and 10 for 243 first babies (predominantly of low-SES white parents) was related to the Bayley scales at 9 months of age (Vaughn et al., 1980). The Mental and Motor scales, and the Infant Behavior Record (based on behaviors during the exam) were used as criteria. The babies' best performances on the NBAS were used to score the AIs a priori clusters. Factor analyses on both scores and clusters yielded five factors, three of which were significantly correlated with the Bayley Mental Scale, but the largest r was .19 (less than 4% of variance accounted for). None of the factors was significantly correlated with motor scores on the Bayley, which replicates Sostek and Anders (1977), but is in contrast to other data (Sepkoski et al., 1990) to be discussed shortly. Ratings of "worrisome" on the a priori dimensions of motor processes and state control were related to significantly lower mental scores than ratings of average or optimal, but the worrisome group (Vaughn et al., 1980) scored at or above the norm (IQs 99 to 118). Sostek and Anders (1977) found state control to be related to 10-week Bayley mental scores. It has been shown to be related to motor development at 8 and 12 months (Risholm-Mothander, 1989).

All 157 infants born from January 1971 to February 28, 1973, in four villages in rural Guatemala were assessed by Lasky, Klein, Yarbrough, and Kallio (1981) using the NAS, an earlier version of the NBAS. The subjects were given a battery of tests at 6, 15, and 24 months, and at 3 and 4 years of age. The researchers report that "the correlations between the NBAS variables and all later assessments of intellectual performance were generally nonsignificant (only 13 of the 294 correlations were significant at the .05 level with no pattern evident)" (p. 851). It had previously been shown by Brazelton et al. (1977) that the NBAS variables had concurrent validity because they were correlated with birth weight and other indices of risk. Neonatal length and weight were significantly related to behavioral development in this population, although the NBAS was not (Lasky, Klein, Yarbrough, & Kallio, 1981). In a middle-class but highly varied sample of infants in the United States, a sample that included premature (in intensive care) and term infants (healthy and hospitalized because of the illness of their mothers), the NBAS had even less predictive value for later IQ. IQ at age 3 was not predicted by the obstetric or postnatal complications, the NBAS, or a combination of these (Reich et al., 1984).

Change scores from one test to another might possibly have more prognostic validity than the scores on the individual tests (Sepkoski et al., 1990). The change scores of prematures tested at 36 and 40 weeks (they had to be off of supplemental oxygen) were related to their PDI scores on the Bayley at 18 months ($r = .46$). When the separate clusters were examined it was the motor and state range clusters that accounted for most of the relation. Swedish data also show that state control capacity on the NBAS in the first 2 weeks predicts motor development on the Griffiths at 8 and 12 months (Risholm-Mothander, 1989).

Separate tests developed for prematures will be discussed shortly. However, the Sepkoski et al. data and those of Rosenblith showing that the strongest prediction to 7 years from her scales was for prematures (muscle tonus to reading) make it appear that the conventional neonatal tests are of use for older prematures.

Neonatal Tests as Dependent Variables

Neonatal tests are also used to provide a dependent measure of the effects of experimental treatment variables, and as outcome measures in correlational studies of the effects of pre- and perinatal factors. Although no such use has been made of the Graham test, to my knowledge, there have been cases where the G/R has been used to assess the effects of stimulation programs of various types.

Neal (1968) used the G/R to assess the effects of a stimulation program in which small premature infants (1 lb, 1 oz, to 3 lb, 9 oz) received a period of rocking in a hammock daily from the fifth day after birth until 36 weeks gestational age. The experimental groups (tested by persons unaware of their treatment group) scored higher on motor strength and coordination, visual following, and some of the other specific items of the G/R. They also gained more weight.

Another study assessed the effect of patterned auditory stimulation (a tape recording of the mother's voice talking to her infant) on the development of 28- to 32-week gestational age prematures randomly assigned to experimental and control (routine care) groups. When assessed at 36 weeks by the G/R, the experimental group had higher general maturation, visual and auditory scores, and muscle tonus ratings, but did not differ in irritability. The tonus ratings differed according to the particular hospital the babies were in, so they are hard to interpret (Katz, 1970).

The use of the NBAS as a dependent variable was encountered in Chapter 5 in the discussion of studies on the effects of maternal medications on babies.

Some of the studies cited found differences and some did not. Even in studies that found differences, they were usually small. The Graham/Rosenblith has sometimes been used in a similar way (e.g., Sostek et al., 1976) with similar results. The use of the NBAS as a dependent variable(s) to assess the effects of maternal methadone addiction on infant behavior was covered in Chapter 4. Those studies will not be reviewed here, nor shall I attempt to cover the myriad such studies.

An unusual use of the NBAS is to compare the performance of chimpanzee and human infants. In particular, Bard et al. (in press) looked for possible differences in responses to social compared with nonsocial stimuli. They found the chimpanzee infants to be indistinguishable from the humans.

TESTING OF PREMATURE NEWBORNS

Younger and smaller prematures are surviving with much more frequency today than in the past, and tools to assess their development and the effects of interventions or changes in their care procedures have become highly desirable.

Assessment of Preterm Infants' Behavior

Als and her colleagues (1982a, 1982b) who had been involved in the NBAS felt the need for a separate assessment tool for use with premature infants, as the NBAS was increasingly inappropriate for use with them. The Assessment of Preterm Infants' Behavior (**APIB**), based on the NBAS, was developed. It focuses on infants' reactivity and threshold of disorganization and stress in response to environmental input. It has an extremely complex scoring system and requires extensive training to administer, hence most work using it has come out of the same laboratory.

The APIB assesses six systems: autonomic, motor, state, attention/interaction, self-regulation, and the degree of examiner or environmental facilitation needed to help the infant maintain or regain an integrated, balanced state. The complex scores are reduced to system scores. The relation of these system scores to conceptional age at time of birth has been studied using the APIB administered at 42 weeks to term infants and infants of varying degrees of prematurity, all selected to be healthy and lacking in medical or home complications (Als et al., 1988a). On all six systems the full-term sample was most well modulated and well functioning, and the very early born prematures (born at 27 to 32 weeks) were most disorganized, with low thresholds to stress and hypersensitive reactions. They continued to show moderate motoric disorganization, autonomic instability, and difficulties in self-regulation, and considerable difficulty in maintaining alertness, and required moderate to considerable facilitation from the examiner in order to regain stabilization. Those born at 33 to 37 weeks were intermediate. A classification system was developed; it was applied to a previously studied group of babies and successfully identified them as term or preterm.

A cluster analysis applied to the data of the above study resulted in three clusters termed nimbuloids (Als et al., 1988b).[10] Nimbuloid I was made up of well-organized infants and Nimbuloid III of the least well organized, with II being intermediate. Infants from each gestational age category were found in each nimbuloid, but disproportionately, as one would expect. Nimbuloid status was independent of SES, ethnicity, and sex. In another study only Nimbuloid II contained both premature and term infants (Als et al., 1989).

The APIB has been used as an outcome measure to determine the effectiveness of an individualized care program for very low birth weight prematures. The care program is devised based in part on the behaviors shown in the APIB (Als et al., 1986). And the long-term continuity (predictive validity) has been evaluated at 5 years of age (Als et al., 1989).[11] Als et al. found that the newborn membership in modulation groups predicted to neuropsychological functioning at 5 years, but the complexity of the variables and level of description do not permit an independent evaluation.

Neurobehavioral Assessment for Preterm Infants

Korner and her colleagues, prompted by the need to assess the effects of intervention on prematures, developed the Neurobehavioral Assessment for Preterm Infants (**NAPI**) for those from 32 weeks conceptional age to term (see Korner, 1990; Korner et al., 1987; Korner & Thom, 1991). Profiting from the problems of all the examinations that started as collections of items that could be quantified in newborns (full-term or premature), they used much more sophisticated procedures to develop their examination. Instead of

determining test-retest reliability or clusters or factors after using the examination, these were built into the examination. Items were clustered on conceptual principles and kept in the examination only if they had test-retest reliability and cohered with the cluster they were in. Clusters were kept only if they cohered statistically as well as conceptually. In addition, a developmental course of response was required. They ended with eight clusters, only two of which (Active Tone/Motor Vigor and Excitation Proneness) were primarily influenced by postconceptional age. This poses an important question regarding all evaluations of the development of preterm infants. It has generally been assumed that development proceeds at about the same pace whether in utero or postbirth, hence that conceptional age should determine the maturity of function. One cluster (Alertness/Orientation) had a developmental course compatible with catch-up, that is, the differences between infants born at different gestational ages disappeared by 3 to 4 postnatal weeks. The remaining five clusters (Inhibition Proneness, Cry Quality, Maturity of Vestibular Response, Scarf Sign, and Popliteal Angle)[12] were highly influenced by postnatal medical course or environment.

State assessments (made 22 times during the NAPI) showed that sleep decreased over time and waking increased, but there was no significant stability of individual differences over time (Korner et al., 1988). The proportion of waking time that was spent in drowse or alert activity both showed changes with age and individual stability across age. The number of state changes during the examination did not change with age, but showed high individual stability. A test of which of these patterns or models would be found for other aspects of functioning assessed on the NAPI was undertaken for those prematures that had three or more assessments (Korner et al., 1989). The data are complicated by the fact that two cohorts were used, one tested with the preliminary and one with the final form of the exam. Results are similar for the two, and some differences found could be due to the fact that the final form is shorter. I will present the findings in general, and not try to deal with the statistical bases for determining the best fitting model.

Motor development (including Tone and/or Vigor) increased with age for 17 of the 19 items tested. Stability for individuals was impressively high with model 2 (.32 to .84) with only 4 out of 30 items below .50. Spontaneous motility was similar. Only items related to auditory, visual, and ocular functioning showed more stability when the third model was used (all stability coefficients above .55). In all cases the first (developmental) model explained the largest part of the

---

10. The extensive statistical work reported in these papers would make them inaccessible to most students.

11. This reference also contains an overview of Als's synactive theory of development and a description of an assessment tool she and her colleagues have developed for use with older infants and young children—the Kangaroo Box.

12. All except Inhibition Proneness are items from clusters that were dropped but where the item itself satisfied all criteria, and hence was kept as a 1-item cluster. The last two are items from neurological examinations.

variance, even though others improved on it. The authors speculate that the unusually high stabilities found, which are atypical in neonatal testing, may stem from the fact that the 32-week fetus is much like that at term, with similar dendritic development in the CNS, and that since they were tested at 3 weeks or more postbirth, they are not making the adaptations that newborns (term or preterm) are.

Like the APIB, the NAPI has not yet been used to show the relations between the stable individual differences found and later outcomes. However, it has been shown to have test-retest reliability in a new population tested by different testers 7 years later (with all the changes in care for prematures) and with one test being the shortened final version and the other the original longer one (Korner et al., 1991). Even the mean scores were highly similar. Excitation proneness and the ratings of the percentage of time crying, which had test-retest reliabilities only in the .40s (a correlation that is often accepted as adequate for neonatal testing), were eliminated as having inadequate reliability. This is indeed a remarkable degree of stability. NAPI has also been shown to have developmental (face) validity (Korner et al., 1991). All clusters increase with conceptional age, except for the percentage of time asleep, which decreases.

Neurobehavioral Assessments From Sleep Monitoring

Before leaving the topic of assessment of prematures, I must call attention to the work of Thoman in automating the collection and analysis of sleep records (Thoman & Glazier, 1987; Thoman & Whitney, 1989). The intent of this work is to make it possible to determine which infants have stable state profiles and which do not, factors that have been shown in earlier work to be related to later outcomes.

INFANT TESTING

Infant tests were developed before the neonatal tests, which owe a great debt to them. Infant tests, in turn, were an outgrowth of the testing movement that started with school-age children. To understand the infant tests, a brief overview of school-age testing is necessary. At the beginning of this century, Binet and Simon (1905) developed tests to screen children to determine who could profit from schooling (English versions followed soon thereafter; see also Kite, 1916). Terman and Merrill (1937, 1960) adapted these tests for use in the United States. They were both at Stanford University at the time, and their adaptation became known as the Stanford-Binet test. Terman, like

Gesell, was a student of G. Stanley Hall, whom many regard as the first American developmental psychologist.

Tests for school-age children (the Binet-Simon and a number of subsequent ones) examined a wide variety of behaviors, all thought to indicate intelligence. They were designed to sample all intellectual functions through "the sinking of shafts at critical points" (Terman & Merrill, 1937, p. 4). In fact, the variety of behaviors is strongly biased toward verbal behaviors. These tests of intellectual functioning arrived at a single score that summarized the child's status. At first this status was expressed as mental age (MA), which was the age at which the child being tested performed as well as the average child of that age. For example, if Samantha passed as many test items as the average 8-year-old, she would be given an MA of 8 years (regardless of her chronological age). The MA allows comparisons of children's mental functioning and permits actions based on functioning. For example, all children functioning at an MA of 8 years can be put into the same classroom, thereby creating a presumably homogeneous group to teach. The functioning of two individuals can also be compared. For example, if Samantha has an MA of 8 and Julia an MA of 6, Samantha is functioning at a higher level than Julia. If Samantha and Julia are of the same chronological age (say, 6 years), then we can say that Samantha is brighter. If, however, Samantha is much older or younger than Julia, then such comparison becomes more difficult and MA does not tell which is brighter. To solve this problem, the intelligence quotient (IQ) was developed early in the history of intelligence testing (Kuhlman, 1912; Stern, 1914/1924). It compares MA to chronological age (CA) and provides a measure of intellectual functioning that is independent of age—that is, that permits comparisons of the brightness or so-called intelligence of children of different ages. In the original IQ measure, MA was divided by CA and the product multiplied by 100. If Samantha were 10, her IQ would be (8/10) x 100 = 80. If Julia were 4, her IQ would be (6/4) x 100 = 133. Thus, although Samantha is functioning at a higher level than Julia, Julia is brighter; Julia is functioning ahead of her years and Samantha is functioning behind hers.

More recently the formula for the IQ has been changed to reflect better the statistical nature of the distribution of scores. For tests scored the new way (such as the various Wechsler tests) and for the Binet tests it is substantially correct to say that the average IQ is between 85 and 115 (or the mean of 100 plus or minus one standard deviation). This means that about 68% of persons tested will have IQs in the average range.

The infant and preschool testing movement grew out of both the school-age testing movement and the enthusiasm for the study of growth and development that characterized the 1930s and led to longitudinal studies of physical and psychological development. In contrast with the tests for school-age children, infant and preschool tests cannot be primarily verbal; indeed, tests in early infancy can only examine sensory, perceptual, and motor development and their linkages, and social interactions. They can include more symbolic material after 1 year.

The Tests

Some of the infant tests that have been used extensively in both research and practical settings will be described briefly, and then the Bayley test will be discussed in detail, because it is probably the most widely used test in infant research in the United States.

Gesell. Arnold Gesell was one of the key figures in understanding the sequencing of development and in the development of infant tests. He has been largely neglected by psychologists in recent years. At first this neglect was probably triggered by many of the same factors that led child psychologists in the United States to neglect the work of Piaget (see Chapter 10). Gesell's work was criticized for lack of rigor and control. However, the data on the developmental sequences of responses to certain stimulus situations that he and his colleagues produced have withstood the test of time. The theories he derived from his data, especially with respect to continuity of development and the biological nature of the growth spiral, are more subject to criticism. For a single source that gives his own presentation of his views and work at a relatively late stage in his life, see Gesell (1954).

Gesell was also a pioneer in the use of the motion picture camera to study infant behavior. Film provides a record that others can study to determine whether they see the same sequences or not. Gesell (1934) used motion pictures (which had only recently become available) because "the wealth and complexity of infant behavior are beyond human description" (p. 20). Movies supplemented by other forms of investigation and inventory are needed to chart such behavioral complexity systematically.

The Sunday supplements of the mid-1930s published not only articles and reviews of Gesell's books, but pages and pages of his pictures. After his initial scientific books, he and his colleagues wrote books designed specifically for parents and child-care workers (a

pattern followed earlier by Preyer; see Chapter 1). Many generations of American children (at least from upper educational levels) were raised by parents who used Gesell norms to see whether their babies were behaving appropriately (normally) or were farther ahead of the norms than their friends' babies.

After a 1919 study charting behavior from birth to age 6, Gesell (1925) codified his developmental schedule and in 1926 started a normative study using movies. Unlike intelligence testers, he did not try to represent the population as a whole in a standardization sample. Rather, he attempted to represent the "most normal" by choosing only full-term infants born after normal pregnancies and from what he considered to be a "homogeneous middle-class population." This population was both considerably varied and rather different from our current perceptions of the middle class. For example, sound sources in the homes included radios (62% of homes), victrolas (old version of record player, in 40%), and pianos (19%). Only 35% had cars, but 52% sent their laundry out.

Detailed observations, including some physiological measures, and extensive movies and history taking took a full half day. Because mothers were asked to choose an optimal time of day, and as a result of Gesell's remarkable skill, only 1 out of 524 examinations of the 107 infants studied had to be continued to another day.

The first form of his examination used seven groups of behaviors to describe the infant. This was later reduced to four major groupings of behaviors: motor, adaptive, language, and personal-social. Maternal reports were largely used for the last two areas. The Gesell test can be used with separate evaluations for each of the four areas of performance, or those scores can be combined and a developmental quotient (DQ) obtained. The latter was done to provide an infant evaluation analogous to that of the IQ. Numerically, it works like the IQ. The average score is 100 and 68% of all babies score between 85 and 115. The DQ is, however psychologically quite different from the IQ. Many of the behaviors that go into the DQ score are decidedly nonintellectual; postural and locomotor behaviors (discussed in the earlier section on motor development) are perhaps the best examples. The DQ and comparable scores on other infant tests are not, in fact, highly related to IQ scores; that is, babies who have relatively high or low DQs may or may not have similarly high or low IQs. Gesell's belief that the DQ and the IQ were highly related is one reason psychologists ignored his work. Nevertheless, with the exception of quick screening tests such as the Denver Developmental Screening Test (Frankenburg, Camp,

& VanNatta, 1971; Frankenburg & Dodds, 1967; Frankenburg, Goldstein, & Camp, 1971), the Gesell has been, and probably continues to be, the infant examination most used by pediatricians in the United States. A revision was issued in 1975 (Knoblock & Pasamanick, 1975).

Other Early Tests. Another early test, by Bühler and Hetzer (1935), included items that assessed phenomena that were not used in other standardized infant tests until recently, when Uzgiris and Hunt (1975a, 1975b) developed tests based on Piaget's research. A good example is an ingenious item that could be said (in current terms) to assess memory or cognitive processing or object constancy, but that can also be well described as a form of delayed-reaction test. The infant is given a rubber ball out of which a chicken pops when the ball is squeezed. After playing with this toy for 1 minute, the infant is engaged by the examiner in other activities for from 1 to 15 or 20 minutes. The infant is then given a ball that looks and feels just like the first one, but nothing pops out when it is squeezed. Expressions of astonishment, questioning looks at the tester, and exploration of the hole from which the chicken "should have popped" are scored as passing the item. At 10 or 11 months of age this item can be passed after a 1-minute interval and at 15 to 16 months children usually pass after a delay of 8 minutes. Delays of 15 minutes are tolerated at 19 to 20 months, and of 17 minutes at 21 to 24 months.

Additional early infant tests include the Mental Measurement of Preschool Children, by Stutsman (1931); the 1933 Bayley scales; and Measurement of Intelligence in Infants and Young Children, by Cattell (1940). The last test attempted to achieve a format like that of the Stanford-Binet. The age range is 2 to 30 months. It is still used, but has never been properly standardized. It does have the advantages of being relatively short and interesting to infants.

Other Currently Used Tests. The rather widely used Denver Developmental Screening Test (DDST) has not been discussed here because information on its diagnostic efficiency is rather mixed. Early reports indicated that it did rather well, but later evidence showed that it may not be so useful (Solomons & Solomons, 1975; Wacker, 1980). Although 94% of children over 3 with good later outcomes had been classified as normal on the DDST, it failed to identify 80% of children with poor outcomes (Greer et al., 1989). It has also been found to be of limited value in screening infants who had been in NICUs (Sciarillo et al., 1986). The DDST appears to be subject to considerable social

class variation, according to both old data from the United States and newer data from an urban Turkish population (Epir & Yalaz, 1984).

Despite these problems, the DDST has been used as a basis for assessments designed to take even less time. One is the Denver Prescreening Questionnaire and its revision (Frankenburg et al., 1987), which identifies 84% of those classed as nonnormal on the DDST. Frankenburg et al. (1988) have also been involved in an effort to determine key items from the DDST (covering ages from birth to 6 years) that would identify those found abnormal or suspect on the full test. They found 39 items that identified 100% of the abnormals and over 90% of those suspect on the DDST. At any one age only 4 items would be needed, a considerable saving in time over the 15 to 20 minutes required to administer the DDST. Unfortunately, neither of these screening tools has been validated against criteria other than the DDST.

A more psychologically oriented effort to assess infants in less time than is required for the Bayley or McCarthy scales (½ hour to 1½ hours) was the Minnesota Child Development Inventory (MCDI) was developed by Ireton et al. (1975). This 320-item maternal report yields developmental levels in eight areas, and was originally used primarily with 2- to 5-year-olds. Its relation to the Bayley has been assessed with infants from 8 to 30 months of age (Saylor & Brandt, 1986). The MCDI summary index correlates with the Bayley MDI at $r = .91$ for the total sample and above .79 for those from 8 to 12 and from 13 to 20 months of age. Each subscale correlates at .55 to .84 for these age groups.

Another assessment tool to predict cognition in infancy is CLAMS (Clinical Linguistic and Auditory Milestone Scale), which is based on parental report of language behaviors, both receptive and expressive, and provides an ordinal scale (Capute et al., 1986). The attainment of 25 linguistic and auditory milestones has been significantly but modestly related to the MDI at 12 months.

Tests From Other Countries. Infant tests developed and primarily used in other countries (that are cited in the literature in the United States) include the Abilities of Babies, developed by Griffiths (1954) in England. It has five subtests: locomotor, personal-social, hearing and speech, hand-eye functions, and performance. It uses a motor and mental DQ. The performance scale is interesting in that it attempts to assess the infant's readiness and ingenuity over a variety of test situations. Like most infant tests, it borrows heavily from the Gesell. Unlike Gesell, Griffiths not only did not feel that her test should predict later IQ, she did not understand why psychologists should expect this to be the case. An interesting screening has been done in Sweden based on the Griffiths. A total of 40 items from the test were transformed into questions that could be answered yes or no by parents. It was mailed to parents of all 18-month-olds living in Stockholm (3,245; 2,791 returned), who were asked to observe their infants for a couple of days and then fill out the questionnaire (Sonnander, 1987). For a subsample tested on the Griffiths, the correlation of the two measures was .87. The Griffiths correctly identified 64% of all cases identified as retarded at 8 and 14 years; the parental questionnaires correctly identified 60%.

Clearly, one could not expect such a rate of compliance in returning questionnaires in the United States without a special effort. Further, an extensive test of the reliability of scoring of the Griffiths items showed the infant items based on maternal report to have low reliability (Hanson et al., 1984). Nevertheless, one wonders whether parents, if given very specific questions to answer, may not be rather good observers of their children's behaviors, and they certainly have access to a much larger sample of those behaviors.

A French infant test, the Brunet-Lézine Test, follows the Gesell scheme of dividing items into four categories, as well as the Binet-Simon (Cattell) scheme of having set numbers of items at each age level (Brunet & Lézine, 1951). It also asks a set number of questions of the mother (caretaker) at each age level. Scoring is based on both the test items passed and the mother's reports. The test is used in Europe.

The Bayley Scales. Now we will take up the test that is most widely used in the United States today and consider it in greater detail. This test was developed by Bayley in connection with the Berkeley Growth Study, which she helped initiate in the late 1920s. It was one of several longitudinal studies of development started in that era. The test was originally called the California First-Year Mental Scale (Bayley, 1933a), but was extended to cover ages from 1 to 30 months. It had originally been standardized on a sample from the Berkeley-Oakland area that was not chosen to be representative and that later turned out to have average IQs of 120. This sample of 61 infants was tested monthly from 1 to 15 months, and at least 46 subjects were tested at each age level.[13] The Bayley scales received a new standardization in the 1960s. The 1969 revision was standardized on a stratified sample of 1,262 infants (Bayley, 1969). It includes both new items and changes in the order of items. Its current norms are quite representative of babies in the United States at the time, and a new standardization is under way. The normative samples were cross-sectional, which is probably a good thing. The Gesell, Cattell, and original Bayley tests all tested the same babies every few weeks or months, so the babies were highly practiced test takers. The examiners were often the same and thus might remember and have expectations of the babies that could well affect both their perceptions of the infants' future behaviors and even the infants' actual behaviors (based on examiner interactions with them). On the Hunt-Uzgiris scales, for example, infants tested longitudinally, compared with those the same age but tested in a cross-sectional design, were advanced two to three steps in an eight-step sequence (Jackson et al., 1978).

The Bayley is really two tests, the MDI and the PDI, and, unlike the Gesell, it does not have a large variety of subscores (though the Gesell is often reported by the single DQ). In addition to the Mental and Motor scales, there is a 30-item scale of infant test-taking behaviors and clinical impressions of the examiner (rated after the MDI and PDI have been administered)—the Infant Behavior Record (IBR). The Motor Scale was described in the earlier section on motor development. The other two will be considered here.

The Mental Scale attempts to elicit the following adaptive responses: attending to stimuli (visual and auditory), manipulation (grasping, manipulating, combining objects, shaking a rattle, and ringing a bell), interaction with the examiner (smiling, cooing, babbling, imitation, following directions), relating to toys in meaningful ways (putting cubes in a cup, banging spoons together), showing memory or awareness of object constancy (looking for a fallen object, uncovering a hidden toy, searching for a hidden toy in a small box), goal-directed tasks requiring perseverance (putting pegs in a peg board, forms in a form board), and ability to follow a complex set of directions that demand knowledge of object names and the meaning of prepositions as well as the concept of "one."

The number of items passed on the Mental Scale is converted to a Mental Development Index (MDI), where, as for IQ, 100 is average, based on the standardization sample. The Psychomotor Development Scale is done the same way to arrive at the PDI index. The IBR's usefulness may depend more on the individual examiners (or teams of examiners) than do the MDI or the PDI (Bayley, personal communication). However, they have been meaningfully used in a number of recent research efforts.

---

13. This is in contrast to Cattell's sample, which was studied less frequently and sometimes had only 20 subjects at a given age.

Many of the studies reported in this book make use of the Bayley, largely because it has the best standardization, but partly because it covers the ages in which much infancy work is done, and partly in the desire to make new research results comparable with those already published using this test. Its use with about 50,000 8-month-olds during a national collaborative project investigating pre- and perinatal factors in development (CPRP) means that there are many trained testers in various parts of the United States.

Ordinal Scales. Other developments in infant testing include an emphasis on **ordinal** scales. Test items that form an ordinal scale must show a progression in difficulty. An infant who can pass the third item should be able to pass the first two, one who passes the fifth item should have passed the first four, and so on. In terms of age, the infant should pass the first item at an earlier age than any of the later items.

There are two examples of tests based on ordinal scales. One is based on 67 of the 163 items on the Bayley test (Kohen-Raz, 1967). These items form five ordinal scales: eye-hand, manipulation, object relation, imitation-comprehension, and vocalization-social contact-active vocabulary. These scales worked equally well (that is, they were equally ordinal) in the three subpopulations studied by Kohen-Raz; hence it is reasonable to assume that the ordinal character of the scales may be generalized to other populations. It was his hope that such ordinal scales would be more effective in predicting later outcomes than the more global measures of the Bayley. We shall return to this question later.

The second example of ordinal scales in infant testing is provided by the Uzgiris and Hunt (1975a, 1975b) scales. They started with a theory (that of Jean Piaget, see Chapter 10). All other tests described here are **empirically based**; that is, their items were selected purely on the basis that they discriminated between what older and younger infants (or children) could do. Because Piaget's theory says that the order of achieving skills is always the same, the tests take the form of ordinal scales. The potential advantage of a theory-based test is that it may select behaviors that are more relevant to intellectual development, and hence could better predict later intellectual behaviors. The possible disadvantage is that the test will be only as good as the theory. Theories may lead a test constructor either to omit aspects of behavior that do not fit the theory or to include items that fit but are in fact not important.

Reliability

The questions addressed above in connection with neonatal tests can also be asked about the reliability of infant tests and their uses. Indeed, a book could be written on the answers to these questions. We shall take a very brief look at them. Two reviews that address these issues for infant tests generally are those by Thomas (1970) and St. Clair (1978). The latter is historical, as is this one to a limited degree.

Bayley (1933a, 1933b, 1935) assessed the reliability of the Bayley tests of mental and motor abilities in her original work. In addition, in connection with the CPRP, this question was addressed on a rather large scale (Werner & Bayley, 1966). Agreement in scoring between well-trained testers and observers was high, indicating good interscorer reliability. In addition, 8-month-old infants who were retested after a week's time tested very similarly, hence test-retest reliability was established. When these results were broken down according to the individual items on the tests, they showed that items from the mental scales that had relatively poor reliabilities were the ones involving social interactions, but even for these items the reliabilities were high compared with neonatal tests. For the Motor Scale items the poorest reliabilities were for items involving assistance from an adult.

Diagnostic Value

Like neonatal tests, infant tests are used as diagnostic aids or as predictors of later development. This was an important aim of Gesell, but because his infants were often either tested by persons who knew their histories or tested repeatedly by the same person, people came to mistrust his findings or at least his strong opinions about the very great predictive value of his tests. Other infant testers, such as Griffiths and Uzgiris and Hunt, have not expected test scores to be predictive. Both Cattell (1940) and Bayley (1955) considered predictability an empirical question to be answered from their longitudinal studies. Both concluded that variability was marked and that the test should not be relied on for long-range prediction. Indeed, at 2 years of age the Bayley results from the Berkeley Growth and Berkeley Guidance studies showed that there were very low correlations (about .30) with IQ at 8 years. Data based on a Stockholm study using the Brunet-Lézine tests are similar (cited in Honzik, 1976). The closer together in time the tests are given (years, not weeks), and the older the child, the closer the correlation between an earlier and a later assessment (Bayley, 1955; Honzik, 1976), but even 5-year IQs did not correlate with 8-year IQs more than .70.

Other studies showed greater predictive value for the infant tests. These studies included larger proportions of damaged or handicapped infants and children or predicted for the retarded portions of their samples (Broman & Nichols, 1975; Honzik, 1962; Illingworth, 1960; Knoblock & Pasamanick, 1960; MacRae, 1955; Reich et al., 1984). Drillien (1961) directly demonstrated that developmental tests, especially in prematures, do a very good job of predicting mental dullness. Of 16 children found unsuitable for ordinary school education at 5 years (IQ less than 70), 12 had performed at this level at 6 months and at all ages up to 5 years. Not a child in this group had scored higher than very dull on any test at any age. Even among the 16 children whose IQs were borderline (70-79) at 5 years, 12 had performed at this level or lower from 6 months on. Werner et al. (1968, 1971) have shown that Hawaiian infants with Cattell IQs below 80 at 20 months are very likely to have low IQs at age 10. An alternative scoring of the MDI to indicate the amount of scatter in performance shows promise of better differentiating groups with problems than does the MDI (Bregman et al., 1988). This needs to be replicated. Predictions of giftedness from early scores on the Bayley scales is modest, and of use only in group comparisons, not for predicting individual gifted children (Shapiro et al., 1989).

Another support for the predictive usefulness of infant tests comes from tests of muscular-motoric development. Although there is little in common between what would be called intelligence in infancy and what would be called intelligence in later childhood, there may be some infant behaviors that are indicators of general biological or maturational functioning. (Recall the discussion of muscle tonus in relation to neonatal testing, for example.) Kangas and colleagues (1966) rescaled the Bayley into three scales: Mental, Fine Motor, and Gross Motor. They found that the 8-month performance on the Fine Motor Scale had by far the highest correlation to 4-year Stanford-Binet IQ scores. In fact, the Fine Motor Scale alone correlated as well as the Fine Motor combined with the Mental Scale.

One study looked directly at the question of which of several infant tests provides the greatest predictive validity. Siegel (1981) administered both the Bayley and the Uzgiris-Hunt scales to 148 infants, 80 of whom were preterm (less than 1,501 g). The preterm infants were matched with the full-term ones on SES, parity, sex, and maternal age. The 10 preterm and 1 full-term infant who were discovered to have serious

disabilities (cerebral palsy, blindness, severe developmental delay) were excluded. The scales were administered at 4, 8, 12, and 18 months. The Bayley was scored both traditionally and by the Kohen-Raz ordinal scaling referred to earlier.

At 24 months the infants were tested again and had a standardized test of language expression and comprehension (the Reynall). These constituted the criterion measures to be predicted. All of the testing was done by testers who had no knowledge of the infants' prenatal history or performance on previous tests.

In this varied sample, the Bayley Mental and Motor indices showed impressive stability. Both were related to language comprehension and expression at 2 years. The Kohen-Raz scoring showed that different scales were related to the Bayley Motor and Mental indices depending on the age at the earlier test. It is impressive to note that the eye-hand coordination and manipulation scale at 4 months was about as much related to the 2-year indices as the Bayley at 18 months was. By 8 months the conceptual ability scale was related to the 2-year measures more strongly than any other scale. By 12 months all five of Kohen-Raz's ordinal scales are related to the 2-year Bayley outcomes and account for 15-36% of the variance. The pattern is similar when the language scores are used as the criteria.

The Uzgiris-Hunt scales showed relations from 4 months to 2 years, except for the gestural imitation scale (which assesses a skill that is poorly developed at 4 months). In general, the 8-month Uzgiris-Hunt scales were no more correlated with the 2-year motor and mental indices than the 4-month results were (except for gestural imitation). At later ages the Uzgiris-Hunt scales do not become more predictive, a fact that might be attributed to an insufficient range at the older ages. Again, a similar pattern holds when the language scores are the criteria. It is interesting to note that the vocal imitation scale from the Uzgiris-Hunt is not related to either language expression or comprehension.

Considering all of Siegel's data (those described here as well as some that are not), we can conclude that which tests will predict better depends on the age at testing and, to a lesser degree, on whether the goal is to predict Bayley performance or language scores. Kohen-Raz's scaling of the Bayley does seem to have achieved some of the better prediction he was hoping for. The results of Uzgiris and Hunt's scaling seem to indicate that they were correct not to expect long-term prediction.

The diagnostic worth of infant tests is not limited to their predictive power. Illingworth (1960) showed their effectiveness in assessing the effects of various damaging conditions such as anoxia, head damage, and viral diseases capable of affecting the brain. Honzik (1962, 1976) has shown that infants diagnosed as having neurological problems are well differentiated from controls at 8 months of age on both the Mental and the Motor scales of the Bayley. Suspect infants were less well identified, but did differ from controls. The Cattell has also been shown to be a useful supplement to pediatric diagnosis at 20 months (Bierman et al., 1964; Werner et al., 1968, 1971).

As noted earlier, the IBR from the Bayley is being used both as a predictor and as an outcome measure. Its 30 items have been reduced to six composite scores—task orientation, motor coordination, activity, audiovisual awareness, affect, and sociability—by Matheny (1980). These scores, together with the MDI and PDI, have been used by Baroni (1989) to examine the outcomes of infants who spent time on apnea monitors and who had varying numbers of apnea episodes. The number of apnea episodes was related to the MDI, the PDI, and five of the six scores from the IBR. Both the frequency of apnea and the IBR scores were related with the other held constant. In a number of instances, they accounted for 25% of the variance.

DiLalla and Fulker (1990) have reduced the IBR to three scales: activity, affect/extraversion, and task orientation. The latter two at 12 and 24 months are significantly related to IQ at 24 and 36 months. These researchers consider the IBR-based scores to be measures of temperament or test-taking behavior. It should be noted that they were studying twins and found that heredity played an important role in these temperamental behaviors during the first year, but less in the second and third years. They also found sex differences in these measures at 24 and 36 months, with girls being more happy, outgoing, and cooperative, as well as more attentive and goal directed.

Infant Tests as Dependent Variables

In the examination of the usefulness of neonatal tests, we looked at their use as a dependent variable to measure the effects of some other factor such as obstetric medication or anoxia. To some extent the work of Illingworth (1960) and Honzik (1976) discussed above follows this model. Infant tests are also used to assess the effects of such variables as malnutrition, institutional life, maternal deprivation, various aspects of parent-child interaction, and aspects of the nature of the home (such as the stimulating factors in it). Siegel's (1981) study that assessed the comparative

value of infant tests also used the infant test at 2 years to look at the effects of various home and maternal factors as measured by the Caldwell Inventory of Home Stimulation (HOME) at 12 months. She found that maternal responsiveness, avoidance of restriction or punishment, and organization of the environment at 12 months were not related to the 2-year outcomes. The provision of stimulation and its variety were related. To a lesser degree, maternal involvement was related to performance on the test but not to the infant's language expression. Indeed, a total score based on all aspects of the HOME inventory was not as highly related to performance as was the single subscale "provision of play materials."

The Bayley has also been used to validate a measure of spontaneous play as an indicator of cognitive development (Hrncir et al., 1985). Spontaneous mastery behavior in play at 12 and 18 months was as much related to the MDI across the 6-month period as the MDI was related to itself.

Summary

PHYSICAL DEVELOPMENT

Knowledge about physical growth and development of the infant is interesting to parents and professionals, both to give a picture of normal growth and to provide an index of potential problems. It also can lead to deeper understanding of historical and social trends, of health and nutritional changes within populations, and of the relationship between genetic inheritance and environmental experiences.

Diet and improved health care over the last 100 or so years has led to an average increase in height (in developed countries) ranging from 2.9 cm (young white males in the United States) to 10.8 cm (Swedish conscripts). Both height and weight at birth have also increased. Difficulties in determining exact measurements were discussed here to indicate that measurement presents problems even when one has well-defined metrics.

Height, weight, and head circumference are most often measured in the infant. One of the most striking features of growth is the fact that there are extreme differences between body parts in rates of growth. The head doubles in length between birth and adulthood, the trunk triples, the arms quadruple, and the legs quintuple. The brain's weight at birth is closer to the adult level than that of other organs (except the eye). However, development of major functional areas within the brain continues until puberty and beyond.

MOTOR DEVELOPMENT

Most development occurs cephalocaudally (from the head down) and from the center to the periphery of the body (proximodistally). Developmental milestones for both gross and fine motor development have been identified. The ages at which babies hold up their heads, sit, stand, walk, and reach for or grasp objects are of great interest to parents and researchers.

One important theoretical issue is that of the relative roles of experience and maturation on motor development. Gesell assumed that motor development was biologically determined and depended primarily on the passage of time to unfold. He studied various aspects of motor development and created a widely used test. There are wide age differences in the acquisition of particular motor skills, depending on a number of factors, including health, nutrition, and genetic, cultural, and familial backgrounds, with their differences in environmental stimulation and opportunities for learning and practice.

Further improvements in the assessment of motor tasks are needed to reveal the quality of motor behaviors: whether accomplished with ease or difficulty, whether coordinated or clumsy, and so forth. Tests of motor behavior should take degrees of competence into account, not just success or failure. Cross-cultural studies add information to the discussion of the effect of different child-rearing patterns on motor development. Current work is yielding exciting detailed descriptions and analyses of the muscle patterns involved in various motor movements and their developmental changes.

The Motor Scale of the Bayley test was summarized to show the normal ages at which various gross motor behaviors are achieved. The youngest and oldest ages at which any baby in a standardization sample demonstrated the behavior were also shown; such ranges emphasize the fact that there are large individual differences among infants.

At birth infants exhibit little or no fine motor behavior, but show many of the gross motor components that will later become coordinated into finely tuned arm, hand, and finger movements. The importance of gross motor control for fine motor behaviors is beginning to be studied.

The infant is born with numerous reflex movements, some of which may fade before reappearing as parts of newly developed skills. Reflex grasping and stepping are examples. The discontinuity found in Western cultures between the reflex and the later coordinated behavior may be a function of the type of experiences babies have. There is exciting new work showing that one reason for the temporary disappearance of reflex behaviors such as walking may be that physical growth places new demands on the muscles.

One of the most important aspects of fine motor coordination that develops during infancy is visually guided reaching. It develops around 4 months of age and allows infants to explore their world much more effectively and thereby to occupy themselves for much longer periods of time. A primitive neonatal form (visually initiated reaching) is largely governed by biological factors and is relatively impervious to environmental deprivation. The 4-month form requires that infants experience visual feedback from their reaching movements. Later in the first year reaching again changes and in a more practiced form demands less visual attention.

Fine motor development has had an explosion of research attention recently. Ingenious techniques have led to the finding of much greater sophistication in the behavior of infants than had been supposed. The current interest is appropriate because fine motor behavior is more related to later outcomes (for example, IQ at age 4) than is gross motor development. Further, it provides a bridge between perceptual and cognitive research.

NEONATAL TESTING

The presence or absence of expected reflex responses in newborns is used to diagnose CNS damage. Various reflexes appear and disappear on varied time schedules. Muscle tonus is also used for diagnostic and predictive purposes. Several neonatal neurological examinations have been developed to identify neurological problems that might presage difficulties in later development, and to determine which sick babies should have a good prognosis. Prechtl, in Holland, and Saint-Anne Dargassies, in France, have presented evidence that neurological difficulties in infancy do not necessarily mean long-term problems. However, repeated abnormal findings on neurological examinations are associated with later problems.

Behavioral tests for newborns include the Graham Behavioral Test for Neonates, the Graham/Rosenblith Behavioral Test for Neonates, and the Brazelton or Newborn Behavioral Assessment Scales. The first two are primarily oriented toward detecting CNS immaturity or damage, and the NBAS is concerned with behaviors that might affect mother-infant interaction.

Interscorer agreement and test-retest reliability (given the fact that newborns make rapid and profound changes during the first days) are satisfactory on all of these tests. However, examiner differences have been found in a number of studies. It is nevertheless doubtful that any neonatal exam should be considered a standardized test in the way that tests given to older children and adults are.

Although the evidence for the relation of the NBAS to other neonatal variables is complex and sometimes contradictory, there is some support for the idea that the NBAS taps temperamental characteristics of infants.

Neonatal tests have also been used successfully as dependent variables in experimental treatment programs. For example, the effects of stimulation activities for prematures have been evaluated with the Graham/Rosenblith. The Brazelton has been shown to be affected by many different antecedent conditions or happenings, including maternal use of drugs and obstetric use of drugs, among others.

The Graham/Rosenblith has demonstrated some long-term predictive validity, although it does not enable predictions to be made for an individual baby. Muscle tonus is strongly related to a number of intellectual, perceptual, and behavioral outcomes. The day on which a baby is tested is relevant to the predictive usefulness of the test, but varies for different behaviors tested.

Special examinations oriented toward testing premature infants have been developed. One such examination (APIB) is based on the NBAS and is very complex. Another (NAPI) was developed in a very sophisticated fashion and is easier to learn and has high reliability and face validity. Sleep and state are also increasingly being used to assess functioning.

INFANT TESTING

The history of tests for intellectual ability (IQ) and developmental level (DQ) was reviewed briefly. The infant and preschool testing movement grew out of the IQ testing movement. However, infant tests measure primarily sensory, perceptual, and motor development, their linkages, and social interaction. Gesell's test was the main basis for all other tests designed to assess infants. A number of American and other tests were mentioned, but the Bayley was discussed in detail because it is best standardized and most widely used.

Some researchers have emphasized ordinal scales, which show a regular progression in difficulty on a variety of tasks. The Bayley scales have been scored in ways that produce ordinal scales (Kohen-Raz) that appear to have greater predictive validity than the Bayley itself, but this has not been replicated. Ordinal scales based on Piagetian theory have been developed by Uzgiris and Hunt, who are less concerned with predic-

tion. These tests are being increasingly used.

Screening tools for more rapid assessment of infants were discussed. Some based on parental reports have considerable promise.

Neonatal and infant tests tend not to have long-range accuracy, except for those babies who have been badly damaged. They are useful for assessing the effects of factors such as malnutrition, drugs, institutional life, maternal deprivation, environmental stimulation, and parent-child interaction.

References

ADAMSON, L., Als, H., Tronick, E., & Brazelton, T. B. (1975). *A priori profiles for the Brazelton Neonatal Assessment.* Unpublished manuscript. (Available from Child Development Unit, Children's Hospital, Boston)

ALS, H. (1978). Assessing an assessment: Conceptual considerations, methodological issues, and a perspective on the future of the Neonatal Behavioral Assessment Scale. In A. J. Sameroff (Ed.), Organization and stability of newborn behavior: A commentary on the Brazelton Neonatal Behavior Assessment Scale. *Monographs of the Society for Research in Child Development, 43*(5-6, Serial No. 177).

ALS, H., Duffy, F. H., & McAnulty, G. B. (1988a). Behavioral differences between preterm and full-term newborns as measured with the APIB system scores: I. *Infant Behavior and Development, 11,* 305-318.

ALS, H., Duffy, F. H., & McAnulty, G. B. (1988b). The APIB, an assessment of functional competence in preterm and full-term newborns regardless of gestational age at birth: II. *Infant Behavior and Development, 11,* 319-331.

ALS, H., Duffy, F. H., McAnulty, G. B., & Badian, N. (1989). Continuity of neurobehavioral functioning in preterm and full-term newborns. In M. Bornstein & N. Krasnegor (Eds.), *Stability and continuity in mental development.* Hillsdale, NJ: Lawrence Erlbaum.

ALS, H., Lawhon, G., Brown, E., Gibes, R., Duffy, F. H., McAnulty, G., & Blickman, J. G. (1986). Individualized behavioral and environmental care for the very low birth weight preterm infant at high risk for bronchopulmonary dysplasia: Neonatal intensive care unit and developmental outcome. *Pediatrics, 78,* 1123-1132.

ALS, H., Lester, B. M., Tronick, E. Z., & Brazelton T. B. (1982a). Manual for the assessment of preterm infants' behavior (APIB). In H. E. Fitzgerald, B. M. Lester, & M. W. Yogman (Eds.), *Theory and research in behavioral pediatrics.* New York: Plenum.

ALS, H., Lester, B. M., Tronick, E. Z., & Brazelton T. B. (1982b). Toward a research instrument for the assessment of preterm infants' behavior (APIB). In H. E. Fitzgerald, B. M. Lester, & M. W. Yogman (Eds.), *Theory and research in behavioral pediatrics.* New York: Plenum.

ALS, H., Tronick, E., Lester, B. M., & Brazelton, T. B. (1977). The Brazelton Neonatal Behavioral Assessment Scale (BNBAS). *Journal of Abnormal Child Psychology, 5,* 215-231.

AMIEL-TISON, C. (1976). A method for neurological evaluation within the first year of life. *Current Problems in Pediatrics, 7,* 1-50.

AMIEL-TISON, C. (1982). Neurological signs, aetiology, and

implications. In P. Stratton (Ed.), *Psychobiology of the human newborn*. New York: John Wiley.

AMIEL-TISON, C., & Grenier, A. (1986). *Neurological assessment during the first year of life*. New York: Oxford University Press.

ANDERSON, R. B., & Rosenblith, J. F. (1964). Light sensitivity in the neonate: A preliminary report. *Biologia Neonatorum, 7*, 83-94.

ANDERSON-HUNTINGTON, R. B., & Rosenblith, J. F. (1971). Sudden unexpected death syndrome: Early indicators. *Biology of the Neonate, 18*, 395-406.

ANDERSON-HUNTINGTON, R. B., & Rosenblith, J. F. (1972). Report on newborns with questionable light sensitivity. *Biology of the Neonate, 20*, 1-84.

ANDERSON-HUNTINGTON, R. B., & Rosenblith, J. F. (1976). Central nervous system damage: A possible component of the sudden infant death syndrome. *Developmental Medicine and Child Neurology, 18*, 480-492.

ANDRÉ-THOMAS, Chesni, C. Y., & Saint-Anne Dargassies, S. (1960). *Neurological examination of the infant* (Clinics in Developmental Medicine, No. 1). London: Spastics International Medical Publications.

AYLWARD, G. P., Verhulst, S. J., & Colliver, J. A. (1985). Development of a brief infant neurobehavioral optimality scale: Longitudinal sensitivity and specificity. *Developmental Neuropsychology, 1*, 265-276.

AZUMA, S. D., Malee, K. M., Kavanagh, J. A., & Deddish, R. B. (1991). Confirmatory factor analysis with preterm NBAS data: A comparison of our data reduction models. *Infant Behavior and Development, 14*, 209-225.

BARD, K. A., Platzman, K. A., Lester, B. M., & Suomi, S. J. (in press). Orientation to social and nonsocial stimuli in neonatal chimpanzees and humans. *Infant Behavior and Development*.

BARONI, M. A. (1989, April). *Bayley Infant Behavior Record (IBR): Relations between behavioral factors, apnea and Bayley test scores*. Paper presented at the Society for Research in Child Development, Kansas City, MO.

BAYLEY, N. (1933a). *The California first-year mental scale*. Berkeley: University of California Press.

BAYLEY, N. (1933b). Mental growth during the first three years: A developmental study of 61 children by repeated tests. *Genetic Psychology Monographs, 14*, 1-92.

BAYLEY, N. (1935). The development of motor abilities during the first three years. *Monographs of the Society for Research in Child Development, 1*(Serial No. 1).

BAYLEY, N. (1954). Some increasing parent-child similarities during the growth of children. *Journal of Educational Psychology, 45*, 1-21.

BAYLEY, N. (1955). On the growth of intelligence. *American Psychologist, 10*, 805-818.

BAYLEY, N. (1969). *Manual for the Bayley Scales of Infant Development*. New York: Psychological Corporation.

BEKEDAM, D. J., Visser, G. H., deVries, J. J., & Prechtl, H. F. (1985). Motor behavior in the growth retarded fetus. *Early Human Development, 12*, 155-165.

BENCH, J., & Parker, A. (1970). On the reliability of the Graham/Rosenblith Behavior Test for Neonates. *Journal of Child Psychology and Psychiatry, 11*, 121-131.

BEAUDREAU, P. R., & Salmoni, A. W. (1990, April). *The development and coordination of prehension skills in 6-7 and 9-10 month-old infants*. Paper presented at the International Conference on Infant Studies, Montreal.

BERTENTHAL, B. I., & Bai, D. L. (1989). Infants' sensitivity to optical flow for controlling posture. *Developmental Psychology, 25*, 936-945.

BIERMAN, J. M., Connor, A. M., Vaage, M., & Honzik, M. P. (1964). Pediatricians' assessments of the intelligence of two-year-olds and their mental test scores. *Pediatrics, 34*, 680.

BINET, A., & Simon, T. (1905). Upon the necessity of establishing a scientific diagnosis of inferior states of intelligence. *L'Annee Psychologique, 11*, 163-190.

BRAZELTON, T. B. (Ed.). (1973). *Neonatal Behavioral Assessment Scale* (National Spastics Society Monograph). Philadelphia: J. B. Lippincott.

BRAZELTON, T. B. (Ed.). (1984). *Neonatal Behavioral Assessment Scale* (Clinics in Developmental Medicine, No. 88). London: Blackwell Scientific.

BRAZELTON, T. B., Nugent, J. K., & Lester, B. M. (1987). Neonatal Behavioral Assessment Scale. In J. D. Osofsky (Ed.), *Handbook of infant development* (2nd ed., pp. 780-817). New York: John Wiley.

BRAZELTON, T. B., Tronick, E., Lechtig, A., & Lasky, R. (1977). The behavior of nutritionally deprived Guatemalan infants. *Developmental Medicine and Child Neurology, 19*, 364-372.

BRAZELTON, T. B., & Tryphonopoulou, Y. A. (n.d.). *A comparative study of the Greek and U.S. neonates*. Unpublished manuscript.

BREGMAN, J., Holmes, D. L., & Reich, J. N. (1988, April). *Use of a scatter index in scoring Bayley MDI performance*. Paper presented at the International Conference on Infant Studies, Washington, DC.

BRILL, B., & Sabatier, C. (1986). The cultural context of motor development: Postural manipulation in the daily life of Babbara babies (Mali). *International Journal of Behavioral Development, 9*, 439-453.

BROMAN, S. (1981). Risk factors for deficits in early cognitive development. In G. G. Berg & H. D. Maillie (Eds.), *Measurement of risks*. New York: Plenum.

BROMAN, S., & Nichols, P. L. (1975, September). *Early mental development, social class, and school-age IQ*. Paper presented at the annual meeting of the American Psychological Association, Chicago.

BRUNER, J. S. (1969). Eye, hand, and mind. In D. Elkind & J. H. Flavell (Eds.), *Studies in cognitive development: Essays in honor of Jean Piaget*. New York: Oxford University Press.

BRUNER, J. S. (1971). The growth and structure of skill. In K. J. Connolly (Ed.), *Motor skills in infancy*. New York: Academic Press.

BRUNER, J. S. (1973). Organization of early skilled action. *Child Development, 44*, 1-11.

BRUNET, 0., & Lézine, P. U. (1951). *Le developement psychologique de la premiere enfance* [Psychological development in early infancy]. Issy-les-Moulineaux: Editions Scientifique et Psycho-techniques.

BÜHLER, C., & Hetzer, H. (1935). *Testing children's development from birth to school age* (H. Beaumont, Trans.). New York: Farrar & Rinehart.

BUSHNELL, E. W. (1985). The decline of visually guided reaching during infancy. *Infant Behavior and Development, 8*, 139-155.

BUSHNELL, E. W., & Boudreau, P. R. (in press). The development of haptic perception during infancy. In M. A. Heller & W. Schiff (Eds.), *The psychology of touch*. Hillsdale, NJ: Lawrence Erlbaum.

CAPUTE, A. J., Palmer, F. B., Shapiro, B. K., Wachtel, R. C.,

Ross, A., & Accardo, P. J. (1984). Primitive reflex profile: A quantitation of primitive reflexes in infancy. *Developmental Medicine and Child Neurology,, 26,* 375-383.

CAPUTE, A. J., Palmer, F. B., Shapiro, B. K., Wachtel, R. C., Schmidt, S., & Ross, A. (1986). Clinical linguistic and auditory milestone scale: Prediction of cognition. *Developmental Medicine and Child Neurology, 28,* 762-771.

CATTELL, P. (1940). *The measurement of intelligence in young children.* New York: Psychological Corporation.

CIONI, G., Ferrari, F., & Prechtl, H. F. (1989). Posture and spontaneous motility in fullterm infants. *Early Human Development, 18,* 247-262.

CLIFTON, R., Perris, E., & Bullinger, A. (1991). Infants' perception of auditory space. *Developmental Psychology, 27,* 187-197.

CONNOLLY, K., & Dalgleish, M. (1989). The emergence of a tool-using skill in infancy. *Developmental Psychology, 25,* 894-912.

COOKE, D. W., & Thelen, E. (1987). Newborn stepping: A review of puzzling infant co-ordination. *Developmental Medicine and Child Neurology, 29,* 394-404.

CROUCHMAN, M. (1986). The effects of babywalkers on early locomotor development. *Developmental Medicine and Child Neurology, 28,* 757-761.

DAMON, A. (1968). Secular trend in height and weight within old American families at Harvard, 1870-1965: I. Within twelve four-generation families. *American Journal of Physical Anthropology, 29,* 45-50.

DENNIS, W. (1938). Infant development under conditions of restricted practice and of minimum social stimulation: A preliminary report. *Journal of Genetic Psychology, 53,* 149-158.

DENNIS, W. (1940). Does culture appreciably affect pattern of infant behavior? *Journal of Social Psychology, 12,* 305-317.

DENNIS, W. (1943). Is the newborn infant's repertoire learned or instinctive? *Psychological Review, 50,* 330-337.

DENNIS, W., & Dennis, M. G. (1940). The effect of cradling practices upon the onset of walking in Hopi children. *Journal of Genetic Psychology, 56,* 77-86.

deSONNEVILLE, L. M., Visser, S. L., Njiokiktjien, C. (1989). Late sequelae of a non-optimal neonatal neurological condition in ERPs at the age of 11-13 years. *Electroencephalography and Clinical Neurophysiology, 72,* 491-498.

DiLALLA, L. F., & Fulker, D. W. (1990, April). *The Infant Behavior Record as a predictor of later IQ.* Paper presented at the International Conference on Infant Studies, Montreal.

DODWELL, P. C., Muir, D., & DiFranco, D. (1976). Responses of infants to visually presented objects. *Science, 194,* 209-211.

DRILLIEN, C. M. (1961). A longitudinal study of the growth and development of prematurely and maturely born children. *Archives of Disease in Childhood, 36,* 233-240.

DUBOWITZ, L., & Dubowitz, V. (1981). *The neurological assessment of the preterm and full-term newborn infant* (Clinics in Developmental Medicine, No. 79). London: Heinemann.

DUNKELD, J., & Bower, T. G. R. (1981). *The effect of wedge prisms on the reaching behavior of infants.* Unpublished manuscript, University of Edinburgh, Department of Psychology.

EMDE, R. N. (1978). Commentary on "Organization and stability of newborn behavior: A commentary on the Brazelton Neonatal Behavior Assessment Scale." *Monographs of the Society for Research in Child Development, 43*(Serial No. 177).

EPIR, S., & Yalaz, K. (1984). Urban Turkish children's performance on the Denver Developmental Screening Test. *Developmental Medicine and Child Neurology, 26,* 632-643.

FELDMAN, H. (1833). *Observations on the normal functioning of the human body.* Bonne: C. Georgie.

FIELD, T. M., Dempsey, J. R., Hallock, N. H., & Shuman, H. H. (1978). The mother's assessment of the behavior of her infant. *Infant Behavior and Development, 1,* 156-167.

FRAIBERG, S. (1971). Interaction in infancy: A program for blind infants. *Journal of the American Academy of Child Psychiatry, 10,* 381-405.

FRAIBERG, S. (1977). *Insights from the blind.* London: Souvenir.

FRANCIS, P. L., Self, P. A., & Horowitz, F. D. (1987). The behavioral assessment of the neonate: An overview. In J. D. Osofsky (Ed.), *Handbook of infant development* (2nd ed., pp. 723-779). New York: John Wiley.

FRANKENBURG, W. K., Camp, B. W., & VanNatta, P. (1971). Validity of the Denver Developmental Screening Test. *Child Development, 42,* 475-485.

FRANKENBURG, W. K., & Dodds, J. B. (1967). The Denver Developmental Screening Test. *Journal of Pediatrics, 71,* 181-191.

FRANKENBURG, W. K., Fandel, A. W., & Thornton, S. M. (1987). Revision of Denver Prescreening Developmental Questionnaire. *Journal of Pediatrics, 110,* 653-657.

FRANKENBURG, W. K., Goldstein, A. D., & Camp, B. W. (1971). The revised Denver Developmental Screening Test: Its accuracy as a screening instrument. *Pediatrics, 20,* 988-995.

FRANKENBURG, W. K., Ker, C. Y., Engelke, S., Schaefer, E. S., & Thornton, S. M. (1988). Validation of key Denver Developmental Screening Test items: A preliminary study. *Journal of Pediatrics, 112,* 560-566.

GANZ, L. (1975). Orientation in visual space. In A. H. Riesen (Ed.), *The developmental neuropsychology of sensory deprivation.* New York: Academic Press.

GEBER, M. (1958). The psycho-motor development of African children in the first year, and the influence of maternal behavior. *Journal of Social Psychology, 47,* 185-195.

GEBER, M., & Dean, R. F. A. (1957). Gesell tests on African children. *Pediatrics, 20,* 1055-1065.

GESELL, A. (1925). *The mental growth of the preschool child.* New York: Macmillan.

GESELL, A. (1934). *An atlas of infant behavior* (Vols. 1-2). New Haven, CT: Yale University Press.

GESELL, A. (1954). The ontogenesis of infant behavior. In L. Carmichael (Ed.), *Manual of child psychology* (pp. 335-373). New York: John Wiley.

GESELL, A., & Amatruda, C. S. (1947). *Developmental diagnosis.* New York: Harper & Row.

GESELL, A., & Thompson, H., with Amatruda, C. S. (1934). *Infant behavior: Its genesis and growth.* New York: McGraw-Hill.

GOLDFIELD, E. C. (1989). Transition from rocking to crawling: Postural constraints on infant movement. *Developmental Psychology, 25,* 913-919.

GORSKI, P. A., Lewkowicz, D. J., & Huntington, L. (1987). Advances in neonatal and infant behavioral assessment: Toward a comprehensive evaluation of early patterns of development. *Developmental and Behavioral Pediatrics, 8,* 39-50.

GRAHAM, F. K. (1956). Behavioral differences between normal and traumatized newborns: I. Test procedures. *Psychological Monographs, 70*(20, Whole No. 427).

GRAHAM, F. K., Ernhart, C. B., Thurston, D., & Craft, M.

(1962). Development three years after perinatal anoxia and other potentially damaging newborn experiences. *Psychological Monographs, 76*(3, Whole No. 522).

GRAHAM, F. K., Matarazzo, R. G., & Caldwell, B. M. (1956). Behavioral differences between normals and traumatized newborns: II. Standardization, reliability and validity. *Psychological Monographs, 70*(21, Whole No. 428).

GREER, S., Bauchner, H., & Zuckerman, B. (1989). The Denver Developmental Screening Test: How good is its predictive validity? *Developmental Medicine and Child Neurology, 31,* 774-781.

GRIFFITHS, R. (1954). *The abilities of babies: A study in mental measurement.* New York: McGraw-Hill.

HADDERS-ALGRA, M., Touwen, B. C. L., & Huisjes, H. J. (1986). Neurologically deviant newborns: Neurological and behavioral development at the age of six years. *Developmental Medicine and Child Neurology, 28,* 569-578.

HALVERSON, H. M. (1931). An experimental study of prehension in infants by means of systematic cinema records. *Genetic Psychology Monograph, 10,* 107-286.

HANSON, R., Smith, J. A., & Hume, W. (1984). Some reasons for disagreement among scorers of infant intelligence test items. *Child Care, Health and Development, 10,* 17-30.

HATWELL, Y. (1987). Motor and cognitive functions of the hand in infancy and childhood. *International Journal of Behavioral Development, 10,* 509-526.

HAY, D. F. (1986). Infancy. *Annual Review of Psychology, 37,* 135-161.

HEIN, A. (1972). Acquiring components of visually guided behavior. In A. Pick (Ed.), *Minnesota Symposia on Child Psychology* (Vol. 6). Minneapolis: University of Minnesota Press.

HEIN, A., & Diamond, R. M. (1971). Contrasting development of visually triggered and guided movements in kittens with respect to interocular and interlimb equivalence. *Journal of Comparative and Physiological Psychology 76,* 219-224.

HEIN, A., & Held, R. (1967). Dissociation of the visual placing response into elicited and guided components. *Science, 158,* 390-391.

HIRSCHEL, A., Pehoski, C., & Coryell, J. (1990). Environmental support and the development of grasp in infants. *American Journal of Occupational Therapy, 44,* 721-727.

HOFSTEN, C. von. (1979). Development of visually directed reaching: The approach phase. *Journal of Human Movement Studies, 5,* 160-178.

HOFSTEN, C. von. (1982). Eye-hand coordination in the newborn. *Developmental Psychology, 18,* 450-461.

HOFSTEN, C. von. (1984). Developmental changes in the organization of prereaching movements. *Developmental Psychology, 20,* 378-388.

HONZIK, M. (1962). *The mental and motor test performance of infants diagnosed or suspected of brain injury.* Unpublished manuscript.

HONZIK, M. (1976). Value and limitations of infant tests: An overview. In M. Lewis (Ed.), *Origins of intelligence: Infancy and early childhood.* New York: Plenum.

HOPKINS, B., & Westra, T. (1989). Maternal expectations of their infants' development: Some cultural differences. *Developmental Medicine and Child Neurology, 31,* 384-390.

HOROWITZ, F. D., Aleksandrowicz, M., Ashton, L. J., Tims, S., McCluskey, K., Culp, R., & Gallas, H. (1973, March). *American and Uruguayan infants: Reliabilities, maternal drug histories and population difference using the Brazelton scale.* Paper presented at the biennial meeting of the Society

for Research in Child Development, Philadelphia.

HOROWITZ, F. D., Ashton, J., Culp, R., Gaddis, E., Levin, S., & Reichmann, B. (1977). The effect of obstetrical medication on the behavior of Israeli newborns and some comparisons with American and Uruguayan infants. *Child Development, 48,* 1607-1623.

HOROWITZ, F. D., & Brazelton, T. B., (1973). Research with the Brazelton Neonatal Scale. In T. B. Brazelton (Ed.), *Neonatal Behavioral Assessment Scale* (National Spastics Society Monograph). Philadelphia: J. B. Lippincott.

HOROWITZ, F. D., Self, P. A., Paden, L. Y., Culp, R., Boyd, E., & Mann, M. E. (1971, April). *Newborn and four-week retests on normative population using the Brazelton Newborn Assessment Procedure.* Paper presented at the biennial meeting of the Society for Research in Child Development, Minneapolis.

HOROWITZ, F. D., Sullivan, J. W., & Linn, P. (1978). Stability and instability in the newborn infant: The quest for elusive threads. In A. J. Sameroff (Ed.), Organization and stability of newborn behavior: A commentary on the Brazelton Neonatal Assessment Scale. *Monographs of the Society for Research in Child Development, 43*(5-6, Serial No. 177).

HRNCIR, E. J., Speller, G. M., & West, M. (1985). What are we testing? *Developmental Psychology, 21,* 226-232.

ILLINGWORTH, R. S. (1960). *The development of the infant and young child: Normal and abnormal.* London: Livingston.

IRETON, H., Thwing, E., & Currier, S. K. (1975). Minnesota Child Development Inventory. *Journal of Pediatric Psychology, 3,* 15-19.

JACKSON, E., Campos, J., & Fischer, K. (1978). The question of decalage between object permanence and person permanence. *Developmental Psychology, 14,* 1-10.

JACOBSON, J. L., Fein, G. G., Jacobson, S. W., & Schwartz, P. M. (1984). Factors and clusters for the Brazelton Scale: An investigation of the dimensions of neonatal behavior. *Developmental Psychology, 20,* 339-353.

JENSEN, A. (1973). *Educability and group differences.* London: Methuen.

KAMM, K., & Thelen, E. (1989, April). *Sitting to quadruped: A developmental profile.* Paper presented at the Society for Research in Child Development, Kansas City, MO.

KANGAS, J., Butler, B. V., &. Goffeney, B. (1966, March). *Relationship between preschool intelligence, maternal intelligence, and infant behavior.* Paper presented at the Second Scientific Session Collaborative Study on Cerebral Palsy, Mental Retardation, and Other Neurological and Sensory Disorders of Infancy and Childhood (U.S. Department of Health, Education and Welfare), Washington, DC.

KATZ, V. (1970). *The relationship between auditory stimulation and the development behavior of the premature infant.* Unpublished doctoral dissertation, New York University.

KAYE, K. (1978). Discriminating among normal infants by multivariate analysis of Brazelton scores: Lumping and smoothing. *Monographs of the Society for Research in Child Development, 43*(Serial No. 177).

KITE, E. S. (1916). *The development of intelligence in children.* Baltimore: Williams & Wilkins.

KNOBLOCK, H., & Pasamanick, B. (1960). An evaluation of the consistency and predictive value of the 40-week Gesell Development Schedule. *Psychiatric Research Reports, 13,* 10-31.

KNOBLOCK, H., & Pasamanick, B. (1975). *Gesell and Amatruda's developmental diagnosis* (3rd ed., rev.). Hagerstown,

MD: Harper & Row.

KOHEN-RAZ, R. (1967). Scalogram analyses of some developmental sequences of infant behavior as measured by the Bayley Infant Scale of Mental Development. *Genetic Psychology Monographs, 76*, 3-22.

KOPP, C. B. (1974). Fine motor abilities of infants. *Developmental Medicine and Child Neurology, 16*, 629-636.

KOPP, C. B., Sigman, M., Parmelee, A. H., & Jeffrey W. E. (1975). Neurological organization and visual fixation in infants at 40 weeks conceptional age. *Developmental Psychobiology, 8*, 165-170.

KORNER, A. F. (1990). Infant stimulation: Issues of theory and research. *Clinics in Perinatology, 14*, 173-184.

KORNER, A. F., Brown, B. W., Dimiceli, S., Forrest, T., Stevenson, D. K., Lane, N. M., Constantinou, J., & Thom, V. (1989). Stable individual differences in developmentally changing preterm infants: A replicated study. *Child Development, 60*, 502-513.

KORNER, A. F., Brown, B. W., Jr., Reade, E. P., Stevenson, D. K., Fernbach, S. A., & Thom, V. A. (1988). State behavior of preterm infants as a function of development, individual and sex differences. *Infant Behavior and Development, 11*, 111-124.

KORNER, A. F., Constantinou, J., Dimiceli, S., Brown, B. W., & Thom, V. A. (1991, October). Establishing the reliability and developmental validity of a neurobehavioral assessment for preterm infants: A methodological process. *Child Development, 62*.

KORNER, A. F., Kraemer, H. C., Reade, E. P., Forrest, T., & Dimiceli, S. (1987). A methodological approach to developing an assessment procedure for testing the neurobehavioral maturity of preterm infants. *Child Development, 58*, 1478-1487.

KORNER, A. F., & Thom, V. A. (1991). *Neurobehavioral assessment of the preterm infant.* Orlando, FL: Harcourt Brace Jovanovich.

KUHLMAN, F. (1912). A revision of the Binet-Simon system for measuring the intelligence of children. *Journal of Psycho-Asthenics* (Monograph Suppl.).

LANCIONE, E., Horowitz, F. D., & Sullivan, J. W. (1980). The NBAS-K: I. A study of its stability and structure over the first month of life. *Infant Behavior and Development, 3*, 341-359.

LASKY, R. E., Klein, R. E., Yarbrough, C., Engle, P. L., Lechtig, A., & Martorell, R. (1981). The relationship between physical growth and infant behavioral development in rural Guatemala. *Child Development, 52*, 219-226.

LASKY, R. E., Klein, R. E., Yarbrough, C., & Kallio K. D. (1981). The predictive validity of infant assessments in rural Guatemala. *Child Development, 52*, 847-856.

LASKY, R. E., Tyson, J. E., Rosenfeld, C. R., Priest, M., Krasinski, D., Hartwell, S., & Gant, N. F. (1983). Principal component analyses of the Bayley Scales of Infant Development for a sample of high-risk infants and their controls. *Merrill-Palmer Quarterly, 29*, 25-32.

LINN, P. L., & Horowitz, F. D. (1983). The relationship between infant individual differences and mother-infant interaction during the neonatal period. *Infant Behavior and Development, 6*, 415-428.

LOCKMAN, J. J., Ashmead, D. H., & Bushnell, E. W. (1984). The development of anticipatory hand orientation during infancy. *Journal of Experimental Child Psychology, 37*, 176-186.

LORENZ, K. Z. (1971). Gestalt perception as a source of scientific knowledge. In K. Z. Lorenz (Ed.), *Studies in animal and human behavior* (Vol. 2, pp. 281-322). Cambridge, MA: Harvard University Press.

MacRAE, J. M. (1955). Retests of children given mental tests as infants. *Journal of Genetic Psychology, 87*, 111-119.

MATHENY, A. (1980). Bayley's Infant Behavior Record: Behavioral components and twin analyses. *Child Development, 51*, 1157-1167.

McDONNELL, P. M. (1975). The development of visually guided reaching. *Perception and Psychophysics, 19*, 181-185.

McGRAW, M. B. (1935). *Growth: A study of Johnny and Jimmy.* New York: Appleton.

McGRAW, M. B. (1977, March). *Theories and techniques of child development research during the 1930s.* Invited address at the biennial meeting of the Society for Research in Child Development, New Orleans.

McNAY, M. B. (1988). Fetal movements. *Developmental Medicine and Child Neurology, 30*, 821-828.

MENKES, J. H. (1984). Malformations of the central nervous system. In M. E. Avery & H. W. Taeusch, Jr. (Eds.), *Schaffer's diseases of the newborn* (5th ed.). Philadelphia: W. B. Saunders.

MITCHELL, S. K., Abbs, M., & Barnard, K. (1977, August). *Intercorrelations between Brazelton Scale scores, perinatal indices, and early behavior.* Paper presented at the annual meeting of the American Psychological Association, San Francisco.

National Center for Health Statistics. (1976). [Growth charts.] *Monthly Vital Statistics Report, 25*(3, Suppl. HRA).

NEAL, M. V. (1968). Vestibular stimulation and developmental behavior of the small premature infant. *Nursing Research Report, 3*, 1, 3-5.

NEUHAUSER, G. (1975). Methods of assessing and recording motor skills and movement patterns. *Developmental Medicine and Child Neurology, 17*, 369-386.

OSOFSKY, J. D. (1976). Neonatal characteristics and mother-infant interaction in two observational situations. *Child Development, 47*, 1138-1147.

OSOFSKY, J. D., & Danzger, B. (1974). Relationships between neonatal characteristics and mother-infant interaction. *Developmental Psychology, 10*, 124-30.

OWEN, G. M., Kram, K. M., Garry, P. J., Lower, L. E., & Lubin, A. H. (1974). A study of status of preschool children in the United States. *Pediatrics, 53*(Part II, Suppl.), 597-646.

PALMER, C. F. (1989). The discriminating nature of infants' exploratory actions. *Developmental Psychology, 25*, 885-893.

PARMELEE, A. H., Jr. (1962). European neurological studies of the newborn. *Child Development, 33*, 69- 180.

PARMELEE, A. H., Jr. (1974). *Newborn neurological examination.* Unpublished manuscript.

PEIPER, A. (1963). *Cerebral function in infancy and childhood* (3rd ed., H. Nagler & B. Nagler, Trans.). New York: Consultants Bureau Enterprises. (Original work published 1961)

PIAGET, J. (1952). *The origin of intelligence in children.* New York: W. W. Norton.

PICK, H. L., Jr. (1989). Motor development: The control of action. *Developmental Psychology, 25*, 867-870.

PIPER, M. C., Byrne, P. J., Darrah, J., & Watt, M. J. (1989). Gross and fine motor development of preterm infants at eight and 12 months of age. *Developmental Medicine and Child Neurology, 31*, 591-597.

PLOOF, D. (1976, April). *The reciprocal effects of maternal perceptions and infant characteristics in the early mother-infant interaction.* Paper presented at the meeting of the Eastern

Psychological Association, New York.

PRECHTL, H. F. R. (1965). Prognostic value of neurological signs in the newborn infant. *Proceedings of the Royal Society of Medicine, 58*(3).

PRECHTL, H. F. R. (1974). The behavioral states of the newborn infant: A review. *Brain Research, 76,* 185-212.

PRECHTL, H. F. R. (1977). *The neurological examination of the full-term newborn infant* (2nd ed., rev.). London: Heinemann.

PRECHTL, H. F. R. (1982). Assessment methods for the newborn infant: A critical evaluation. In P. Straton (Ed.), *Psychobiology of the human newborn.* New York: John Wiley.

PRECHTL, H. F. R. (1990). Qualitative changes of spontaneous movements in fetus and preterm infant are a marker of neurological dysfunction. *Early Human Development, 23,* 151-158.

PRECHTL, H. F. R., & Beintema, D. J. (1964). *The neurological examination of the full-term infant* (Clinics in Developmental Medicine, No. 12). London: Heinemann.

PRECHTL, H. F. R., & Dijkstra, J. (1960). Neurological diagnosis of cerebral injury in the newborn. In B. S. ten Berge (Ed.), *Prenatal care.* Groningen: Noordhoff.

PRECHTL, H. F. R., & Nolte, R. (1984). Motor behavior of preterm infants. In H. F. R. Prechtl (Ed.), *Continuity of neural functions from prenatal to postnatal life* (Clinics in Developmental Medicine, No. 94) (pp. 79-92). Oxford: Basil Blackwell.

PROVINE, R. R., & Westerman, J. A. (1979). Crossing the midline: Limits of early eye-hand behavior. *Child Development, 50,* 437-441.

QUETELET, L. A. J. (1835). *Sur l'homme et le developpement de ses facultes: un essai de physique sociale* [About man and the development of his faculties: An essay on social physique]. Paris: Bachdier.

REICH, J. N., Holmes, D. L., Slaymaker, F. L., Lauesen, B. F., & Gyurke, J. S. (1984, April). *Infant assessments as predictors of 3-year IQ.* Paper presented at the International Conference on Infant Studies, New York.

RICHARDSON, G. A., Day, N. L., & Taylor, P. M. (1989). The effect of prenatal alcohol, marijuana, and tobacco exposure on neonatal behavior. *Infant Behavior and Development, 12,* 199-209.

RISHOLM-MOTHANDER, P. (1989). Predictions of developmental patterns during infancy: Assessments of children 0-1 years. *Scandinavian Journal of Psychology, 30,* 161-167.

ROCHAT, P. (1987). Mouthing and grasping in n: Evidence for the early detection of what hard and soft substances afford for action. *Infant Behavior and Development, 10,* 435-449.

ROCHAT, P. (1989). Object manipulation and exploration in 2- to 5-month-old infants. *Developmental Psychology, 25,* 871-884.

ROCHAT, P., & Senders, S. J. (1990, April). *Sitting and reaching in infancy.* Introduction to the symposium Posture and Action in Infancy, presented at the International Conference on Infant Studies, Montreal.

ROCHAT, P., & Senders, S. J. (in press). Active touch in infancy: Action systems in development. In M. J. Weiss & P. R. Zelazo (Eds.), *Biological constraints and the influence of experience.* Norwood, NJ: Ablex.

ROCHAT, P., & Stacy, M. (1989, April). *Reaching in various postures by 6- and 8-month-old infants: The development on monomanual grasp.* Paper presented at the meeting of the Society for Research in Child Development, Kansas City, MO.

ROCHE, A. F. (1979). Secular trends in human growth, malnutrition, and development. *Monographs of the Society for Research in Child Development, 44*(Serial No. 179).

ROSENBLITH, J. F. (1961a). *Manual for behavioral examination of the neonate.* Manuscript published privately by Brown University. (Available from the author)

ROSENBLITH, J. F. (1961b). The modified Graham behavior test for neonates: Test-retest reliability, normative data, and hypotheses for future work. *Biologia Neonatorum, 3,* 174-192.

ROSENBLITH, J. F. (1973). Prognostic value of neonatal behavioral tests. *Early Child Development and Care, 3,* 31-50.

ROSENBLITH, J. F. (1974). Relations between neonatal behaviors and those at 8 months. *Developmental Psychology, 10,* 779-792.

ROSENBLITH, J. F. (1979a). The Graham/Rosenblith behavioral examination for newborns: Prognostic values and procedural issues. In J. Osofsky (Ed.), *Handbook of infant development.* New York: John Wiley.

ROSENBLITH, J. F. (1979b, June). *Relations between behaviors in the newborn period and intellectual achievement and IQ at 7 years of age.* Paper presented at the International Society for the Study of Behavioral Development, Lund, Sweden.

ROSENBLITH, J. F., & Anderson, R. B. (1968). Prognostic significance of discrepancies in muscle tonus. *Developmental Medicine and Child Neurology, 10,* 322-330.

ROSENBLITH, J. F., Anderson, R. B., & Denhoff, E. (1970). Hypersensitivity to light, muscle tonus discrepancies: A follow-up report. *Biology of the Neonate, 15,* 217-228

ROSENBLITH, J. F., & Lipsitt, L. P. (1959). Interscorer agreement for the Graham Behavior Test for Neonates. *Journal of Pediatrics, 54,* 200-205.

RUBIN, R. A., & Balow, B. (1980). Infant neurological normalities as indicators of cognitive impairment. *Developmental Medicine and Child Neurology, 22,* 336-343.

RUFF, H. S., & Halton, A. (1978). Is there directed reaching in the human neonate? *Developmental Psychology, 14,* 425-426.

SAINT-ANNE DARGASSIES, S. (1972). Neurodevelopmental symptoms during the first year of life. *Developmental Medicine and Child Neurology, 14,* 235-246.

SAINT-ANNE DARGASSIES, S. (1977a). Neuro-developmental symptoms during the first year of life: Part 1. Essential landmarks for each rey-age. Part II. Practical examples and the application of this assessment method to the abnormal infant (analytical charts, synthetic evolutive profiles). *Developmental Medicine and Child Neurology, 19,* 462-478.

SAINT-ANNE DARGASSIES, S. (1977b). *Neurological development in the full term and premature neonate.* Amsterdam: Elsevier. (Original work published 1974)

SAINT-ANNE DARGASSIES, S. (1983). Developmental neurology from the fetus to the infant: Some French works. In W. Hartup (Ed.), *Review of child development research* (Vol. 6). Chicago: University of Chicago Press.

ST. CLAIR, K. L. (1978). Neonatal assessment procedures: A historical review. *Child Development, 49,* 280-292.

SAMEROFF, A. J., Krafchuk, E. E., & Bakow, H. A. (1978). Issues in grouping items from the Neonatal Behavioral Assessment Scale. In A. J. Sameroff (Ed.), *Organization and stability of newborn behavior: A commentary on the Brazelton Neonatal Assessment Scale. Monographs of the Society for Research in Child Development, 43*(5-6, Serial No. 177).

SAYLOR, C. F., & Brandt, B. J. (1986). The Minnesota Child Development Inventory: A valid maternal-report form for assessing development in infancy. *Developmental and Behavioral Pediatrics, 7,* 308-313.

SCIARILLO, W. G., Brown, M. M., Robinson, N. M., Bennett, F. C., & Sells, C. J. (1986). Effectiveness of the Denver Developmental Screening Test with biologically vulnerable infants. *Journal of Developmental and Behavioral Pediatrics, 7,* 77-83.

SEPKOSKI, C., Corwin, M., Lourie, A., & Golub, H. (1990, April). *Predicting developmental outcome from changes in NBAS performance of preterm infants.* Paper presented at the meeting of the International Society for Infant Studies, Montreal.

SHAPIRO, B. K., Palmer, F. B., Antell, S. E., Bilker, S., Ross, A., & Capute, A. J. (1989). Giftedness: Can it be predicted in infancy? *Clinical Pediatrics* (Philadelphia), *28,* 205-209.

SHIRLEY, M. M. (1931). *The first two years: A study of twenty-five babies: Vol. 1. Postural and locomotor development.* Minneapolis: University of Minnesota Press.

SIEGEL, L. S. (1981). Infant tests as predictors of cognitive and language development at two years. *Child Development, 52,* 545-557.

SIGMAN, M., Kopp, C. B., Littman, B., & Parmelee, A. H. (1975, April). *Infant visual attentiveness in relation to birth condition.* Paper presented at the biennial meeting of the Society for Research in Child Development, Denver.

SIGMAN, M., Kopp, C. B., Parmelee, A. N., & Jeffrey, W. E. (1973). Visual attention and neurological organization in neonates. *Child Development, 44,* 461-466.

SOLOMONS, G., & Solomons, H. G. (1975). Motor development in Yucatecan infants. *Developmental Medicine and Child Neurology, 17,* 41-46.

SONNANDER, K. (1987). Parental developmental assessment of 18-month-old children: Reliability and predictive value. *Developmental Medicine and Child Neurology, 29,* 351-362.

SOSTEK, A. M., & Anders, T. F. (1977). Relationships among the Brazelton Neonatal Scales, and early temperament. *Child Development, 48,* 320-323.

SOSTEK, A. M., Brackbill, Y., Broman, S. H., & Rosenblith, J. F. (1976). *Effects of barbiturates on newborn behavior: Short and long term effects on the offspring.* Contribution to a symposium on maternal medication presented at the annual meeting of the American Psychological Association, Washington, DC.

STERN, W. (1924). *Psychology of early childhood: Up to the sixth year of age* (3rd ed., rev., A. Barwell, Trans.). New York: Holt. (Original work published 1914)

STOFFREGEN, T. A., Schmuckler, M. A., & Gibson, E. J. (1987). Use of central and peripheral optical flow in stance and locomotion in young walkers. *Perception, 16,* 113-119.

STRAUSS, M. E., & Rourke, D. L. (1978). A multivariate analysis of the Neonatal Behavioral Assessment Scale in several samples. In A. J. Sameroff (Ed.), Organization and stability of newborn behavior: A commentary on the Brazelton Neonatal Behavioral Assessment Scale. *Monographs of the Society for Research in Child Development, 43*(5-6, Serial No. 177).

STREISSGUTH, A. P., & Barr, H. M. (1977, August). *Neonatal Brazelton assessment and relationship to maternal alcohol use.* Paper presented at the annual meeting of the American Psychological Association, San Francisco.

STUART, H. C., & Meredith, H. V. (1946). Use of body measurements in school health programs. *American Journal of Public Health, 36,* 1365-1386.

STUTSMAN, R. (1931). *Mental measurement of preschool children with a guide for the administration of the Merrill-Palmer Scale of Mental Tests.* Yonkers-on-Hudson, NY: World.

SUPER, C. M. (1976). Environmental effects on motor development. *Developmental Medicine and Child Neurology, 18,* 561-567.

TANNER, J. M. (1962). *Growth at adolescence* (2nd ed.). Oxford: Basil Blackwell.

TANNER, J. M. (1970). Physical growth. In P. H. Mussen (Ed.), *Carmichael's manual of child psychology* (Vol. 1). New York: John Wiley.

TANNER, J. M. (1978). *Foetus into man.* Cambridge MA: Harvard University Press.

TANNER, J. M., Healy, M. J. R., Lockhart, R. D., MacKenzie, J. D., & Whitehouse, R. H. (1956). Aberdeen growth study: I. The prediction of adult body measurement from measurements taken each year from birth to 5 years. *Archives of Diseases in Childhood, 31,* 372-381.

TANNER, J. M., & Thomson, A. M. (1970). Standards for birth weight at gestation periods from 32 to 42 weeks allowing for maternal height and weight. *Archives of Diseases in Childhood, 45,* 566-569.

TANNER, J. M., Whitehouse, R. H., Marshall, W. A. Healy, M. J., & Goldstein, N. (1975). *Assessment of skeletal maturity and prediction of adult height.* London: Academic.

TERMAN, L. M., & Merrill, M. A. (1937). *Measuring intelligence.* Cambridge, MA: Houghton Mifflin.

TERMAN, L. M., & Merrill, M. A. (1960). *Stanford-Binet Intelligence Scale.* Cambridge, MA: Houghton Mifflin.

THELEN, E. (1984). Learning to walk: Ecological demands and phylogenetic constraints. In L. P. Lipsitt (Ed.), *Advances in infancy research* (Vol. 3, pp. 213-250). Norwood, NJ: Ablex.

THELEN, E. (1985). Developmental origins of motor coordination: Leg movements in human infants. *Developmental Psychobiology, 18,* 1-22.

THELEN, E. (1986). Treadmill-elicited stepping in seven-month-old infants. *Child Development, 57,* 1498-1506.

THELEN, E. (1989). The (re)discovery of motor development: Learning new things from an old field. *Developmental Psychology, 25,* 946-949.

THELEN, E., & Cooke, D. W. (1987). Relationship between newborn stepping and later walking: A new interpretation. *Developmental Medicine and Child Neurology, 29,* 380-393.

THELEN, E., & Fisher, D. M. (1982). Newborn stepping: an explanation for a "disappearing reflex." *Developmental Psychology, 18,* 760-775.

THELEN, E., Fisher, D. M., & Ridley-Johnson, R. (1984). The relationship between physical growth and a newborn reflex. *Infant Behavior and Development, 7,* 479-493.

THELEN, E., Fisher, D. M., Ridley-Johnson, R., & Griffin, N. (1982). The effects of body build and arousal on newborn stepping. *Developmental Psychobiology, 15,* 447-453.

THELEN, E., Skala, K. D., & Kelso, J. S. (1987). The dynamic nature of early coordination: Evidence from bilateral leg movements in young infants. *Developmental Psychology, 23,* 179-186.

THELEN, E., Ulrich, B. D., & Niles, D. (1987). Bilateral coordination in human infants: Stepping on a split-belt treadmill. *Journal of Experimental Psychology, Human Perception and Performance, 13,* 405-410.

THOMAN, E. B., & Glazier, R. (1987). Computer scoring of motility patterns for states of sleep and wakefulness: Human infants. *Sleep, 10,* 122-129.

THOMAN, E. B., & Whitney, M. (1989). Sleep states of infants monitored in the home: Individual differences, developmental trends, and origins of diurnal cyclicity. *Infant Behavior and Development, 12,* 59-75.

THOMAS, H. (1970). Psychological assessment instruments for use with human infants. *Merrill-Palmer Quarterly, 16,* 179-223.

TREVARTHEN, C. (1974). The psychobiology of speech development. In E. Lennenberg (Ed.), Language and brain: Developmental aspects [Special issue]. *Neurosciences Research Program Bulletin, 12,* 570-585.

TRONICK, E., & Brazelton, T. B. (1975). Clinical uses of the Brazelton Neonatal Behavioral Assessment. In B. Friedlander, G. M. Sterritt, & G. E. Kirk (Eds.), *Exceptional infant* (Vol. 3). New York: Brunner/Mazel.

UZGIRIS, I. C., & Hunt, J. M. (1975a). *Assessment in infancy.* Champaign: University of Illinois Press.

UZGIRIS, I. C., & Hunt, J. M. (1975b). *Toward ordinal scales of psychological development in infancy.* Champaign: University of Illinois Press.

VAUGHN, B. E., Taraldson, B., Crichton, L., & Egeland, B. (1980). Relationships between neonatal behavioral organization and infant behavior during the first year of life. *Infant Behavior and Development, 3,* 47-66.

VISSER, G. H., Laurini, R. N., deVries, J. J., Bekedam, D. J., & Prechtl, H. F. (1985). Abnormal motor behavior in anencephalic fetuses. *Early Human Development, 12,* 173-182.

WACKER, D. (1980, September). *Diagnostic efficiency of the Denver Developmental Screening Test.* Paper presented at the annual meeting of the American Psychological Association, Montreal.

WALK, R. D., & Bond, E. K. (1971). The development of visually guided reaching in monkeys reared without sight of the hands. *Psychonomic Science, 23,* 115-116.

WARREN, N. (1972). African infant precocity. *Psychological Bulletin, 78,* 353-367.

WERNER, E. E. (1972). Infants around the world: Cross-cultural studies of psychomotor development from birth to two years. *Journal of Cross-Cultural Studies, 3,* 111-134.

WERNER, E. E., & Bayley, N. (1966). The reliability of Bayley's revised scale of mental and motor development during the first year of life. *Child Development, 37,* 39-50.

WERNER, E. E., Bierman, J. M., & French, F. E. (1971). *The children of Kauai: A longitudinal study from the prenatal period to age 10.* Honolulu: University of Hawaii Press.

WERNER, E. E., Honzik, M. P., & Smith, R. S. (1968). Prediction of intelligence and achievement at 10 years from 20 month pediatric and psychological examinations. *Child Development, 39,* 1063-1075.

WHITE, B. L. (1971). *Human infants: Experience and psychological development.* Englewood Cliffs, NJ: Prentice-Hall.

WHITE, B. L., Castle, P., & Held, R. (1964). Observations on the development of visually-directed reaching. *Child Development, 35,* 349-364.

WHITE, B. L., & Held, R. (1966). Plasticity of sensorimotor development in the human infant. In J. F. Rosenblith & W. Allinsmith (Eds.), *The causes of behavior: Readings in child development and educational psychology* (2nd ed). Boston: Allyn & Bacon.

WOROBEY, J. (1986). Neonatal stability and one-month behavior. *Infant Behavior and Development, 9,* 119-124.

WOROBEY, J. (1990). Behavioral assessment of the neonate. In J. Colombo & J. W. Fagan (Eds.), *Individual differences in infancy: Reliability, stability and prediction* (pp. 137-154). Hillsdale, NJ: Lawrence Erlbaum.

WOROBEY, J., & Blajda, V. M. (1989). Temperament ratings at two-weeks, two-months and one year: Differential stability of activity and emotionality. *Developmental Psychology, 25,* 257-263.

ZELAZO, P. R. (1983). The development of walking: New findings and old assumptions. *Journal of Motor Behavior, 15,* 99-137.

ZELAZO, P. R. (1984). "Learning to walk": Recognition of higher order influences? In L. P. Lipsitt (Ed.), *Advances in infancy research* (Vol. 3, pp. 213-250). Norwood, NJ: Ablex.

ZELAZO, P. R., Zelazo, N. A., & Kolb, S. (1972). "Walking" in the newborn. *Science, 176,* 14-15.

Chapter 9

The Basic Mechanisms

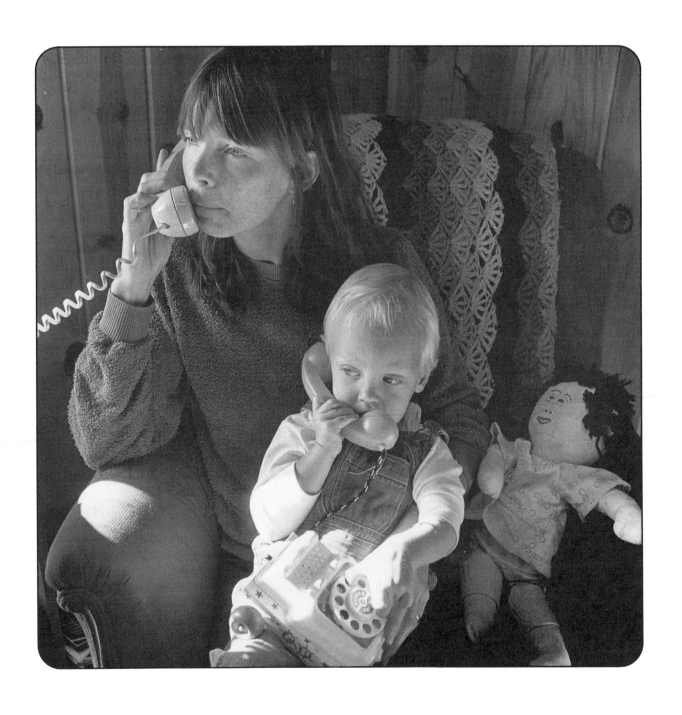

Most topics in infant development involve learning in the broad sense or relatively permanent changes in behavior as a result of environmental events. This chapter will discuss research that attempts to determine the extent to which young babies are able to learn about and remember their world. Research in this area has focused primarily on when babies can first use particular mechanisms to acquire knowledge about the world. Researchers have explored the onset in infants of some of the processes that operate in learning and memory in older humans and in many other species. These processes are habituation, conditioning, imitation, and memory.

Habituation of the Orienting Response

All mammals have a very general response to a change in stimulation; this is called the **orienting response (OR)**, and it reflects attention to the stimulus. Whenever stimulation changes—whether from no stimulation to stimulation (stimulus onset), from stimulation to no stimulation (stimulus offset), or from one kind of stimulation to another—and regardless of whether the level of background stimulation is high or low, we orient to the change. The OR can take the forms of such responses as looking, listening, a slower heart rate, or changed breathing. The OR is the most general mechanism of attention and has even been found in anencephalics (Graham et al., 1978).

If the stimulus continues unchanged for a while, we gradually stop paying attention to it. This decrease in response is called habituation, and it must be distinguished from sensory adaptation or fatigue or from a change in arousal level. Habituation is a primitive kind of learning based on exposure, and it implies a variety of perceptual and cognitive mechanisms. If, after habituation occurs to one stimulus, a new one is presented, orienting again occurs; this renewed OR to a newly changed stimulus is called dishabituation (because it reverses the previous habituation). In evolutionary terms, the orienting response is a very adaptive characteristic, for it causes us to attend to any change in the world around us. We can then investigate the cause of the change and respond appropriately.

Many criteria have been used to measure the OR. Some, such as evoked cortical potentials, measured by electrophysiological apparatus, and cortisol responses, measured biochemically, require relatively elaborate equipment. Others, such as heart and respiration rates, are easily measured internal responses. Still others, such as the length of time babies look at a stimulus or cease to turn their heads toward a stimulus, are exter-

nally observable, as is resuming sucking (babies often stop sucking when they orient to a change in stimulation and gradually resume as they habituate). Habituation as measured by one of these indices does not necessarily equate with habituation as measured by a different one.

USE IN RESEARCH

Habituation of the OR is one of the most widely used experimental techniques in infant research today. It is of interest for its own sake, in the study of perception, as a possible index of cognitive functioning, and also to test memory (discussed later in the chapter). But the habituation paradigm requires careful attention to methodology.

First, each dependent variable used to index habituation has its own set of measurement problems that must be addressed. Both heart rate (HR) and its change are related to behavioral state. The amount of change in heart rate depends in part on its rate prior to the presentation of the stimulus (Steinschneider et al., 1966). Heart rate also reflects movement. Movements such as startle responses or sucking may be triggered by the stimulus or may be mere random arm or leg movements; either way, they will change heart rate.

Second, the methodology used to study habituation makes a difference in the results. Prior to the introduction of the infant-control procedure (Horowitz et al., 1972), all procedures used were those in which the experimenter determined a fixed number of trials; their duration and the interval between exposures (or the number of trials) were allowed to vary until a fixed level of decrease in responding was reached. This method had serious flaws. Infants did not necessarily have equal "study" time, since one did not know whether the infant was really looking during all of a trial. The infant-control procedure is designed to make sure the infant is looking toward where the stimulus will appear before it is shown, and the stimulus is turned off when the infant no longer looks. This enables individual differences to be assessed in terms of that infant's actual looking time (using percentages).

The two methods produce very different amounts of infant cooperation. In the original infant-controlled habituation study (Horowitz et al., 1972), babies 3 to 14 weeks of age cried and fussed less, so that experimenters were able to complete 93% of the testing sessions (compared with 70% completions in the fixed-presentation mode), and subject loss was only 28% (versus 40%). In addition, babies often looked longer at the stimulus than most researchers would have believed. The longest single look was 1,073 seconds (more than 17 minutes) and looks of greater than 2 minutes' duration were common. Subsequent research suggests that infants in the first several months of life can process stimuli much better than had previously been thought, but can do so only after much longer inspection times than had often been offered (e.g., Slater et al., 1984; see also the description of face perception in Chapter 7).

Third, in order to rule out the possibility that a response decrement might actually be due to fatigue of sensory receptor cells or to fatigue in the motor system, or even to changes in the baby's state, dishabituation must be determined even when, as in memory studies, the focus is on habituation. If fatigue explained habituation, one should not find dishabituation.

Inasmuch as visual habituation is most studied, most of the discussion presented here centers on it.

DEVELOPMENT OF THE ORIENTING RESPONSE AND ITS HABITUATION

Early researchers found that the OR, measured by changes in heart rate, seemed to develop at around 2 months of age (Graham & Clifton, 1966; Lipton et al., 1966). Younger babies' heart rates speeded up when they were presented with a novel stimulus, whereas the HRs of babies 2 months and older slowed down, the typical OR response at all later ages. Many subsequent studies have been limited to infants 3 months old or older, on the assumption that the HR data meant that younger infants do not have ORs. We now know that newborns and even fetuses exhibit ORs, although under more circumscribed conditions than do older infants or adults. To exhibit ORs, both newborns and older infants must be alert, and must have been so for more than a few minutes. Resumption of sucking can serve as a measure of habituation in very young infants, but if infants are sucking they do not exhibit HR deceleration, another possible index of the OR. In general, HR deceleration appears not to be a good measure to use very early: Only a few studies have found it, and it occurs only in response to pulsed, not continuous, sounds. (For reviews of this research, see Berg & Berg, 1979; Von Bargen, 1983.)

Habituation of head turning to sound can be found neonatally. Inasmuch as a new, softer sound will produce dishabituation, receptor adaptation or fatigue cannot be the explanation for the habituation (Tarquinio et al., 1990). Habituation and dishabituation have been demonstrated in newborns for movements of eyes, mouth, head, and arms (Kisilevsky & Muir, 1984). Habituation of looking responses to visual

stimuli is easily found with older infants, but is more difficult to obtain with younger ones (see the review in Werner & Perlmutter, 1979). Some earlier inconsistencies have been resolved by identifying circumstances under which habituation can be obtained (Slater et al., 1984). In general, it appears easier to obtain habituation in infants under 2 months of age if the exposure depends on infant responses or if contingent procedures are used for stimulus presentation.

It is possible to obtain habituation in the 28- to 37-week-old fetus without any contingency. Ultrasound was used to assess movement responses of the fetus to a vibratory stimulus applied to the mother's abdomen (Madison et al., 1986). All fetuses responded to the stimulus, and all but one showed habituation within 40 trials (mean 18 or 22 trials, depending on the frequency of the vibration). Furthermore, the number of trials needed was not related to the age of the fetus.

DOES THE ORIENTING RESPONSE REFLECT CORTICAL FUNCTION?

The OR generated a great deal of interest because Sokolov (1963) hypothesized that it represented the cortical processing of information. Three important implications of this hypothesis are as follows: (a) It would make the OR an important mechanism by which mammals learn about the world; (b) study of the OR could yield information about the development of cortical functioning in newborns; and, more generally, (c) the OR might serve as a marker variable for cortical dysfunction in infants. Others have argued that the OR reflects the operation of the autonomic nervous system (ANS) (Lipton et al., 1966). This disagreement is still not resolved. Although the current emphasis is primarily on the CNS and cognitive aspects of the OR and its habituation/dishabituation, there is increasing work being done on the relation of autonomic system functioning to infant behaviors, including those of orienting and habituation.

One way to study whether the OR is cortical or autonomic is to see in what states it occurs. Inasmuch as it occurs primarily in awake, alert states, which are optimal for functioning of the central nervous system, one might conclude that it is CNS mediated, but what about its occurrence in an anencephalic infant (a baby lacking a cerebral cortex)? Habituation of the OR by newborns has been shown during sleep (Field et al., 1979; Kisilevsky & Muir, 1984), which is the optimal state for autonomic nervous system functioning, because metabolic demands are minimal. However, if we accept Maurer and Maurer's (1988) contention that young babies are conscious during sleep, the CNS is not ruled out as the mediator. Variations in the type of stimulation affect the OR and do so increasingly with age, as would be expected for a cortical, but not for an autonomic, function (Berg & Berg, 1979).

STABILITY OF THE OR AND HABITUATION/DISHABITUATION BEHAVIORS

In view of the current interest in these behaviors as markers for cognitive processes, one has to ask whether they are characteristic of the individual; that is, are the infants who are slow or fast to habituate on one day also slow or fast a day, week, or month later? If a test is designed to predict future performance, we must know whether it has reliability. Both specific measures of habituation/dishabituation and patterns of habituation have been examined for stability. The patterns are addressed first in this discussion.

Different researchers have categorized infants in different ways: into slow and fast to habituate (DeLoache, 1976); into fast, who increased their responses before habituating, and idiosyncratic (McCall, 1979); and, most recently, into those who show exponential decreases, those who decrease after first increasing, and those who fluctuate (Bornstein & Benasich, 1986). Bornstein and Benasich (1986) used infant-control procedures with 5-month-old infants and found 60% to be exponential decreasers, 30% first to increase, and 10% to fluctuate. The stimuli used (red geometric figures or color slides of female faces) affected this distribution somewhat, with more fluctuators in those habituated to geometric figures. (The importance of having stimuli appropriate to the ages studied complicates the problem of finding reliability across long time spans.) These patterns of responding were stable over a 10-day period for two-thirds of the infants, but *only* in the female face group. Other workers using faces as stimuli (but different infant age groups) have not found stability (Colombo, Mitchell, et al., 1987b). The basic facts of habituation were the same for infants in each pattern and for those exposed to both types of stimuli (Bornstein & Benasich, 1986). Infants recovered significantly when exposed to a stimulus from the other class and did not differ in the degree of recovery. These authors estimate the mean test-retest reliability of habituation across studies by several researchers to have an r of .44.

Different measures do not all behave alike. For example, in a study conducted by Pêcheux and Lécuyer (1983), 4-month-olds in an infant-controlled procedure showed reliability in looking time, but not in the number of trials required for habituation. The same

researchers later found stability in accumulated looking time between 3 and 5 or 5 and 8 months, but none across the total span (i.e., from 3 to 8 months) (Pêcheux & Lécuyer, 1989). Some reliability has been found from 3 to 9 months (Colombo, O'Brien, et al., 1987). But the fact that the greatest reliability over a 1- to 2-week period was at 4 and 9 months, with considerably less reliability at 3 and 7 months, lacks a rationale. Questions of what systems were evolving most rapidly at the different times or of differential attractiveness of the stimuli to infants of the different ages might be raised.

Of the 12 measures Colombo et al. examined, duration of fixation and magnitude of habituation were most stable, but only for 4-month-olds was there 33% of the variance in common between the testings. Dishabituation was not stable at any of the ages, a finding that needs to be better understood. The stability of duration of fixation and magnitude of habituation is further attested to by data on 3-year-olds (Colombo, Mitchell, et al., 1987a).

The Colombo group has suggested that durations of fixation variables, which are not central to traditional visual habituation models, may provide more understanding of processes that determine infant visual behavior (whether they turn out to be cognitive or motivational). However, this may be an artificial distinction, given that the fixation durations are part of the OR. In any event, long looking at a visual stimulus in infancy is related to poorer performance on preschool intelligence tests and IQ at 8 years (Sigman et al., 1986). This finding is not obvious to the layperson, who is apt to suppose that high attentiveness in infancy should be related to high intelligence.

One issue that has not been directly addressed in these studies is the role of the nature of the stimuli in controlling visual attention. E. J. Gibson (1988) has proposed that as new motor abilities or action capabilities unfold there should be shifts in attention to information relevant to the new abilities. Preliminary data confirming this possibility have been reported by Eppler et al. (1990).

Another issue that has not been addressed is that of whether we know anything about the characteristics of infants who fail to complete habituation tasks. Is it a question of random fluctuations in state? Or do they differ from those who do complete the task, thus limiting the generalizability of findings from those who do? The latter appears to be the case. Wachs and Smitherman (1985) found that at 11, 18, and 28 weeks, girls were less likely to complete habituation tasks, and those who failed to complete them were more likely to have been earlier rated by their mothers as fussy and unadaptable.

A final consideration about a possible fundamental aspect of orienting and habituation calls attention to work examining a dual process model of infant visual attention. According to this model, changes in response to repeated presentations of a stimulus reflect two processes: (a) the decremental process of habituation, and (b) an incremental process resulting from **sensitization** to a general state-dependent arousal or activation.[1] According to the dual hypothesis, dishabituation to the original, familiar stimulus should occur after dishabituation to a novel stimulus is followed by a re-presentation of the original stimulus. The novel stimulus should serve to sensitize, and hence energize the response to any subsequent stimulus; that is, it should enhance attention. Such visual dishabituation (called Thompson-Spencer dishabituation) has been demonstrated in 4-month-olds, and the role of timing of presentation of stimuli has been clearly shown (Kaplan & Werner, 1987). The elapsed time between the stimuli must not be too great, or the sensitization will have waned. Kaplan and Werner (1987) point out that sensitization may affect not only duration of fixation but the information processing that occurs during fixation (facilitation of associative learning, maintenance of attention). Further work studying this dual process model is called for.

In sum, it appears that while there is some continuity or test-retest reliability for measures of habituation and attention, it is hardly overwhelming, or of the order considered adequate for psychological tests.

ATTENTION MEASURES AS PREDICTORS OF INTELLECTUAL DEVELOPMENT

I noted in Chapter 6 that we would return to attention as a topic, because it is being used to predict later cognitive development. Indeed, it has even been called a test of infant intelligence.

Decrements in and recovery of attention (that is, habituation and dishabituation) in infancy show moderate but significant relations to measures of cognitive competence in later childhood. Decrements in the habituation paradigm reflect a situation in which stimuli are presented one at a time, sequentially. Recovery of attention (necessary to ensure that habituation rather than fatigue caused the decrement) can be defined as novelty preference. However, novelty preference is usually studied by presenting two stimuli simultane-

ously, after the infant has been familiarized to one of them. Response to novelty is determined by responses to stimuli shown one at a time after familiarization or habituation to one.

Overall, one can say that decrement and recovery of attention usually predict childhood intellectual outcomes better than infant tests, and that these predictions should improve if the infant measures are made more reliable. However, these measures fail to account for very much variance in later cognitive outcomes. These conclusions were reached by Bornstein and Sigman (1986), and they accurately represent my own current view as well.

Some Evidence

A number of researchers in the 1980s showed that patterns of attention in infancy seemed to reveal meaningful individual differences (e.g., Lewis & Brooks-Gunn, 1981; Caron et al., 1983, Rose & Wallace, 1985b). Also, the rate and amount of habituation in infancy were related to later intelligence in a number of studies (for example, Bornstein & Ruddy, 1984; Miller et al., 1980). Even fetal habituation was shown to be related to the Bayley MDI at 4 months (Madison et al., 1986). All of this led to the conclusion that speed and degree of visual processing in infancy might have some bearing on intellectual capacities in childhood.

Now let us turn to some of the findings in more detail. Cohen and Parmelee (1983) showed that premature infants at term date had measures of visual attention (a composite of duration of fixations, length of first fixation, and number of fixations) that significantly related to their IQ at age 5. This measure was more strongly related than any of their other risk indices. Sigman et al. (1986) found that specific attention measures were also related to IQ at age 8. However, the largest of the correlations was .42, indicating only 16% common variance, and significant correlations were as small as .27. Infants at term age, who continued to look at a stimulus shown for 1 minute and who looked repeatedly for a total exposure time of 1 minute at 4 months of age, performed less well on later IQ tests. The capacity to turn off attention seems to be especially important here. However, the results are not strong enough to justify their clinical use. In all events, the continuity found could stem from either cognitive or motivational/temperamental characteristics.

Novelty preference is found in 6- to 8-month-old infants, and has some stability over time (Rose & Feldman, 1987). Using three pairs of abstract forms

---

1. One is reminded of the fact that in some schemes, some infants were classified as increasing their looking time after the first presentation, then habituating, a behavior not dealt with by the dual hypothesis.

and three pairs of faces that differed markedly, these researchers showed that the stability over time was modest on any one pair of stimuli, but, summing across all six pairs, 7-month scores correlated .51 with 8-month scores (25% of variance shared). Some 60-70% (depending on the measure) of infants who showed novelty preferences at 6 months did so at 7 or 8 months. There was moderate stability in the exposure times needed to reach the predetermined amount of looking time (*r*s ranged from .24 to .42). These stability figures are very similar to those found by Bornstein for recovery to a novel dishabituation stimulus.

Fagan and Singer (1983) reviewed 25 studies and report a median *r* of .40 between novelty scores in the first months of life and later mental outcomes. Bornstein and Sigman (1986) report a median *r* of .46 between later mental outcome and infant measures of habituation, dishabituation, and response to novelty.

Further work is needed to assess the role of biological maturity in the finding of stability. Head circumference (physiological maturity) at birth of full-term infants has been related to attention and to greater response decrement to faces when the infants were 15 to 29 weeks old (Camp et al., 1990). This demands further exploration.

For prematures, novelty preference scores at 6 months correlated between .45 and .66 with measures of outcome over the period of 2 to 6 years in a study by Rose and Wallace (1985a). Visual recognition memory at 12 months was correlated with outcomes through 6 years (Rose & Wallace, 1985b). In new samples of full-term and preterm low-SES infants, visual scores at 7 months have been related to 3-year IQ (Rose et al., 1989). Measures were more strongly related to 3-, 4-, and 5-year IQ test scores than to earlier Bayley MDI scores, which are based more on sensorimotor performances. The relations between visual scores and 3- to 5-year IQs were higher for preterm than for term infants. For prematures the visual summary score, together with the Bayley MDI and maternal education, accounted for 52% of the variance in 1-year MDIs (35% in the 1½-year MDI), but vision score alone accounted for only 1% and 9% of the variance at the two ages. The 7-month MDI was most strongly related to the outcomes at ages 1 and 1½. From 2 years on, the 7-month visual summary score contributes unique variance, and the amount is substantially the same for both preterm and full-term infants (9-24% and 9-32%). Rose et al. (1989) conclude: "These results suggest that the processes involved in early recognition memory and attention are important

to later outcome. It is currently unclear, however, what these processes are and how they are related to IQ" (p. 573).

Bornstein and Sigman (1986) conclude that infant attention (measured by either decrements or recovery) should not to be considered a cognitive index without taking account of experimental considerations of stimulus, method, state, and subject populations. They consider statements such as "Habituation predicts IQ" or "Novelty preference predicts IQ better than habituation" to be meaningless, a conclusion with which I agree. At the same time, this is certainly a line of research that should be pursued, both to create more reliable measures and to look at relations to more specific aspects of cognitive functioning later in childhood, not just at IQ.

We turn now from learning of the primitive type evidenced by habituation to conditioning, a more traditional learning topic.

Conditioning

The big question that has intrigued researchers for many decades is, Are newborns equipped to learn immediately after birth, or do they develop learning abilities only at later ages? If they develop these abilities later, how much later? What kinds of things can newborns learn earliest and what sorts of learning must wait for later development? Researchers' orientations influence the methods they use to answer these questions. Learning psychologists have made a unique contribution, in that they have asked what the specific mechanisms are by which learning can occur. They have focused on infants' abilities to form new associations, either between stimuli and responses or between stimuli, rather than on their ability to make sense of the world (for example, to recognize faces or to categorize objects), which is in the domain of cognitive psychology. They have used the paradigms of classical and operant conditioning to ask the following questions:

(1) When (at what age) can classical conditioning beobtained? What kinds of unconditioned and conditioned stimuli are effective? What responses can be conditioned?

(2) When (at what age) can operant conditioning be obtained? What responses can be conditioned? What events can serve as reinforcers?

CLASSICAL CONDITIONING

Classical conditioning, developed by Pavlov early in this century, begins with a naturally occurring stimulus-response connection. The stimulus, an environmental event, **elicits** (brings forth or produces) a response from the organism. In infant studies, an innate stimulus-response connection, such as the rooting reflex (stroking the infant's cheek stimulates head turning), is typically used. This stimulus-response connection occurs before conditioning takes place, so it is called unconditioned. The stroking is the **unconditioned stimulus** (UCS) and the head turning is the **unconditioned response** (UCR). The purpose of classical conditioning is to train a new stimulus-response connection, the conditioned association. This is done by pairing a neutral stimulus (e.g., a buzzer) with the UCS. The neutral stimulus is called the **conditioned stimulus** (CS). The CS and UCS are repeatedly presented together, most often with the CS (buzzer) preceding the UCS (stroking). If classical conditioning occurs, the subject eventually responds to the CS alone.

In the rooting reflex example, after a number of trials in which the buzzer is sounded (CS) and the baby's cheek is stroked (UCS), the baby should turn its head when only the buzzer is sounded. This head-turning response is called the **conditioned response** (CR). Even though the UCR and CR are similar (both are head turning in this instance), subtle differences—in intensity or duration, for example—can be demonstrated, so they are given different names. The process of classical conditioning is diagrammed in Figure 9.1.

What is learned in classical conditioning is an association between two events: that the CS always signals the occurrence of the UCS. A further demonstration that the subjects have learned such an association is to reverse the process and break the association after it has been learned. This procedure, called **extinction**, occurs after initial testing for conditioning. The CS is presented alone again and again, and subjects gradually cease to make the CR. At that point their responses are said to have been extinguished.

Can Newborns Be Classically Conditioned?

The purpose of much of the research on classical conditioning in infancy is to discover whether newborns can learn associations that are new to them.

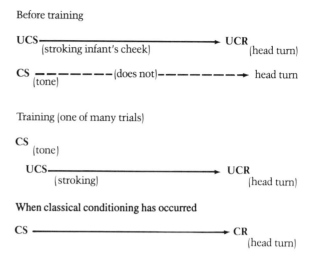

Figure 9.1. The course of classical conditioning. Before conditioning, infants make no association between the CS and the UCS-UCR sequence. After conditioning, the CS acts as a signal that the UCS will follow and hence triggers the CR.

There is a long history of attempts to demonstrate such conditioning in newborns, which is understandable because classical conditioning was the earliest form of learning demonstrated experimentally. In 1931, Marquis tried to condition newborns to suck a nipple in response to a buzzer. During each session a buzzer sounded for 5 seconds, followed by the insertion of the nipple of a milk bottle into the baby's mouth. Marquis found conditioning effects; that is, the babies learned to start sucking when the buzzer sounded. Later studies, however, demonstrated that such a result may really be due to other phenomena. This sort of apparent, artifactual conditioning is now called **pseudoconditioning**.

The first study to demonstrate the existence of pseudoconditioning was done by Wickens and Wickens (1940). Their UCS-UCR sequence was another newborn reflex: mild electric shock (UCS) producing foot withdrawal (UCR).[2] They paired a buzzer with the shock in the effort to get the CS-CR sequence, buzzer-foot withdrawal. It worked: The sound of the buzzer came to elicit foot withdrawal. Wickens and Wickens would have concluded that conditioning had taken place except for the fact that they had a control group in which the shocks alone were given during conditioning. During the subsequent test procedure the buzzer, which the babies in the control group had not experienced, was presented alone. It elicited foot withdrawal even though it had never been paired with shock. Although the babies may have learned something, it was not the association of the buzzer with shock. Because

---

2. The phrase *electric shock* often sounds startling to students; however, the intensities of shocks used in research are such as to produce only mild prickling sensations.

Marquis (1931) did not have control groups that would have eliminated alternative interpretations of her results, they have not been accepted as evidence that classical conditioning occurs in newborns.

Subsequent attempts to demonstrate classical conditioning in newborns have been equally problematic. The choice of a UCS-UCR connection is difficult. In newborns all such connections are reflexes, but not all reflexes are appropriate. The response must be one that can come under voluntary control. The foot withdrawal reflex chosen by Wickens and Wickens is not a good candidate for study. Because development proceeds from head to foot (the cephalocaudal principle of development), foot withdrawal would not be expected to win a race to be conditionable earliest. By the late 1960s most investigators had begun to use responses at the head of the body: sucking (used by Marquis in 1931) and head turning. Since then, it has become clear that choosing prepotent responses presents its own problems. Sucking, for example, is such a strong response that it often occurs naturally in response to what are supposed to be conditioned stimuli. For example, auditory stimuli innately elicit sucking responses (Keen, 1964; Semb & Lipsitt, 1968). Therefore, complex controls are necessary in studies of classical conditioning of sucking.

Successful classical conditioning that did not involve sucking, but did utilize a response of the head, has been demonstrated by Kaye (1965). The Babkin reflex involves the wide opening of the mouth and a tendency to turn the head from its usual tonic-neck reflex position toward midline in response to having the palms of the hands pressed. Kaye raised infants' arms over their heads (the CS) before pressing on their palms (the UCS) and was able to demonstrate conditioning and extinction.

The state of infants being tested has been shown to be a powerful variable in their conditionability. There is a clear relation between state of wakefulness and the probability of obtaining even the UCR in response to the UCS (Clifton, Siqueland, & Lipsitt, 1972). Because newborns drift in and out of sleep, even in experimental situations, state has to be carefully controlled.

In spite of improved methodology, based on increased sophistication in both experimental design and electronic technology, it is not yet clear whether newborns can be classically conditioned in the purest sense of that term—that is, that an arbitrary CS can be associated with any UCS through a gradual process of "stamping in" the association (a process that has limits at any age). It does appear, however, that there are three circumstances under which classical conditioning

or a variant can be achieved. The first is when the behaviors and the contingencies between CS and UCS are biologically adaptive ones that newborns are "prepared" to learn (e.g., Blass et al., 1984; see also discussions by Fitzgerald & Brackbill, 1976; Lipsitt et al., 1977; Rovee-Collier & Lipsitt, 1982; Sameroff, 1971; Sameroff & Cavanagh, 1979). There is ample evidence from conditioning studies in other domains that such associations are more easily conditioned than ones that are not biologically prepotent (Seligman, 1970). One classic example is that rats learn to associate taste with poisoned food in one trial, rather than learning the association slowly over repeated trials. Fitzgerald and Brackbill (1976) argued that tactile, auditory, and visual CSs are more readily conditioned to motoric responses (such as head turning), whereas temporal CSs are more readily linked to autonomic responses (such as the pupillary reflex).

The second circumstance is found in three methodologically sophisticated studies—by Clifton (1974), Crowell et al. (1976), and Stamps and Porges (1975)—that show evidence of learning within a classical conditioning paradigm, although not in the usual sense of a gradual increase in the strength of the conditioned response followed by a gradual decrease during extinction. All of these studies found evidence that newborns reacted differently to the CS during extinction (after they had been conditioned) than they did before. Their response to the omission of the CS indicated that the CS had become associated with the UCS. In two of the studies, the response shown on extinction was heart rate deceleration rather than conditioned acceleration (Clifton, 1974; Stamps & Porges, 1975). Heart rate deceleration is a typical response mammals make to a change in the environment; that is, it is a response indicating interest or orienting to a novel stimulus. That these infants showed the orienting response means that they noticed the change in stimuli. In other words, they must have learned to expect the UCS. When it was no longer presented, it violated their expectation and they responded to the change. To call this kind of learning classical conditioning may be misleading, however, because this "What happened?" response is different from the anticipatory response of adults.

The third circumstance under which something like classical conditioning has been demonstrated in newborns involves a paradigm developed by Papoušek (1961, 1967a, 1967b) that uses components of both operant and classical conditioning. His UCS was a tactile stimulus to the side of the mouth, which elicits the UCR of head turning (the rooting response) about 25% of the time. An auditory stimulus was used as the

CS and was paired in standard classical conditioning fashion with the UCS. Papoušek's innovation was to reward the head-turning response with milk. This introduces operant conditioning (to be discussed next), in which a reward increases the probability that the subject will make a future response. Thus success at conditioning might be due to the influence of the reward. Papoušek's procedure did succeed with newborns, but only after an average of 177 trials over a 3-week period.

The interpretation of these results is clouded in two ways. First, as already mentioned, the results might be due to the effectiveness of the reward or to the specific combination of operant and classical techniques. Second, by the time the newborns had learned the response, they were no longer newborns. Subsequent attempts to demonstrate conditioning in one session using Papoušek's techniques have met with some success (Clifton, Meyers, & Solomons, 1972; Clifton, Siqueland, & Lipsitt, 1972; Siqueland & Lipsitt, 1966), but alternative interpretations are still possible (see Sameroff & Cavanagh, 1979). At best, it is possible to conclude that a combination of classical and operant conditioning is possible at birth; at worst, we can conclude that even this combined conditioning is not clearly demonstrated until 3 weeks of age.

Researchers seem to accept that this is the way things are and do not seem to be trying to obtain classical conditioning in newborns currently. Admittedly, doing so is a procedure that has few rewards for the researcher. Evidence for this current neglect may be found in the fact that it is barely mentioned in a recent review article by Lipsitt (1990) on learning and memory in infants.

Later Development

Most research on classical conditioning has been designed to discover the earliest age at which it is possible. Explorations of classical conditioning in older infants are extremely limited. Papoušek (1967a) is one of the few researchers who has used the same procedure with babies of different ages. He used the combined procedure described above with newborns and with 3- and 5-month-old babies. He found that older

babies learned more rapidly. The number of trials to the criterion chosen as a proof of conditioning decreased from 177 for newborns to 42 for 3-month-olds to 28 for 5-month-olds. Once babies learned the response, they all, regardless of age, took the same amount of time to extinguish (stop responding) when the CS was presented alone. This indicates that what develops with age is the speed of learning, not the nature of the response once it is learned (Papoušek would call the latter "the neurological mechanisms"). Perceptual studies of babies' ability to recognize their mothers show a similar phenomenon in that young babies need a longer time to examine the faces, but, when given that time, they can distinguish their mother from a stranger.

Recently, Donohue et al. (1991) have shown that 7-month-old infants presented with an interesting visual stimulus during the late phase of an auditory stimulus show signs of anticipatory HR responses after 12 pairings, a pattern also found for adult subjects. Responses to trials where the visual stimulus was omitted (the "What happened?" response) also occurred. While anticipatory responses have been found in younger infants (Haith et al., 1988), Donohue and Berg have provided the first clear evidence of anticipatory HR responses.

While it is not strictly a case of classical conditioning, it is interesting to note that Reardon and Bushnell (1988) have shown that 7-month-old infants can learn an arbitrary pairing of color and taste. In their study, after three trials each of sweet or tart applesauce from red or blue paper cups, 11 of 14 infants chose the color associated with sweet.

OPERANT CONDITIONING

Operant conditioning starts with a spontaneous or **emitted response**, that is, one that the subject makes or emits rather than one elicited by a stimulus. The subject's response is followed by a **reinforcer** (reward or desirable environmental event). The effect of reward is that the subject is more likely to emit the response again. We say that **operant conditioning** has occurred if the probability of the subject's response increases when it has been followed by a reward. During extinction the response is no longer rewarded, and the probability of the subject's making it decreases.[3]

Early Operant Conditioning

Operant conditioning of newborns has been well demonstrated, most often with two response systems, sucking (described earlier) and head turning. The

---

3. Students of operant conditioning investigate not only whether it occurs, but the effects of delayed reinforcement, and whether reinforcement (or contingency) occurs on all trials. If not, the schedule of reinforcement may be studied. Performance when the contingency occurs on a given proportion of trials (fixed ratio) and the effects of different ratios may be studied. These topics are beyond the scope of this discussion.

latter has been demonstrated and replicated (reported in Sameroff & Cavanagh, 1979). In these studies, a band that allowed continuous recording of head turns was placed on the newborns' heads. Any turn greater than 10 degrees in any direction was followed by (rewarded by) insertion of a nonnutritive nipple to suck on for 5 seconds. Head turning quickly increased. Common wisdom has it that newborns do not condition easily. However, recent data show that 3- to 7-week-old infants can be "taught" not to have colic through the reinforcement of quiet alertness with music and parental attention and not attending to crying for a period (Larson & Ayllon, 1990). The learning was reversible and rereversible.

Infants are most likely to respond during active, awake periods, which constitute a small proportion of their day. As babies mature, they spend more and more time in active, awake periods and are thereby more often available for learning.

The variety of responses that can be operantly conditioned in newborns is also limited. The response must be in their behavioral repertoire, and there must be a natural relation between the response (sucking or head turning) and the reward (milk, a drop of sweet water, or nonnutritive sucking). These are biologically prepotent associations that newborns are "prepared" to learn.

Young babies also condition relatively slowly. Babies 8-9 weeks of age often require two sessions before conditioning is evident, whereas babies 12 weeks of age exhibit reliable conditioning in the first 3 to 6 minutes of training (Davis & Rovee-Collier, 1983; Gekoski, 1977; Sullivan, 1982). A similar development has been found in preweanling versus postweanling rats (Spear & Parsons, 1976).

Later Operant Conditioning

Studies of operant conditioning in older infants have been successful in a greater range of situations (see Figure 9.2), but some response-reward pairings are easier to condition than others. Further, some infants condition differently than others. For example, the speed with which 2- to 3-month-olds learn an operant task is related to their rhythmicity and persistence as rated by their mothers (Dunst & Lingerfelt, 1985). Social responses, such as vocalization, are more effectively conditioned by social reinforcement, such as mommy saying "peekaboo," than they are by comparable nonsocial reinforcement (Ramey & Watson, 1972; Weisberg, 1963). Social reinforcement works better for social than for nonsocial responses (Millar, 1976). Nonsocial responses (for example, auditory lo-

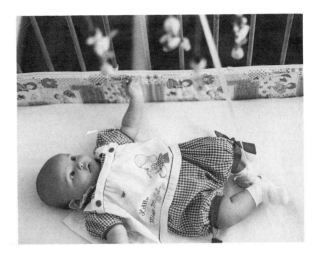

Figure 9.2. An infant participating in the operant conditioning developed by Rovee-Collier and described in the section on memory later in this chapter. A ribbon is attached to the infant's leg. She has learned that when she kicks her leg, the mobile moves. The intent look on her face as she watches the mobile shows how rewarding it is to her. (Photograph courtesy of Carolyn Rovee-Collier.)

calizations) are learned more easily when the reinforcer is a complex nonsocial stimulus (animated toy) than when it is either a social or a simple nonsocial stimulus (a blinking light).

Operant conditioning reveals other interesting aspects of infant behavior. The emotional expressions of 4- and 6-month-old infants are varied during learning. Sullivan and Lewis (1989) found that these expressions in infants receiving contingent reinforcement (i.e., reinforcement contingent on prior response) are different from those in infants who receive noncontingent reinforcement (i.e., the same number of reinforcements, but they do not depend on their behavior). The authors interpret this in terms of a model that links emotion and cognition as interdependent processes. During extinction, the violation of the expectation that has been developed temporarily yields increased responding prior to extinction in infants from 2 to 8 months of age (Alessandri et al., 1990). It also is apt to lead to emotional behaviors of crying and attacking the apparatus, as I have noted in my observations of various conditioning studies.

Operant conditioning has been shown to be a very useful form of intervention or therapy with a variety of profoundly handicapped infants (Dunst et al., 1985). One recent example is that contingent social reinforcement has been shown to increase vocalization rates in Down syndrome infants (Poulson, 1988).

Response Elicitation

In many, but not all, operant conditioning studies, the infant makes the target response even when that response has not been paired with a reward. This phenomenon, in which some aspect of the situation results in an increase in the frequency of the target response, is called **response elicitation**. It is both a methodological problem, in that it represents a form of pseudoconditioning, and an interesting phenomenon in its own right.

Response elicitation can be demonstrated by the use of a **noncontingent reinforcement** control condition, in which the environmental event that serves as a reinforcer in the experimental group is presented to the control group but not timed in relation to the subjects' responses. A good example of this is found in a study by Cavanagh and Davidson (1977) in which 6-month-old infants who pressed a clear Plexiglas panel were rewarded by seeing a multicolored light display behind the panel and hearing a bell. Those in the contingent reinforcement (experimental) group received the reward only after they had pressed the panel, whereas the noncontingent reinforcement group received the reward at random—sometimes after they had pressed the panel and sometimes not. Each infant in the experimental group was **yoked** to one in the noncontingent control group (i.e., the control infant received the same number of rewards, distributed similarly in time, as the experimental infant to which he or she was yoked). In every other way each pair of babies was treated exactly the same. The frequency of panel pressing increased for both groups during training, but more for the contingent group. Conditioning was demonstrated by the increased frequency of responses for the contingent group. Response elicitation was shown by the increase for the noncontingent group, who received no rewards for the responses. Response elicitation is a form of pseudoconditioning. That is, the infants' responses change as if they were being conditioned, but the cause is response elicitation, not conditioning. To determine whether true conditioning has occurred, it must be shown that contingent reinforcement results in greater response change than does noncontingent reinforcement.

Response elicitation is an adaptive mechanism, inasmuch as it keeps infants actively interacting with the environment. Such interaction results in an increased likelihood that they will make a response that is rewarded, and hence provides a basis on which reward contingencies can be learned. It is a very general phenomenon that may result from innate connections (such as an auditory stimulus that elicits sucking) or

from a learned connection. An example of the latter is that babies may kick when they see an interesting event because in their experience prior to the present situation, they learned that kicking was followed by (reinforced by) interesting events. Response elicitation also occurs with social responses such as vocalization (Bloom & Esposito, 1975) and smiling (Zelazo, 1971).

Learning theory research has become less fashionable in child psychology as interest in Piaget and cognitive psychology has dominated the field for some years. However, the operant conditioning paradigm is a powerful technique used for studying other aspects of infant development. Its use in perception has been discussed; later in this chapter its use in the study of memory is described, and Chapter 12 reports on its use in the study of attachment. In addition, it should be noted that it has been used continuously to teach older children with varying problems or handicaps to modify their behavior or to learn important skills (see, e.g., Dunst et al., 1985).

Imitation

One of the more frequent and noticeable behaviors of older babies and young children is their tendency to imitate. Imitation in infancy has long attracted the interest of child psychologists. Historically, it was thought to be a behavior that developed after the first half year of life. Furthermore, it was considered to depend on conscious effort on the part of the infant, or, in today's usage, to be purposive. (For a good brief review of this history, see Anisfeld, 1991; Piaget considered the topic in detail, some of which will be covered in Chapter 10.)

This section focuses on the issues of whether babies imitate in the first 2 months of life and how such early imitation develops. Also considered are how imitation facilitates learning, problem solving, and parent-infant relationships. Chapter 10 discusses in greater detail the development of increasingly sophisticated forms of imitation during infancy and its relation to cognitive development.

In 1977, Meltzoff and Moore completely restructured thinking and research about when imitation begins by showing imitation of several facial and one manual gesture by 2- and 3-week-old babies. Many studies followed, a number of which failed to find imitation. Before considering the research, let us examine some questions of method and definition.

Studies of newborn imitation all use behaviors that babies can exhibit spontaneously, such as crying, sticking out the tongue, and opening and closing the hands. Imitating a commonly performed action does not demonstrate the ability to learn new actions, which is sometimes considered a criterion for true imitation. Only imitating an unfamiliar action would show that.

The procedures used to study imitation may involve a model performing an act and waiting for the infant to imitate, or the model may perform the act a number of times before waiting for the infant's response (as in Meltzoff's work). Nothing but the model may be visible in the environment (as in Meltzoff's work), or there may be a normal room environment or something less "visually busy" than a normal room. Scoring may be by someone who knows what the stimulus is or by someone who does not (who is "blind" to the stimulus). Criteria for scoring an act as imitation may call for a strict reproduction of the modeled behavior (exact imitation) or may accept what might be called pseudoimitation, or inexact imitation. These are called **same-class responses**. For example, a parent may say "aah" to the baby and the baby may say "ehh." The response is in the same class of behavior as the parent's (a vocalized vowel sound), but does not match it (it is not the same vowel).

Next, one must consider the question of what is accepted as proof that imitation has occurred. In general, this has been to show that the gesture occurs with greater frequency when it is modeled than in control conditions. In some developmental research, such as in psychophysics, the criterion is often more strict, and a response is judged reliable only if it occurs on at least 66% or 75% of the trials. (For example, in a study of orientation toward the source of a sound, infants were described as doing so if they turned correctly on 75% of the trials.) In addition, the question of the time between when an act is modeled and when it is imitated is an important one, with implications for memory and for cognitive development.

Finally, the theoretical implications of a successful demonstration of imitation differ depending on whether the babies can see or hear their own actions. Babies could match hand gestures by watching their hands and those of the model until they produced a match. Babies cannot see their own faces, so in order to imitate a facial gesture it is thought that they must have a mental representation of that gesture that permits them to recognize the similarity between their facial gesture and that of the model. If newborns can truly imitate actions they cannot see themselves perform, this is presumed to be evidence that their innate cognitive equipment is much more sophisticated than many psychologists believe it to be. A related concep-

tual issue pertains to the question of whether any imitative behaviors found are purposeful or not.

EARLY IMITATION

Imitative Crying

With this background, let us look at some of the data. The first behavior investigated as neonatal imitation was crying. Newborns in hospital nurseries cry in response to the cries of other newborns. As long ago as 1928, Bühler and Hetzer found that 84% of babies in their first 2 weeks of life cried when exposed to the sound of another crying infant. When researchers again became interested in imitation in the 1970s, they introduced conditions that demonstrated that this sort of crying is not simply a response to a noxious noise. Several studies have now found that newborns cry more in response to cries of other newborns than they do to cries of older infants, synthetic cries, cries of a chimpanzee, or silence (Martin & Clark, 1982; Sagi & Hoffman, 1976; Simner, 1971). If imitative crying were simply part of the newborn's basic tendency to cry at loud noises, then all three situations should increase crying similarly. Furthermore, a tape of another newborn crying increased crying both when the target infants were calm and when they were excited, but a tape of their own crying had no effect when they were calm. If they were already crying, they stopped (Martin & Clark, 1982).

It seems clear that newborns respond to something rather specific when they cry in response to the cries of other newborns, but whether this indicates that they imitate is still in question. The response is exact imitation in the sense that crying is triggered by the specific stimulus of another crying newborn. However, if other arousal responses, such as activity level, increase as much as crying, it would suggest that crying triggers general arousal, not imitation specifically. (I am unaware of any research undertaken to answer this question.) Imitation does not fully explain why distress is part of the response. Several researchers have argued that a better explanation for this phenomenon of sympathetic crying is that it is a rudimentary empathic response to distress (Martin & Clark, 1982; Sagi & Hoffman, 1976).

The imitation of sounds other than crying will not be addressed here, but I do want to call to your attention to this as a possible subfield of imitation. To give two brief examples, infants in the first 6 months of life have been shown significantly (but not consistently) to imitate pitch (Kessen et al., 1979). While 3- to 4-

Table 9.1

Imitative Responses of Young Infants[a]

Scored Responses	Gestures Shown to Infants			
	Lip Protrusion	Mouth Opening	Tongue Protrusion	Sequential Finger Movements
Lip protrusion	27 (21%)[b]	17	15	19
Mouth opening	11	24 (18%)	17	19
Tongue protrusion	21	20	30 (22%)	26
Sequential finger movements	14	13	16	27 (20%)
Hand opening	22	24	28	24
Finger protrusion	18	19	10	8
Passive hand	18	16	18	13
Total	131	133	134	136

SOURCE: The figures in the first four rows are from Figure 2 of Meltzoff and Moore (1977). The rest of the figures were obtained from A. N. Meltzoff. Data also obtained from Anisfeld (1979).
NOTE: Entries in boldface indicate matching responses.
a. Distribution of responses across the four gestures shown to the infants.
b. Percentages have been added after the exact match cases.

month-olds will imitate their mothers' sounds if the sounds are in their repertoire, it is not until after 5 months that they modify their own sounds to resemble those of others, and not until after 9 months that they imitate new sounds and gestures.

Imitation of Facial and Manual Gestures

Although there is a conceptual difference between imitation of facial gestures and of manual gestures in terms of whether the infant can use vision to monitor matching, the two are considered here together because of the nature of the research that has been conducted. Meltzoff and Moore (1977) demonstrated imitation of lip and tongue protrusions, mouth openings (own action unseen), and sequential finger movements (own action seen) in 12- to 21-day-old babies. Although they have replicated their earlier findings (Meltzoff & Moore, 1983a, 1983b, 1989), several others have failed to do so (Hayes & Watson, 1981; Koepke et al., 1983b; McKenzie & Over, 1983b). Meltzoff and Moore (1983a, 1983b, 1989) argue that imitation can be elicited only under certain conditions, and they blame procedural differences for others' failures. Indeed, Meltzoff and Moore's conditions are far from naturalistic: The baby was in a darkened area with nothing to look at except the model's face, the baby had never seen the face of the model before, and the model's face was in a spotlight. Under these conditions, and in a generally well-controlled study with blind scoring, the babies satisfied the criterion of performing the modeled act significantly more often when it and not another gesture had been modeled.

The gesture modeled occurred more often when it, not another, was modeled. Tongue protrusions occurred 7.1 times when modeled and 5.4 times when not, and mouth openings occurred 9.9 times when modeled compared with 6.5 times when another gesture was modeled. Another study using the same procedures for tongue protrusions and head movements had similar results (Meltzoff & Moore, 1989). The means were 6.7 for tongue protrusions and 8.3 for head movements when they had been modeled, and 4.7 for each when the other had been modeled.

The actual data from Meltzoff and Moore's 1977 experiment are presented in Table 9.1, in the restructured form provided by Anisfeld (1979). Whether the babies' responses look like imitation or not depends, in part, on what aspects of the data we focus on. Meltzoff and Moore compared the numbers in boldface (the diagonals) to the other entries in the same rows and found that the infants were more likely to make any of the modeled gestures after the adult had made it than when the adult had made another gesture. In contrast, the vertical columns that list infant responses to each adult gesture show that in many instances the infant did something different from what the adult modeled. Arguments can be made for either comparison as the criterion of whether imitation has occurred. Anisfeld argues for the column comparisons, Meltzoff and Moore for the row comparisons. Regardless of one's focus, the column comparisons make it clear that exact imitation is not a common response. In fact, in no instance did the imitative response exceed 22% of the total number of responses made. For example, in modeled tongue protrusion, an action infants cannot

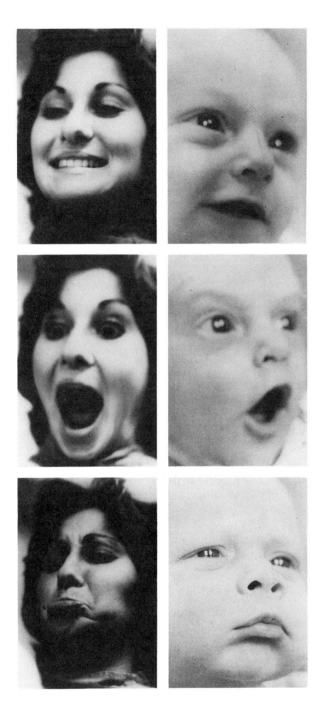

Figure 9.3. Newborns imitating happy and surprised facial expressions in the experiment by Field and her colleagues (1982). The controversy over neonatal imitation does not hinge on whether such sequences ever occur; rather, the question is whether this is true imitation rather than a striking coincidence. (From "Discrimination and Imitation of Facial Expressions by Neonates" by T. Field et al., October 1982 in *Science*, *218*, p. 179. Copyright 1982 by the AAAS. Reprinted with permission. Photographs courtesy of Tiffany Field.)

see themselves perform, hand opening (not the same class) was almost as frequent as tongue protrusion (exact), and it was much more frequent than lip protrusion (same class). Nevertheless, some infants under these circumstances imitate or match gestures they cannot see themselves make. In sequential finger movements, an action infants can see themselves perform, tongue protrusions were essentially as frequent as exact imitations. Hence infants' seeing their own acts does not seem to enhance matching of responses.

In another type of study conducted by Field et al. (1982), the ability of judges standing behind the modeling adult to guess whether a baby is responding to a face expressing joy, sadness, or surprise (see Figure 9.3) was the criterion for imitation. Judges identified the modeled expression at better than chance levels. They also noted facial configurations appropriate to the emotion (widened lips in happiness, pouting lips in sadness, and wide-open mouth in surprise trials) at better than chance levels. Anisfeld (1991) notes that differences in the patterns of gaze reported by Field and her associates could account for the judges' ability to identify surprise, which is the expression for which they were most accurate (76% correct judgments).

How Many Imitate? Why have I said that *some* infants imitate? Many babies who are studied do not complete the procedures; of those who do, only some imitate, even by lenient criteria. Using healthy, middle-class babies, Meltzoff and Moore began with 107 and 93, respectively, to get the 40 who completed each of the 1983 and 1989 studies. Of the 40 who finished in 1983, 65% showed imitation for both gestures, but 17-30% (depending on the gesture) produced more gestures that had not been modeled. In the 1989 study, 50% of the 40 who completed the study produced both gestures more often when they had been modeled. Heimann (1989) has also found 60-70% of neonates and 3-week-olds to imitate tongue protrusions (compared with 40-45% who imitated mouth opening). In a review of 19 studies of imitation, Anisfeld (1991) reports that the loss of subjects varied from 11% to 74%, with a median loss of 47%. Between the loss of subjects and the fact that not all who completed the studies showed imitation, the generality of any conclusions is somewhat tentative. (See Anisfeld, 1991, for a detailed examination of other possible sources of bias in the experiments.)

Other research has addressed the question of whether or not imitation is exact (Abravanel & Sigafoos, 1984; Gardner & Gardner, 1970; Jacobson, 1979; Jacobson & Kagan, 1979). The results indicate that even for 6-week-old infants, imitation may be same class rather than exact. Studies by Gardner and Gardner (1970) and Jacobson (1979) showed that the response of protruding or opening might be made with an organ that is different from that modeled. For example, the model opening her hand might lead to the infant opening her mouth. Jacobson found that inanimate objects moved toward and away from the infant elicited tongue protrusions as effectively as did their being modeled. That is hardly what is generally meant by imitation. She did not find even same-class imitation for hand movements.

Data from several studies suggest that these facial and manual gestures become more difficult to elicit as babies reach 3 or 4 months of age (e.g., Field et al., 1986; Heimann, 1989). Whether this is due to less optimal eliciting conditions being used or to the behaviors that infants imitate becoming less prepotent in their behavior repertoires is unclear. One possibility is that a reflexive type of imitation exists at birth only to drop out and be replaced by intentional imitation later, similar to the stepping reflex and walking. A similar hypothesis tying the behaviors to different neural processes has been advanced by Bjorklund (1987; see also Vinter, 1986). The early imitation does seem to be linked to one later behavior, gaze aversion in interaction with the mother at 3 months (Heimann, 1989). Heimann (1991) has shown that imitation in the first 3 months is not related to imitation on a variety of tasks (object manipulation, social gestures, facial gestures) at 1 year of age. However, imitation of tongue protrusion at 3 months is related to imitation of sounds at 1 year ($r = .42$). With that exception, Heimann's data would seem to support the idea of imitation at later ages being a different process from that early in life.

What Is Imitated?

This discussion does not go into detail on the results for different gestures, but concentrates on the one for which there is the most positive evidence—tongue protrusion. As Anisfeld's (1991) review makes clear, tongue protrusion is more likely to produce effects than are other modeled behaviors. Anisfeld analyzed imitation in the various studies in relation to the duration of the demonstration and found that it existed in all cases in which the demonstration exceeded 60 seconds. The burst of modeled faces followed by the pause for imitations in the Meltzoff and Moore studies makes it impossible to say on how many trials the infants imitated. However, Anisfeld calculated the rate at which the various imitative responses were produced and found that the rate of tongue protrusions, but not that of other responses, was higher when it had been modeled.

Moving Versus Static Stimuli. I would like to call attention to one stimulus variable that may be of great importance. Most studies of imitation have used a moving stimulus or model (with the exception of those by Field et al., whose static face may not have been an optimal eliciting procedure). Vinter (1986) showed that moving displays of gestures were more effective in eliciting imitation (exact and same-class responses were both counted as imitations) than were static models. Given the greater effectiveness of moving stimuli in various studies of visual perception, this hardly seems surprising. Vinter hypothesized that kinetic information is processed in peripheral vision, which is mediated subcortically, but static information is processed in central vision, which is cortically mediated. There should be ways of studying this with current EEG technology.

Conclusions

What can we conclude from all this? Imitation or response matching, at least of tongue protrusion, exists in the neonatal period at above chance levels. But is the cup of neonatal imitation half full or half empty? Is the imitation found part of the same phenomenon that has historically been called imitation, with a purposeful, conscious component? Should we expect more than just statistical significance between groups before we talk about purposiveness? Should we expect that more than half of the half that completes an experiment should show a behavior before that age group is described as being able to imitate? Are there indeed different imitative processes in later infancy from those in the first months?

Meltzoff and Moore describe the phenomenon they have demonstrated as powerful, a conclusion with which I cannot agree. I do agree that they have shown response matching of tongue protrusion to exist. But does this imitation require the kind of cognitive skill (the abstract, cross-modal representation present at birth) that Meltzoff and Moore postulate? Or, despite their arguments to the contrary, can it be explained by appeal to simpler mechanisms? I do not think we have the data to rule out other hypotheses yet.

Tongue protrusion, which is the only gesture that has been shown to be reliably elicited by modeling, is also elicited by inanimate stimuli that protrude. Could tongue protrusion, which is part of the sucking reflex, be released by protruding stimuli because they are innate releasers for sucking?

Meltzoff and Moore (1983b, 1989) note that modeling is not effective in naturalistic settings; they assert that this argues against an innate releaser hypothesis.

But if modeling is not effective in naturalistic settings, how can one say that neonatal imitation is a powerful and important phenomenon? Ineffectiveness in naturalistic situations also seems to argue against Bjorklund's (1987) hypothesis that tongue protrusions, and possibly other matching responses, are innate responses in the service of promoting interaction between parent and newborn. A new possibility has been raised by Anisfeld (1991)—namely, that the data could be accounted for by competition with attentional responses during the demonstration period, which is decreased during the response period, resulting in response release. This has some similarity to Meltzoff and Moore's discussions of turn-taking in relation to their data.

The conservative explanation of the newborn research, particularly in light of studies with somewhat older babies, is that adult modeling of both seen and unseen familiar actions produces response elicitation. But it is possible to be too conservative; rudimentary imitative abilities may exist in the newborn period. Which position researchers accept often depends on their theoretical biases. Those who believe that babies are born with a set of well-developed cognitive structures are likely to believe that newborns are imitating. Those who believe in Piaget's theory of cognitive development are more likely to believe that newborns are exhibiting response elicitation and that 6-week-olds have developed same-class imitation. Those of us who believe in Occam's razor want to withhold attributing higher-order functions to newborns if simpler explanations are available.

Whatever conclusion is accepted, it is clear that newborns imitate only the types of actions that newborns spontaneously emit. It has not been demonstrated that newborns will imitate unfamiliar actions, that is, that imitation is a basis for learning new actions in the newborn period.

The debates will be settled only when attention is diverted from attempts to prove that imitation exists to attempts to clarify the conditions under which it occurs. Would other imitative responses be found if the exposure times to the model were increased? If stimuli were always kinetic, not static? If there were no stimuli in the environment competing for attention? Could we look at what parts of the nervous system react differently (e.g., using EEG responses from different areas of the brain) during imitative responses?

My personal conclusion at this stage of knowledge is that although matching behaviors occur, they are not highly reliable and do not seem to resemble the behaviors discussed under the heading of imitation in children nearing their first birthday.

LATER DEVELOPMENT OF IMITATION

Most research on imitation in infancy has focused on very young babies. Piagetian research, which examines imitation as the development of increasingly sophisticated steps toward mature imitation, has studied it later in the first year. Major discussion of Piaget's theory and the research designed to test it appears in Chapter 10. A brief summary of some studies that support Piaget's account of imitation is included here.

According to Abravanel et al. (1976), same-class imitation of actions already in the infant's behavioral repertoire develops during months 1 to 4. By 4 to 8 months infants can imitate actions that are familiar to them (not necessarily in their repertoire) and do so frequently. Kaye and Marcus (1981) found that by 8 to 12 months infants can imitate actions that are unfamiliar to them, and from 6 to 12 months their imitation becomes increasingly exact.

Other studies seem to indicate that, far from a steady improvement in imitation with increasing age, imitation may get worse, or, at best, be far less effective than has generally been thought. For example, imitation has been found to be poor prior to 16-18 months (Killen & Uzgiris, 1981; McCall et al., 1977). Killen and Uzgiris (1981) used very simple tasks such as shaking and banging, similar to some of the 22 acts modeled in the earlier study by Abravanel et al. (1976), only 8 of which had led to imitation. However, the sheer number of acts modeled in that study might have confused the infants. For both studies, I wonder whether the tasks were appropriate for the stage of development of the infants. In visual research, the stimuli that effectively hold infants' attention are more complex as infants become older. Why should an infant bother to imitate an act that is firmly established in his or her behavioral repertoire? Acts that are in the process of being learned, or that call for a new action in the context of familiar elements, might be more appropriate targets for imitation. Indeed, Harnick (1978) showed that toddlers from 14 to 28 months of age imitated only irrelevant behaviors of intermediate difficulty, not behaviors that were too easy or too hard. Task-related behaviors were less affected.

Meltzoff (1985) used a novel task that would seem to address the above concerns (with excellent control conditions and blind scoring) to investigate the apparent low ability of older infants to imitate. Imitation occurred in 80% of 2-year-olds who received modeling of the act of pulling a toy apart; only 20% of infants in the various control conditions performed the same act. Furthermore, the imitators started to do so in only 2 sec. The same procedure used with 14-month-olds yielded

75% who imitated, compared with less than 8% in the control conditions. The latencies were higher for the younger children (4 sec) and for those who performed the action when it had not been modeled (10 sec).

Meltzoff (1988b) extended the range of ages down to 9 months and the number of acts modeled to three. The 9-month-olds produced the modeled acts significantly more than any of the control groups, but only half successfully modeled at least two acts. It would have helped to have the tasks more comparable across studies. Data on the easier tasks used earlier with younger infants and data on three tasks for the older infants would enable more clear-cut judgments about ease of imitating at different ages. If imitation declines after the neonatal period, it would appear to increase again at a slightly later age.

All of the research reviewed thus far was concerned with immediate imitation, in which the imitative response is made immediately after the modeled act. **Delayed imitation**, in which the imitation occurs at a later time, appears to be more sophisticated. It is characteristic only of highly intelligent animals, such as chimpanzees, monkeys, and humans (Yando et al., 1978), which is consistent with the Piagetian view that delayed imitation develops only at the end of the second year of life (Piaget, 1945/1962; Uzgiris & Hunt, 1975). However, Figure 9.4 shows delayed imitation by an infant just entering the second year of life.

Meltzoff's (1985) studies of 14- and 24-month-old infants reviewed above also looked at delayed imitation. One group of subjects in each study received the demonstration or control procedure one day and were not allowed to handle the objects that day. They came back the next day and the objects were placed in front of them with no new modeling. Of this group, 70% of the 2-year-olds and 45% of the 14-month-olds pulled the toy apart. This did not involve trial-and-error behavior, as they started to do it within 5 sec. Even the 9-month-olds performed the modeled acts after the 24-hour delay significantly more than did the controls. Half of them imitated at least two of the three modeled acts, and 20% of subjects in both immediate and delayed imitation groups reproduced all three acts.

In a further study conducted by Meltzoff (1988a), all but 1 of 12 14-month-old infants given their first opportunity to imitate after 1 week performed three or more of the six behaviors modeled. Only 3 of 24 infants in control groups performed these acts. The proportion of infants imitating varied depending on

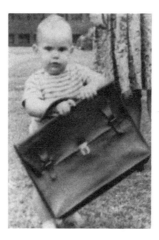

Figure 9.4. Delayed imitation of a frequently seen adult action.

the act, but a novel act was imitated by two-thirds of the infants. The finding of much shorter latencies for performing modeled acts than for doing the same act without its having been modeled is congruent with the idea of intentionality. Furthermore, Hanna and Meltzoff (1991) have shown the efficacy of a 2-year-old model at a day-care center in producing imitation at home 2 days later when the same toys were presented. Infants (14 to 18 months of age) who had seen the model performed three of the child-modeled acts, compared with only one act performed by infants who had not seen the demonstration.[4]

These data indicate stable, large-scale effects and suggest that researchers need to rethink the course of imitation over the period of infancy. The data reinforce the possibility that, as was believed earlier, imitation can be a powerful source for acquiring and coordinating new behaviors over the course of infancy. The delayed imitation work is pertinent to the study of memory in infancy, which will be discussed shortly.

MECHANISMS BY WHICH IMITATION DEVELOPS

Reinforcement psychologists (such as Baer et al., 1967; Gewirtz, 1971a, 1971b; Gewirtz & Stingle, 1968) believe that imitation develops by means of reinforcement training. They argue that infants' apparently imitative responses are reinforced in many different situations, and that through this repeated training a general tendency to imitate develops. The basic mechanism by which such general response tendencies develop through specific training with a large number of exemplars (learning sets) was demonstrated

---

4. Meltzoff (1988a) presents an extensive discussion of the relation of his data to other data and to Piagetian theory, but it is not appropriate to consider that here.

in monkeys many years ago by Harlow (1949). A recent longitudinal study by Poulson and Kymissis (1988) has demonstrated such development. Even very young infants can be trained to imitate using reinforcements. Generalized imitation can be painstakingly developed in severely retarded children (Baer & Sherman, 1964) and in the context of behavior therapy (Baer & Deguchi, 1985).

Other psychologists argue that just because it is possible to develop a generalized imitative tendency by means of reinforcement, this does not mean that it normally develops this way. They believe that imitation is as much a natural characteristic of humans as is the tendency to respond to rewards. Four arguments used to defend this position are as follows:

(1) Some imitation occurs prior to there being much reinforcement history.
(2) The development of imitation follows closely that of cognition (see Chapter 10).
(3) The significance of external reinforcers is subordinate to apparent intrinsic satisfactions.
(4) Reinforcement may not be necessary for development of imitation.

With respect to the third of these, Baer and his colleagues have argued that similarity between the behavior of the model and that of the infant is a sufficient reinforcer (Baer & Deguchi, 1985; Baer et al., 1967; Baer & Sherman, 1964). Bruner (1972) underlines the intrinsic aspects by noting that animals, like children, lose interest in the goal of the act being performed and become preoccupied with the means. A good example of this is Rumbaugh's (1970) account of a chimpanzee named Lana, who saved her banana reinforcements and then returned them to the experimenter, one per trial, in the next part of the experiment. Had the bananas been rewards in the traditional learning theory sense of that term, Lana would have eaten them. Rather, she became preoccupied with the means—the use of bananas as rewards.

With respect to the fourth argument, Waxler and Yarrow (1975) found that while reinforcement operates in a straightforward way in some children's imitation, similar imitation occurs in children who do not experience reinforcement, a finding with which Poulson and Kymissis's (1988) data could be said to agree.

ROLES OF IMITATION IN
INFANT DEVELOPMENT

Imitation is one of the very fundamental human abilities. It plays important roles both in learning about the world and in social development. Whatever view they take of its origins, psychologists agree on the importance of imitation and that it is the source of much learning. When one sees what a handicap the lack of generalized imitation is to learning in the profoundly retarded, who do not imitate adult behaviors to anything like the degree to which normal or mildly retarded children do, one gains a new appreciation for its importance.

One way in which imitation is important is in its role in learning through reinforcement. A behavior must occur before it can be reinforced. Some infant behaviors are highly likely to occur (to be emitted) spontaneously or are easy to elicit for biological reasons (such as sucking), and these behaviors can easily be controlled by reinforcement. Other behaviors are rarely emitted spontaneously. Eliciting them by providing a model to be imitated is often very effective. Learning psychologists have developed techniques other than imitation to encourage individuals to produce such behaviors, but they tend to be either time-consuming (e.g., shaping, see below) or unpleasant. But it is usually easy for adults to model a desired response and obtain imitation. Voilà! The behavior occurs and the adult can now reinforce it. Thus imitation is a powerful method by which children can be induced to behave in a particular way, and that behavior can then become subject to control through reinforcement. Because imitation evidently develops with age, one can ask at what age it can first become an effective mechanism by which to elicit behaviors to be reinforced.

Modeling plus reinforcement forms an important part of Brazelton's (1974) approach to toilet training. He suggests that an older child or parent demonstrate to the 2-year-old the correct procedures for using a toilet. Then, when the child imitates the behaviors, this performance can be reinforced. Learning by modeling plus reinforcement is very common throughout childhood. It is used by parents in child rearing (e.g., see the review of its role in the development of prosocial behaviors in Mussen & Eisenberg-Berg, 1977), as well as in the development of such diverse skills as tennis, spear throwing, and American Sign Language. In fact, Cole and Scribner (1974) report that imitation is the major form of teaching in nontechnological cultures. However, it should also be noted that asking 15- to 21-month-old infants to perform familiar actions has been shown to be as effective as modeling those actions (Murray, 1987). When the task is unfamiliar, males perform better when it is modeled and girls perform better given verbal instructions.

Imitation does not need to be exact in order to aid in learning. Inexact imitation may also be useful to the person who wishes to train through reinforcement; it can provide a basis for **shaping**. This is the process whereby reinforcement is initially given for a crude approximation of a desired behavior and subsequently is given only for behaviors that are more and more like the desired behavior. For example, consider teaching an infant to play "so big." In this game, the parent says, "How big is the baby?" and the baby responds by raising her hands at the same time the adult says, "So big." The parent models the hand raises. On the first few trials any hand movement is rewarded. After several trials the parent stops rewarding just any movement and rewards only movements toward the ceiling. The process is repeated; again the parent ceases to reward the previously acceptable response, and rewards only responses more like the desired arm raises. After several cycles of this procedure, the infant raises her arms fully in response to the parent's query and model of the arm raise. In this way inexact imitations may be used as the basis for developing exact imitations.

Shaping can also be used effectively to teach an unfamiliar action on the basis of a familiar action, provided the shaper can build successive approximations from the familiar action to the unfamiliar one. Thus imitation can be an effective learning device for some activities by 6 weeks of age, when it is clear that babies exhibit same-class imitation of familiar and prepotent actions. Imitation may become even more effective later in infancy, when infants exhibit exact imitation of unfamiliar actions.

Psychologists interested in the development of reasoning and problem solving have identified a second role that imitation plays in the acquisition of knowledge. Imitation of unfamiliar actions is considered by Piaget to be a primary way children incorporate new behavior patterns into their cognitive structures (see Chapter 10). This imitative learning may occur while the infant is trying to solve a problem, or it may occur in the context of play in which no obvious problem is being solved. An example of the latter may occur when an older sibling moves a stool to the sink and stands on it to brush her teeth. The toddler, imitating, takes the stool and carries it from place to place. At each place he puts it down, steps on it, and then steps off; he then picks it up and takes it to another place. Never during this entire sequence does the toddler use this action to reach something. At some later time, however, the toddler wishes to reach a light switch that is too high and fetches the stool to stand on. Bruner (1972) reports an identical pattern for chimpanzees.

This pattern, in which a behavior developed through imitation is later applied to a problem-solving situation, is an example of a more general relation between play and problem solving that has been found repeatedly in psychological research. Animals, from rats to chimps to humans, will engage in exploratory play when they are not hungry. Later, when they have a problem (for instance, they are hungry and want to obtain food), they will use the knowledge of the environment gained in play to find food. Acquiring problem solutions through imitation, either in intentional problem solving or in the context of play, should occur only when the infant can imitate unfamiliar actions, an ability that first develops between 8 and 12 months of life.

Imitation also plays a role in the development of the caretaker-infant relationship. Adults like and are warmer toward children who imitate them (Bates, 1975), and children find being imitated by an adult rewarding (Fouts, 1972, 1975; Thelen et al., 1975). Infants need not exhibit true imitation for it to facilitate the caretaker-infant relationship. Parents are typically delighted with any response from young infants, and they are likely to be rewarded by inexact imitation and by response elicitation as well as by exact matches. Likewise, if parents can successfully train their infants to imitate, mutually rewarding interaction should occur even though the imitation was not spontaneous. Indeed, evidence exists that mothers and infants engage in prolonged reciprocal imitation that involves inexact and trained imitations as well as true imitations. In these sequences the infant and mother trade similar responses back and forth in a sort of dance (Papoušek & Papoušek, 1975, 1977; Stern, 1977). It is also clear from this research that both participants enjoy the interaction; the sequence is continued so long as both participants continue to imitate, which may be a long time, and is stopped when one participant makes another kind of response. Such interactions might serve as an important mechanism in the development of attachment, a topic discussed in Chapter 12.

Memory

In the most general sense, **memory** is the ability of living organisms to store and use past experience. Thus all learning implies memory. In a stricter sense (Piaget & Inhelder, 1973), memory is the ability to **recall** past experience in the absence of original elements of that experience. Regardless of how broadly one defines memory, it can be described as involving three processes:

(1) **encoding**, or acquiring and organizing elements of experience through perceptual and cognitive processes

(2) **retention**, or storage of the acquired elements

(3) **retrieval**, or location and extraction of retained elements

Retrieval is usually achieved by way of cues, which are stimuli that initiate and guide the search for stored elements. The most basic form of retrieval is **recognition**, in which the cue is a reoccurrence of the stored item.

NEONATAL MEMORY

Memory in the neonatal period has been demonstrated in the habituation and conditioning studies discussed above. In order to habituate or to change behaviors of sucking or head turning in conditioning studies, the baby must remember something about the stimuli or the contingencies. So memory has to exist for the few moments of the experiment.

Zelazo et al. (1987) conducted direct study of the length of time information can be remembered by 3-day-olds, using habituation of head turns to single words repeated by a strong voice. After habituation, the experimenters used different delay intervals before testing for dishabituation. The retention interval was about 1 minute.

Memory for longer periods of time, such as several hours or a day, has not been demonstrated experimentally in newborns. For example, Sameroff (1968) has shown that conditioning of sucking in one feeding session does not carry over to the next. This outcome is particularly convincing, because Sameroff used a response that is presumably biologically prepotent (sucking), and because conditioning involved many repeated trials. Thus his procedure should have been optimal to produce long-term memory. However, ecologically relevant research suggests hours-long retention of some naturalistic stimulus dimensions, such as smell (see Chapter 7). DeCasper's research suggests that capacity for limited long-term auditory memory may be present even in utero (DeCasper & Fifer, 1980; DeCasper & Spencer, 1986).

Neonatal memory, therefore, exists, but is limited in (a) the stimulus dimensions that can be encoded, (b) retention intervals, and (c) the range of effective retrieval cues. The stimulus dimensions must be sensory elements (e.g., odors, words). The retention interval may be longer for frequent, naturalistic elements such as a mother's voice, but is brief at best for other stimuli. The only retrieval cues that elicit memory are

complete reoccurrences of the stimulus, such as the word itself rather than a part of it or some other element of the learning context.

However, memory develops rapidly. Long-term memory can be demonstrated in babies under 1 month of age. Ungerer et al. (1978) had mothers repeat a single word 60 times a day for 13 days to their 2-4-week-old babies, at which time the babies exhibited recognition of the familiar stimulus (primarily by moving or widening their eyes, or both) after delays of 15 and 42 hours. However, the same babies failed to recognize their own names, which they had probably heard more frequently during this same period. Thus it appears that infants of this age are unlikely to exhibit enduring memory for most of the stimuli they normally experience.

MEMORY DEVELOPMENT IN EARLY INFANCY

Memory development in this period has been studied using the habituation and operant conditioning paradigms.

Research Using the Habituation Paradigm

The habituation paradigm is used to measure memory for events that are much less frequently experienced than in Ungerer et al.'s (1978) study of repeated words. These studies repeatedly expose infants to a stimulus in one session until they habituate, and then test for long-term memory by rehabituating the babies at a later time. If rehabituation requires fewer trials than original habituation, then something of their earlier experience must have been retained. This is a measure of **savings**, one of the classic measures of memory for past learning. By 3½ months babies exhibit savings in trials needed for rehabituation for more than 24 hours after the original habituation session (Martin, 1975; Topinka & Steinberg, 1978). By 5½ months, savings last for up to 48 hours. Memories for photographs of faces, which are presumably easier to retain because they are more familiar, can be retained for up to 2 weeks (Fagan, 1973). By 7½ months babies exhibit memory for novel stimuli for between 1 and 2 weeks (Topinka & Steinberg, 1978).

Habituation has also been used to study specific memory processes. In visual habituation, Haaf and Lundy (1991) found that encoding was slower in 6-month-olds when the context around the stimulus varied (e.g., context was a colored geometric pattern around the stimulus of a snowman), but later recognition accuracy was not influenced by the presence of a familiar surround. These authors infer that the context was initially encoded as part of the stimulus, but then identified as irrelevant across numerous habituation trials.

Encoding of young infants is influenced by the sensory modalities in which the stimulus is experienced. Infants in the second half of the first year exhibited memory only when the mode(s) of exploration at encoding matched the mode(s) of exploration at test (MacKay-Soroka et al., 1982; Ruff, 1981). In a subsequent study, Ruff (1982) demonstrated why this occurred: When infants explored visually and manually they were more likely to encode shape and texture information, whereas when they explored only visually they tended to encode only two-dimensional stimulus characteristics. Integration of such multimodal information can be achieved by 5-month-olds, who perform better on a visual anticipation task when given both aural and visual location cues during training (Loboschefski et al., 1991). Integration may be limited to particular stimulus dimensions. In a study by Burnham et al. (1988), 4-, 7-, and 10-month-olds who were visually habituated to stimuli that varied along three dimensions remembered all color-shape compounds, but more remembered compounds that also moved. The researchers argue that young infants have encoding and retention capacitors that are limited to a few salient stimulus features that best "go together."

Young infants' memory processes may operate on categories instead of on specific items. When 3- and 10-month-olds were visually familiarized with a set of either dot patterns or schematic animals, both age groups looked longer at the original set than at novel prototypes of the stimuli (Younger, 1990; Younger & Gotlieb, 1988). This is consistent with the view that even young infants abstract and retain categorical information from a set of familiar stimuli. (For further description of this work, see Chapter 10.) Five-month-olds tested for memory for hue remembered the exact hue on an immediate test, but only the color category on a 5-minute-delayed test in which the hue was paired with itself or with one from the same or a different color category (Catherwood et al., 1987). The researchers conclude that memory for hue is like memory for orientation (Quinn et al., 1985), in that unique item information decays more rapidly than category information. Retrieval processes may also be categorical in early infancy. Ten-month-olds habituated to sets of one, two, or three pictures of common objects looked longer at familiar stimuli on test trials as the set size increased, suggesting a sequential retrieval of the pictures retained in memory (de Saint Victor and Hull-Smith, 1991).

Research Using Operant Conditioning

The most fruitful method for studying early memory development has been operant conditioning. By 8 weeks of age babies can remember a stimulus and response when they have not reexperienced it for 2 weeks, but only under special circumstances. Rovee-Collier and her collaborators have studied memory for previously learned operant responses in babies 2 and 3 months old (see reviews in Rovee-Collier, 1987; Rovee-Collier & Fagen, 1981). In these researchers' mobile conjugate reinforcement paradigm (MCRP), infants first learn to move an overhead mobile by kicking their legs, which are attached to the mobile by a ribbon, as shown in Figure 9.2. The babies are brought back to the experimental situation weeks later. The mobile is visually present, but is neither attached to the leg nor in motion. If the babies resume a high rate of kicking, they demonstrate that they have remembered the situation. After 15 minutes' training on 2 consecutive days, 2-month-olds remember for 1 day, but not for 3 (Greco et al., 1986); 3-month-olds remember for 8 days, but not for 13 (Fagen & Rovee-Collier, 1983; Sullivan et al., 1979); and 7-month-olds remember for 14 days, but not 21 (Hill et al., 1988). Thus memory for operant learning increases rapidly after 2 months of age.

A more sensitive version for testing memory with the MCRP uses **reactivation** or **reinstatement** to look at the role of cuing in recall. A day before the long-term memory test, babies are put back into the experimental crib, but the ribbon is not attached to their feet. The mobile is moved for a few minutes by a hidden experimenter, so that the babies experience part of the experimental situation. If this reactivates their memories, they will kick their feet when the ribbon is reattached the next day. This technique has shown that 2- and 3-month-old babies exhibit memory for the response learned 2 weeks earlier, but only do so consistently if their memories have been reactivated (Davis & Rovee-Collier, 1983; Rovee-Collier et al., 1980; Sullivan, 1982; Sullivan et al., 1979). This technique also found reactivated memory in 3-month-olds tested 4 weeks after initial conditioning.

Overall, this is fairly convincing evidence that 2- to 6-month-old babies show evidence of memory over a matter of days and even weeks, and that at a given age memories can be elicited after longer delays when the experimenters provide reactivation cues.

Manipulating variables in various phases of the reactivation MCRP allows investigation of how and when specific memory processes and contents develop. Variations in the amount and distribution of stimulus exposure during training have been shown to affect encoding differently for 2-month-olds (Vander Linde et al., 1985) than for 3-month-olds (Ohr et al., 1989). As for other visual habituation (Rose, 1981), extending the training time has improved long-term memory for the kicking response to the mobile. Previous research had shown that the very young of various species have better retention when training time is distributed over multiple sessions rather than massed into one long session (Coulter, 1979). Ohr et al. (1989) have shown that 2-month-olds did indeed benefit from receiving distributed rather than massed training; however, 3-month-olds remembered the contingency for 1 week after two short episodes, but for 2 weeks after one long training episode. The researchers attribute this variant pattern of a massed training episode to the "distinctiveness" of the stimulus created in one long session.

Differences in 2- and 3-month-olds' visual inspection patterns may account for age differences in memory (Vander Linde et al., 1985). During a long training episode, 2-month-olds tend to fixate (and encode) only a few features of the mobile that could serve as retrieval cues, but 3-month-olds engage in greater visual exploration. With repeated presentations, the younger infants fixate more parts (and encode more features). Support for this interpretation comes from the fact that 1-day retention by 2-month-olds could be improved from zero to perfect by highlighting features of the stimulus (each block hanging from the mobile had a unique picture on each surface instead of each block having the same picture on all sides). This allowed 2-month-olds to encode all key stimulus features while fixating only one rotating block (Rovee-Collier et al., 1989). The 3-month-olds were not affected by the manner in which the pictures were presented.

The question of what is retained in young infants' memories of the MCRP operant situation has been addressed by manipulating dimensions of the mobiles (form, color, and number of objects) presented during various phases of the task. Babies initially kicked less when the mobiles were changed, thus indicating recognition of the change (Fagen, 1984; Fagen et al., 1981; Hill et al., 1988; Mast et al., 1980; Rovee-Collier & Fagen, 1976; Rovee-Collier & Sullivan, 1980). Studies that manipulated the number of familiar items in the reactivation mobile found that even 2-month-olds had perfect retention and complete generalization, but only if no more than one of five objects was novel; otherwise there was no evidence of memory (Hayne et al., 1986; Rovee-Collier et al., 1985). This demonstrated that the infants had encoded and re-

tained specific visual aspects of the stimulus. If infants were tested with a changed mobile more than 3 days after reactivation, kicking resumed at a high rate (Fagen, 1984; Rovee-Collier & Sullivan, 1980). This suggests that with more delay they forgot the details of the stimulus, but remembered the general situation well enough to resume their conditioned kicking response.

Context, as an influence on memory, was also studied by varying the crib liner patterns. The effects depended upon the training procedures. When training was with only one crib liner, even small changes in the pattern caused lower responding (Borovsky & Rovee-Collier, 1990). But if training incorporated multiple contexts (Rovee-Collier & Dufault, 1991) or a reactivation in a novel context (Boller & Rovee-Collier, 1991), then young infants' memory was excellent, even in a novel testing context.

The Rovee-Collier group also found that young infants can remember the stimulus categorically. Babies can learn to expect a new mobile (with different colored and shaped objects) on each day of training (Fagen et al., 1984). When trained with a new mobile every session, babies showed less memory (kick less) for the mobile used in their first session than for another new mobile. Thus these babies had learned to expect the category "new mobile" and remembered that expectation at testing. When 3-month-olds were presented with cube mobiles with a different color on each side as background for either an A or a 2 they could discriminate both color and form (Hayne et al., 1987). (This is also found in 5-month-olds; see Strauss & Cohen, 1980.) Surprisingly, in both a 1-day test and in reactivation after 2 weeks, a novel exemplar of a training category (e.g., blue 2), established by training with other colors of 2, elicited responding, but a novel exemplar from a novel category (e.g., blue A) did not (Hayne et al., 1987). The authors argue that this long-term retention of category-specific information is best explained by retrieval of information about individual exemplars. This interpretation is at odds with the conclusions of habituation studies on categorization (cited earlier), which infer the loss of information about individual exemplars. This discrepancy may be due to differences in methodology: In contrast to the single long sessions used in habituation, shorter multiple sessions of the MCRP operant procedure may facilitate more distinct encoding—and retrieval—of specific stimuli (Hayne et al., 1987). The question of how best to account for infants' memory for categories remains open.

Forgetting

Fagen and collaborators have directly addressed processes of forgetting. Only the 3- to 4-month-olds who cried when their well-learned mobile was replaced by one reduced in number of components showed forgetting during a retention test 1 week (but not 1 day) later (Fagen et al., 1985). Forgetting at 1 week depends on the training procedure (Fagen et al., 1989): When the interval between the last training presentation of the familiar mobile and presentation of the reduced mobile that led to crying was increased from 0 to 30 minutes, there was again significant retention 1 week later. The investigators conclude that crying caused retrograde amnesia (or retrieval failures) due to the absence at testing of cry-related cues (hormonal, neural, visceral, affective) encoded at the end of the learning experience (Fagen et al., 1989). This may be an example of state-dependent learning and memory in infants. However, affect did not appear to influence preschool memory in a study that specifically manipulated it during both learning and testing (Duncan et al., 1985). Caution in interpretation is required until the studies are replicated and the events at the two ages better understood.

Memories From Early Infancy

Some research on infant memory in the first year reveals retention over durations of months or even years. In a naturalistic study, Ashmead and Perlmutter (1980) had 11 parents keep 6-week diaries of memory-related behaviors of their 7- to 11-month-olds. Although fewer than one episode per day was recorded, all infants exhibited behaviors such as searches for absent objects and initiations of social interactions based on previous experiences (such as peekaboo games). Toddler diary data (Nelson & Ross, 1980) and crib speech analyses (Nelson, 1984) reveal recall of information about episodes occurring months and even a year earlier. Similarly, when Hudson (1990) asked 2-year-olds and their mothers to recall past events, the children recalled some novel events and family activities from 10 months earlier. In one study, five 2½-year-olds were invited to return to a unique laboratory setting in which they had repeatedly been tested some 2 years earlier (Myers et al., 1987). Neither controls nor the returning subjects recognized or explicitly named particular objects, but returning subjects were more likely to interact with stimuli as they had in the laboratory 2 years earlier. Thus, in familiar contexts rich in retrieval cues, preschoolers are capable of remembering actions and interactions encoded in infancy and retained over a very extended interval.

Conclusions

Newborns and perhaps even fetuses are capable of limited memory, which develops rapidly during the first year. Encoding initially depends upon repeated exposures to simple stimuli with features highlighted by laboratory procedures or ecological context. Fewer and less focused exposures to stimuli are needed by only a few months of age, when multidimensional stimuli may be remembered categorically. Young infants can remember their own learned responses to stimuli, but not the observed behavior of others, as can older infants in delayed imitation tasks (discussed below). Duration of retention increases rapidly from a few minutes to weeks, months, and even longer during the first year. Memory loss, or decay, occurs first for the specific stimuli and then for features common across stimuli. Retrieval may be the memory process that develops least at the outset; young infants are able only to recognize cues from the original stimulus situation and demonstrate little ability to recall in a way that requires active memory search.

MEMORY DEVELOPMENT IN OLDER INFANTS

Toward the end of the first year, developmental changes in motoric abilities (Chapter 8), cognition (Chapter 10), and language (Chapter 11) enable infants to remember new kinds of content and to remember more efficiently. These changes afford researchers new methodological windows on infant memory processes.

Memory as Seen Using Delayed Search Tasks

One such window is the delayed search task. In this paradigm an infant observes the hiding of one or more interesting objects and then, after a delay, is allowed to search for the objects. The most studied of these tasks is Piaget's (1936/1954) famous object permanence task (see Chapter 10), which elicits the puzzling 8- and 9-month-old "Stage IV error" of searching where an object was momentarily first hidden rather than where it was finally placed. Although many have attributed this error to a variety of memory failures (Bruner et al., 1966; Diamond, 1985; Kagan, 1974; Wellman et al., 1987), recent research by Baillargeon and by Meltzoff supports the position that 8-month-olds are capable of remembering another person's manipulation of an object that they observed earlier. They look longer at "impossible events" (e.g., when a hand recovers a hidden object from behind the wrong screen) even after delays of 70 seconds. This implies that they do remember the object's location (Baillargeon et al., 1989; Baillargeon & Graber, 1988).

In his studies of delayed imitation, Meltzoff (1985, 1988a, 1988b) has also shown that babies remember actions performed on objects. In these studies, a model repeated single actions with unique objects (e.g., folding a large hinge), and later the objects were presented to the infant. It was found that 9-month-olds imitated such actions after a 1-day delay and 14-month-olds did so after 1 week, even though they had no opportunity to imitate immediately and no intermediate contact with the objects. McDonough (1991) found that 11-month-olds not only imitated familiar actions (e.g., "feeding" a wooden block to a teddy bear) after a 24-hour delay, but also remembered the modeled action (feeding) independent of what was fed. Thus it appears that search task failures by infants nearing 1 year of age are not due to problems in remembering single objects, actions, or locations, but to limits on infants' ability to combine memory components.

Memory for Events

A recent burst of work illuminates the combination issue by assessing infants' memory for observed sequences of actions, referred to as *events*. The precursors of preschoolers' excellent event memories have been identified (Nelson, 1986) in the delayed recall of action sequences by infants (Bauer & Mandler, 1989; Bauer & Shore, 1987) sometimes as young as 13 months (Hertsgaard & Bauer, 1991). In these studies, infants observe repetitions of events comprising actions in a sequence (e.g., "make a rattle" by first putting a button in a box and then shaking the box after a delay). Imitation is elicited by verbal and physical cues (the button or the box). Studies vary in the number of repetitions, number of actions, lengths of delays, familiarity of objects and actions, and type of relationship among actions (e.g., temporally invariant, causal, or arbitrary). Results show that after a 1-week delay 13-month-olds can reproduce a two-action sequence modeled twice, even when the actions are novel. But they can do this only if they are given verbal and physical cues, and if the actions are causally related (Hertsgaard & Bauer, 1991). Causal relationships among actions continue to predict memory performance in tasks of this type throughout infancy and preschool (Price & Goodman, 1990), perhaps because memory processes can be organized around the hierarchical goal structure created by the causal relationship (Travis, 1991). For example, in the studies just described, the cause (a button in the box) and effect (the sound when shaking the box) elements would be unitized, or **chunked** into a single memory unit ("make a rattle") that is retained and retrieved as a whole. Then the chunk can be broken into its sequential action elements. This hypothesis is plausible in view of the emergence of means-end planning in two-step tasks at about 9 months of age (Willats, 1990; Willats & Rosie, 1991).

Performance improves rapidly on delayed memory for events. By 16 months of age infants can imitate three-action sequences modeled only once. They can do so for familiar, routine events ("clean the table"), as well as for causally organized sequences, after as long as 6 weeks (Bauer & Mandler, 1989). They can recall the objects and actions in arbitrarily ordered events (e.g., "make a picture"; Dow & Bauer, 1991), but they cannot remember the temporal order (Bauer & Mandler, 1989; Bauer & Thal, 1990; Dow & Bauer, 1991; Hertsgaard & Bauer, 1991). At 16 months, infants also can reproduce events with new props. For example, a "bedtime" event modeled with a small, hard plastic teddy bear can be elicited a week later with a large, stuffed Big Bird (Dow & Bauer, 1991). By 18 to 20 months of age, infants recall event sequences at above chance levels after a 6-week delay (Bauer & Mandler, 1989; Bauer & Shore, 1987). Reactivation analogous to that used in operant conditioning with younger infants can produce recall of once-experienced novel activities (e.g., "feeding fish") after an 8-week delay (Hudson, 1991).

Conclusions

Converging evidence indicates that between 8 and 18 months infants rapidly develop the ability to encode infrequently observed actions, objects, and locations, and to retain that information over long intervals. During this period they also begin to encode relationships among observed phenomena. Memory becomes less tied to specific objects; for example, retrieval is elicited by verbal labels for whole events, indicating better recall memory.

THE LATE INFANCY TRANSITION

Up to 18 months of age, infants' memory processes are dependent largely upon encoding and retrieval cues provided by context. During the last phase of infancy there is a move toward rapid encoding of more abstract dimensions of the context. Employing a paired comparison, looking preference paradigm, Greco and Daehler (1985) found that after a week's delay 2-year-olds recognized a member of a category (e.g., birds) even if they previously had seen only one exemplar of that category. Development also progresses toward more systematic retention and retrieval processes.

Delayed search tasks illustrate this development. Infants of 18 months can successfully search for hidden objects after substantial delays. DeLoache and Brown (1979, 1983) found performance in such search tasks significantly higher when the objects were hidden in obvious spots in the infants' homes than when they were hidden in metal boxes. Similarly, the memory of 24-month-olds in a search for objects hidden in metal boxes was improved when there was a picture of the hidden object on the box (Ratner & Myers, 1980), but not when there was a picture of an unrelated object (Horn & Myers, 1978). It also improved when the boxes were of different sizes (Daehler et al., 1976). There appears to be rapid increase in the range of contextual cues that facilitate memory between the ages of 18 months and 3 years (DeLoache & Brown, 1983; Horn & Myers, 1978). By 3 years children can use rather arbitrary contextual cues such as unrelated pictures on the boxes or the locations of the boxes in the room.

Recent variations in delayed search methodology show that 2-year-olds also encode conceptually related cues and even use metamemory strategies to improve memory performance. **Metamemory** entails the processes or strategies used by the individual to guide encoding, retention, and retrieval. When metamemory involves a self-conscious, systematic strategy, such as a rhyme scheme ("Thirty days hath September . . . "), this is called a **mnemonic** device. Daniel and Jurden (1991) found that children between 24 and 28 months of age not only could use the picture of the hidden object itself as the cue for which box to open, but they performed better even if there were picture cues of conceptually related items (e.g., table-chair). DeLoache et al. (1985) demonstrated that when 18- to 24-month-olds were faced with a difficult memory-for-location task (find a toy) in an unfamiliar setting, they were likely to talk about the object or its hiding place or to point at the hiding place during the delay. Such behaviors rarely occurred when task demands were lessened, but when they did occur they predicted better memory test performance. The authors suggest that these behaviors are precursors of the later-developing covert mnemonic strategies of rehearsal (e.g., subvocal repetition) and monitoring (e.g., periodic checks on availability of memory items). By the end of infancy, children's memory processes are becoming more conceptual and more active.

DEVELOPMENTAL NEUROLOGY OF INFANT MEMORY

Recent methodological and empirical advances in the anatomical and physiological assessment of neurological development during infancy have stimulated provocative speculation and theory regarding infant memory.

Methodological Advances

The possibility of recording event-related potentials (ERPs), which are stimulus-elicited electrical patterns in the brain in awake, active infants, is one such advance. They can be measured with contact electrodes on the scalp. Specific ERP wave patterns over the occipital and frontal areas have been found during visual recognition tasks in 4- to 6-month-olds infants (Nelson & Collins, 1991; Nelson & Salapatek, 1986; Odegaard et al., 1991). The relationship between these patterns and specific memory processes is as yet unclear (Karrer & Hunter, 1991). A second methodology explores the relationship between cardiac vagal tone and visual recognition memory in 6-month-olds. Linnemeyer and Porges (1986) found, for example, that only the infants who showed visual recognition memory also had a heart rate deceleration when inspecting the stimuli. Methodologies like these may eventually offer new indices of infant encoding, retrieval or other memory processes. However, some reviewers argue that infant recognition memory itself is the best index in early infancy of neurodevelopmental well-being (e.g., Butterbaugh, 1988; Fagen, 1985; see McCall, 1989, for an overview).

The Two-Memory Hypothesis

Some of the most provocative empirical and theoretical work comes from the cross-species behavioral and neuroanatomical studies conducted by Mishkin and Appenzeller (1987). Another intriguing approach comes not from infancy studies, but from the life-span and adult organic amnesia research of Moscovitch and colleagues (e.g., Moscovitch, 1985). Despite their differences, these two types of research converge in proposing that two memory systems develop during infancy, one early, perhaps even prenatally, the other just before 1 year of age.

There are several empirical bases for this conjecture. Neuroanatomical studies reveal two distinct brain pathways in lower species and in adult humans. One pathway includes sensory projections into the evolutionarily "older" brain center, which matures early, perhaps even prenatally. This "early" memory pathway is behaviorally associated with memory for stimulus-response repetition, as in operant conditioning and habituation in human infants younger than 8 months. It also operates in adult organic amnesia patients whose lesions are to the higher brain areas, which are phylogenetically associated with the "late" memory system and include "newer" brain areas. Behaviorally, this later maturing system is associated with single-exposure memory, as in memory for an event, in older infants. When this system is damaged, as in organic amnesia patients, there is loss of conscious recollection of specific objects and events.

The two-memory hypothesis is conceptually powerful. It not only encompasses the comparative neuroanatomic data, but the life-span and pathology data bases upon which it is founded. It also fits the patterns of findings in much recent literature on infant memory. For example, in the literature reviewed above, one major transition in memory performance seems to occur around the first birthday. The transformation is from repetition-based memory for self-produced responses (usually elicited by features of the original stimulus) to memory for single exposures to multiple actions of others (often elicited by words only indirectly related to the observed actions and objects). Such a transition fits the two-memory model.

The two-memory hypothesis also is pertinent to the relation between cognition and memory. Those issues are clearly delineated by Piaget's (1945/1962) assertion that "the memory of a two or three year old child is still a medley of made-up stories and exact but chaotic reconstructions, organized memory developing only when speech and the system of concepts exist" (pp. 187-188). A central issue in infant memory research continues to be the relationship between mental representation and memory (see Chapter 10). Clearly, Piaget was convinced—and his evidence and logic are convincing to many others—that mental representation must precede memory-in-the-strict-sense, because representations are the only contents of memory. Objects cannot be recalled until they can be conceptualized. Moscovitch (1985) indirectly challenges this truism by showing that organic amnesia patients, who still have adult representational capacities, perform much like 8-month-old infants on object permanence tasks, making the "Stage IV error" described earlier. He argues that, like organic amnesiacs, 8-month-old infants may fail an object permanence task because they lack a later-developing memory system rather than because of a representational deficit. In contrast to Piaget, Moscovitch conjectures that it may be that objects cannot be fully conceptualized until

they can be recalled. He views memory (both early and late) and representation as separate mental and neurological systems that are interdependent in their development.

The two-memory hypothesis is attractive in its synthesis of diverse lines of research, but it must be treated as preliminary, because it relies heavily on generalizations from other species, from a few tasks, and from atypical populations. Moreover, in a recent review, Rovee-Collier (1987) makes a similarly powerful case for a different two-memory model in infancy, based on the classical distinction between short-term and long-term memory. **Short-term memory** refers to minutes-long memory within one session of a learning paradigm (as in habituation) and **long-term memory** to the between-sessions, days-long memory for a new association (as in the MCRP). Whatever the final outcome, these recent theories and controversies have been exceptionally fruitful in stimulating research at a rate that may soon lead to major advances in our understanding of the development of infant memory and its relationship to other developmental processes.

Summary

This chapter has explored several mechanisms by which infants acquire knowledge of their world and by which researchers are able to determine what they have observed, processed, or learned.

HABITUATION

Habituation is a basic mechanism, both physiological and psychological. To understand it, we must know that what are habituated are orienting responses, such as looking at a visual stimulus, turning toward a sound, and changing heart rate in response to any type of new stimulation. In the habituation paradigm, researchers expose an infant to a stimulus until there is no longer a response. To ensure that sensory or muscular fatigue did not cause the cessation of response, dishabituation is obtained. That is, a new stimulus is presented, which should cause responding to increase.

Whether habituation represents cognitive (or CNS) or autonomic nervous system functioning is unclear. Habituation is difficult to obtain in newborns, but easier to obtain and more stable after 2 months. There is moderate stability of habituation over weeks and months, but findings vary considerably from one study to another. Measures of attention times and patterns during habituation are modestly predictive of later intellectual development for both premature and term infants.

CONDITIONING

The second basic mechanism by which infants acquire knowledge is conditioning. Classical conditioning is extremely difficult to obtain in newborns and can be accomplished only if special techniques or biologicallly prepotent stimuli are used. It is a more tedious procedure than operant conditioning, even with older infants. In operant conditioning a response is reinforced by some positive form of stimulation. This results in the response being made more frequently. Only a response that is emitted or that can be made to occur through shaping can be reinforced. Reinforcers occur contingent upon the baby's having made the desired response. Operant conditioning is also limited, because newborns and young infants have few behaviors that can be reinforced, and they are not awake and alert for long periods. Operant conditioning can be used to modify undesirable behaviors in infants, and is very useful in teaching skills to infants or children with various handicapping conditions.

IMITATION

Imitation is the third basic mechanism. There is a lively debate as to how early infants can imitate, and as to whether the early forms of imitation indicate intent, which is part of some definitions. Newborns do imitate tongue protrusions under some circumstances and some of the time. Imitation by young infants is often not exact, but what is called same-class imitation. By 3 to 4 months, infants' imitations appear to have more intent; from 4 to 8 months they imitate familiar actions, and unfamiliar by 8 to 12 months. Imitation plays an important role in the interactions and social relationships of infants and caregivers.

Severely retarded children can be taught to imitate enough actions (using operant conditioning) that a generalized tendency to imitate, such as normal infants have, develops.

MEMORY

All of the above mechanisms require that the organism remember something, at least for a short time, and all of them are used to study memory.

Newborns and even fetuses have limited memory, and capacity for memory develops rapidly over the first year. What is remembered, and for how long, changes rapidly over the first year. Cuing is important for retrieval. Both encoding and retrieval become more advanced in the period from 8 to 18 months, but become abstract only at the latter time. A transition to

still more advanced processes (metamemory and mnemonic devices) takes place around 2 years.

Methodological advances have led to new ways of studying what goes on in physiological systems during memory. Neuroanatomic and cross-species studies as well as work on clinical cases with memory problems have led to a two-memory hypothesis (early and late) based on different brain pathways. This is different from concepts of short- and long-term memory, which are often conceived as different processes. The two-memory hypothesis is relevant to the relations between mental representation (cognition) and memory as discussed by Piaget.

References

ABRAVANEL, E., Levan-Goldschmidt, E., & Stevenson, M. B. (1976). Action imitation: The early phase of infancy. *Child Development, 47*, 1032-1044.

ABRAVANEL, E., & Sigafoos, A. D. (1984). Exploring the presence of imitation during early infancy. *Child Development, 55*, 381-392.

ALESSANDRI, S. M., Sullivan, M. W., & Lewis, M. (1990). Violation of expectancy and frustration in early infancy. *Developmental Psychology, 26*, 738-744.

ANISFELD, M. (1979). Interpreting "imitative" responses in early infancy. *Science, 205*, 214-215.

ANISFELD, M. (1991). Neonatal imitation. *Developmental Review, 11*, 60-97.

ASHMEAD, D. H., & Perlmutter, M. (1980). Infant memory in everyday life. In M. Perlmutter (Ed.), *Children's memory*. San Francisco: Jossey-Bass.

BAER, D. M., & Deguchi, H. (1985). Generalized imitation from a radical-behavioral point of view. In S. Reiss & R. Bootzin (Eds.), *Theoretical issues in behavior therapy* (pp. 179-217). New York: Academic Press.

BAER, D. M., Peterson, R. F., & Sherman, J. A. (1967). The development of imitation by reinforcing behavioral similarity to a model. *Journal of Experimental Analysis of Behavior, 10*, 405-416.

BAER, D. M., & Sherman, J. (1964). Reinforcement control of generalized imitation in young children. *Journal of Experimental Child Psychology, 1*, 37-49.

BAILLARGEON, R., De Vos, J., & Graber, M. (1989). Location memory in 8-month-old infants in a non-search AB task: Further evidence. *Cognitive Development, 4*, 345-367.

BAILLARGEON, R., & Graber, M. (1988). Evidence of location memory in 8-month-old infants in a nonsearch AB task. *Developmental Psychology, 24*, 502-511.

BATES, J. E. (1975). Effects of a child's imitation versus nonimitation on adult's verbal and nonverbal positivity. *Journal of Personality and Social Psychology, 31*, 840-851.

BAUER, P., & Mandler, J. (1989). One thing follows another: Effects of temporal structure on 1- to 2-year-olds' recall of events. *Developmental Psychology, 25*, 197-206.

BAUER, P., & Shore, C. (1987). Making a memorable event: Effects of familiarity and organization on young children's recall of action sequences. *Cognitive Development, 2*, 327-338.

BAUER, P., & Thal, D. (1990). Scripts or scraps: Reconsidering the development of sequential understanding. *Journal of Experimental Child Psychology, 50*, 287-304.

BERG, W. K., & Berg, K. M. (1979). Psychophysiological development in infancy: State, sensory function, and attention. In J. D. Osofsky (Ed.), *Handbook of infant development* (pp. 283-343). New York: John Wiley.

BJORKLUND, D. F. (1987). A note on neonatal imitation. *Developmental Review, 7*, 86-92.

BLASS, E. M., Ganchrow, J. R., & Steiner, J. E. (1984). Classical conditioning in newborn humans 2-48 hours of age. *Infant Behavior and Development, 7*, 223-235.

BLOOM, K., & Esposito, A. (1975). Social conditioning and its proper control procedures. *Journal of Experimental Child Psychology, 20*, 51-58.

BOLLER, K., & Rovee-Collier, C. (1991, July). *The plasticity of context-specific memories of 6-month-olds.* Paper presented at the biennial meeting of the International Society for the Study of Behavioral Development, Minneapolis.

BORNSTEIN, M. H., & Benasich, A. A. (1986). Infant habituation: Assessments of individual differences and short-term reliability at five months. *Child Development, 57*, 87-99.

BORNSTEIN, M. H., & Ruddy, M. (1984). Infant attention and maternal stimulation: Prediction of cognitive and linguistic development in singletons and twins. In H. Bouma & D. G. Bouwhuis (Eds.), *Attention and performance X: Control of language processes.* London: Lawrence Erlbaum.

BORNSTEIN, M. H., & Sigman, M. D. (1986). Continuity in mental development from infancy. *Child Development, 57*, 251-274.

BOROVSKY, D., & Rovee-Collier, C. K. (1990). Contextual constraints on memory retrieval at six months. *Child Development, 61*, 1569-1583.

BRAZELTON, T. B. (1974). *Toddlers and parents: A developmental perspective.* New York: Dell.

BRUNER, J. S. (1972). Nature and uses of immaturity. *American Psychologist, 27*, 687-708.

BRUNER, J. S., Oliver, R., & Greenfield, P. (1966). *Studies in cognitive growth.* New York: John Wiley.

BÜHLER, C., & Hetzer, H. (1928). Das erste Verständnis von Ausdruck im Ersten Lebensjahre [The first understandings from their expression in the first year of life]. *Zeitschrift für Psychologie, 107*, 50-61.

BURNHAM, D. K., Vignes, G., & Ihsen, E. (1988). The effects of movement on infants' memory for visual compounds. *British Journal of Developmental Psychology, 6*, 351-360.

BUTTERBAUGH, G. (1988). Selected psychometric and clinical review of neurodevelopmental infant tests. *Clinical Neuropsychologist, 2*, 350-364.

CAMP, B. W., Jamieson, D.-K., Hansen, R., & Schmidt, B. (1990). Growth parameters and attention to faces at 4 and 6 months of age. *Journal of Developmental and Behavioral Pediatrics, 11*, 229-233.

CARON, A. J., Caron, R. F., & Glass, P. (1983). Responsiveness to relational information as a measure of cognitive functioning in nonsuspect infants. In T. Field & A. Sostek (Eds.), *Infants born at risk.* New York: Grune & Stratton.

CATHERWOOD, D., Crassini, B., & Froberg, K. (1987). The nature of infant memory for hue. *British Journal of Developmental Psychology, 5*, 385-394.

CAVANAGH, P., & Davidson, M. L. (1977). The secondary circular reaction and response elicitation in the operant learning of six-month-old infants. *Developmental Psychology, 13*, 371-376.

CLIFTON, R. K. (1974). Heart rate conditioning in the newborn infant. *Journal of Experimental Child Psychology, 13*, 43-57.

CLIFTON, R. K., Meyers, W. J., & Solomons, E. (1972). Methodological problems in conditioning the headturning response of newborns. *Journal of Experimental Child Psychology, 13*, 29-42.

CLIFTON, R. K., Siqueland, E. R., & Lipsitt, L. P. (1972). Conditioned headturning in human newborns as a function of conditioned response requirements and states of wakefulness. *Journal of Experimental Child Psychology, 13*, 43-57.

COHEN, L. B. (1973). A two-process model of infant visual attention. *Merrill-Palmer Quarterly, 19*, 157-180.

COHEN, S. E., & Parmelee, A. H. (1983). Prediction of five-year Stanford-Binet scores in preterm infants. *Child Development, 54*, 1242-1253.

COLE, M., & Scribner, S. (1974). *Culture and thought: A psychological introduction.* New York: John Wiley.

COLOMBO, J., Mitchell, D. W., O'Brien, M., & Horowitz, F. D. (1987a). The stability of visual habituation during the first year of life. *Child Development, 58*, 474-487.

COLOMBO, J., Mitchell, D. W., O'Brien, M., & Horowitz, F. D. (1987b). Stimulus and motoric influences on visual habituation to facial stimuli at 3 months. *Infant Behavior and Development, 10*, 173-181.

COLOMBO, J., O'Brien, M., Mitchell, D. W., Roberts, K., et al. (1987). A lower boundary for category formation in preverbal infants. *Journal of Child Language, 14*, 383-385.

COULTER, X. (1979). The determinants of infantile amnesia. In N. Spear & B. Campbell (Eds.), *The ontogeny of learning and memory* (pp. 245-270). Hillsdale, NJ: Lawrence Erlbaum.

CROWELL, D. H., Blurton, L. B., Kobayashi, L. R., McFarland, J. L., & Yang, R. K. (1976). Studies in early infant learning: Classical conditioning of the neonatal heart rate. *Developmental Psychology, 12*, 373-397.

DAEHLER, M., Bukatko, D., Benson, K., & Myers, N. (1976). The effects of size and color cues on the delayed response of very young children. *Bulletin of the Psychonomic Society, 7*, 65-68.

DANIEL, D., & Jurden, F. (1991, April). *The use of categorically related picture cues: Memory for hidden-object locations in 2-year-olds.* Paper presented at the biennial meeting of the Society for Research in Child Development, Seattle.

DAVIS, J. M., & Rovee-Collier, C. K. (1983). Alleviated forgetting of a learned contingency in 8-week-old infants. *Developmental Psychology, 19*, 353-365.

DeCASPER, A., & Fifer, W. P. (1980). Of human bonding: Newborns prefer their mothers' voices. *Science, 208*, 1174-1176.

DeCASPER, A., & Spencer, M. (1986). Prenatal maternal speech influences newborns' perception of speech sounds. *Infant Behavior and Development, 9*, 133-150.

DeLOACHE, J. S. (1976). Rate of habituation and visual memory in infants. *Child Development, 47*, 145-154.

DeLOACHE, J. S., & Brown, A. L. (1979). Looking for Big Bird: Studies of memory in very young children. *Quarterly Newsletter of the Laboratory of Comparative Human Cognition, 1*, 53-57.

DeLOACHE, J. S., & Brown, A. L. (1983). Very young children's memory for the location of objects in a large-scale environment. *Child Development, 54*, 888-897.

DeLOACHE, J. S., Cassidy, D., & Brown, A. (1985). Precursors of mnemonic strategies in very young children. *Child Development, 56,* 125-137.

DE SAINT VICTOR, C., & Hull-Smith, P. (1991, April). *Isolating a retrieval process in infant visual recognition memory.* Paper presented at the biennial meeting of the Society for Research in Child Development, Seattle.

DIAMOND, A. (1985). Development of the ability to use recall to guide action, as indicated by infants' performance on AB. *Child Development, 56,* 868-883.

DONOHUE, R. L., Berg, W. K., & Landis, F. (1991, April). *Seven-month-olds display anticipatory HR decelerations and head position changes in a differential conditioning paradigm.* Paper presented at the meeting of the Society for Research in Child Development, Seattle.

DOW, G., & Bauer, P. (1991, April). *Very young children's event representations: Specifics are generalized, but not forgotten.* Poster presented at the biennial meeting of the Society for Research in Child Development, Seattle.

DUNCAN, S., Todd, C., Perlmutter, M., & Masters, J. (1985). Affect and memory in young children. *Motivation and Emotion, 9,* 391-405.

DUNST, C. J., Cushing, P. J., & Vance, S. D. (1985). Response-contingent learning in profoundly handicapped infants: A social systems perspective. In Early intervention [Special issue]. *Analysis and Intervention in Developmental Disabilities, 5,* 33-47.

DUNST, C. J., & Lingerfelt, B. (1985). Maternal ratings of temperament and operant learning in two- to three-month-old infants. *Child Development, 56,* 555-563.

EPPLER, M. A., Gibson, E. J., & Adolph, K. E. (1990, March). *Infants' attention to objects in the development of object manipulation skills.* Paper presented at the Conference on Human Development, Richmond, VA.

FAGAN, J. F., III. (1973). Infant's delayed recognition memory and forgetting. *Journal of Experimental Child Psychology, 16,* 424-450.

FAGAN, J. F., & Singer, L. T. (1983). Infant recognition memory as a measure of intelligence. In L. P. Lipsitt (Ed.), *Advances in infancy research* (Vol. 2, pp. 31-78). Norwood, NJ: Ablex.

FAGEN, J. W. (1984). Infants' long-term memory of stimulus color. *Developmental Psychology, 20,* 435-440.

FAGEN, J. W. (1985). A new look at infant intelligence. *Current Topics in Human Intelligence, 1,* 223-246.

FAGEN, J. W., Morrongiello, B. A., Rovee-Collier, C., & Gekoski, M. J. (1984). Expectancies and memory retrieval in three-month-old infants. *Child Development, 55,* 936-943.

FAGEN, J. W., Ohr, P., Fleckenstein, L., & Ribner, D. (1985). The effect of crying on long-term memory in infancy. *Child Development, 56,* 1584-1592.

FAGEN, J. W., Ohr, P. S., Singer, J. M., & Fleckenstein, L. K. (1987). Infant temperament and subject loss due to crying during operant conditioning. *Child Development, 58,* 497-504.

FAGEN, J. W., Ohr, P. S., Singer, J. M., & Klein, S. (1989). Crying and retrograde amnesia in young infants. *Infant Behavior and Development, 12,* 13-24.

FAGEN, J. W., & Rovee-Collier, C. K. (1983). Memory retrieval: A time locked process in infancy. *Science, 222,* 1349-1351.

FAGEN, J. W., Yengo, L. A., Rovee-Collier, C. K., & Enright, M. K. (1981). Reactivation of a visual discrimination in early infancy. *Developmental Psychology, 17,* 266-274.

FIELD, T. M., Dempsey, J. R., Hatch, J., Ting, G., & Clifton, R. K. (1979). Cardiac and behavioral responses to repeated tactile and auditory stimulation by preterm and term neonates. *Developmental Psychology, 15,* 406-416.

FIELD, T. M., Goldstein, S., Vega-Lahr, N., & Porter, K. (1986). Changes in imitative behavior during early infancy. *Infant Behavior and Development, 9,* 415-421.

FIELD, T. M., Woodson, R., Greenberg, R., & Cohen, D. (1982). Discrimination and imitation of facial expressions by neonates. *Science, 218,* 179-181.

FITZGERALD, H. E., & Brackbill, Y. (1976). Classical conditioning in infancy: Development and constraints. *Psychological Bulletin, 3,* 353-376.

FOUTS, G. T. (1972). Imitation in children: The effect of being imitated. *Catalog of Selected Documents in Psychology, 2,* 105.

FOUTS, G. T. (1975). The effects of being imitated and awareness on the behavior of introverted and extroverted youth. *Child Development, 46,* 296-300.

GARDNER, J., & Gardner, H. (1970). A note on selective imitation by a six-week-old infant. *Child Development, 41,* 1209-1213.

GEKOSKI, M. J. (1977). Visual attention and operant conditioning in infancy: A second look. *Dissertation Abstracts International, 38,* 875B. (University Microfilms No. 77-17, 533)

GEWIRTZ, J. L. (1971a). Conditional responding as a paradigm for observational, imitative learning and vicarious reinforcement. In H. W. Reese (Ed.), *Advances in child development and behavior* (Vol. 6). New York: Academic Press.

GEWIRTZ, J. L. (1971b). The roles of overt responding and extrinsic reinforcement. In R. Glaser (Ed.), *The nature of reinforcement.* New York: Academic Press.

GEWIRTZ, J. L., & Stingle, K. G. (1968). Learning of generalized imitation as the basis for identification. *Psychological Review, 75,* 374-397.

GIBSON, E. J. (1988). Exploratory behavior in the development of perceiving, acting, and the acquiring of knowledge. *Annual Review of Psychology, 39,* 1-44.

GRAHAM, F. K., & Clifton, R. K. (1966). Heart-rate change as a component of the orienting response. *Psychological Bulletin, 65,* 305-320.

GRAHAM, F. K., Leavitt, L. A., Strock, B. D., & Brown, J. W. (1978). Precocious cardiac orienting in a human, anencephalic infant. *Science, 199,* 322-324.

GRECO, C., & Daehler, M. (1985). Immediate and long-term retention of basic-level categories in 24-month-olds. *Infant Behavior and Development, 8,* 459-474.

GRECO, C., Rovee-Collier, C., Hayne, H., Griesler, P., & Early, L. (1986). Ontogeny of early event memory: I. Forgetting and retrieval by 2- and 2-month-olds. *Infant Behavior and Development, 9,* 441-460.

GUILLAUME, D. (1971). *Imitation in children* (E. P. Halperin, Trans.). Chicago: University of Chicago Press. (Original work published 1926)

HAAF, R., & Lundy, B. (1991, April). *Context, attention, and recognition memory in 6-month-old infants.* Paper presented at the biennial meeting of the Society for Research in Child Development, Seattle.

HAITH, M. M., Hazen, C., & Goodman, G. S. (1988). Expectation and anticipation of dynamic visual events by 3.5-month-old babies. *Child Development, 59,* 467-479.

HANNA, E., & Meltzoff, A. N. (1991, April). *Learning from others in infant daycare: Remembering and imitating the ac-*

tions of another. Paper presented at the biennial meeting of the Society for Research in Child Development, Seattle.

HARLOW, H. F. (1949). Formation of learning sets. *Psychological Review, 56,* 51-65.

HARNICK, F. S. (1978). The relationship between ability level and task difficulty in producing imitation in infants. *Child Development, 49,* 209-212.

HAYES, L. A., & Watson, J. S. (1981). Neonatal imitation: Fact or artifact. *Developmental Psychology, 17,* 655-660.

HAYNE, H., Greco, C., Early, L., Griesler, P., & Rovee-Collier, C. (1986). Ontogeny of early event memory: II. Encoding and retrieval by 2- and 3-month-olds. *Infant Behavior and Development, 9,* 461-472.

HAYNE, H., Rovee-Collier, C., & Perris, E. (1987). Categorization and memory retrieval by three-month-olds. *Child Development, 58,* 750-767.

HEIMANN, M. (1989). Neonatal imitation, gaze aversion, and mother infant interaction. *Infant Behavior and Development, 12,* 495-505.

HEIMANN, M. (1991, April). *Imitation during the first three months of life and at 12 months of age: Findings from a follow-up.* Paper presented at the biennial meeting of the Society for Research in Child Development, Seattle.

HERTSGAARD, L., & Bauer, P. (1991, April). *Thirteen- and sixteen-month-olds' long-term recall of event sequences.* Paper presented at the biennial meeting of the Society for Research in Child Development, Seattle.

HILL, W., Borovsky, D., & Rovee-Collier, C. (1988). Continuities in infant memory development. *Developmental Psychobiology, 21,* 43-62.

HORN, H., & Myers, N. A. (1978). Memory for location and picture cues at ages two and three. *Child Development, 49,* 845-856.

HOROWITZ, F. D., Paden, L. Y., Bhana, K., & Self, P. (1972). An infant control procedure for studying infant visual fixations. *Developmental Psychology, 7,* 90.

HUDSON, J. (1990). The emergence of autobiographic memory in mother-child conversation. In R. Fimmsh & J. Hudson (Eds.), *Knowing and remembering in young children.* New York: Cambridge University Press.

HUDSON, J. (1991, April). *Effects of reenactment on toddlers' long-term memory for a novel event.* Paper presented at the biennial meetings of the Society for Research in Child Development, Seattle.

JACOBSON, S. W. (1979). Matching behavior in the young infant. *Child Development, 50,* 425-430.

JACOBSON, S. W., & Kagan, J. (1979). Interpreting "imitative" responses in early infancy. *Science, 205,* 215-217.

JENKINS, J. J. (1980). Can we have a fruitful cognitive psychology? *Nebraska Symposium on Motivation, 28,* 211-238.

KAGAN, J. (1974). Discrepancy, temperament, and infant distress. In M. Lewis & A. Rosenblum (Eds.), *The origins of fear* (pp. 229-248). New York: John Wiley.

KAPLAN, P. S., & Werner, J. S. (1987). Sensitization and dishabituation of infant visual fixation. *Infant Behavior and Development, 10,* 183-197.

KARRER, R., & Hunter, S. (1991, July). *Event-related potentials during a recognition memory task: Effects of stimulus duration on infant responses.* Poster presented at the biennial meeting of the International Society for the Study of Behavioral Development, Minneapolis.

KAYE, H. (1965). The conditioned Babkin reflex in human newborns. *Psychonomic Science, 2,* 287.

KAYE, K., & Marcus, J. (1981). Infant imitation: The sensory-motor agenda. *Developmental Psychology, 17,* 258-265.

KEEN, R. (1964). Effects of auditory stimuli on sucking behavior in the human neonate. *Journal of Psychology, 1,* 348-354.

KESSEN, W., Levine, J., & Hendrich, K. A. (1979). The imitation of pitch in infants. *Infant Behavior and Development, 2,* 93-99.

KILLEN, M., & Uzgiris, I. C. (1981). Imitation of actions with objects: The role of social meaning. *Journal of Genetic Psychology, 138,* 219-229.

KISILEVSKY, B. S., & Muir, D. W. (1984). Neonatal habituation and dishabituation to tactile stimulation during sleep. *Developmental Psychology, 20,* 367-373.

KOEPKE, J. E., Hamm, M., Legerstee, M., & Russell, M. (1983a). Methodological issues in studies of imitation: Reply to Meltzoff and Moore. *Infant Behavior and Development, 6,* 113-116.

KOEPKE, J. E., Hamm, M., Legerstee, M., & Russell, M. (1983b). Neonatal imitation: Two failures to replicate. *Infant Behavior and Development, 6,* 97-102.

LARSON, K., & Ayllon, T. (1990). The effects of contingent music and differential reinforcement on infantile colic. *Behaviour Research and Therapy, 28,* 119-125.

LEWIS, M., & Brooks-Dunn, J. (1981). Visual attention at three months as a predictor of cognitive functioning at two years of age. *Intelligence, 3,* 131-140.

LINNEMEYER, S., & Porges, S. (1986). Recognition memory and cardiac vagal tone in 6-month-old infants. *Infant Behavior and Development, 9,* 43-56.

LIPSITT, L. P. (1990). Learning and memory in infants. *Merrill-Palmer Quarterly, 36,* 53-66.

LIPSITT, L. P., Mustaine, M. G., & Zeigler, B. (1977). Effects of experience on the behavior of the young infant. *Neuropaediatrie, 8,* 107-133.

LIPTON, E. L., Steinschneider, A., & Richmond, J. B. (1966). Autonomic function in the neonate: VII. Maturational changes in cardiac control. *Child Development, 37,* 1-16.

LOBOSCHEFSKI, T., Hull-Smith, P., & Bennett, K. (1991, April). *Structure and modality: Differential impacts on infants' recall memory.* Paper presented at the biennial meeting of the Society for Research in Child Development, Seattle.

MacKAY-SOROKA, S., Trehub, S. E., Bull, D. H., & Corter, C. M. (1982). Effects of encoding and retrieval conditions on infants' recognition memory. *Child Development, 53,* 815-818.

MADISON, L. S., Madison, J. K., & Adubato, S. A. (1986). Infant behavior and development in relation to fetal movement and habituation. *Child Development, 57,* 1475-1482.

MARQUIS, D. (1931). Can conditioned responses be established in the newborn infant? *Journal of Genetic Psychology, 39,* 479-490.

MARTIN, G. B., & Clark, R. D., III. (1982). Distress crying in neonates: Species and peer specificity. *Developmental Psychology, 18,* 3-9.

MARTIN, R. M. (1975). Effects of familiar and complex stimuli on infant attention. *Developmental Psychology, 11,* 178-185.

MAST, V. K., Fagen, J. W., Rovee-Collier, C. K., & Sullivan, M. W. (1980). Immediate and long-term memory for reinforcement context: The development of learned expectancies in early infancy. *Child Development, 51,* 700-707.

MAURER, D., & Maurer, C. (1988). *The world of the unborn.* New York: Basic Books.

McCALL, R. (1979). The development of intellectual functioning in infancy and the prediction of later IQ. In J. D. Osofsky (Ed.), *Handbook of infant development*. New York: John Wiley.

McCALL, R. (1989). Commentary. *Human Development, 32,* 177-186.

McCALL, R. B., Kennedy, C. B., & Dodds, C. (1977). The interfering effects of distracting stimuli on the infant's memory. *Child Development, 48,* 79-87.

McDONOUGH, L. (1991, April). *Infant recall of familiar actions with decontextualized objects.* Poster presented at the biennial meeting of the Society for Research in Child Development, Seattle.

McKENZIE, B., & Over, R. (1983a). Do neonatal infants imitate? A reply to Meltzoff and Moore. *Infant Behavior and Development, 6,* 109-111.

McKENZIE, B., & Over, R. (1983b). Young infants fail to imitate facial and manual gestures. *Infant Behavior and Development, 6,* 85-95.

MELTZOFF, A. N. (1985). Immediate and deferred imitation in fourteen- and twenty-four-month-old infants. *Child Development, 56,* 62-72.

MELTZOFF, A. N. (1988a). Infant imitation after a 1-week delay: Long-term memory for novel acts and multiple stimuli. *Developmental Psychology, 24,* 470-476.

MELTZOFF, A. N. (1988b). Infant imitation and memory: Nine-month-olds in immediate and deferred tests. *Child Development, 59,* 217-225.

MELTZOFF, A. N., & Moore, M. K. (1977). Imitation of facial and manual gestures by human neonates. *Science, 198,* 75-78.

MELTZOFF, A. N., & Moore, M. K. (1979). Interpreting "imitative" responses in early infancy. *Science, 205,* 217-219.

MELTZOFF, A. N., & Moore, M. K. (1983a). Methodological issues in studies of imitation: Comments on McKenzie & Over and Koepke et al. *Infant Behavior and Development, 6,* 103-108.

MELTZOFF, A. N., & Moore, M. K. (1983b). Newborn infants imitate adult facial gestures. *Child Development, 54,* 702-709.

MELTZOFF, A. N., & Moore, M. K. (1989). Imitation in newborn infants: Exploring the range of gestures imitated and the underlying mechanisms. *Developmental Psychology, 25,* 954-962.

MILLAR, W. S. (1976). Social reinforcement of a manipulative response in six and nine month old infants. *Journal of Child Psychology and Psychiatry, 17,* 205-212.

MILLER, D., Spridigliozzi, G., Ryan, E. B., Callan, M. P., & McLaughlin, J. E. (1980). Habituation and cognitive performance: Relationships between measures at four years of age and earlier assessment. *International Journal of Behavioral Development, 3,* 131-146.

MISHKIN, M., & Appenzeller, T. (1987). The anatomy of memory. *Scientific American, 256*(6), 80-89.

MOSCOVITCH, M. (1985). Memory from infancy to old age: Implications for theories of normal and pathological memory. *Annals of the New York Academy of Sciences, 444,* 78-96.

MURRAY, P. (1987, April). *Infants' responsiveness to modeling vs. instruction.* Paper presented at the meeting of the Society for Research in Child Development, Baltimore.

MUSSEN, P., & Eisenberg-Berg, N. (1977). *Roots of caring, sharing, and helping: The development of prosocial behavior in children.* San Francisco: W. H. Freeman.

MYERS, N., Clifton, R., & Clarkson, M. (1987). When they were very young: Almost-threes remember two years ago. *Infant Behavior and Development, 10,* 123-132.

NELSON, C., & Collins, P. (1991). Event-related potential and looking-time analysis of infants' responses to familiar and novel events: Implications for visual recognition memory. *Developmental Psychology, 27,* 50-58.

NELSON, C., & Salapatek, P. (1986). Electrophysiological correlates of infant recognition memory. *Child Development, 57,* 1483-1497.

NELSON, K. (1984). The transition from infant to child memory. In M. Moscovitch (Ed.), *Infant memory: Its relation to normal and pathological memory in humans and other animals* (pp. 103-130). New York: Plenum.

NELSON, K. (1986). *Event knowledge: Structure and function in development.* Hillsdale, NJ: Lawrence Erlbaum.

NELSON, K., & Ross, G. (1980). The generalities and specifics of longterm memory in infants and young children. *New Directions for Child Development, 10,* 87-102.

ODEGAARD, R., Nelson, C., & Gould, P. (1991, April). *Electrophysiologic correlates of visual recognition memory in four month old infants.* Paper presented at the biennial meeting of the Society for Research in Child Development, Seattle.

OHR, P., Fagen, J., Rovee-Collier, C., Hayne, H., & Vander Linde, E. (1989). Amount of training and retention by infants. *Developmental Psychobiology, 22,* 69-80.

PAPOUŠEK, H. (1961). Conditioned head rotation reflexes in infants in the first months of life. *Acta Pediatrica, 50,* 565-576.

PAPOUŠEK, H. (1967a). Conditioning during postnatal development. In Y. Brackbill & G. G. Thompson (Eds.), *Behavior in infancy and early childhood* (pp. 259-284). New York: Free Press.

PAPOUŠEK, H. (1967b). Experimental studies of appetitional behavior in human newborns and infants. In H. W. Stevenson, E. H. Hess, & H. L. Rheingold (Eds.), *Early behavior: Comparative and developmental approaches* (pp. 249-278). New York: John Wiley.

PAPOUŠEK, H., & Papoušek, M. (1975). Cognitive aspects of preverbal social interactions between human infants and adults. In *Parent-infant interaction* (CIBA Foundation Symposium 33, New Series). Amsterdam: Elsevier.

PAPOUŠEK, H., & Papoušek, M. (1977). Mothering and the cognitive head-start: Psychobiological considerations. In H. R. Schaffer (Ed.), *Studies in mother-infant interaction.* London: Academic Press.

PECHEUX, M. G., & Lécuyer, R. (1983). Habituation rate and free exploration tempo in 4-month-old infants. *International Journal of Behavioral Development, 6,* 37-50.

PECHEUX, M. G., & Lécuyer, R. (1989). A longitudinal study of visual habituation between 3, 5 and 8 months of age. *British Journal of Developmental Psychology, 7,* 159-169.

PIAGET, J. (1954). *The construction of reality in the child* (M. Cook, Trans.). New York: Basic Books. (Original work published in 1936)

PIAGET, J. (1962). *Play, dreams and imitation in childhood* (C. Gattegno & F. M. Hodgson, Trans.). New York: W. W. Norton. (Original work published 1945)

PIAGET, J. (1968). *On the development of memory and identity.* Barre, MA: Clark University Press.

PIAGET, J., & Inhelder, B. (1973). *Memory and intelligence.* Basic Books: New York.

POULSON, C. L. (1988). Operant conditioning of vocalization rate of infants with Down syndrome. *American Journal on Mental Retardation, 93,* 57-63.

POULSON, C. L., & Kymissis, E. (1988). Generalized imitation in infants. *Journal of Experimental Child Psychology, 46,* 324-336.

PRICE, D., & Goodman, G. (1990). Visiting the wizard: Children's memory for a recurring event. *Child Development, 61,* 664-680.

QUINN, P., Siqueland, E., & Bomba, P. (1985). Delayed recognition memory for orientation by human infants. *Journal of Experimental Child Psychology, 40,* 293-303.

RAMEY, C. T., & Watson, J. S. (1972). Nonsocial reinforcement of infants' vocalizations. *Developmental Psychology, 6,* 538.

RATNER, H. H., & Myers, N. A. (1980). Related picture cues and memory for hidden-object location at age two. *Child Development, 51,* 561-564.

REARDON, P., & Bushnell, E. W. (1988). Infants' sensitivity to arbitrary pairings of color and taste. *Infant Behavior and Development, 11,* 245-250.

ROSE, S. A. (1981). Developmental changes in infants' retention of visual stimuli. *Child Development, 52,* 227-233.

ROSE, S. A., & Feldman, J. F. (1987). Infant visual attention: Stability of individual differences from 6 to 8 months. *Developmental Psychology, 23,* 490-498.

ROSE, S. A., Feldman, J. F., Wallace, I. F., & McCarton, C. (1989). Infant visual attention: Relation to birth status and developmental outcome during the first 5 years. *Developmental Psychology, 25,* 560-576.

ROSE, S. A., & Wallace, I. F. (1985a). Cross-modal and intramodal transfer as predictors of mental development in full-term and preterm infants. *Developmental Psychology, 21,* 949-962.

ROSE, S. A., & Wallace, I. F. (1985b). Visual recognition memory: A predictor of later cognitive functioning in preterms. *Child Development, 56,* 843-852.

ROVEE-COLLIER, C. (1987). Learning and memory in infancy. In J. Osofsky (Ed.), *Handbook of infant development* (2nd ed., pp. 98-148). New York: John Wiley.

ROVEE-COLLIER, C., & Dufault, D. (1991). Multiple contexts and memory retrieval at three months. *Developmental Psychobiology, 24,* 39-49.

ROVEE-COLLIER, C., Early, L., & Stafford, S. (1989). Ontogeny of early event memory: III. Attentional determinants of retrieval at 2 and 3 months. *Infant Behavior and Development, 12,* 147-161.

ROVEE-COLLIER, C. K., & Fagen, J. W. (1976). Extended conditioning and 24-hour retention in infants. *Journal of Experimental Child Psychology, 21,* 1-11.

ROVEE-COLLIER, C. K., & Fagen, J. W. (1981). The retrieval of memory in early infancy. In L. P. Lipsitt (Ed.), *Advances in infancy research.* Norwood, NJ: Ablex.

ROVEE-COLLIER, C. K., & Lipsitt, L. P. (1982). Learning, adaptation, and memory in the newborn. In P. Stratton (Ed.), *Psychobiology of the human newborn.* New York: John Wiley.

ROVEE-COLLIER, C. K., Patterson, J., & Hayne, H. (1985). Specificity in the reactivation of infant memory. *Developmental Psychobiology, 18,* 559-574.

ROVEE-COLLIER, C. K., & Sullivan, M. W. (1980). Organization of infant memory. *Journal of Experimental Psychology: Human Learning and Memory, 6,* 798-807.

ROVEE-COLLIER, C. K., Sullivan, M. W., Enright, M., Lucas, D., & Fagen, J. W. (1980). Reactivation of infant memory. *Science, 208,* 1159-1161.

RUFF, H. A. (1981). Effect of context on infants' responses to

novel objects. *Developmental Psychology, 17,* 87-89.

RUFF, H. A. (1982). Role of manipulation in infants' responses to invariant properties of objects. *Developmental Psychology, 18,* 682-691.

RUFF, H. A., Lawson, K. R., Parrinello, R., & Weissberg, R. (1990). Long-term stability of individual differences in sustained attention in the early years. *Child Development, 61,* 60-75.

RUMBAUGH, D. M. (1970). Learning skills of anthropoids. In L. A. Rosenblum (Ed.), *Primate behavior: Developments in field and laboratory research.* New York: Academic Press.

SAGI, A., & Hoffman, M. L. (1976). Empathic distress in the newborn. *Developmental Psychology, 12,* 175-176.

SAMEROFF, A. J. (1968). The components of sucking in the human newborn. *Journal of Experimental Child Psychology, 6,* 607-623.

SAMEROFF, A. J. (1971). Can conditioned responses be established in the newborn infant? *Developmental Psychology, 5,* 1-12.

SAMEROFF, A. J., & Cavanagh, P. J. (1979). Learning in infancy: A developmental perspective. In J. D. Osofsky (Ed.), *Handbook of infant development* (pp. 344-392). New York: John Wiley.

SELIGMAN, M. E. P. (1970). On the generality of the laws of learning. *Psychological Review, 77,* 406-418.

SEMB, G., & Lipsitt, L. P. (1968). The effects of acoustic stimulation on cessation and initiation of non-nutritive sucking in neonates. *Journal of Experimental Child Psychology, 6,* 585-597.

SIGMAN, M. D., Cohen, S. E., Beckwith, L., & Parmelee, A. H. (1986). Infant attention in relation to intellectual abilities in childhood. *Developmental Psychology, 22,* 788-792.

SIMNER, M. L. (1971). Newborns' response to the cry of another infant. *Developmental Psychology, 5,* 136-150.

SIQUELAND, E. R., & Lipsitt, L. P. (1966). Conditioned head-turning in human newborns. *Journal of Experimental Child Psychology, 3,* 356-376.

SLATER, A., Morison, V., & Rose, D. (1984). Habituation in the newborn. *Infant Behavior and Development, 7,* 183-200.

SOKOLOV, E. N. (1963). *Perception and the conditioned reflex.* New York: Macmillan.

SPEAR, N. E., & Parsons, P. G. (1976). Analysis of reactivation treatment: Ontogenetic determinants of alleviated forgetting. In D. L. Medin, W. A. Roberts, & R. T. Davis (Eds.), *Processes of animal memory.* Hillsdale, NJ: Lawrence Erlbaum.

STAMPS, L. E., & Porges, S. W. (1975). Heart rate conditioning in newborn infants: Relationships among conditionability, heart rate variability, and sex. *Developmental Psychology, 11,* 424-431.

STEINSCHNEIDER, A., Lipton, E. L., & Richmond, J. B. (1966). Auditory sensitivity in the infant: Effect of intensity on cardiac and motor responsivity. *Child Development, 37,* 233-252.

STERN, D. (1977). *The first relationship: Infant and mother.* Cambridge, MA: Harvard University Press.

STRAUSS, M. S., & Cohen, L. B. (1980, April). *Infant immediate and delayed memory for perceptual dimensions.* Paper presented at the International Conference on Infant Studies, New Haven, CT.

SULLIVAN, M. W. (1982). Reactivation: Priming forgotten memories in human infants. *Child Development, 53,* 516-523.

SULLIVAN, M. W., & Lewis, M. (1989). Emotion and cognition in infancy: Facial expressions during contingency learning. *International Journal of Behavioral Development, 12,* 221-237.

SULLIVAN, M. W., Rovee-Collier, C. K., & Tynes, D. M. (1979). A conditioning analysis of infant long term memory. *Child Development, 50,* 152-162.

TARQUINIO, N., Zelazo, P. R., & Weiss, M. J. (1990). Recovery of neonatal head turning to decreased sound pressure level. *Developmental Psychology, 26,* 752-758.

THELEN, M. H., Dollinger, S. J., & Roberts, M. C. (1975). On being imitated: Its effects on attraction and reciprocal imitation. *Journal of Personality and Social Psychology, 31,* 467-472.

TOPINKA, C. V., & Steinberg, B. (1978, March). *Visual recognition memory in 3½ and 7½ month old infants.* Paper presented at the International Conference on Infant Studies, Providence, RI.

TRAVIS, L. (1991, April). *Recall of events by two-year-olds: Causal relations and temporal invariance provide separate sources of facilitation.* Poster presented at the biennial meeting of the Society for Research in Child Development, Seattle.

UNGERER, J., Brody, L. R., & Zelazo, P. R. (1978). Long-term memory for speech in 2- to 4-week-old infants. *Infant Behavior and Development, 1,* 127-140.

UZGIRIS, I. C., & Hunt, J. M. (1975). *Assessment in infancy.* Urbana: University of Illinois Press.

VANDER LINDE, E., Morrongiello, B., & Rovee-Collier, C. (1985). Determinants of retention in 8-week-old infants. *Developmental Psychology, 21,* 601-613.

VINTER, A. (1986). The role of movement in eliciting early imitations. *Child Development, 57,* 66-71.

VON BARGEN, D. M. (1983). Infant heart rate: A review of research and methodology. *Merrill-Palmer Quarterly, 29,* 115-150.

WACHS, T. D., & Smitherman, C. H. (1985). Infant temperament and subject loss in a habituation procedure. *Child Development, 56,* 861-867.

WAXLER, C. Z., & Yarrow, M. (1975). An observational study of maternal models. *Developmental Psychology, 11,* 485-494.

WEISBERG, P. (1963). Social and non-social conditioning of infant vocalizations. *Child Development, 34,* 377-388.

WELLMAN, H., Cross, D., & Bartsch, K. (1987). Infant search and object permanence: A meta-analysis of the A-not-B error. *Monographs of the Society for Research in Child Development, 51*(3).

WERNER, J. S., & Perlmutter, M. (1979). Development of visual memory in infants. In H. W. Reese & L. P. Lipsitt (Eds.), *Advances in child development and behavior* (Vol. 14, pp. 1-56). New York: Academic Press.

WICKENS, D. D., & Wickens, C. (1940). A study of conditioning in the neonate. *Journal of Experimental Psychology, 25,* 94-102.

WILLATS, P. (1990). Development of problem-solving strategies in infancy. In D. Bjorkund (Ed.), *Children's strategies: Contemporary views of cognitive development.* Hillsdale, NJ: Lawrence Erlbaum.

WILLATS, P., & Rosie, K. (1991, April). *A longitudinal study of planning in young infants.* Poster presented at the biennial meeting of the Society for Research in Child Development, Seattle.

YANDO, R., Seitz, V., & Zigler, E. (1978). *Imitation: A developmental perspective.* Hillsdale, NJ: Lawrence Erlbaum.

YOUNGER, B. (1990). Infant categorization: Memory for category-level and specific item information. *Journal of Experimental Child Psychology, 50,* 131-155.

YOUNGER, B., & Gotlieb, S. (1988). Development of categorization skills: Changes in the nature or structure of infant form categories? *Developmental Psychology, 24,* 611-619.

ZELAZO, P. R. (1971). Smiling to social stimuli: Eliciting and conditioning effects. *Developmental Psychology, 41,* 32-42.

ZELAZO, P. R., Weiss, M., Randolph, M., Swain, I., & Moore, D. (1987). The effects of delay on neonatal retention of habituated head-turning. *Infant Behavior and Development, 10,* 417-434.

PART III

The Fundamental Processes

Cognitive Development

JUDITH E. SIMS-KNIGHT

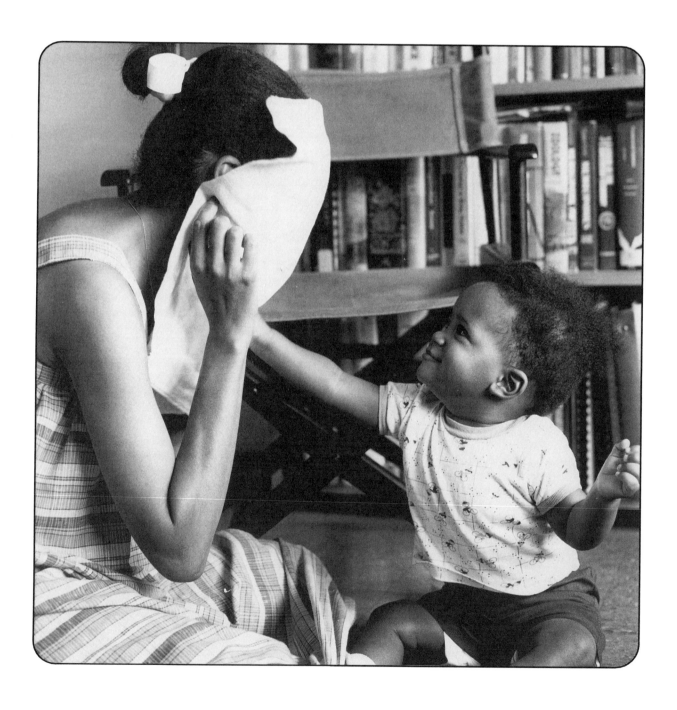

This chapter examines what and how infants understand about their world and how that understanding develops. The discussion first addresses the historical context from which the research developed. Next is presented in some detail the theory of Jean Piaget, who developed what is currently the most extensive theory of cognitive development, and who has been the major impetus for research in this area over the last two decades. Piaget's theory is very broad and complex, with many interpretations that go far beyond the data. In writing about his work, I have several goals. First, I want to describe the phenomena Piaget identified in terms of everyday behaviors of infants so that readers can identify these behaviors in informal observations. Second, I want to describe the theory and phenomena in a way that shows how he arrived at his highly inferential theory. Third, I want to evaluate the theory in a way that will help students cope with the complexity of the issues and the research. The strategy used to accomplish these goals is as follows: First, I present Piaget's theory more or less as he developed it, sprinkling the description liberally with "homey" examples. Included in the discussion are both those aspects of his theory that have been replicated and those about which there is a lot of controversy. The controversial aspects are mentioned along with the general description, but I will not attempt to deal with them at that time. After the theory has been presented, some of the work it has inspired will be examined, starting with the large-scale studies that have replicated the behavioral sequences described by Piaget and studies of sensorimotor development in other species. Next, the areas that have generated the most research are discussed: imitation and the object search tasks of the object permanence sequence. This is followed by a review of Fischer's theory, which is designed to incorporate the best of both Piagetian and learning theory. Finally, the chapter turns to the research on categorization, to which Piaget contributed little but which psychologists with other orientations have explored.

Perception researchers have learned that even newborns can see, hear, taste, smell, and feel—not always as well as adults, but surely well enough to be able to learn about the world (see Chapter 7). That immediately raises the question, What do the environmental events that infants see, hear, and so forth mean to

them? For example, infants can detect light-dark contours, but does that mean they can know what a rattle or a human being is? Infants have biologically adaptive responses such as avoidance responses to looming objects and rooting responses to a touch on the cheek, but what do such responses imply about the infants' knowledge about the stimuli that trigger them? Do such responses mean that babies know that objects are objects? Do they understand what separates one object from another? Do they know, for example, that the features of a face all belong to one object and that the hat above the face is an object in its own right rather than part of the face object? Do they know that objects are stable and enduring and exist even when people cannot see, hear, touch, smell, or taste them? Do they know that certain objects are similar to each other and different from others and that those patterns of similarities and differences identify an object—what its function is, how it is related to other kinds of objects, which aspects of it are important and which unimportant?

Historical Perspective

How humans come to know all this about their environment has been a subject of speculation at least since the time of the ancient Greeks. Philosophers who study epistemology have subjected these issues to reasoned arguments that form the context from which much of the psychological research in infant cognition has developed. Indeed, Jean Piaget, one of the foremost cognitive researchers, called himself a **genetic epistemologist**—that is, one who studies the basis of knowledge by studying development. The epistemological questions that have been most often pursued through infant research are the following two related questions:

(1) Are infants born with knowledge about the world?
(2) How is knowledge structured or organized?[1]

To understand the research on these questions, it is important to know something about the historically important philosophical positions.

THE ASSOCIATIONIST VIEW

In a very real sense, the associationist theory is the traditional theory of knowledge against which all others argue (Bolton, 1972). Aristotle first formulated it; it flowered again in the British associationist

1. This is not to imply that all philosophers would accept such research as an appropriate way to approach epistemological questions. Many philosophers consider questions about the basis of knowledge to be independent of questions about actual cognitive processes.

school of the seventeenth and eighteenth centuries—Hobbes, Locke, Hume, James Mill, and John Stuart Mill; and it was reborn in psychology in the learning theories of the twentieth century. To understand infancy research, it is necessary to understand two basic principles common to most associationist theories. First, they reflect a belief in empiricism (see Chapter 7). Babies at birth know nothing and have no preconceived notions, such as what an object is or who mother is. The second basic principle, which gives associationism its name, is that everything humans know (e.g., who mother is, what time is, and how to reason logically), they learn by associating sense impressions. Aristotle argued for three principles of association: (a) contiguity—things are associated because they are experienced at the same time and place; (b) similarity—things are associated because they are alike; and (c) contrast—things are associated because they are opposites. It is easy to see how learning psychology fits in. Both classical and operant conditioning occur when two events, previously not associated by an organism, become associated. Imitation also fits into associationism if an imitation is assumed to be an association of another's behavior with one's own (see Chapter 9). The only mental ability that is innate in associationism is the ability to receive sense impressions and to form associations among them.

NATIVISM

Nativism is the belief that certain structures of knowledge exist independent of sensations and thus of experience. (They may also exist independent of minds, but that aspect of the issue will not be considered here.) This view was described in Chapter 7, but an understanding of the issues in this chapter requires a more in-depth look at its historical development in psychology. Nativism has a long, illustrious past, starting with Plato, continuing with Kant, and currently represented by Gestalt psychologists, ethologists, and those linguists and psychologists who follow Chomsky's views about language. Kant, for example, believed that the concepts of objects, space, time, and causality are given a priori; that is, they do not have to be learned. Gestalt psychologists believe that people automatically impose organization on their perceptual world. For example, if they see dots arranged in a circle, they perceive a circle. Ethologists believe that through evolution animals have become biologically prepared to recognize certain classes of things that have survival value for them. For example, precocial birds (those that can walk at birth, such as geese,

chickens, and ducks) appear to recognize predators at their first exposure to them or to reasonable facsimiles. A baby chick will avoid a hawklike figure even though it has never seen, let alone been attacked by, a hawk. Chomsky argues that human knowledge of the structure of language is innate, and that young children need only hear language in order to actualize that knowledge.

Piaget's Interactionist Theory

Piaget was unhappy with both the associationist and the nativist solutions to the question of how humans know. He wished to reconcile the two approaches by demonstrating that the laws of logic and the Kantian categories can be derived from experience, something that associationists were never able to do convincingly. To do this he adopted an empirical approach; that is, he used the scientific method to investigate how humans' knowledge actually develops, rather than using argumentation as the sole basis for his opinion. This approach motivated him to engage in intensive naturalistic studies of his own three babies, which were described in Chapter 1. He concluded that babies are born with the potential to form Kantian categories, but they must construct their knowledge of the world from their interactions with the world beyond themselves. Newborns are equipped with reflex structures that permit them to interact with the world, for example, to suck, look, and grasp. Those reflex structures develop (by the process of adaptation) into cognitive structures. These cognitive structures form the basis of both knowledge of the physical world and understanding of general principles. Let us see how Piaget proposes this comes about.

MODEL OF ADAPTATION

The concept of adaptation is Piaget's model to explain the process whereby children come to know about their world. Rather than proposing that people make associations among events (stimuli and responses, or two stimuli, in learning terms), Piaget believed that people incorporate each new event into the structure of what they already know, so that experiencing new events enlarges and changes what they know. At the center of children's ability to learn about the world is their knowledge about the world. Children assimilate (take in, understand) new information when it fits what they already know. When they cannot fit new information into what they already understand (or, in the case of infants, when they do not know how to act upon it), they will do one of two things. They will ignore it, if it is just too far from anything they understand, or they will accommodate (modify their understanding) so that they can act upon the stimulus. The latter will presumably happen when some aspect of the environmental event or object is similar enough to their current understanding that they can stretch or modify that understanding to fit the new stimulus.

Assimilation, then, is the process of incorporating an environmental event into one's understanding of the world. **Accommodation** is the process of modifying one's understanding to embrace novel aspects of an environmental event, and it occurs when the event cannot be assimilated (directly incorporated into one's understanding) without changing the way one understands things like that object or event. The mutual functioning of assimilation and accommodation is what Piaget calls **adaptation**.

Assimilation and accommodation always occur relative to what a person understands. Piaget believed that a person's understanding of an event is organized into **cognitive structures**, which are structures of the mind analogous to the structures of a building. In other words, the structure provides the framework of understanding on which humans hang information from the world. Infants understand and organize their world through physical acts such as looking, grasping, shaking, and sucking. The motor act itself is the means by which the infant learns about the world. Repetition of these motor acts forms infants' cognitive structure, the framework by which they organize their understanding. The structure is not the act itself but is the general form abstracted from the repetition of actions. The structure is the means by which the meaning of environmental events becomes codified and remembered. These cognitive structures of infancy are called **action schemes** and are individually labeled by the respective acts, such as the sucking scheme or the grasping scheme. Central to Piaget's theory is his belief that infants actively construct their knowledge of the world by means of their cognitive structures. Piaget did not believe that infants are passive responders to environmental contingencies.

As an example of how the cognitive system operates in concrete situations, consider a 10-month-old infant who has been given a new rattle. She has played with rattles before and has learned to shake them, which produces the rattle noise. Today she looks at the new rattle, mouths it, feels its contours, and finally shakes it. It rattles and she breaks into a smile and shakes it again and again (see the top part of Figure 10.1). She has assimilated this object into her things-that-can-be-

shaken-and-make-noise scheme. Next, the baby is given a stuffed animal that makes a noise when a key on its back is turned. She mouths the key, feels its contours, shakes the animal—but she does not turn the key. The object is simply too different to be accommodated into her scheme, because shaking it does not produce a noise and she cannot change her shaking action to a turning movement. She can, however, accommodate to a less different object. She picks up a pull toy that has a long handle attached to an egg-shaped plastic container half filled with marblelike balls. She cannot hold the container in one hand and shake it like a rattle because it is too large. She cannot hold the handle and shake the toy like an oversized rattle, because she lacks the strength. She can, however, accommodate to the object: She grabs the handle (the egg is on the ground) and moves the hand and arm holding the handle up and down. This causes the ball to move back and forth on the floor, and it rattles (second part of Figure 10.1). Thus the baby has been able to accommodate her rattle scheme to the new object—to change her scheme to match the requirements of the new object—and she can then assimilate that object to her rattle scheme. Note that assimilation and accommodation are mutually interacting modes. The child must accommodate to certain environmental events if she is to assimilate them into her scheme. Likewise, she must have assimilated enough objects to have a smoothly functioning scheme before she can accommodate new things or events to it (broaden the scheme to include variants).

Cognitive change occurs through this mechanism. When the child accommodates to a scheme, that scheme becomes, at the very least, more developed, because it can handle a new kind of object. The scheme does not lose specificity through this process; that is, the distinctions between rattles and pull toys are not masked. Observers know this because in subsequent development the baby shakes rattles and her pull toy in different ways. Other, greater, kinds of cognitive change also occur through adaptation. New, differentiated schemes sometimes develop, such as shaking rattles and pulling toys. Schemes also can become intercoordinated: The pull toy can be shaken and pulled.

Finally, adaptation is the process through which the child changes from one kind of functioning to another; that is, moves from one stage of development to the next. Piaget's theory is a stage theory. He divides all of development into three major periods. The first period is infancy, or the period of sensorimotor development, and it lasts for the first 2 years of life. This period is the one with which we are

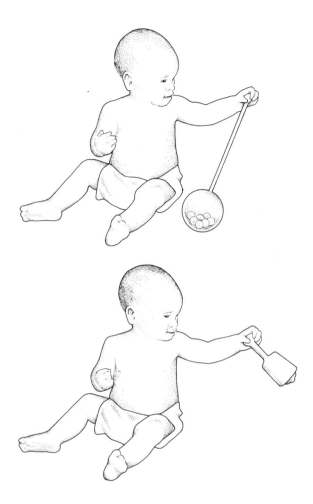

Figure 10.1. This baby accommodates her rattle shaking scheme (above) to an object that is only somewhat like the rattles she has previously experienced (below). (Figures drawn from movies provided by Judith E. Sims-Knight.)

In considering the problems of duration or rate of succession of the stages, we can readily observe that accelerations or delays in the average chronological age of performance depend on specific environments (e.g., abundance or scarcity of possible activities and spontaneous experiences, educational or cultural environment), but the order of succession will remain constant. (p. 713)

Underlying this statement is Piaget's belief that children actively construct their cognitive structures through their interactions with the environment. He did not believe that each stage unfolds according to fixed biological laws, as did Gesell. This is clear in the following quotation:

The stages always appear in the same order of succession. This might lead us to assume that some biological factor such as maturation is at work. But it is certainly not comparable to the hereditary neurophysiological programming of instincts. Biological maturation does nothing more than open the way to possible constructions (or explain transient impossibilities). It remains for the subject to actualize them. (Piaget, 1970, p. 712)

This means that children must interact with the environment to develop, and that the speed with which they move through the cognitive stages depends on the quality of the environment. It does not mean that poor environments will permanently prevent cognitive development, at least not in the infancy period. All except the most profoundly retarded (who lack the biological prerequisites) do proceed through all six stages of infancy.

STAGE I: REFLEX STRUCTURES
(0-1 MONTH)

Piaget believed that infants are born with the potential to develop complex cognitive structures culminating in the understanding of formal logic at around 14 years of age. At birth, however, they have no cognitive structures. They do have precursors to cognitive structures, which Piaget calls reflex structures. These are sucking, grasping, crying, looking, and so forth.

concerned in this book on infancy.[2] Through adaptation the infant's action schemes (the structures of the sensorimotor period) begin, become more complex, and gradually change into the next, more sophisticated form. The sensorimotor period itself is subdivided into six stages, and the infant progresses through the stages in an invariant sequence (that is, Stage I is always before Stage II, which is always before Stage III, and so forth). In each stage the infant's cognitive understanding is distinctly different from that in the other stages.

Before describing the infant at each of these stages, I should note that although Piaget gives ages for each stage, they are only approximate. Humans are the most variable of creatures and will often progress at different rates. Piaget (1970) notes:

---

2. The other periods are II, preparation for and development of concrete operations with substages of preoperational and concrete operational periods; and III, formal operations (alternatively, the middle period is sometimes subdivided into two periods, so there are four periods in all—II, preoperations; III, concrete operations; and IV, formal operations).

These reflex structures exhibit the tendency to function spontaneously and repeatedly. People who watch newborns when they are awake quickly become convinced that they do use these reflex structures and that they use them with increasing frequency as the first month passes.

Piaget always asked what infants of a certain stage of development know—and how they know it. Stage I infants know very little. True, they can see, hear, grasp, suck, taste, and smell, but these provide them with little meaningful information. Even though infants have a number of innate responses to environmental events, this does not mean that they understand those events as adults do. Consider auditory localization. That infants look in the direction from which a sound emanates does not mean that they know objects have both visual and auditory characteristics. It is just as reasonable to conclude that infants have a biological predisposition to orient toward sounds, but they do not make the inference that the sound-making object is seeable. Although either view might be correct, it is safer to conclude that the infant is unaware that the noise-producing stimulus is an object, because this does not require as many assumptions about what the newborn innately knows (this is an example of the principle of parsimony, also known as Occam's razor). Such additional assumptions—that newborns know what an object is, that they know how to differentiate among objects, that they know that objects exist in three-dimensional space, and so forth—would be reasonable only if there were additional evidence to support these assumptions. Although extensive research addressing the validity of these assumptions has been conducted (e.g., newborns imitate, perceive patterns, particularly faces, have intersensory coordination, and perceive objects in three-dimensional space; see Chapters 7 and 9), in none of these areas have researchers been able to convince the majority of experts in the field that newborns know what objects are.

STAGE II: PRIMARY CIRCULAR REACTIONS— THE FIRST ACQUIRED ADAPTATIONS (1-4 MONTHS)

Gradually, through repeated use, reflex structures are transformed into sensorimotor cognitive structures called action schemes. Piaget identifies these first cognitive structures by a new kind of behavioral sequence.

In this sequence, called a **circular reaction**, a baby does something (such as sucks or looks), repeats the behavior several times rapidly, gradually slows down the frequency of repetition, and finally stops altogether. An example from one of Piaget's observations of his children illustrates this reaction:

Observation 53—From 0;2(3) Laurent evidences a circular reaction which will become more definite and will constitute the beginning of systematic grasping; he scratches and tries to grasp, lets go, scratches and grasps again, etc. On 0;2(3) and 0;2(6) this can only be observed during the feeding. Laurent gently scratches his mother's bare shoulder. But beginning 0;2(7) the behavior becomes marked in the cradle itself. Laurent scratches the sheet which is folded over the blankets, then grasps it and holds it a moment, then lets go, scratches it again and recommences without interruption. At 0;2(11) this play lasts a quarter of an hour at a time, several times during the day. At 0;2(12) he scratches and grasps my fist which I placed against the back of his right hand. He even succeeds in discriminating my bent middle finger and grasping it separately, holding it a few moments. At 0;2(14) and 0;2(16) I note how definitely the spontaneous grasping of the sheet reveals the characteristics of circular reaction— groping at first, then regular rhythmical activity (scratching, grasping, holding, and letting go), and finally progressive loss of interest.

But this behavior grows simpler as it evolves in that Laurent scratches less and less, and instead really grasps after a brief tactile exploration. Thus already at 0;2(11) Laurent grasps and holds his sheet or handkerchief for a long time, shortening the preliminary scratching stage. So also at 0;2(14) he pulls with his right hand at a bandage which had to be applied to his left. (Piaget, 1936/1963, pp. 91-92)[3]

Other typical Stage II circular reactions are pumping the arm up and down, sucking the thumb, and sticking out the tongue. Piaget concluded that infants must be learning something through circular reactions because they repeat the reactions at various times with different objects and because the circular reactions change as they become more practiced, as described in the observation of Laurent's grasping.

The circular reaction in Stage II marks the beginning of learning ability, but it is a very primitive beginning and Piaget emphasizes that by calling Stage II circular reactions "primary circular reactions" (later-developing types of circular reactions will be discussed shortly). Primary circular reactions are distinctive in

---

3. Piaget's style of age notation shows years, months, and (days) of age. For example, in the first line of this extract, it is noted that Laurent was 0 years, 2 months, and 3 days old.

that infants focus on the action itself; in later versions they focus more and more on the object. In fact, primary circular reactions often do not involve objects at all (see Figure 10.2). Babies can be seen opening and closing their hands on thin air as well as on blankets or shoulders or any available object. Furthermore, they do not explore characteristics of the object involved in circular reactions, such as size, shape, or differences from other objects. When they are no longer acting upon (looking, grasping, sucking, and so forth) the object, Stage II babies act as if the object no longer exists. They do not search for objects when they drop them, for example. These three characteristic behaviors suggest that infants of this age know objects only as extensions of their actions and not as independent things-in-the-world.

When a circular reaction begins, infants often appear to be concentrating intensely. After the repetitions become rapid and smooth (it is tempting to say, "After they get the problem firmly in hand"), their expressions often become more relaxed. They are full of smiles and often laughter and gleeful screams ensue. Such expressions strengthen Piaget's interpretation that circular reactions are the way cognitive structures develop. He also notes that this is the earliest kind of play; he calls it **"functional play"** because through it infants develop the means to operate intellectually (adapt).

Piaget observed circular reactions in infants beginning at about 1 month of age. Papoušek's studies of conditioning (see Chapter 9) found that newborns

could be conditioned, but it took about a month to do, and infants already 1 month old conditioned much more rapidly. A convergence such as this, using two disparate kinds of evidence (experimental and naturalistic observation) strengthens the conclusion that a real development in learning ability occurs around this time.

Two other major advances occur during Stage II. First, Piaget believed that Stage II marks the very beginnings of imitation. For example, when someone coos (makes vowel sounds), infants of this age will also coo. Piaget believed this response to be a very primitive approximation to imitation because (a) an infant will imitate behaviors only if a model has just imitated them (that is, the sequence is baby emits behavior, adult imitates baby, baby imitates adult), and (b) the infant's responses do not usually match the adult's behaviors exactly. Piaget believed that infants are assimilating the modeled behavior to their own schemes, thus sparking their own circular reactions. This means that imitation at this stage is a learning device in the same sense that circular reactions are: a means of assimilating. Later imitation will become a way of changing, expanding, and differentiating schemes: a way of accommodating. This interpretation of imitation in young infants is controversial, as noted in Chapter 9. Some researchers believe that neonatal imitation is exact imitation, which requires more innate knowledge than Piaget was willing to attribute to young infants.

Finally, during Stage II the various schemes—look-

Figure 10.2. Humans are not the only primates to exhibit the behavioral sequences described by Piaget. Gorillas develop in very similar ways to humans. Here, in three frames of a sequence, an infant gorilla, Mkumbwa, repeatedly grasps his foot with his hand. It is a circular reaction in that it is repetitive; it is primary in that the infant focuses on the actions of his own body. (Photographs courtesy of Dr. Suzanne Chevalier-Skolnikoff.)

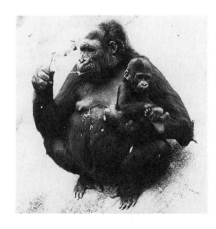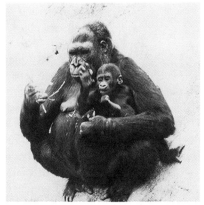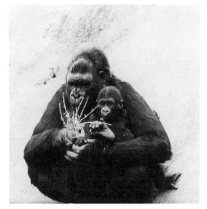

ing, sucking, grasping—become coordinated. The last intercoordination is visually guided reaching (discussed in Chapter 8), which develops around 4 months of age. Piaget used the development of these intercoordinations as crucial evidence that young infants construct their understanding of objects through actions. He argued that through the gradual intercoordination of schemes, Stage II infants learn that a single object can be explored in all modalities (visual, oral, and so forth) at the same time, and thereby they learn that these multimodal characteristics inhere in one object. Thus the object is no longer merely an extension of one action. As an object becomes distinct from any particular action, a step is taken toward its becoming one object with an existence separate from the infant and his or her actions. Some researchers believe that intersensory coordination (and its implication—that an object has visual, auditory, and tactile characteristics) is innate (e.g., Bower, 1982).

The increase in exploratory skills and the intercoordination of schemes that occurs at 4 months of age (or reintercoordination, in Bower's view) has implications for parents and others who play with babies. One of the first coordinations is between hand and mouth, which allows infants to find their fingers to suck. Those babies who suck their fingers or thumbs have a ready means to calm themselves. Visually guided reaching provides infants with a marvelous means by which they can entertain themselves and also get into trouble—they can grab everything in sight. Babies who can reach for things to explore also seem to become more human to many parents. For infants, mouthing is an extremely important exploratory tool that seems to develop at the time the schemes are being coordinated. Before this time babies tend to suck vigorously at every object put into their mouths (unless they are hungry, at which time they refuse nonnutritive objects), but once visually guided reaching develops, the sucking changes to mouthing (the mouth is not pursed and no vacuum is created), and for months afterward exploration includes putting all possible objects into the mouth.

STAGE III: SECONDARY CIRCULAR
REACTIONS (4-8 MONTHS)

Two effects of the accomplishments of Stage II are that (a) infants' abilities to explore their world are vastly improved because they can look at what they grasp, and (b) objects are by now things that have visual, auditory, and tactile features. These developments mark the onset of secondary circular reactions. Secondary circular reactions are quite striking behav-

iors, perhaps because the object plays a much more important role than it did in Stage II. A good example is dropping and picking up. Infants in this stage often drop toys they have grasped, and this action often results in a secondary circular reaction in which they grasp and then drop the toy repeatedly. Such sequences have all the characteristics of circular reactions: The first several repetitions are done slowly and with expressions of intense concentration; the repetitions then increase in speed, and are often accompanied by smiles and gleeful squeals; the repetitions are rather rhythmic; and they peter out gradually. Secondary circular reactions are more advanced than primary ones in that infants seem to be repeating or maintaining an interesting environmental event. In the above example, the dropping of the object is the interesting event. Other such interesting events that secondary circular reactions repeat or maintain are the sounds of rattles being shaken, objects being rubbed against others, objects being swung in the air, and of course that all-time favorite, "dump the bowl" (this last can be a circular reaction only with the patient help of an older human, who must refill the bowl so that it can be dumped again).

Notice that secondary circular reactions are described in terms of action-object sequences (e.g., dump is the action and bowl is the object in the dump-the-bowl scheme). Although in secondary circular reactions the object or event plays a larger role than in primary circular reactions, Piaget believed that infants' understanding of the world is still firmly tied to their own actions. Note also that the first instance of a secondary circular reaction occurs by chance. That is also characteristic.

One reason Piaget believed that secondary circular reactions are attempts to reproduce interesting events is that infants attend more to the objects they are manipulating than they did in primary circular reactions. The circular reaction of dropping is a good example of this because the baby's eyes follow the falling object, which is direct evidence of interest in the object. In some circular reactions, such as rattle shaking, we cannot see babies' interest directly. Nonetheless, we know they are interested, because, for example, they often smile and squeal when they cause the rattle noise and they then repeat their actions, thus continuing the circular reaction.

A second behavioral phenomenon that led Piaget to conclude that Stage III infants are more aware of and interested in environmental events is a special case of the secondary circular reaction that he calls "procedures for making interesting spectacles last." These procedures occur when babies in this stage are confronted with new events that they find interesting. Rather than attending to the novel aspects of the objects or events (which would lead older infants to play with the objects appropriately), Stage III infants simply apply their habitual schemes. This sometimes results in procedures that would have to be magical to be effective. For example, consider a Stage III infant who knows how to pump his arms up and down to shake rattles. An adult stands beyond his reach with a string of bells. The adult shakes the bells and the infant looks toward the bells and reaches for them. When he fails to grasp them, he immediately starts pumping his arm up and down. He stops when the adult rings the bells again and repeats the action when the bells stop ringing. During the course of Stage III these procedures become more and more obviously magical and look less like regular circular reactions (which differ from procedures for making interesting spectacles last in that in regular circular reactions the babies' actions do make the environmental events occur). Here is an example from Piaget's (1936/1963) observations of his son Laurent that shows the procedures at their colorful, magical best:

> At 0;7(7) he looks at a tin box placed on a cushion in front of him, too remote to be grasped. I drum on it for a moment in a rhythm which makes him laugh and then present my hand (at a distance of 2 cm. from his, in front of him). He looks at it, but only for a moment, then turns toward the box; then he shakes his arm while staring at the box (then he draws himself up, strikes his coverlets, shakes his head, etc.; that is to say, he uses all the "procedures" at his disposition). He obviously waits for the phenomenon to recur. Same reaction at 0;7(12), at 0;7(13), 0;7(22), 0;7(29) and 0;8(1) in a variety of circumstances. (p. 201)

The procedures for making interesting spectacles last indicate clearly that Stage III infants are aware of environmental events and wish to perpetuate them.

Secondary schemes are also infants' first system for classifying and relating objects. When infants of this age are given familiar objects, they can immediately comprehend the objects' uses because of their secondary schemes. They know whether the objects can be shaken, thrown, mouthed, and so forth. They can explore possible classifications of new objects by actions such as mouthing, fingering, and kicking. Thus Stage III infants demonstrate that objects are similar—to them—by acting upon them in the same way. All objects that can be put into their mouths are assimilated to the mouthing schemes and therefore can be

said to be in the same class. Piaget believed that this primitive organization is the precursor of that most basic intellectual pursuit, logical classification. Two aspects of this description have been widely investigated. One is the general question of how infants' abilities to form concepts develop, and the second is whether early concepts of objects are based on action schemes. Research in both of these areas will be discussed later in this chapter.

In describing how Stage III marks the onset of the ability to form relations among events, Piaget focuses on relations between means and ends. Stage III infants repeat behaviors that are the means to reach an end, such as pulling a cord to make an attached object move. These are the earliest instances Piaget found (and he was looking hard to find them) in which infants relate two events (for example, a pull and the subsequent movement of a toy). This is not true means-end problem solving, however, because the infants discovered the means to the end by chance and simply became able to repeat the means action.

Piaget (1936/1963) further notes that infants seem to vary the intensity of their actions and the intensity of the subsequent reaction in a systematic way. For example:

> Jacqueline, too, at 0;9(5) shakes while holding a celluloid rattle in the form of a parrot which she has just been given. She smiles when the noise is slight, is anxious when it is too loud and knows very well how to gradate the phenomenon. She progressively increases the noise until she is too frightened and then returns to the soft sounds. Furthermore, when the rattle is stuck at one of the ends, she shakes the parrot by turning it in another direction and thus knows how to reestablish the noise. (pp. 166-167)

Piaget infers from such examples that Stage III infants not only relate two events, but also discover quantitative relations. This is another first in Stage III, and Piaget claims that this primitive forming of relations provides the basis from which all later relation making comes. Included in the later forms are Piaget's famous seriation tasks (making sequential orderings along a dimension, such as ordering 10 sticks by size) and understanding of number (which is based on understanding "greater than" and "less than").

Stage III infants show early signs of development of **object permanence**, which is the knowledge that objects continue to exist even when the observer is not interacting with them. The topic of object permanence includes two questions:

(1) Do infants know that an object exists when they are not acting upon it? (For Piaget this is equivalent to the question, Can infants mentally represent an absent object?)

(2) How do infants conceive of objects? (For Piaget this means, Do objects exist as entities in the world separate from the infants' actions and separate from other objects?)

Piaget infers that for infants of Stages I and II, objects do not exist when the infants are not acting upon them and that objects are merely a part of their action, not independent entities. Only when they reach Stage III do infants look at the place where they just dropped an object. They also reach for objects they have been playing with when they are partly, but not wholly, covered; that is, the part signals the presence (and the existence) of the whole object. Piaget used these behaviors to argue that infants of this age have a primitive notion that an object continues to exist when they are not acting upon it. The sequence of behaviors describing the development of object permanence is one of the most reproducible parts of Piaget's infancy work, yet his theoretical conclusions from this sequence are among the most challenged portions of this work. The

research addressing this controversy is discussed later in the chapter.

Another phenomenon that Piaget found to appear first in Stage III is motor recognition, in which babies perform their secondary schemes, but in abbreviated form and with no apparent attempt actually to act upon the object. For example, he concluded that Lucienne shook herself in recognition of events involving shaking, because he saw her shake herself when she was presented with several objects that she had previously shaken in circular reactions (spools hanging on elastic bands, two celluloid parrots). These movements were always abbreviated and always in response to situations that in the past had elicited more extensive shaking of the objects. At least some instances of motor recognition develop later into gestural symbols, which will be discussed later.

Piaget believed that imitation in Stage III acts as a procedure to make interesting events last. If, for example, the model makes a sound, infants will go through several verbal schemes to maintain the event. If the model requires exact imitation, infants can provide it, with the limitations that (a) they must have a scheme that closely corresponds to it, and (b) it must be an act they can see themselves make (which eliminates facial

Figure 10.3. Two examples of typical secondary circular reactions, exhibited during a single interaction with the toy. The actions are very different from the ones an older infant would exhibit with this toy. (left) Lifting the arm. This develops from a primary circular reaction of moving the arm up and down repeatedly. In its reappearance as a secondary scheme it is part of the baby's exploration of the object. If this were a rattle, it would shake during this response and the baby would recognize it as a thing-that-can-be-shaken-and-make-noise. (right) Mouthing the object. This is part of the typical exploration sequence of look-reach-grasp-put-into-mouth. Most objects are explored in this way. Notice that the baby is mouthing the wheel rather than running the wheel along the table top as would be appropriate for the toy. (Figures drawn from movies provided by Judith E. Sims-Knight.)

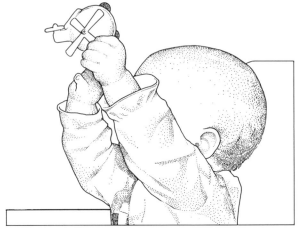
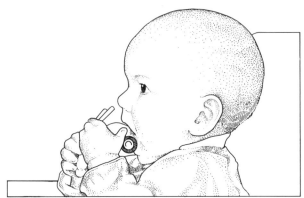

gestures). Thus, while exact imitation is possible, it has no interest for the infant other than as a way to maintain an interesting event. As was discussed in Chapter 9, and as I will review later in this chapter, this conclusion is challenged by the research on neonatal imitation.

Although secondary schemes are a great cognitive advance, they are still quite limited. The secondary scheme is an unanalyzed action-object sequence in which the particular characteristics of the object are not noticed. Given a new object, infants run through their typical schemes in typical fashion. By so doing, they must ignore novel features. This characteristic is very obvious to adults when they give babies of this age a marvelous toy and watch the baby play with it "all wrong"—such as mouthing the handle of a pull toy rather than pulling it or fingering the various protuberances of a toy truck rather than pushing it along the ground (see Figure 10.3).

This tendency to ignore novel characteristics of an object in favor of applying typical schemes (Piaget would say that infants of this age assimilate more than they accommodate) also limits the quality of classification. Because objects are so undifferentiated from actions in Stage III, the precision of classification must also be extremely rough. As the object becomes more differentiated from action in later stages, infants can better judge when two objects are in equivalent classes (for example, two toys are for shaking).

Finally, Stage III infants' ability to conceive of an object independent of their own action is limited. Looking for an object that has disappeared is possible only when the search immediately follows the infant's action, and uncovering a hidden object is possible only when part of it is visible.

STAGE IV: COORDINATION OF SECONDARY SCHEMES (8-12 MONTHS)

The major development in Stage IV is that babies become able to coordinate secondary schemes. Thus they are able to use one scheme as a means of obtaining their desired goal (of using another scheme). Such means-end behaviors are the prototypes of all problem solving. These are the first infant behaviors that Piaget calls truly intelligent. Here is an example of Laurent during this stage:

Observation 130.—Laurent, at 0;10(3) utilizes as a "means" . . . a behavior pattern which he discovered the previous day. . . . By manipulating a tin of shaving cream he learned, at 0;10(2), to let this object fall intentionally. Now, at 0;10(3) I give it to

him again. He at once begins to open his hand to make it fall and repeats this behavior a certain number of times. I then place, 15 cm. from Laurent, a large wash basin and strike the interior of it with the tin in order to make Laurent hear the sound of the metal against this object. It is noteworthy that Laurent, already at 0;9(0), had, while being washed, by chance struck a small pot against such a basin and immediately played at reproducing this sound by a simple circular reaction. I therefore wanted to see if Laurent was going to use the tin to repeat the phenomenon and how he was going to go about it.

Now, at once, Laurent takes possession of the tin, holds out his arm and drops it over the basin. I moved the latter as a check. He nevertheless succeeded, several times in succession, in making the object fall on the basin. Hence this is a fine example of the coordination of two schemes of which the first serves as "means" whereas the second assigns an end to the action: the schema of "relinquishing the object" and that of "striking one object against another." (Piaget, 1936/1963, p. 225)

Other common means-end behaviors seen at this stage are pushing an obstacle away to get at a goal object, pulling a string to get the object attached to it (see Figure 10.4), and trying to reproduce an interesting event by having the person who first produced that event repeat it (such as putting a whistle in a parent's mouth to be blown).

Means-end behaviors are the first behaviors that Piaget thought were intentional beyond a doubt. Two advances convinced him of this. First, in Stage III Laurent could not have abstracted the means (dropping the tin) from its original context and applied it to a new goal (making the metallic clink against the basin). Second, Stage III infants often get caught by the means behaviors and forget the original goal. For example, once they pick up the cloth covering a desired toy, they play with the cloth, not the toy. Stage IV infants, in contrast, typically return to the goal after performing the means scheme. Thus by using a scheme as a means in a new situation, Stage IV infants demonstrate that they have produced the means behavior on purpose rather than by accident. Also, by consistently stopping the means scheme when it has served its purpose and by engaging in the goal behavior, they demonstrate that they really were interested in that goal. This is a conservative use of the term *intentional*. In contrast, Bruner (1973) called visually guided reaching intentional because infants make anticipatory adjustments in order to reach accurately.

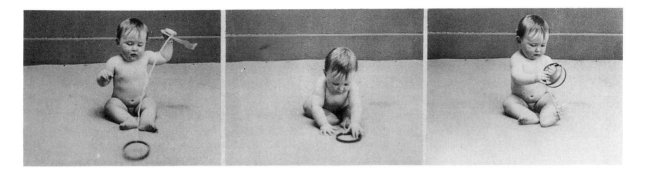

Figure 10.4. Means-end behavior. This 40-week-old baby pulls a string to get the ring toy attached to it. (From A. L. Gesell, *Atlas of Infant Behavior.* New Haven, CT: Yale University Press, 1934. Used by permission.)

Understanding that a behavior can be the means to an end is a major step toward understanding causality. For example, Jacqueline must attribute a causal role to Piaget's hand when she places it against a swinging doll that she wishes to activate (Piaget, 1937/1954, p. 260). She is now free from her earlier magical assumption that her actions were responsible for all environmental events, including procedures for making interesting spectacles last. Furthermore, Stage IV babies begin to discover that other objects (in addition to themselves) can act as causal agents, an achievement that helps infants to conceive of one independent force acting upon another. Their notion of causality is not yet mature, however, because they still appreciate an external causality only when their own actions intervene (as when Jacqueline placed Piaget's hand on the doll).

Also appearing in Stage IV is the ability to anticipate actions of objects and of other people on the basis of a sign. For example, babies of this age often cry when they see the white-coated doctor who has inflicted pain on them in the past or protest when parents put their coats on to go out. Piaget considered these true signs compared with the more primitive signals that first appear in Stage III, because a sign is an anticipation of an event that is independent of the infant, whereas a signal forms part of an undifferentiated action scheme. Signs can be distinguished from signals in that signs become independent of their original contexts. Piaget gives the example of a creaking chair being a sign for a person's disappearance. This occurred first at the dinner table, but was quickly generalized to Piaget's creaking his desk chair (1936/1963, p. 252). This development is important theoretically because signs are another indication that infants are separating actions of objects from their own actions to a greater extent than in previous stages.

The coordination of secondary schemes makes other advances possible. When schemes are coordinated they are extracted from their original circumstances. They can then be applied to all sorts of new situations, so they are more effective instruments of exploration. Through this more extensive exploration, Stage IV children become able to attend more closely to the characteristics of objects and thus can apply their schemes more appropriately.

An advance in object permanence is also related to the coordination of secondary schemes. Infants can now search for an object that has disappeared and can remove a screen that completely covers an object. These are both means-end behavioral sequences (doing something to retrieve an object the infant is interested in acting upon). Because all means-end sequences require that infants know that they will be able to execute their goals (such as touching, shaking, dropping the object) before they actually do, they must know something about the object even when the object is completely absent (and they are not engaged in acting upon it in any way, even looking at it). This means that Stage IV infants possess some incipient representation of objects, but, Piaget argues, that representation is still tied to the infants' actions. His evidence for this interpretation is the occurrence of A-not-B error. This error occurs when an object is put first under one cover (A) and then, in full view of the infant, under a second (B). Stage IV babies often look under the first cover rather than the second even though from an adult point of view the object is clearly under the second. Everyday examples are also easy to find. For example, if an infant is playing with a ball and it rolls under a chair, she can retrieve it (a single cover). If she continues to play with it and it now rolls out the door of the room and out of sight, she is likely to look under the chair for it (see Figure 10.5).

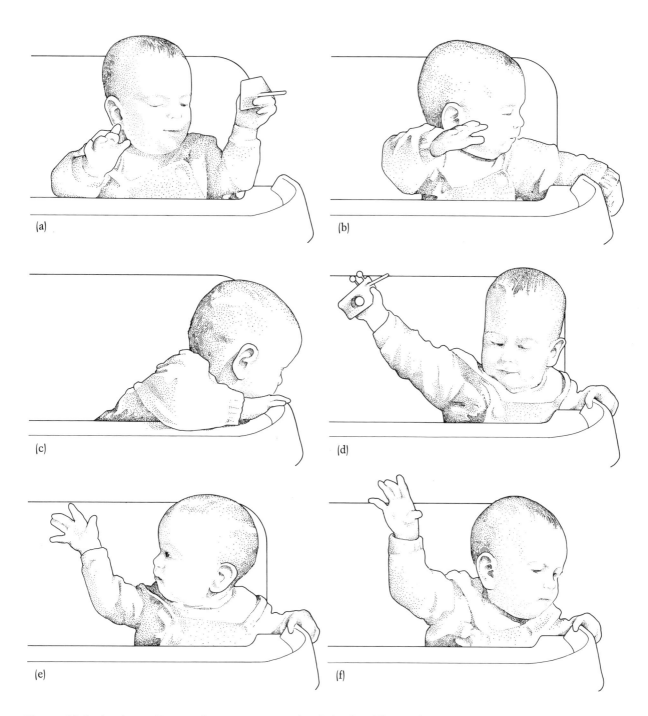

Figure 10.5. An A-not-B error in spontaneous play behavior. These pictures are drawn from a movie sequence of an infant playing with his toys in his home. (a) and (b) He drops the toy car over the right side (A) of his high chair. (c) He looks after the toy he has just dropped. (d) He drops the car over the left side (B) of the high chair. (e) He looks at his empty hand as if noting the absence of the car. (f) He looks over the right side (A-not-B) of the high chair. (Figures drawn from movies provided by Judith E. Sims-Knight.)

Piaget (1937/1954) interprets the error as indicating that

> there would not be one chain, one doll, one watch, one ball, etc., individualized, permanent, and independent of the child's activity, that is, of the special positions in which that activity takes place or has taken place, but there would still exist only images such as "ball-under-the-armchair," "doll-attached-to-the-hammock," "watch-under-a-cushion," "papa-at-his-window," etc. Certainly the same object reappearing in different practical positions or contexts is recognized, identified, and endowed with permanence as such. In this sense it is relatively independent. But, without being truly conceived as having several copies, the object may manifest itself to the child as assuming a limited number of distinct forms of a nature intermediate between unity and plurity, and in this sense it remains a part of its context. (pp. 62-63)

This phenomenon has been replicated many times over, although babies only sometimes make the error. Whether Piaget's interpretation needs modification is a matter of opinion, as we will see later.

This stage marks the beginning of the use of imitation as a means of accommodation, a development that fits in with the general characterization of Stage IV as the first stage in which assimilation and accommodation become differentiated. Piaget's evidence for this claim is that for the first time infants are able to imitate behaviors of others even when those behaviors are not already in their repertoires. They can also imitate behaviors of another person when that person is matching actions of the infants that the infants cannot see themselves perform (for example, biting the lip; see Figure 10.6). This is accomplished by the same mechanism as that of means-end behaviors. Infants first run through the familiar schemes that are similar to the model's behavior (for example, all the ways of moving their mouths). Then, if the modeled behavior is new to them, they combine (coordinate) schemes in their attempt to match the new behavior. Thus imitation becomes intentional, albeit limited. Such a mechanism for learning new things provides an important impetus to cognitive growth.

Although Stage IV advances are quite impressive, they of course have their limitations. Means-end behaviors do represent truly intelligent behavior, but the efficiency of the Stage IV version is quite limited because these infants can employ only familiar schemes as means in their problem solving. If a typical way of interacting is not successful, they simply cannot solve the problem. Because they are limited to applying familiar schemes, their exploration of new objects is limited to a search for ways in which those objects operate in the same ways as familiar objects. Likewise, they are able to imitate new behaviors only when those behaviors are very similar to familiar behaviors, and then only through a rather lengthy process of trying familiar schemes and combinations of familiar schemes. Finally, their understanding of objects and events is still tied to their actions.

STAGE V: TERTIARY CIRCULAR REACTIONS (12-18 MONTHS)

Piaget calls Stage V the stage of the elaboration of the object because infants' interactions with objects are much more reality-oriented than in earlier stages. Stage V babies actively investigate the novel properties of objects rather than running roughshod over unusual features in their attempts to assimilate the objects to their familiar schemes. They can learn accurately the spatial and causal relations among objects. In short, objects have become conceptually separated from and independent of infants' actions upon them. The mechanism of these advances is the tertiary circular reaction. As with all circular reactions, Stage V reactions are repetitions of an action upon an object with the apparent goal of reproducing the effect. As in earlier forms of circular reactions, the new goal is always discovered by chance. Unlike in earlier forms, however, in tertiary circular reactions the infant varies his or her actions upon the object to explore its nature. (Piaget concludes that the purpose is exploration because the infant attends carefully to the object during the varying actions.) A classic example is dropping things:

> At 0;10(11) Laurent is lying on his back but nevertheless resumes his experiments of the day before. He grasps in succession a celluloid swan, a box, etc., stretches out his arm and lets them fall. He distinctly varies the positions of the fall. Sometimes he stretches out his arm vertically, sometimes he holds it obliquely, in front of or behind his eyes, etc. When the object falls in a new position (for example on his pillow), he lets it fall two or three times more on the same place, as though to study the spatial relation; then he modifies the situation. At a certain moment the swan falls near his mouth; now, he does not suck it (even though this object habitually serves this purpose), but drops it three times more while merely making the gesture of opening his mouth. (Piaget, 1936/1963, p. 269)

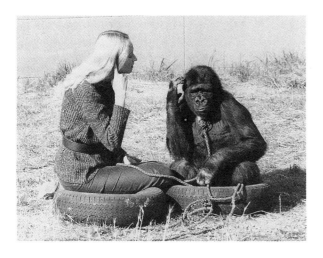

Figure 10.6. The Piagetian sequence of imitative development is also seen in gorillas. Here Koko shows Stage IV imitation of body parts she is unable to see on herself. This sort of behavior first develops in gorillas at about the same age as it does in human infants, but Koko is much older in this photograph. (Photograph courtesy of Dr. Suzanne Chevalier-Skolnikoff.)

The net effect of such exploration is that infants can discover properties of objects that they could not discover in earlier stages. They also discover relations among objects. Stage V babies spend hours putting objects into, on top of, and beside other objects. They explore how spoons fit into certain containers and not others, how tops fit onto certain containers, fall into other containers, and fall off still other containers. They find out that some objects make loud noises when they are thrown on the ground, some objects bounce or roll, and some objects make the most satisfying splat (see Figure 10.7 for another example). At first it may seem difficult to distinguish tertiary circular reactions from the secondary version, because in both cases infants systematically vary the effects. Recall the example of Jacqueline in Stage III, shaking her parrot rattle with different degrees of vigor, which produced rattle sounds of varying intensities. Such gradations of secondary circular reactions produce variations of a single effect (in this case the rattle sound), but those of the tertiary circular reactions produce different effects. Contrast the parrot rattle example with the following example of a tertiary circular reaction:

Observation 146.—At 1;2(8) Jacqueline holds in her hands an object which is new to her: a round, flat box which she turns all over, shakes, rubs against the bassinet, etc. She lets it go and tries to pick it up. But she only succeeds in touching it with her index finger, without grasping it. She nevertheless makes an attempt and presses on the edge. The box then tilts up and falls again. Jacqueline, very much interested in this fortuitous result, immediately applies herself to studying it. Hitherto it is only a question of an attempt at assimilation analogous to that of Stage IV and of the fortuitous discovery of a new result, but this discovery, instead of giving rise to a simple circular reaction, is at once extended to "experiments in order to see."

In effect, Jacqueline immediately rests the box on the ground and pushes it as far as possible (it is noteworthy that care is taken to push the box far away in order to reproduce the same condition as in the first attempt, as though this were a necessary condition for obtaining the result). Afterward Jacqueline puts her finger on the box and presses it. But as she places her finger on the center of the box she simply displaces it and makes it slide instead of tilting it up. She amuses herself with this game and keeps it up (resumes it after intervals, etc.) for several minutes. Then, changing the point of contact, she finally again places her finger on the edge of the box, which tilts it up. She repeats this many times, varying the conditions, but keeping track of her discovery: now she only presses on the edge! (Piaget, 1936/1963, p. 272)

In this Stage V example, when Jacqueline discovered by chance that the box sometimes tilted and sometimes slid, she was interested in both effects and groped through various actions to see what action caused each effect. In Stages III or IV she would have been unable to understand that variations of her actions could lead to two different kinds of movement of the boxes.

Piaget called tertiary circular reactions "experiments in order to see" for two reasons. First, infants in tertiary circular reactions are pursuing novelty for its own sake—in order to see—because they attend closely to the varying results and repeat the actions that lead first to one outcome and then to another. Younger babies do not actively investigate novelty. Stage III babies completely ignore aspects of objects that cannot readily be assimilated to their secondary schemes. Stage IV babies discover novelties only because, during their persistent groping to explore objects and events, they must cope with the novel aspects of those objects and events; that is, they must accommodate in order to assimilate. In contrast, Stage V infants seek out the novelty; that is, accommodation becomes an end in itself.

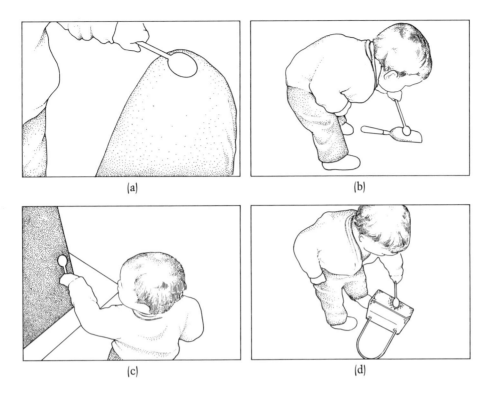

Figure 10.7. During spontaneous play, this baby is doing an "experiment in order to see." This toddler is playing with a "banger" (to adults, a honey dipper) for the first time. She explores what objects are "bangable" and what the consequences of this banging are. (a) On daddy's knee the banger makes little noise and does not bounce much. (b) In a scoop the banger makes a tinkling noise and sets the scoop rocking. (c) On a loudspeaker the banger produces a thud, a moderate give and bounce back, and a parental admonition. (d) On a purse the banger sinks in and makes little noise. (Figures drawn from movies provided by Judith E. Sims-Knight.)

The second reason Piaget calls tertiary circular reactions "experiments in order to see" is that they are experiments. Infants of this age explore the nature of objects by trying them out. For example, they explore the nature of chalk by writing first on a chalkboard, then on the floor, the wall, their clothes, their friends' faces, and so forth.

Tertiary circular reactions provide the mechanism for another advance, the discovery of new means through active experimentation. Means-end behaviors in Stages IV and V are very similar. They occur when babies want to play with an object or reproduce an interesting event, and that goal can be reached only by an intermediate action. They reach the goal by forming a new coordination between behaviors that serve as the means and the goal action. Stage IV infants are limited to using familiar schemes as means, but Stage V infants can find new means through tertiary circular reactions, that is, by varying their behaviors and observing the effects upon the goal.

There are really two steps to discovering new means. First, infants must realize that the familiar means are not adequate; second, they must be able to discover the new means. Younger infants try to do something to maintain interesting events (procedures to make interesting spectacles last in Stage III and familiar means in Stage IV), but they do not really understand the physical principles involved and so they do not know exactly how their behaviors are related to the goal.

Piaget describes quite a few examples of discovery of new means through active experimentation. Babies discover how to use a stick to nudge objects toward them; this is the earliest tool use Piaget observed. They learn that when an object rests on a support such as a blanket or cardboard, they can reach the object by pulling the support. They discover how to tilt long, skinny objects to bring them in between the bars of their playpens or cribs. They discover how to open various containers and how to put peculiar objects, such as watch chains, into small receptacles. Solving all these problems requires that infants understand the relation between variations of their actions and the differing effects so that they can discard ineffective actions, improve upon partially effective actions, and repeat successful ones.

Infants' notion of causality thus takes a giant step forward in Stage V, because they can explore the nature of the physical relations among objects in a much more precise way than before. Another advance in the understanding of causality is that babies of this age begin to treat themselves as objects and therefore they can serve as effects as well as means. Piaget gives the example of Jacqueline at 1;3(10) letting herself fall down in a sitting position. Her goal is the dropping of herself. This was a new behavior for her at the time; before that she would not let go of the bars of her playpen until she was seated (Piaget, 1937/1954, p. 291).

Imitation of new behaviors becomes much more extensive and systematic in Stage V. As with the discovery of new means, infants grope through various new actions in their attempts to imitate. Thus they can imitate behaviors that are much more unfamiliar than those they could imitate in Stage IV, when they were limited to familiar schemes and combinations of familiar schemes. Notice also that the success of Stage V groping toward accurate imitation requires that the infant be able to decide when he or she has produced a behavior that matches the model's action. Doing so requires that the infant assimilate the new action to the framework provided by his or her schemes. Piaget gives the example here of Jacqueline recognizing that she has correctly imitated Piaget touching his hair by touching her own hair and recognizing it by its texture (a previously learned tactile scheme).

Recall that Piaget calls this the stage of the elaboration of the object. Let us review the discussion of tertiary circular reactions to see how those phenomena demonstrate development of the object concept. First, because Stage V infants focus on novel aspects of objects and can investigate novel effects of objects, they can find out how a new object differs from familiar objects as well as how it is similar. Stage IV babies' interactions with novel aspects of objects are limited to searching for ways in which those novel aspects are assimilable to familiar schemes. For example, Stage IV infants presented with a toy car notice those peculiar protuberances adults call wheels and run through their typical action patterns of shaking, touching, mouthing, and so forth to find out how the wheels look, feel, taste, sound, and so forth. Stage V infants do not stop there, because novelty itself fascinates them. They vary their action patterns while paying close attention to the resulting behav-

iors of the wheels. Through such experimentation they discover that the wheels go around in a unique fashion, and eventually they rub those wheels along the floor and the car moves in its conventional way. Thus experimentation leads to a more accurate understanding of the object. A second way that tertiary circular reactions lead to the elaboration of the object is the advance in the precision of understanding causal behaviors. Consider how Stage V babies learn about the properties of sticks by trying to pull them through the bars of playpens or cribs. Finally, a third indication of the maturation of the object concept is found in infants' ability to treat themselves as objects of causal actions. This indicates that they are able to consider themselves as separate objects among other objects.

The Stage V step in the object permanence sequence demonstrates additional aspects of the elaboration of the object. In Stage V the A-not-B error disappears. Infants at this stage can watch an object being hidden successively under three screens and will pick up the last screen to find the object underneath. This ability shows that infants no longer consider the object to be embedded in the global action-object sequence. They now know that the object is a thing that is different from themselves, although their ability to conceptualize movements of objects independent of themselves is still limited. Piaget hypothesized this because an infant of this age can follow an object through three displacements only if the examiner makes the object visible to the infant between each screen. The infant will look under the first screen if the displacements are invisible. This phenomenon suggests that Stage V infants' ability to represent an absent object is still limited.

This final limitation to object permanence fits with Piaget's belief that Stage V infants have not yet achieved mature mental representation, the ability to think about objects or events when they are absent. Children of this age can solve problems only through actions. In both experiments to see and discovery of new means, infants try different behaviors and observe the effects. For example, when trying to fit a stick through the bars of a playpen, they must actually try all physical displacements that occur to them—horizontal and vertical, with or without tilt—until they hit upon one that works. They cannot simply examine the stick and the playpen bars and after some pause execute the correct movement. Solution of problems by thinking rather than acting has not yet developed.

STAGE VI: INVENTION OF NEW MEANS
THROUGH MENTAL COMBINATIONS
(18 MONTHS)

Mental representation develops fully in Stage VI. Piaget considers this achievement so important that he describes Stages I-V as five parts of one large stage characterized by the absence of representation.

Problem solving in Stage VI involves the same process as in Stage V except that the actual experimentation is absent. Instead, the infant pauses for a brief period and then solves the problem.

The following description is of Jacqueline discovering through Stage V active experimentation how to make a watch chain enter a narrow opening. Notice that after 22 attempts she still achieves success only with some difficulty.

At 1;7(25) Jacqueline holds a rectangular box, deep and narrow whose opening measures 34 x 16 mm. (for this purpose I use the cover of a match box which is three quarters open), and she tries to put my watch chain into it (45 cm. long). During the first fifteen attempts, she goes about it in the following way: First she grasps the chain about 5 cm. from this end and thus puts a second segment into the box. She then gets ready to do the same with a third segment when the chain, no longer supported by the child's hand, slides out of the box and falls noisily. Jacqueline recommences at once and fourteen times in succession sees the chain come out as soon as it is put in. It is true that, around the tenth attempt, Jacqueline has tired of it and was about to give up; but I placed the chain in the box (without the child's seeing how) and then she regained hope by noting that such a result was not impossible.

At the sixteenth attempt, a new phenomenon: Jacqueline having grasped the chain nearer the middle, the chain no longer lengthened as before at the time when the child raises it but takes the form of two entwined cords. Jacqueline then understands the advantage she can take of this new presentation and tries to make the two ends enter the box together (more precisely, one immediately after the other, the second following shortly after the first). She no longer lets the chain go after putting one of the ends into the box, as was the case in attempts 1-15, but tries to put all of it in. But, as always occurs when a child of this age manipulates flexible objects, Jacqueline considers the chain as being rigid and lets go the whole of it when both extremities have been put in the box. The chain then comes out again

somewhat, but Jacqueline gently reintroduces the part that hangs (the middle part).

Attempt 17: Jacqueline distinctly tries to repeat the preceding movement. At first she does not grasp the chain at one end but pulls it together somewhat and grasps the middle part (without of course trying to find the actual middle).

Attempt 18: resumes the initial procedure and fails.

Attempt 19: rediscovers the procedure of attempts 16 and 17.

Attempt 20: same reaction, but this time Jacqueline encounters some difficulty in putting the second end in. Not succeeding, she recommences trying to put in a single end first. But as the chain slides out, she resumes the procedures of attempts 16, 17 and 19.

Attempts 21-22: same hesitations, but with ultimate success. (Piaget, 1936/1963, pp. 318-319)

Lucienne solved the same problem in Stage IV through mental combinations. She is trying to put the chain in the box:

She begins by simply putting one end of the chain into the box and trying to make the rest follow progressively. This procedure, which was first tried by Jacqueline, Lucienne finds successful the first time (the end put into the box stays there fortuitously), but fails completely at the second and third attempts.

At the fourth attempt, Lucienne starts as before but pauses, and after a short interval, herself places the chain on a flat surface nearby (the experiment takes place on a shawl), rolls it up in a ball intentionally, takes the ball between three fingers and puts the whole thing in the box.

The fifth attempt begins by a very short resumption of the first procedure. But Lucienne corrects herself at once and returns to the correct method.

Sixth attempt: immediate success. (Piaget, 1936/1963, pp. 336-337)

Problem solving in Stage VI often happens very rapidly and without distinctive behaviors. The above examples demonstrate that the absence of behavioral experimentation marks the advance. This makes it difficult for adults to detect when Stage VI infants are solving problems, particularly because they are often solving problems of such an elementary nature that adults often fail to see them as problems. Sometimes the only indication that a child is solving a problem rather than engaging in typical actions is a brief pause before the problem-solving action. Occasionally, however, Stage VI children give a positive indication that they are actually thinking through a problem. Here is an example:

> I put the chain back into the box and reduce the opening to 3 mm. It is understood that Lucienne is not aware of the functioning of the opening and closing of the matchbox and has not seen me prepare the experiment. She only possesses the two preceding schemes: turning the box over in order to empty it of its contents, and sliding her finger into the slit to make the chain come out. It is of course this last procedure that she tries first: she puts her finger inside and gropes to reach the chain, but fails completely. A pause follows during which Lucienne manifests a very curious reaction bearing witness not only to the fact that she tries to think out the situation and to represent to herself through mental combination the operations to be performed, but also to the role played by imitation in the genesis of representations. Lucienne mimics the widening of the slit.
>
> She looks at the slit with great attention; then, several times in succession, she opens and shuts her mouth, at first slightly, then wider and wider! Apparently Lucienne understands the existence of a cavity subjacent to the slit and wishes to enlarge that cavity. The attempt at representation which she thus furnishes is expressed plastically, that is to say, due to inability to think out the situation in words or clear visual images she uses a simple motor indication as "signifier" or symbol. . . .
>
> Soon after this phase of plastic reflection, Lucienne unhesitatingly puts her finger in the slit and, instead of trying as before to reach the chain, she pulls so as to enlarge the opening: She succeeds and grasps the chain. (Piaget, 1936/1963, pp. 337-338)

In this example Lucienne used a motoric or gestural symbol to represent the solution to the problem. It is clearly a symbol and not a sign, because it represents. This is a positive indication that she is really able to represent an absent object mentally. She does so with a motoric gesture because she is not yet able to use language. Infants often use private symbols, both motoric and verbal, before they are able to use conventional language. Piaget's observations indicate that these private forms of representation nevertheless fulfill the criterion for mental representation: They act as referents for absent objects or events.

The advent of mental representation permits infants to achieve object permanence. Stage VI infants can follow an object as it is hidden sequentially under three screens even when it is hidden in the examiner's hand between screens, because they are able to represent objects mentally even when the objects are invisible. They therefore assume that the object is not annihilated during its displacements and they infer its movement from the movements of the hand of the examiner.

The ability to represent the world mentally is clearly an extraordinary advance in problem solving and in children's understanding of objects. It is, however, equally important in the development of other domains. Advances in three other areas—causality, imitation, and play—are described in turn below.

Mental representation makes possible two advances in infants' ability to understand causality. First, they can infer causes when they see effects. Piaget gives the example of Laurent being able to remove an armchair that was holding a gate closed. He experienced the effect, that the gate would not open, and inferred the cause, that something must be blocking its path (1937/1954, p. 296). Second, they can infer effects when given causes. Piaget (1937/1954) describes an example in which Jacqueline infers the effect of expressing a need to go to the bathroom:

> Observation 160—At 1;4(12) Jacqueline has just been wrested from a game she wants to continue and placed in her playpen from which she wants to get out. She calls, but in vain. Then she clearly expresses a certain need, although the events of the last ten minutes prove that she no longer experiences it. No sooner has she left the playpen than she indicates the game she wishes to resume!
>
> Thus we see how Jacqueline, knowing that a mere appeal would not free her from her confinement, has imagined a more efficacious means, foreseeing more or less clearly the sequence of action that would result from it. (p. 297)

A particularly important advance is that of deferred imitation. Stage VI infants for the first time imitate events that occurred in the past. For example, Piaget (1945/1962, p. 63) describes Jacqueline imitating a temper tantrum that she had seen a little boy perform a day earlier. She could do this only if she had some way of mentally representing that past event. Note also that deferred imitation demonstrates that infants can now remember specific past events when no sign of the event remains (see Chapter 9). Imitation that follows right after a model's action also changes in Stage VI. It becomes both more direct and immediate and is less embedded in a context of other actions. The immediacy results from the fact that infants no longer have to try out imitative actions; they can do so mentally. Thus imitation at this stage is more obviously imitation.

Finally, the emergence of mental representation marks the onset of make-believe or symbolic play. Children of this age and older children use donkey tails to represent their pillows, broomsticks to represent horses, sand to represent bread dough, and blocks to represent houses. For the younger infant a pillow can be a sign for sleep, because it is part of the original action scheme, but a donkey tail cannot signify ("stand in" for) the pillow because it is not part of the action scheme itself. In Stage VI, however, the signifier can be separate from the action pattern and thus very disparate objects, including donkey tails, can be assimilated to the action scheme.

Research Testing Piaget's Theory

It should be obvious by now that Piaget's analysis of infant development is integrated, complex, and extensive. Piaget's epistemological approach—both a strength and a weakness—provided a framework for his investigations. He looked for behaviors relevant to such questions as how infants come to understand causality and whether they are born with certain kinds of knowledge about the nature of the world. Because he was looking for evidence that would resolve these questions, he noticed behaviors and developmental sequences of behaviors that other infant observers had not noticed. The danger of this approach is that one is more likely to notice evidence supporting one's theory and less likely to notice disconfirming evidence than is someone who does not believe that theory. This is a particularly troublesome problem for Piaget's research, because it lacks the kind of controls that would minimize the effect of experimenter bias. Nonetheless, Piaget partly compensated for the weakness of his method by his attempts to gather evidence for and against alternative hypotheses (see Chapter 1).

REPLICATION OF BEHAVIORAL SEQUENCES

It is a tribute to Piaget's skill as a scientist that the behavioral sequences he describes have been confirmed by studies using methods far more controlled than his

own. There have been several large-scale replications (Corman & Escalona, 1969; Decarie, 1965; Uzgiris, 1973; Uzgiris & Hunt, 1975) and many small-scale studies. The most extensive well-controlled study was that conducted by Uzgiris and Hunt. Their goal was to develop standardized Piagetian infant tests, and in that pursuit they collected data on all the aspects of Piaget's theory described above (object relations or the development of schemes, object permanence, means-end behaviors, imitation, and causality) plus one more (spatial relations).

The first step in verifying Piaget's formulations concerning infancy is to establish that the behaviors he describes can be reliably observed. Piaget's work clearly fulfills this requirement by two criteria: interobserver agreement and test-retest reliability. Uzgiris and Hunt found that two observers agreed on their assessments of more than 90% of infants' reactions. They also found that on the average 80% of the responses infants gave on one day were the same as those they gave 48 hours later. This demonstrates that Piaget did discover real behaviors and that they were typical and consistent infant behaviors.

The second step in evaluating Piaget's work is to determine whether the behaviors develop in the order described by Piaget. By definition, stage sequences must occur in an invariant order: Stage I must always precede Stage II, which must always precede Stage III, and so on. Although they used a finer analysis than the six stages (their scales had from 7 to 14 levels), Uzgiris and Hunt found remarkable consistency in development within each scale. Other studies that have used the six stages have also found the sequences to be as Piaget describes. The stages have been corroborated by both cross-sectional and longitudinal studies. Indeed, of dozens of studies that have tested the hypothesis of invariant order of development, only one major study, by Miller et al. (1970), found clear disconfirmatory evidence (in the object permanence sequence). Even those authors, when repeating their study with a shortened test series (Kramer et al., 1975), failed to replicate their original findings; in the second study they found the order predicted by Piaget.[4]

Although it seems clear that infant cognitive development in each domain (such as sensorimotor schemes, imitation, object permanence) does proceed in an invariant order, the domains do not always develop together (e.g., Corrigan, 1979; Uzgiris & Hunt, 1975; Watson & Fischer, 1977). Thus a baby may exhibit Stage IV behaviors with respect to object permanence, but Stage III behaviors with respect to imitation. Although Piaget provides a term to describe such uneven development (horizontal décalage), he does not allow

---

4. Keep in mind that these are group data. The majority of infants do show perfect ordinality (58% of the subjects in Kramer et al., 1975, showed perfect ordinality over a 6-month period), but there are exceptions. Piaget would claim that the exceptions are either measurement error or anomalies due to particular environmental experiences.

such noncorrespondences to interfere with his tendency to describe children as if all aspects of their development proceeded in lockstep. Such a practice is often inaccurate, given the frequency with which any given baby may be in one stage in one domain and a different stage in another domain. Thus it is probably preferable to specify the task domain when describing infants' cognitive development; for example, "Johnny is in Stage IV of imitation," rather than "Johnny is in Stage IV."

SENSORIMOTOR DEVELOPMENT IN OTHER SPECIES

The sensorimotor sequence of development has also been demonstrated in primates. The great apes, whose evolution and biology are most like that of humans, show remarkably similar progression through the sensorimotor stages. Research on great apes (most frequently gorillas and chimpanzees, but also including orangutans; see the review by Doré & Dumas, 1987) has found consistent evidence that they progress through each stage sequentially in the same invariant sequences as humans. They do not skip stages, nor do they exhibit characteristics of two or more stages in a single domain (see, e.g., Chevalier-Skolnikoff, 1982). There are also differences in development that seem to reflect the unique biology of each species. First, great apes proceed through the stages more rapidly than humans because of their earlier locomotion (Doré & Dumas, 1987). Second, great apes interact with physical objects less than do humans, and thus the circular reactions are displayed in fewer modalities and contexts (Doré & Dumas, 1987). Third, only humans exhibit sensorimotor development in the realm of vocal gestures (Chevalier-Skolnikoff, 1977). If the development of vocal schemes presages language development, this species difference is consistent with the rather extensive research in language training in great apes. Chimpanzees and gorillas seem readily able to learn to use tokens or signs as symbols (a sensorimotor Stage VI achievement), but they have not demonstrated (to the satisfaction of many researchers) that they can master the more specifically linguistic aspects of language, that is, grammar (for example, see Premack, 1976; Seidenberg & Petitto, 1979; Terrace, 1979, 1985). These variations are in no way inconsistent with the conclusion that the sensorimotor development of great apes is in general quite like that of humans.

Other animals also show sensorimotor development, although not as similarly to humans as is true for great apes. In particular, monkeys show some, but by no means all, the sensorimotor phenomena (Doré &

Dumas, 1987). Perhaps most important, monkeys apparently exhibit tertiary circular reactions only socially and not with objects, which means that their problem-solving skills are severely limited, and it is not clear that they reach Stage VI (although Mathieu et al., 1976, have found Stage VI behaviors in a single white-throated capuchin). This research demonstrating sensorimotor development in different primates is further evidence that the developmental sequences (particularly as standardized by Uzgiris and Hunt) tap real, biologically based developmental progressions, and/or that the basic environmental experiences necessary for Piagetian development are found across an enormous range of environments, from that of apes in the wild to urban humans.

EVALUATION OF PIAGET'S THEORY

The studies just described, both with humans and with other primates, have demonstrated that there are invariant sequences of development within each of the specific behavioral domains, such as sensorimotor schemes, imitation, and object permanence. This degree of confirmation is quite impressive in an area in which the methodology is as difficult as it is in infant studies. This research does not, however, demonstrate that Piaget's theory is the best explanation of infant cognition. Just because the behavioral sequences exist does not mean that Piaget's interpretation of them is correct. Observers may agree that infants exhibit certain behaviors, but may disagree about their meaning and about the causes of those behaviors. In addition, investigators with different theoretical orientations may discover different behavioral phenomena. Piaget may have selected behaviors that fit the interpretations that he favored. Furthermore, the traditional Piagetian procedures may produce results that are different from those produced by other, similar, procedures. Therefore, establishing the validity of Piaget's behavioral sequences is not sufficient.

A critical evaluation of a theory of the scope of Piaget's is an extremely complex task. It typically proceeds in saltatory fashion, testing each derived hypothesis or set of hypotheses separately. For each of these separate enterprises researchers must develop clever research designs to differentiate Piaget's theory from alternative explanations. Finally, if and when a research area yields definite conclusions, it must be integrated with other, related, research for evaluation. This kind of work is going on for a number of different aspects of Piaget's theory. Work on two of these aspects, imitation and the development of the object concept in secondary circular reactions (Stages III and IV), is discussed below.

IMITATION

Research on imitation tackles Piaget's major premise that imitative ability is part of and dependent on cognitive development. Two aspects of that belief can be delineated. The first is that imitation develops in the same sequence and at the same pace as general cognitive development. The second is the role imitation plays in the acquisition of new knowledge. Piaget believed that imitation, once developed, primarily involved accommodation; that is, when one imitates, one must stretch or modify one's understanding to be able to understand the modeled behavior. Thus imitation is a major mechanism for adaptation. It does have limits in that children should be unable to imitate a behavior that is totally unfamiliar to them, because they lack the requisite cognitive basis for understanding.

Research that challenges Piaget's description of the early development of imitation is first discussed below, and then research on the relation between imitation and acquiring new knowledge is addressed. As noted above, studies of the general sequence of behaviors as described by Piaget have supported his findings (Uzgiris, 1972; Uzgiris & Hunt, 1975).

Imitation in Young Babies

As an example of research on development of imitation that challenges Piaget, we will consider the nature of early imitative responses. There are three relevant issues. First is the question of whether there is imitation before the onset of primary schemes, which occurs at about 1 month of age. Second is whether developmental changes in imitation between birth and 4 months reflect the development of primary schemes. Third is whether babies can imitate actions they cannot see themselves do (e.g., tongue protrusion) earlier than Piaget claimed.

Research on the first issue, neonatal imitation, was discussed in Chapter 9. Those who believe there is neonatal imitation consider the evidence as tending toward their position, whereas those who are inclined toward a Piagetian position are not convinced by the evidence. This is largely because the two groups have different requirements for establishing the existence of imitation. Those who wish to demonstrate neonatal imitation are impressed by any demonstration that neonates ever exhibit anything akin to imitation. They then focus on the positive findings in Meltzoff and Moore's (1977) original demonstration of imitative tongue protrusion rather than the negative findings. They are impressed that Martin and Clark (1982)

found that newborns cry more in response to the crying of other newborns than to other kinds of cries and noises. They are not convinced by the alternative interpretation that the crying represents an innate response to distress. Piagetians, in contrast, require the more stringent criterion for exact imitation and conclude that neither exact nor same-class imitation in newborns has been demonstrated. They are unconvinced that the neonatal crying phenomenon is imitation; alternative interpretations such as the innate response to distress interpretation or several proposed by Piaget (1945/1962) seem more feasible.

Second, whether one believes in developmental changes in imitation in the first 4 months of life depends on one's interpretation of neonatal imitation. Those who believe in neonatal imitation do not typically address the issue of developmental change. Those influenced by Piaget accept the evidence that 6-week-olds exhibit same-class imitation and are not convinced by the evidence for younger babies (see Chapter 9). This fits with Piaget's theory: Same-class imitation is a developmental phenomenon that is contingent upon the development of primary schemes and thus should develop only after the first month of life. Piaget describes same-class imitation in babies this age for other responses, such as vocalization.

Third, Piaget claims that before Stage IV, babies cannot imitate actions of body parts that they cannot see. A number of studies have found that Stage II infants imitate tongue protrusions, which are unseen. Abravanel and Sigafoos (1984), Jacobson (1979), and Maratos (1973) all found that babies imitated tongue protrusions (unseen) in Stage II and Kaye and Marcus (1978) showed imitation of mouth opening in Stage III. Although this seems at first glance to be clear disconfirmation of Piaget's theory, it actually is a difference of interpretation. Piaget (1945/1962) notes similar phenomena (including tongue protrusions and mouth opening, which are unseen responses), but he does not see them as instances of true imitation. He claims that these "pseudoimitations" can be distinguished from true imitations because the former cannot be consistently elicited and because they do not last "unless the training is prolonged and consistently kept up" (p. 27). The data support that claim. All these studies found that imitative tongue protrusions became less frequent around 3 months of age, except in Jacobson's experimental group of babies whose mothers regularly modeled tongue protrusions.

Piaget would consider the research on the early development of imitation to confirm his theory. He considered these early phenomena to be unrelated to what to him were the more interesting later-developing forms of imitation, those he called "true imitation." Of course, he might have been wrong about their lack of importance. To demonstrate that they are important, researchers could show (a) that these early imitative responses are related to later forms; (b) that early forms clearly show greater cognitive competence than Piaget granted them, an argument made by Bower (1976) and Meltzoff and Moore (1977), and argued against by Anisfeld (1979), Cohen (1981), and Masters (1979); or (c) that Piaget's interpretations of the later forms are wrong.

Today, the studies of early imitation are intriguing to many workers. Although Piaget (1945/1962, p. 18) himself refused to offer an explanation for such pseudoimitation, others have tried (Bower, 1976; Cohen, 1981; Jacobson, 1979; Meltzoff & Moore, 1977; Smillie, 1980; Trevarthen, 1978). One particularly interesting interpretation is that the early imitation of unseen actions represents the same sort of intersensory unity that has been found with vision-audition and visually guided reaching. As with visually guided reaching, the early form of imitation seems to be distinct from the later form. Early forms wane during Stage II and the later forms wax during Stage III (see Cohen, 1981, for an excellent discussion of this view and Poulson et al., 1989, for a recent review). In addition, the early forms of imitation are not accompanied by well-formed orienting and vocalizing behaviors, as later forms are (Trevarthen, 1978).

The Function of Imitation

The second aspect of Piaget's account of imitation that has been investigated in some detail by others is the role imitation plays in cognitive development. Three disparate ways in which this relation has been explored will be described here. First are two studies of the development of the imitative response itself. Kaye and Marcus (1978, 1981) reasoned that if Piaget's description of imitation is correct, then studies that test imitation of only one or two modeled acts are insufficient to test it. They made a longitudinal study of development of six different imitative responses in babies 6 to 12 months old by modeling each action repeatedly for periods of up to 10 minutes, stopping each task when the infant cried or turned away permanently. They found that generally the infants' imitations became more and more exact over time. For example, in response to a model clapping her hands four times, babies exhibited the following behaviors in a consistent order from less to more exact: touching experimenter's hand, touching own hands together, pulling experimenter's hands together in clapping motion, clapping

once own hands, clapping four times. Kaye and Marcus interpret this to mean that the babies successively assimilated features of the modeled behavior until they successfully accommodated to the modeled behavior.

The second research strategy explores the relation of types of imitations to children's cognitive level on other tasks. In Piaget's account, children imitate behaviors at or just above their typical level of cognitive ability. They do not imitate behaviors either too advanced or too primitive with respect to their current cognitive functioning. Watson and Fischer (1977) examined this relation. They elicited pretending behaviors by modeling both less and more cognitively mature instances of the behaviors they wanted. Both the spontaneous and the elicited imitations demonstrated by their toddlers were at or near their highest cognitive capacity, and they did not imitate behaviors that reflected skills they had mastered much earlier. In language also, imitation reflects the child's cognitive level. When children imitate adults' utterances, they change the utterances into their own more primitive grammatical structures.

The other side of this relation between imitation and understanding of modeled acts is that modeling is an effective teaching tool only when children are cognitively ready to learn. For example, it should be impossible to teach a Stage II infant to solve invisible displacements (a Stage VI achievement), but training might be effective for a Stage V infant. This third research strategy of training subjects at different developmental levels has been employed primarily with older children. It suggests that the most effective kinds of training, including modeling, are effective with children who are just one step below the level described (for a review of this literature, see Yando et al., 1978). Comparable research with infants would have to be designed to consider their limited imitative ability, but that could be done.

In summary, the research generally supports Piaget's proposal that what children imitate depends on their cognitive skills. It also supports the notion that imitation does develop over time and becomes more frequent and more exact, although at least some of the details of Piaget's developmental sequence may need revision. There is still controversy of whether newborns can imitate, whether young infants can imitate unfamiliar actions, and the nature of early development of imitation. Current evidence is conflicting, but if such imitation is demonstrated in the future, it would seriously question Piaget's major tenet that newborns have no innate epistemological categories and must construct their own reality. In addition, although the research has not been discussed here, attempts to validate Piaget's claims about deferred imitation have yielded inconsistent conclusions (see the review by Poulson et al., 1989).

EXPLORATIONS OF THE UNDERLYING PROCESSES INVOLVED IN OBJECT SEARCH TASKS

Piaget's work on infants' object concept during Stages III and IV has generated many sophisticated tests of his theory, particularly with respect to the A-not-B error. The research has focused on the following issues:

(1) Is the A-not-B phenomenon real?
(2) Can associative memory principles account for the A-not-B error?
(3) Is infants' object concept really tied to their reaching actions, or can it be developed by visual exploration?
(4) Do infants know more about the object than Piaget claimed?

Is the A-not-B Error Real?

Studies of the A-not-B error are numerous and confusing. Fortunately, Wellman et al. (1986) have recently analyzed the extant literature by means of a mathematical method of summarizing across studies known as meta-analysis. A **meta-analysis** uses statistical tests to see whether a particular effect was consistently found by the studies that examined it. Generally, Wellman et al. found clear evidence for the existence of A-not-B error in Stage IV infants and for its waning in older infants, as predicted by Piaget.

Is the A-not-B Error Based on Associative Memory?

The Wellman et al. meta-analysis provided several tests of alternative explanations based on associative memory. Let us first review the relevant predictions. If infants are allowed to search immediately after the experimenter has hidden the object under B, infants will search under B, because they will retain the event in their short-term memory, a well-established temporary memory system. If infants are prevented from immediate search, short-term memory will fade, and they must rely on their long-term memory. In the A-not-B situation their long-term memory has stored two events—the object being hidden under A (earlier trial or trials) and the object being hidden under B (the last trial). If they have experienced each event equally (one trial of each), then they should respond randomly—50% of the time at each place. If the

experimenter has presented more A trials than B trials, the infants should search under A.

Let us compare these predictions against the consistent findings Wellman et al. document with their meta-analysis. First, 9-month-old infants are likely to correctly choose B if allowed to search immediately after the object is hidden. Thus short-term memory seems to play a role. Second, in none of Wellman et al.'s analyseis did infants respond at chance levels, which indicates that something other than association was influencing their responses. Third, the meta-analysis found that infants who had searched under A for several trials were no more likely to make the A-not-B error than were those who had fewer A trials. These latter two findings disconfirm the long-term memory predictions, but are consistent with Piaget's theory.

Just because inadequate motoric ability cannot account for the object permanence sequence by itself does not mean that Piaget's cognitive theory must be true. Another possibility is that infants fail these tasks only because their memories are so limited. This hypothesis may seem confusing, because Piaget would certainly agree that memory is a necessary condition for object permanence; that is, object permanence cannot occur until infants' memories are adequate. He did not believe, however, that memory development is a sufficient explanation for the development of object permanence. Piaget hypothesized that babies make the A-not-B error because their understanding of an object is tied to their actions, and so they will remember incorrectly. The studies described in the section on motoric ability are also relevant to determining the role of memory limitations. A transparent screen eliminates the necessity of remembering the object because it can still be seen. Thus if memory limitations are responsible for failure to complete object permanence tasks, using transparent covers should permit infants to pass the test. Both the studies using the single cover task (Bower & Wishart, 1972; Gratch, 1972) and others using the AB situation (Butterworth, 1977; Harris, 1974) found that transparent covers made the task easier than opaque covers, but they did not eliminate infants' errors. This demonstrates that memory limitations are involved, but that they cannot account for all errors. In research using other variations of the AB situation, Harris (1973) found evidence supporting this conclusion; he demonstrated that when experimental conditions minimized memory requirements, Stage IV infants were less likely to commit A-not-B errors.

Cummings and Bjork (1981a, 1983) also demonstrated that memory limitations are involved in performance on object search tasks. They argue that past research fails to support Piaget's interpretation of the

A-not-B error because in many studies the error rate is around 50%, which is what would be expected if babies could not remember where the object was and so chose a position randomly. A greater number of positions in the experimental situation would permit a more adequate test of Piaget's interpretation that babies return to A because their conception of the object is tied to their previous actions upon it. If babies choose to respond to A (the first hiding position) regardless of how many positions away from B (the second hiding position) it is, Piaget's position would be confirmed. If they choose positions close to B regardless of where A is, that would demonstrate that they remember the general location, although they may be unable to remember B specifically. The latter results were found in a series of studies with both Stage IV and Stage V versions of the A-not-B error (visible and invisible displacement tasks). The evidence clearly demonstrates that infants' memory for hiding places is only approximate, but it is not clear whether this constitutes disconfirmation of Piaget's theory of secondary schemes for two reasons, one conceptual and one evidential. First, a situation with five possible hiding places might simply confuse the subjects so much that they would be unable to use their action-based memories of A and so would be limited to their more recent memory of the object at B. Second, infants in a replication study (Schuberth & Gratch, 1981) exhibited A-not-B errors in Bjork and Cummings's situation (but see Cummings & Bjork, 1981b, for their objections to Schuberth and Gratch's article).

What can we conclude about the role of memory in object search tasks? First, memory is clearly involved. Second, memory alone cannot account for all the phenomena exhibited in the research. Third, whether memory is of action-object sequences remains unclear. Additional research relevant to this issue is described in the next sections.

The two contrasting views of the meaning of action—reaching to grasp a toy under a cover in infancy versus reasoning through mental representation—are considered by some to be consistent because they represent cognitive structures at different periods.

The Relative Roles of Action and Visual Exploration

Because of his reliance on naturalistic observation, Piaget focused on infants' reaching behaviors as his indicators of the development of object concept. As researchers have learned more about the sophistication of the neonatal visual system and its rapid development (see Chapter 7), it has become clear that visual exploration may provide the basis for considerable development of the object concept, particularly before the onset of visually guided reaching.

Several avenues of research support that conclusion. For example, Stage IV infants make the A-not-B error even when they are just observing and are not themselves reaching (Butterworth, 1974). Babies born without limbs (primarily victims of their mothers' prenatal use of thalidomide) evidently develop cognitively in a relatively normal fashion even though they obviously have little or no grasping experience (Kopp & Shaperman, 1973). In fact, vision appears predominant in the development of the object permanence sequence in Stages III and IV. Blind babies develop reaching behaviors much later than sighted infants, apparently because they have to rely on auditory cues. Sighted babies generally develop object permanence to the sound of objects later than they do to the sight of objects (Bigelow, 1981, 1983; Freedman et al., 1969; Uzgiris & Benson, 1980). In fact, the general tenor in infancy research that involves sucking, grasping, looking, and hearing is that the visual modality is the primary modality for cognitive development in babies.

Some experts consider the evidence of the importance of visual exploration to be a serious challenge to Piaget's theory, because they equate Piaget's claim that action schemes underlie cognitive development with reaching schemes. In contrast, other experts agree that he probably seriously overestimated the importance of reaching and mouthing and underestimated the importance of looking, but would include visual and auditory exploration as types of action that would result in action schemes.

Do Infants Know More About the Object Than Piaget Claimed?

According to Piaget, Stage V is the age of elaboration of the object, the first age at which infants can explore objects as they really are. Many researchers have challenged this claim by exploring what Stage III and IV infants (4-12 months) know about objects.

The first way this question was asked was to explore whether infants understand aspects of the A-not-B situation other than those that are tied to their own actions. The answer is clearly yes. When perceptual aspects, such as distinctive colors of the covers, consistently cue the presence of the object (for example, the object is always under the blue cover), infants are less likely to make the A-not-B error than when no such cues exist (see Wellman et al.'s 1986 meta-analysis). Likewise, when the perceptual cues conflict with the placement of the object, infants do worse than when there is no such conflict (Butterworth et al., 1982). Infants also apparently notice if the object changes under successive hidings (for single-cover tasks, see LeCompte & Gratch, 1972; Ramsay & Campos, 1975; for the A-not-B situation, see Moore & Clark, 1979; Schuberth et al., 1978; but not Evans & Gratch, 1972). Thus infants assimilate visually perceptible features of the situation.

Research in experimental situations beyond the traditional object search task also strongly supports the conclusion that infants know more about objects than would be expected from a strict interpretation of the Piagetian concept of action-object sequences. Baillargeon (1987, 1991) and her colleagues have shown that babies in Stage III understand that a screen should not be able to rotate through space that is currently occupied by an object. This research demonstrates that babies know that the object has size and solidity without ever touching it. This knowledge evidently develops around the beginning of Stage III. Baillargeon has found that only some 3½-month-old babies (the fast habituators; see Chapter 9) exhibit the phenomenon, whereas it is typical of 4½-month-olds. Her research has also suggested that 6½-month-olds have a quantitative understanding of the size of the object being occluded and perhaps this quantitative understanding develops from 4½ to 6½ months.

Another area of research that demonstrates that babies in the middle age range understand more about objects than would be expected from Piaget's accounts is that demonstrating that young infants can identify objectness for moving objects at younger ages than they can for stationary objects (see the description of this research in Chapter 7). This is true even when the object is novel and the infants watch only the movement (see Spelke, 1988, for a very nice review of her work in this area and its theoretical implications).

These three areas of research—Piagetian object permanence tasks, Baillargeon's object occlusion tasks, and Spelke's moving object tasks—all lead to the same conclusion. Stage III babies understand aspects of the object in its context beyond that assimilated through reaching. Thus to explain how infants of this age understand objects, we must go beyond a simple description of their concept as an undifferentiated action-object sequence.

Coordination of Schemes

According to Piaget, Stage IV infants are able to remove a barrier to reach an object because they can coordinate two schemes (the scheme that governs removing the barrier with the one that governs reaching for the desired object). They commit the A-not-B

error because the first coordination they form (remove-barrier-at-A and grasp-object-previously-hidden-at-A) interferes with their being able to form the second (remove-barrier-at-B and grasp-object-previously-hidden-at-B). Frye (1980) tested this interpretation in an ingenious pair of experiments. He argued that if Piaget's interpretation is correct, then having infants form a novel coordination of schemes after they form the coordination involving A and before they form the coordination involving B should help to break the influence of the first coordination (involving A) and prevent its intrusion into the B situation. He found this to be the case for two of three interposed tasks (hiding at a third place and pulling a support to get to an object, but not for pulling a string to get at an object). In addition, he included other experimental groups to permit comparisons of the predictive power of several other explanations. Only the intercoordination hypothesis predicted the results.

Frye's findings are consistent with the findings in Wellman et al.'s meta-analysis of the A-not-B error that infants were more likely to respond correctly and less likely to make the A-not-B error when there were more than two search locations. These findings are intriguing, but clearly not conclusive.

Conclusions

Research on the object search tasks has clearly confirmed some of Piaget's claims and disconfirmed others. It has confirmed his claim that the first indications of object permanence appear around 4 months of age and that major improvements occur around 8 months and around 12 months (all ages are approximate). It also confirms Piaget's assertions that during these ages babies' concepts of objects are developing and babies show definite limitations in how they understand the world.

What is in dispute is how best to describe understanding of the object in Stage III and IV infants (for currently viable alternative hypotheses, see Baillargeon, 1991; Harris, 1986; Spelke, 1988; Wellman et al., 1986; and, in a broader context, work in skills theory, which is described below). Piaget claims that infants' understanding is not of objects independent of the actions being performed upon them, but rather of action-object amalgams. Subsequent research has made it quite clear that he is wrong if the actions in action-object sequences refer only to the physical reaching movements that underlie most of the Piagetian tasks. Objects' movements that are caused by environmental events other than the infants' own reaching actions appear to play an equally strong role. Moreover, it is clear that other aspects of the situation (e.g., characteristics of the objects and covers) are both processed and incorporated into their concepts. Thus at the least we need to describe the object concept during secondary circular reactions as situation-object amalgams rather than as action-object sequences. Such a description is consistent with the subsequent development of tertiary circular reactions, in which the object is clearly abstracted from its situation. A more complete, specific, and generally accepted explanation must await further research.

Skills Theory

In science a new theory takes hold when it proves to be a powerful heuristic device by which research can be guided. Associative learning theory provided such an impetus to the study of infants in the 1950s and 1960s, and Piagetian theory did the same in the 1960s and 1970s. A third successful point of view is information processing. In this view, information from the environment is processed by the organism, who then acts upon it. Information-processing approaches are derived from analogies to machines, most prominently the computer.

As knowledge from research inspired by each of these theories accumulates, instances in which the data do not fit the theory also increase. This has happened to all these theories. Fischer (1980) has recently developed skills theory, which attempts to integrate the positive findings from these other theories. It pays specific attention to infancy and has inspired several nice research tests.

Fischer developed his skills theory from American learning theory and Piagetian research and theory; it can be classified as a process-oriented theory. As is true of most process-oriented psychologists, Fischer assumes that the cognitive structures of the organism interact with the environment to determine the organism's behavior at a given time. Although he acknowledges that the role of the organism includes inherited and constitutional factors, skills theory does not focus on the biology-experience issue.

In one sense, Fischer takes the same interactionist stance with respect to innate ideas as does Piaget: He believes that, rather than being innate, the first sensorimotor structures develop through experience acting upon the reflex structures, and he cites some evidence to support that belief (Bullinger, 1977). In spite of this similarity, Fischer has a different answer to the question of the basic nature of the categories of mind, a matter we will return to shortly. His theory also differs from that of Piaget in that he attributes less of development to maturation. Like learning theories,

Fischer's theory focuses on the role the environment plays in producing cognitive structures and their development. He starts from the general notion of adaptation in the sense that "the cognitive organism is constantly adapting skills to the world, and this adaptation provides the foundation for cognitive development and learning" (Fischer, 1980, p. 525).

The skills mentioned in this quotation are the heart of Fischer's theory. Their role is analogous to that of schemes in Piaget's theory. They develop through the infant's acting (motorically or perceptually) on the environment. Like Piaget's schemes, Fischer's skills are the basic cognitive structures for knowing; that is, they are procedures by which infants come to know their world. They are different from Piaget's schemes in two very important ways. First, schemes are organized by particular actions, such as a scheme for scratching versus a scheme for shaking, but skills are developed from initial global situations, such as shaking and hearing a rattle. Whereas for Piaget each scheme develops in its own modality and must be coordinated with the schemes of other senses, for Fischer the set of actions in a particular environmental situation is globally linked in a basic skill set, and later will be differentiated and then interrelated in a more sophisticated fashion.

The second way Fischer's skills differ from Piaget's schemes is related to the first. Piaget assumes that the sensory and motoric action patterns derive from the infant's biological substrate, and therefore will develop as cognitive structures of wide generality regardless of the particular environment in which the baby grows up. Fischer assumes the opposite. Skills develop from the particular situations infants encounter, and the course of each infant's development may be somewhat different from that of others because of the particular situations he or she encounters. This means that (a) babies will not develop at the same rate, (b) they will develop along somewhat different pathways, and (c) individual babies will be more advanced in some task domains than in others. Fischer's theory here is a response to many data that have shown unevenness in development, both within a given child and from one child to another. Although Uzgiris and Hunt (1975) found clear developmental sequences within a particular domain, such as object permanence or imitation, they found only low correlations from one domain to another (some correlation would be expected, because development in each domain is correlated with age). Fischer argues that unevenness is the norm in development because the particular skills infants develop are the result of both the particular environments they experience and their own levels of understanding with respect to those skill domains.

In skills theory each child has an optimal level of skills development. This is the highest level the child can reach at any particular time. For example, if a baby's optimal level is still sensorimotor rather than representational, then that baby is not able to reach full understanding of object permanence. Fischer does not specify what determines optimal level. It can be governed by maturation or by experience or by both without affecting the theory.

Fischer's theory can also be compared with learning theory. Skills can be conceived of as operants (emitted behaviors that are changed by environmental contingencies). This means that skills are more likely to recur if they have been followed by a reinforcement. It is also consistent with learning theory to suggest that uneven development is normal, because the opportunity to practice skills is what determines whether and how rapidly particular skills develop. Skills are unlike operants in one very important way. The concept of operant does not include a system that describes how operants are related to each other or how those relations change with learning and development. Skills theory provides such a system. The baby acquires specific skills; these become more complex, differentiated, and integrated, and they become intercoordinated with other skills.

Fischer accepts Piaget's division of development into three broad periods, which he calls tiers. His first tier corresponds to Piaget's sensorimotor period; like Piaget's, it ends when the baby develops mental representations. Within each tier, Fischer identifies four levels of development. The first three levels of the first tier correspond, roughly, to Piaget's primary, secondary, and tertiary schemes, and the fourth is equivalent to Piaget's Stage VI. Piagetian phenomena will be used here to demonstrate the first four levels of skills theory.

Level 1 skills are simple sets of sensorimotor actions. Actions coalesce in a set because they occur in a certain situation, such as interaction with particular people, objects, or events. Unlike Piaget's primary schemes, these sets may involve two sensory modalities, such as vision and audition. Fischer argues this way because many of the studies of conditioning in young infants may involve such multimodality sets (see Papoušek, 1967; Sameroff, 1971). This concept also, of course, fits Bower's theory of innate intercoordination of senses.

Level 2 is reached when one sensorimotor set is mapped (related element by element) onto another. A good example of a mapping is visually guided reaching, in which looking at an object becomes integrated with grasping it. Many, but not all, of Piaget's secondary circular reactions are Level 2 mappings.

Level 3 involves more complex mappings in which two or more components of one sensorimotor set are mapped onto analogous components of a second set, producing what Fischer calls a system. The tertiary circular reactions, in which variations of infants' actions produce interesting variations in results (remember Piaget's description of Jacqueline exploring how the box moved) are an example of Level 3 mapping.

Level 4 is when two systems become intercoordinated, which results in a simple representational set. For example, a child's sensorimotor system by which he manipulates a toy car becomes intercoordinated with a system derived from watching his older brother play with the toy car. This final intercoordination of systems frees children from the sensorimotor limitation of objects being tied to specific sets of actions. They can now represent simple properties of objects, events, and people independent of their own actions. Armed with these simple representational sets, 2-year-olds start on another tier of development that parallels the first—but that is a story for another book.

Fischer bases his description of sensorimotor development on the phenomena discovered by Piaget, but he provides a different theoretical basis, one that eliminates the following controversial aspects of Piaget's theory: (a) the assumption of general developmental synchrony, (b) Piaget's belief that infants actively invent their understanding of the world rather than learn about the environment, and (c) Piaget's belief that young infants cannot coordinate sensory information from several modalities and therefore have only fragmented knowledge of a single stimulus situation. Most of the infant research Fischer and his coworkers have produced has been centered on finding asynchronies in development that are predictable from skills theory (Bertenthal & Fischer, 1978; Corrigan, 1979; Jackson et al., 1978; Pipp et al., 1987; Watson & Fischer, 1977). In addition, Bertenthal and Fischer (1983) have applied the skills theory approach to the invisible search task (Stage VI object permanence) and have demonstrated that its development does not reflect systematic search (which should not develop this early, according to skills theory), but it does reflect the development of mental representation (as both theories would predict). Thus research stemming from skills theory clearly has heuristic value (i.e., it promotes new discoveries), which is exactly what a new theory should do.

Categorization

The terms *category*, *class*, and *concept* all refer to a group of objects or events that are considered to belong together. Traditionally, children's abilities to form categories (classes, concepts) have been studied through observation of how children sort objects into groups. Children were said to be capable of logical classification only when they could sort objects into two groups (circles and triangles, or circles and all noncircles) without error and then put all the objects back together and sort them on a different basis (such as all large, all medium, all small). Success in such tasks is usually achieved in the late preschool years.

By accepting other, less stringent, criteria and by using sensitive experimental techniques, researchers have been able to detect categorization much earlier. Much of the research has used techniques developed in perceptual studies, particularly habituation/dishabituation, conditioning, and tracking of visual stimuli. Research that uses these techniques to study concepts that can be represented visually is described first below, followed by discussion of the few studies that have used object sorting with infants. Finally, a review of the research that has related developing categorization to development of symbols is offered.

EARLY DEVELOPMENT: VISUAL CONCEPTS

To investigate how babies classify, we must demonstrate that babies (a) perceive a visual configuration as a whole (an object or an integrated pattern) and (b) can process a series of pictures as exemplars of a class and distinguish those exemplars from pictures that are not members of the target class. The first issue has been a major focus of perception research, which was discussed in Chapter 7; its conclusions are summarized below. Discussion of the second issue follows.

Configurations

It is clear that newborns can make many of the discriminations needed to form concepts. They can perceive contours that demarcate the boundaries between objects. They can discriminate straight lines from curves, vertical lines from horizontals or diagonals, and patterns with high density from patterns with low density, and they can detect color and brightness. With the possible exception of perception of faces, the evidence consistently supports the view that infants younger than 2 months of age do not use such discriminations to form concepts.

The first indication that infants perceive a configuration of such discriminable elements as a unit is found in the research on face perception. At 2 months infants seem to discriminate between faces and scrambled faces. By 3 months of age infants discriminate their

mothers' faces from strangers' faces. This demonstrates that they have learned to recognize a particular configuration in contrast to others. Babies of this age also show evidence of perceiving other configurations as concepts: (a) They perceive an angle as the relation between two lines, whereas infants 6 weeks old perceive the same angles as lines of differing orientation (Cohen & Younger, 1984); (b) they treat triangular patterns of dots of various sizes and in varying positions in their field of vision as similar to each other and different from dots in a straight line (Milewski, 1979); and (c) they recognize objects from various orientations as similar (what is called shape constancy; see Bornstein, 1984, for a review of the research).

At 4 months infants develop visually guided reaching, the last of the intersensory coordinations (Piaget, 1936/1963). After this age, if not before, infants conceive of objects as things that have mass in a three-dimensional world and that have visual, tactile, and sometimes auditory attributes. Infants 4 and 5 months old make other perceptual discriminations that demonstrate their increasing knowledge of objects in the world and that could conceivably provide the basis for classification. At 5 months infants can discriminate between two strange faces and between a photograph of a person or doll and the actual person or doll. This capability evidently reflects, in part, infants' changing abilities to process multidimensional stimuli. Bower (1966) found that 4-5-month-old babies respond to complex patterns as integrated wholes, whereas younger infants seem to respond to complex patterns as collections of separate parts. It has also been shown that 5-month-old infants can detect a single dimension within a complex pattern as well as compounds of such dimensions (Cohen et al., 1971; Cornell, 1975; Fagan, 1977), although these studies did not test younger babies and so have not demonstrated conclusively that such abilities do not develop until this age. Finally, infants of this age can use movement cues to classify what they see into various objects, as discussed in Chapter 7 (see also Spelke, 1988).

Concepts

The second developmental phenomenon to be demonstrated is that babies can treat a group (class) of stimuli as forming a category and recognize that other stimuli do not belong to that category. The most common paradigm used to demonstrate this is a habituation/dishabituation paradigm (see Chapter 9). When using this paradigm to test concept formation, researchers present several different exemplars of the concept during habituation trials. If babies habituate

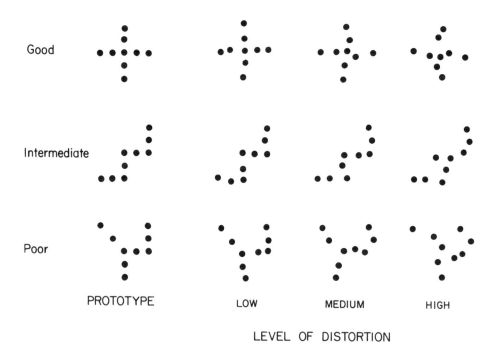

Figure 10.8. The top rows are all members of the good category in Younger and Gotlieb's (1988) study. The leftmost cross is the best exemplar of the class (the prototype) and the other three in the row are distortions at randomly chosen distances and in randomly chosen directions. After being presented a series of the crosslike figures (but not the prototype cross), 3-month-old babies recognized the prototype as a member of the category and distinguished it from a similar form from another category (not shown). The middle row shows the comparable stimuli for the intermediate forms, which 5-month-olds could categorize. The bottom row are comparable stimuli for the poor forms, which only the 7-month-olds could categorize.

to these multiple stimuli, it suggests that they are responding to the exemplars as a class. Dishabituation trials can verify that interpretation. If babies are forming a concept they should dishabituate to stimuli that are not in that class and should fail to dishabituate (that is, continue to show little response) to stimuli that are new instances of the habituated concept.

Research of this sort has been developed relatively recently, so there are still many unanswered questions. Nonetheless, some generalizations are possible:

- The youngest age at which categorization has been demonstrated is 3-4 months (Bomba & Siqueland, 1983; Younger & Gotlieb, 1988).
- Babies 3-4 months old categorize only with carefully selected stimuli. Younger and Gotlieb (1988) have shown that 3-month-olds will categorize "good" forms, 5-month-olds will categorize both "good" and "intermediate" forms, and 7-month-olds will categorize "poor" forms as well (see Figure 10.8). The concepts used in this study were of

the type known as prototypic; that means these young babies did not simply remember the exact stimuli they had seen, but they abstracted the general form (e.g., the cross) and then remembered that. When more complex stimuli such as imaginary animals or faces in various orientations are used, 4- and 5-month-olds do not show evidence of categorization (Cohen & Strauss, 1979; Oakes et al., 1989; Younger & Cohen, 1982, 1983, 1986). Note, however, that all of the research cited here used stationary stimuli. Since Spelke's research (1988) suggests that 4-month-olds perceive "objectness" in moving stimuli and not in stationary stimuli, it may be that they can form more sophisticated habituation-type concepts with moving stimuli than have been found at this time.

- Babies 7 months old can form habituation-type categories to different orientations of a face versus a new face (Cohen & Strauss, 1979), but they still do not form categories for visual representation of unfamiliar or complex stimuli (Oakes et al., 1989; Younger & Cohen, 1982, 1983, 1986; Younger & Gotlieb, 1988).

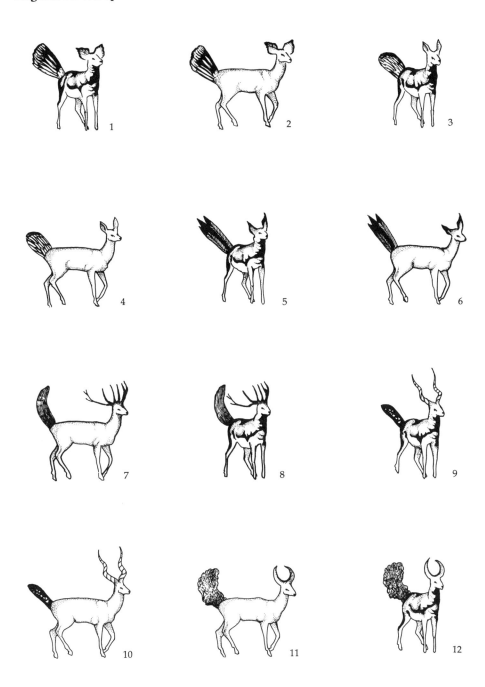

Figure 10.9. The set of 12 habituation stimuli used in Younger (1990). These stimuli included exemplars of two classes: deer bodies with ears and feathered tails (stimuli 1-6), and deer bodies with antlers and furry tails (stimuli 7-12). These figures were actual photographs that had been cut up and pasted in imaginary combinations. These pictures were presented in random order (not as shown here) until the infants habituated. Then the infants were shown three test stimuli: a new exemplar of one of the categories, an animal that violated the rules of the habituation set (e.g., one with feathers and antlers), and a monkey. The infants showed that they had formed a category by ignoring the new exemplar but dishabituating to the other two stimuli.

- By 10 months infants are able to form categories using a variety of stimuli—imaginary cartoon and lifelike animals (Roberts, 1988; Roberts & Horowitz, 1986; Sherman, 1985; Strauss, 1979; Younger, 1985, 1990; Younger & Cohen, 1982, 1983, 1986) and toy trucks versus toy animals (Oakes et al., 1989). They can even form two distinct categories for a set of pictures if attributes are correlated (see Figure 10.9 for an example). And remember that they are forming these categories merely by looking sequentially at a series of pictures of exemplars of both classes (e.g., Younger, 1985, 1990).
- By 12 months (and maybe earlier) infants can form abstract concepts of objects, that is, concepts whose defining attributes are not perceptible, such as dogs versus antelopes (Cohen & Caputo, 1978), men versus other animals, and food versus furniture (Ross, 1980).

Among the questions still to be answered are two raised by Ross's (1980) study. First, she found no changes in children 12, 18, and 24 months of age. Because the second year is notable for improvement in communication skills, particularly in language, it is striking that by Ross's technique (habituation/dishabituation) knowledge of concepts in a nonverbal context does not appear to be developing as well. Second, she found that the subjects did not habituate to some concepts, although they still distinguished between novel exemplars and nonexemplars. The exemplars of the concepts for which this was true—animals, food, and furniture—were all more varied than for those that habituated—men and the letters M and O. Thus the more abstract (less perceptually based) concepts elicited different behaviors. Whether this has any important implications for development is unclear.

LATER DEVELOPMENT

Sorting Into Categories

None of the studies of conceptual development described so far used that classic method of testing children's concepts, the sorting task. By 6 months of age infants are good at reaching for objects they see, and therefore it is possible to lay out a group of toys and watch what infants do with them. Starkey (1981) did just that, using a procedure highly congenial to the ages he studied (see Figure 10.10). He found that 6-month-old infants neither sorted into groups nor sequentially touched more than two similar objects. After selecting one or two of a kind, they would start to reach for a third, only to stop in the middle and move to another

object that had caught their attention. Thus their behaviors showed no evidence of categorization even though the stimuli were clearly no more complex than the face and animal pictures used in the habituation studies discussed earlier, which infants of this age did categorize. The object sorting task, however, is probably more difficult for two reasons. First, it requires that infants maintain their activity with respect to a single category in the face of possibilities of alternative classification criteria. In habituation/dishabituation paradigms, there are no alternative categories to be ignored. Throughout development, problems that present a conflict between two alternative solution strategies are more difficult and the ability to solve them develops later than it does for comparable tasks without such conflicts. Second, the grouping task also often involves sophisticated reaching, particularly reaching while already holding an object. Such complex reaching skills develop later than 6 months of age (Bruner, 1969, 1973).

By 9 months infants show signs of overcoming the problems 6-month-olds have. More than 80% of Starkey's 9-month-old babies tended to pick sequentially at least three or four similar objects from a group of toys and to put at least two of them into a separate pile. Infants advance rapidly after this initial achievement. By 12 months around 40% of infants, on at least one occasion, picked out all four instances of one class and put those objects together. Whether this sequential selection requires true classification skills is not clear. Sugarman (1982) argues that infants may successively select similar objects only because the objects interest them, not because they note that a similarity relation exists among them. Both Sugarman's (1981) data and Starkey's (1981) support this notion. Infants younger than 1 year showed successive selection of exemplars in a class primarily when the stimuli in one class were more likely to interest the infants and when the two sets were easily distinguishable. Sugarman (1981; see also 1982 for additional analyses) argues that infants have established true classes when they select all of one class and then all of a second class. This develops between 18 and 24 months and is soon followed by another advance. At 2½ years infants begin to group into two classes at once; for example, they will pick up two dolls and put them in one place, then put a circle in a second place, next place another doll with the other dolls, and so on.

Gestures

At about the same time the more complex forms of concepts discussed above are apparently developing, the

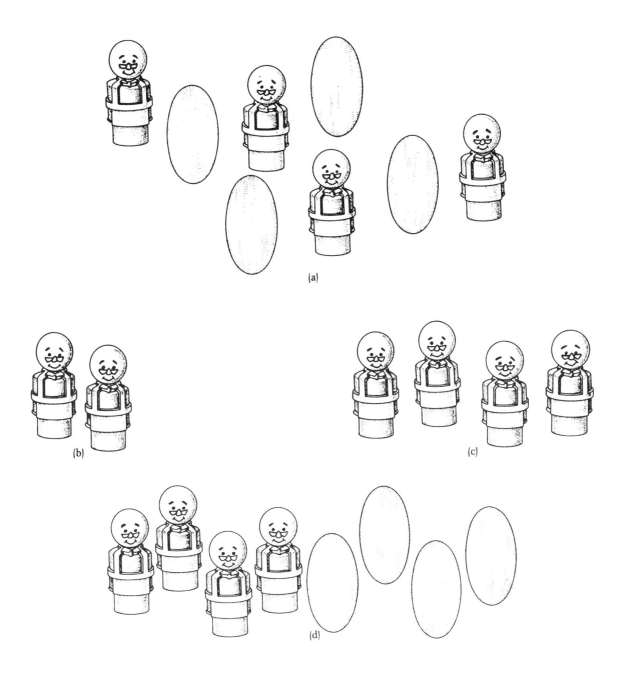

Figure 10.10. The stimulus situation and typical responses of infants in object sorting tasks. (a) A tray with the stimuli spread out was placed in front of the infants without verbal instructions or modeling and the infants were permitted to play with them as they wished. Parts b, c, and d represent infant responses of varying sophistication. (b) Selecting two of a kind. About 33% of 6-month-old babies and 80% of 9-month-old infants do this on occasion. (c) Selecting all four of a kind. About 40% of 12-month-olds do this on occasion. (d) Both classes of objects separated into distinct groups. This ability develops between 1½ and 2½ years of age.

use of symbols (perhaps more accurately called presymbols) is beginning. A symbol is an activity or object that can refer to something that is not present. A narrower definition reserves the term **symbol** for instances in which the signifier and the referent are arbitrarily related. For example, words are arbitrarily related to their referents because they do not in any way resemble the objects to which they refer. However, the term *symbol* will be used here to include both abstract signifier-signified relations and those in which the signifier does resemble its referent, because the focus here is on what toddlers' developing symbol use can reveal about their knowledge of concepts. Much of the work that sheds light on this question concerns language development, which is described in Chapter 11. This chapter will deal with some of the burgeoning research that investigates the developing use of symbols through representational systems other than language.

Bates, Bretherton, and their colleagues have been studying the development of gestural schemes in relation to verbal schemes. In gestural schemes infants represent knowledge of an object by involving it in a conventional action in a pretend fashion. For example, an infant shows by gesture that she knows something about a telephone if she puts the receiver of a play telephone to her ear. Likewise, an infant knows something about soap if he pretends to wash his hands when he sees a bar of soap. Gestural schemes occur frequently by 10 to 12 months of age. When gestural schemes are used with their original objects, they show that the infant knows something about the objects, but they do not demonstrate that the infant has demarcated a class of objects. When infants also exhibit these schemes with new and similar objects, they can be said to know the concept. In addition, as children develop, they exhibit their gestural schemes with substitute objects that "stand for" the original objects. Piaget calls this development "symbolic play"; it is characteristic of Stage VI. The substitute object serves as a symbol for the object in the gestural scheme, and, according to Piaget, indicates that the scheme has become representational.

When these gestural schemes first develop, they are closely tied to their original contexts. For example, gestural schemes are less likely to be made when the object is abstract (same basic shape and criterial attribute) than when the object is realistic (Bretherton et al., 1981). Objects used as signifiers in symbolic play are likely to be similar, both perceptually and in function, to the signified object (Ungerer et al., 1981). With time, these schemes become more widely applied and applied in an increasing number of different circumstances ("decontextualized," in Werner & Ka-

plan's, 1963, terminology). For example, a child might develop a telephone gesture in a game with her mother, and first apply it only to that toy telephone, then to other toy telephones, outside game contexts, and later still to a spoon (Bates et al., 1975; Volterra et al., 1979). Through decontextualization children's concepts clearly become more refined, because the essential characteristics become abstracted from the original context in which they were learned and can be applied to a range of appropriate exemplars.

Gestural schemes serve two important functions in addition to helping observers infer children's concepts. First is symbolic play, in which children use one object to symbolize another. Use of the spoon as a telephone is one example. Children 2 years and older are more likely than younger children to use symbolic objects (Elder & Pederson, 1978; Fein, 1975; Watson & Fischer, 1977; Ungerer et al., 1981).

Second, gestures serve a communicative function. Acredolo and Goodwyn (1988) demonstrated this in a study of the later, more abstracted type of gestures, that is, those gestures that are applied in consistent and often abbreviated fashion to varying instances of the object (e.g., panting to indicate different dogs, and/or pictures of dogs). Such gestures develop at 14-15 months of age. They seem to serve the same purpose as words, to develop at the same time as infants' first words, and to be used only until infants learn the appropriate words. Some communicative gestures develop in the same general social context as words do—from repeated interactions with parents about objects. Other communicative gestures are infant originals—they develop from infants' experiences outside of parent-infant routines. Particularly for the infant-original gestures, communicative gestures more often reflect the actions of the referent (e.g., throwing to represent ball) than they do the perceptible characteristics (the roundness of the ball). These findings are consistent with the view of gestures developing from action schemes. They also fit with Bretherton et al.'s (1981) finding that gestural schemes start to decline by 20 months of age, when language is developing rapidly.

The development of gestural schemes has an interesting parallel in the development of infants' use of American Sign Language (ASL), which is for adults a shared symbol system. Bonvillian and his colleagues studied the development of the use of ASL in children of deaf parents (Bonvillian, Orlansky, & Novack, 1983; Bonvillian, Orlansky, Novack, & Folven, 1983; Orlansky & Bonvillian, 1985). Although signs in ASL are gestural, they are quite different from gestural schemes. Gestural schemes often develop from the sensorimotor schemes of the babies themselves, whereas ASL signs are taught by the parents. Therefore ASL might be expected to develop the same way spoken language does. Because the fine motor coordination necessary to sign evidently develops earlier than motoric control of the articulatory apparatus, signing should develop earlier than language, so long as infants' concepts are sufficient.

This is the question that such a study investigates: Do infants have the concepts necessary to be able to attach symbols to them at an earlier age than they can in language? According to Bonvillian and his colleagues, they do. The average age at which the children in their study produced their first recognizable sign was 8.6 months, when they scored primarily in sensorimotor Stages III and IV (by Uzgiris and Hunt norms). Nevertheless, these early signs were not necessarily used in a completely symbolic fashion. During their home visits Bonvillian and his collaborators were seldom able to elicit signs for objects that were not present or for events that had not just happened. They therefore made a separate judgment on the basis of parents' diaries and discussions with them as to when such signs were made in clear symbolic fashion (a procedure often used in assessing language development). The babies did not use their signs symbolically until after they had developed 10 signs (13.2 months) and sometimes not until they had started to combine signs (17.1 months) and had reached Piagetian Stages V or VI. Thus ASL signs show the same developmental course as gestural schemes. Early use is not fully symbolic, in that signs initially occur only in context, as do gestural schemes. This is also consistent with Sugarman's interpretation of sequential selection of same-class objects in a display; that is, infants of this age are able to note similarities among objects within a class, but have not yet developed the representational skills necessary to conceptualize classes independent of the particular exemplars in the particular situation.

The research in these three areas (development of gestural schemes, development of communicative gestures, and development of ASL) provides three windows on the development of mental representation. The studies show that (a) the earliest forms of gestures occur at 10-12 months of age, (b) gestures are used symbolically at 13-14 months of age, and (c) gestures wane—and are replaced by formal language—toward the end of the second year of life.

This research is consistent with the general Piagetian framework, in which mental representation and symbols develop from action schemes. In specifics it is only partly consistent—presymbolic gestures (what Piaget calls signs) do develop in Stage IV, as Piaget claims, but truly symbolic gestures have been demon-

strated in both hearing and deaf infants in Stage V, whereas Piaget claims symbols develop in Stage VI.

CONCLUSIONS

By the end of their first 2 years, children are still a long way from the sort of mature classification behaviors seen in late preschool and elementary school children. Nevertheless, infants are beginning to form concepts and thereby distinguish between exemplars and nonexemplars of such concepts during these 2 years. The description of this developmental sequence is still extremely sketchy, and care must be used in interpreting the data. Nonetheless, it seems clear that there are several phases. Before 2 months of age babies seem capable only of discriminating among stimuli and show little ability to make similarity judgments in response to repeated patterns. Simple examples of recognizing such similarity in visual configurations appear at 2-3 months. By 3-4 months babies can categorize, as operationally defined by the habituation/dishabituation paradigm, but only with particular kinds of stimuli. For the next few months their ability to categorize more difficult pictures develops gradually, until at 12 months, they can even form abstract categories. Shortly after this age, they can produce decontextualized gestures to represent concepts even when the referent is not present. It is not until the last half of the second year, however, that they can show comparable skill at sorting objects.

Summary

Because of my desire to show how knowledge about infants is discovered as well as the knowledge itself, I felt it was important to present the research in this chapter in its scientific context. However, the complexities of that context make it difficult to see what a baby at each age is like. Therefore, this section is devoted to a chronological summary of the sequence of cognitive development in infancy. This summary includes the most firmly established and least controversial evidence, and not those aspects about which there is substantial disagreement. Also included are developmental phenomena discussed in earlier chapters when they elucidate cognitive development.

At birth infants can respond to limited sorts of changes in their world. They can change their sucking behaviors to meet the world's requirements, such as adapting to fast- or slow-flowing nipples. They also exhibit behaviors such as grasping, sucking, and looking in the absence of an obvious eliciting stimulus: They just seem to act.

In the first month of life more sophisticated abilities begin to develop. By the end of that first month babies are able to learn new, previously unknown connections, ones that are not just responses to immediate changes in the environment. They can learn arbitrary associations such as that footsteps in the hall occur just before they receive milk and they can remember the connection so that the next time they hear those footsteps they know food will arrive. Furthermore, babies 1 month old have acquired a primitive means by which to explore their world actively, the primary circular reactions.

During the second and third months of life (Piaget's Stage II) infants advance in several ways. They can detect perceptual invariants, the mark of true perceptual processing (see Chapter 7), and they can distinguish their mothers from strangers. They can imitate in a general, same-class fashion. They can recognize previous events for at least 24 hours without prompting and for several weeks if their memories are reactivated before presentation of the stimulus.

At 4 months infants develop the mature form of visually guided reaching, which greatly improves their ability to explore the world. Infants of this age (entering Stage III) are more responsive to environmental events and objects than are younger infants, and they can often make a happening recur through their own actions (secondary circular reactions). They imitate frequently, albeit still with limitations. They can form a concept by seeing a set of varying exemplars with a common attribute, although their success is limited to particularly "good" stimuli. Their understanding of the world is still very limited.

During the 4-6-month period infants show improved ability to discriminate among multidimensional stimuli. They clearly have intercoordinated objects' visual, auditory, and tactile characteristics, and apparently see objects in depth. These developmental phenomena suggest that babies of this age understand the nature of three-dimensional objects.

By 8-9 months (entering Stage IV) infants have developed truly intentional behaviors. They can set aside an obstacle to reach an object and pull a string to get what is attached to it. They are beginning to develop object permanence in that they search for objects that are out of their sight, including objects that they left in another room several minutes earlier. Their concept of the object, however, is not yet mature, although the nature of their object concept is in dispute. They sometimes commit the A-not-B error, looking for an object in a previous hiding place even though they have seen it put into a new hiding place. Infants of this age clearly use imitation to learn about their environ-

ment, because they imitate unfamiliar actions and their imitation seems intentional. They also show evidence of reconstructive memory.

By 10 months infants show evidence that they can categorize on the basis of presentation of exemplars in a variety of settings. During this period they often use gestures (or signs for those learning ASL) to communicate.

By around 12 months of age (the beginning of Stage V) infants have learned that objects are independent of their own actions on them. Because of this they can focus on the characteristics of an object to a greater degree than in previous stages and they become particularly interested in novel aspects of their environment. They pay close attention to distinctive features of objects. They vary events such as the height from which they drop objects so that they can note the varying actions of the falling object. They can recognize abstract concepts, ones that have no common perceptual attributes or configurations.

The problem solving of infants in Stage V also takes a major step forward. Not only can they use means to achieve ends, they can invent new means; that is, they can figure out how to solve means-end problems by new, untried means. Their problem-solving ability is still limited, however, and they have to try out the means behavior to see if they will achieve the desired end.

Although it has been developing gradually throughout infancy, particularly in Stages IV and V, representational thought is not clearly developed until the last half of the second year. By that time infants (a) achieve mature object permanence, (b) can solve problems through mental combinations, (c) classify two classes at a time (Sugarman's 1982 criterion of true representation in classification), and (d) use language symbolically.

References

ABRAVANEL, E., & Sigafoos, A. D. (1984). Exploring the presence of imitation during early infancy. *Child Development, 55*, 381-392.

ACREDOLO, L., & Goodwyn, S. (1988). Symbolic gesturing in normal infants. *Child Development, 59*, 450-466.

ANISFELD, M. (1979). Interpreting "imitative" responses in early infancy. *Science, 205*, 214-215.

BAILLARGEON, R. (1987). Object permanence in 3½- and 4½-month-old infants. *Developmental Psychology, 23*, 655-664.

BAILLARGEON, R. (1991). Reasoning about height and location. *Cognition, 38*, 13-42.

BATES, E., Camaioni, L., & Volterra, V. (1975). The acquisition of performatives prior to speech. *Merrill-Palmer Quar-*

terly, 21, 205-226.

BERTENTHAL, B. I., & Fischer, K. W. (1978). The development of self-recognition in the infant. *Developmental Psychology, 14*, 44-50.

BERTENTHAL, B. I., & Fischer, K. W. (1983). The development of representation in search: A social-cognitive analysis. *Child Development, 54*, 846-857.

BIGELOW, A. (1981). Object permanence for sound-producing objects: Parallels between blind and sighted infants. *Journal of Genetic Psychology, 139*, 11-26.

BIGELOW, A. E. (1983). Development of the use of sound in the search behavior of infants. *Developmental Psychology, 29*, 317-321.

BOLTON, N. (1972). *The psychology of thinking*. London: Methuen.

BOMBA, P. C., & Siqueland, E. R. (1983). The nature and structure of infant form categories. *Journal of Experimental Child Psychology, 35*, 294-328.

BONVILLIAN, J. D., Orlansky, M. D., & Novack, L. L. (1983). Developmental milestones: Sign language acquisition and motor development. *Child Development, 54*, 1435-1445.

BONVILLIAN, J. D., Orlansky, M. D., Novack, L. L., & Folven, R. J. (1983). Early sign language acquisition and cognitive development. In D. R. Rogers & J. A. Sloboda (Eds.), *Acquisition of symbolic skills* (pp. 207-214). New York: Plenum.

BORNSTEIN, M. H. (1984). A descriptive taxonomy of psychological categories used by infants. In C. Sophian (Ed.), *Origins of cognitive skills* (pp. 313-338). Hillsdale, NJ: Lawrence Erlbaum.

BOWER, T. G. R. (1966). Heterogeneous summations in human infants. *Animal Behavior, 14*, 395-398.

BOWER, T. G. R. (1976). Repetitive processes in child development. *Scientific American, 235*, 38-47.

BOWER, T. G. R. (1982). *Development in infancy* (2nd ed.). San Francisco: W. H. Freeman.

BOWER, T. G. R., & Wishart, J. G. (1972). The effects of motor skill on object performance. *Cognition, 1*, 165-172.

BRETHERTON, I., Bates, E., McNew, S., Shore, C., Williamson, C., & Beeghly-Smith, M. (1981). Comprehension and production of symbols in infancy: An experimental study. *Developmental Psychology, 17*, 728-736.

BRUNER, J. S. (1969). Eye, hand, and mind. In D. Elkind & J. H. Flavell (Eds.), *Studies in cognitive development: Essays in honor of Jean Piaget* (pp. 223-235). New York: Oxford University Press.

BRUNER, J. S. (1973). Organization of early skilled action. *Child Development, 44*, 1-11.

BULLINGER, A. (1977). Orientation de la tete du nouveau ne en presence d'un stimulus visuel [Orientation of the head of the newborn in the presence of a visual stimulus]. *L'Annee Psychologique, 77*, 357-364.

BUTTERWORTH, G. (1974). *The development of object permanence*. Unpublished doctoral dissertation, Oxford University.

BUTTERWORTH, G. (1977). Object disappearance and error in Piaget's Stage IV tasks. *Journal of Experimental Child Psychology, 23*, 391-401.

BUTTERWORTH, G., Jarrett, N., & Hicks, L. (1982). Spatiotemporal identity in infancy: Perceptual competence or conceptual deficit? *Developmental Psychology, 18*, 435-449.

CHEVALIER-SKOLNIKOFF, S. (1977). A Piagetian model for describing and comparing socialization in monkey, ape, and human infants. In S. Chevalier-Skolnikoff & F. E. Poirier (Eds.), *Primate bio-social development: Biological, social, and ecological determinants* (pp. 159-187). New York: Garland.

CHEVALIER-SKOLNIKOFF, C. (1982). A cognitive analysis of facial behavior in Old World monkeys, apes, and human beings. In C. T. Snowdon, C. H. Brown, & M. R. Petersen (Eds.), *Primate communication* (pp. 302-368). Cambridge: Cambridge University Press.

COHEN, J. S. (1981, May). *Neonatal imitation: A critical analysis of its implications for Piagetian theory*. Paper presented at the meeting of the Jean Piaget Society, Philadelphia.

COHEN, L. B., & Caputo, N. (1978, March). *Instructing infants to respond to perceptual categories*. Paper presented at the International Conference on Infant Studies, Providence, RI.

COHEN, L. B., Gelber, E. R., & Lazar, M. A. (1971). Infant habituation and generalization to differing degrees of stimulus novelty. *Journal of Experimental Child Psychology, 11*, 379-389.

COHEN, L. B., & Strauss, M. S. (1979). Concept acquisition in the human infant. *Child Development, 50*, 419-424.

COHEN, L. B., & Younger, B. A. (1984). Infant perception of angular relations. *Infant Behavior and Development, 7*, 37-47.

CORMAN, H. H., & Escalona, S. K. (1969). Stages of sensorimotor development: A replication study. *Merrill-Palmer Quarterly, 15*, 351-360.

CORNELL, E. H. (1975). Infants' visual attention to pattern arrangement and orientation. *Child Development, 46*, 229-232.

CORRIGAN, R. (1979). Cognitive correlates of language: Differential criteria yield differential results. *Child Development, 50*, 617-631.

CUMMINGS, E. M., & Bjork, E. L. (1981a). The search behavior of 12 to 14 month-old infants on a five-choice invisible displacement hiding task. *Infant Behavior and Development, 4*, 47-60.

CUMMINGS, E. M., & Bjork, E. L. (1981b). Search on a five-choice invisible displacement hiding task: A rejoinder to Schuberth and Gratch. *Infant Behavior and Development, 4*, 65-67.

CUMMINGS, E. M., & Bjork, E. L. (1983). Search behavior on multi-choice hiding tasks: Evidence for an objective conception of space in infancy. *International Journal of Behavioral Development, 6*, 71-87.

DECARIE, T. G. (1965). *Intelligence and affectivity in early childhood*. New York: International Universities Press.

DORÉ, F. Y., & Dumas, C. (1987). Psychology of animal cognition: Piagetian studies. *Psychological Bulletin, 102*, 219-233.

ELDER, J., & Pederson, D. (1978). Preschool children's use of objects in symbolic play. *Child Development, 49*, 500-504.

EVANS, W. F., & Gratch, G. (1972). The stage IV error in Piaget's theory of object concept development: Difficulties in object conceptualization or spatial localization? *Child Development, 43*, 682-688.

FAGAN, J. F., III. (1977). An attention model of infant recognition. *Child Development, 48*, 345-359.

FEIN, G. (1975). A transformational analysis of pretending. *Developmental Psychology, 11*, 291-296.

FISCHER, K. W. (1980). A theory of cognitive development: The control and construction of hierarchies of skills. *Psychological Review, 87*, 477-531.

FREEDMAN, D. A., Fox-Kolenda, B., Margileth, D A., & Miller, D. H. (1969). The development of the use of sound as a guide to affective and cognitive behavior. *Child Develop-

ment, 40, 1099-1105.

FRYE, D. (1980). Stages of development: The Stage IV error. *Infant Behavior and Development, 3,* 115-126.

GESELL, A. L. (1934). *Atlas of infant behavior.* New Haven, CT: Yale University Press.

GRATCH, G. (1972). A study of the relative dominance of vision and touch in six-month-old infants. *Child Development, 43,* 615-623.

HARRIS, P. L. (1973). Perseverative errors in search by young children. *Child Development, 44,* 28-33.

HARRIS, P. L. (1974). Perseverative search at a visibly empty place by young children. *Journal of Experimental Child Psychology, 18,* 535-542.

HARRIS, P. L. (1986). Bringing order to the A-not-B error: Commentary on Wellman, H. M., Cross, D., & Bartsch, K. (1986). Infant search and object permanence: A meta-analysis of the A-Not-B error. *Monographs of the Society for Research in Child Development, 51*(3, Serial No. 214), 52-61.

JACKSON, E., Campos, J., & Fischer, K. W. (1978). The question of the décalage between object permanence and person permanence. *Developmental Psychology, 14,* 1-10.

JACOBSON, S. W. (1979). Matching behavior in the young infant. *Child Development, 50,* 425-430.

KAYE, K., & Marcus, J. (1978). Imitation over a series of trials without feedback: Age six months. *Infant Behavior and Development, 1,* 141-155.

KAYE, K., & Marcus, J. (1981). Infant imitation: The sensory-motor agenda. *Developmental Psychology, 17,* 258-265.

KOPP, C. B., & Shaperman, J. (1973). Cognitive development in the absence of object manipulation during infancy. *Developmental Psychology, 9,* 430.

KRAMER, J. A., Hill, K. T., & Cohen, L. B. (1975). Infant's development of object permanence: A refined methodology and new evidence for Piaget's hypothesized ordinality. *Child Development, 46,* 149-155.

LeCOMPTE, G. K., & Gratch, G. (1972). Violation of a rule as a method of diagnosing infants' levels of object concept. *Child Development, 43,* 385-396.

MARATOS, O. (1973, April). *The origin and development of imitation in the first six months of life.* Paper presented at the annual meeting of the British Psychological Society, Liverpool.

MARTIN, G. B., & Clark, R. D., III. (1982). Distress crying in neonates: Species and peer specificity. *Developmental Psychology, 18,* 3-9.

MASTERS, J. C. (1979). Interpreting imitative responses in early infancy. *Science, 205,* 215.

MATHIEU, M., Bouchard, M. A., Granger, L., & Herscovitch, J. (1976). Piagetian object-permanence in Cebus capucinus, Lagothrica flavicauda and Pan troglodytes. *Animal Behavior, 24,* 585-588.

MELTZOFF, A. N., & Moore, M. K. (1977). Imitation of facial and manual gestures by human neonates. *Science, 198,* 75-78.

MILEWSKI, A. E. (1979). Visual discrimination and detection of configural invariance in 3-month infants. *Developmental Psychology, 15,* 357-363.

MILLER, D., Cohen, L. B., & Hill, K. T. (1970). A methodological investigation of Piaget's theory of object concept development in the sensory-motor period. *Journal of Experimental Child Psychology, 9,* 59-85.

MOORE, M. K., & Clark, D. E. (1979, April). *Piaget's Stage IV error: An identity theory interpretation.* Paper presented at the biennial meeting of the Society for Research in Child Development, Denver.

OAKES, L. M., Madole, K. L., & Cohen, L. B. (1989, April). *Object exploration in infancy: Habituation and categorization.* Paper presented at the biennial meeting of the Society for Research in Child Development, Kansas City, MO.

ORLANSKY, M. D., & Bonvillian, J. D. (1985). Sign language: Language development in children of deaf parents and implications for other populations. *Merrill-Palmer Quarterly, 31,* 127-143.

PAPOUSEK, H. (1967). Experimental studies of appetitional behavior in human newborns and infants. In H. W. Stevenson, E. H. Hess, & H. L. Rheingold (Eds.), *Early behavior: Comparative and developmental approaches.* New York: John Wiley.

PIAGET, J. (1954). *The construction of reality in the child* (M. Cook, Trans.). New York: Basic Books. (Original work published 1937)

PIAGET, J. (1962). *Play, dreams and imitation in childhood* (C. Gattegno & F. M. Hodgson, Trans.). New York: W. W. Norton. (Original work published 1945)

PIAGET, J. (1963). *The origins of intelligence in children* (M. Cook, Trans.). New York: W. W. Norton. (Original work published 1936)

PIAGET, J. (1970). Piaget's theory. In P. H. Mussen (Ed.), *Carmichael's manual of child psychology* (Vol. 1, 3rd ed., pp. 703-732). New York: John Wiley.

PIPP, S., Fischer, K. W., & Jennings, S. (1987). Acquisition of self- and mother knowledge in infancy. *Developmental Psychology, 23,* 86-96.

POULSON, C. L., Nunes, L. R. P., & Warren, S. F. (1989). Imitation in infancy: A critical review. In H. W. Reese (Ed.), *Advances in child development and behavior* (Vol. 22, pp. 271-299). Orlando, FL: Academic Press.

PREMACK, D. (1976). Language and intelligence in ape and man. *American Scientist, 64,* 674-683.

RAMSAY, D. S., & Campos, J. J. (1975). Memory by the infant in an object notion task. *Developmental Psychology, 11,* 411-412.

ROBERTS, K. (1988). Retrieval of a basic-level category in prelinguistic infants. *Developmental Psychology, 24,* 21-27.

ROBERTS, K., & Horowitz, F. D. (1986). Basic level categorization in seven- and nine-month-old infants. *Journal of Child Language, 13,* 191-208.

ROSS, G. S. (1980). Categorization in 1- to 2-year-olds. *Developmental Psychology, 16,* 391-396.

SAMEROFF, A. J. (1971). Can conditioned responses be established in the newborn infant? *Developmental Psychology, 5,* 1-12.

SCHUBERTH, R. E., & Gratch, G. (1981). Search on a five-choice invisible displacement hiding task: A reply to Cummings and Bjork. *Infant Behavior and Development, 4,* 61-64.

SCHUBERTH, R. E., Werner, J. S., & Lipsitt, L. P. (1978). The stage IV error in Piaget's theory of object concept development: A reconsideration of the spatial localization hypothesis. *Child Development, 49,* 744-748.

SEIDENBERG, M. S., & Petitto, L. A. (1979). Signing behavior in apes: A critical review. *Cognition, 7,* 177-215.

SHERMAN, T. (1985). Categorization skills in infants. *Child Development, 56,* 1561-1573.

SMILLIE, D. (1980). *Evaluating Piaget's theory of the origin of imitation.* Paper presented at the International Conference on Infant Studies, New Haven, CT.

SPELKE, E. S. (1988). Where perceiving ends and thinking begins: The apprehension of objects in infancy. In A. Yonas

(Ed.), *Perceptual development in infancy: The Minnesota Symposium on Child Psychology* (Vol. 20, pp. 197-234). Hillsdale, NJ: Erlbaum.

STARKEY, D. (1981). The origins of concept formation: Object sorting and object preference in early infancy. *Child Development, 52,* 489-497.

STRAUSS, M. S. (1979). Abstraction of prototypical information by adults and 10 month old infants. *Journal of Experimental Psychology: Human Learning and Memory, 6,* 618-632.

SUGARMAN, S. (1981). The cognitive basis of classification in very young children: An analysis of object-ordering trends. *Child Development, 52,* 1172-1178.

SUGARMAN, S. (1982). Developmental change in early representational intelligence: Evidence from spatial classification strategies and related verbal expressions. *Cognitive Psychology, 14,* 410-449.

TERRACE, H. S. (1979, November). How Noam Chomsky changed my mind. *Psychology Today,* pp. 65-76.

TERRACE, H. S. (1985). In the beginning was the "name." *American Psychologist, 40,* 1011-1028.

TREVARTHEN, C. (1978). Modes of perceiving and modes of acting. In H. L. Pick & E. Saltzman (Eds.), *Modes of perception and processing information.* Hillsdale, NJ: Lawrence Erlbaum.

UNGERER, J. A., Zelazo, P. R., Kearsley, R. B., & O'Leary, K. (1981). Developmental changes in the representation of objects in symbolic play from 18 to 34 months of age. *Child Development, 52,* 186-195.

UZGIRIS, I. C. (1972). Patterns of vocal and gestural imitation in infants. In F. J. Monks, W. H. Hartup, & J. DeWit (Eds.), *Determinants of behavioral development* (pp. 467-471). New York: Academic Press.

UZGIRIS, I. C. (1973). Patterns of cognitive development in infancy. *Merrill-Palmer Quarterly, 19,* 181-204.

UZGIRIS, I. C., & Benson, J. (1980, April). *Infants' use of sound in search for objects.* Paper presented at the International Conference on Infant Studies, New Haven, CT.

UZGIRIS, I. C., & Hunt, J. M. (1975). *Assessment in infancy.* Urbana: University of Illinois Press.

VOLTERRA, V., Bates, E., Benigni, L., Bretherton, I., & Camaioni, L. (1979). First words in language and action: A qualitative look. In E. Bates (Ed.), *The emergence of symbols: Cognition and communication in infancy.* New York: Academic Press.

WATSON, M. W., & Fischer, K. W. (1977). A developmental sequence of agent use in late infancy. *Child Development, 48,* 828-835.

WELLMAN, H. M., Cross, D., & Bartsch, K. (1986). Infant search and object permanence: A meta-analysis of the A-not-B error. *Monographs of the Society for Research in Child Development, 51*(3, Serial No. 214).

WERNER, H., & Kaplan, B. (1963). *Symbol formation.* New York: John Wiley.

YANDO, R., Seitz, V., & Zigler, E. (1978). *Imitation: A developmental perspective.* Hillsdale, NJ: Lawrence Erlbaum.

YOUNGER, B. A. (1985). The segregation of items into categories by ten-month-old infants. *Child Development, 56,* 1574-1583.

YOUNGER, B. A. (1990). Infants' detection of correlations among feature categories. *Child Development, 61,* 614-620.

YOUNGER, B. A., & Cohen, L. B. (1982). Infant perception of correlated attributes. *Infant Behavior & Development, 5,* 262.

YOUNGER, B. A., & Cohen, L. B. (1983). Infant perception of correlations among attributes. *Child Development, 54,* 858-867.

YOUNGER, B. A., & Cohen, L. B. (1986). Developmental change in infants' perception of correlations among attributes. *Child Development, 57,* 803-815.

YOUNGER, B. A., & Gotlieb, S. (1988). Development of categorization skills: Changes in the nature or structure of infant form categories? *Developmental Psychology, 24,* 611-619.

Early Communicative and Language Behavior

PAULA N. MENYUK

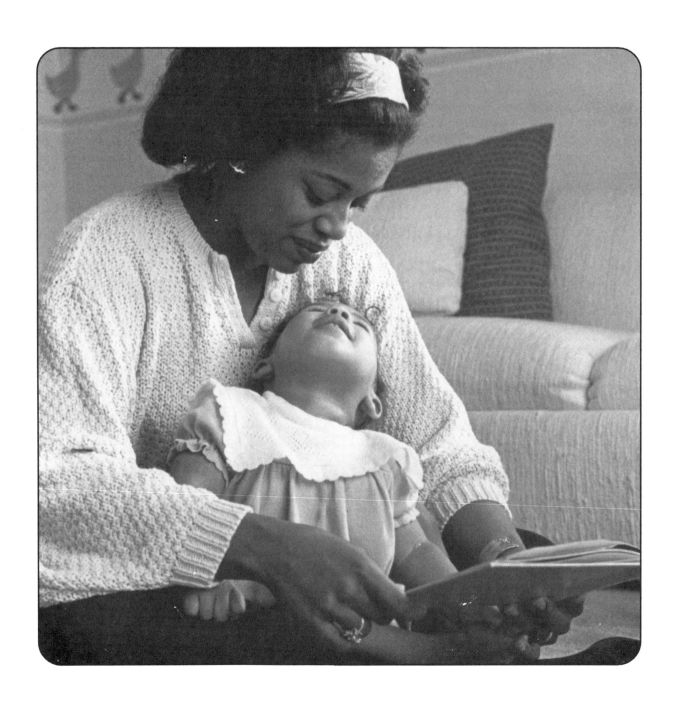

Chapter 11

Introduction and Overview

Language development has received a great deal of attention over the years. Early studies primarily cataloged the types of sounds, words, sentences and errors produced by children as they matured, and simple explanations were provided to account for development and errors. Over the last two decades researchers have attempted both to describe the developmental process more adequately and to explain it. Now there are linguistic descriptions of these early behaviors that allow us to see the relations between early and later language knowledge. Current explanations for infant language development attempt to take into account the readiness of infants to acquire language, the functions of their early communicative and linguistic behavior, the role of the input they receive, and the processing abilities needed to acquire linguistic categories and relations. These efforts have resulted in a more integrated picture of language development and more information about the details of this development from birth on. This information indicates that the infant is much more linguistically sophisticated than had previously been thought.

One of the most exciting developments that takes place during infancy is the child's acquisition of the community's language. Parents greet the production of first words with overt joy and often state, prior to its occurrence, that they wished the child would communicate with them. As we shall see, infants communicate long before the appearance of words. Further, they learn a great deal about the structure and function of language during the so-called preword or **babbling period**, when infants produce a variety of sounds, but not words. Many caregivers behave as if infants communicate during this period, and this may play a very important role in infants' acquisition of language. In some instances, the expected first words do not appear during infancy because of known or suspected physiological causes. In these cases, language acquisition is either delayed or both delayed and different.

A brief overview of the general language acquisition accomplishments of infancy follows. Infancy was once thought of as being composed of prelinguistic and linguistic phases that were held to be unrelated. The prelinguistic phase, cooing and babbling, was thought to end with a period of silence before the onset of the linguistic phase, the production of words (Jakobson, 1968). This view of complete discontinuity between behaviors is no longer accepted, although the exact relations between them are still matters for research. Continuities between the behaviors of these two phases are discussed below. We now know that the infant learns much about language and communicates a great deal during this so-called prelinguistic phase.

During much of the first year of life, language production consists of cooing, babbling, and use of gesture, facial expression, and intonation and stress on babbled utterances to express emotions; during the second year, word and word combinations are used to express ideas. The infant's comprehension of language over this period cannot be so clearly defined. Studies have indicated that very young infants, 1 to 2 days of life, can discriminate between speech and nonspeech sounds, and at 1 to 2 months of age, can discriminate between sets of speech sound contrasts (see Chapter 7). Observational data indicate that infants can comprehend a small set of words some months before they produce recognizable words. Experimental data indicate that infants 8 to 12 months of age can learn to associate objects with words or nonsense syllables if they are specifically taught to do so, and do associate very familiar objects with words at 12 months. Nevertheless, the extent of and the basis for recognition of the meaning of words during these early months is open to question. Babies at the end of the first year may also understand a few short sentences, but they are probably using the concrete context to interpret the language they hear rather than understanding the language as such. This primitive understanding of short sentences and phrases precedes the ability to produce them. During the second year babies begin to understand longer and more complex sentences and can do this out of context.

It is also during the second year that babies begin to produce words and phrases. At around 2 years most children produce utterances that often are composed of at least two words. A few still produce one-word utterances that some call holophrases (complete messages), and some produce lengthier utterances. As the above summary indicates, babies make very dramatic strides in language development during infancy, from cry and vocalization to sentence comprehension and production. In general it is thought that comprehension precedes production of both words and sentences, but little is known about the length of the gap between the aspects of language the child comprehends and those that are produced. In fact, the length of the gap may vary for individual infants. There is some agreement that production does not faithfully follow the developmental progression of comprehension. That is, the course of comprehension may not dictate the course of production. Thus the bases for comprehension and production of the units of language may differ.

In this chapter, communicative behavior, the perception and production of aspects of language during infancy, and the effects of biological, environmental, and cognitive factors on early acquisition of language are discussed. The chapter concludes with some of the vital unanswered questions about language acquisition during this period of development.

COMMUNICATIVE BEHAVIOR

During the first year of life, babies acquire knowledge of how to communicate with others in the environment. Their communication abilities diverge from those of other animals during this first year. During the second half of the first year they also learn a great deal about how to convey their intentions through vocalizations. How human infants' communication differs from that of other animals and how their communications abilities develop are discussed in turn below.

Human Compared With Other Animal Communication

Most definitions of communication mention its purposes. These include expression of needs and feelings and indication of needs, feelings, and ideas by symbolic means. Many animal species, ranging from the social insects (bees, wasps, ants, and termites) to chimpanzees, have elaborate communication systems. These systems, while extremely complex and effective as communication devices, have limited purposes (expression of needs, primarily, and sometimes feelings) and seem to be different in kind from human language (Fromkin & Rodman, 1974). The most important characteristics of human language that are not part of the communication systems of other animals are as follows:

(1) *Creativity or generativity:* Rearrangements of parts (sounds, words, and sentences) can create totally new messages. (Example: "The girl kissed the boy" and "The boy kissed the girl.")
(2) *Arbitrariness:* Words stand for objects and events but are neither the objects and events themselves (such as a cry of fear) nor graphic representations of them (such as a picture of a tree).
(3) *Discreteness:* Parts are separated into units, such as sounds, words, and sentences.
(4) *Displacement:* Language can be used to refer to things that are remote in time or space.

Communication during the earliest phases of infancy seems to share the purposes of nonhuman communication systems, mere expression of needs and feelings. However, some of the above differences between human language and other systems begin to appear at a very early age. Vocalization during the early months of life, when the child does not understand the meanings of words and sentences and does not produce them, is not generally considered to be language, but communication. Nevertheless, this communication has begun to take on some of the purposes of purely human systems, and it uses the means by which these purposes are conveyed by humans.

The structured aspects of language present in early infancy are those relating to speech sounds. At about 6 to 9 months of age, infants can produce articulated speech sounds, and the sound sequences they produce begin to resemble words. It is interesting to note that at this age deaf infants produce hand movements that resemble signs much more than do the hand movements of hearing infants (Petitto & Marentette, 1990). Thus it is not speech per se that differentiates between other animal and human communication. These sequences of articulated sounds are produced with intonational contours that do more than simply communicate needs and feelings, they request and declare. It had been thought that only when ideas are expressed in terms of words and phrases do human and animal systems diverge (Vygotsky, 1962). However, this divergence may come at an earlier stage.

The Use of Sounds to Convey Intentions

Very young infants are sensitive to certain communications carried by the sequences of speech sounds. Spoken sentences carry information in addition to the meanings of the individual words and the meaning carried by the relations among the words in the sentence. Information concerning the age, sex, and identity of speakers is carried by the tone qualities of their voices. The pattern of rise and fall of pitch and loudness of words in sentences, which are called **intonation contours**, also carry meaning. Intonation contours differ as a function of speakers' emotions (such as anger or friendliness). They also tell us whether speakers are making statements, asking questions, or demanding something. In English statements, speakers' voices rise gradually and then fall; in requests, their voices rise gradually at the end of the sentence; and in commands, there is a sharply rising and then falling contour. Speakers also emphasize certain parts of sentences by increasing loudness (called stress). These different kinds of information, which are carried by the sequence of speech sounds in sentences, not by the words and relations among words, are called **prosodic** or **suprasegmental cues**.

The ability to use suprasegmental cues to convey needs and feelings and to understand communicative intent develops very early in infancy and remains fairly stable throughout life. Comprehension of affect may not, however, be a uniquely human characteristic. Other mammals (for example, dogs) may also comprehend affect from the suprasegmental cues in humans' voices. However, humans who can hear both perceive and produce suprasegmental cues that first convey affect and then intent. Humans also differ from other animals in the variability of meanings attached to these suprasegmental cues. In nonhuman species the meaning of these cues is typically ritualized and innately determined, but in humans the particular meanings given to a cue can vary across cultures, as can the meanings of facial expressions and gestures. Despite these possibilities, the purpose and form of the communication system during early infancy does not vary across different linguistic environments. It is initially used by young human infants to convey needs and feelings and to socialize and only later to convey intent.

Development of Communication

Let us now turn to the development of prelinguistic communication in infants. The generalizations that can be made about the comments to follow are limited by the following facts. Most of the information available about communicative behavior during this period is based on data obtained in Western, urbanized, primarily middle-class cultures. Many of the data on language development in other cultures deal with developments in periods later than infancy (Schieffelin & Ochs, 1986) or are concerned with speech sound perception and production (Kuhl, 1990). Further, the infant-caregiver pairs studied are few in number, and there are large differences among pairs. Nevertheless, it is possible to discern general trends as well as individual differences in communication development; this discussion will focus on the general trends.

From birth, infants engage in both cry and noncry vocalizations, although crying is the most frequent vocalization in the first 5 or 6 months. In general, vocalizations are initially only expressions of infants' physiological state, that is, comfort or discomfort. Little control of air flow can be observed. At about 6 to 8 weeks both cries and noncries begin to take on the structure of human speech. This is the result of the infant's achievement of much greater control of the ex-

penditure of air and movement of parts of the vocal mechanism during vocalizations (Stark, 1986; Truby et al., 1965). Phonation, or sound making, is superimposed on the infant's normal respiratory cycle, and one phonation is much longer than one normal respiration (Nakazima, 1962). By about 3 months of age patterned vocalizations that are vowellike (ah, ee, and so forth) are produced.

At about the same time, so-called **pseudoconversations** between caregiver and infant have been observed (Bateson, 1969). The adult vocalizes, waits for a vocal response from the infant, and then vocalizes again, either in reply to the infant's vocalization or to elicit a response if one is not forthcoming (see Figure 11.1). Although imitation of vocalization and attempts to elicit responses are primarily caregiver behaviors in early "conversations," infants occasionally attempt to elicit vocal responses to their vocalizations if their caregivers do not respond. In urban groups in Western cultures, these vocal exchanges are a very frequent occurrence in interactions between 3-month-old infants and their caregivers, regardless of the socioeconomic status of the dyad or mother-infant pair (Lewis & Freedle, 1972). These behaviors have been called the beginning of conversational turn-taking.

Sensitivity to cues that mark whose turn it is in a conversation and prompt participation once the cues are given are presumably evidence of mature communicative behavior. Evidence of this sensitivity appears very early in life. Conversational turn-taking appears to begin when the infant indicates readiness by the nature of the vocalizations produced and by being quietly alert for longer periods of time. Caregivers appear to be cued by the infant's behaviors to engage them in vocal-social interactions. Thus both readiness on the part of the infant and caregiver sensitivity to readiness cues contribute to the establishment of communicative interaction at this early period in the child's life.

In addition to taking turns, which, after all, fulfills a general social obligation, infants communicate needs and feelings by vocalization, facial expression, and gesture. These means have been termed **paralinguistic**. Infants modify the intonation contours of their babbles in a manner that is quite similar to that used by adults. In a study of the vocalizations of infants in American-English- and Japanese-speaking environments, Nakazima (1962) found that both groups of infants start to imitate sentence intonational contours (rising or falling patterns) in their babbled utterances at about 6 to 8 months of life. The prosodic patterns of their babbling during the last quarter of the first year have the characteristics of their native language (Boysson-Bardies et al., 1986). During this period their babbled utterances

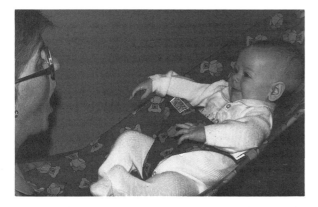

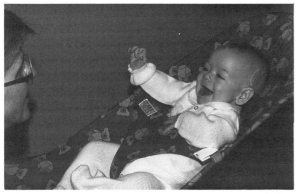

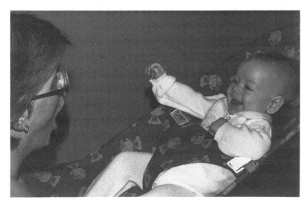

Figure 11.1. A pseudoconversation. The adult makes a sound and waits. The infant then responds, and the adult makes the same or another sound. (Photographs courtesy of Judith E. Sims-Knight.)

have the intonational contours of statements (slowly rising and falling contour), requests (slowly rising, falling, and rising again) and commands (sharply rising and falling). Data on perception of contours indicate that infants discriminate between utterances with rising contours and those with falling contours at approximately 1 month, and they respond differently to the emotional qualities of voice alone (that is, without visual cues) shortly thereafter (Menyuk, 1972). They are

upset by angry voices and soothed by friendly voices. Thus the use and understanding of different intonational contours is not only a very early language acquisition but precedes knowledge of any other aspect of language (Siegler, 1986).

At about 10 months, infants begin to use specific gestures to indicate intent (Bates et al., 1975). They show objects to adults (the declarative use of action) or they seek aid with objects from adults (command or request). By use of intonational patterns, gestures, and facial expressions, infants convey both negative and positive affect, and, in addition, indicate or state, command, and request. These behaviors begin after the sixth month of life. The research on turn-taking in conversation and on the use of suprasegmental features, gestures, and facial expressions to convey intent and emotion indicates that these basic principles of communicative interaction appear to be well established during the first year of life.

In the postbabbling period some developmental changes occur in both turn-taking behavior and the use of suprasegmental features. A longitudinal study of conversational turn-taking in four mother-toddler dyads was carried out by Donahue (1978). The toddlers ranged in age from 12 to 19 months at the beginning of the study and were observed at biweekly intervals for 8 months. The principal findings were that patterns of turn-taking behavior changed over that time, becoming almost adultlike. The infants developed from merely taking turns to engaging in true conversation.

Recall that early turn-taking behavior consists primarily of responding to vocalization with vocalization. Donahue (1978) notes that in the transition from this behavior to communicative exchanges, particular strategies were used to indicate that a turn was being taken. These strategies were different for the girls than for the boys. The two girls took turns by imitating the intonational contours of the mothers' utterances. The two boys responded with a set question phrase ("wuzzis" or "wuzzat"). Still later in the transition period the girls responded by using intonational contours that contrasted with those of the mothers' utterances (falling to rising or rising to falling), whereas the boys provided acknowledgments ("Oh!" "Uh huh"). These latter behaviors gave the impression that real understanding was taking place, but the behaviors were, in fact, random. The final period was marked by appropriate responses to the content of the mothers' utterances.

In a study by Liebergott et al. (1985), conversational interactions of some 50 infants and their mothers indicated that at 25 months 25% of the infants' conversational turns were appropriate responses and 15% were elicitations from the infant to start a conversation. These changes in conversational behavior have led some researchers to conclude that the primary impetus to and basis for further language development stems from interaction between caregiver and infant. However, it is not clear how interaction alone can lead to acquisition of knowledge of language structures, because these interactions are not tutorial. Mothers seem to accept whatever infants provide.

What is remarkable is that from a very early age (3 months) infants take turns when pauses are provided by their caregivers. They use gesture, facial expression, intonation, and stress to communicate their affect, needs, and feelings. Altogether, the communicative behavior of prelinguistic infants indicates how ready they are to participate in conversation and to receive linguistically important inputs. They seem ready to go beyond the kind of communication most animals engage in and to make the transition from communication to language.

From Prelanguage to Language Behavior

Toward the end of the first year, babbling decreases and wordlike approximations are more frequently produced. After babbling decreases, a large proportion of the utterances produced are recognizable words or recognizable words within stereotyped or babbled utterances (Branigan, 1976). The different intonational contours used with babbled utterances (assertion, narration, command, and request) are now used with words and phrases (Menyuk & Bernholtz, 1969). Thus there is continuity in development in that strategies developed earlier to convey needs and feelings (gesture, facial expression, and suprasegmental features) continue to be used in the same form during the postbabbling or real word production phase. Turn-taking in communicative interaction also continues. In addition, there are new developments. Needs and feelings are now specified by references to the particular objects and actions wanted or rejected or liked, because recognizable words and phrases are now being used. Conversational turn-taking is no longer simply participation in an exchange by any vocal response, it involves response appropriate to the nonlinguistic context and the content of the utterance heard. In summary, the general purpose of communication and some of the means by which communicative intent is conveyed remain unaltered from the purpose and means established during the very early months of life. It is the content of utterances produced and under-

stood that changes. Infants' ability to understand and produce words and phrases in the language of the community is the basis of the change. These developments are traced below.

SPEECH SOUND DISCRIMINATION

The ability to produce speechlike sounds is a function of the particular vocal mechanism of the human. It has been concluded that efforts to teach chimpanzees to speak were doomed to failure, not simply because of possible intellectual limitations, but because their vocal mechanisms do not permit the production of speech (Lieberman, 1974). Some studies of infant speech sound discrimination have raised the question of whether the infant has a species-specific sensitivity to certain sound differences. These sound differences are those that make up the features of speech sounds.

In a pioneering study using synthetic speech (speech generated by a computer), 1- and 4-month-old infants discriminated between speech sounds in an adultlike manner (Eimas et al., 1971). The stimuli used were speech sounds that ranged, in a continuum of gradual change, from a minus voice stop and vowel (/pa/) to a plus voice stop and vowel (/ba/). The distinction between /pa/ and /ba/ in terms of sound is the **voicing onset time** (**VOT**) of the vowel that follows the burst of the stop consonant. The stop burst and transition to the vowel is immediate for /b/ (the + voice sound) and delayed for /p/ (the - voice sound). Adults given stimuli that range across a set of VOTs categorize stimuli at one end of the range as /pa/ and at the other end as /ba/, but do not notice sound differences of stimuli that vary in VOT within each end (as in the categorical perceptions discussed in Chapter 7). In like fashion, infants conditioned to suck when presented with a stimulus in one end of the range and habituated to the sound dishabituate only to a stimulus from the other range, not to an acoustically different stimulus from the same range. Figure 11.2a shows two typical stimuli that are not differentiated by infants or adults and 11.2b shows two stimuli that are differentiated by both. Since this behavior is observed in infants at an age when little learning of the phonological or speech sound categories of any language can have occurred, it has been suggested that the human infant is biologically programmed to discriminate among speech sounds, that is, that infants come biologically "prewired" with speech sound feature detectors.

Speech sounds vary from each other on a number of acoustic dimensions. These dimensions have been called **distinctive features** (Jakobson et al., 1963). For example, some sounds are consonants and others

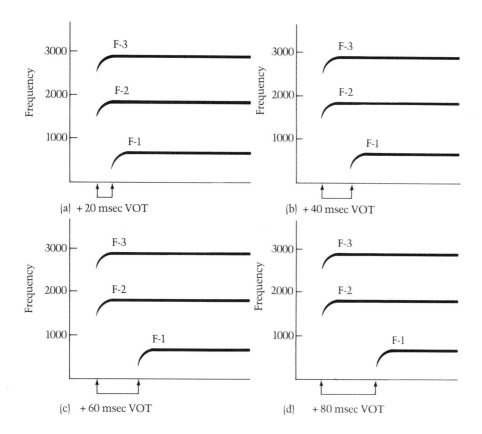

Figure 11.2. A visual representation of auditory speech stimuli. The vertical axis represents frequency of sound waves (pitch) and the horizontal axis represents time. As a consonant is uttered, sound is produced in a series of waves, called *formants*, represented here by thick black lines. The relative time of onset of the first two formants (F-1 and F-2) distinguishes between the /b/ and /p/ sounds and is called voice onset time (VOT). (a) If the formants start fewer than 25 msec after the burst (the VOT in the figure is 40 msec), an unvoiced consonant, /p/, is heard. (c) and (d) Discrimination of speech sounds is categorical, because all differences in VOT within a speech sound category are heard as the same speech sound. Thus the stimuli in parts c and d are both perceived as /p/. Their VOTs (60 msec and 80 msec, respectively) are both greater than 25 msec, the cutoff between /b/ and /p/. Notice that the difference between the VOTs in parts c and d (60 and 80) is physically the same as the difference between the VOTs in parts a and b (20 and 40). Thus, although the physical difference between the two stimuli in c and d is exactly the same as that between a and b, humans (adults and babies) can hear a difference between a and b but not between c and d.

vowels. Some consonants are nasal (e.g., m and n) and others oral (e.g., b and g); some are continuants (e.g., s and sh) and others are stops (e.g., p, t, and k). These features are determined by particular articulatory movements that produce different acoustic consequences. Some sounds vary from each other in terms of one feature (/p/ is a minus voice sound and /b/ a plus voice sound; /b/ is nonnasal and /m/ is nasal) or in terms of several features (/t/ is minus voice, noncontinuant, and coronal—made with tongue tip touching roof of mouth; /r/ is voiced, continuant, noncoronal). Thus some sounds differ from each other more markedly than others; in addition, some features are presumably more perceptually salient than others because they are more easily detected by the human auditory system. For example, the presence or absence of nasality is an easily detectable feature. Some types of feature distinctions are found in all languages and some in only a subset of languages. For example, there is a subset of languages in which the voicing distinctions are like those found in English and a subset in which these distinctions are like those found in Spanish. The distinctions are somewhat different in the two named languages.

Since the time of the initial study of infant speech discrimination, there have been many studies that have examined a variety of speech and nonspeech sound contrasts and have used different response measures to test discrimination. Eimas et al. (1971) used the non-nutritive sucking response. Cardiac rate change and conditioned head turning have also been used. Studies comparing infants' abilities to discriminate between speech and nonspeech stimuli indicate that infants differentiate categorically between nonspeech sounds if they have certain acoustic characteristics such as frequency, rate of change, complexity, and others that are similar to speech (Aslin et al., 1983). Thus early speech sound discrimination is based on *acoustic*, not particular speech, features. Studies examining speech sound discriminations have found that other animals behave the way human infants do with speech stimuli: Across-category is better than within-category discrimination (Kuhl, 1986). Thus categorical speech sound discrimination is not species specific, and it seems highly unlikely that infants' auditory systems are equipped with special speech detectors.

It was once thought that any speech sound feature contrast that could be found in any human language would be discriminable by infants until words were acquired. This would support the notion that innate abilities, not learning, are involved in infant speech sound discrimination. However, this does not appear to be the case. At 6 months, American and Swedish babies learn to discriminate vowels that are in their own languages more rapidly than those that are not (Kuhl, 1990). Between 6 and 12 months infants appear to become more and more sensitive to the speech sound contrasts of their native language and less sensitive to those in other languages (Werker & Lalonde, 1988). They may be sensitive to distinctions among native and nonnative vowels first and then to distinctions among consonants. Thus learning takes over at an early age. Nevertheless, infants have the ability to discriminate among speech sounds categorically, which is a good beginning for getting from the acoustic signal to meaning (inasmuch as words are composed of speech sounds). In the earliest months of life they also have the ability to discriminate among all possible speech sound contrasts in all languages. Both of these facts indicate that human infants *are* biologically programmed to process the speech signal in special ways,

an ability they may share with other animals. It has been suggested that this biological programming can be thought of as special processing of speech by the infant because of the inherent salience of such sounds for the human infant. The latter has been referred to as an innately guided learning process (Jusczyk & Bertoncini, 1988). (Further discussions of speech sound discrimination in infants can be found in Aslin et al., 1983; Perkell & Klatt, 1986.)

SPEECH SOUND PRODUCTION

The relation between early speech sound discrimination and babbling is unclear. Linguists once thought that infants babbled all possible human sounds randomly throughout the babbling period. Research has now revealed that babies begin to babble some speech sounds earlier than others, and there is evidence that the same developmental sequence in production of sounds is found in children of differing language communities (Menyuk, 1972).

The actual content of babbled utterances is difficult to determine. In addition to listening and coding these utterances into phonetic symbols (such as /pa/ and /ba/), researchers have carried out spectrographic analyses of samples of utterances. Spectrograms provide a graph of vocalizations that can then be analyzed in terms of whether or not particular features of sound formation are present. Examples of the kinds of information spectrograms can provide are shown in Figure 11.2, which illustrates the between-category characteristics of two speech sounds (plus voice /ba/ and minus voice /pa/).

There is a great deal of argument about the validity of both human and spectrographic analysis of speech sounds. Spectrograms can provide more objective information about the speech sound content of an utterance than can the ear of a human coder, because human coders tend to perceive their own native speech sound categories regardless of the actual content of the vocalizations. However, it is sometimes difficult to see characteristics of speech sounds in the spectrograms of infant vocalizations. Researchers often use both techniques and see how each relates to the other, and computer-assisted analysis of speech signals has recently been used to help obtain meaningful measures from spectrograms and speech signals.

The pioneering work of Irwin (1947) using phonetic coding of infant utterances indicated that the infant did not produce all possible sounds in the language with the same relative frequency throughout the babbling period. The proportional representation of different sounds changed over the babbling period, so that toward the end of it, the frequency of occurrence of the different sounds produced accurately reflected their actual frequency of occurrence in the native language. These developmental changes in the sounds produced may be a product of the infant's achieving increasingly greater control of the articulators (Menyuk, 1972). The changes seem to reflect differences in ease of articulation of various sounds, with those that are easiest to articulate being produced with much greater frequency at the beginning of the babbling period, more difficult sounds occurring with increased frequency toward the middle, and the most difficult toward the end. Even at the end not all sounds of the language occur in babblings, and those missing require very subtle adjustments of the articulators. At the end of the babbling period the repertoire of sounds produced seems to reflect the speech sound characteristics of a particular language (Boysson-Bardies et al., 1984; Locke, 1986). This evidence, along with research that indicates that infants of approximately the same age (10 months) are no longer sensitive to speech sound contrasts outside their own language, indicates that the baby is probably now listening for specific linguistic information and not just to an acoustic signal. If so, a shift occurs in what the infant attends to some time during the second half of the first year. This shift may occur because the infant begins to understand that the sounds produced by others are related to real-world objects and events and are not just expressions of affect, needs, and feelings. (For additional discussions of developmental changes in vocalizations and speech sound production, see Kent & Hodge, 1990; Stark, 1986.)

Infant vocalizations in American-English-speaking environments have been studied in sizable samples and have included both spectrographic analysis and phonetic coding. In one such study, Oller (1980) lists the following changes and the approximate ages at which they occur:

(1) *phonation* (0-1 month): nonsyllabic and primarily vocalic

(2) *cooing* (2-3 months): nonsyllabic, partially repetitive, vowel and velar (made in the back of the mouth) consonant productions (such as /h/ or gargles)

(3) *expansion* (4-6 months): a variety of vocalizations, including vowellike elements; raspberries, squealing, growling, yelling, ingressive-egressive sequences, and marginal babbling ("shaky or slow transitions between vowel and consonant")

(4) *canonical babbling* (7-10 months): syllabification and reduplication of the same consonant and

vowel (CV) such as (/ba/ /ba/ /ba/)

(5) *variegated babbling* (11-12 months): variation in CV (/babi/, /bada/)

It has been hypothesized that because the sequence of speech sound production appears to reflect increasing control of the vocal mechanism, and because the general sequence of motor development is universal over this period, there should be similarities in the patterns of sounds babbled by children acquiring different languages. Such cross-linguistic similarity was found in a study that used spectrographic analysis to compare vocalizations of infants in Japanese- and American-English-speaking environments (Nakazima, 1962). Until data have been collected from many language environments, no conclusions can be reached about universality in the sequence of babbling.

The questions that remain are as follows: Does acquisition of a particular language affect the sequence of sounds babbled at about the same age as cross-linguistic differences in speech sound perception begin to be observed (6 months), or are the sequences universal? Or is speech discrimination nonuniversal and speech production universal? If the latter is the case, then it might be concluded that the discrimination and production of speech sounds are not intimately related during this period of development. However, such conclusions must await more data collected in a variety of linguistic settings.

PERCEPTION AND PRODUCTION OF LANGUAGE

The infant's tasks in acquiring the grammar or rules of a language are to determine the meaningful units in language (vocabulary or lexicon) and the meaning of the relations of these units when they are combined (grammar). The most important step in getting from speech perception and production to language perception and production is to relate words to categories and word combinations to relations among categories. For example, the child must relate the word *cookie* to the object cookie and the combination "give cookie" to someone giving a cookie to someone else.

A first and crucial step is to decide how the speech signal should be segmented into these meaningful units and how they should be grouped together in utterances. Infants' preferential listening behavior indicates that they are sensitive to cues that correspond to clausal units at approximately 4 to 6 months of age, to those cues that correspond to phrase units at approximately 9 months, and to those that correspond to word units at 11 months (Hirsh-Pasek, 1989; Hirsh-

Pasek & Golinkoff, in press). The cues that mark boundaries in a language are prosodic cues: intonation patterns, stress, and pause. As noted above, infants are able to process such speech information very early in life. The sequence of segmentation of clause first and then word makes sense given the research results discussed in previous sections. The first units that infants appear to attend to and reproduce are the communicative messages, and these are contained within the clause. Attention to word length units is necessary for the transition from communicative behavior to language behavior. Some infants approach the task primarily word by word, while others do so primarily phrase by phrase. The infant may be getting ready to make the transition from speech to language at about 6 months. The first unit of segmentation, the clause, conveys the intent of the utterance. Then parts of the message (perhaps the actor, action, and object) are segmented by the phrase boundaries. Finally, the words are segmented. However, one should be very cautious in interpreting the findings in this way. There is little evidence to suggest that the infant is treating the signal in any way other than as a communicative message until lexical items are comprehended and then produced.

At about 8 months, the infant has been observed to recognize a small repertoire of words as indicated by head turning toward or reaching for a named object or person (Murai, 1960). Toward the end of the babbling phase, utterances begin to take on the shape of words. Long babbled utterances are reduced to one syllable or reduplicated syllable length. These syllables sound like words because they contain well-formed consonant-vowel sequences. This change occurs at about 1 year. Infants at 13 months of age give evidence of associating a small set of objects with their names (Thomas et al., 1981). Thus some months before the infant produces wordlike approximations, he or she recognizes a few words. There have been few studies of infants' comprehension of words during the latter months of the first year of life, so the types of words usually recognized are unknown. Menyuk et al. (1991), in a study of 53 infants about whom mothers kept diary data, found that the average ages at which given numbers of words were recognized were 12 months for 10 words, 14 months for 50 words, and 16 months for 100 words. At about 12 months recognizable words begin to be produced and are used appropriately to express needs and feelings about particular objects and actions. It is logical to conclude that a baby has begun the task of relating speech sound sequences, heard and understood, to objects and events perceived before 12 months. After the production of words and their refer-

ential use has begun comes the next phase of language development: understanding of how words are combined to express relations between objects and actions and attributes of objects and actions.

Language Behavior

When lexical items are acquired and when basic semantax (word combination) relations are understood and produced, the infant is said to be in the linguistic phase of language development. Developments in the linguistic phase are discussed in this section. Development of indication and referencing by the use of words is discussed first, followed by development of comprehension and production of semantactic relations.

ACQUISITION OF WORD MEANING

As the diary data cited above indicate, the number of words comprehended doubles in a 2-month period, from 50 words at 14 months to 100 words at 16 months. There is also a sudden spurt in word production that occurs in many, but not all, infants when 50 words are acquired (Goldfield & Reznick, 1990). On average, this happens at about 18 months. Individual differences in language development begin to become very evident when first words appear. Those infants who exhibit this rapid spurt primarily acquire nouns. Infants who acquire words more slowly show a balance of word classes in their vocabularies. Further, Bloom and Capatides (1987) found that the more frequently children express positive and negative affect, the later their first words appear, and the later the vocabulary spurt occurs. These researchers conclude that more neutral affect supports early transfer to language by *allowing* a reflective stance.

In addition to differences in the timing and pattern of lexical development, there are individual differences in the proportion of types of forms used at the beginning of this period. Some children appear to go about the task of acquiring a lexicon primarily by using one word at a time, while others tend to produce jargon phrases (Peters, 1983). All children use some mixture of both. Differences in lexicon acquisition appear to be related to differences in the primary purposes for which children use language and in the syntactic classes they use to express relations (Bates et al., 1987). Some children are "expressers" (that is, they use language primarily to express needs and feelings), while others are primarily "referrers." The former children label most frequently by using pronouns, the latter by using nouns (Nelson, 1980).

Mama	Sheep	Picture
Dada	Cup	Book
Baby	Bee	See
Car	Tea	Wa-wa (as in water)
Tree	Shoes	Bye-bye
Bow-wow	Button	Pig
Cow	Tick-tock	Hi
Turkey	Light (pronounced yight)	Hello
Chicken	Cheese	Up
Duck	Choo-choo (as in train)	Cracker

Figure 11.3. The first 30 words spoken by one child. The child was 14 months old when the thirtieth word was added to the vocabulary. At that time the addition of new words became so rapid that keeping track was no longer feasible for the parents. The animals probably represent exposure to picture books as well as to a small-town environment. In addition to using "bye-bye" to indicate a desire to go out, this infant would also bring galoshes to indicate that she wanted to go out.

Several aspects of early acquisition of word meaning have been studied. The first words produced appear to be limited to either labels or expression of needs and feelings about particular objects and actions. For example, action words that can carry out functions, such as *want, give, no, like, up,* and *see* are acquired early. Nelson (1973) found that the first 50 words produced by a group of 18 children could be categorized as specific nominals (mama, papa), general nominals (toy, doggie), actions (go, up), attributes (more, all gone), and social or affective words (okay, please). The specific nominals were most frequently produced by referrers, and the social affective words were most frequently produced by expressers. Figure 11.3 lists the first 30 words of one child. This list is quite typical of infants in middle-class families in U.S. culture.

The meanings of nominals appear to change over time. A number of researchers have found that the first 10 words are usually applied to specific items. For example, "cup" means only "the cup I drink out of." Shortly thereafter, word usage or production is overgeneralized. This indicates that some of the semantic features of word meaning have been acquired and that words are being used to denote classes, not just specific items. It was initially hypothesized that one word was applied to several objects that shared certain perceptual features, because infants only encoded a small set of features for the words they produced (Clark, 1973). "Doggie," therefore, was applied to all objects that shared the features *animal + four legged* (which could apply to dogs, cows, horses, cats, and so on). As additional features were added to the meanings of words (for example, the feature of size), new words

were acquired to mark this differentiation (horse and cow as distinct from dog). This early behavior did not mean that infants perceived dogs, horses, cows, and cats as having the same observable features, or that they had difficulty in comprehending the meanings of the words *dog, horse,* and *cow*. It merely meant that early on only the most salient or general perceptual features were associated with the meanings of words produced. Infants added to their productive lexicons when they added features to the meanings of the words they produced.

The hypothesis that new words are acquired by adding features to the meanings of words has now been rejected in favor of what has been called the principle of contrast (Clark, 1987) or the principle of mutual exclusivity (Markman, 1987). Thus new words are acquired as the child observes that different objects should be referred to by different names. Some researchers suggest that as infants acquire lexicons, they first use the principle that an object can have only one label, and that as they begin to expand their lexicons, they use the principle that different objects have different labels. When overextensions occur at a later time ("doggie" for "kitty"), they are not the result of the baby's lack of knowledge of the meanings for the words used. Rather, they occur because the baby does not have a word available to mark an observed difference. The baby must learn what a word unit represents, and, therefore, must use some principle or set of principles to do this, otherwise the task would be impossible (Golinkoff & Hirsh-Pasek, 1990).

As more data are collected on both the perception and production of words, these principles and the sequence of development of word meaning become clearer. Some additional data indicate that at the earliest period of development there may be some overlapping of perceptual and functional features in the comprehension of the meaning of lexical items. Behrend (1988) carried out a study with infants aged 11 to 13 months. In the first of two experiments, the paradigm used by Thomas et al. (1981) was employed, and the findings were similar. Objects that mothers said their children knew or did not know the names for and real and nonsense words were used. Infants looked significantly longer at objects with known names versus those with unknown names, including both real and nonsense names. In the second experiment, it was found that when items were paired (for example, truck and car, ball and orange, dog and cat), infants extended their looking time significantly when looking at perceptually similar items but not when looking at distractor items. Thus at the earliest stages there are overextensions in the comprehension of words. Somewhat later, perceptual extensions do not occur. Labels are then applied to specific items for a short time following the principle of contrast, and then productive extensions occur. This happens, as stated previously, because the infant is stretching available vocabulary (Clark, 1983).

In summary, the sequence of development of lexical items appears to be as follows:

(1) overextension in comprehension of the scope of application of a lexical item

(2) application of the principle that different objects should have different labels, and, therefore, no overextension in the comprehension of the meaning of lexical items or in the production of lexical items

(3) initially and briefly, labels produced for specific items only

(4) overextensions in use because of limited vocabulary

(5) end of occurrence of productive overextensions

It is important to note that overextensions of labels occur only within the same syntactic class (nouns are substituted only for other nouns, not prepositions) and for members of the same class of objects (animal labels are overextended only to other animals, not to inanimate objects). Infants, however, constantly exercise the principle that different objects should have different labels. They are helped in this by the fact that the environment provides different labels for different objects (Baldwin & Markman, 1989).

The above description does not address the issue of how the infant goes about the task of determining that phonological sequences (words) are related to their categorizations of the objects and events the infant has perceived. There have been several scenarios written to account for that development. All of them include the notion that object permanence (see Chapter 10) must play some role in this accomplishment. That is, objects must remain in mind and be separated from other objects if labels for them are to be acquired. From that point, explanations for sequences of development diverge. For a long time it was held that there is a constant sequence of, first, development of cognitive and then linguistic categorization. Later there was a shift to the position that cognitive and linguistic categorization occur simultaneously or nearly simultaneously (Gopnik & Meltzoff, 1986). At present, some hold, with Vygotsky (1962), that linguistic labels shape cognitive categorizations (Bowerman, 1988). These positions will be discussed at greater length in the section below on cognitive factors that affect language development. Also, imitation or shared attention, which are discussed below as well, may play some role in word learning.

COMBINING SOUNDS INTO WORDS

Comprehension of words (or utterances) requires relating speech sound sequences to objects and events in the environment. Production requires retrieving from memory and articulating a speech sound sequence that relates to these objects and events. As stated previously, this behavior requires segmentation of the stream of speech and categorization of segments into utterances, words, and speech sounds. The data available on speech sound production in words and utterances indicate that, just as in babbling, there are developmental changes in the speech sound sequences produced over the period of early word acquisition. In contrast to babbling, which produces nonsense syllables, the target for production during this period is the word or phrase that has meaning (Menyuk, 1990). The sequence of development during this period reflects how individual infants map what they hear into meaningful units. The development of these mapping rules has been the focus of much research (e.g., Ferguson, 1986; Ingram, 1990).

Given the speech sound sequences produced during this phase, it has been hypothesized that words are initially produced as unsegmented wholes and not as a sequence of speech sound segments. Later behavior indicates that infants attempt to match syllables, rather than single sounds or distinctive features of sounds (Menyuk et al., 1986). The infant's vocabulary is still small during the second year of life, hence it is not unreasonable to think that words are initially stored in memory as whole syllables and not simply retrieved as syllables for production. Once the vocabulary of the child grows into thousands of words, these words *may* be stored in terms of patterns of sequences of sound, rather than as wholly different and unique sound sequences. Evidence for this can be found in the older child's ability to segment a word into separate sounds and relate sounds to symbols in reading.

Some of the early mapping rules appear to be universal (Ingram, 1990). These types of rules suggest that most infants attempt to preserve those distinctions in word production that they hypothesize will allow others to understand what they are saying. Sometimes they accomplish this goal, and at other times they do not. Some early strategies are (a) syllable repetition (*mommy* produced as "mama"), (b) weak syllable reduction (*umbrella* produced as "bella" or "brella"), (c) cluster reduction (*stop* produced as "top"), (d) metathesis (*top* produced as "pop" or "tot"), and (e) stopping of continuants (*this* and *that* produced as "dis" and "dat").

In addition to these universal strategies, there are particular language strategies that have to be developed because of differences among dialects and languages in the speech sound distinctions that have to be made. Also, individual infants develop unique mapping rules. For example, some children avoid some sounds and prefer others (Menn, 1981). These word production behaviors indicate that they are perceiving parts of words, but the perceptual basis for their behavior is unclear.

The task for infants is to map what they perceive into distinguishable meaningful lexical items. Three models have been proposed to explain this mapping process (Menyuk, 1990). One model suggests that speech production is only a subset of what the child perceives and that the child perceives distinctions the way an adult does (Smith, 1973). For example, the child might perceive the differences between the words *tie* and *die* in the way an adult does, but have difficulty in producing the two as distinct words, because the motor movements required are beyond the capabilities of the infant. For example, some infants will protest when they have said "die" when in fact they meant tie if an adult asks, "die?" Because of difficulties in obtaining evidence, there is little to suggest that infants perceive distinctions among speech sounds in words exactly the way adults do.

A second model suggests that all that is perceived is mapped into speech sound productions, but that the perception of the child is distorted in some way. The distinction between *tie* and *die* might be made by the child, but the parameters used for the distinction would be different from those used by the adult. There is some evidence that children may distinguish among speech sounds on the basis of acoustic cues that are different from those used by older children and adults (Nittrouer et al., 1989). There is little evidence that children's unique productions are always based on these hypothesized unique perceptions.

A third model suggests that infants' speech production and perception are governed by the limits of their information-processing abilities (Ferguson, 1986). Perceiving the distinction between *tie* and *die* might not create difficulties for the processing abilities of the infant, but translating what is perceived into motor movements might do so because of the timing controls on the vocal mechanism that are required. Other distinctions might be both difficult to perceive and to produce, but for different reasons. For example, the distinction between *gas* and *grass* might be difficult for infants to perceive because of the amount of information that needs to be processed to make that distinction. The contrast between the words might be difficult to produce because of the rapid motor movements that are required in consonant clusters such as /gr/. If this is the case, perception and production of lexical items need not be related. This model does not account for the fact that infants must rely on their speech perception to produce lexical items that are either recognizable or consistent enough to be recognized by others.

In addition to the problems mentioned above, none of the models discussed addresses the issue of what may occur in speech sound perception when processing meaningful words and phrases in context. In summary, there is some evidence that speech sound sequences are analyzed in terms of prosodic characteristics into phrases and, possibly, words or syllables. At the earliest stage of development of the lexicon there is no evidence that differences between lexical items are perceived in terms of segmental differences (the difference between /t/ and /d/) or in terms of distinctive feature differences (+/- voicing) among segments, but rather as differences between whole syllables. However, there are some data that indicate that when final segment cues are filtered out, infants have difficulty in perceiving word boundaries (Hirsh-Pasek & Golinkoff, in press). At some point such distinctions must be made, but much of the evidence for them is based on speech production, not perception. Both the universal lexical production rules that many children use and the idiosyncratic phonological rules that individual children employ in the mapping process indicate that they are using information about the segments in words. This is a logical extrapolation from the production data. Although a wealth of information exists on the speech discrimination abilities of babies during the first year of life, few data are available on the development of speech perception in the lexical acquisition period.

COMBINING WORDS INTO UTTERANCES

To acquire words, the infant must relate a speech sound sequence to categorizations of objects and actions. To acquire a grammar, the child must relate word combinations to relations of objects and actions. The functions of language at this stage of development are to express needs, feelings, and ideas. The form in which these purposes are carried out describe relations among objects and actions ("give cookie") and attributes of both objects ("red" or "funny hat") and actions ("fall there" or "put on table"). To develop language, the infant must acquire knowledge of the structural properties of language needed to convey the functions and forms of language.

It is because language is composed of several nested structures that the infant must learn to segment a stream of speech into several categories. These categories can then be filled or combined in different ways to convey different meanings. A basic unit is the sentence, and it is composed of phrases. The sentence "The cat chased the dog" is composed of two phrases: the subject phrase ("the cat") and the predicate phrase ("chased the dog"). A different subject and predicate would convey a different meaning, as in the sentence "The cat saw the bird." Each sentence and phrase is composed of **morphemes**, the grammatical and meaningful segments of words. The sentence "The cat chased the dog" consists of six (not five) such segments—the five words and the past-tense segment "ed" of chase. The "ed" conveys the time at which the action took place. Parts of words, as well as whole words, can also be replaced, as in "The cat chases the dog" or "The cats chased the dogs." The meaning changes each time. Relations can be negated, as in "The cat didn't chase the dog," or questioned, as in "Did the cat chase the dog?" or action commanded, as in "Chase that dog." Morphemes themselves are composed of speech sounds. Changing a single segment in a morpheme can change its meaning, as in *boy* versus *toy*, *pop* versus *pot*, and *big* versus *bag*.

During the language acquisition process, children learn the variety of ways in which their language allows morphemes, phrases, and sentences to be formed. This is termed *acquisition of knowledge of the grammar of the language*. There are **morphophonological rules** that govern how sounds are put together to create morphemes and **semantactic rules** that govern how words are put together to create sentences. As children mature, their knowledge of the rules not only grows, but changes. For example, at one period the child may have no rule for making plurals and may say "foot" for one or more feet. Later, plural is marked by generalizing a rule, and more than one foot is "foots." Still later the generalization changes and the word may be expressed as "feets" and finally as "feet." Similar changes occur in forming sentence types. To express negation initially the child says "no," then "no bed" and "no go." Later the negative morpheme is inserted in a sentence ("He no can go") and finally the rules for producing negative sentences in English are applied ("He can't go"). The changes are from no rule to express a relational meaning, to some rule or rules, to finally the appropriate rule (Menyuk, 1988).

What Is Comprehended in Word Combinations

There is some real evidence that children understand two-part relations while they themselves produce only holophrases (single words that convey a relation) and jargon phrases. Sachs and Truswell (1978) studied the ability of holophrastic children to carry out actions on objects that describe a relation (for example, "Kiss Teddy"). It was found that a significant proportion of the children's responses were related to the utterances (70%) and that 75% of the related responses were correct. The older children in the group (20 months to 2 years) responded more frequently and more correctly than the younger. Children appear to comprehend two-part relations while producing only single words themselves.

Additional support for the claim that linguistic relational knowledge is available to the holophrastic child is provided by two studies. Horgan (1976) found that during this period children could successfully identify pictures that describe a three-part relation of subject, object, and action. Holophrastic infants tested using the preferential looking paradigm shown two different actor-action-object relations (e.g., Big Bird kissing Cookie Monster on one screen and Cookie Monster kissing Big Bird on the other) watched the screen that matched the utterance they were listening to significantly longer than the screen that did not (Hirsh-Pasek et al., 1985). A replication, using children who said practically nothing, found that phrases containing two-part relations could be understood (Hirsh-Pasek & Golinkoff, in press). Thus preferential looking provided evidence of comprehension of two-part relations at an earlier age than did asking infants to move objects (as in

Sachs & Truswell, 1978). The evidence indicates that two-part relations are understood even when no or few words are produced, and three-part relations are understood as infants produce holophrases.

All of these findings indicate that knowledge of semantactic relations (how words are put together to describe relations among objects, actions, and their attributes) is acquired very early in the lexical acquisition period. Babies in this phase apparently cannot produce combinations of words, although they can produce long babbled utterances. They initially produce one word marked with an intonational contour or an unsegmented phrase. Later they produce two single words with large pauses between them (Branigan, 1976). Nevertheless, babies indicate comprehension of two-part and three-part relations long before they express two-part relations.

Studies by Hirsh-Pasek and Golinkoff (in press), Hirsh-Pasek et al. (1985), Horgan (1976), and Sachs and Truswell (1978) provide some evidence that children not only acquire knowledge of semantic relations, but also have some basic semantactic knowledge during the holophrastic and transitional stages. That is, they have knowledge of such fundamental word-order rules in the English language as action precedes the object (Kiss Teddy), subject precedes the action (Teddy kiss), the attribute precedes the noun (Dirty baby), and the actor or subject precedes action, which precedes object (Daddy kiss Teddy). Unless these ordering rules were understood by the infants studied, incorrect responses would have occurred; for instance, they would have looked at Teddy kissing Daddy in response to "Daddy kiss Teddy."

What Is Produced in Utterances

During the early stages of the word combination period, the child produces utterances that have been labeled *holophrastic*. As stated, this implies that the single words produced by the child ("mommy," "shoe," "sit") convey more than merely the name of an object or action. As we have seen, infants convey different intentions by the use of different intonational contours with the same word. Thus they can request, demand, or state the presence of an object or event using a single word with different intonational contours. During this same period they produce jargon phrases as well. Some of these phrases may contain more than one unit. In addition, infants presumably convey relations between attributes, objects, and events by use of situational context, gesture, and facial expression.

Greenfield and Smith (1976) carried out a detailed study of the utterances of two children over a period of several months. During this time the children produced primarily one-word utterances. The technique used to code these utterances was to have two adults (the mother and an observer) indicate the communicative intent of the utterance, that is, the relation intended. When there was agreement, an utterance was coded as expressing a particular relation. On the basis of such clear cases, the investigators concluded that after a short initial period in which words are used in imitative routines, naming games, and calls to others (called *vocatives*, e.g., "Mama"), all holophrastic utterances express a two-part relation. Although only one part of the relation is, in fact, expressed, the second part is intended. For example, when the infant says "dirty" and points to an object, his or her intention is to state that the object is dirty.

The relations expressed change in time, and Greenfield and Smith (1976) suggest that these changes come about because of cognitive maturation. The cognitive maturation cited to account for the change is the process of decentering, or taking the perspective of another. This, the authors state, is reflected in the child's expressing the relation action of object before state of object and talking about self as actor before others as actors. Greenfield and Smith's findings have suggested to some that, in addition to expressing needs and feelings with single words by the use of intonation and gesture, young children can convey semantic relations with single words. However, a great deal of rich interpretation is needed to come to that conclusion, and some have argued against it for that reason and because of Greenfield and Smith's small sample size.

Data obtained with older children may shed some light on the issue. By 2 years of age many children produce two-word utterances that describe a range of semantic relations, and some produce utterances with three or more words in which the basic structure of English sentences (actor + action + object) is expressed. A few children at this age produce what are called *embedded* sentences, such as "I want to go." This sentence contains two relations: I want and I go. Over the age of 2 to 3 years a number of children further develop such complex sentences by using such epistemic verbs as *think* and *know* (Bloom et al., 1989). In addition, the basic sentence types of declaration, negation, question, and imperative are produced with two words and lengthier utterances. Nevertheless, there are still many structural gaps in the utterances produced. Table 11.1 gives examples of the relations and sentence types produced at the two- and three-word sentence stages. The list shows that three-word utterances represent combinations of relations produced during the two-word phase. This indicates that development from two- to three-word sentence production may be a function of the ability to say more in one utterance, rather than acquisition of new knowledge about semantax. In like fashion, one might argue that although the child is only producing holophrases and jargon phrases during the period studied by Greenfield and Smith, development from one- to two-word sentences may also simply be a function of the ability to say more in one utterance rather than acquisition of new knowledge about semantax.

Even when two-word utterances are produced, rich interpretation is often needed to understand them. Figure 11.4 demonstrates the variety of different relations a single two-word utterance can express. It shows that adults and older children often have to use the context of the utterance to guess which of these relations the toddler wishes to express.

In summary, there is a body of data available on the language structures (semantic, syntactic, and phonological) produced by the child in the second year of life. There are still comparatively few data on what the child perceives. It has been assumed that perceptual development precedes productive development. The productive data indicate that 2-year-olds have at least acquired knowledge of how to express basic semantic relations in the correct syntactic (word order) form of a particular language. Word meanings and phonological realizations are in the beginning stages of acquisition. How far perceptual knowledge exceeds productive knowledge at age 2 is still unclear, but there is some indication that perceptual abilities exceed the abilities displayed in production. Given the data on comprehension of relations in sentences, the distance between the

two types of knowledge seems remarkable. Children give evidence of understanding actor-action-object relations while they are still producing single words or jargon phrases.

Factors That Affect Language Development

Various theoreticians have taken dramatically opposing views about the effects of environmental factors on language behaviors observed during infancy and later. In one view, the development of language during infancy is primarily a function of the types of inputs the infant receives from caregivers. The opposite view is that these language developments are primarily a function of the biological structure of the human infant. Similarly, some theorists suggest that language development is almost totally a product of cognitive development, while others suggest that language development is special and is not dependent on cognitive development. All of these positions highlight important factors in the process of language development, but no one of them explains all of language acquisition. What seems to be the case is that there are obvious biological factors that affect the course of development over this period, and there are environmental factors that affect it as well. There are general cognitive factors that appear to affect both language and other development (for example, both early speech and visual perception), and there are aspects of some areas of development that seem to require special types of processing that are not shared with other areas of development. The research concerning biological and environmental factors that might affect development during infancy is discussed

Table 11.1
Early Relations and Sentence Types Produced in Two- and Three-Word Utterances

Two Words		Three Words	
Agent + action	Baby run.	Agent + action + present participle	Baby running.
Action + object	Push truck.	Agent + action + object	Mommy push truck.[a]
Agent + object	Daddy truck.		Daddy drive truck.[a]
Possessor + possessed	Daddy hat.	Demonstrative + possessor + possessed	That daddy hat.
Demonstrative + noun	That fish.		
Attributive + noun	Dirty baby.	Location + attributive + object	Here dirty baby.
Location + object	Here ball.	Location + copula + object	Here be ball.
Action + location	Put chair	Action + object + location	Put sweater chair.[a]
Negation	No/not wash.	Negation	Me no wash.
	No/not fish.		That no fish.
Question	Where daddy?	Question	Where daddy go?

a. These utterances are either comments on actions observed or commands.

first below, followed by discussion of research concerning the relation between cognition and language.

BIOLOGICAL FACTORS

The biological factors that have been cited as affecting the course of language development in infancy include the special nature of the central nervous system and of the auditory and vocal mechanisms of the human infant (Menyuk, 1988). Structural and functional differences in the two hemispheres of the brain have indicated that the association area of the cortex in the left hemisphere of the neonate is larger than in the right. Initially it was found that when speech and nonspeech sounds are presented to an infant there is greater electrical activity in response to speech in the left hemisphere and to nonspeech in the right (Molfese, 1973). Later findings indicated that there is specialization of function in the two hemispheres for particular aspects of auditory discrimination, which is the basis for speech functioning (Molfese & Molfese, 1985). These findings have led to the conclusion that the human infant is biologically preprogrammed to acquire language because specific areas of the hemispheres are involved in discrimination of specific parameters of speech sound discrimination, and this specialization of function appears to be present at birth.

Additional evidence cited for biological preprogramming is the structure and functioning of the vocal mechanism. The human vocal tract is different from that of other animals even at birth. The structure of the pharynx, the location of the vocal cords in the pharynx, and the size and shape of the mouth, tongue, and lips and their relation to each other allow for the production of articulated sounds. No other animal's vocal mechanism has the same characteristics, and this is one of the reasons that all attempts to teach great apes to talk have been doomed to failure. The course of maturation of the vocal tract is said to account for the sequence and organization of vocal behavior during babbling; these vocal behaviors may be universal.

The structure of the auditory mechanism of the human infant is not different from that of other animals. Nevertheless, the data obtained from studies of infant speech sound discrimination have led some researchers to conclude that the infant is both biologically preprogrammed to be sensitive to certain acoustic feature differences and to process the acoustic information in speech in special ways. The acoustic features that infants can discriminate among are the same as those required to discriminate among speech sounds in any language, and, as discussed, these features may

be particularly salient for the human infant. Like babbling, then, the sequence of development of speech sound discrimination should be universal. Despite the fact that some studies show very early effects of a particular linguistic environment on these discriminations, the possibility that speech and that particular universal aspects of speech are very salient to the infant (which allow rapid development of speech perception) is not excluded.

A special argument has been made that the infant's use of gesture to indicate or demand an object might be the innate biological ability that distinguishes humans from other animals. Gesturing is an indication that the human infant can refer, and, therefore, is not only a prerequisite of language acquisition but also distinguishes the human infant from other animals (Bates et al., 1987; Vygotsky, 1962). A similar argument might be made about the use of other paralinguistic cues, such as prosody (intonation and stress) and facial expression, to indicate reference and request. These abilities are also absent in other animals. Finally, it is clear that the information-processing capacities of the human infant differ from those of other animal infants. This fact has also been cited as evidence for biological preprogramming for language acquisition. However, there is nothing about these capacities, as such, that indicates that they are specially designed for language acquisition. They simply allow the acquisition of all types of human knowledge, linguistic and nonlinguistic.

Data obtained in studies of handicapped children shed some light on the biological prerequisites of language acquisition and thus on the role of special biological structures in language acquisition. Children who are born deaf have enormous difficulty in acquiring oral language, but not sign language. It has been suggested that deaf youngsters who are not exposed to sign language and have profound hearing loss invent a symbol system that is quite similar in structure (that is, in semantic relations and order of gesture) to the system developed by young hearing children (Feldman et al., 1978; Goldin-Meadow & Mylander, 1990). Therefore, speech discrimination abilities are not crucial for the acquisition of language, only speech. Children who become deaf after the second year of life have much less difficulty with oral language, although problems still exist. Exposure to vocal language, even if only for the first 2 years, provides a foundation of basic knowledge that allows further, though very slow, development of this knowledge (Lenneberg, 1967). This evidence is used to support the notion that the human infant is biologically preprogrammed specifically to acquire language.

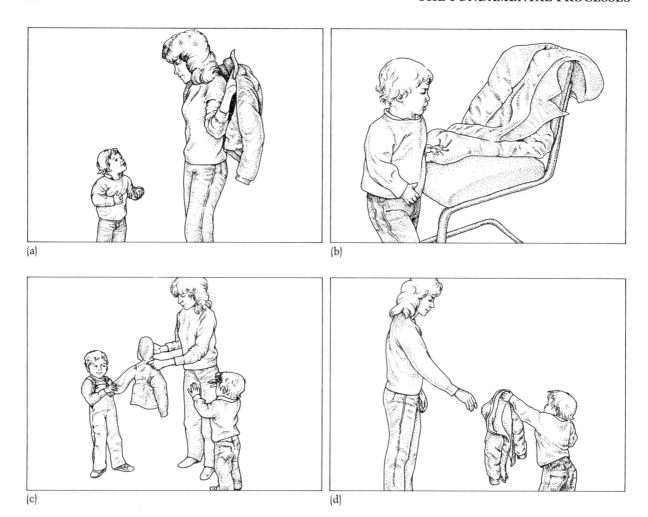

Figure 11.4. When a toddler says "Mommy coat," the utterance may have any of a number of meanings. (a) If this is what the child means, the two-word utterance can be described as agent (Mommy) + object (coat). The intent is to describe Mommy's action. (b) If this is what the child means, the two-word utterance is possessor (Mommy) + possessed (coat). (c) If this is what the child means, the two-word utterance would be agent (Mommy) + object (coat). Notice that the sentence type is the same as that in a, but the implied action is different. The action here is "get," not "put on." A three-word sentence, "Mommy get coat," would make the toddler's intent clear. (d) If this is what the child means, the two-word utterance is again agent (Mommy) + object (coat). The unuttered action in both a and d is "put on," so a three-word utterance would not distinguish between the two meanings. The adjective specifying which coat distinguishes a from d: In a, the action is Mommy putting on her coat; in d, Mommy is putting the child's coat on the child. Notice that in d the child's intonation might give a clue as to the meaning of the utterance. The word *Mommy* operates as an appositive, and in adult language would be followed by a pause. If such a pause exists in the toddler's utterance, it would suggest meaning d rather than a or c. Likewise, the child's intonation in d is likely to be a command rather than a simple declarative.

The language development of blind children has been found to be very similar to that of sighted children, with minor deviations (Landau & Gleitman, 1985). There is no evidence that children who are born without limbs, or who suffer loss of limbs or lack of motor control (that is, they cannot gesture, walk, or even sit up) have any difficulty in acquiring language. All of these findings indicate that sensorimotor deficits or losses do not prevent the acquisition of language. Hence we conclude that language development is independent from other developmental processes and, therefore, that the human infant is biologically predisposed to acquire language. If this is the case, then the question still remains: What structures or functions in the infant cause this predisposition? This question is not a simple one to answer.

Lesions in the brain, not sensorimotor deficits, appear to constitute a biological factor that can affect language acquisition. They can either enormously delay the process of language acquisition (to the point where it is suspected that language knowledge, when acquired, is different for these children) or cause differences in the acquisition of particular aspects of language (semantactic, morphophonological, or pragmatic). Such lesions do not always, if ever, cause *only* language difficulties. Severely retarded children show enormous delay in language development, but they may be delayed in all aspects of development. However, not all mentally retarded children acquire language at an enormously slow rate, and their rate and level of learning development, at least in the range of moderate retardation, are not wholly reflected by IQ. Children labeled as dysphasic (so called because they have not lost language, like adult aphasics, but failed to develop it normally) show specific difficulties in either comprehending or producing certain categories and relations in the language rather than overall delay, but it is not clear that they are deficient only linguistically. These children do vary in their language behaviors, and this variation seems quite similar to that observed in adult aphasics who have suffered injury in different parts of the brain (Menyuk, in press). The differences within these populations in patterns of language behavior lead to a suspicion that different parts and functions of the central nervous system are affected in different children in the same diagnostic category.

Given the above findings of differences in language behavior, it is also reasonable to suppose that different parts of the brain control different aspects of language behavior. It is known, or at least it is highly likely, that such lesions existed prenatally or were caused by birth trauma. This leads to the reasonable assumption that organization of parts and functions of the brain takes place prenatally, at least in terms of readiness to begin processing linguistic information. Nevertheless, there is probably a great deal of redundancy in the nervous system, which allows for compensation for some types of damage. In other instances, as in the populations described above, compensation may not take place at all, or not to a degree sufficient to allow for normal language development.

In conclusion, data on the language development of handicapped children indicate that such development is highly resistant to peripheral sensory losses. Differing central losses or deviations affect different aspects of language development. All of these data suggest that the biological specialization of the human infant to acquire language lies in the structure and organization of the brain, but whether or not this biological specialization is different for language processing compared with other types of cognitive processing is still open to question.

ENVIRONMENTAL FACTORS

A reasonably intact nervous system is a necessary condition for language development, but it is not sufficient. It is clear that communicative interaction with other humans is also necessary (see Figure 11.5). The question is, What role does this interaction play in language development? There are few theoreticians now who suggest that the environment teaches language to the infant by modeling and shaping behavior. Also, there are few who suggest that simple exposure is all that is necessary to get the presumably innate language acquisition device going. Some hypothesize that the environment tunes language input to the capacities of the infant and thus provides the infant with appropriate data to work on (Gleitman et al., 1984). Conversely, others suggest that it is the infant who tunes the environment and elicits from adults the appropriate data to keep the language acquisition device going (Sherrod et al., 1977).

There is clear evidence that caregivers talk to their infants and young children in a way that is different from that they use in talking to their older children and to adults. When they talk to infants, their voices are higher pitched, they often end clauses and phrases with rising intonation, and they use more varied intonational patterns, which convey intent more clearly (Fernald, 1989). These prosodic cues affect the listening preferences of young infants. Kemler-Nelson et al. (1989) gave 8- to 9-month-old infants four types of tapes to listen to: adult-directed speech with pauses at clause boundaries, such speech with pauses within boundaries, child-directed speech with pauses at clausal boundaries, and such speech with pauses within clauses. The infants preferred to listen to child-directed speech with pauses at the clause boundaries significantly more than to any other category of speech. The researchers suggest that marked attention to clausal boundaries in child-directed speech can make a substantial contribution to the learning of syntax.

It has also been found that caregivers use simpler sentences and phrases when they talk to infants than when they talk to older children and adults (Ochs & Schieffelin, 1984). They appear to tune their utterances to what they think the child knows about language, but it is also the case that the primary functions of communication to young children are quite limited and simple. Thus it is not clear whether caregivers speak in simple structures in order to provide appropriate language data or because what they wish to say requires only simple structures.

A number of studies indicate that there is a marked shift in the structure of maternal utterances once the mother believes that her utterances might be at least partially understood. For example, in a study of vocal interactions of 4-, 6-, and 8-month-old infants with their mothers, the age of the infant had a significant effect on the mean length of utterances and on the complexity of the mothers' utterances (Sherrod et al., 1977). They were shorter and simpler (often parts of sentences rather than whole sentences) to 8-month-old infants than to 4- and 6-month-old infants. A number of studies indicate that at a later age, when the infant can respond by action, a large proportion of the mother's utterances are simple directions ("Wash your hands"), but there are also frequent indirect requests ("Your hands are dirty") that require inferential abilities for understanding. It is difficult to see how language input of this kind can teach language structures directly, because such differing structures are used to convey similar meanings. It is also not clear that mothers intend their communicative interactions to teach language. Maternal utterances seem to be a product of trying to communicate with a much less able partner.

The most important question about the effect of input on language development concerns not what caregivers do and why they do it, but rather what effect what they do has on language development. A carefully designed longitudinal study found little correlation between what mothers and their infants do linguistically (Newport et al., 1977). What mothers said had little effect on the development of what is called the *propositional content* of utterances (i.e., numbers and types of noun phrases and verb phrases in utterances). There was some effect on the use of

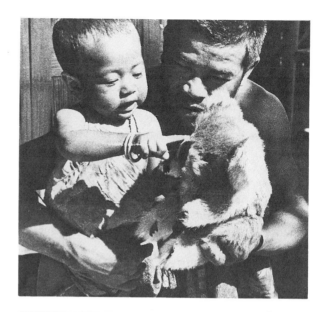

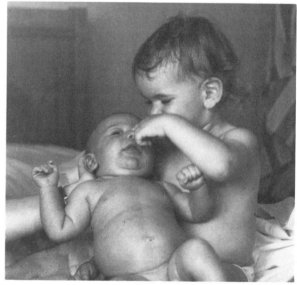

Figure 11.5. In very different cultures young infants learn to identify and label body parts on humans or animals. The American baby is saying "nose" (pronounced "noce"). (Photograph of Balinese baby courtesy of the Library of Congress; that of American baby courtesy of Judy F. Rosenblith.)

auxiliary verbs (am going) and plural markers on nouns (cakes), which are both grammatical markers. The way mothers promoted the development of grammatical markers was not direct. Mothers whose children acquired them more rapidly did not differ significantly from mothers of children who were slower in acquiring them in the frequency of usage of these structures. Rather, they provided more instances in which these aspects were presented clearly. For example, mothers who asked more yes/no questions in which the auxiliary verb was fronted (i.e., appeared at the beginning, as in "Is he going?") had children who developed auxiliary verbs more quickly. Thus the teaching was very indirect and was limited to specific kinds of grammatical knowledge. These results have been replicated in a number of studies (Menyuk, 1988).

More recent studies have been concerned with the effect of communicative interaction on language development rather than with the form of the input. A study of 56 infants and their mothers found that the grammar of the language that mothers used with their children had little effect on the rate of their children's structural language development, but that the ways in which they conversed with their infants did (Liebergott et al., 1985). The number of opportunities that mothers provided for their babies to take turns in conversations, and their degree of acknowledgment of those turns, had an effect on how early their children adequately participated in conversation. From the 1950s to the 1970s, children who came from socioeconomically deprived families were cited as proof that lack of environmental input affects language development. A long history of research appeared to indicate language deficits in these children. However, more recent studies do not indicate marked differences in the amount of input provided infants during the early months of life that is dependent on sociocultural background or SES. Rather, there are differences in the types of communicative interactions that take place in adult-child dyads that are dependent on such sociocultural factors (Ochs & Schieffelin, 1984). Studies of these children's language knowledge have not indicated deficits, but rather differences in language knowledge that are due to the particular dialects and rules of use of language to which the children are exposed. These differences in styles of communicative interaction can, however, lead to differences in the ways language is used to communicate. Such differences in the rules of use of language can lead to problems in school when the communicative style that a child is accustomed to varies from that of the school (Heath, 1982).

ROLE OF IMITATION

From the research on the effect of language input on language development, it is clear that children need to hear language and that the nature of the language children hear is different for babies of different ages and for children of different sociolinguistic backgrounds. The exact relation between type of input and acquisition of linguistic knowledge is still unclear. One aspect of input that has received some attention is imitation. The notion is that the environment provides the models that the infant imitates and then stores in memory. Thus there is interaction between the role of input and cognitive factors, such as memory, on the child's acquisition of language. Some researchers suggest that imitation of a structure in the language is necessary for its acquisition. Several studies have examined the role of imitation in language acquisition and have come up with conflicting conclusions. In summary, some findings indicate that imitation plays no role, because children do not imitate what they do not produce spontaneously. Other findings indicate that imitation may be used to test hypotheses about the production of categories and relations in the language, but it plays no role in comprehension.

Two studies point up the complexities of assessing the role of imitation in acquisition. Over a period of 12 months, Ninio and Bruner (1978) observed one child who was provided with the names of objects while being read to. They found that the rate of repetition of words by the child was not increased either by the mother's imitation of the child's utterances or by the mother's providing a model. They conclude that participation in ritualized dialogue, rather than imitation, is the major mechanism through which word acquisition is achieved. Folger and Chapman (1978) studied the effect of types of speech acts or purpose of communication on spontaneous imitation by six children aged 1 year, 7 months, to 2 years, 1 month. They found that (a) children imitated when cued to do so— that is, when they heard their own utterances repeated or when the referent was described or talked about; (b) elicited imitation was an infrequent occurrence; (c) spontaneous imitation occurred most frequently in particular speech act situations, such as when the mother described referents or when the baby asked for information about a referent; and (d) there was a significant correlation between the percentage of infant utterances imitated by mothers and the percentage of maternal utterances imitated by the infants. That is, children who imitated had mothers who imitated.

Both studies indicate that little direct modeling or imitation of a model goes on in acquisition of words. However, the studies differed both in type and in terms of their findings concerning indirect modeling. The first study found no positive effect of repetition of the child's utterance by the mother leading to repetition on the part of the child; the second did. The first study was longitudinal; the second, cross-sectional. These conflicting findings underscore the difficulty of making generalizations about the role of imitation in language acquisition. The amount of imitation varies from situation to situation and, indeed, from child to child (Nelson, 1973). Some children imitate a great deal, and others do not. Imitation is another instance of early language learning behavior in which individual variation is observed. Nevertheless, it is clear that mothers do not strive to elicit imitation (that is, to teach words directly by modeling) and that imitation does not play a direct role in the acquisition of even such likely candidates as words. Thus it is highly unlikely that imitation plays a direct role in the acquisition of semantic and syntactic categories and relations.

Another way of looking at imitation is suggested by a study that examined the role of joint attention in communication interaction (Tomasello & Farrar, 1986). Interactions of 24 mothers and their children were videotaped when the babies were 15 and 20 months of age. Episodes of joint attention were identified. Within these episodes, there were more utterances produced by both the mothers and their infants, mothers used shorter sentences, and dyads engaged in longer conversations than the individual members did outside the dyads. Maternal references to objects that were already the child's focus of attention were positively correlated with vocabulary acquisition, while references that attempted to redirect attention were negatively correlated. No measures from episodes without joint attention were related to child language. Again, there is evidence that imitation of a model per se does not play the crucial role in lexical acquisition. Rather, the crucial role appears to be played by a combination of factors that add up to positive social interaction between caregiver and infant that caters to the infant's processing limitations.

COGNITIVE FACTORS

Research on the role of cognitive development in language acquisition has also led to many more questions than answers and to conflicting views on the subject. One view is that each linguistic development is dependent on some cognitive development. For example, object permanence is said to lead to referencing (Brown, 1973), and combinatory abilities in symbolic play to word combination (McCune-Nicolich & Bruskin, 1982). These positions suggest that the sequence of acquisition is first some cognitive product and then a related language product. However, the evidence obtained on the sequence of acquisition of language used and cognitive behaviors is not clear. Three infants ages 9 to 11 months at the beginning of study and 27 to 29 months at the end were examined for the

relation between object permanence and word acquisition (Corrigan, 1978). Both abilities matured, but when age was partialed out statistically there were no significant correlations between the two abilities. Thus, in this small sample, word acquisition and object permanence developed as a function of age, but the two were not dependent on each other. To complicate the issue further, in another study, conducted by Gopnik and Meltzoff (1986), infants approximately 15 months of age acquired the word *gone* after the ability to solve simple displacement problems, as would be predicted, but they acquired the word before serial invisible displacements in object permanence tasks. They acquired *no, uh,* and *oh* after the use of insight to solve the string problem, but before the use of insight to solve more difficult means-ends problems. The researchers suggest that there are specific relations between acquisition of the meanings of types of words and particular cognitive achievements of the sensorimotor period, but that word acquisition is not dependent on the achievement of object permanence.

An opposite view is that word acquisition is necessary for concept development (Vygotsky, 1962). Most researchers who take this position are referring to the cognitive developments that take place after age 2. Prior to that age linguistic and cognitive developments are presumably independent. During infancy, adults use language to socialize with the baby, and the baby uses vocalization to socialize with adults. Still another point of view is that both the cognitive and the linguistic accomplishments in the first 2 years of life are dependent on developmental changes in infants' ability to process the information that reaches their senses (Menyuk, 1980). The exact nature of these changes is unknown at present. Data from infant visual processing (Haith, 1979) and speech sound processing (Eilers et al., 1977) indicate that as maturation takes place both the amount and type of information that the infant can process change. For example, in speech sound perception larger chunks of speech sound sequences (more than one syllable) can be processed and different distinctions within the speech sound stimuli can be detected as the infant matures. These maturational changes probably govern observed developmental changes in linguistic and nonlinguistic behavior, rather than behaviors in one domain causing changes in behavior in the other domain, at least during the early months of life. The perceptual salience, simplicity of structure of the information, plus its usefulness in terms of outcomes for the infant, probably affect, respectively, the rate and sequence of acquisitions in either domain.

It is possible that specific information-processing

abilities are required in language acquisition. Slobin (1985) makes such a suggestion. He presents evidence from studies of language development in a number of different languages that indicates that infants use particular linguistic processing strategies to acquire the grammar of these languages. He terms these strategies "operating principles." One such strategy or operating principle is to pay attention to the ends of words, a strategy that is useful in acquisition of the morphophonology of a language. The ends of words mark number and tense in English; case markers in a number of languages, such as Russian, are also at the ends of words. General information-processing abilities may also be required. A series of general information-processing strategies to acquire morphophonological knowledge have been suggested by MacWhinney (1978), with rote memorization first, then analogies used to generalize, and, finally, rules generated when required.

At this point neither the types of information-processing abilities needed nor their specificity for acquisition of structural linguistic knowledge has been determined. However, it is clear that linguistic processing strategies, guided by principles of strategy application, within a context that makes clear to the baby what the data to be processed are, in positive affective situations of joint attention, must all play a very important role in language acquisition.

Summary

It was long held that the period in infancy before words are produced was unrelated to subsequent language development, and the term *prelinguistic* was applied to babies during this time. This view has now changed, largely due to studies that indicate that babies know a great deal about communication and learn a great deal about the structure of language before they acquire words.

Infants communicate with their caregivers in different ways over the first year of life. They begin with cry and noncry vocalizations to convey affect, needs, and feelings, and they then use different patterns of intonation, stress, gesture, and facial expressions with vocalizations to convey these same things. They appear to comprehend the meanings of these different patterns when they are used by others. How to convey intent and emotion are well established in the first year. These features are then applied to holophrases and phrases over the next half year. Infants begin taking their turns in conversational interaction by 3 months. After words appear there is a continuation of turn-tak-

ing, but the content of the child's turn changes, and it becomes a meaningful response to the caregiver's utterance.

As far as knowledge of the structure of language is concerned, the different phases of language production in infancy can be characterized as the cooing, then babbling, phase, followed by the word and word combination phases. Perception of speech grows from single-syllable discrimination (/pa/ versus /ba/) to discrimination of larger speech chunks such as multisyllables. Along with single-syllable discrimination, the infant is able to discriminate between rising and falling intonations of these syllables and perceive clause and phrase and word boundaries. Along with multisyllable discrimination the infant is able to distinguish between statement and question intonation contours of sentences. At the end of the first year of life there is evidence that babies know what words for a small set of objects mean even when the words are presented in isolation.

The apparent ability of young infants to discriminate speech sounds in the same fashion as adults raises the question of whether there are detectors in the auditory system that are particularly sensitive to acoustic differences relevant to speech sound discrimination in any language (as with early sensitivity to color categories or movement differences). Speech sounds vary in several acoustic dimensions or distinctive features. The language experience of infants modifies their ability to discriminate among sounds at about 6 months. Further, infants discriminate among sounds on the basis of acoustic dimensions that are not limited to speech sounds, and other animals can be taught to discriminate among speech sounds. Hence the existence of innate *speech* feature detectors in the infant's central nervous system is questionable.

The production of speech sounds in babbling appears to develop in the same order in children from different language communities. Certain consonant sounds occur earlier than others; for example, those formed by the lips occur ahead of those formed by the tip of the tongue. This order seem to be a reflection of ease of articulation. Unlike earlier views that babbling contained all possible speech sounds of the language, the current view is that sounds produced during the babbling period are a reflection of the development of motor skills, and that sounds requiring subtle articulatory muscle control have not occurred even by the end of this period. This motor skill aspect of speech sound production would imply a universal pattern of acquisition across all language communities. The data collected thus far support this implication. The universal repertoire, however, becomes more specific to particular language experiences toward the end of the first year.

Over the first year the infant evidences the ability to segment the stream of speech heard or seen. First, clause boundaries are detected, then phrase and, finally, word boundaries. There are data that indicate that comprehension of words out of context begins at about 12 months. Knowledge of word meaning develops in a nonrandom fashion. The types of words used first refer to persons, objects, and actions that are important to the infant. Words are first used in an underextended manner and then are overextended to refer to more than one object in a category. Data on comprehension of word meaning are limited, but it appears that infants first generalize, then are specific, and then generalize again in the process of comprehension of word meaning. There is some evidence that this may be the case in both perception and production, because very early word use may be a generalization, but there is little evidence to support this conclusion.

At first, productions are holophrases, single words or phrases that express needs or feelings about objects or actions. These needs and feelings are conveyed by the use of intonation, stress, gesture, and facial expressions. Such utterances are used in particular situational contexts with particular gestures and facial expressions. Several sources indicate that infants may understand utterances that describe relations between objects and actions, or objects and attributes, or even relations among actor, action, and object while they can produce only one part of a relation at a time. Later comes the use of utterances to describe relations between objects and actions and attributes of objects and actions. Thus at 14 to 15 months some infants indicate comprehension of some word-order syntactic rules of the language as well as semantic knowledge of the meanings of words, and can do this many months before they produce two- and three-word sentences.

There are differences among infants in their patterns of language development. There appear to be at least two strands of development that occur. Some infants show a rapid spurt in lexical development, producing lexical items that largely refer to objects. These infants use language primarily to refer, and they use a high proportion of nouns when they begin to produce two-part utterances. Other infants acquire words more slowly, show a more even balance in their acquisition of word classes, initially use language primarily to express needs and feelings, and use a high proportion of pronouns when they begin to combine words. Some infants spend much more time listening than they do imitating or speaking.

The factors that affect language development in-

clude biological factors. An intact CNS and appropriate hemispheric specializations in the brain, intact vocal structures (and muscle control mechanisms, not discussed), and a sufficiently intact auditory system to discriminate speech sounds are necessary for acquisition of oral language. Research indicates, however, that deafness, blindness, and loss of the ability to manipulate the vocal mechanism do not prevent or even seriously retard acquisition of language, either oral or signed. Language acquisition is independent of peripheral sensorimotor abilities, but damage to the CNS does seriously affect the process. This suggests that the biological predisposition to acquire language lies in the structure and function of the brain. Whether this specialization for language differs in any meaningful way from that of other forms of cognitive processing is still open to question.

Language acquisition also depends on communicative interaction with other language users. The role of this environmental input is interpreted very differently by different researchers. Some see it as teaching language to the child, while others see it as providing the data the child uses to learn language. There is no evidence that what caregivers do affects the child's acquisition of the structures of language. Specific types of mother input, or variations in this input due to sociocultural differences, appear to have little effect on the acquisition of such knowledge, but they do have a marked effect on how children use language. Providing babies with opportunities to take turns, and acknowledging these turns, has a positive effect on their conversational abilities.

The relation of language development to general cognitive development (questioned previously in relation to biological factors) needs more study. The research results to date indicate that language and cognitive development may be two sides of a single coin: the information-processing abilities of the infant. These abilities, however, may account only for acquisition of the structures of language, not for the child's communicative use of these structures. Other factors, such as affect and social pressures, may better account for the development of this aspect of language.

References

ASLIN, R., Pisoni, D., & Jusczyk, P. (1983). Auditory development and speech perception in infancy. In M. Haith & J. Campos (Eds.), *Handbook of child psychology* (Vol. 2, 4th ed.). New York: John Wiley.
BALDWIN, D., & Markman, E. (1989). Establishing word-object relations: A first step. *Child Development, 60,* 381-398.
BATES, E., Camaioni, L., & Volterra, V. (1975). The acquisi-

tion of performatives prior to speech. *Merrill-Palmer Quarterly, 21,* 205-226.

BATES, E., O'Connell, B., & Shore, C. (1987). Language and communication in infancy. In J. Osofsky (Ed.), *Handbook of infant development* (2nd ed., pp. 149-203). New York: John Wiley.

BATESON, M. (1969). The interpersonal context of infant vocalization. *Quarterly Progress Reports, Research Laboratory of Electronics, MIT, 100,* 170-176.

BEHREND, D. (1988). Overextensions in early language comprehension: Evidence from a signal detection approach. *Journal of Child Language, 15,* 63-75.

BLOOM, L., & Capatides, J. (1987). Expression of affect and the emergence of language. *Child Development, 58,* 1513-1522.

BLOOM, L., Ripoli, M., Gartner, B., & Hafitz, J. (1989). Acquisition of complementation. *Journal of Child Language, 16,* 101-120.

BOWERMAN, M. (1988). *The role of meaning in grammatical development: A continuing challenge to theories of language acquisition.* Paper presented at the Thirteenth Annual Boston University Conference on Language Development.

BOYSSON-BARDIES, B., Sagart, L., & Durand, C. (1984). Discernible differences in the babbling of infants according to target language. *Journal of Child Language, 11,* 1-15.

BOYSSON-BARDIES, B., Sagart, L., Halle, P., & Durand, C. (1986). Acoustic investigations of cross-linguistic variability in babbling. In B. Lindblom & R. Zetterstrom (Eds.), *Precursors of early speech* (pp. 113-126). New York: Stockton.

BRANIGAN, G. (1976). *Organizational constraints during the one word period.* Paper presented at First Annual Boston University Conference on Language Development.

BROWN, R. (1973). *A first language.* Cambridge, MA: Harvard University Press.

CLARK, E. (1973). What's in a word. In T. Moore (Ed.), *Cognitive development and the acquisition of language* (pp. 65-100). New York: Academic Press.

CLARK, E. (1983). Meanings and concepts. In J. Flavell & E. Markman (Eds.), *Handbook of child psychology* (Vol. 3, pp. 787-840). New York: John Wiley.

CLARK, E. (1987). The principle of contrast: A constraint on language acquisition. In B. MacWhinney (Ed.), *Mechanisms of language acquisition.* Hillsdale, NJ: Lawrence Erlbaum.

CORRIGAN, R. (1978). Language development as related to stage 6 object permanence development. *Journal of Child Language, 5,* 173-189.

DONAHUE, M. (1978). *Form and function in mother-toddler conversational turn-taking.* Unpublished doctoral dissertation, Boston University.

EILERS, R., Wilson, W., & Moore, J. (1977). Developmental changes in speech discrimination. *Journal of Speech and Hearing Research, 20,* 766-780.

EIMAS, P., Siqueland, F., Jusczyk, P., & Vigorito, J. (1971). Speech perception in early infancy. *Science, 171,* 303-306.

FELDMAN, H., Goldin-Meadow, S., & Gleitman, L. (1978). Beyond Herodotus: The growth of language by linguistically deprived deaf children. In A. Locke (Ed.), *Action, gesture and symbol* (pp. 351-414). New York: Academic Press.

FERGUSON, C. (1986). Discovering sound units and constructing sound systems: It's child's play. In J. Perkell & D. Klatt (Eds.), *Invariance and variability in speech production and speech perception* (pp. 36-50). Hillsdale, NJ: Lawrence Erlbaum.

FERNALD, A. (1989). Intonation and communicative intent in mothers' speech to infants: Is the melody the message? *Child Development, 60,* 1497-1510.

FOLGER, J., & Chapman, R. (1978). A pragmatic analysis of spontaneous imitations. *Journal of Child Language, 5,* 25-38.

FROMKIN, V., & Rodman, R. (1974). *An introduction to language.* New York: Holt, Rinehart & Winston.

FURROW, D., & Nelson, K. (1984). Environmental correlates of individual differences in language acquisition. *Journal of Child Language, 11,* 523-534.

GLEITMAN, L., Newport, E., & Gleitman, H. (1984). The current status of the motherese hypothesis. *Journal of Child Language, 11,* 43-79.

GOLDFIELD, B., & Reznick, J. (1990). Early lexical acquisition: Rate, content and the vocabulary spurt. *Journal of Child Language, 17,* 171-183.

GOLDIN-MEADOW, S., & Mylander, C. (1990). Beyond the input given: The child's role in the acquisition of language. *Language, 66,* 323-355.

GOLINKOFF, R., & Hirsh-Pasek, K. (1990). Let the mute speak: What infants can tell us about language acquisition. *Merrill-Palmer Quarterly, 36,* 67-92.

GOPNIK, A., & Meltzoff, A. (1986). Relations between semantic and cognitive development in the one word stage: The specificity hypothesis. *Child Development, 57,* 1040-1053.

GREENFIELD, P., & Smith, J. (1976). *The structure of communication in early language development.* New York: Academic Press.

HAITH, M. (1979). Visual cognition in early infancy. In R. Kearsley & I. Sigel (Eds.), *Infants at risk: Assessment of cognitive functioning* (pp. 23-48). Hillsdale, NJ: Lawrence Erlbaum.

HEATH, S. (1982). What no bedtime story means: Narrative skills at home and school. *Language and Society, 11,* 49-77.

HIRSH-PASEK, K. (1989). *Infants' perception of fluent speech: Implications for language development.* Paper presented at the biennial meeting of Society for Research in Child Development, Kansas City, MO.

HIRSH-PASEK, K., & Golinkoff, R. (in press). Skeletal supports for grammatical learning: What the infant brings to the language learning task. In C. E. Rovee-Collier (Ed.), *Advances in infancy research* (Vol. 10). Norwood, NJ: Ablex.

HIRSH-PASEK, K., Golinkoff, R., Beaubien, F., Fletcher, A., & Cauley, K. (1985). *In the beginning: One word speakers comprehend word order.* Paper presented at the Tenth Annual Boston University Conference on Language Development.

HORGAN, D. (1976). *Linguistic knowledge at Stage I: Evidence from successive single word utterances.* Paper presented at the Child Language Research Forum, Stanford University.

INGRAM, D. (1990). Toward a theory of phonological acquisition. In J. Miller (Ed.), *Research on child language disorders: A decade of progress* (pp. 55-72). Austin, TX: Pro-Ed.

IRWIN, O. (1947). Infant speech: Consonant sounds according to the manner of articulation. *Journal of Speech Disorders, 12,* 397-401.

JAKOBSON, R. (1968). *Child language, aphasia and phonological universals.* The Hague: Mouton.

JAKOBSON, R., Fant, G., & Halle, M. (1963). *Preliminaries to speech analysis.* Cambridge: MIT Press.

JUSCZYK, P., & Bertoncini, J. (1988). Viewing the development of speech perception as an innately guided learning process. *Language and Speech, 31,* 217-238.

KEMLER-NELSON, D., Hirsh-Pasek, K., Jusczyk, P., & Cassidy, K. (1989). How the prosodic cues in motherese might assist language learning. *Journal of Child Language, 16,* 55-68.

KENT, R., & Hodge, M. (1990). The biogenesis of speech: Continuity and process in early speech and language development. In J. Miller (Ed.), *Research on child language disorders: A decade of progress* (pp. 25-54). Austin, TX: Pro-Ed.

KUHL, P. (1986). Reflections on infants' perception and representation of speech. In J. Perkell & D. Klatt (Eds.), *Invariance and variability in speech production and speech perception* (pp. 19-29). Hillsdale, NJ: Lawrence Erlbaum.

KUHL, P. (1990). Toward a new theory of the development of speech perception. In S. Furui (Ed.), *Proceedings of the International Conference on Spoken Language Processing* (Vol. 2, pp. 745-748). Tokyo: Acoustical Society of Japan.

LANDAU, B., & Gleitman, L. (1985). *Language and experience.* Cambridge, MA: Harvard University Press.

LENNEBERG, E. (1967). *Biological foundations of language.* New York: John Wiley.

LEWIS, M., & Freedle, R. (1972). *Mother-infant dyad: The cradle of meaning.* Princeton, NJ: Educational Testing Service.

LIEBERGOTT, J., Schultz, M., & Menyuk, P. (1985). *A prescriptive manual for parents and teachers of children at risk for language disorder* (Final report on Field-Initiated Research Grant G008006727). Washington, DC: U.S. Department of Education, Office of Special Education and Rehabilitative Services.

LIEBERMAN, P. (1974). *On the origins of language.* New York: Macmillan.

LOCKE, J. (1986). The linguistic significance of babbling. In B. Lindblom & R. Zetterstrom (Eds.), *Precursors of early speech* (pp. 143-162). New York: Stockton.

MacWHINNEY, B. (1978). The acquisition of morphophonology. *Monographs of the Society for Research in Child Development, 43*(1-2, Serial No. 174).

MARKMAN, E. (1987). How children constrain the possible meanings of words. In U. Neisser (Ed.), *Concepts and conceptual development: Ecological and intellectual factors in categorization.* Cambridge: Cambridge University Press.

McCUNE-NICOLICH, L., & Bruskin, C. (1982). Combinatorial competency in play and language. In K. Rubin (Ed.), *The play of children: Current theory and research.* Basel, Switzerland: Karger.

MENN, L. (1981). Theories of phonological development. In H. Winitz (Ed.), Native language and foreign language acquisition [Special issue]. *Annals of the New York Academy of Science, 379,* 130-137.

MENYUK, P. (1972). *Speech development.* Indianapolis: Bobbs-Merrill.

MENYUK, P. (1980). Non-linguistic and linguistic processing in normally developing and language disordered children. In N. J. Lass (Ed.), *Speech and language: Advances in basic research and practice* (Vol. 4, pp. 1-97). New York: Academic Press.

MENYUK, P. (1988). *Language development: Knowledge and use.* New York: HarperCollins.

MENYUK, P. (1990). Relationship between speech perception and production in language acquisition. In S. Furui (Ed.), *Proceedings of the International Conference on Spoken Language Processing* (Vol. 2, pp. 733-737). Tokyo: Acoustical Society of Japan.

MENYUK, P. (in press). Developmental dysphasia: Linguistic aspects. In G. Blanken, J. Dittman, H. Grimm, J. Marshall, & C. Wallesch (Eds.), *Linguistic disorders and pathologies: An*

international handbook. Berlin: Walter de Gruyter.

MENYUK, P., & Bernholtz, M. (1969). Prosodic features and children's language. *Quarterly Progress Reports, Research Lab of Electronics, MIT, 93,* 216-219.

MENYUK, P., & Flood, J. (1981). Linguistic competence, reading, writing problems and remediation. *Bulletin of the Orton Society, 31,* 13-28.

MENYUK, P., Liebergott, J., Schultz, M., Chesnick, M., & Ferrier, L. (1991). Patterns of early lexical and cognitive development in premature and full-term infants. *Journal of Speech and Hearing Research, 34,* 88-94.

MENYUK, P., Menn, L., & Silber, R. (1986). Early strategies for the perception and production of words and sounds. In P. Fletcher & M. Garman (Eds.), *Language acquisition: Studies in first language development* (pp. 198-222). Cambridge: Cambridge University Press.

MOLFESE, D. (1973). Cerebral asymmetry in infants, children and adults: Auditory evoked responses to speech and music stimuli. *Dissertation Abstracts International, 34*(3-B), 1298.

MOLFESE, D., & Molfese, V. (1985). Electrophysiological indices of auditory discrimination in newborn infants: The bases for predicting later language development? *Infant Behavior and Development, 8,* 197-211.

MURAI, J.-I. (1960). Speech developments of infants. *Psychologia, 3,* 27-35.

NAKAZIMA, S. (1962). A comparative study of speech developments of Japanese and American English childhood. *Studia Phonologica, 2,* 27-39.

NELSON, K. (1973). Structure and strategy in learning to talk. *Monographs of the Society for Research in Child Development, 38.*

NELSON, K. (1980). *Individual differences in language development: Implications for development and language.* Paper presented at the Fifth Annual Boston University Conference on Language Development.

NEWPORT, E., Gleitman, H., & Gleitman, L. (1977). Mother, I'd rather do it myself: Some effects and non-effects of maternal speech style. In C. Snow & C. Ferguson (Eds.), *Talking to children* (pp. 109-149). Cambridge: Cambridge University Press.

NINIO, A., & Bruner, J. (1978). The achievement and antecedents of labelling. *Journal of Child Language, 5,* 1-15.

NITTROUER, S., Studdert-Kennedy, M., & McGowan, R. (1989). The emergence of phonetic segments: Evidence from the spectral structure of fricatives in novel syllables spoken by children and adults. *Journal of Speech and Hearing Research, 32,* 120-132.

OCHS, E., & Schieffelin, B. (1984). Language acquisition and socialization: Three developmental stories. In R. Schweder & R. Levine (Eds.), *Culture theory: Essays on mind, self and emotion.* Cambridge: Cambridge University Press.

OLLER, K. (1980). The emergence of the sounds of speech in infancy. In G. Yeni-Komshian & C. Ferguson (Eds.), *Child phonology* (Vol. 1, pp. 93-112). New York: Academic Press.

PERKELL, J., & Klatt, D. (Eds.). (1986). *Invariance and variability in speech production and speech perception.* Hillsdale, NJ: Lawrence Erlbaum.

PETERS, A. (1983). *The units of language acquisition.* Cambridge: Cambridge University Press.

PETITTO, L., & Marentette, P. (1990). *The timing of linguistic milestones in sign language acquisition: Are first signs acquired earlier than first words?* Paper presented at the Fifteenth Annual Boston University Conference on Language Development.

SACHS, J., & Truswell, L. (1978). Comprehension of two-word instructions by children in the one-word stage. *Journal of Child Language, 5*, 17-24.

SCHIEFFELIN, D., & Ochs, S. (Eds.). (1986). *Language socialization across cultures.* Cambridge: Cambridge University Press.

SHERROD, H., Friedman, S., Crawley, S., Drake, D., & Devieux, J. (1977). Maternal language to prelinguistic infants. *Child Development, 48*, 1662-1663.

SIEGLER, R. (1986). *Children's thinking.* Englewood Cliffs, NJ: Prentice-Hall.

SLOBIN, D. (1985). Cross-linguistic evidence for the language making capacity. In D. Slobin (Ed.), *The cross-linguistic study of language acquisition* (pp. 1157-1256). Hillsdale, NJ: Lawrence Erlbaum.

SMITH, N. (1973). *The acquisition of phonology: A case study.* Cambridge: Cambridge University Press.

STARK, R. (1986). Prespeech segmental feature development. In P. Fletcher & M. Garman (Eds.), *Language acquisition: Studies in first language development* (pp. 149-173). Cambridge: Cambridge University Press.

THOMAS, D., Campos, J., Shucard, D., Ramsay, D., & Shucard, J. (1981). Semantic comprehension in infancy: A signal detection analysis. *Child Development, 52*, 798-803.

TOMASELLO, M., & Farrar, M. (1986). Joint attention and early language. *Child Development, 57*, 1454-1463.

TRUBY, H., Bosma, J., & Lind, J. (1965). Newborn infant cry. *Acta Paediatrica Scandinavica* (Suppl. 163).

VYGOTSKY, L. S. (1962). *Thought and language.* Cambridge: MIT Press.

WERKER, J., & Lalonde, C. (1988). Cross-language speech perception: Initial capabilities and developmental change. *Developmental Psychology, 24*, 672-683.

Social Development of the Infant

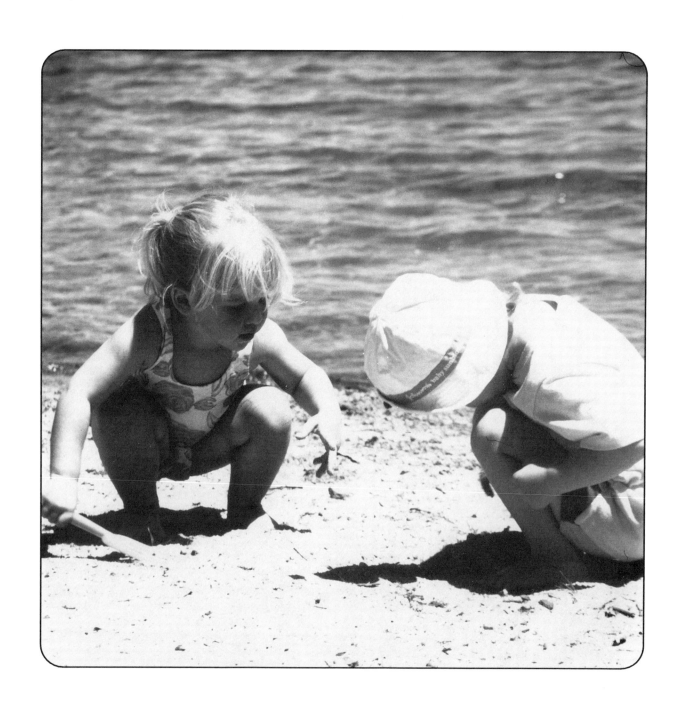

Chapter 12

This discussion of social development starts with the topic of the development of an infant's love relationship, called **attachment** by psychologists. This topic has been a strong focus of the field for a considerable period of time. Most theorists and researchers have considered infants' attachment to their mothers to be of primary importance, so that topic is addressed first. The discussion then moves to the topic of mother-infant interactions in early infancy, which are considered by many to be the major determinant of "good attachment." A description then follows of infants' developing relationships with their fathers, a topic that has only recently received much attention. Finally, a brief overview of infants' social interactions with peers is offered.

Attachment

HISTORY AND THEORIES OF THE CONCEPT

Psychoanalytic theory is the source of much of the belief that infants' initial attachment to their mothers is of the utmost importance. Freud (1905/1938) believed that the mother-infant relationship is "unique," with the mother established for a lifetime as the child's first and strongest love object. The relationship between mother and child, in Freud's view, is the prototype of all later love relations. He believed that the infant develops what he called an **object relation** with the mother through the feeding relationship and that, as sucking is the primary means of gratification available to the infant in the first year of life, the person who provides that gratification becomes a love object (the primary object relation). Weaning denies infants gratification, thus producing a conflict in the mother-infant relationship. Only if weaning is neither too severe nor too lenient—neither too rapid nor too prolonged—will the baby develop the ability to establish adequate interpersonal relationships.

Because Freud was interested in psychopathology and studied only adults, he contributed little to the verification of his theory about infant attachment. His

ideas, however, appealed to psychiatrists, psychologists, and laypeople alike, and influenced not only the study of attachment, but the study of infants' separations from their mothers as well.

Erik Erikson (1963) extended and revised Freud's theory, incorporating knowledge gained between Freud's time and his own. He hypothesized that children who have had a good mother-infant relationship develop a basic trust in people and institutions, while children who do not experience a satisfactory attachment develop basic mistrust. The trust-mistrust dimension is the infants' general emotional reaction to events in their world. Trust implies a positive and accepting reaction, while mistrust is a negative and rejecting reaction. Erikson hypothesized that mother-infant interactions other than sucking also contribute to the relationship.

Both men believed the prototypical mother-child relationship set the child's way of interacting with others for life (if not altered by specific experiences), and hence that inadequate attachment would result in interpersonal difficulties throughout life, especially in marital and parental difficulties. As if these two kinds of dire consequences were not enough to blame on the nature of the attachment relationship, Erikson's notion of basic trust includes consequences for the development of instrumental competence (competence with things rather than with people). This happens in two ways. Children develop trust in themselves and in their own competence and trust in institutions (from the family to government and religion). The mechanism by which the trust in one's own competence might develop from attachment is clear. Mothers of toddlers who are securely attached serve as a secure base from which their toddlers can explore, and toddlers develop competence through exploration. Trust in institutions is a reasonable extrapolation. Basic trust is a pervasive emotional tendency to respond positively and in an accepting fashion, so it would be reasonable to predict that this acceptance would extend to abstract institutions as well as to people and oneself.

The term *attachment* was first used not by Freudians, but by Sears, in his 1943 survey of objective studies of psychoanalytic concepts. He used it to describe children's differential relationships to parents (or, in psychoanalytic terms, their differential cathexes). The term was not widely used, however, until 15 years later, when Bowlby (1958) adopted it, both to get away from the learning theorists' concept of dependency and because it seemed more congruent with some of the ideas about affectional ties that were being developed by animal ethologists.[1] Thus psychoanalytic instinct theory was reformulated or updated in

---

1. The dependency notion was that some children developed a general tendency to seek help, attention, or emotional support from adults. This was conceived to be a generalized individual trait that one would expect the child to exhibit in many situations and with many different adults. It was often hypothesized to develop because the mother reinforced her child for such behaviors during infancy and later childhood.

the new ethological context, which views behavior (including human social behavior) in terms of Darwinian evolutionary theory. Ethological theory, developed by zoologists rather than by psychologists, focuses on those environmental events and infant response systems that are specific to each species. Many of the original formulations of ethologists were based on studies of **imprinting** in precocial birds (birds that can walk at hatching), such as ducks, geese, and chickens. For these species, attachment develops during a critical period that occurs shortly after birth. The duckling or gosling follows the first moving object it encounters (normally the mother) and becomes imprinted on it. That which the infant first follows "becomes" its mother and, at sexual maturity, the preferred sex object. Since Lorenz's initial work, imprinting has been studied extensively. It has been determined that "mother" is a stimulus moving away at a particular rate and that the effects of this early experience typically are long lasting.

Ethologists appreciate the great differences that exist among species, and recognize that since humans cannot follow at birth, something else must play the crucial role in the development of attachment in humans. They do see infants as biologically set to learn to recognize their "mothers" (analogous to being set to follow an object moving away) and to respond to them by a strong, enduring bond, such as that found in birds.

Bowlby found five behavioral response systems in human infants that he thought functioned to develop the attachment relationship. *Following* is of course an obvious first choice; *clinging* may serve the same function for many primates (monkeys and apes) that following does for precocial birds, and hence is a good second choice. Human newborns, however, do not show the universal and intense clinging to their mothers that monkeys do, so clinging is unlikely to be a predominant response for humans. Bowlby proposed that *crying, smiling,* and *sucking* play important roles in human infants' development of attachments. All three systems are present in at least primitive form in early infancy (see Chapter 6), and they all have the effect of bringing or keeping the adult in contact. Bowlby viewed the five behavioral systems as initially independent of each other, with different times and rates of development; with time, the systems become integrated and focus on the mother. They then form the basis of attachment, which develops by about 7 months of age.

Consistent with his ethological viewpoint, Bowlby considered the development of the specific attachment to mother to be biologically based. That does not mean that it unfolds solely due to maturation or that the environment is irrelevant. Rather, Bowlby proposed that each of the five systems needs environmental stimulation to develop and depends on both experience and maturation.[2] Experience and maturation both play roles in developing and integrating the systems, which then provide the basis for attachment. Unfortunately, some followers of this approach have often talked about stages as if they were entirely dependent on maturation.

Much of the early interest in attachment came from studies of the reactions of infants and young children to being separated from their mothers by being hospitalized. However, the "threats" to the infant in a hospital far exceed those of separation from the mother, hence the effects of hospitalization will be omitted from this discussion. It should be noted, however, that this work has had a profound influence on hospital practice with respect to parental visiting of infant and child patients.

Ainsworth, who modified and introduced Bowlby's ideas in the United States, did extensive research that has been a major contribution to understanding individual differences in attachment and the antecedent mother-infant interactions that seem to produce these differences, as shall be seen in the material to follow.

ATTACHMENT TO THE MOTHER

Before presentation of discussion of the ways in which attachment is and has been measured, a general historical overview of the concept and a description of the stages of attachment are in order.

There are three (or four, if we go beyond infancy) stages to the development of specific attachments. Very young babies cannot identify their mothers and therefore cannot exhibit differential emotional responses to them. Such infants do, however, show what is called **undiscriminating social responsiveness**. During the first 2 or 3 months infants can use their basic capacities to orient to people (as well as to things). They orient to salient features of the environment, which increasingly are human, through such responses as visual fixation, visual tracking, listening, rooting, and postural adjustments when held. They can also gain or maintain contact with other humans

---

2. Although sucking is one of the behaviors in his group, he did not consider feeding to play an important role in attachment. This conclusion was concurrently being demonstrated empirically by the Harlows (e. g., Harlow, 1958), who found that, in monkeys, clinging (contact comfort) was a far more important ingredient for attachment to artificial mothers than was feeding.

in a limited way through sucking or grasping, although they do not do these behaviors in order to maintain social contact (remember from Chapter 10 that they have not yet developed the capacity for means-ends behaviors). They also have special signaling behaviors (again presumably not intentional)—smiling, crying, and vocalizing. As described earlier, some stimuli are more attractive than others. Included in the more attractive group are several that commonly emanate from adults—faces, voices, and parents' imitations of the infant, particularly vocal imitation. (Piaget's explanation for the effectiveness of the latter is that infants can assimilate parents' vocalizations and similar behaviors to their own schemes.) This early experience with humans presumably provides the basis on which young infants can learn to discriminate one human from another. Recall from Chapter 7 that newborn babies probably cannot distinguish their mothers' faces, although they can distinguish their mothers' odors. By 8 weeks they can discriminate their mothers' faces, but only if given ample time. It is not until 3-4 months that babies can easily and quickly recognize particular faces.

Once such discriminative ability develops, the infant has the basis for the second phase, that of **discriminating social responsiveness**, during which infants respond differently (e.g., in vocalizing, smiling, and crying) to one (or a few) familiar figure(s) than they do to strangers. Ainsworth subdivided this into an early stage, in which infants differentiate only between the attachment figure and another person when they are in close contact, and a later phase, in which they differentiate at a distance (e.g., when the figure enters or leaves the room). Babies who exhibit discriminating social responsiveness not only are able to discriminate their mothers' faces from other faces, but they also exhibit positive affective responses. These suggest that they have become familiar with their mothers' caretaking and social behaviors. This familiarity has undoubtedly been developing throughout their young lives, because newborns are able to learn at birth, and their learning abilities increase rapidly in the first few months (recall Chapter 9). Thus they are more and more able to learn their mothers' ways of interacting and to respond to them in ways that will lead to rewards and will be rewarding to their mothers.

---

3. In Freud's theory attachments to inanimate objects should appear later than social attachments, but should share characteristics with them. The only study I know of concerning object attachment did not find this to be the case (Jones et al., 1990). Rather, object attachments were related to some aspects of temperament.

Most attachment research has not studied these two early phases, but has focused on the third phase, **active initiative in seeking proximity and contact**, which has been described as follows by Ainsworth (1973):

During this phase all the earlier attachment behaviors are still present and differential, but there is a striking increase in the baby's initiative in promoting proximity and contact. His signals are no longer merely expressive or reactive; they often are intended to evoke a response from the mother or other attachment figure. Locomotion facilitates proximity seeking, and voluntary movements of hands and arms are conspicuous now in attachment behavior. Greeting responses become more active and effective. Following, approaching, clinging, and various other active contact behaviors become significant. The median age for attaining this phase is about seven months.

Bowlby (1969) suggests that "goal-corrected" sequences of behavior emerge in this third phase: Sequences that are guided by a constant stream of feedback, so that the baby alters the direction, speed, and nature of his behavior in accordance with that of the figure to whom he has become attached. This is also when psychoanalytic theorists judge "true object relations" to emerge. Further, the onset of the third stage coincides with Piaget's fourth stage of sensorimotor development, in which the child first begins to search for hidden objects and thus manifests the beginnings of the concept of an object as permanent despite its not being present to perception. (p. 12)[3]

Clearly, the timing of the action-initiation phase in attachment is dependent on certain motoric and cognitive developments occurring. Infants are beginning to move on their own, so that they can seek proximity to mother much more effectively. Further, as described in Chapter 10, infants of this age are developing intentionality (means-ends behaviors) and the beginnings of object permanence (successful search for an object hidden under a single screen). An example of the newly developed intentionality is infants lifting their hands to be picked up. A secondary scheme—hand lifting—has been subordinated to the goal of being picked up. Object permanence also means that infants now understand that mother still exists when they are not interacting with her. In the previous Piagetian stage, part of the object (mother) would have to be present for the infant to initiate any action toward it (her).

A fourth phase, **goal-corrected partnership**, was

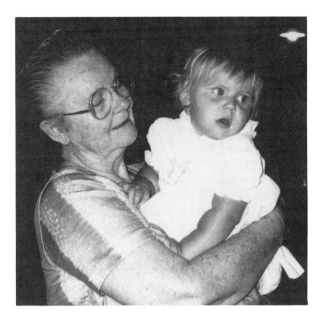

Figure 12.1. A departing attachment figure (father) evokes anxious looks when the infant is left in the arms of her grandmother, whom she has not seen for several months. (Photograph courtesy of Judy F. Rosenblith.)

suggested by Bowlby (1969). During this phase children come to understand the factors that influence their mothers' behaviors and can therefore be more sophisticated in their efforts to modify their mothers' behaviors to fit their own needs. This probably starts at about 3 years, and hence will not be covered here.

The first three stages are well documented by Ainsworth (1967) and others. All children, whether in Uganda or the United States, apparently go through each stage in the same sequence, although not at the same ages. This invariance of stage development supports the ethological notion of the maturational unfolding of stages (given the prior activation of the infant's behavior systems by the environment). However, this invariant stage sequence might reflect perceptual, motor, or cognitive development, which also tend to unfold on a maturational timetable. Infants make social responses to social stimuli from birth (see the discussions of smiling in Chapter 6, imitation in Chapters 9 and 10, early verbal communication in Chapter 11, and early social responsiveness later in this chapter). However, they cannot respond differentially to their mothers versus strangers until they can discriminate perceptually between the two. Thus they cannot move from Phase 1 to Phase 2 until they have learned something about mommies and strangers. The relative roles of maturation and experience in percep-

tual, motor, and cognitive development are still unknown, but the data suggest that attachment phases themselves are not directly controlled by maturational mechanisms.

Although each of these stages is qualitatively distinct from the other, that does not mean that the transitions between them are abrupt. Infants develop gradually, and there may be occasional signs, say, of preferential looking at mother long before one sees preferences expressed in other behaviors (such as smiling and waving) or in more than one context (arrival *and* departure of mother). Only at the height of each phase would the phenomena described be strong and clear to the casual observer. Even then, babies do not behave consistently in all situations. For example, they are more likely to protest separation from the attachment figure (mother) in a strange place than at home, after a previous separation than at first separation, and when left with a stranger than when left with another attachment figure. Technically, attachment behaviors are context specific.

WHAT IS THIS THING CALLED ATTACHMENT?

Because most research on the development of infants' attachment has focused on the phase of active initiative in seeking proximity and contact, the term *attachment* often refers specifically to that phase. The first measures used to study attachment were infants' protests on being separated from mother and their fear of strangers. This was based on the Freudian notion, developed in this context by Spitz (1950), that the underlying motivating force behind attachment is infants' fear of losing their mothers. Thus the best measures of this love force should be protest at separation from the mother (crying and fussing), measured either in the laboratory or in natural situations, and fear of strangers (see Figure 12.1), and for a period many studies were made of these phenomena. The reason protest at separation reflects infants' fear of losing mother is obvious, but the relation to stranger anxiety is more indirect.

Both protest at separation from the mother and stranger anxiety have been questioned as adequate measures of attachment. Consider protest at separation: Babies who exhibit intense protest at separation could be either more positively attached or less secure in their attachment or their overall feelings of security. Babies who exhibit little separation protest might not be less attached; rather, they may be more secure, or they may have mothers who have discovered specific techniques for solving protest at separation (Weinraub

& Lewis, 1977). Protest by itself is also a less sensitive measure than the ones discussed next, in that infants will sometimes show equal protest at separation from two attachment figures, but will show greater attachment to one of those two in other ways (e.g., Fox, 1977).

Ainsworth (1963) became convinced that indications of attachment that included more positive behaviors were needed. With Wittig, she developed a laboratory procedure called the **Strange Situation**. Following an introductory period in which the infant becomes acquainted with the room, the toys, and a stranger, the parent twice leaves the room and twice returns to it. This provides measures of the infant's behavior before, during, and after separation from the mother, and when with a stranger, thus permitting measurement of such positive attachment behaviors as heightened proximity-seeking and contact-maintaining behaviors during the reunions. Infants also show anger, resistance, or avoidance, are easy or difficult to comfort, have their play greatly or slightly disrupted, and so on. Use of the Strange Situation is appropriate for infants between 9 months and 2 years.[4]

Before turning directly to studies using the Strange Situation or returning to the theory of what attachment is, it may be useful to examine the question of the validity of stranger anxiety as a measure of attachment. Ainsworth (1973) concludes that stranger anxiety is not a valid measure of developing attachment because (a) not all babies who are attached to their mothers display fear of strangers with any consistency, and (b) stranger anxiety first develops at a different time from other attachment measures and cannot therefore be part of the same process (Ainsworth cites six studies to support her claims). Not only is fear of strangers inconsistently found, but Ainsworth and Wittig (1969) found that strangers served to comfort some 1-year-olds by picking them up after the mother left. Some even protested when put down by the stranger and tried to maintain the contact by clinging to her. Other studies supporting Ainsworth's claims include those by Solomon and Décarie (1976) and Sroufe and Waters (1977). The latter found that infants who responded positively to strangers were consistent in doing so.

If fear of strangers is not fear of losing mother, then what is it? A plausible answer to this question is that it

is part of the general fear of the unknown that is typical of infants. Such general fear seems to be a biologically adaptive response. It is found in chimpanzees (Hebb & Riesen, 1943), rhesus monkeys (Harlow, 1958), and many other species (see Bronson, 1968; Sluckin, 1965). This explanation also accounts for the lack of stranger anxiety in some babies. If a baby encounters many strangers daily, he or she will not see them as strange, and they will not elicit fear. For example, one baby kept in his mother's campus office three days a week for the first 9 months of his life experienced dozens of strangers weekly, both in her office and around campus. During this period he never exhibited stranger anxiety. On one occasion, at a party attended by about 50 adults, he spent most of the time surrounded by strangers at the opposite end of a large room from his mother. The only stranger anxiety he ever exhibited was when he was left with an older adult (strange person) in the stranger's yard (strange setting).

But what about attachment? Its significance as measured by behaviors such as protest at separation and proximity seeking has also been questioned. These behaviors, say the critics, may be valid as measures of the onset of attachment, but they do not fulfill our requirements of a construct. If there were such a construct as attachment, infants who scored high on one measure (e.g., protest at separation) should also score high on other measures (e.g., proximity seeking). Furthermore, infants should exhibit long-term stability (e.g., infants who show high proximity seeking at 10 months should do so at 18 months). Finally, infants who are strongly attached in one context, such as under the stress of an unfamiliar situation, should show that same strong attachment in other contexts, such as at home. None of these is the case. Critics have suggested that it makes no sense to call some infants more attached than others. The only appropriate use of attachment measures is to study the influence of the environment on specific behaviors within the mother-infant pair (Cairns, 1972; Gewirtz, 1972a, 1972b; Rosenthal, 1973).

In direct opposition to the above views are those of Ainsworth (1972, 1973, 1974) and Sroufe (1979; Sroufe & Waters, 1977). They agree that attachment as measured by the behaviors described above is not a stable individual trait, but they argue that this should not lead us to conclude there is no such construct as attachment. Attachment has meaning beyond the specific behaviors studied, they say, but only if one conceptualizes both its meaning and the way one measures it differently from that of an internal personality trait. It is not a characteristic of an individual in-

---

4. Recent early work using newly available measures of stress hormones (salivary cortisol) indicates that a 30-minute separation from the mother produces an elevation compared with play with the mother (Larson et al., 1991). It would be interesting to see if the separations used in the Strange Situation have an effect.

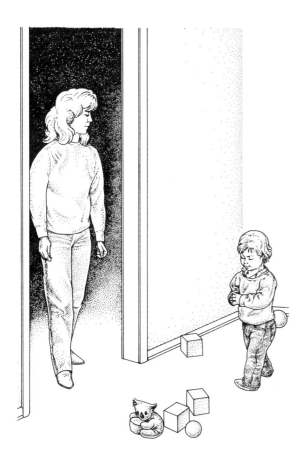

Figure 12.2. The ambivalent reactions some toddlers (12- to 18-month-olds) have when their mothers return after a brief absence. This toddler is approaching his mother (a positive reaction), but his head is turned down (a negative reaction).

fant, but of an infant's interactions with a particular individual. Second, the reality of the attachment lies not in specific behaviors, even if positive, but rather in qualitative patterns of behaviors.

To get away from counts of specific behaviors that occur in the Strange Situation and to tap the qualitative patterns, Ainsworth and her colleagues developed a tripartite classification scheme for patterns of attachment (Ainsworth et al., 1971; Ainsworth & Wittig, 1969; S. M. Bell, 1970). In this scheme, **securely attached** infants (about 70%) exhibit increased positive reunion behaviors with few proximity-avoiding, angry, or resistant behaviors. **Resistant** (or ambivalently attached) infants (about 10%) show heightened positive reunion behaviors, but in addition display angry, resistant behaviors (e.g., kicking, hitting, and pushing). When reunited with their mothers, **avoidant** infants (about 20%) avoid and ignore them or mix avoiding and approach behav-

iors, for example, moving toward the mother, then stopping and looking away (see Figure 12.2).

This approach espoused by Ainsworth and Sroufe predicts that the three qualitatively different patterns of reunion behavior should be stable, although the more discrete behaviors are not. Infants who are securely attached at 12 months should still be securely attached at 18 months if their living situations have been stable. Waters (1978) found that 48 out of 50 infants remained in the same attachment category, even though they did not show stability on concrete behaviors. For example, a particular avoidant infant may have turned her head away when picked up at 12 months and not at 18 months. She may have ignored her mother at 18 months, but not at 12 months. Both turning one's head away and ignoring mother are avoidant, but in different ways, and the infant would have been classified as stably avoidant. Although the stability Waters found is truly impressive, it must be interpreted carefully. Waters deliberately selected as subjects babies from advantaged, stable, middle-class homes. Only 62 of 100 economically disadvantaged babies tested were assigned to the same class at both 12 and 18 months (Vaughn et al., 1979). Infants who changed from secure to anxious attachments came from higher-stress homes than those who exhibited stable secure patterns. Thompson et al. (1982; see also Thompson & Lamb, 1984) reported similar findings. They correlated stability in attachment to changes in family circumstances within a broad range of middle-class families (from semiskilled workers to professionals). Only 53% of their infants were in the same attachment category at both 12 and 19 months. Changes in attachment classification were more common for babies whose mothers took jobs, although these babies were as likely to go from insecure to secure attachment as vice versa. The authors suggest that maternal employment requires renegotiation of the mother-infant relationship, which could be for better or for worse.

The above-cited studies on stability of attachment, considered together, show that (a) the tripartite classification of babies' *patterns* of attachment leads to more stability of measurement than do measures of individual behaviors, but (b) although there is substantial stability, there is also substantial instability when infants' life situations are changed. This state of affairs is common in the study of stability of children's behaviors, be they those of attachment or those assessed by the MDI or DQ. Usually when researchers argue that a behavioral pattern or trait is stable, they mean that children show more stability than we would expect on the basis of chance alone. They do not mean that all individuals are stable.

The tripartite classification of quality of attachment suggests other hypotheses. A few that have been supported experimentally are as follows:

(1) Securely attached infants exhibit more friendly, cooperative behaviors toward peers and adults (Pastor, 1980).
(2) Securely attached infants exhibit less fear of strangers than do ambivalent or avoidant infants (Sroufe, 1977).
(3) The negative feelings avoidant infants have toward their mothers interfere with the infants' seeking and maintaining contact with them. Avoidant infants played with their mothers during the initial period before their mothers left, but their play did not include expressions of emotion, expressions one would expect in babies who feel securely attached (Waters et al., 1979).

All of the measures of reactions to mothers' leaving and returning—protest at separation, positive reunion behaviors, and qualitatively different patterns of reunion behaviors—have been used successfully in research concerning the role of attachment in infants' development and in its relation to maternal variables hypothesized to be important to the development of the mother-infant relationship. Unfortunately, these different measures of attachment often yield different conclusions about the same hypothesis.

Subsequent to the early work, the three basic types of attachment have been broken down into subtypes: two types of avoidant, two types of resistant, four types of secure, and a new type, **disorganized** (see Main & Solomon, 1986). This discussion will use the original tripartite labels without specifying subtypes unless they are the basic point of the research. Many studies also combine avoidant and resistant infants into one group called "insecurely attached" and compare them with securely attached infants.

A behavioral system as derived from ethology should have a CNS control mechanism for regulating the behaviors of the system. This aspect of attachment has not been explored until recently. For example, Fox and others have been looking at different patterns of EEG activity in relation to infants' behavior in stranger-approach, mother-approach, and mother-leave situations (e.g., Fox & Davidson, 1987). Another example is work looking at heart rate correlates of both infant and maternal reactions in the Strange Situation (e.g., Donovan & Leavitt, 1985). This promising approach is still in its infancy.

Challenges to the Concept of Attachment

Attachment, as we have seen, is conceptualized as resulting from the infant's interactions with another person (mother, father, or other). However, some have proposed that it really is, or reflects, a temperamental characteristic of the infant. Sroufe (1985) reviewed a great deal of evidence counter to this hypothesis. The facts that infants have different types of attachments to different people and that attachment classification is unstable when life circumstances change were viewed as in favor of the interaction view or counter to the temperament view. However, temperament could be made to account for these differences. It is not usually seen as immutable, and some studies find relatively little difference between attachment to mother and to father. In fact, a recent meta-analysis of 11 studies that assessed attachment to both mothers and fathers found that assignment as secure/insecure was similar for the two parents, as was assignment to types of insecurity and to subtypes of security (Fox et al., 1991).

Belsky and Rovine (1987) have tried to achieve a rapprochement between the temperament and interaction views of infant attachment behaviors by redividing the categories according to subcategories. However, other work from the same laboratory complicates the interpretation of the subdivisions (Braungart et al., 1990). During separation avoidant infants appeared more distressed than, but engaged in as much toy play as, B1 and B2 secure infants. They were less distressed than B3s and B4s, and played significantly longer with the toys, but showed similar amounts of negative affect. In short, different B classifications were more or less similar to avoidant or resistant classifications, a result the researchers felt stemmed from temperamental differences.

Finally, Jones (1985, 1987) has challenged the idea that attachment is a unitary phenomenon or concept. She has pitted exploratory motivation against attachment motivation and found that different aspects of contacting the mother are affected. Although her 1987 studies replicated her 1985 findings, it is too early to fit this work into the total picture.

THE FUNCTIONS OF ATTACHMENT

The discussion thus far has addressed what attachment is and how it develops. Attachment is obviously an area of great interest and concern for parents, who find their children's developing love to be exciting and rewarding. It also serves some very important roles in children's development, and it has stimulated a great deal of research.

The Theoretical Context

Attachment is a biological mechanism for survival. The theory of evolution tells us that those organisms that manage to produce offspring that in turn survive to reproduce are more successful because their genes survive across generations. The famous phrase *survival of the fittest* refers to the survival of an organism's genes and therefore of that organism's species. Successful adaptation, then, requires that organisms survive until they are old enough to mate and then that they mate successfully and parent in such a way as to maximize the probability that their offspring will survive.

One important difference among species is the extent to which learning plays a role in the life of the individual. For example, mating and parenting behaviors are instinctive in some species, but must be learned in others. In some bird species, individuals raised from birth to reproductive age in isolation from others of their species are able to mate and parent normally. But rhesus monkeys raised in isolation are unable to mate and parent normally, which means that they need to learn something in their own life spans to enable them to engage in these basic functions. Those species for which extensive learning is necessary typically are born at a quite immature stage of development and have long childhoods. In contrast, those species in which the basic behavioral systems are "prewired" or innate typically are born better able to fend for themselves and have short childhoods.

Basic behavioral systems (such as mating and raising young) that can involve learning or are modifiable are biologically adaptive traits, because many species have so evolved. But the long period of immaturity after birth poses substantial survival risks to the offspring. Perhaps the biggest danger in the wild for both humans and other animals is the threat of predators. While predators are not a major problem in most modern human cultures, substantial threats to survival exist for toddlers in the forms of mechanical/electrical monsters, such as cars, electrical outlets, stoves, and hot water faucets, and chemical monsters, such as lye, bleach, insecticides, pills, and lead paint. One role of caretakers is to protect babies from such dangers. Babies' attachments to their mothers serve to help their mothers provide such protection. Attached offspring are secure near mother and afraid when far from her. Therefore, they tend to stay close to mother, where she can protect them, particularly in new, strange surroundings. This desire for maintaining proximity develops at the time infants are beginning to locomote and do not yet know what is dangerous. Thus it is maximally adaptive.

Functions During Infancy

As noted earlier, relatively little research has been concerned with the infant prior to the locomotor stage of development, except to look at mother-infant interactions then in relation to later measured attachment. The biological functions discussed in the section above indicate that the sucking, crying, smiling, and clinging behaviors Bowlby saw as relevant to attachment during early infancy serve to see that the infant receives food and necessary care to survive.

Secure Base for Laboratory (Outside the Home) Exploration. In the locomotor period attachment figures function as secure bases for exploration. Because learning is very important in animals with long childhoods, it is important for babies to explore in order to learn. But if toddlers were to explore far and wide without maternal supervision, they would encounter increased threats to their survival. The attachment relationship serves as an effective device because it provides a way to balance exploration with security needs. Novel situations often elicit fear in toddlers, which is reduced by the security provided by a mother to whom the infant is attached. This allows the infants to explore strange situations. Thus we would expect toddlers to explore a strange, presumably anxiety-invoking situation more readily when the mother is present than when she is not. This phenomenon has been well established in different contexts and in different groups, including humans (Ainsworth & Bell, 1970; Arsenian, 1943; Cox & Campbell, 1968; Gershaw & Schwartz, 1971; Lester et al., 1974; Maccoby & Feldman, 1972; Rheingold, 1969; Rheingold & Eckerman, 1970; Ross et al., 1975; Schaffer & Emerson, 1964), monkeys (Harlow & Zimmerman, 1959), and chimpanzees (Bard, 1991). This pattern develops in the second half of the first year of life, or in what has been called the locomotor period (Ainsworth, 1974), and is waning by the second birthday (Cox & Campbell, 1968). This is why the use of the Strange Situation is appropriate only within that age frame. Furthermore, infants show less wariness of strangers (and hence can explore relationships with them) in standard stranger-approach studies when near their mothers or on their laps (Bronson, 1972; Campos et al., 1975; Morgan & Ricciuti, 1969).

When mother is present, the basic pattern of exploration (monkey and human) is an alternation between exploring the environment and a kind of checking in with mother, which may involve eye contact, proximity, or clinging. The confidence with which toddlers explore new situations when their mothers are present is both delightful and somewhat surprising. Toddlers often move away from their mothers immediately after they enter strange environments; an infant will often leave the room the mother is sitting in to explore neighboring areas, and may even allow the mother to go into a nearby room, out of sight and hearing, especially if the child has something interesting to explore.

It seems clear that in such situations infants leave their mothers in order to explore. Rheingold and Eckerman (1969) had mothers sit in a small unfurnished room that adjoined a larger unfurnished room (called the "open field" room). All 24 of the 10-month-old infants left the mother's room without fussing or crying. When a toy was in the open field room, the children spent less time with their mothers than when there was no toy. Children who had access to three toys, rather than one, in the open field room went further from their mothers and stayed away longer. In short, the more there was to explore, the more time the infants spent away from their mothers exploring.

When the mothers left their infants in the first room, either with or without a toy, those without a toy quickly followed their mothers and reached the threshold between rooms in an average of 23 seconds. Infants with a toy took 215 seconds (Corter et al., 1972). When an infant in the toy group did go to the mother, the infant touched her more quickly (average latency to touch was 69 seconds compared with 123 seconds for the no-toy group). It appears that the infants' desire to explore the toy was powerful enough to delay following, but when they followed they seemed more intent on making contact. The no-toy babies seemed, in contrast, to be following mother to find stimulation; they were not eager to establish or to maintain physical contact.

Ross et al. (1972) found that 12-month-old infants preferred going to a room with a novel toy over going to a room with a familiar toy. The infants spent more time with the novel toy and spent relatively little time in contact with their mothers (averages were 66 and 76 seconds out of 5 minutes for each of two trials); however, there were great individual differences (range 1 to 198 seconds on trial 1 and 15 to 262 seconds on trial 2). It is unfortunate that these individual differences were not examined in relation to differences in attachment classifications. Securely attached infants might be expected to spend less time with their mothers.

In these studies, the exploration carried out by toddlers seems remarkably courageous. They leave their mothers, and even tolerate their mothers' moving out of sight and hearing, with remarkably little anxiety. The more interesting the environment, the more readily the infant leaves the mother. Nonetheless, these studies show only one side of the coin—the high-quality exploration that occurs when mother is nearby or easily reachable. Conditions that emotionally stress infants decrease their exploration and increase their need for their mothers. For example, in the paradigm described above, when a strange person, rather than a toy, was in the adjoining room, infants were much less likely to enter that room. Of 10 infants in the person group, 5 entered, compared with 9 of 10 in the toy group (Eckerman & Rheingold, 1974). Those infants in the stranger group who entered the second room did so much more slowly.

In an even more stressful situation, when a stranger confronted the infants in the same room, 12-month-olds tended to move toward their mothers and visually explore the stranger from that "safe" vantage point (Bretherton & Ainsworth, 1974; Feldman & Ingham, 1975). Those few infants who were brave enough to touch the stranger were highly likely to run back to their mothers immediately afterward (Bretherton & Ainsworth, 1974).

When toddlers experience successive anxiety-arousing experiences, there is a cumulative effect. Ainsworth and Bell (1970) found that the amount of exploration 1-year-olds exhibited decreased when a stranger entered the room in which mother and infant had been playing, declined further when mother left the room, revived somewhat when mother returned, but declined to a new low when the mother left for a second time, and did not revive when she returned. This situation was taken advantage of in the design of the Strange Situation.

The developed attachment relationship is what provides the security. Rheingold (1969) showed that when the mother was gone, neither toys nor the presence of a stranger encouraged exploration any more than an empty room. Overt signs of support from the mother are not necessary. Carr et al. (1975) found that toddlers 18-30 months of age played with toys more if their mothers were readily in visual contact (seated on the other side of the toys rather than behind the child or behind a screen). They did not actually interact with their mothers more when they were in sight, but having the opportunity evidently gave them the necessary base from which to explore the toys in the room.

Secure Base for Home Exploration. The above-mentioned reports concern laboratory behaviors. Secure attachment as measured by the Strange Situation was originally shown to be related to secure-base behaviors in the home, but this was not studied again until recently. To report the recent findings, I must first note that Waters has developed another methodology that can be used to assess attachment.

Another measure of attachment: The Q-sort. The **Q-sort** is a psychometric technique for assigning ratings of a large number of items to a seminormal distribution. In the Attachment Q-set, 90 or 100 items of behavior are sorted into nine piles depending on the degree to which they are characteristic of an infant's behavior. This can be done by the researcher on the basis of home or laboratory observations or by the mother or teachers on the bases of their total observations of the infant (for a discussion and description, see Waters & Deane, 1985). The Attachment Q-set can be scored for security, dependency, and sociability (current version, Waters, 1989). Using this methodology, infants classified as secure in the Strange Situation had higher scores on security and sociability on the Q-set than did insecure infants (Vaughn & Waters, 1990). They differed on security after statistical controls for sociability were applied, but they did not differ on dependency, thus enhancing Bowlby's view that attachment and dependency are different. The specific items that discriminated are consistent with the Bowlby/Ainsworth conceptualization of the secure-base phenomenon (see Waters et al., 1990).

While Waters and his colleagues describe this technique as an adjunct to the Strange Situation, it seems well worth using independently.[5] Q-sort methodology offers the advantage that items appropriate to any age level can be developed, whereas the Strange Situation may not be appropriate after the age of 2 years. It is a technique that has possibly been underused in developmental psychology (see Block, 1961/1978). It has many advantages over rating scales and behavior coding in terms of focusing observers on details of behavior in ways that may be analogous to the process of moving from the specific behaviors noted in the Strange Situation to the classifications (Pederson et al., 1990).

Attachment Figures as Playmates. The third function attachment figures serve in infancy is that of providing a source of stimulation—being a playmate. For example, in a study described earlier (Corter et al., 1972), the babies in the toy group apparently followed their mothers to touch base—that is, for security reasons—but the no-toy babies seemed to be seeking stimulation from their mothers.

The playmate relationship of toddlers to their mothers is demonstrated by the fact that they share toys with their mothers. In a study by Rheingold et al. (1976), three related kinds of behavior were exhibited frequently: (a) showing by pointing or holding up an object, (b) giving (i.e., putting an object in a person's hand or lap), and (c) manipulating an object the child had given the adult, who was still in contact with it. In a 10-minute period 15- and 18-month-old toddlers showed and gave objects approximately six times and engaged in partner play about three times. These data suggest that toddlers use their mothers not only as secure bases for exploration, but also as playmates.[6] It has not yet been clearly demonstrated that such sharing is necessarily an aspect of differential attachment to a particular person rather than simply one facet of social development. Nevertheless, there is some support for the idea that sharing is related to attachment. In one of the experiments, children shared more with fathers (to whom specific attachments have also formed) than with strangers.

An interesting light is shed on the functions of attachment by findings from the Gusii tribe in Kenya, in which infants are cared for primarily by child caretakers. These infants are securely attached to both their caretakers and their mothers (54% and 61%, respectively). Kermoian and Leiderman (1986) found that those securely attached to their mothers (the primary feeders) had better nutritional status, and those securely attached to their child caretakers had higher scores on the Bayley MDI.

The playmate role of mother can be fulfilled by others. Harris et al. (1991) have shown that whether baby-sitters are given the role of caretakers or of baby-sitters affects the stress responses of 9-month-old infants. Neither signs of negative affect nor the cortisol levels of infants were increased over what they were with their mothers *if* the adults they were with had the role of playmate, but were higher if the adults' role was that caretaker.

In summary, three functions of attachment that operate during the period of infancy are as follows: (a) It keeps infants close to their mothers, who provide safety; (b) it enables babies to explore the inanimate

---

5. The Attachment Q-set has recently been used for diverse purposes. Parents' ratings for ideal attachment have been compared with a theory-based standard and found similar (Goff & Britt, 1990). Maternal Attachment Q-set sorts have been used to compare attachment in Down syndrome infants with that in normally developing infants (Hron-Stewart et al., 1989). There is considerable evidence that the Strange Situation may not be appropriate for use with Down infants because of their lower levels of arousal. A good description of differences in emotional responses can be found in Thompson et al. (1985), although they found the Strange Situation useful.

6. This could be seen as analogous to the role of mother-infant interaction in language acquisition, as discussed in the previous chapter.

world within that safe context; and (c) it affords an opportunity for the attachment figure to provide stimulation through playful interactions.

LONG-TERM CONSEQUENCES OF ATTACHMENT

None of the functions of attachment discussed above addresses the belief, important to clinicians and evolutionists, that the early maternal-infant relationship forms the basis for all later interpersonal relationships. For Freud and Erikson, attachment served as the prototype for all later personal relationships (of which mating and parenting are the most important). For evolutionary theorists, attachment is what allows the young to learn the social interactions necessary for later mating and parenting. Bowlby shared this view and has been extremely important in promulgating these beliefs.

These views all assume a critical period: Events that occur within a restricted period of infancy (the first year of life for Freud and Erikson; from 6 months to 1½ years for Bowlby) have permanent, long-term consequences, and the period of susceptibility or sensitivity is determined by biological mechanisms. Freud and Erikson both believed that reliving infancy experiences in therapy could undo or ameliorate the bad effects. Erikson also believed that, while basic trust is most easily developed during infancy, negative outcomes from infancy could be overcome by a good environment in later stages. Thus attachment (effects induced over a relatively long time span and not necessarily lasting) can be seen as related to a **sensitive period** hypothesis as distinguished from the less flexible, more permanent notions of a critical period.

Most research designed to test hypotheses concerning long-term consequences of attachment has used the strategy of studying children deprived of their mothers, and has not tested specific personality outcomes. This research, together with some tests of critical period hypotheses, is discussed in Chapter 13.

After Ainsworth (1985) developed her tripartite classification of the quality of attachment, a frequent research strategy was to follow children for 1 to 2 years after they had been classified (usually between 12 and 18 months). The criterion behaviors measured at the time of follow-up have varied widely across the few studies and at present do not provide a coherent picture of exactly what sorts of cognitive, emotional, and social characteristics are related to quality of attachment. These studies do, however, consistently show relations of some variables to quality of attachment.

Several research findings indicate the kinds of vari-

ables for which relations have been found. Main (1973) found that infants securely attached at 12 months had higher Bayley scores at 21 months than did resistant children (avoidant children were in between). Resistant children also showed less intense play with toys, more restless changing of activity, and less enjoyment than the other two groups (as is typically true of play within the Strange Situation). Matas et al. (1978) found that securely attached 2-year-olds clearly enjoyed a situation that called for problem solving using a standard set of tools. These children followed instructions easily, and, when frustrated by failure, seldom cried, fussed, or became angry. When they needed help, they asked nearby adults with little discomfort. Insecurely attached infants (either avoidant or resistant) became frustrated easily, reacted strongly to the frustration, and quickly gave up trying to solve the problems. They seldom asked for help, even when they needed it, and ignored or rejected directions from adults. In a study by Waters et al. (1979), nursery school children (3½-year-olds) securely attached as infants tended to be social leaders—they initiated and participated actively in group activities and were sought out by other children. Teachers rated them as curious, eager to learn, and more self-directed and forceful than others. Insecurely attached children were more likely to be socially withdrawn and to hesitate about participating in activities. Teachers rated them as less curious and less forceful in pursuit of their activities. Lutkenhaus et al. (1985) found that 3-year-olds securely attached as infants interacted more smoothly with strangers. If they failed in a competitive game, they were likely to increase their effort, whereas the insecurely attached decreased theirs. This replicates Matas et al.'s (1978) findings with 2-year-olds. Maternal, but not paternal, attachment has been found to be slightly related to the breadth of interests and behaviors in emotional situations in late childhood, but Grossmann (1989) has found that the relations for boys are very different from those for girls. Sex differences have also been found in predictability of psychopathology at age 6 from attachment at age 1, according to Lewis et al. (1984). Insecurely attached males (but not females) showed more psychopathology than securely attached males; however, demographic and life-stress variables were important.

Clearly, there are many later differences between securely and insecurely attached children. Notice, however, that most of the differences found in the studies cited above have been between securely attached infants and the two groups of insecurely attached infants. Few long-term differences have yet been found between avoidant and resistant infants, even though as infants and toddlers they appear quite different.

Until the advent of the Q-sort technique there was no way to look for relations between attachment in infancy and that in childhood. Using it, Main and Cassidy (1987) developed a coding for reunion behaviors of 6-year-olds with their mothers after a one-hour separation that shows remarkable stability from infancy to age 6 (Main & Cassidy, 1988), a result that has been replicated in Germany (Wartner & Grossmann, 1987). The long-term stability does not answer the question of whether it is caused by concurrent maternal behaviors or earlier attachment and antecedent maternal behaviors.

Remember that correlations do not prove causality. It may be that secure attachment provides the basis for later positive development, as proposed by the Freudians and others. But it is just as likely that mothers whose parenting behaviors produce secure attachment in infancy continue to behave in successful ways when their children are preschoolers. Thus maternal behaviors at later ages may be the cause of later good development. Indeed, attachment at age 6 is related to maternal behaviors (from extensive home observations) at that age. Solomon et al. (1987) found that security is related to mothers' current supportive acceptance and active encouragement of learning and competence in the home; ambivalence is related to their overinvolvement, indulgence, and discouragement of independence; and avoidance is related to their rejection, hostility, and discouragement of dependence. Of course, it also may be that maternal behaviors are not causal variables in themselves. Babies who are easy and rewarding to take care of may encourage responsivity, acceptance, and even sensitivity in their mothers, as discussed in Chapter 6 and later in this chapter. Thus the stability of these behaviors might be caused by infants' stable temperamental characteristics or by the interaction of these characteristics with their mothers' rearing preferences and techniques, rather than by any specific infant-care techniques mothers or other caretakers might have used.

MOTHERS' ROLE IN THE DEVELOPMENT OF ATTACHMENT

Most of the research exploring this question has focused, naturally enough, on the role mothers play in determining the degree and quality of their infants' attachment. The three systems that have been most studied are sucking-feeding, contact comfort, and maternal sensitivity or responsivity. Each is discussed in turn below.

Sucking-Feeding

The maternal-infant interaction that both Freudian and learning theories hypothesized to be crucial in the development of infants' love for their mothers is the feeding situation. Certainly young infants spend a large proportion of their waking hours feeding, and mothers spend much of their caretaking time in feeding interactions. Two related hypotheses are derived from these theories. One is that the person who feeds the infant should be the object of attachment: If mother is not the primary food provider, then she will not be the primary object of the infant's affection. Freudian theory stresses the idea that a mother who provides either too much or too little sucking gratification disrupts the quality of her infant's attachment and emotional health. Weaning, in Freudian theory, is a time of major crisis for infants, because the gratification of their sucking need is threatened, and thus the severity and suddenness of weaning should affect the quality of the attachment relationship.

Schaffer and Emerson (1964) provide evidence (expanding on that presented in Chapter 6) on the limited role of feeding. They conducted a short-term longitudinal study of 60 normal working-class infants from intact families in Glasgow, Scotland. Infants were studied every 4 weeks until 1 year of age and again at 18 months. Attachment was measured both by direct observation and by mothers' reports of infants' reactions to normally occurring separations. In the direct observation, a stranger made a six-step graduated approach to the infant, starting with appearing in the infant's visual range but doing nothing else and ending with picking up the infant and placing him or her on his knee. Mothers were asked about their infants' reactions to seven situations: (a) being left alone in a room, (b) being left with other people, (c) being left in a baby carriage outside the house, (d) being left in a carriage outside shops, (e) being left in a crib at night, (f) being put down after being held in an adult's arms or lap, and (g) being passed by while in a crib or chair. Scores on the two measures agreed 92% of the time. Mothers were also interviewed about their socialization practices with respect to feeding, weaning, and toilet training. (Toilet training is related to development in the second year of life in psychoanalytic theory.) The feeding and weaning variables were not related to intensity of attachment as indexed by the researchers' measures. Schaffer and Emerson also failed to find relations between attachment and toilet training variables. These data do not support Freudian theory or attachment theory, but, combined with the evidence on sucking and oral behaviors in Chapter 6, they make it unlikely that sucking-feeding plays a key role in later development.

Contact Comfort

A second variable that has been compared with feeding as a major determinant of attachment by people who are either ethologically oriented or who have been influenced by Harlow's research is **contact comfort** (or comforting tactile contact between mother and child). Ethologists have noted that in many primate species the young spend much time clinging to their mothers and that this often serves an adaptive purpose in allowing mothers to move around without needing to provide much support for their babies. While human infants do not need to cling to survive, they nevertheless do cuddle. Remember that cuddling is a behavior measured on the NBAS (Chapter 8). Advocates of Leboyer deliveries and those who believe in maternal bonding emphasize the value of skin-to-skin contact immediately after birth. And advocates of breast-feeding often talk about the importance of the body contact involved. There are two specific hypotheses one would like to test, as was true for feeding. One is that contact comfort is necessary for the development of attachment; the second is that the quality of contact comfort or cuddling is related to the quality of attachment.

Trying to test these, or other, hypotheses concerning the role of the mother in attachment is very difficult. Researchers cannot randomly assign human babies to different maternal rearing conditions and watch the results. We can, however, do experimental animal studies and compare their results with those obtained from correlational studies using humans. Fortunately, findings from the two kinds of studies fit together nicely, and so we can have more confidence in our conclusions than is often the case when we have only correlational studies with humans.

The animal research, done primarily with rhesus macaque monkeys, was begun by Harry and Margaret Kuenne Harlow. Rhesus monkeys are a good choice for this research because, like humans, they are mammals, and their infants are born singly and in an immature state that requires substantial maternal care. Furthermore, their intellectual and emotional systems are highly complex and vulnerable to environmental deprivation.

To manipulate the role the mother plays in the development of attachment, the Harlows built surrogate monkey mothers that were essentially angled stands (see Figure 12.3). Surrogates could have nipples or not (be feeders or not), and they could be covered with terry cloth or made of wire (provide contact

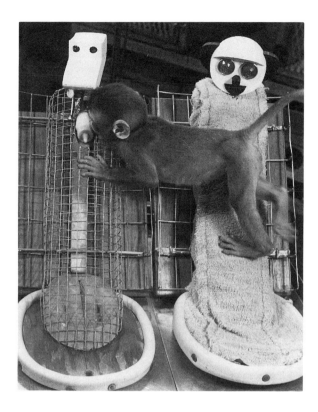

Figure 12.3. Surrogate mothers used in Harlow's studies of the development of attachment in baby rhesus monkeys. The baby can choose either the soft nonfeeding mother or the wire feeding mother. She spends most of her time on the soft mother who cannot feed her and becomes attached only to it. (Photograph courtesy of the University of Wisconsin Primate Laboratory.)

comfort or not). Both feeding and contact comfort played roles. If baby monkeys had access to two surrogate mothers, one with a working nipple and one without, they spent more time on the feeding mother. If the babies had available a terry cloth and a wire mother, they spent more time on the terry cloth mother. But which was more important, food or contact comfort?

To determine this, the researchers provided baby monkeys with a wire mother with a nipple and a cloth mother with no nipple, so that they had to choose between their pleasures—food or contact comfort. The babies overwhelmingly chose contact comfort. They would stay on the nonfeeding cloth mother for most of the time, switching to the wire mother only to feed. If they could reach, they would stay on the cloth mother even when feeding (see Figure 12.3).

Is the amount of time spent clinging an adequate measure of attachment? Even baby monkeys might

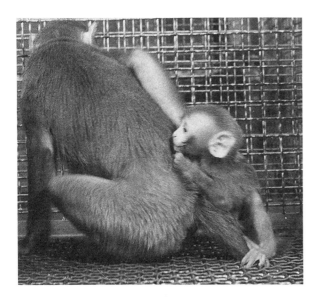

Figure 12.4. A monkey mother who had been reared on a surrogate mother. Her baby clings to her, even though the mother tries to push the baby away. (Photograph courtesy of the University of Wisconsin Primate Laboratory.)

prefer a soft to a hard seat, and yet that might not be attachment. Luckily, Harlow and Harlow went on to measure the infants' use of their surrogate mothers as bases for exploration. They put the infants and the "mothers" into a strange room filled with many scary things, such as a wooden block, a doorknob, and a cootie toy. Monkeys raised with cloth mothers or with both cloth and wire mothers would rush to their cloth mothers and cling, subsequently venturing out to explore. They derived no comfort from the wire feeding mother and would cower in a corner and act as if no mother at all were there. Even infants who had known only a nursing wire mother from birth derived no comfort from her in this open-field test. Finally, babies who had nursing and nonnursing mothers showed no long-term preference between the two (although they did show preference for the nursing mother prior to 100 days of age). Thus it is clear that the nursing aspect of mothering did not provide an adequate basis for the development of the secure base phenomenon (remember Benjamin's data on sucking in Chapter 6).

The attachment these infant monkeys developed to their cloth mothers was maintained even after long separations. One group was separated from the surrogate mothers at 180 days of life, and they still showed positive responses to them at 2 years. Thus, for rhesus monkeys, it appears that nursing plays only a small role in the initial development of attachment and is of no

importance to its longer-term function as a secure base for exploration. Contact comfort, in contrast, is a powerful and long-term influence on the monkey infants' developing bond. That contact comfort is so powerful a determinant of attachment in baby monkeys should not lead us to believe that there is nothing more to mothering than providing a soft surface. Contact comfort was sufficient to establish attachment; it was not sufficient to enable development into normal adults. When cloth-reared monkeys grew up, they were unable to mate properly, and if a female was made pregnant, she was unable to mother properly. Figure 12.4 shows such a mother rejecting her offspring.

The relative importance of feeding and contact comfort, then, is quite clear in the case of monkeys, but what about humans? One of the very early observers of infant development, Tiedemann (1787/1927), noticed a similar relation between feeding and nonfeeding caretakers:

> Whenever the weather permitted, his nurse took him out upon the streets, which gave him inordinate pleasure and a great desire for this type of diversion, despite the cold air. Therefore, he was loath to leave his nurse, and even preferred her to his mother except when he was hungry. (p. 217)

Exploring the role of contact comfort in humans is complicated, both theoretically and methodologically. On purely theoretical grounds, one might expect contact comfort to be more important in monkeys than in humans. Rhesus monkeys cling to their mothers' bodies so strongly that the mother needs only one limb to support the young infant when she is traveling through the trees. Clinging in humans does not have direct survival value, since mothers provide full support for their infants when the pair move through space. In our culture infants spend less of their time in contact with their mothers than in many cultures. In contemporary Western cultures babies typically sleep in cribs or carriages, separated from their parents, and spend much of their waking time in infant seats, playpens, and other devices that do not promote contact. Methodologically, it is difficult to investigate contact comfort in humans, since experimenters would not deny tactile contact to human infants to satisfy their intellectual curiosity.[7] Therefore, when we study

---

7. Indeed, in one of Harlow's samples of isolated monkeys, their behaviors were rather normal. It was later discovered that a student caretaker had felt sorry for them and had taken them out at night and played with them.

contact comfort in humans, we cannot compare its presence to its absence. Since all humans, generally speaking, are soft, all infants in the normal process of caretaking are exposed to what is probably adequate contact comfort. We can study the amount and quality of contact comfort infants receive experimentally through an analog study. That is, when a study one would like to do is too difficult or ethically impossible to do, an **analog study** (one that is somewhat similar) may be done.

Roedell and Slaby (1977) did an analog study of the development of 5-month-old infants' relationships with female strangers during eight sessions spread out over three weeks. The infants' reactions to the roles played by three different women, seen one at a time, were evaluated. One woman (called the proximal interacter) patted, rocked, and carried the infant around the room, but did not smile, speak, or play eye-contact games. Another, the distal interacter, did not touch the infant, but smiled at, talked to, played peekaboo with, and in other ways kept eye contact with the infant. The third woman was simply present and did not interact with the baby. Each of the women played each of the roles (with different babies), so that there was no confounding between individuals and roles; therefore effects were due to the roles, not to differences in the women's personalities. The infants' feelings toward the women were gauged by the amounts of time the infants spent near each of them. The amount of time spent near the distal interacter increased over the three weeks, while the amount of time near the proximal interacter decreased. The amount of time near the neutral interacter remained the same.

At first glance, the conclusions from this study seem directly opposite to those from the contact comfort work with monkeys. Like surrogate monkey "mothers," the proximal interacters did not respond socially, through visual or oral means, to the infants. They merely provided contact comfort. The human infants, however, were living in a world in which the normal behavior to be expected from adult "toys" is that they provide social interaction in a variety of ways, including talking to, looking at, and responding to the infant. Thus the proximal interacter violated the infants' expectations. We would not want to argue from these data that contact comfort is unimportant or undesirable, but that in the normal world of human infants, contact comfort takes place either when the infant signals a desire for it or when the mother deems it necessary, and is usually accompanied by other types of social interaction. Providing proximal contact when the baby neither wants it nor needs it might be aversive, at least when the infant has alternatives. In Har-

low and Harlow's monkey research, contact comfort and/or feeding were the only "social" responses the monkey infants received. It is therefore difficult to conclude that humans are less needful of or responsive to contact comfort. We can, however, study contact comfort in what is perhaps a more ecologically valid context (i.e., in a context more appropriate to the natural environment). In humans, the natural situation is when contact comfort provides a response to infants' signals for caretaking and/or attention and stimulation.

The importance of context, including social expectations, although recognized long before Roedell and Slaby's (1977) study, is suggested by it. Their major conclusion is that babies like to be near adults who socially interact with them. The relative ineffectiveness of the proximal interacters in their study can be attributed to two factors: (a) that contact comfort will be desirable to human infants only when it occurs in response to infants' needs for caretaking, comfort, and social interaction; and (b) contact comfort isolated from social interaction may so violate the infant's expectations as to be disturbing. In the attachment context these conclusions would suggest that babies become more (or more securely) attached to mothers who provide social stimulation. Furthermore, mothers' sensitivity and responsivity to their infants' needs should also be related to intensity and/or quality of their infants' attachment.

The ideal study to bridge the subjects of contact comfort and maternal sensitivity is a recent one by Anisfeld et al. (1990), in which a group of low-SES mothers were randomly assigned to receive either a soft baby carrier (Snugli), modeled on the way some African groups carry their babies (close chest-to-chest contact), or a plastic infant seat. All the mothers had agreed in advance to use whichever they received on a daily basis. The babies' times in various situations were determined, and pedometers also recorded the use of the Snuglis. At 3½ months the Snugli mothers were more contingently responsive to their infants' vocalizations, and at 13 months their infants were more likely to be securely attached than were those in the infant seat group—83% compared with 39%. The latter figure is similar to that of other studies of other low-SES infants. The use of the Snugli was significantly related to attachment even after differences in maternal sensitivity were statistically controlled for. Infant behaviors at 3½ months had also differed. Snugli infants looked more frequently at their mothers, and only half as many as in the control group had daily crying episodes at 2 months, but they smiled later. Infants in the two groups did not differ in their Bayley scores or in the number who were "difficult" on ratings of temperament. If these findings are replicated, they have profound implications for positive intervention in the lives of low-SES infants. Certainly no bonding studies have produced results of this magnitude.

Maternal Sensitivity/Responsivity

Mothers' 3½-month sensitivity scores were higher for the securely attached infants in the Anisfeld et al. (1990) study described above. This is a recent example of a long series of such findings. Schaffer and Emerson (1964) rated mothers on their tendencies to interact and to be responsive. Interaction referred to the mother's tendency to initiate interaction of any sort. Responsivity referred to the consistency and speed with which mothers responded to their infants' crying. Both variables were related to infants' intensity of attachment (e.g., mothers who were highly responsive tended to have babies who protested strongly to separation). The type of interaction—whether mothers initiated contact sports (picking up, fondling, and kissing), noncontact social interactions (talking, cooing, singing, smiling), or impersonal interactions (presenting toys, food, and other objects)—did not matter. What did matter was that the mother initiated interaction. Thus it appears that contact comfort is desirable when it serves the function of providing social stimulation, but that it is no more effective than other forms of social stimulation.

Subsequent studies have confirmed these findings using somewhat different maternal ratings and including Strange Situation measures of attachment. Ainsworth et al. (1971) rated mothers on four dimensions, all having to do in some way with sensitivity/responsivity:

(1) *Sensitivity-insensitivity:* Sensitive mothers perceive their infants' needs and respond to their signals. Insensitive mothers interact on their own schedules and according to their own needs.

(2) *Acceptance-rejection:* Accepting mothers in general accept the problems and limitations imposed by the responsibility of having an infant. While they sometimes become irritated with their babies, they generally enjoy the infants' good moods and accept their bad moods. Rejecting mothers feel so angry and resentful that these negative feelings outweigh their affection for their babies. These feelings may be expressed through complaints about the baby's irritating behaviors, frequent opposition to the infant's wishes, scolding, or all of these.

(3) *Cooperation-interference:* Cooperative mothers allow their babies autonomy and avoid interrupt-

ing their activities or exerting direct control. When they have to exert control, they try to do so in a way that will be congenial to the child. Interfering mothers impose their wills on their babies with little concern for their moods or current activities. They attempt to force the children to their standards, often doing so in an abrupt manner.

(4) *Accessibility-ignoring:* Accessible mothers pay attention to their infants' signals, even when distracted. Ignoring mothers are preoccupied with their own activities and thoughts. They do not notice their infants' signals, and tend to them only during scheduled times or when the infants demand it.

Mothers of securely attached 12-month-old infants scored above average on all four of these dimensions; they were sensitive, accepting, cooperative, and accessible. Mothers of avoidant infants were rejecting and insensitive; those of resistant (ambivalent) infants were rejecting and either interfering or ignoring (Ainsworth et al., 1971).

In a similar procedure carried out by Clarke-Stewart (1973), mothers' behaviors were rated on three dimensions when their babies were 11 months old. Responsiveness was indexed by the proportion of the infants' calls and cries to which the mothers responded. Expression of positive emotion was measured by the mother's frequency of affectionate touching, smiles, praise, and social speech per hour of her infant's waking life. Social stimulation was assessed by the average number of times the mother came close to, smiled at, talked to, or imitated the child per hour of the child's time awake. Thus the first dimension measured mother's responsivity, the second measured maternal warmth or acceptance, and the third measured mother as playmate. When the infants were 12 months old they were assessed with the Strange Situation and were classified into one of three patterns similar to those designated by Ainsworth. Consistent with many studies, securely attached babies had mothers who scored high on all three dimensions, while mothers of unattached and malattached infants (Clarke-Stewart's system) were low on all three dimensions.

Clarke-Stewart considered infants to be intensely attached if they frequently looked at, smiled at, stayed close to, followed, or gave objects to their mothers. Thus her measure is one of active interaction rather than of protest at separation. Mothers who received high scores on all three dimensions tended to have intensely attached babies.

Goldberg et al. (1986) have examined attachment of prematures in relation to mother-infant behaviors at

6 weeks and at 3, 6, and 9 months. Maternal, but not infant, behaviors at each of those ages was related to attachment classifications at 1 year. The least optimal behaviors were found in mothers whose infants became As (resistant) or Cs (avoidant), intermediate optimality for those infants classified in the secure attachment subcategories of B1 and B4, and most optimal for those who were B2s and B3s. One exception to this was that the least responsive mothers were more frequent in the marginally secure group (B1 and B4), not the As or Cs.

Because the relation of the mother's social support to security of attachment has been established primarily in lower-SES samples, Zaslow et al. (1988) examined the interactions of middle-class mothers with their infants in relation to attachment and support. They assessed mothers of 12-month-olds, twice when alone with their infants, and once with the fathers present. Mothers of avoidant infants had not differed in their interactions with their infants 2½ months earlier from those of secure infants when the father had been present, but they showed less playful interaction and more expression of negative affect, smiled less, and engaged in less mutual looking when alone with their infants than those of secure infants. For the 22% of babies who became avoidantly attached, being alone with mother may not be optimal.

A new aspect of attachment research is its extension to measuring attachment across the life span. One study relevant to infancy found that measures of adults' attachment were related to the behaviors of their infants in the Strange Situation (Crowell & Feldman, 1991).

The research reviewed above is impressive in that different ways of measuring maternal and infant characteristics have produced similar results. Nevertheless, it is problematic in that all the relationships found have been correlational. It would be nice to be able to make causal statements such as "Mothers who are sensitive provide good environments in which babies can establish secure attachments," but correlational data do not permit this. Researchers cannot do experimental research with humans, and manipulating maternal

sensitivity in monkey mothers would be extremely difficult.[8] One can, however, approach the problem in a different way. One can look at maternal characteristics or maternal reactions to infants in early infancy (prior to the development of attachment). Ainsworth and her colleagues have consistently found that ratings of maternal sensitivity early in infancy predict security of attachment when it subsequently develops (see, e.g., Ainsworth, 1973). Such findings make a causal explanation more plausible, but they still are not conclusive. Some babies might have ways of interacting that appeal to their mothers. These more appealing babies are then responded to more promptly, more often, and more positively. The ultimate cause of their subsequent secure attachment may be the babies' ability to reward their mothers, rather than the mothers' ability to respond to and stimulate them. There is also the possibility that characteristics of maternal interaction at the time of measuring attachment are what cause differences in attachment behaviors. (See also Grossmann et al., 1989.)

If we, like most researchers in this field, accept early maternal behaviors as causing attachment, we can draw some interesting conclusions about the importance of different maternal characteristics for the development of attachment. Whether and how mothers feed their babies and whether they spend a lot of time holding them do not seem to be important determinants of attachment. Rather, what seems to be important is whether mothers meet their babies' needs, not only of being kept fed, dry, and warm, but also of being stimulated, of having power over their environment by being able to get adults to respond to them, of being given autonomy of action, and of being accepted. Mothers who fulfill one of these latter needs also tend to fulfill the others.

The strength of the relation between maternal sensitivity and attachment security has been questioned subsequent to the work of Ainsworth and her colleagues (Goldsmith & Alansky, 1987; Lamb et al., 1985). However, Smith and Pederson (1988) correctly distinguished between securely and anxiously attached infants with 94% accuracy using maternal behaviors as predictor variables. Subsequently, Pederson et al.'s (1990) similar findings using Q-sort measures have reinforced the role of maternal sensitivity in producing secure attachment. In both of the above studies maternal sensitivity was assessed when the mother had competing tasks—a questionnaire to fill out and her child to monitor. The authors suggest that assessing sensitivity during play situations or face-to-face interactions, when all of the mother's attention is focused on the infant, may provide a less

---

8. One can imagine an analog study in monkeys in which surrogate mothers would be equipped with robotic capabilities such that they would respond with appropriate gestures of padded arms and head or body movements to appropriate auditory, tactile, and motor cues of infant monkeys. For example, an infant's approach might close a circuit (as happens in automatic doors) that would activate the surrogate's arms to reach out to hold the infant.

sensitive measure of her ability to tune in to her infant's needs.

However, studies assessing mother-infant interactions when mothers were instructed to go about their usual routines have also shown sensitivity to be related to later attachment classifications (Isabella & Belsky, 1991; Isabella et al., 1989). Insecure attachments have been related to asynchronous interactions at both 3 and 9 months. Mother-infant interactions involving infants who later were insecure-avoidant were shown to be high in co-occurrences suggestive of maternal intrusiveness, and the mothers tended to be overinvolved with their infants. The mother-infant interactions of future resistant infants were characterized by poorly coordinated interactions and minimal maternal involvement (as in Lewis & Feiring, 1989; Smith & Pederson, 1988). Overall, the findings suggest that insecure-resistant relationships result not only when mothers are underinvolved, but also when they tend to time their interactive bids poorly.

We can now reconsider whether feeding is an important determinant of attachment. It appears that being the person who feeds the baby (at least in monkeys) does not produce attachment. Nevertheless, it would be wrong to conclude that what happens in feeding is irrelevant to the mother-infant attachment process. The same maternal characteristics of sensitivity and responsivity operate in the feeding situation as in the general context of mother-infant interaction, and sensitivity in feeding (e.g., allowing babies to decide when they have finished, or waiting until they open their mouths before feeding the next spoonful) is strongly related to quality of attachment (Ainsworth & Bell, 1969). This suggests that feeding is not different in kind from other situations, although it may be particularly important in the early months, because such a large amount of time is spent feeding.

Mothers' Role as "Teacher"

The above discussion has all been oriented to the theories that dominate the field of attachment. This is true partly because almost all research is so oriented. Learning, which, as we have seen in many contexts, is used as a tool to study all types of problems, dropped out of fashion as a general approach to behaviors in developmental psychology, replaced on one side (cognitive) by the Piagetians and their successors and on the other (social-emotional) by the ethological/Freudian thinkers. One could argue, as do Gewirtz and his colleagues, that when we talk about mother-infant interaction as a source of attachment behaviors, we are talking about the learning contingencies that

have developed between mother and infant—about what behaviors mothers have reinforced in their infants in separations and reunions, hence in what behaviors were strengthened in the infant. Similarly, we could talk about what behaviors in the infant rewarded the mother for her behaviors. Do infants who cling and whine during separation reinforce some mothers in their feelings of importance, or in their feelings of being loved (missed)?

Gewirtz and Peláez-Nogueras (1991) have studied separation protests in the laboratory by having mothers give extra attention to signs of protest or give extra attention when there are no signs of protest or when play is ongoing. They showed that infants will learn to protest and, conversely, they will learn not to protest when the contingencies are changed. Furthermore, this occurs in infants who are younger than those usually studied in the Strange Situation, hence enhancing an interpretation of these behaviors being learned over a lengthy period of interaction. Gewirtz and Peláez-Nogueras point out that Schaffer and Emerson (1964) called attention to the fact that mothers might, by their consistent, rapid responses to their infants' protests, have led to the infants' learning of the cued protest response on which their attachment index was based. However, they do not pursue this explanation. It is to be hoped that Gewirtz and Paláez-Nogueras will study reunion behaviors to round out the possible relations of learning and attachment.

This leads us to the general observation that there has been a great deal of emphasis in the field of infancy on putting more and more infant behaviors into the wired-in (biological, innate) category, without seriously looking for other mechanisms or processes to explain them. As pointed out earlier in connection with the sense of smell, built-in, innate responses could be very maladaptive, especially in a species with a long period of development. The discussions of attachment behaviors and their antecedents (and consequents) are discussions of correlations; they have never really been concerned with the mechanisms by which the effects are achieved. Perhaps it is time that more researchers return to study of possible mechanisms.

ATTACHMENT IN OTHER CULTURES, SUBCULTURES, AND SPECIAL GROUPS

Data from other countries show marked differences in the distribution of the three classifications from that found in the United States (Grossmann & Grossmann, 1989, 1990). Studies in other cultures (with two exceptions) are similar to those in the United States in having about 70% classified as securely attached (As), but differ markedly in how the remainder are divided between resistant (Bs) and avoidant (Cs).

Some 40% or less have been classified as secure in Bielefeld, Germany (Grossmann et al., 1981), and on an Israeli kibbutz (Sagi et al., 1985). Such findings have led to challenges to the validity of the Strange Situation as a tool for use cross-culturally. However, a meta-analysis of data from 32 samples from eight countries has shown that the differences between cultures are small compared with differences within cultures (Van IJzendoorn & Kroonenberg, 1988). Hence it would seem more important to understand attachment in those cultures that produce deviant distributions than it is not to use the Strange Situation in cross-cultural research. It is also necessary to address the question of possible differences in coding in different studies (Van IJzendoorn & Kroonenberg, 1990).

When the proportion of As and Cs in different countries is examined, there is a suggestion that As are relatively more frequent in Western Europe and Cs more frequent in Japan (Miyake et al., 1985) and Israel (Sagi et al., 1985), but nonexistent in a Chinese sample (Trnavsky, 1988). It is easy to hypothesize about cultural differences in child rearing and exposure to strangers as explanations for the differences in distributions. In some cultures the Strange Situation may not fulfill Ainsworth's definition that it should be strange enough to encourage exploration but not so strange as to cause initial fear.

The Strange Situation may be more novel to children in some cultures than in others. This idea is borne out by one study in which negative behaviors prior to the separation episodes predicted classification as a C (Ujiie & Chen, 1985). To test this idea, a meta-analysis of infants' reactions to the initial situation (that is, prior to the mother's leaving) was conducted (Sagi et al., 1991). If infants showed resistant or avoidant behaviors prior to mothers' first leaving the room, they were apt to be classified that way on the basis of the entire procedure. Other interactive behaviors were only modestly related to classification. Cross-cultural differences did not depend on differences in the infants' initial reactions to the situation, except in the kibbutz sample (in which the infants had been exposed to multiple caretakers, but to very few strangers). Nor did procedural variations from the Ainsworth and Wittig formula account for differences in initial appraisal. In short, infants in countries with different classification rates made similar appraisals of the Strange Situation with only a few exceptions (Sagi et al., 1991). (For further discussion of these issues, see Main, 1990; Van IJzendoorn, 1990.)

So far, only a few of the world's cultures have been studied in this way. Nevertheless, the apparent stability exhibited cross-culturally in attachment behaviors as measured by the Strange Situation is supportive of Bowlby's and the ethologists' view that it is a biologically based phenomenon.

Other findings from special populations and subcultures are consistent with this view:

(1) Infants adopted in the first 6 months do not differ from nonadopted infants (Singer et al., in press). Interracial adoptees show a higher incidence of insecure attachment than nonadoptees, but not higher than intraracial adoptees. This finding could be due to the documented greater insecurity and lesser support their mothers felt.

(2) The distribution of attachment categories of infants with cystic fibrosis do not differ from the norms or from a control group (Fischer-Fay et al., 1988). However, those with insecure attachments are apt to have been diagnosed earlier and to have been smaller at testing, indicating their greater health problems.

(3) Nutritional status is related to attachment classifications. Chronically malnourished infants have a large proportion of anxious attachments and disorganized attachments are most frequent in the most severely malnourished (Valenzuela, 1990). The effects of various illnesses and of nutritional status on attachment need further exploration.

(4) Attachment distributions in very low birth weight infants (singletons and twins) appear the same as in the normative population, unless one looks at the different subcategories of secure attachments, where one finds an excess of B1s and B4s (Goldberg et al., 1986).

(5) The distribution of attachment classifications is the same for chimpanzees reared in a nursery by humans and tested with their favorite caretaker in the role of "mother" (Bard, 1991).

Studies in our own culture have used primarily Caucasian samples or have used mixed samples in which ethnic status was not examined. Preliminary results on a study of attachment in black American families conducted by Randolph (1989) have shown that the proportions of securely and insecurely attached are similar to those for Caucasian samples. However, birth order was found to be very important to attachment classification in this study, while it has not been so in other samples. All insecurely attached infants in Randolph's sample were firstborns, although first- and later-born infants were equally represented in the securely attached group.

The data on the resilience of the attachment system within an assortment of environments and specially defined groups lead to a consideration of possible resilience in the face of mother-infant interactions that differ from the norms. Infants reared by blind or deaf parents (or mothers) lack many of the interactions that are considered optimal for attachment. Normal infants appear able to adapt to the available interaction patterns, albeit with initial negative behaviors and delays. An example involving blind parents can be found in Adamson et al. (1977), and a study involving deaf parents found this to be the case (Meadow-Orlans et al., 1986). We clearly know little about the compensatory behaviors or mechanisms that can buffer the effects of "nonoptimal" interaction patterns.

Early Social Interactions

For many infancy experts, social responses are by definition responses made differentially to one or a few individuals, that is, attachment responses. That is why attachment relationships have received our first and most extensive attention. Nevertheless, infants respond to humans long before they differentially respond to specific humans.

NATURE OF EARLY SOCIAL INTERACTIONS

Early "social responses" are less clearly social in nature than later ones, because young infants respond in the same ways (e.g., by smiling) to both social and nonsocial stimuli. Whether there are uniquely patterned social responses or the apparently social responses are simply part of the general set of processes by which infants come to respond to both the social and nonsocial worlds is unclear. The latter is what Papoušek and Papoušek (1975) call the fundamental cognitive response system. Those who believe there are unique social responses are generally ethologically or biologically oriented, while those who believe that social responses are not basically different from other responses are often interested in infants' abilities to learn or perceive. Two relevant instances of this controversy were addressed earlier in this book. One was in Chapter 6, in discussion of how a smile can be elicited in the first month of life first by auditory stimulation, then by visual stimulation, and later by a combination of the two. Both human and nonhuman sources of stimulation are effective. According to ethological theory, stimulation from mother should be uniquely effective in eliciting smiling. The human voice, especially a high-pitched one, is an effective stimulus (Eisenberg, 1969; Wolff, 1959), but the

range of stimuli, social and nonsocial, tested has been inadequate to allow a general statement.

The ability to perceive faces appears to develop in the same way as the ability to make perceptual discriminations of nonhuman stimuli (see Chapter 7). This would support the beliefs of those who hypothesize that social responsivity develops from the general adaptation of the infant. Ethologists tend to believe that infants have an innate ability to perceive that most human of stimuli, the face, and, as noted in Chapter 7, there is some, albeit as yet unconvincing, evidence in favor of this view.

While the controversy is unresolved, some investigators have circumvented the whole problem by looking at the issue somewhat differently. They do not require that the infant understand the distinction between social and nonsocial stimuli or give unique "social" responses to "social stimuli." Rather, they regard any response made to a social stimulus as a social response. This allows them to go on to their major interest: How do the babies' responses interact with those of their mothers, and what effects do such interactions have on the infants' subsequent social development? These questions coincide with those asked by parents, who are rarely concerned with the niceties of the definition of *social*. If a mother of a 2-week-old can elicit a smile in response to her voice, she is not concerned with the possibility that a bicycle bell might also elicit a smile. Rather, she is excited and glad that her baby is responding—socially—to her. A whole new area of research has evolved in this context of watching infants respond within a natural social situation, usually in face-to-face (or *en face*) situations. The role of tactile components of interaction has received relatively little direct study. Recently, Stack and Muir (1990) asked mothers to keep their faces immobile when looking at their infants (the still-face paradigm) and examined the role of tactile behaviors in this context. Given the importance of the tactile modality in early infancy, this area would seem to deserve more study.

The following discussion will catalog those infant responses that seem to be important in these *en face* situations. The earliest ages at which such responses are found will be covered, as well as the roles they probably play in the developing social relationship. Before presenting this information, however, I would like to note that face-to-face interactions may constitute a more valid measuring tool between 3 and 5 months of age than earlier or later, as shown by Lamb et al. (1987). Indeed, these researchers challenge its usefulness as a tool for studying the emergence of infant social expectations, a caution that has not yet received much response.

Newborn babies seem remarkably asocial to many people. They do interact with adults by sucking, crying, and molding their bodies when held front-to-front, but these responses often encourage caretaking rather than social responses. But by the end of the first month three very strong elicitors of maternal social responses have begun to develop—sustained visual regard, smiling, and vocalizations. The first means that babies will focus on a stimulus (which is sometimes a person) for relatively long times. One stimulus they like to gaze at is eyes (although not eyes in unsmiling and unmoving faces; Brackbill, 1958; Stechler & Latz, 1966). The onset of eye-to-eye contact helps mothers feel less strange with their babies (Robson, 1967) and gives them a feeling that their babies are real social beings (Klaus et al., 1970; Robson & Moss, 1970). The second infant behavior that elicits social responses from others is smiling. Babies' increased smiling to the sights and sounds of parents and others by the end of the first month helps parents perceive their infants as social beings. The third elicitor of social responses begins to appear by the fourth week, when infants respond to vocalizations of others with gurgles. By the fifth week they vocalize in response to the vocalizations of others (although not necessarily the same sounds) and will engage in exchanges of 10-15 vocalizations (Wolff, 1963, 1969).

Thus it is clear that very early in life babies do things that reward their mothers. It has already been demonstrated that mothers do things that interest babies. Even newborns are attracted to contours such as the human hairline, to visual movement, to sounds, and to tactile stimulation (Chapter 7). Chapters 9 and 10 charted the development of imitation, noting that infants' earliest imitations are of adult imitations of infants' own vocalizations. Mothers' imitations also reward babies, and they frequently repeat behaviors over and over, particularly if their infants respond positively to them (Papoušek & Papoušek, 1977; Schoetzau & Papoušek, 1977; Stern et al., 1977). This is highly rewarding to infants in two ways. First, infants respond positively to familiarization from repeated stimulation (Lewis & Goldberg, 1969; McCall & Kagan, 1967). Second, infants are rewarded by events that occur contingent on their own responses; in other words, when their own actions make things happen (Papoušek, 1967; Papoušek & Bernstein, 1969). Mothers and babies thus are mutually rewarding. A special form of repetition is that which is rhythmic, in which both infant and mother contribute to the rhythm. Koester et al. (1989) see the mother's behavior as part of what they call "intuitive parenting" (e.g., use of baby talk, exaggerated facial and vocal expressions, distance regulation, and repetitious behaviors), all of which effectively elicit, sustain, and reinforce the infant's attentiveness. Lester et al. (1985) note the differences in rhythmic interaction with premature and term babies and question whether they may explain later linguistic differences between the two groups.

Sears (1951), in his presidential address to the American Psychological Association, noted that mutually rewarding behaviors form the basis of mother-infant interactions. In the framework of learning theory, he described the way in which one person's actions are stimuli (or environmental events or rewards) for the other person. He made a plea in this address for psychologists to combine individual and social behavior into a single theoretical system concerned with interacting pairs, or dyads. Unfortunately, only in the late 1960s and early 1970s did researchers use approaches that treated the mother and infant as a mutually interacting dyad (R. Q. Bell, 1968, 1971; Harper, 1971; Yarrow et al., 1971). One reason it has been hard for researchers to shift to this type of research is the lack of a statistical basis for analyzing the data of such sequences or of analyzing the dependencies of one actor's behavior upon that of the other actor. There have been recent attempts to develop ways of dealing with the complexities.

Different investigators describe the nature of these interactions differently, depending on their interests. Papoušek and Papoušek (1975), like Sears, describe it in a learning context:

> The most impressive feature of the interaction between infant and mother is the continuous sequence of short scenes in which the two members mutually stimulate and reinforce one another. Thus, the mother is not just a source of rich external stimulation or a selective reinforcing agent of behavioural expressions of her child. The child's spontaneous behaviour engages her too, and sets the occasion for her responding. The interaction of these two, therefore, tends to be reciprocal. Besides mutual stimulation and reinforcement, both members also learn how each can influence the other with his or her own behaviour. In sum, it is not simply the quantitative aspects of stimulation, but the structure, sequence and causal relations between individual components of behaviour which play the decisive roles. The discovery and mastery of the active and adaptive manipulation of a partner is a more decisive feature of mother-infant interaction than passive behavioural modification which is acquired through external reinforcement. (p. 254)

Trevarthen (1977) describes early mother-infant interactions as prespeech conversations. He emphasizes their turn-taking nature—that first one partner is active and the other quiet, and then they reverse. He sees the beginning of language behavior in these interactions. Thoman (1981a) also views early mother-infant interactions as being communicative, but she sees their underlying nature as affective rather than cognitive. On the basis of neurological as well as other evidence she concludes that "the behaviors of mother and infant are integrated through the expression, reception, and reaction to affective behaviors of each member of the dyad." She cites a number of studies that have shown evidence of affect in facial expressions and in sucking patterns. Whether or not all of these behaviors or facial expressions have meaning (a very real question), mothers react to them as if they do.

Brazelton et al. (1975), like Thoman, consider mother-infant interactions to be basically social-emotional phenomena. They describe the interactions as "a sequence of phases, each representing different states of the partner's mutual attentional and affective involvement" (p. 142). They are impressed with a different sort of rhythm than the turn-taking described by Trevarthen. They describe alternation between social interactions (which often involve activity by both participants) and what they call disengagement—a sort of a rest period between interactions. Following is an example of a description of an interaction between a 60-day-old infant and his mother. It shows this sort of alternation:

Baby is looking off to side where mother will come in. He lies completely quiet, back in his baby seat, face serious, cheeks droopy, mouth half open, corners down, but there is an expectant look in his eyes as if he were waiting. His face and hands reach out in the same direction. As his mother comes in, saying, "Hello" in a high-pitched but gentle voice, he follows her with his head and eyes as she approaches him. His body builds up with tension, his face and eyes open up with a real greeting which ends with a smile. His mouth opens wide and his whole body orients toward her. He subsides, mouths his tongue twice, his smile dies and he looks down briefly, while she continues to talk in an increasingly eliciting voice. During this, his voice and face are still but all parts of his body point toward her. After he looks down, she reaches for and begins to move his hips and legs in a gentle containing movement. He looks up again, smiles widely, narrows his eyes, brings one hand up to his mouth, grunting, vocalizing, and begins to cycle his arms and legs out toward her. With

this increasing activity, she begins to grin more widely, to talk more loudly and with higher-pitched accents, accentuating his vocalizations with hers and his activity with her movements of his legs. The grunting vocalizations and smiles, as well as the cycling activity of his arms and legs come and go in two-second bursts—making up small cycles of movement and attention toward her. She contains his hips with her hands as if to contain the peaks of his excitement.

Meanwhile, with her voice and her face, as well as with her hands, she both subsides with and accentuates his behavior with her own. He looks down again, gets sober at 40 seconds, makes a pouting face. She looks down at his feet at this point, then comes back to look into his face as he returns to look up at her. She lets go of his legs, and they draw up into his body. He bursts out with a broad smile and a staccato-like vocalization for three repetitions. Each time, his face broadens and opens wide, his legs and arms thrust out toward her. She seems to get caught up in his bursts, and smiles broadly, her voice getting brighter, too. After each burst, he subsides to a serious face, limbs quiet, and her quieting response follows his.

At 70 seconds, he subsides completely, and looks down at his feet with a darkly serious face. She gets very still, her face becomes serious, her voice slows down and almost stops, the pitch becomes low. Her mouth is drawn down, reflecting his serious mouth. After three seconds, he begins to brighten again into a wide, tonguing smile. This time, he is more self-contained, holding back on the movement of his extremities and his excitement. She responds immediately, cocks her head coyly, smiles gently and her voice gently begins to build up again. He builds up to two more staccato vocalizations with smiles and jerky, cycling movements of his legs out toward her. She contains his hips, and this time her voice doesn't build up to a peak of excitement with him. She looks down after 6 seconds to pick up his arms with her hands as if to keep control over his build-up. He follows her downward look about ten seconds later, by looking down, too. His movements subside and his face becomes serious. She is quite serious also, at 90 seconds. (Brazelton et al., 1975, pp. 141-142)

These interactions occur very rapidly (90 seconds for the above sequence). The particular behaviors that occur are not constant. For example, turn-taking might occur with smiles, nods, grunts, coos, or a variety of other responses and might change within an interaction. This is similar to the problem we encountered when talking about attachment responses. The particular discrete responses, although easier to measure, are not necessarily meaningful psychologically.

Thoman has also focused on patterns of behaviors between mothers and infants that occur over longer time spans (days, weeks, or months). She believes that any one sequence of interactions may be trivial and that the behaviors of both mother and infant are determined by all of their interactive experiences prior to the particular one in question. Thus she recorded large numbers of behaviors using a coding system of about 75 categories that has a language structure with "nouns," "verbs," and "modifiers," which can be combined to identify meaningful interactions that differ between dyads (mother-infant pairs). For example, this system can describe the proportion of time the infant fusses during a social interaction or when the mother is looking at him or her. Thoman's goal is to characterize stable individual patterns among dyads rather than in infants or mothers.

In Thoman's view, the potential for these early communications between mothers and infants is biologically determined; that is, the interactive capabilities of infants have developed through evolution and provide a critical form of early adaptation that assures their survival. Even Papoušek and Papoušek (1975), who describe the interactions in learning terms, argue that mothers are not systematically providing stimulation or reward to their infants. Rather, they argue, mothers' behaviors are by their nature social responses (as in intuitive parenting).

IMPORTANCE OF EARLY
SOCIAL INTERACTIONS

The task of finding ways to characterize early social interactions is so immense that most researchers' efforts have been centered on this important first step. Nevertheless, it appears that the researchers in this area are making progress toward exploring the meaning of the early interaction patterns between mothers and young infants.

Reciprocal Influences Between Mother and Infant

Osofsky and Danzger (1974) found that babies' auditory responses were related to both the frequency and the quality of maternal auditory stimulation during the feeding interaction. The correlations were substantial, accounting for about 25-50% of the variance. Infants' visual and motor responsivity was moderately correlated (accounting for more than 20% of the vari-

ance) with the mothers' attentiveness and sensitivity to their babies and to mothers' facial movements and tactile or handling stimulation. A second, larger study found similar patterns of correlations (but smaller) between maternal sensitivity and infant responsiveness (Osofsky, 1976).

Thoman (1981b) has described individual pairs who exhibited synchrony or asynchrony in their interactions in the first 5 weeks of life. In one pair, the more optimal baby with asynchronous interactions had problems at ages 1 and 2 years, including impaired cognitive functioning and the most crying of any of the 10 infants in the study. This latter was particularly striking since the infant had cried very little early in life. The less optimal baby with synchronous interactions was doing very well. Mother-infant interactions were still synchronous or asynchronous as in early infancy and could be the proximal cause of infant behaviors.

Although it is not possible to base firm conclusions on two infants, the sampling bias in this study is not as severe as in traditional case studies. Thoman initially selected her 10 infants randomly from a normal population and then selected clear cases of her variables of interest. Furthermore, her conclusions match those of research done in another context. Thomas and Chess (1977) have found that mutual adaptations (whether babies and parents fit each other's needs), rather than parent style or infant characteristics, often determine the outcome, especially for babies somewhat outside the usual pattern of behavior. This finding also supports the synchrony position and adds a new ingredient, that synchrony may be more important for some babies than for others.

Correlational studies can tell us only that two behaviors (or classes of behaviors) are associated with each other, not whether one causes or leads to the other. The correlations Osofsky found may mean that attentive, sensitive mothers can more easily get their babies to be responsive than less attentive, less sensitive mothers, or that responsive babies tend to elicit attentive, sensitive behaviors from their mothers. In addition, it is likely that some newborn behaviors that elicit differential caretaking are constitutional. One such factor is cuddliness of the infant, which Osofsky (1976) assessed as part of the Brazelton exam (see Chapter 8, Table 8.7). Mothers' attempts to aid cuddling and to use eye contact in cuddling were negatively related to cuddling in their infants. Also, the greater the arousal of the infant, the more effort was required from the mother to achieve cuddling. The negative relation between cuddliness and both state and overall reactivity supports Osofsky's interpretation that babies requiring greater effort to cuddle were behaviorally, and possibly constitutionally, less cuddly. Indeed, there is some danger that cuddliness in the Brazelton scale is confounded with a low arousal state and poor muscle tone.

Richards (1971) noted that some mothers respond to quiet babies by continuing to try to stimulate them, while others wait for the infant to "reply." The former overwhelm their babies and the babies "turn off" (crying, turning away, or lying motionless with nonconverging, staring eyes and sleeplike respiration). Babies of the latter type of mothers are able to continue interactions for longer periods of time.

It is, of course, the case that infants have interactions with people other than mothers. Except for attachment, these have been much less studied. One study found that among a large group of caregivers in a variety of day-care situations, those who smiled the most elicited not only more smiles from their charges, but more reciprocal affection (Zanolli et al., 1990). Differential smiling was the only teacher behavior that seemed to have an influence.

Should Mothers Attempt to Change Their Babies' Styles?

If some babies are constitutionally noncuddlers, and if attempts to cuddle them result in their cuddling less, then perhaps mothers who insist on cuddling are creating difficulties. Mothers who allow their infants to quiet by themselves may be promoting a synchronous mother-infant relationship. The position that babies should be allowed to exert as much autonomy in their early days as possible is a popular one today. It may, however, be quite wrong. We lack the data to say whether mothers should or should not encourage their babies to develop just those aspects of temperament that they initially lack. However, the research on secure attachment shows that mothers who are sensitive and responsive to their babies in a general way are likely to have securely attached babies. The attachment research (though only indirectly relevant) would argue that mothers should focus on establishing a synchronous relationship by permitting their babies to express their own needs and to control themselves and their environment as much as possible. Indeed, monkey data show that infant monkeys that were allowed to control their own getting of food or even the flashing of lights in their environments were less fearful, explored more, and coped better with separations from peers than monkeys that received the same food or lights, but not contingent on their own behavior (yoked to experimentals), or than controls (Mineka et al., 1986).

Learning theorists would say that if mother wants a cuddly baby she can, by sensitively reinforcing the baby's slight bits of cuddling, increase the cuddling's frequency and strength. In fact the positions are not really antithetical, because the learning approach does not mean that one should force behavior on the infant.

Long-Term Outcomes Related to Early Social Interactions

In the Thoman work cited above we saw that synchrony or its lack appeared to influence outcome in two babies. It has been shown that longer-term outcomes (IQ and academic assessments at age 12) are influenced by the reciprocity of parent-infant interactions at 21 months ($r=.44$) for prematures (Beckwith & Cohen, 1989; Cohen, 1988). Furthermore, the outcomes were more highly related to 21-month reciprocity than to SES or maternal education (variables that often account for the most variance, among those measured, in outcomes).

A number of studies have found relations between interactions and later language development. For example, Smith et al. (1988) found that mother-infant interactions in 15-month-olds (taped during play at home) are related to the variety of words used by the infants at 18 months.

THE ROLE OF MATERNAL PERCEPTIONS IN EARLY SOCIAL INTERACTIONS

The research described above was all based on observations of mothers actually interacting with their babies. Adults are also affected by their perceptions of situations independent of reality. It is likely that mothers' perceptions of their infants and of mother-infant interactional patterns also influence the developing relationship. Perhaps the first question to ask is how clearly mothers' perceptions match infants' behaviors. If mothers are always accurate in their perceptions of their babies, we need not concern ourselves with maternal perceptions at all; they have no effect independent of the infants' behaviors. But the research suggests that mothers' perceptions reflect both their ideas of what babies in general are like and their knowledge of their own babies in particular. For example, Ploof (1976) found that mothers' perceptions of their second-born babies became more similar to the babies' behaviors as they got to know the babies (during the first 4 months of the babies' lives) and less like their perceptions of average babies or of their firstborns. In addition, the mothers' perceptions of their infants were related to the infants' behaviors at the time of rating and also to their earlier behaviors. Ploof interprets her results to mean that the mothers' perceptions of their infants at 4 months are based on the infants' particular characteristics as experienced over the first 4 months of interaction. This view is strengthened by Broussard and Hartner's (1971) finding that mothers' perceptions of their infants at birth were not related to their adjustment at 4 years of age, although their perceptions of the infants at 1 month were.

This evidence also suggests that mothers' perceptions of a baby are influenced by their knowledge of other babies, including their own. Ploof found direct evidence that mothers' perceptions of their firstborns were related to actual behaviors of their second-borns at 4 months. Those who had given high evaluations to their first children had second children who were more alert, more rhythmic, and had good temperaments at 4 months. Those whose mothers had low evaluations of their firstborns were unalert, arhythmic, and difficult at 4 months. It is not likely that the mothers' perceptions that arose from their experiences with their firstborns were the cause of the second infants' behaviors. Perhaps the most obvious alternatives are that the mothers may produce genetically or constitutionally easy or difficult babies or that the mothers are equally effective or ineffective with both children.

Research on maternal perceptions demonstrates that they are a factor to be dealt with. Whether maternal perceptions actually cause different infant behaviors is still an open question, one that will likely become a hot research topic in the next decade. To answer this question properly we need to find some way of separating out the influence of mothers' perceptions from the reality of their infants' behaviors. In other words, we may find that maternal perceptions are related to later infant outcomes, but only because these perceptions are related to early infant outcomes; the real operative factor might be the early infant behaviors, rather than the maternal perceptions. So far we have evidence only that perceptions are related to infant outcomes; there is no evidence that it is the maternal perceptions themselves that are the real cause.

LATER SOCIAL INTERACTIONS

One later social interaction usually initiated by the infant is **social referencing**. This is the process in which the infant uses information from others (usually a parent) to appraise events or regulate behavior. This has become a topic of study in the last few years. Most studies have been of affective referencing, but some have included instrumental social referencing. The presence of a stimulus that is ambiguous or that generates uncertainty is thought by some to enhance this

form of behavior, but not all research evidence supports this. This behavior emerges late in the first year and appears to change rapidly in the second.

Responses to toys have been investigated after teaching mothers a routine for reacting positively, negatively, or neutrally to a toy that is presented to the infant. The reactions of 12-month-old infants to toys tend to mirror those of their mothers and to carry over to a second presentation of the toy when the mother does not react. Negative maternal affect appears to have a greater immediate effect (Hornik et al., 1987).

Mothers who provided either positive or neutral messages to their 12-month-olds when a stranger approached affected the infants' behavior. Infants receiving the positive message were friendlier, cried less, and smiled more (not directed to anyone). The effect was greatest at the stage of approach when the stranger tried to make friends, and the effect was found for temperamentally more difficult as well as easier infants (Feinman et al., 1986).

Hornik and Gunnar (1988) exposed 12- and 18-month-olds to a large caged rabbit in the presence of their mothers, who had been told to encourage their infants to like the rabbit. They first sat without talking, but smiled when their infants glanced at them, then they showed positive emotion and talked about the rabbit while still sitting, and finally approached the cage. The infants were classified as bold or wary on the basis of their initial reactions. Referencing glances increased after the mothers started talking about the rabbit, and the bold referenced as much as the wary. The 18- but not the 12-month-olds changed their behavior more after referencing looks to mother than after other types of looks. Referencing was instrumental, as well as affective, and the 18-month-olds used language for referencing, not just looks. However, 16% never referenced.

Age differences have also been shown in infants' relations to toys. In a study by Walden and Ogan (1988), social referencing had a regulatory effect in 10- to 13-month-olds, but not in 6- to 9- or 14- to 22-month-olds. Only those in the oldest group were inhibited touching the toy until they had referenced the parent, but they sometimes preferred a toy despite a fearful message associated with it (see also Feinman, 1985).

Using an attachment figure as a secure base from which to explore is basic to the idea of attachment theory. Using a parent for social referencing would seem to be a highly related behavior. Dickstein and Parke (1988) found that 11-month-old infants left with one parent in a room that a stranger entered used that parent as a reference equally regardless of whether the parent was the father or mother. The sex of the infant did not affect the referencing.

The data are not yet adequate to allow us to chart the path of social referencing, but it certainly exists. Gewirtz and Paláez-Nogueras (in press) have shown that social referencing of maternal facial expressions can be taught, as can its unlearning.

Fathers' Role in Infants' Social Development

Most of the discussion so far in this chapter has concerned mother-infant social relationships. Father-infant interactions aroused little interest for a long time, although research in the 1960s demonstrated that babies also develop attachment to their fathers. Schaffer and Emerson (1964) showed this for crying when fathers (and other adults) left their babies, and Pedersen and Robson (1969) showed it for positive greeting behaviors. The reason father-infant interactions were rarely studied is that in our culture and in the theories of our culture (psychoanalytic, behavioristic, and ethological) mothers have been considered the primary (or only important) influence on infants. Fathers traditionally have been considered to have little interest or involvement in the care and nurture of infants. Indeed, J. Nash (1965), in a review of fathers in contemporary literature and the then-current psychological literature, concluded that there was virtually no research concerning the role of fathers in infant development. Since Nash's review there has been considerably more study of the relations between fathers and their infants and of the roles fathers may play in the social and cognitive development of their infants. However, it seems to have diminished again despite feminism and the increased numbers of working mothers of young infants and single-parent homes, which one would think would make this topic very "in." The results of the research conducted to date are difficult to present with confidence, because so many of the studies have been done with rather small samples and it is difficult to assess how typical the babies and the fathers in these small samples are. As Yogman (1982) points out in his review, this topic has perhaps led to more writing than research.

FATHERS AND CHILDBIRTH

The maternal bonding studies led to a mushrooming of reports about the effects of father presence, much of it not carefully documented. This in turn led to widespread acceptance of the importance of pater-

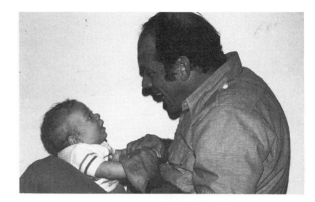
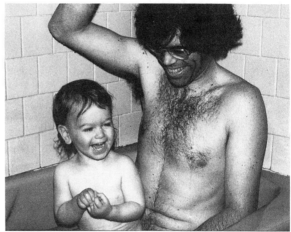
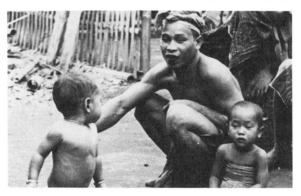

Figure 12.5. Parent-infant love is not limited to mothers and babies. (top) An American father plays with his young infant. (center) An American father enjoys a bath with his son. (bottom) A Balinese father serves as a secure base for exploration. (American photographs courtesy of Judith E. Sims-Knight; Balinese photograph by G. Bateson, courtesy of the Library of Congress.)

nal bonding as documented by Palkovitz (1984).

As noted in Chapter 5, fathers are increasingly involved in the birth process in our society and generally feel very positive about it. Entwisle and Doering

(1981) found that 95% of men felt positive about being in the delivery room at the birth of their babies, and about 25% reported it as a "peak experience." Fathers who spent time in the waiting room were generally neutral in their reactions. Although it is tempting to use these data to suggest that such experiences strengthen the involvement of fathers with their babies, such a conclusion may not be warranted for a number of reasons.

One reason is that presence at birth may be confounded by early contact. In a study of 30 fathers of first sons, half of whom were present at delivery, Greenberg and Morris (1974) found that early contact with their babies may affect fathers more than actual presence at birth. Lind (1974) found that fathers who were permitted to feed and diaper their babies in the hospital continued to do more caretaking at home 3 months later. Similarly, fathers of babies delivered by cesarean section, who presumably spent more time caring for their babies while the mothers were in the hospital, spent more time in caretaking when their babies were 5 months old (Pedersen et al., 1980). These studies are extremely suggestive, but far too limited to permit confident conclusions. In a critical review of the effects on fathers of birth attendance and early and extended contact with their newborns, Palkovitz (1985) concludes that no conclusive statements can be made. It does not appear that the literature since then has changed that conclusion.

A second reason for caution in interpreting the findings lies in the fact that it may be the father's attitude toward fathering, not his presence at the birth, that affects later behaviors. The father's desire to be present at birth is more important than his actual presence to his later behaviors with his infant. Palkovitz (1982) found that fathers who attended the birth did not differ from those who had intended to, but were not there. Actually, the latter were more interactive with their babies if, and only if, the mother was also there, a behavior Palkovitz attributes to guilt. A German study found that the desire to be present was associated with more willingness to baby-sit, more knowledge of feeding needs, and more ability to make a game out of a potentially annoying baby behavior (throwing the pacifier to the ground repeatedly) (Grossmann & Volkmer, 1984). It did not affect the time spent with the infant. Presence at delivery, regardless of attitude, led to more frequent taking of infants on pram walks. These data highlight a problem with some bonding research: Fathers (or mothers) who choose to be involved with their babies during and immediately after delivery may differ in important ways from those who do not so choose. Only experimental research can de-termine whether and which of fathers' experiences during their babies' birth and early life affect their later relationships.

HOW FATHERS INTERACT WITH THEIR BABIES

Our cultural stereotype of fathers, reflected in Parsons and Bales's (1955) social role theory, has been that fathers are disciplinarians, socializers, and teachers of instrumental activity for their children. It was long considered inappropriate for them to be nurturant toward their infants (Josselyn, 1956), and their influence on their children was expected to begin only after infancy.

Whether fathers share this cultural stereotype seems to depend on what fathers are sampled. An Australian study found that only 34% of fathers felt they had the ability to care for children, although 60% of mothers felt their husbands had such ability (Russell, 1980). In addition, most fathers felt that their parental role began after infancy. Other samples fit the stereotype less well. Cordell (1978) interviewed a subset of Parke and Sawin's (1977) sample. Although the majority of these men (14 of the sample of 25) accepted the stereotypical roles of provider, disciplinarian, and socializer, they did not accept the other stereotypic characteristics. Most of these fathers (16 of the 25) felt their functions as parents included emotional support in the sense of both being responsive to their infants' needs and sharing their infants' activities and joys. They all included routine care as part of their function. Furthermore, they did not perceive their role to be teacher or male role model.

Consistent with the stereotype, several studies have found that fathers tend to be little involved in infant caretaking (Kotelchuck, 1976; Richards et al., 1977). For example, Kotelchuck (1976) found that only 7.5% of the fathers in his sample shared caretaking equally with their wives, and only 25% had regular caretaking responsibilities. As we would expect from this large difference in caretaking responsibilities, fathers tend to spend much less time with their babies than do mothers (Kotelchuck, 1976; Pedersen & Robson, 1969). Kotelchuck (1976) found that fathers spent an average of 3.2 hours per day with their infants versus mothers' 9.0 hours. Those figures are at the high end. German data indicate that fathers spend between 1 and 2 hours per day with their infants on weekdays and 1½ to 4½ hours on weekends.

Nevertheless, although fathers are less involved quantitatively with their infants, many do interact with them throughout infancy in ways that are more similar to mothers than different. Parke and his collaboratories, in extensive behavioral observations of the sample described above (who conformed less well to the fathering stereotype), found that, overall, the fathers were as affectionate, sensitive, and responsive as mothers, although in somewhat different ways (Parke & O'Leary, 1976; Parke & Sawin, 1975, 1977). Mothers engaged in more routine caregiving (e.g., wiping faces, grooming) and more frequent kissing, whereas fathers provided more visual and auditory stimulation through toys and through imitating their infants' facial expressions and mouth movements. Interestingly, the fathers perceived their newborns as needing more affection than did the mothers, but there were no related behavioral differences. Thus, in terms of meeting the emotional needs of their babies, which appears to be the crucial ingredient in the development of attachment, these middle-class, white fathers appear to be as motivated and adequate as mothers.

Parke and Tinsley's (1987) finding that fathers stimulate their infants in different ways from mothers has been corroborated both early in infancy (Yogman et al., 1977) and later. Fathers engage in proportionately more play and less caregiving than mothers, although in overall quantity mothers play more with their infants than do fathers simply because they are available for more hours per day. Furthermore, fathers play more physical games and mothers more quiet, non-physical games (Belsky, 1979b; Clarke-Stewart, 1978, 1980; Field, 1978; Lamb, 1977a, 1977b; Power & Parke, 1979). Playing and stimulation of infants has been found to be more frequent for Israeli fathers than for mothers (Levy-Shiff et al., 1989).

When infants were 11, 14, and 17 months, fathers were less likely to enforce household rules than were mothers. Both parents socialized their infants differently depending on the sex of the infant. They were more likely to discourage aggression and encourage prosocial behavior in girls, and to encourage household responsibilities and turn-taking games in boys (Power & Parke, 1986). However, there were only four children of each sex at each age in this sample.

There is evidence that the stereotype may be more adhered to in practice than in intent. Palkovitz (1988) reports that couples interviewed prior to birth expected the mothers to do twice as much caretaking as fathers, but at 3 weeks after birth the mothers were doing four times as much. Fathers were doing less caretaking in every category (feeding, diapering, bathing, and dressing) than they had projected. Palkovitz speculates that this might be partly due to the fact that the mothers were still on maternity leave.

Fathers' Interactions With Their Premature Infants

It was noted in Chapter 5 that fathers interact differently and more with their infants if they were born by cesarean (e.g., Vietze et al., 1980). Premature infants also elicit different behaviors from their fathers than do full-term infants, and different behaviors from those they elicit from their mothers. Harrison (1990) found that at 3 months fathers of premature infants had more favorable interactions with them than did fathers of term infants. In contrast, mothers of prematures had less favorable interactions. The mothers' satisfaction with the fathers' participation in child care was related positively to responsive paternal behavior with both term and premature infants.

When fathers of Israeli preterm and carefully matched term infants were compared during the initial period of the infants' being at home, the fathers of preterms were more involved in caretaking and holding (Levy-Shiff et al., 1989). Both mothers and fathers played with and stimulated their preterm infants more than did parents of term infants. They both also perceived the preterm infants as more difficult. For both term and preterm fathers higher education led to greater paternal involvement, stimulation, and caregiving.

Effects of Early Father Caretaking on Later Behaviors

Middle-class fathers who had had contrasting amounts of experience in caring for their infants in the absence of the mother during the first year were compared for their interactions with their infants at 12 months (Pedersen et al., 1987). The amount of such experience varied from 21 to 962 hours, with a median of 143. Those below the median (average 90 hours) did not differ from those above the median (average 319 hours) on any background characteristics or on the total duration of all mother-infant separations. (Overall, paternal care accounted for 38% of all time of maternal separations.) After controlling for individual differences in interactions at 3 months of age, when the fathers had little experience in independent infant care, the researchers found that the fathers with the most caregiving experience had more eye-to-eye contact with their infants, more often held their infants close, and presented and manipulated objects with them more than did the fathers with less experience. They also tended to verbalize, touch, and smile more at their infants, but not significantly so.

BABIES' ATTACHMENTS TO THEIR FATHERS

Most of the traditional theories of infant development assumed that infants first form a single exclusive attachment to mothers and only later and secondarily (if at all) would they form attachments to fathers. We now know that this is not true. Two aspects of attachment that have been documented as occurring between infants and fathers have already been mentioned—crying at separation (Schaffer & Emerson, 1964) and greeting on return (Pedersen & Robson, 1969). These were both based on reports of naturalistic situations. What about responses in the laboratory or home to the Ainsworth-Wittig Strange Situation or similar tasks? Kotelchuck (1976) showed that infants at 12 months or older tended to cry when either the mother or the father left the room, but not when a stranger did. They also stayed near the door regardless of which parent left and touched the parent who returned to the room, but did neither for the stranger. Other studies showing attachment to both parents at different ages between 8 and 30 months, whether measured in home or laboratory, are too numerous to mention. Furthermore, Yogman and his collaborators have found that by 2 months of age babies are responding more positively to their fathers than to strangers, which shows the early beginnings of this responsiveness (see Yogman, 1982; Yogman et al., 1976a, 1976b).

The fact that babies attach to both parents does not mean that there are no differences. Evidence about differences is somewhat conflicting. A meta-analysis of 11 studies of attachment did not find the independence attachment theorists would expect between an infant's attachment classification with the mother and with the father (Fox et al., 1991). It is not clear to what degree the dependence of classifications with one parent depended on those with the other leaves room for some differences. Other studies have found differential reactions, but often not in the classifications per se or behavior in the original strange situation. The degree of stress in the situation may be one determining factor in whether or not differences are found. Under high stress it appears there may be more preference for (or effectiveness of) the mother (e.g., Lamb, 1976a, 1976b). A six-episode situation (infants first in a playroom with both parents, then joined by a stranger who later stayed when the parents left, parents returned and stranger left, parents left, parents returned) was studied with 12- to 19-month-olds. In all episodes, which parent the child sought out was noted. As the stressfulness increased, so did the aver-

age preference for the mother (Colin, 1987). In particular, greater stress led to many fewer infants with no real preference. While it led to more infants who preferred the mother, more than one-third still preferred the father. Preference for the mother was not affected by her working, and that for the father was not affected by the number of hours he spent at home or in child care, but was affected by the variety of types of child care he engaged in.

Toddlers have been found to prefer their fathers as playmates (Clarke-Stewart, 1978; Lamb, 1976a, 1976c), although these preferences are not universal (Lamb et al., 1983) and they may only represent responses to the father's own behaviors (Belsky, 1979b; Clarke-Stewart, 1978; Lamb, 1977b). Male toddlers judged as securely attached (18 and 21 months of age at time of testing with one or the other parent) directed more affiliative behavior to the stranger in the strange situation when the father was present (Kromelow et al., 1990). This is another indication that the father may play a different role in early social development from that of the mother.

Fathers are, of course, not the only adults other than mothers to whom infants become attached. Infants (15-23 months) studied with grandparents in a modification of the Strange Situation behaved in the same way with their maternal grandmothers as with their mothers (Myers et al., 1987). Their behavior with their paternal grandmothers was not as similar (see Figure 12.6).

Recent data indicate that in a racially mixed, low-SES sample the degree of the father's participation in child care at 4 months predicted attachment to mother at 1 year (Camfield et al., 1991). Maternal interaction with her infant at 4 months was also influenced by paternal child care, but it, her marital satisfaction, and the degree of social support she had were all controlled for. Maternal interaction at 4 months did not predict attachment at 1 year, nor did support variables that had played a role in studies with middle-class families.

SOURCES OF DIFFERENCES BETWEEN FATHERS AND MOTHERS

A large part of the cultural stereotype of fathers stems from a belief in "maternal instinct," that is, that mothers are biologically equipped to care effectively for infants and fathers are not. In Russell's (1980) study of attitudes of Australian parents, 51% of the mothers and 71% of the fathers believed in this maternal instinct.

A convincing demonstration of the truth or falseness of a biologically based sex difference is a difficult

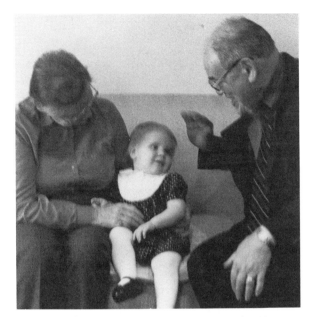

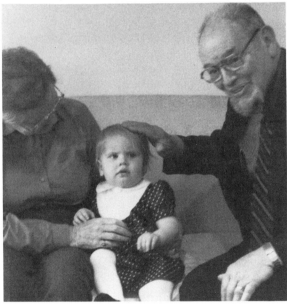

Figure 12.6. Attachment to this paternal grandmother is sufficient for distal, but not for close (touching) interaction with the more unfamiliar grandfather. (Photograph courtesy of Judy F. Rosenblith.)

endeavor, and evidence that would convince doubters (on either side) is not likely to appear in the near future. It is, however, safe to say that no strong evidence exists to support a conviction that biological factors are of overriding importance in explaining parenting. Examinations of fathering in other species and other human cultures reveals that paternal roles vary widely.

One can find species within most categories of animals (primates, mammals, fishes, invertebrates) in which fathers play an active or even predominant role in parenting (see, for example, Bailey, 1982; Earls & Yogman, 1978). Thus it is difficult to argue that females are evolutionarily adapted to be exclusive parents. Also, although it is possible that maternal hormones produced during pregnancy and childbirth may influence maternal behaviors, no strong evidence exists for this in humans (remember the discussion of bonding in Chapter 5). It is possible that interaction with his infant might stimulate hormone production related to caregiving in the male, too; this occurs for such species as stickleback fish, after all. Moreover, there is evidence that certain personality traits are more important than biological sex in determining responsivity to infants. Bem et al. (1976) found that college students who were classified as more expressive (a stereotypically female trait) exhibited more affectionate behaviors to an infant than did other students, regardless of whether they were male or female. Their sex did not influence their behaviors, nor did their scores on a typically masculine trait, instrumental orientation. Consistent with these findings are those of Russell (1978), who found that men who scored high on both feminine (expressive) and masculine (instrumental) behaviors took more caretaking responsibility than "masculine" males. Thus the personality of the parent, rather than biological sex, may turn out to be the most important determinant of parenting.

Related to this are the results of a study by Easterbrooks (1982), who correlated an array of father variables with toddlers' behaviors (including responses to Ainsworth and Wittig's Strange Situation). She found that individual differences in fathers' attitudes and perceptions were more related to toddlers' attachment and task-oriented behaviors than was the time fathers spent alone with their toddlers. As with mothers, it is not just the presence or absence of the father that determines his relationship with his infant (although that is clearly important; see review by Belsky, 1981), but his personal characteristics and reactions to the infant.

Another line of evidence concerning the hypothesis that there is a maternal instinct is the research on whether fathers and mothers respond differentially to infants' cries, discussed in Chapter 6. The evidence overall does not lend strong support to the hypothesis that females are genetically programmed to respond to babies' cries and males are not. Some superior sensitivity found in females is likely a joint result of women's greater expressiveness (the culturally approved norm) and their greater experience with caretaking.

The power of cultural context is obviously strong in

parenting. Parke and Sawin's fathers were responding to their subcultural norm as surely as the more traditional males were responding to the traditional norms. We must, however, be careful not to see these as two monolithic norms—traditional, masculine (instrumental) noncaretakers versus nontraditional, egalitarian, expressive (feminine or androgynous) males who are indistinguishable from mothers. The situation is much more complex. For example, a series of studies of fathering in Sweden found that, unlike American fathers, Swedish fathers did not engage in more active and physical play with their babies than did Swedish mothers (Lamb, Frodi, Frodi, & Hwang, 1982; Lamb, Frodi, Hwang, et al., 1982; Lamb et al., 1983). This was true even of fathers who were obviously involved with their babies, since they took paternity leave of at least one month. Different aspects of fathering— amount of caretaking, degree to which responsibility for care is assigned to father, amount and kind of emotional support father provides, differences in behaviors with sons versus daughters, mothers' view of proper paternal role, and many more—may all operate in different ways in different families. Until the research reflects the complexity, we are likely to make slow progress in isolating differences between mothers and fathers. Another aspect that needs to be considered is that the father's interaction with his infant outside of the home (at the zoo, on a picnic, and so on) may be more active than that in the home (see Mackey, 1985). The reverse may be true for mothers.

THE FAMILY CONTEXT

Fathers and infants do not interact in a vacuum. The parents' marital relationship, their individual parenting styles, and the individual characteristics of their babies all influence each other in a complex family system. Little research has addressed the issues involved in this system, but a few scattered studies and one integrative review (Belsky, 1981) have appeared. The bulk of the available research has examined the influence one parent has on the way the other interacts with the infant (see, e.g., Pedersen, Andersen, & Cain, 1977, 1979; Pedersen, Rubenstein, & Yarrow, 1979). These studies have found that when fathers were negative concerning their wives, the wives were less competent at feeding their newborns and were more negative toward their 5-month-olds. In contrast, when fathers were impressed with their wives as mothers, the mothers exhibited more feeding skill. Mothers' interactions with their husbands also are related to fathering. Belsky (1979a) found that when the mother and father talked to each other about the baby, the father was more in-

volved with the baby, even when the father and baby were alone together.

Low-SES mothers living in extended families were more likely to respond contingently to their 3½-month-old infants' vocalizations and reacted more sensitively to them than similar mothers living in nuclear families (Anisfeld et al., 1990).

SUMMARY AND CONCLUSIONS

The research on fathering, although limited, has accomplished a major task of dispelling some of the untested assumptions about fathers in our culture. It is clear that many fathers are actively involved in the development of their infants even when they are not major caretakers. In response to such involvement, infants generally become attached to their fathers, who then serve as secure bases in much the same way mothers do (even though often as supplements to mothers).

Infant-mother and infant-father interactions differ in a variety of ways, and presumably for a variety of reasons. Research has only begun to reveal some of the many factors that influence these two kinds of interactions. It is clear that the cultural roles of father and mother are a major influence, but so too are the parents' personalities, which are at least partially independent of their biological sex. Furthermore, father, mother, and infant all operate within a complex family system, so that interactions between any two members can change the functioning of that system. Finally, the sex of the infant adds another layer of complexity. Both mothers and fathers treat boy and girl babies in different ways. Since all of these factors operate together, we can expect wide variability in the results that are found. Single studies of small samples made up of upper-middle-class families are likely to yield results that are very restricted in their generalizability. The prediction we offered in the 1985 edition of this text, that research in the next 10 years would focus on these components and provide us with a more complete picture of the role of the father, has not been borne out. The amount of research on fathers seems to have declined again. Research on fathering within family systems has continued (see e.g., Belsky & Volling, 1987; Berman & Pedersen, 1987; Bronstein & Cowan, 1988; and, while not focused on infants, Lewis & Salt, 1986). In addition, people are beginning to address the great variety of patterns of fathering, both in Western cultures and others (Lamb, 1987). Books are also being written on the personal experiences of fathering (Kort & Friedland, 1986). Despite all this, actual knowledge about the impacts of fathering and its variations in different family patterns is still minimal.

Peer Relations and Play

Two topics that have received far too little attention in both infancy and early childhood research are the development of play behaviors and relations with peers. This limited discussion begins with peer relations, but note that the two topics can overlap.

PEER RELATIONS

Social behavior in the infant does not develop only in relation to adults. Many infants are born into families with one or more older siblings. Infants are increasingly in contact with persons outside of the nuclear family as they reach the latter half of the first year, and many infants are in contact with both nonfamilial adults and peers in various day-care settings. Much attention has focused on the effects of day care on infants (which will be discussed in Chapter 13), but little of it has focused on the effects of peers.

Lee (1975) wrote about social competence being acquired by the same process as cognitive competence, a process in which social schemes are constructed. These are more difficult to construct than physical schemes because of the inconsistencies of social compared with physical objects. She saw peers as important to these constructions. However, much of the intervening peer research has been rather atheoretical. Currently, play is beginning to be looked at from a perspective similar to Lee's (Roggman et al., 1990). The usefulness of play as an indicator of the developmental level of mother-infant play and the use of play by the infant as a means of making contact with the attachment figure led to Roggman's interest in play as a possible tool for assessing attachment (Roggman et al., 1987, 1990).

Both old and new research shows the readiness of infants in their second year to be sociable with peers. They interact freely with other infants with whom they were previously unacquainted, smiling, laughing, vocalizing, gesturing, showing and offering toys to each other, imitating each other, and struggling and engaging in reciprocal play (Eckerman et al., 1975). They do this in a strange room and, indeed, even a strange peer leads to faster leaving of the mother and greater exploration at a distance from the mother at 18 months of age (Eckerman et al., 1975; Gunnar et al., 1984). While cooperative play increases from 16 to 24 months, it rises sharply at 28 months (Eckerman et al., 1989). Uncooperative play also increases at that time. Imitation increases steadily from 16 to 32 months and constitutes the majority of cooperative communicative

acts. When a dyad is at the same toy, imitation occurs every 10 seconds. Eckerman et al. have characterized the infant below 16 months of age as being able to assume and maintain complementary roles in familiar ritualized games. In contrast, the 16- to 24-month-old can imitate nonverbal acts as a general strategy for coordinating action in contexts that are not ritualistic. Interactions at the latter age are characterized by widespread imitation of the acts of others, resulting in imitative games and games with both imitative and complementary roles. A case study of development of friendship between toddlers who met once a week for almost a year provides a description of the stages found: attraction, exploration, explorative aggression, explorative passivity, cooperative play refereed by an adult, reciprocal and imitative play not needing a referee, early cooperative representational play, and finally enlargement of the friendship circle (Press & Greenspan, 1985).

Recently some attention has focused on comparisons of infant-peer with infant-mother interactions. New interactive abilities have been thought to emerge with supportive partners such as mothers and then to be used with peers (Adamson & Bakeman, 1985; Bakeman & Adamson, 1984). An example is that nonverbal imitation was found with an adult at 20 months but only at 22 months with a peer (Eckerman et al., 1989). This is sometimes referred to in relation to what is called maternal scaffolding, or the mother's ability to structure the situation to bring out the highest-level behaviors of her infant. (An interesting model of the skills that must emerge to achieve coordinated play behaviors can be found in Eckerman & Didow, 1989.)

The role of maternal behavior in encouraging peer interaction appears anomalous. Fourteen-month-olds stayed closer to their peer partners, and interacted more frequently and for longer times with them, when both mothers were busy filling out questionnaires than when they tried to encourage interaction (A. Nash, 1989). But competency of relations of 2-year-olds with peers has been related to the interactive competencies of the mothers (Parke & Bhavnagi, 1989). Bakeman and Adamson (1984) found that mothers provided qualitatively different support for drawing infants into a state of coordinated joint engagement.

Sex differences have been found in both toddler (15-, 18- and 21-month-olds) and maternal behaviors in a study where each infant was taped in his or her own home interacting with the mother, a known peer, and the peer's mother. By 21 months females initiated more appeals to their mothers when interacting with either of the other partners than earlier, but the appeals of males did not change in frequency with age (Walters et al., 1989). In general, mothers did more stage setting (scaffolding?) for boys than for girls. The toddlers were less engaged, and appealed more to their mothers, when interacting with other partners. The fact that the toddlers used more glances to their mothers when interacting with the peers' mothers and more proximity seeking/maintaining when playing with peers is in agreement with the idea that social referencing and proximity seeking are separate mechanisms (Dickstein et al., 1984).

As one might expect, smooth later relations with peers have been held to be more likely in securely attached infants or in infants whose mothers had characteristics typical of those with securely attached infants. Both engagement with peers and competence of play with mother are positively related to secure attachment (measured using Q-sort for child-care arrival and departures) both with mother and with caregiver (Howes et al., 1988). Seyen et al. (1989) found that peer competence at 12 and 24 months is related to maternal behaviors, both at home and in the peer interaction situation. Cooperation between peers is related to the mother's responsiveness and her *noninterference* with her child's ongoing activity. In this study, dominance in social relations (assessed with different peers every week for four weeks) was related to the mother's unprovoked initiatives toward her child. Both the more cooperative and the more dominant left the mother's vicinity more easily, but the more dominant more often kept an eye on her. Cooperation and dominance remained only slightly similar from 12 to 24 months. However, a number of specific behaviors were related over the year—total initiatives, positive initiatives, physical initiatives, positive reactions, proximity to mother and to peer, and looking at mother and partner ($rs > .50$), and exploration. Two temperamental traits were more strongly related over the 1-year time span—activity and laughter/pleasure ($rs=.68$ and $.63$, respectively)—but not related to dominance and cooperation. Overall, maternal interaction appears more important than peer contacts in determining the nature of interaction with peers. It seems that infants copy the style of interaction practiced by the mother.

PLAY

Play is a spontaneous, self-initiated, meaningful activity of children by which they explore the world and organize concepts about how it works (Bruner, 1972; Piaget, 1962; Vygotsky, 1978). Early in the study of children, play was categorized into descriptive categories that had no theoretical underpinnings. (For a comprehensive, relatively nontechnical, look at research on play in early life, see Gottfried & Brown, 1986.)

A study by Rothstein-Fisch and Howes (1988) that combined play, peers, and environmental settings found that toddlers (16 to 23 months old) in family day care with access to a variety of ages of children oriented to 2-year-olds more often than to infants or older children. They engaged in more, and more complex, play with same-age and 2-year-old children than with infants, but they watched preschoolers more often. They imitated 2-year-olds more often than infants, same-age partners, or preschoolers. They also used emerging language skills more often with 2-year-olds than with other ages, but babbled and gestured more to their age-mates. Their play with peers was affected by the degree of arousal in the environment. Solitary play, supposedly immature, was highest in environments with a low arousal level. Both the amount of time spent playing with peers and the complexity of that play were greater when the amount of motion or activity was anywhere from above average to constant. The toddlers engaged in more complex peer play when the caregiver was engaged in other activities than when she was interacting with them. The role of the 2-year-olds calls to mind Vygotsky's idea that someone only slightly ahead of a child is appropriate for eliciting growth (in his terms, they create an appropriate zone of proximal development). These data suggest two things for those interested in child care at this age range:

(1) Having children in a group of age-mates may not be optimal for the development of social interactions with peers, nor are children who are 2 or 3 years older (as many siblings are) necessarily the best models.
(2) Having a quiet, well-behaved setting is not optimal for learning to play with peers.

Game play with adults shows an increasing capability from 9 to 18 months of age (Ross & Lollis, 1987). As early as 9 months, infants' behavior during interruptions of games shows their understanding of the game and their ability to request their partners to continue, skills that become more frequent with age.

Play reveals something about the central organization of the infant or young child. It has been shown to be related to intellectual development and to degree of biological risk (Bédard et al., 1990), and it has recently been used to assess the functioning of toddlers who were exposed prenatally to drugs (Rodning et al.,

1989). Competence of play with toys was assessed both for those exposed to drugs prenatally and for a control group of premature babies at considerable biological risk. This was done at 18 to 20 months in a playroom with the primary caretaker.[9] Representational play (e.g., combing hair, putting lid on pot) was greater in the preterm than in the drug-exposed toddlers, whose play was disorganized and contained little fantasy play, curious exploration, or combining of toys. Their play was not only disorganized, but impoverished. The range of play events was 2-38 for the prematures, but 0-10 for the drug-exposed infants (the infant with 10 play events had a DQ of 144 and was securely attached). The deficits of the drug-exposed infants were much more dramatic in their play than in their DQs, suggesting that they can function better with a lot of external structure than in unstructured play situations. Within the drug-exposed group, but not in the premature controls, securely attached toddlers had significantly more representational play then the insecurely attached (who made up 61% of the group). Drug-exposed infants raised by extended families or foster mothers had the same attachment patterns as the prematures, but 88% of those reared by their biological mothers were insecurely attached. These negative outcomes were found despite the fact that all of these infants were involved in intervention programs that provided toys and help to families, and that ensured the infants were well nourished even though all but one of their biological mothers were still on drugs.

Much more study is needed in these areas, as well as studies that tie peer interaction styles not only to parenting but to cognitive development and play behaviors. These studies in turn need to be anchored in development in ways similar to those in which the relation of motor behaviors and especially visually guided reaching are being tied to physical development and postural control. Finally, infants' social behaviors generally need to be seen as occurring within a social network that consists of a variety of adults (relatives, family friends, teachers, store clerks), peers, and siblings. They need to be studied in these networks, and the networks need to be studied (see, e.g., Feinman & Roberts, 1986).

Summary

ATTACHMENT

Belief in the importance of infants' early attachment to their mothers was first popularized by Freud's the-

ory and has been maintained. Freud and Erikson both believed that the mother-infant relationship is the prototype for all subsequent relationships (Freud through sucking experiences; Erikson included other aspects of mother-infant relationships).

Bowlby integrated Freudian and ethological views in his theory of attachment. He believed that five behavioral systems within the infant (following, clinging, crying, smiling, sucking) are focused on the mother and form the basis of attachment. Development of each of these systems depends on both experience and maturation. Bowlby described four stages of attachment, three in infancy that have been documented by Ainsworth's work:

(1) Undiscriminating social responsiveness, in which infants orient to salient features of the environment, including human faces and voices, gain and maintain contact with humans, and use special signaling behaviors but do not show consistent preference for one or a few individuals.

(2) Discriminating social responsiveness, in which infants respond differently to familiar figures than they do to relative strangers. Transition to this stage requires development of perceptual and learning abilities.

(3) Active initiation, facilitated by locomotion and control of body movements in seeking proximity and contact with the attachment figure.

As for Piagetian stages, all infants apparently go through each stage in the same sequence, although not at the same ages. Since transitions between stages are both gradual and uneven, an infant's attachment behaviors at any particular time may include behaviors characteristic of earlier and of still-developing stages. They are also, of course, influenced by the specific situation.

Most current studies of attachment are concerned with active initiative in seeking proximity contact, which develops around 7 months of age. Early work primarily used as a measure of attachment the child's protests when separated from the mother and indications of fear of strangers. Later work deemphasized stranger anxiety as a measure because it waxes and wanes on a developmental timetable different from that for protest at separation. Ainsworth's tripartite classification of quality of attachment, based on reunion behaviors, has been selected by many re-

---

9. Some infants had had eight changes in primary caregiver in their first year.

searchers as their measure of attachment. These global patterns of attachment are often stable over time.

FUNCTIONS OF ATTACHMENT

Attachment is seen by its theorists as a biological mechanism for survival whereby infants stay close to mother, and hence can be protected from dangers in the environment. The security mothers provide affords a secure base from which infants can explore the world around them. Between 6 months and 2 years, a toddler typically explores strange situations more readily when mother or another attachment figure is present. The attachment figure serves as an emotional support, a source of stimulation, and a playmate.

Both Freud and Erikson believed that poor attachment in infancy would prevent children from ever forming healthy interpersonal relationships. Erikson further believed that trust in institutions would be negatively affected. Both Erikson and Bowlby argued that the negative effects of poor early attachment experiences can be ameliorated later through therapy or an improved environment. Thus these two theories hypothesize that infancy is a sensitive period rather than a critical period.

Short-term longitudinal studies have found that babies who are securely attached are more likely than insecurely attached infants to exhibit desirable cognitive and social characteristics in later preschool years. Because of the correlational nature of these studies, however, interpretations other than that the mother-infant relationship in infancy caused them are possible. The same maternal behaviors that fostered security may also support the development of social competence in young children, or babies who are easy and rewarding to mothers may stimulate responsiveness and acceptance (maternal characteristics that promote attachment) in mothers, teachers, and peers.

Work using another measure of attachment, the Q-set sort, which is applicable at any age, is commencing and allows comparison of attachment in infancy/toddlerhood to be compared with that in childhood or later. In addition, work looking at the role of mothers and caretakers as playmates is getting started.

THE MOTHER'S ROLE

Feeding and weaning behaviors, as well as the infant's need for contact comfort, have been studied and tested rigorously in monkeys. Contact comfort has been shown to be more important than nursing in developing a secure base in artificially mothered monkeys. Sucking or feeding also appear unimportant for humans. Contact comfort may be important for human babies if it is an appropriate response to the infant at the time. Indeed, it is mothers' responsiveness to their infants' needs (whether for handling or for being left alone) that seems to be most related to the quality of their infants' attachment.

Ainsworth et al. (1971) have proposed that sensitivity-insensitivity, acceptance-rejection, cooperation-interference, and accessibility-ignoring are crucial dimensions. Mothers of securely attached infants have been found to be above average on all four; mothers of avoidant infants were rejecting and insensitive, and those of resistant (ambivalent) infants were rejecting and either interfering or ignoring. Other research supports the hypothesis that the crucial maternal characteristics involve acceptance of one's infant as an independent individual with rights, needs, and power.

The mother's role as teacher of protest behaviors at separation has only recently been studied. Mothers can bring protest behaviors under experimental control (either strengthened or diminished) by reinforcing particular infant behaviors. It will be interesting to see whether reunion behaviors can be similarly influenced.

With a few exceptions (e.g., the kibbutz), attachment classifications seem similar in many different cultures and in subcultures and special groups (e.g., in infants with cystic fibrosis).

EARLY SOCIAL INTERACTIONS

Some researchers believe that newborns exhibit biologically based specifically social responses. Others believe that newborns are incapable of differentiating between social and nonsocial stimuli and so their responses to people are no different (to the babies) from their responses to nonsocial stimuli. A third group feels that this argument is unimportant, because in either case newborn infants do respond to other people and these interactions can thus be studied.

During the first few months, babies become increasingly effective in eliciting social responses from caretakers. Beginning at birth with sucking, crying, and molding their bodies when held front-to-front, they move on to sustained visual regard, smiling, wriggling, cooing, gurgling, and responsive vocalization—all behaviors that are rewarding to their mothers.

Babies also respond positively to adult imitations of their own vocalizations and to other enjoyable behaviors that are repeated over and over again. Familiarization through repetition and making things happen through their own actions are both rewarding to infants.

Mothers and infants are now being looked at as

dyads in which both partners can synchronize their activities to stimulate and reinforce each other. Early mother-infant interactions have been described as prespeech conversations between active turn-taking partners. Other investigators have described social interactions between mother and infant as pulsing engagement and disengagement, and still others in terms of the rhythms and the congruence of interactions. All of these view the infant as an important determiner of the course of interaction. The lack of statistical tools for analyzing the data of such rapid sequential behaviors has handicapped these types of research. One promising hypothesis that needs further research is that dyads whose interactions result in babies' "turning off" may be at risk for future difficulties, while pairs who consistently have synchronized interactions may become securely attached.

The question of whether mothers should try to change their babies' interactive styles has a *no* answer for attachment theorists and a *why not?* answer for learning-oriented researchers. The latter are careful to point out that it needs to be done sensitively.

FATHERS AND INFANT SOCIAL DEVELOPMENT

Because of the strong traditional belief that only mothers are important to infants' development, the nature of father-infant interactions and the role fathers play in infants' development were little studied before the 1970s. Fathers vary greatly in the extent to which they conform to traditional norms; those who reject the traditional role of paternal non-involvement spend more time with their babies. Regardless of their later roles, fathers today are much more involved in childbirth than were earlier fathers, although apparently their desire to be involved is more important than their actual involvement in relation to their later behaviors with their infants.

Studies exploring differences between fathers and mothers find widely varying results. Some find fathers very similar to mothers in their interactions with infants; others find that fathers do less caretaking and engage in more games and rough-and-tumble play. Fathers' and mothers' interactions with prematures differ from those with term infants, and fathers appear more positively involved with their prematures.

Under stress, infants often prefer their mothers. Fathers do not appear to have a single clearly defined role to play, as one would expect if paternal behavior were biologically determined. In fact, it appears that personality is a greater determinant of parenting behavior than is biological sex. Finally, it is clear that fathers, mothers,

and infants constitute a dynamic interactive system in which each influences both others and the relationship between each pair affects the third.

PEERS AND PLAY

This much-neglected topic is beginning to get attention. Studies of day care have focused on other topics (see Chapter 13), but should consider the role of peers in social development. There are indications that peers can serve as secure bases for exploration and that peers who are only slightly older then target infants may evoke the most mature play behaviors and interactions.

Play is a potential index of adequacy of functioning, both biological and cognitive. Finally, the role of mother or other caretaker as playmate is important and deserves much more study.

References

ADAMSON, L. B., Als, H., Tronick, E., & Brazelton, T. B. (1977). The development of social reciprocity between a sighted infant and her blind parents: A case study. *Journal of the American Academy of Child Psychiatry, 16,* 194-207.

ADAMSON, L. B., & Bakeman, R. (1985). Affect and attention: Infants observed with mothers and peers. *Child Development, 56,* 582-593.

AINSWORTH, M. D. S. (1963). The development of infant-mother interaction among the Ganda. In B. M. Foss (Ed.), *Determinants of infant behaviour* (Vol. 2, pp. 67-112). London: Methuen.

AINSWORTH, M. D. S. (1967). *Infancy in Uganda: Infant care and the growth of love.* Baltimore: Johns Hopkins University Press.

AINSWORTH, M. D. S. (1972). Attachment and dependency: A comparison. In J. L. Gewirtz (Ed.), *Attachment and dependency* (pp. 97-137). Washington, DC: Winston.

AINSWORTH, M. D. S. (1973). The development of infant-mother attachment. In B. M. Caldwell & H. N. Ricciuti (Eds.), *Review of child development research* (Vol. 3, pp. 1-94). Chicago: University of Chicago Press.

AINSWORTH, M. D. S. (1974). Infant-mother attachment and social development: Socialization as a product of reciprocal responsiveness to signals. In M. Edwards (Ed.), *The integration of the child into the social world.* Cambridge: Cambridge University Press.

AINSWORTH, M. D. S. (1985). Patterns of attachment. *Clinical Psychologist, 38,* 27-29.

AINSWORTH, M. D. S., & Bell, S. M. V. (1969). Some contemporary patterns of mother-infant interaction in the feeding situation. In J. A. Ambrose (Ed.), *Stimulation in early infancy* (pp. 133-170). London: Academic Press.

AINSWORTH, M. D. S., & Bell, S. M. V. (1970). Attachment, exploration, and separation: Illustrated by the behavior of one-year-olds in a strange situation. *Child Development, 41,* 49-67.

AINSWORTH, M. D. S., Bell, S. M. V., & Stayton, D. J. (1971).

Individual differences in strange-situation behavior of one-year-olds. In H. R. Schaffer (Ed.), *The origins of human social relations* (pp. 17-52). New York: Academic Press.

AINSWORTH, M. D. S., & Wittig, B. A. (1969). Attachment and exploratory behavior of one-year-olds in a strange situation. In B. M. Foss (Ed.), *Determinants of infant behaviour* (Vol. 4, pp. 111-136). London: Methuen.

ANISFELD, E., Casper, V., Nozyce, M., & Cunningham, N. (1990). Does infant carrying promote attachment? An experimental study of the effects of increased physical contact on the development of attachment. *Child Development, 61,* 1617-1627.

ARSENIAN, J. M. (1943). Young children in an insecure situation. *Journal of Abnormal and Social Psychology, 38,* 225-249.

BAILEY, W. T. (1982, March). *Affinity: An ethological theory of the infant-father relationship.* Paper presented at the International Conference on Infant Studies, Austin, TX.

BAKEMAN, R., & Adamson, L. B. (1984). Coordinating attention to people and objects in mother-infant and peer-infant interaction. *Child Development, 55,* 1278-1289.

BARD, K. A. (1991, June). *Distribution of attachment classifications in nursery chimpanzees.* Paper presented at the meeting of the American Society of Primatologists, Veracruz, Mexico.

BECKWITH, L., & Cohen, S. E. (1989). Maternal responsiveness with preterm infants and later competency. In M. H. Bornstein (Ed.), *Maternal responsiveness: Characteristics and consequences* (New Directions for Child Development, No. 43). San Francisco: Jossey-Bass.

BÉDARD, R., Laplante, D. P., Stack, D. M., & Zelazo, P. R. (1990, August). *Directed functional play behaviors of normal, moderate, and high risk infants.* Paper presented at the annual meeting of the American Psychological Association, Boston.

BELL, R. Q. (1968). A reinterpretation of the direction of effects in studies of socialization. *Psychological Review, 75,* 81-95.

BELL, R. Q. (1971). Stimulus control of parent or caretaker behavior by offspring. *Developmental Psychology, 4,* 63-72.

BELL, S. M. (1970). The development of the concept of object as related to infant-mother attachment. *Child Development, 41,* 291-311.

BELSKY, J. (1979a). The interrelation of parental and spousal behavior during infancy in traditional nuclear families: An exploratory analysis. *Journal of Marriage and the Family, 41,* 62-68.

BELSKY, J. (1979b). Mother-father-infant interaction: A naturalistic observational study. *Developmental Psychology, 15,* 601-607.

BELSKY, J. (1981). Early human experience: A family perspective. *Developmental Psychology, 17,* 3-23.

BELSKY, J., & Rovine, M. (1987). Temperament and attachment security in the Strange Situation: An empirical rapprochement. *Child Development, 58,* 787-795.

BELSKY, J., & Volling, B. L. (1987). Mothering, fathering, and marital interaction in the family triad during infancy: Exploring family systems' processes. In P. Berman & F. Pedersen (Eds.), *Men's transition to parenthood* (pp. 37-63). Hillsdale, NJ: Lawrence Erlbaum.

BEM, S. L., Martyna, W., & Watson, C. (1976). Sex typing and androgyny: Further explorations of the expressive domain. *Journal of Personality and Social Psychology, 34,* 1016-1023.

BERMAN, P., & Pedersen, F. A. (Eds.). (1987). *Men's transition to parenthood.* Hillsdale, NJ: Lawrence Erlbaum.

BLOCK, J. (1978). *The Q-sort method in personality assessment and psychiatry research.* Palo Alto, CA: Consulting Psychologists Press. (Original work published 1961)

BOWLBY, J. (1958). The nature of the child's tie to his mother. *International Journal of Psychoanalysis, 39,* 350-373.

BOWLBY, J. (1969). *Attachment and loss: Vol. 1. Attachment.* New York: Basic Books.

BRACKBILL, Y. (1958). Extinction of the smiling response in infants as a function of reinforcement schedule. *Child Development, 29,* 115-124.

BRAUNGART, J. M., Stifter, C. A., & Belsky, J. (1990, April). *Avoidance in the Strange Situation: Independence or regulation?* Paper presented at the International Conference on Infant Studies, Montreal.

BRAZELTON, T. B., Tronick, E., Adamson, L., Als, H., & Wise, S. (1975). Early mother-infant reciprocity. In M. A. Hofer (Ed.), *Parent-infant interaction.* London: Ciba.

BRETHERTON, I., & Ainsworth, M. D. S. (1974). Responses of one-year-olds to a stranger in a strange situation. In M. Lewis & L. Rosenblum (Eds.), *The origins of fear* (pp. 131-164). New York: John Wiley.

BRONSON, G. W. (1968). The year of novelty. *Psychological Bulletin, 69,* 350-358.

BRONSON, G. W. (1972). Infants' reactions to unfamiliar persons and novel objects. *Monographs of the Society for Research in Child Development, 37*(3, Serial No. 148).

BRONSTEIN, P., & Cowan, C. P. (Eds.). (1988). *Fatherhood today: Men's changing role in the family.* New York: John Wiley.

BROUSSARD, E. R., & Hartner, M. S. S. (1971). Further considerations regarding maternal perception of the first born. In J. Hellmuth (Ed.), *Exceptional infant: Studies in abnormalities* (Vol. 2, pp. 432-449). New York: Brunner/Mazel.

BRUNER, J. S. (1964). The course of cognitive growth. *American Psychologist, 19,* 1-15.

BRUNER, J. S. (1972). The nature and uses of immaturity. *American Psychologist, 27,* 1-22.

CAIRNS, R. B. (1972). Attachment and dependency: A psychobiological and social learning synthesis. In J. L. Gewirtz (Ed.), *Attachment and dependency* (pp. 29-80). New York: Winston.

CAMFIELD, E., Brownell, C., Taylor, P., Day, N., Brown, E., & Kratzer, L. (1991, April). *Mediators of relations between maternal behavior at 4 months and infant attachment at 12 months.* Paper presented at the meeting of the Society for Research in Child Development, Seattle.

CAMPOS, J., Emde, R., & Gaensbauer, T. (1975). Cardiac and behavioral interrelationships in the reactions of infants to strangers. *Developmental Psychology, 11,* 589-601.

CARR, S., Dabbs, J., & Carr, T. (1975). Mother-infant attachment: The importance of the mother's visual field. *Child Development, 46,* 331-338.

CLARKE-STEWART, K. A. (1973). Interactions between mothers and their young children: Characteristics and consequences. *Monographs of the Society for Research in Child Development, 38*(6, Serial No. 153).

CLARKE-STEWART, K. A. (1978). And daddy makes three: The father's impact on mother and child. *Child Development, 49,* 466-478.

CLARKE-STEWART, K. A. (1980). The father's contribution to children's cognitive and social development in early childhood. In F. A. Pedersen (Ed.), *The father-infant relationship: Observational studies in a family setting.* New York: Holt, Rinehart & Winston.

COHEN, S. E. (1988, April). *Parent-infant interaction: Ten years later.* Paper presented at the International Conference on Infant Studies, Montreal.

COLIN, V. L. (1987, April). *Infants' preferences between parents before and after moderate stress activates attachment behavior.* Paper presented at the meeting of the Society for Research in Child Development, Baltimore.

CORDELL, A. S. (1978). *The father-infant relationship.* Unpublished doctoral dissertation, University of Chicago.

CORTER, C. M., Rheingold, H. L., & Eckerman, C. O. (1972). Toys delay the infant's following of his mother. *Developmental Psychology, 6,* 138-145.

COX, F. N., & Campbell, D. (1968). Young children in a new situation with and without their mothers. *Child Development, 39,* 123-131.

CROWELL, J. A., & Feldman, S. S. (1991). Mothers' working models of attachment relationships and mother and child behavior during separation and reunion. *Developmental Psychology, 27,* 597-605.

DICKSTEIN, S., & Parke, R. D. (1988). Social referencing in infancy: A glance at fathers and marriage. *Child Development, 59,* 506-511.

DICKSTEIN, S., Thompson, R., Estes, D., Malkin, C., & Lamb, M. (1984). Social referencing and the security of attachment. *Infant Behavior and Development, 5,* 507-516.

DONOVAN, W. L., & Leavitt, L. A. (1985). Physiologic assessment of mother-infant attachment. *Journal of the American Academy of Child Psychiatry, 24,* 65-70.

EARLS, F., & Yogman, M. (1978). The father-infant relationship. In J. Howells (Ed.), *Modern perspectives in the psychiatry of infancy.* New York: Brunner/Mazel.

EASTERBROOKS, M. A. (1982, March). *Father involvement, parenting characteristics and toddler development.* Paper presented at the International Conference on Infant Studies, Austin, TX.

ECKERMAN, C. O., Davis, C. C., & Didow, S. M. (1989). Toddlers' emerging ways of achieving social coordinations with a peer. *Child Development, 60,* 440-453.

ECKERMAN, C. O., & Didow, S. M. (1989). Toddlers' social coordination: Changing responses to another's invitation to play. *Developmental Psychology, 25,* 794-804.

ECKERMAN, C. O., & Rheingold, H. L. (1974). Infants' exploratory responses to toys and people. *Developmental Psychology, 10,* 255-259.

ECKERMAN, C. O., Whatley, J. L., & Kutz, S. L. (1975). Growth of social play with peers during the second year of life. *Developmental Psychology, 11,* 42-49.

EISENBERG, R. B. (1969). Auditory behavior in the human neonate: Functional properties of sound and their orthogenetic significance. *International Audiology, 8,* 34-44.

ENTWISLE, D. R., & Doering, S. G. (1981). *The first birth.* Baltimore: Johns Hopkins University Press.

ERIKSON, E. H. (1963). *Childhood and society.* New York: W. W. Norton.

FEINMAN, S. (1985). Emotional expression, social referencing and preparedness for learning in infancy: Mother knows best—but sometimes I know better. In G. Zivin (Ed.), *The development of expressive behavior: Biology-environment interactions* (pp. 291-318). New York: Academic Press.

FEINMAN, S., & Roberts, D. (1986, April). *Frequency and duration of social contact during the first year: Basic patterns, age effects, and infant temperament differences.* Paper presented at the International Conference on Infant Studies, Los Angeles.

FEINMAN, S., Roberts, D., & Morissette, L. (1986, April). *The effects of social referencing on 12-month-olds' responses to a stranger's attempts to "make friends."* Paper presented at the International Conference on Infant Studies, Los Angeles.

FELDMAN, S., & Ingham, M. (1975). Attachment behavior: A validation study in two age groups. *Child Development, 46,* 319-330.

FIELD, T. (1978). Interaction patterns of primary versus secondary caretaker fathers. *Developmental Psychology, 14,* 183-185.

FISCHER-FAY, A., Goldberg, S., Simmons, R., & Levison, H. (1988). Chronic illness and infant-mother attachment: Cystic fibrosis. *Journal of Developmental and Behavioral Pediatrics, 9,* 266-270.

FOX, N. (1977). Attachment of kibbutz infants to mother and metapelet. *Child Development, 48,* 1228-1239.

FOX, N. A., & Davidson, R. J. (1987). Electroencephalogram asymmetry in response to the approach of a stranger and maternal separation in 10-month-old infants. *Developmental Psychology, 23,* 233-240.

FOX, N. A., Kimmerly, N. L., & Schafer, W. D. (1991). Attachment to mother/attachment to father: A meta-analysis. *Child Development, 62,* 210-225.

FREUD, S. (1938). Three contributions to the theory of sex. In A. A. Brill (Ed.), *The basic writings of Sigmund Freud* (pp. 553-629). New York: Modern Library. (Original work published 1905)

GERSHAW, N. J., & Schwartz, T. C. (1971). The effects of a familiar toy and mother's presence on exploratory and attachment behaviors in young children. *Child Development, 42,* 1662-1666.

GEWIRTZ, J. L. (1972a). Attachment, dependence, and a distinction in terms of stimulus controls. In J. L. Gewirtz (Ed.), *Attachment and dependency* (pp. 139-177). Washington, DC: Winston.

GEWIRTZ, J. L. (1972b). On the selection and use of attachment and dependence indices. In J. L. Gewirtz (Ed.), *Attachment and dependency* (pp. 179-215). Washington, DC: Winston.

GEWIRTZ, J. L., & Paláez-Nogueras, M. (in press). Infant social referencing as a learned process. In S. Feinman (Ed.), *Social referencing and the social construction of reality in infancy.* New York: Plenum.

GEWIRTZ, J. L., & Paláez-Nogueras, M. (1991). Infants' separation difficulties and distress due to misplaced maternal contingencies. In T. Field, P. McCabe, & N. Schneiderman (Eds.), *Stress and coping in infancy and childhood.* Hillsdale, NJ: Lawrence Erlbaum.

GOFF, D. M., & Britt, G. C. (1990, March). *An empirical comparison of parents' and published criteria for a secure attachment.* Paper presented at the Conference on Human Development, Richmond, VA.

GOLDBERG, S., Perrota, M., & Minde, K. (1986). Maternal behavior and attachment in low birthweight twins and singletons. *Child Development, 57,* 34-46.

GOLDSMITH, H., & Alansky, J. (1987). Maternal and infant temperamental predictors of attachment: A meta-analytic review. *Journal of Consulting and Clinical Psychology, 55,* 805-816.

GOTTFRIED, A. W., & Brown, C. C. (1986). *Play interactions: The contribution of play materials and parental involvement to children's development.* Lexington, MA: Lexington.

GREENBERG, M., & Morris, N. (1974). Engrossment: The newborn's impact upon the father. *American Journal of Or-*

thopsychiatry, 44, 520-531.

GROSSMANN, K. (1989, July). *Differential effects of attachment quality to mother and father on boys and girls.* Paper presented at the meeting of the International Society for the Study of Behavioural Development, Jyväskyla, Finland.

GROSSMANN, K. E., & Grossmann, K. (1989). *Preliminary observations on Japanese infants' behavior in Ainsworth's Strange Situation.* Unpublished manuscript.

GROSSMANN, K. E., & Grossmann, K. (1990). The wider concept of attachment in cross-cultural research. *Human Development, 33*, 31-47.

GROSSMANN, K. E., Grossmann, K.,, Huber, F., & Wartner, U. (1981). German children's behavior toward their mothers at 12 months and their fathers at 18 months in Ainsworth's Strange Situation. *International Journal of Behavioral Development, 7*, 157-181.

GROSSMANN, K. E., Scheuerer-Englisch, H., & Stephan, C. (1989, July). *Attachment research: Lasting effects and domains of validity.* Paper presented at the meeting of the International Society for the Study of Behavioural Development, Jyväskyla, Finland.

GROSSMANN, K. E., & Volkmer, H.-J. (1984). Fathers' presence during birth of their infants and paternal involvement. *International Journal of Behavioral Development, 7*, 157-165.

GUNNAR, M. R., Senior, K., & Hartup, W. W. (1984). Peer presence and the exploratory behavior of eighteen- and thirty-month-old children. *Child Development, 55*, 1103-1109.

HARLOW, H. F. (1958). The nature of love. *American Psychologist, 13*, 673-685.

HARLOW, H. F., & Zimmerman, R. R. (1959). Affectional responses in the infant monkey. *Science, 130*, 421-432.

HARPER, L. V. (1971). The young as a source of stimuli controlling caretaker behavior. *Developmental Psychology, 4*, 73-88.

HARRIS, M., Buhr, S., Ahles, B., Sorenson, D., Loesch, A., & Beyer, J. (1991, April). *Quality of care effects on infant stress reactions to separation.* Paper presented at the meeting of the Society for Research in Child Development, Seattle.

HARRISON, M. J. (1990). A comparison of parental interactions with term and preterm infants. *Research in Nursing and Health, 13*, 173-179.

HEBB, D. O., & Riesen, A. H. (1943). The genesis of irrational fears. *Bulletin of the Canadian Psychological Association, 3*, 49-50.

HORNIK, R., & Gunnar, M. R. (1988). A descriptive analysis of infant social referencing. *Child Development, 59*, 626-634.

HORNIK, R., Risenhoover, N., & Gunnar, M. (1987). The effects of maternal positive, neutral, and negative affective communications on infant responses to new toys. *Child Development, 58*, 937-944.

HOWES, C., Rodning, C., Galluzzo, D. C., & Myers, L. (1988). Attachment and child care: Relationships with mother and caregiver. In Infant day care: II. Empirical studies [Special issue]. *Early Childhood Research Quarterly, 3*, 403-416.

HRON-STEWART, K., Weintraub, D., & Clark, W. (1989, April). *A comparison of maternal assessments of attachment using the Attachment Q-sort for Down syndrome and normal children.* Paper presented at the meeting of the Society for Research in Child Development.

ISABELLA, R. A., & Belsky, J. (1991). Interactional synchrony and the origins of infant-mother attachment: A replication study. *Child Development, 62*, 373-384.

ISABELLA, R. A., Belsky, J., & von Eye, A. (1989). Origins of infant-mother attachment: An examination of interactional synchrony during the infant's first year. *Developmental Psychology, 25*, 12-21.

JONES, S. S. (1985). On the motivational bases for attachment behavior. *Developmental Psychology, 21*, 848-857.

JONES, S. S. (1987, April). *Is attachment unitary?* Paper presented at the meeting of the Society for Research in Child Development, Baltimore.

JONES, S. S., Ridge, B., & Bates, J. E. (1990, March). *On the origins and significance of young children's attachments to inanimate objects.* Presented at the Conference on Human Development, Richmond, VA.

JOSSELYN, I. M. (1956). Cultural forces, motherliness, and fatherliness. *American Journal of Orthopsychiatry, 26*, 264-271.

KERMOIAN, R., & Leiderman, P. H. (1986). Infant attachment to mother and child caretaker in an East African community. *International Journal of Behavioral Development, 9*, 455-469.

KLAUS, M. H., Kennell, J. H., Plumb, N., & Zuehlke, S. (1970). Human maternal behavior at first contact with her young. *Pediatrics, 46*, 187-192.

KOESTER, L. S., Papoušek, H., & Papoušek, M. (1989). Patterns of rhythmic stimulation by mothers with three-month-olds: A cross-modal comparison. *International Journal of Behavioral Development, 12*, 143-154.

KORT, C., & Friedland, R. (Eds.). (1986). *The fathers' book: Shared experiences.* Boston: G. K. Hall.

KOTELCHUCK, M. (1976). The infant's relationship to the father: Experimental evidence. In M. E. Lamb (Ed.), *The role of the father in child development* (pp. 329-344). New York: John Wiley.

KROMELOW, S., Harding, C., & Touris, M. (1990). The role of the father in the development of stranger sociability during the second year. *American Journal of Orthopsychiatry, 60*, 521-530.

LAMB, M. E. (1976a). Interactions between eight-month-old children and their fathers and mothers. In M. E. Lamb (Ed.), *The role of the father in child development* (pp. 307-327). New York: John Wiley.

LAMB, M. E. (1976b). The role of the father: An overview. In M. E. Lamb (Ed.), *The role of the father in child development* (pp. 1-63). New York: John Wiley.

LAMB, M. E. (1976c). Twelve month olds and their parents: Interaction in a laboratory playroom. *Developmental Psychology, 12*, 237-244.

LAMB, M. E. (1977a). The development of mother-infant and father-infant attachments in the second year of life. *Developmental Psychology, 13*, 639-649.

LAMB, M. E. (1977b). Father-infant and mother-infant interaction in the first year of life. *Child Development, 48*, 167-181.

LAMB, M. E. (Ed.). (1987). *The father's role: Cross-cultural perspectives.* Hillsdale, NJ: Lawrence Erlbaum.

LAMB, M. E., Frodi, A. M., Frodi, M., & Hwang, C.-P. (1982). Characteristics of maternal and paternal behavior in traditional and nontraditional Swedish families. *International Journal of Behavioral Development, 5*, 131-141.

LAMB, M. E., Frodi, M., Hwang, C.-P., & Frodi, A. M. (1983). Effects of paternal involvement on infant preferences for mothers and fathers. *Child Development, 54*, 450-458.

LAMB, M. E., Frodi, A. M., Hwang, C.-P., Frodi, M., & Steinberg J. (1982). Mother- and father-infant interactions involving play and holding in traditional and nontraditional

Swedish families. *Developmental Psychology, 18,* 215-221.

LAMB, M. E., Morrison, D. C., & Malkin C. M. (1987). The development of infant social expectations in face-to-face interaction: A longitudinal study. *Merrill-Palmer Quarterly, 33,* 241-254.

LAMB, M. E., Thompson, R., Gardner, W., & Charnov, E. (1985). *Infant-mother attachment: The origins and developmental significance of individual differences in Strange Situation behavior.* Hillsdale, NJ: Lawrence Erlbaum.

LARSON, M. C., Gunnar, M. R., & Hertsgaard, L. (1991). The effects of morning naps, car trips, and maternal separation on adrenocortical activity in human infants. *Child Development, 62,* 362-372.

LEE, L. C. (1975). Toward a cognitive theory of interpersonal development: Importance of peers. In M. Lewis & L. Rosenblum (Eds), *Friendship and peer relations.* New York: John Wiley.

LESTER, B. M., Hoffman, J., & Brazelton, T. B. (1985). The rhythmic structure of mother-infant interaction in term and preterm infants. *Child Development, 56,* 15-27.

LESTER, B. M., Kotelchuck, M., Spelke, E., Sellers, M. J., & Klein, R. E. (1974). Separation protest in Guatemalan infants: Cross cultural and cognitive findings. *Developmental Psychology, 10,* 79-85.

LEVY-SHIFF, R., Sharir, H., & Mogilner, M. B. (1989). Mother- and father-preterm infant relationship in the hospital preterm nursery. *Child Development, 60,* 93-102.

LEWIS, M., & Feiring, C. (1989). Infant, mother, and mother-infant interaction behavior and subsequent attachment. *Child Development, 60,* 831-837.

LEWIS, M., Feiring, C., McGuffog, C., & Jaskir, J. (1984). Predicting psychopathology in six-year-olds from early social relations. *Child Development, 55,* 123-136.

LEWIS, M., & Goldberg, S. (1969). Perceptual-cognitive development in infancy: A generalized expectancy model as a function of mother-infant interaction. *Merrill-Palmer Quarterly, 15,* 81-100.

LEWIS, R. A., & Salt, R. E. (Eds.). (1986). *Men in families.* Beverly Hills, CA: Sage.

LIND, J. (1974, October). *Observations after delivery of communications between mother-infant-father.* Paper presented at the International Congress of Pediatrics, Buenos Aires.

LUTKENHAUS, P., Grossman, K. E., & Grossman, K. (1985). Infant-mother attachment at twelve months and style of interaction with a stranger at the age of three years. *Child Development, 56,* 1538-1542.

MACCOBY, E., & Feldman, S. (1972). Mother-attachment and stranger-reactions in the third year of life. *Monographs of the Society for Research in Child Development, 37*(1, Serial No. 146).

MACKEY, W. C. (1985). *Fathering behaviors: The dynamics of the man-child bond.* New York: Plenum.

MAIN, M. (1973). *Exploration, play, and cognitive functioning as related to child-mother attachment.* Unpublished doctoral dissertation, Johns Hopkins University.

MAIN, M. (1990). Cross-cultural studies of attachment organization: Recent studies, changing methodologies, and the concept of conditional strategies. *Human Development, 33,* 48-61.

MAIN, M., & Cassidy, J. (1987). *Reunion-based classifications of child-parent attachment organization at 6 years of age.* Unpublished scoring manual, University of California, Berkeley, Department of Psychology.

MAIN, M., & Cassidy, J. (1988). Categories of response to reunion with the parent at age 6: Predictable from infant attachment classifications and stable over a 1-month period. *Developmental Psychology, 24,* 415-426.

MAIN, M., & Solomon, J. (1986). Discovery of an insecure-disorganized/disoriented attachment pattern. In T. B. Brazelton & M. Yogman (Eds.), *Affective development in infancy.* Norwood, NJ: Ablex.

MATAS, L., Arend, R., & Sroufe, L. (1978). Continuity in adaptation in the second year: Quality of attachment and later competence. *Child Development, 49,* 547-556.

McCALL, R. B., & Kagan, J. (1967). Stimulus-schema discrepancy and attention in the infant. *Journal of Experimental Child Psychology, 5,* 381-390.

MEADOW-ORLANS, K. P., Erting, C., Prezioso, C., Bridges-Cline, F., & MacTurk, R. H. (1986, August). *Effects of deafness on mother-infant interaction.* Paper presented at the annual meeting of the American Psychological Association, Washington, DC.

MINEKA, S., Gunnar, M., & Champoux, M. (1986). Control and early socioemotional development: Infant rhesus monkeys reared in controllable versus uncontrollable environments. *Child Development, 57,* 1241-1256.

MIYAKE, K., Chen, S. J., & Campos, J. J. (1985). Infant temperament, mother's mode of interaction, and attachment in Japan: An interim report. In I. Bretherton & E. Waters (Eds.), Growing points in attachment theory and research. *Monographs of the Society for Research in Child Development, 50*(Serial No. 209), 276-297.

MORGAN, G. A., & Ricciuti, H. N. (1969). Infant's responses to strangers during the first year. In B. M. Foss (Ed.), *Determinants of infant behaviour* (Vol. 4, pp. 253-272). London: Methuen.

MYERS, B. J., Creasey, G. L., Jarvis, P. A., & Resnik, J. (1987, April). *Paternal grandmothers and their infant grandchildren: Interaction in a strange situation.* Paper presented at the meeting of the Society for Research in Child Development, Baltimore.

NASH, A. (1989, April). *The role of adults in infant-peer interactions.* Paper presented at the meeting of the Society for Research in Child Development, Kansas City, MO.

NASH, J. (1965). The father in contemporary culture and current psychological literature. *Child Development, 36,* 261-297.

OSOFSKY, J. D. (1976). Neonatal characteristics and mother-infant interaction in two observational situations. *Child Development, 47,* 1138-1147.

OSOFSKY, J. D., & Danzger, B. (1974). Relationships between neonatal characteristics and mother-infant interaction. *Developmental Psychology, 10,* 124-130.

PALKOVITZ, R. (1982). Fathers' birth attendance, early extended contact, and father-infant interaction at five months postpartum. *Birth: Issues in Perinatal Care and Education, 9,* 173-177.

PALKOVITZ, R. (1984). [Lay attitudes concerning fathers and "bonding."] Unpublished raw data.

PALKOVITZ, R. (1985). Fathers' birth attendance, early contact, and extended contact with their newborns: A critical review. *Child Development, 56,* 392-406.

PALKOVITZ, R. (1988, March). *Who does what revisited: Projected and actual division of child care tasks across the transition to parenthood.* Paper presented at the Conference on Human Development, Charleston, SC.

PAPOUŠEK, H. (1967). Experimental studies of appetitional behavior in human newborns and infants. In H. W. Stevenson, E. H. Hess, & H. L. Rheingold (Eds.), *Early behavior: Comparative and developmental approaches* (pp. 249-277). New York: John Wiley.

PAPOUŠEK, H., & Bernstein, P. (1969). The functions of conditioning stimulation in human neonates and infants. In A. Ambrose (Ed.), *Stimulation in early infancy* (pp. 229-252). London: Academic Press.

PAPOUŠEK, H., & Papoušek, M. (1974). Mirror image and self recognition in young human infants: A new method of experimental analysis. *Developmental Psychology, 7,* 149-157.

PAPOUŠEK, H., & Papoušek, M. (1975). Cognitive aspects of preverbal social interaction between human infants and adults. In R. Porter & M. O'Connor (Eds.), *Parent-infant interaction* (pp. 241-260). Amsterdam: Elsevier.

PAPOUŠEK, H., & Papoušek, M. (1977). Mothering and the cognitive head-start: Psychobiological considerations. In H. R. Schaffer (Ed.), *Studies in mother-infant interaction.* London: Academic Press.

PARKE, R. D., & Bhavnagi, N. P. (1989). Parents as managers of children's peer relationships. In D. Bell (Ed.), *Children's social networks and social supports* (pp. 241-259). New York: John Wiley.

PARKE, R. D., & O'Leary, S. E. (1976). Family interaction in the newborn period: Some findings, some observations and some unresolved issues. In K. F. Riegel & J. A. Meacham (Eds.), *The developing individual in a changing world: Vol. 2. Social and environmental issues* (pp. 653-663). Chicago: Aldine.

PARKE, R. D., & Sawin, D. B. (1975, April). *Infant characteristics and behavior as elicitors of maternal and paternal responsibility in the newborn period.* Paper presented at the biennial meeting of the Society for Research in Child Development, Denver.

PARKE, R. D., & Sawin, D. B. (1977, March). *The family in early infancy: Social interactional and attitudinal analyses.* Paper presented at the biennial meeting of the Society for Research in Child Development, New Orleans.

PARKE, R. D., & Tinsley, B. J. (1987). Family interaction in infancy. In J. D. Osofsky (Ed.), *Handbook of infant development* (2nd ed., pp. 579-641). New York: John Wiley.

PARSONS, T., & Bales, R. F. (1955). *Family, socialization and interaction process.* New York: Free Press.

PASTOR, D. L. (1980, April). *The quality of mother-infant attachment and its relationship to toddler's initial sociability with peers.* Paper presented at the International Conference on Infant Studies, New Haven, CT.

PEDERSEN, F. A., Anderson, B. J., & Cain, R. L. (1977, March). *An approach to understanding linkages between the parent-infant and spouse relationships.* Paper presented at the biennial meeting of the Society for Research in Child Development, New Orleans.

PEDERSEN, F. A., Anderson, B. J., & Cain, R. (1979, March). *Parent-infant interaction observed in a family setting at age 5 months.* Paper presented at the biennial meeting of the Society for Research in Child Development, San Francisco.

PEDERSEN, F. A., & Robson, K. S. (1969). Father participation in infancy. *American Journal of Orthopsychiatry, 39,* 466-472.

PEDERSEN, F. A., Rubenstein, J., & Yarrow, L. J. (1979). Infant development in father-absent families. *Journal of Genetic Psychology, 135,* 151-161.

PEDERSEN, F. A., Suwalsky, J. T. D., Cain, R. L., Zaslow, M. J., & Rabinovich, B. A. (1987). Paternal care of infants during maternal separations: Associations with father-infant interaction at one year. *Psychiatry, 50,* 193-205.

PEDERSEN, F. A., Zaslow, M. T., Cain, R. L., & Anderson, B. J. (1980, April). *Caesarean birth: The importance of a family perspective.* Paper presented at the International Conference on Infant Studies, New Haven, CT.

PEDERSON, D. R., Moran, G., Sitko, C., Campbell, K., et al. (1990). Maternal sensitivity and the security of infant-mother attachment: A Q-sort study. *Child Development, 61,* 1974-1983.

PIAGET, J. (1962). *Play, dreams and imitation in childhood.* New York: W. W. Norton.

PLOOF, D. (1976, April). *The reciprocal effects of maternal perceptions and infant characteristics in the early mother-infant interaction.* Paper presented at the meeting of the Eastern Psychological Association, Washington, DC.

POWER, T. G., & Parke, R. D. (1979, March). *Toward a taxonomy of father-infant and mother-infant play patterns.* Paper presented at the biennial meeting of the Society for Research in Child Development, San Francisco.

POWER, T. G., & Parke, R. D. (1986). Patterns of early socialization: Mother- and father-infant interaction in the home. *International Journal of Behavioral Development, 9,* 331-341.

PRESS, B. K., & Greenspan, S. I. (1985). Ned and Dan: The development of a toddler friendship. *Children Today, 14,* 24-29.

RANDOLPH, S. M. (1989). Infant attachment in black American families: An interim report. In J. L. McAdoo (Ed.), *The Twelfth Conference on Empirical Research in Black Psychology.* Washington, DC: National Institute of Mental Health.

RHEINGOLD, H. L. (1969). The effect of a strange environment on the behavior of infants. In B. M. Foss (Ed.), *Determinants of infant behaviour* (Vol. 4, pp. 137-166). London: Methuen.

RHEINGOLD, H. L., & Eckerman, C. O. (1969). The infant's free entry into a new environment. *Journal of Experimental Child Psychology, 8,* 217-283.

RHEINGOLD, H. L., & Eckerman, C. O. (1970). The infant separates himself from his mother. *Science, 168,* 78-83.

RHEINGOLD, H. L., Hay, D. F., & West, M. J. (1976). Sharing in the second year of life. *Child Development, 47,* 1148-1158.

RICHARDS, M. P. M. (1971). A comment on the social context of mother-infant interaction. In H. R. Schaffer (Ed.), *The origins of human social relations* (pp. 187-193). New York: Academic Press.

RICHARDS, M. P. M., Dunn, J. F., & Antonis, B. (1977). Caretaking in the first year of life: The role of fathers, and mothers' social isolation. *Child: Care, Health, and Development, 3,* 23-26.

ROBSON, K. S. (1967). The role of eye-to-eye contact in maternal infant attachment. *Journal of Child Psychology, 8,* 13-25.

ROBSON, K. S., & Moss, N. A. (1970). Patterns and determinants of maternal attachment. *Journal of Pediatrics, 77,* 976.

RODNING, C., Beckwith, L., & Howard, J. (1989). Characteristics of attachment organization and play organization in prenatally drug exposed toddlers. *Development and Psychopathology, 1,* 277-289.

ROEDELL, W. C., & Slaby, R. G. (1977). The role of distal and proximal interaction in infant social preference formation.

Developmental Psychology, 13, 266-273.

ROGGMAN, L. A., Carroll, K. A., Pippin, E. A., & McCool, D. E. (1990, April). *Toddler play in relation to social and cognitive competence.* Paper presented at the International Conference on Infant Studies, Montreal.

ROGGMAN, L. A., Langlois, J. H., & Hubbs-Tait, L. (1987). Social play and attachment: A study in construct validation. *Infant Behavior and Development, 10,* 233-237.

ROSENTHAL, M. (1973). Attachment and mother-infant interaction: Some research impasses and a suggested change in orientation. *Journal of Child Psychology and Psychiatry and Allied Disciplines, 14,* 201-207.

ROSS, G., Kagan, J., Zelazo, P., & Kotelchuk, M. (1975). Separation protest in infants in home and laboratory. *Developmental Psychology, 11,* 256-257.

ROSS, H. S., & Lollis, S. B. (1987). Communication within infant social games. *Developmental Psychology, 23,* 241-248.

ROSS, H. S., Rheingold, H. L., & Eckerman, C. O. (1972). Approach and exploration of a novel alternative by 12-month-old infants. *Journal of Experimental Child Psychology, 13,* 85-93.

ROTHSTEIN-FISCH, C., & Howes, C. (1988). Toddler peer interaction in mixed-age groups. *Journal of Applied Developmental Psychology, 9,* 211-218.

RUSSELL, G. (1978). The father role and its relation to masculinity, femininity and androgyny. *Child Development, 49,* 1174-1181.

RUSSELL, G. (1980, July 15-17). *Fathers as caregivers: Possible antecedents and consequences.* Paper presented at a study group on Fathers and Social Policy, University of Haifa, Israel.

SAGI, A., Lamb, M. E., Lewkowicz, K. S., Shoham, R., Dvir, R., & Estes, D. (1985). Security of infant-mother, -father, and -metapelet attachments among kibbutz-reared Israeli children. In I. Bretherton & E. Waters (Eds.), Growing points in attachment theory and research. *Monographs of the Society for Research in Child Development, 50*(Serial No. 209), 257-275.

SAGI, A., Van IJzendoorn, M. H., & Koren-Karie, N. (1991). Primary appraisal of the Strange Situation: A cross-cultural analysis of preseparation episodes. *Developmental Psychology, 27,* 587-596.

SCHAFFER, H. R., & Emerson, P. E. (1964). The development of social attachments in infancy. *Monographs of the Society for Research in Child Development, 29*(3, Serial No. 94).

SCHOETZAU, A., & Papoušek, H. (1977). Mothers' behavior in making eye contact with newborn infants. *Zeitschrift für Entwicklungspsychologie und Pädagogische Psychologie, 9,* 231-239.

SEARS, R. R. (1943). *Survey of objective studies of psychoanalytic concepts.* New York: Social Science Research Council.

SEARS, R. R. (1951). A theoretical framework for personality and social behavior. *American Psychologist, 6,* 476-483.

SEYEN, E. van, Lieshout, C. F. M. van, Baay-Knoers, M. deB., & Roos, S. de. (1989, July). *Antecedents of peer competence in the first two years.* Paper presented at meeting of the International Society for the Study of Behavioural Development, Jyväskylä, Finland.

SINGER, L. M., Brodzinsky, D. M., Ramsay, D., Steir, M., & Waters, E. (in press). Mother-Infant attachment in adoptive families. *Child Development.*

SLUCKIN, W. (1965). *Imprinting and early learning.* Chicago: Aldine.

SMITH, C. B., Adamson, L. B., & Bakeman, R. (1988). Interactional predictors of early language. *First Language, 8,* 143-156.

SMITH, P. B., & Pederson, D. R. (1988). Maternal sensitivity and patterns of infant-mother attachment. *Child Development, 59,* 1097-1101.

SOLOMON, J., George, C., & Ivins, B. (1987, April). *Mother-child interaction in the home and security of attachment at age 6.* Paper presented at the meeting of the Society for Research in Child Development, Baltimore.

SOLOMON, R., & Décarie, T. (1976). Fear of strangers: A developmental milestone or an overstudied phenomenon? *Canadian Journal of Behavioral Science, 8,* 351-362.

SPITZ, R. A. (1950). Anxiety in infancy: A study of its manifestations in the first year of life. *Journal of Psychoanalysis, 31,* 132-143.

SROUFE, L. A. (1977). Wariness of strangers and the study of child infant development. *Child Development, 48,* 731-746.

SROUFE, L. A. (1979). Socioemotional development. In J. D. Osofsky (Ed.), *Handbook of infant development* (pp. 462-516). New York: John Wiley.

SROUFE, L. A. (1985). Attachment classification from the perspective of infant-caregiver relationships and infant temperament. *Child Development, 56,* 1-14.

SROUFE, L. A., & Waters, E. (1977). Attachment as an organizational construct. *Child Development, 48,* 1184-1199.

STACK, D. M., & Muir, D. W. (1990). Tactile stimulation as a component of social interchange: New interpretations for the still-face effect. *British Journal of Developmental Psychology, 8,* 131-145.

STECHLER, G., & Latz, E. (1966). Some observations on attention and arousal in the human infant. *Journal of the American Academy of Child Psychiatry, 5,* 517-525.

STERN, D. N., Beebe, B., Jaffe, J., & Bennett, S. L. (1977). The infants' stimulus world during social interaction: A study of caregiver behaviors with particular reference to repetition and timing. In H. R. Schaffer (Ed.), *Studies in mother-infant interaction.* New York: Academic Press.

THOMAN, E. B. (1981a). Affective communication as the prelude and context for language learning. In R. L. Schiefelbusch & D. Bricker (Eds.), *Early language: Acquisition and intervention.* Baltimore: University Park Press.

THOMAN, E. B. (1981b). Early communication as the prelude to later adaptive behaviors. In M. J. Begab, H. C. Haywood, & H. L. Garber (Eds.), *Psychosocial Influences in retarded performance: Vol. 2. Strategies for improving competence.* Baltimore: University Park Press.

THOMAS, A., & Chess, S. (1977). *Temperament and development.* New York: Brunner/Mazel.

THOMPSON, R. A., Cicchetti, D., Lamb, M. E., & Malkin, C. (1985). Emotional responses of Down syndrome and normal infants in the Strange Situation: The organization of affective behavior in infants. *Developmental Psychology, 21,* 828-841.

THOMPSON, R. A., & Lamb, M. E. (1984). Infants, mothers, families, and strangers. In M. Lewis (Ed.), *Beyond the dyad.* New York: Plenum.

THOMPSON, R. A., Lamb, M. E., & Estes, D. (1982). Stability of infant-mother attachment and its relationship to changing life circumstances in an unselected middle-class sample. *Child Development, 53,* 144-148.

TIEDEMANN, D. (1927). Tiedemann's observations on the development of the mental faculties of children (S. Langer & C. Murchison, Trans.). *Pedagogical Seminary and Journal of Genetic Psychology, 34,* 205-230. (Original work published 1787)

TREVARTHEN, C. (1977). Descriptive analyses of infant communicative behaviour. In H. R. Schaffer (Ed.), *Studies in mother-infant interaction*. New York: Academic Press.

TRNAVSKY, P. (1988, August). *Attachment characteristics in a sample of infants from the People's Republic of China*. Paper presented at the International Congress of Psychology, Sydney, Australia.

UJIIE, T., & Chen, S.-J. (1985, April). *Affective state and attachment behavior in the Strange Situation in Japanese infants*. Paper presented at the meeting of the Society for Research in Child Development, Toronto.

VALENZUELA, M. (1990). Attachment in chronically underweight young children. *Child Development, 61*, 1984-1996.

VAN IJZENDOORN, M. H. (1990). Development in cross-cultural research on attachment: Some methodological notes. *Human Development, 33*, 3-10.

VAN IJZENDOORN, M. H., & Kroonenberg, P. M. (1988). Cross-cultural patterns of attachment: A meta-analysis of the Strange Situation. *Child Development, 59*, 147-156.

VAN IJZENDOORN, M. H., & Kroonenberg, P. M. (1990). Cross-cultural consistency of coding the strange situation. *Infant Behavior and Development, 13*, 469-486.

VAUGHN, B., Egeland, B., Sroufe, L. A., & Waters, E. (1979). Individual differences in infant-mother attachment at twelve and eighteen months: Stability and change in families under stress. *Child Development, 50*, 971-975.

VAUGHN, B. E., & Waters, E. (1990). Attachment behavior at home and in the laboratory: Q-sort observations and Strange Situation classifications on one-year-olds. *Child Development, 61*, 1965-1973.

VIETZE, P. M., MacTurk, R. H., McCarthy, M. E., Klein, R. P., & Yarrow, L. J. (1980, April). *Impact of mode of delivery on father- and mother-infant interaction at 6 and 12 months*. Paper presented at the International Conference on Infant Studies, New Haven, CT.

VYGOTSKY, L. (1978). *Mind in society*. Cambridge, MA: Harvard University Press.

WALDEN, T. A., & Ogan, T. A. (1988). The development of social referencing. *Child Development, 59*, 1230-1240.

WALTERS, A. S., Adamson, L. B., & Bakeman, R. (1989, April). *Interacting with a new partner: Toddler appeals and maternal stage-setting*. Paper presented at the meeting of the Society for Research in Child Development, Kansas City, MO.

WARTNER, U. B., & Grossmann, K. (1987). *Stability of attachment patterns and their disorganizations from infancy to age 6 in South Germany*. Unpublished manuscript.

WATERS, E. (1978). The reliability and stability of individual differences in infant-mother attachment. *Child Development, 49*, 483-494.

WATERS, E. (1989). *Attachment Q-set (version 4.0)*. Stony Brook: State University of New York.

WATERS, E., & Deane, K. (1985). Defining and assessing individual differences in attachment relationships: Q-methodology and the organization of behavior in infancy and early childhood. In I. Bretherton & E. Waters (Eds.), Growing points in attachment theory and research. *Monographs of the Society for Research in Child Development, 50*(Serial No. 209), 41-65.

WATERS, E., Kondo-Ikemura, K., Posada, G., & Richters, J. (1990). Learning to love: Mechanisms and milestones. In M. Gunnar (Ed.), *Minnesota Symposia on Child Psychology* (Vol. 24, pp. 217-255). Hillsdale, NJ: Lawrence Erlbaum.

WATERS, E., Wippman, J., & Sroufe, L. A. (1979). Attachment, positive affect, and competence in the peer group: Two studies in construct validation. *Child Development, 50*, 821-829.

WEINRAUB, M., & Lewis, M. (1977). The determinants of children's responses to separation. *Monographs of the Society for Research in Child Development, 42*(4, Serial No. 172).

WOLFF, P. H. (1959). Observations on newborn infants. *Psychosomatic Medicine, 21*, 110-118.

WOLFF, P. H. (1963). Observations on the early development of smiling. In B. M. Foss (Ed.), *Determinants of infant behaviour* (Vol. 2, pp. 113-138). London: Methuen.

WOLFF, P. H. (1969). The natural history of crying and other vocalizations in early infancy. In B. M. Foss (Ed.), *Determinants of infant behaviour* (Vol. 4, pp. 81-109). London: Methuen.

YARROW, M. R., Waxler, C. Z., & Scott, P. M. (1971). Child effects on adult behavior. *Developmental Psychology, 5*, 300-311.

YOGMAN, M. W. (1982). Development of the father-infant relationship. In H. E. Fitzgerald, B. M. Lester, & M. W. Yogman (Eds.), *Theory and research in behavioral pediatrics* (Vol. 1, pp. 221-279). New York: Plenum.

YOGMAN, M. W., Dixon, S., Tronick, E., Adamson, L., Als, H., & Brazelton, T. B. (1976a, April). *Development of social interaction*. Paper presented at the meeting of the Eastern Psychological Association, New York.

YOGMAN, M. W., Dixon, S., Tronick, E., Adamson, L., Als, H., & Brazelton, T. B. (1976b, May). *Parent-infant interaction*. Paper presented at the meeting of the American Pediatric Society—Society for Pediatric Research.

YOGMAN, M. W., Tronick, E., Dixon, S., Keefer, C., Als, H., & Brazelton, T. B. (1977, March). *The goals and structure of face-to-face interaction between infants and fathers*. Paper presented at the biennial meeting of the Society for Research in Child Development, New Orleans.

ZANOLLI, K., Saudargas, R., & Twardosz, S. (1990). Two-year-olds' responses to affectionate and caregiving teacher behavior. *Child Study Journal, 20*, 35-54.

ZASLOW, M. J., Rabinovich, B. A., Suwalsky, J. T. D., & Klein, R. P. (1988). The role of social context in the prediction of secure and insecure/avoidant infant-mother attachment. *Journal of Applied Developmental Psychology, 9*, 287-299.

PART IV

The Social Context

Chapter 13

Influence of Environment: Deprivation and Enrichment

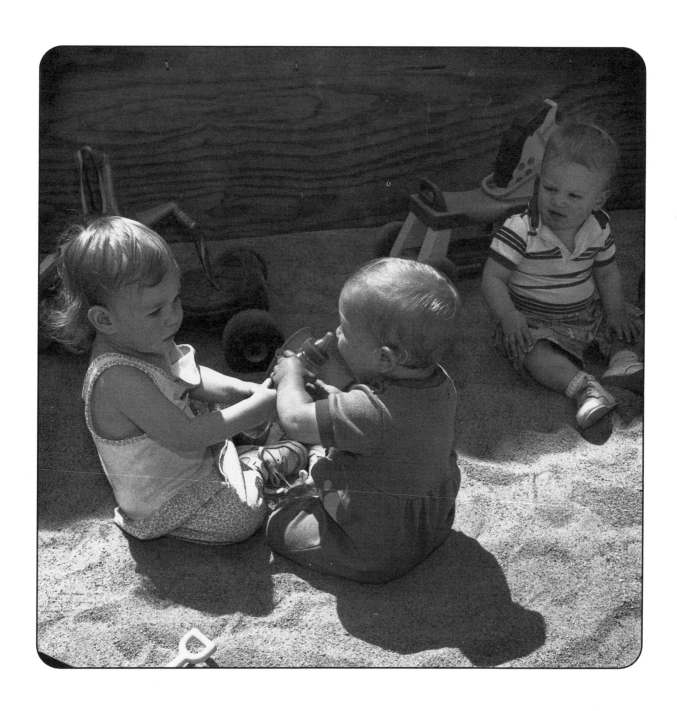

Chapter 12 described the common critical periods hypothesis that babies must develop their affectional relationships with their mothers during infancy or they will be unable to develop normally. The primary focus of this chapter will be research that examines this hypothesis by looking at the effects of various types of deprivation and its timing. One way of testing such a hypothesis is to examine the lives of children who were deprived of that maternal bond. Because researchers would not want to deprive babies of their mothers for the sake of science, they must look at so-called experiments of nature, unavoidable occurrences in the natural world that provide the deprivation conditions whose effects they are interested in. The most severe case of maternal deprivation probably occurs in orphanages. Because care in orphanages is provided by paid caretakers who often have a large number of babies to care for and who work in shifts, the substitute care seems to be quite different from that a mother would provide. Thus researchers have been interested in studying the effects of deprivation during the presumed critical period of infancy by studying institutionalized infants. A related set of experiments of nature occurs when institutionalized children leave institutions for adoptive homes or other settings. By studying these children at different ages, researchers can examine the long-term effects of deprivation. If, indeed, there is a critical period for the formation of attachment, or for cognitive or linguistic development, infants adopted after that critical period should show long-term effects of their early deprivation.

By studying or manipulating the environments of orphanages and the subsequent placements of orphanage children, researchers can get some idea of whether maternal deprivation itself produces ill effects. While, indeed, orphanage children are deprived of their mothers, they are also often deprived of other sorts of environmental stimulation that home-reared infants enjoy. In some institutions, children are not played with, taken places, or provided with toys to anywhere near the extent that home-reared infants are. Improvements in physical environment and caretaking arrangements lead to improved development in orphanage children, thus suggesting that deprivations other than that of the mother are important. In general, the research finds few permanent deficits from even severe early deprivation, so long as an adequate environment is provided by 2 years of age.

Other natural experiments that permit examination of the effects of early maternal deprivation (or at least alternative child-care arrangements) are studies of communal child rearing in other cultures and of day care in the United States. The argument goes like this:

Mother is the crucial source of early psychological growth in the child, therefore partial deprivation of mother, whether from multiple mothering in communal care or from being in day care, should have deleterious effects. Studies of multiple mothering in situations in which infants experience adequate stimulation—things to look at, touch, play with, and so forth—provide a good test of the effect of the mother herself. This research is quite consistent in showing that multiple mothering is not harmful, even when the biological mother spends much less time with her baby than the other caretaker or caretakers do.

The opposite of deprivation—enrichment—can also add to our understanding of the role of early experience. Research on enrichment has focused on the societally important goal of preventing or ameliorating the negative effects of deprivation by providing enriching experiences. Unlike human deprivation research, that on enrichment can be done experimentally. The limited research available has found intervention moderately successful, which suggests that deprivation effects are both preventable and correctable.

Finally, this chapter examines a small part of the vast animal literature on the effects of early experience. The research reviewed suggests that deprivation and enrichment affect various aspects of brain functioning and of behavior and that various kinds of early experience affect animals of varying genetic constitutions differently.

Institutionalization

EARLY STUDIES

The great interest in studying institutionalized infants stems from the early to mid-1940s, when several studies pointed to the dire consequences that institutionalization had for infants. Spitz (1945, 1946) coined the term **hospitalism** for the syndrome shown by these infants: They failed to gain weight, many died in a measles epidemic, they had great trouble in relationships with people, and they reached normal developmental milestones (sitting, walking, talking) very late. Goldfarb (1945a, 1945b) presented similar data and later presented a reanalysis (1955).

At about the same time, Skodak and Skeels (1945, 1949) published the initial follow-up of their series of studies that suggested that dire consequences were not an inevitable result of institutionalization. This experiment of nature began at overcrowded, unstaffed, poorly equipped orphanages in Iowa (Skeels, 1936; Skodak, 1939). Skeels served as staff psychologist for these orphanages and for several institutions for the retarded. His experiment began by accident. Two little girls, 13 and 16 months of age, had been committed to the orphanage because of neglect by their relatives. They were malnourished and had developmental levels of 6 and 7 months, respectively (DQs=46 and 35), but had no physical defects. Because they clearly seemed to be retarded, they were transferred to a home for the retarded, where they were placed in a ward of mentally deficient women. On Skeels's visit to that institution 6 months later, he found that the two little girls were alert and responsive and not recognizable as the two children with the hopeless prognosis he had seen earlier. When he retested them he found them close to normal, but he did not believe the tests could be valid, so the girls were left in the institution. New tests 12 months later and again when they were 35 and 40 months old showed development well within the normal range. The girls were transferred back to the orphanage and shortly afterward were adopted.

To find out why their development had changed so radically, Skeels examined their daily living situation and found that they had been made pets of the ward:

The older and brighter girls became very attached to the children and would play with them during most of their waking hours. Moreover, the attendants on the ward took a great fancy to the babies, and took them with them on their days off, took them to the store, bought them toys, picture books, and play materials. (Skeels & Dye, 1939, p. 5)

In the total program of the orphanage at that time, children whose development was so delayed that adoptive placement was out of the question remained there awaiting eventual transfer to an institution for the retarded. In light of the experience with the two little girls, Skeels was able to get such children accepted as "house guests" in the state school for the retarded. For the most part only one guest child was assigned to each elite ward (wards with the highest grades of retardates), but sometimes there were more children than elite wards. Periodic reevaluations were to be made and the children committed to the institution only if they did not improve. A total of 13 children became house guests, at an average age of 19 months (range, 7 to 36 months). Their IQs averaged 64 (range, 35 to 89). A number showed severe motor retardation or other abnormal behaviors. Most spent 1 to 2 years as house guests (range, 6 months to 52 months). The development of these 13 children was varied but positive. All showed gains in IQ, ranging from 7 to 58 points; 11 showed gains of

more than 17 points (which is greater than one standard deviation).

Skeels was able to select a comparison group from among the children who had remained at the orphanage until placement or institutionalization. Their initial IQs were higher (range, 50 to 103), but their ages at first assessment were similar and their home backgrounds were as poor as those transferred to the institution for the retarded. The mothers of both groups had averaged only eighth-grade education, and the mothers' IQs (when known) were, with one exception, below normal (mean of 70 for the experimental group and 63 for the contrast group).

Although the comparison group started off somewhat more advantaged, their subsequent development was markedly inferior to that of the experimental group. Only 1 child maintained his IQ (2 points gained); the rest lost an average of 26 IQ points (range, 9 to 45 points). Of the 12, 10 lost more than 15 points (or changed one standard deviation in the opposite direction from that of the experimental group).

What happened to the experimental children after their "visits" in the institution for the retarded? Of the 13 guests, one remained in the institution until adulthood, 11 were adopted, and 1 was returned to the orphanage for some years and later committed to the institution for the retarded. The adoptive homes were lower middle class, but somewhat better than the children's natural homes.

About 2½ years after the adopted children were placed in their new homes, all 25 children were evaluated. The average IQ for the experimental group was 96, and for those adopted it was 101. Only 1 of the adoptees, who was in the poorest of the adoptive homes, had a loss (5 points). The two children who were not adopted lost IQ points (17 points for the child returned to the orphanage and 9 for the child kept in the home for the retarded). The average IQ of the contrast group was 66, and 8 of the 12 had dropped markedly. Two were transferred at 41 months to the state school for the retarded and treated like the original experimental group. The IQ of one of these two children improved from 54 to 80. The other child failed to improve.

IQ is not the most important measure of people's adaptation in this world. Skeels (1966), in a rare show of persistence, and perhaps prodded by increased emphasis on mother-infant relations, followed these individuals when they reached adulthood. Of the 13 experimental children, not one was in an institution. All were self-supporting, in skilled or semiskilled jobs. Of the 12 contrast children, 5 ended up in institutions, and 5 of the 6 who worked were in unskilled jobs (the twelfth had died). The median grade completed by the experimental group was twelfth; by the contrast group, third. Of the experimental group, 4 had attended college, and 1 had graduated and then earned a Ph.D. at a major university. None of the contrast group attended college. Of the 13 former "house guests," 11 had married and 9 were parents. Their children had an average IQ of 105 and were progressing satisfactorily in school. Of the contrast group, only 2 had married, and only one of these marriages had lasted.

Although there are many methodological problems with this study (small number of subjects, lack of random assignment of subjects to groups, extreme diversity of the sample), the results are so striking that its conclusions are difficult to ignore. They suggest that early deprivation effects can be overcome by the provision of a more stimulating environment. They also suggest that such enrichment needs to be continued; the children who returned to the earlier, less stimulating environment again declined in IQ.

The Skeels and Skodak studies did not systematically examine differences between the orphanages and the institution for the retarded. Skeels attributed the effect of the latter to an abundance of attention and experiential stimulation from many sources and a one-on-one relationship with a loving adult (because the older retarded girls tended to "adopt" one baby). An equally good claim could be made that these babies were being raised by multiple mothers, because there was a whole ward for them to play with and receive contact from, as well as attendants.

WHAT PRODUCES THE RETARDATION EFFECTS OF INSTITUTIONS?

Skeels's study was greatly criticized for its methodological defects (e.g., see Longstreth, 1981), and so it had little impact on social policies. Nevertheless, subsequent research has confirmed that deprived children's development improves dramatically when their environment becomes more stimulating. The later studies have also helped to clarify conditions under which children institutionalized during infancy can later develop within the normal range. Dennis (1960) compared the development of infants in two institutions in Tehran. (Neither is necessarily representative

of institutions in Tehran, which had many institutions for foundlings, orphans, half orphans, and others needing care.) Children in the poorer institution showed profoundly retarded motoric development: 85% of them were not yet walking in their fourth year, and scooting rather than creeping was the modal pattern of prewalking locomotion. Nevertheless, they did not show the profound marasmus (or wasting away) from psychological causes that Spitz had described. Children from the better institution did not even show marked retardation in motor skills.

A comparison of the two institutions suggests some possibly crucial environmental differences. The better institution was a new demonstration institute set up to provide more adequate stimulation, with one trained attendant for every three to four infants, compared with one untrained attendant for every eight infants in the first institution. Infants in the poorer orphanage were fed lying in bed, were never placed in a prone position (lying face down), and were never propped up, although they were placed on the floor once they could sit up. Infants in the demonstration project, in contrast, were held while being fed, were placed in the prone position (which leads to better motoric organization in newborns), were propped in their cribs, and were placed in playpens after 4 months. The motoric retardation at the first institution, then, very likely resulted from lack of practice and use of appropriate muscles.

Further evidence concerning the causes of institutional retardation has been provided by Hunt and his collaborators, who explored the importance of the number of children per caregiver (child:caregiver ratio), what caregivers might do to foster cognitive development, and the role of visual and auditory stimulation independent of caregivers (Hunt et al., 1975, 1976; Paraskevopoulos & Hunt, 1971). These researchers explored the child:caregiver ratio in two studies. First, they investigated two institutions in Athens, Greece, that appeared to differ mainly in the child:caregiver ratio (Paraskevopoulos & Hunt, 1971). The babies at an orphanage with a 10:1 ratio were much slower to develop cognitively (as measured by the Hunt and Uzgiris ordinal scales of Piagetian-based cognitive development) than were babies at a demonstration institution with a 3:1 ratio.[1]

Second, Hunt et al. (1976), working at the same institution in Tehran that Dennis had found to foster retardation, introduced various experimental changes and assessed their effects. One intervention was to change the ratio from 10:1 to 10:3 (they called it 10:3 rather than 3:1 to emphasize that each infant received care from about 3 caregivers, not 1). The caregivers

---

1. Demonstration programs in institutions in this country are often discontinued despite their successes, due to lack of continued funding.

were not specially tutored in any way. The increase in the infants' motoric development was quite spectacular. They stood and "cruised" around their cribs holding on to the edge about 30 weeks earlier than infants in the same institution who had experienced the 10:1 ratio. Time-sampling observations suggested that the caregivers in the low child:caregiver ratio carried the babies in their arms and put them in strollers (where their feet could touch the floor) much more frequently. Hunt et al. surmised that this increase in muscular practice was what fostered motoric development. The effects of the better ratio on cognitive development were less clear. When the infants in the 10:3 condition were 11 to 13 months old, they were still quite retarded cognitively, but during the second year they made spectacular gains. They reached top-level performance in all the Uzgiris-Hunt scales much earlier than infants with the 10:1 ratio. On some scales, they were within the range of home-reared infants. However, this improvement cannot necessarily be attributed to the child:caregiver ratio. When Hunt visited the babies at the end of their first year and found them so cognitively retarded, he introduced an informal experiment in eliciting vocal imitation and managed to get two of the infants to advance on that scale. The caregivers, who watched this procedure, instituted it with the other infants, who also showed sudden development in vocal contagion. The sudden improvement in cognitive development in the second year may have stemmed from this intervention and its consequences. The caregivers were surprised that imitating the infants had such good effects and may subsequently have watched the testing procedures to get more ideas of ways to stimulate their charges.[2]

The second manipulation (Hunt et al., 1976) introduced visual and auditory experiences in a progression designed to increase both in complexity and in the extent to which the infants were allowed to exert control. These conditions fostered earlier development in the intermediate steps of the Hunt-Uzgiris scales (the first year of life) relative to the 10:3 ratio condition, but approximately the same developmental progress for the final steps of sensorimotor development.

Hunt's (1981, 1982) last manipulation involved trained caregivers in a 3:1 ratio. The training included Badger's (1973, 1977) program for training mothers of infants and toddlers, which involves teaching mothers (a) to recognize and respond to early signs of distress in their infants; (b) to recognize their infants' reactions of interest, boredom, and distress to environmental stimuli; and (c) to provide playthings and actions that bring forth interest rather than boredom or distress. In addition, to improve on Badger's program,

Hunt taught the caregivers to foster vocal imitation and to talk to the infants about what the caregivers were doing when caring for them. This program was the most successful of all. These babies achieved both the intermediate and final steps on the Uzgiris-Hunt scales earlier than those in any other conditions. They even achieved the final steps on five of the seven scales earlier than the offspring of professional parents in the United States.

Regardless of methodological problems that prevent clear interpretation of the cause of improvement, Hunt's data show that motoric and cognitive retardation need not be an inevitable consequence of institutionalization. The interventions these researchers instituted were relatively simple, yet they had profound effects. Their work also reveals something about the kinds of early experience that foster development. The presence of enough caretakers to enable activities other than essential caretaking has a strong effect, but it is not enough. What is enough for the first year is perceptual stimulation that increases in complexity as the infant develops and that is responsive to the infant's behaviors. More is necessary for the second year if development is to be normal. What that something is, is not entirely clear from Hunt's research. The best results were obtained when there had been both systematic and extensive cognitive stimulation and a deep affectional relationship with a caregiver (when these babies were adopted, their caregivers were demonstrably sad at losing "their" infants). Thus the infants' advancement may have been due to either factor or to the combined effects of both.

Broussard and Décarie (1971) carried out an experiment similar to, but much more limited, than Hunt's. Four groups of 12 institutionalized infants were matched on sex, age (at 2 to 2.1 months), and developmental quotients. The control group received normal institutional treatment. The three experimental groups received 15 minutes per day, 5 days per week, of systematic stimulation. The extra stimulation of one group was perceptual: They were exposed to a mobile that could be seen, touched, and made to make noise and a series of nonhuman everyday sounds from a tape recording. The second group was socially stimulated: One of two adults (each adult assigned to half the babies) sang, talked to, smiled at, caressed, carried, and rocked the babies in a strict sequence. The third group received half of each stimulation program.

---

2. In an earlier intervention study, Dennis (1960) had failed to find significant effects and then had found that the caregivers of the control group were copying the experimental procedures.

The babies were evaluated by the Griffiths Mental Development Scale, a Piagetian object concept scale, observational records of spontaneous behavior and interaction patterns, and records of gross motor activity. Table 13.1 presents the DQs for the babies at the onset of the experiment, after 5 weeks, and after 10 weeks (when the babies were 4-5 months old). The DQs of the control group decreased, which shows that this institution did not provide an adequate environment for normal psychological development. Both the perceptual stimulation and social stimulation groups were higher than the controls after 10 weeks of stimulation (when the babies were 4-5 months of age), but had not differed after 5 weeks. Thus even small doses of either perceptual or social stimulation in the first year of life prevent the development of retardation that would otherwise be the lot of these institutionalized babies.

Contrary to Broussard and Décarie's expectations, the mixed stimulation group was not only not superior to either single type of stimulation alone, it was, in fact, inferior to them. The inferior results of the mixed stimulation condition may be an artifact of Broussard and Décarie's method. The social and perceptual stimulations were isolated from each other, and the babies received less than 10 minutes per day of each. Hunt's trained caregiver condition was also a mixed condition: The caregivers were trained to be responsive socially and to provide playthings appropriate to the babies' immediate needs. Either the more extensive nature of this intervention or the embedding of the perceptual stimulation within the context of a responsive relationship, or the combination, may have been the key to its success.

Hunt and colleagues and Broussard and Décarie found that specific interventions had specific effects. The trained caregiver condition (Hunt, 1981, 1982) was designed to overcome the fact that the Badger training program, while leading to more advanced performance on the object permanence scale for poverty and Tehran orphanage babies did not lead to normal vocal imitation in either. Improvement in object permanence seemed to result from the types of playthings given and the timing of their introduction. As a result of their early data, Hunt et al. included vocal imitation in their final training program. Their Tehran interventions produced specific effects, usually in the predicted direction: Infants exposed to perceptual stimulation were somewhat retarded motorically compared with infants who had additional (but untrained) caregivers, but they were advanced in the first year on cognitive scales and on the final levels for scales involving language. Babies who were carried around would be ex-

Table 13.1
DQs of Babies in Broussard and Décarie's Experimental Situation

Stimulation Group	Prior to Intervention	5 Weeks Later	10 Weeks Later
Perceptual	104	86	103
Social	102	89	102
Mixed	110	91	94
Control	102	86	83

pected to have had more motoric exercise, and those experiencing auditory stimulation matched to their progress (without training, caregivers generally tended not to talk to their charges) would be expected to have improved more on relevant cognitive scales. The babies exposed to tutored caregivers were advanced in the domains relevant to the training, but retarded in untrained areas such as demonstrating knowledge of the whereabouts of familiar others and in the spontaneous naming of familiar objects.

The meaning of the specificity of the effects is not clear. Many are pure specificity effects; that is, babies advance in an area when they are exposed to specific experiences relevant to it. Other effects do not seem to conform to predictions, perhaps because we do not know the necessary specific experiences for these achievements. (If so, a wonderful goal for future intervention research could be to figure out what experiences are relevant for different achievements.) But they may represent part of unknown nonspecific patterns.

HIGH-QUALITY INSTITUTIONS

The research in inadequate orphanages clearly shows the importance of stimulation in infancy and demonstrates that rather simple environmental interventions can make great inroads against retardation. "Institutionalization effects" depend on the quality of the institution. In high-quality institutions infants apparently are not at intellectual or social risk. One well-documented study has demonstrated this quite well. Tizard (1977) studied children who spent their first 2 years in a group of British orphanages designed to provide optimal physical environments and stimulation in the provision of both toys and social interactions with staff and other infants. Children were read to and taken on outings regularly; they had at least one caregiver for every three children for most of the time (and for many of the children, all of the time). Generally, these orphanages attempted to provide homelike environments in level and quality of stimulation, but with one major exception: Close personal relationships between caregivers and children were discouraged. Care for each child was divided among the staff, and the staff were discouraged from spending too much time with any one child. By the age of 24 months the average child had been looked after for at least a week by 24 different people, and by 4½ years, by 50.

Tizard first studied these children at 2 years of age. Their IQs were measured, and their general development was compared with that of a control group of working-class children in two-parent families. Intellectual development of the nursery children was slightly retarded (mean MA 22 months) compared with that of home-reared controls (mean MA 25 months). Most of this retardation was in language development, which was independently observed during play. The institutionalized children spoke less frequently and used more limited vocabulary than their working-class counterparts.

Social development of the institutionalized group seemed normal. None was grossly disturbed or unhappy, and so-called institutional behaviors, such as rocking and head banging, were rare. But Tizard was struck by the children's infantile attachment behaviors. When their nurse entered the room, 60% of the institutionalized children ran to be picked up, but no home-reared children did so when their mothers entered the room. The institutionalized children were also more likely to protest at separation, exhibit stranger anxiety, suck their thumbs, wet their pants, and cry over minor mishaps. They were also very reluctant to share toys (characteristic of 90% of institutionalized and 53% of home-reared children). However, the institutionalized children seemed more mature in some ways: Most occupied themselves well on their own (compared with about half the home reared), and only 3% woke during the night (compared with one-third of the home reared).

Thus children being reared in a high-quality institution seem developmentally and emotionally quite similar to home-reared children. The few differences might reflect specifics of the institutional setting. The orphanage children might have been more insecure in attachments because they were discouraged from putting their trust in any one caregiver. They might have had more difficulty in getting along with peers because the staff did not teach them to cooperate. Indeed, the way the staff dealt with competition for adult attention among the children was to avoid the situation by not spending a concentrated period of time with any one child.

Taken in their totality, these studies make it clear that being raised in an institution does not necessarily condemn a child to a life of motoric, intellectual, and linguistic retardation or to profound inability to relate to people. They also provide guidelines for the design of institutions and care of children in institutional settings. Good orphanages always seem to have low child:caregiver ratios, and always seem to provide sensory and intellectual stimulation. They do not, however, necessarily provide a child a continuing relationship with a significant other person.

LONG-TERM EFFECTS OF INSTITUTIONALIZATION DURING INFANCY

Naturally, interest in the effects of institutionalization is not limited to the period during infancy. People are also interested in what happens to these children as they grow up, particularly when they leave the institution. They want to know whether initial deficits can be overcome by later development and whether infants reared in high-quality institutions are nonetheless at risk for later developmental problems.

Experiments of nature allow investigation of these questions. Researchers can study children who moved from one institutional setting to another or who were adopted, as Skeels and Skodak did. Studies of children who have left a deprived environment provide a good test of whether or not infancy is a critical period for later development. According to a strict version of the critical periods hypothesis, normal postinfancy environments would not be sufficient to overcome the permanent deficiencies produced by early deprivation. Studies of children who have been adopted from good institutional environments can help to pinpoint aspects of institutionalization that might produce the effects found.

Most of the studies relevant to long-term effects have used intellectual development as the major dependent variable. Emotional development is rarely measured, partly because of less adequate measures. Failure to get expected results can as easily be due to low reliability or validity of the measures used as to a false hypothesis. If consistent effects on intellectual development can be shown, at least the argument can be made that some psychological (rather than physical or medical) function is affected.

Long-Term Effects on Intellectual Development

One of the best research projects on the topic of permanence of early deprivation is the series of studies on the Crèche, a Lebanese orphanage run by French nuns (Dennis, 1973). Children stayed in the Crèche from infancy to the age of 6 years. The Crèche provided good physical care—the children were adequately fed, clothed, and kept warm and dry—but there was only 1 caregiver for every 10 infants, and caregivers were often of below-average intelligence (many were raised in the Crèche). Thus the infants received little stimulation. They were laid on their backs in cribs with white crib bumpers. The ceilings were white. They stayed in these cribs except for changing and daily baths, thus there was little perceptual variation in their environment (see Figure 13.1). They were fed and changed on a schedule, and crying was not responded to. The attendants rarely talked to them. Thus the infants had little control over their environment. It should be no surprise that these circumstances led to extreme retardation of motoric, linguistic, and intellectual development. The children often did not sit up until 1 year of age or walk until 4 or 5 years. At 6 years, when they left the Crèche, they had IQs of approximately 50, which is well into the retarded range.

What happened after they left the Crèche provides a relatively neat experiment of nature. The girls and boys were transferred to separate institutions. Girls were transferred to a home staffed by low-level workers and trained to do low-level work. This institution was as unstimulating as the original one. At age 16 the girls had an average IQ of 50, with most being between 30 and 60. In contrast, boys were sent to an institution with many opportunities for stimulation. They received training to become workers in the outside world and were regularly taken on outings. At 15 their average IQ was 80.

In 1956 a new experiment of nature began at the Crèche. Adoption became legal in Lebanon in that year, and children of all ages were swooped out of the Crèche and into homes. Dennis followed up children who had been adopted at various ages, from shortly after birth to 8 years. He then compared those who had been adopted early (before 2 years) with those adopted later (2-4 years or 4-8 years).

Children adopted by 2 years of age regained normal IQs. Their IQs at the time of adoption were 50, but within several years their average IQ increased to almost 100. Similar recovery has been found in other studies of deprived children adopted within the first several years of life (Clark & Hanisee, 1982; Scarr & Weinberg, 1976).

In contrast, the Crèche children adopted later showed permanent deficits; the later the adoption, the greater the permanent retardation. This retardation was a residue from the earlier institutionalization and

was not caused by later inability to learn or progress intellectually. These children's rate of development once they left the Crèche was normal, exactly like that of home-reared children, regardless of their age at adoption (that is, they gained one year of mental age for each year of chronological age). Because the children adopted at later ages developed at a normal rate once they left the Crèche, their permanent deficit was caused by their failure to show catch-up in intellectual growth, as the children adopted as infants did. The older children had suffered more initial deficit in terms of mental age. For example, a 4-year-old with an IQ of 50 has a mental age of 2 years, but an 8-year-old with an IQ of 50 has a mental age of 4. By 12 years of age, the child adopted at 4 had 8 years of normal growth, and hence 8 additional years of mental age. Thus he had a mental age of 10 (2 + 8=10) and hence an IQ of 83 (10 ÷ 12 x 100=83). The child adopted at 8, in contrast, had only 4 additional years of normal mental growth, resulting in a mental age of 8 (4 + 4=8) and hence an IQ of 67 (8 ÷ 12 x 100=67). Thus neither of these late-adopted children reached a normal IQ, and the one adopted later had a lower IQ.

These data demonstrate that deprivation during the first 2 years can be overcome, so long as the later environment is normal. Therefore, if there is a critical period for intellectual development, it is not in the first 2 years. That leaves the possibility that there is a critical period sometime between 2 and 8 years.

The environment necessary to promote sensorimotor development is relatively simple to obtain. Babies need objects to see, to hear, and to manipulate. The emotional needs of infants, particularly in the first year of life, may be equally easy to meet. Responding to babies' distress and providing appropriate stimulation seem to be the keys. Only the most deprived environments (some orphanages and homes) fail to fulfill these basic needs. In institutions it is relatively easy to overcome these deficits by providing toys and other environmental supports and enough staffing to allow some noncaretaking stimulation. By 18 months to 2 years of age, children are developing language and other forms of mental representation. At this time the amount and quality of language and communication through language become important (Atkin et al., 1977). Furthermore, the increased cognitive power brought about by mental representation makes children more responsive to many other aspects of their environment, such as picture books and make-believe toys (see Chapter 10).

The ensuing cognitive development may well have a snowball effect in that, as children assimilate more complex aspects of their environment, their understanding develops, and they need ever more complex environments. It is right at the 18-24-month period that day care (which will be discussed shortly) and other forms of early intellectual intervention (Levenstein, 1977; Levenstein et al., 1968, 1973; White & Watts, 1973) begin to have an effect on intellectual development.[3]

Naturally, researchers have speculated about processes of development underlying these phenomena. The developing abilities of symbol formation and their cognitive consequences may actually operate in a critical periods fashion, a hypothesis that is made plausible by Epstein's (1974a, 1974b) evidence that spurts in head size independent of physical growth occur between 2 and 4 years, during the onset of mental representation, and between 6 and 8 years, during the onset of Piaget's concrete operational period.[4] Epstein infers that these spurts reflect similar spurts in brain growth, and he has found that they occur at the same ages as spurts in IQ. Both spurts lie within the ages for which Dennis found permanent effects and strengthen the argument for a postinfancy critical period. The clearest demonstrations of critical periods have involved physiological mechanisms (recall the prenatal critical periods described in Chapter 4 and the critical periods of perception described in Chapter 7). Although finding such physiological growth spurts makes the critical periods hypothesis more plausible, we have seen no follow-up work on this hypothesis, and the evidence is not compelling. Not all biological growth operates according to the principles of critical periods. The phenomenon of catch-up growth after deprivation-produced retardation has been documented for physical growth and is closer to Piaget's model for intellectual growth than is a critical periods notion.

Dennis's data are also consistent with an interpretation that it is the length of deprivation, not its timing, that determines the possibility of catch-up growth. Dennis's data suggest that deprivation must last longer than 2 years to have a permanent effect, and that after 2 years the degree of retardation increases regularly (in a linear fashion) as the duration of deprivation increases.

Regardless of whether the later critical period or the duration interpretation is correct, this experiment of nature does not necessarily mean that those who were institutionalized for longer than 2 years could under no circumstances overcome their deficits. The postinfancy experiences of the boys transferred to a more enriching institution and of the children adopted into normal homes cannot be considered optimal. With optimal experiences (perhaps provided by trained or

especially understanding parents, or special school experiences), these seemingly permanent deficits might be overcome. The available research on the effects of enrichment on noninstitutionalized children will be discussed later in this chapter.

Luckily, there is corroborative evidence for Dennis's finding that retardation in infancy is not necessarily permanent. Kagan (1976b) studied children in an isolated, subsistence-level farming village in northern Guatemala. These children spent the first year of their lives (until they become mobile at 13-16 months) inside windowless bamboo huts, with little light, few objects, and no conventional toys. An infant typically spent about one-third of the time in a sling on the mother, a third on a straw mat, and a third asleep in a hammock. Parents, relatives, and older children played or talked to the infants only 10% of their awake time (compared with 25-40% in homes in the United States; Clarke-Stewart, 1973). At 1 year of age these infants were 3-4 months behind U.S. children on various measures of development, including Piagetian object permanence and stranger anxiety. Their overall appearance was also quite different from that of toddlers in the United States. The Guatemalan babies were quiet, nonsmiling, minimally alert, motorically flaccid, and temperamentally passive. (The comparable profile for middle-class U.S. toddlers is that they are highly vocal, smiling, alert, and active.) Despite this rather severe retardation, by preadolescence these children were essentially normal on a variety of cognitive tasks, including tests of memory and inferential abilities. Here, then, is a second case in which early environmentally produced retardation is not permanent. In both cases, the subsequent environment was not optimal. Kagan's study was not an exact replication of Dennis's, since the Guatemalan children were deprived of sensory and intellectual stimulation, and, in large measure, of a responsive social environment, but not of the opportunity to form one-to-one relationships with their mothers.

Tizard (1977), in the study described in part earlier, also explored the effects of early institutionalization and late adoption. The children had spent the first 2 to 7 years of life in good orphanages. Most were adopted or returned to their own homes (restored) at between 2 and 4 years, but some went to private

3. It should be pointed out that White and Watts (1973) concluded from their data that the critical period is between 10 and 18 months because differences between treatment groups are evident by 18-24 months.

4. There are also later spurts, but they are not relevant to either Dennis's data or this book.

homes only when they were between 4 and 7 years of age. These restored and adopted children experienced markedly different environments, and the differential effects on the children reveal something about the role of the later environment on their development. To assess the effects of early institutionalization, Tizard needed a control group of home-reared children. Because the children in the orphanages came primarily from working-class homes, Tizard used a working-class home-reared group as a control. However, because most adoptive parents were middle-class, a middle-class home-reared group was also used for comparisons.

This study differed from those of Dennis and Kagan in that the early institutional experiences of these children did not result in gross retardation. Thus it is not a good test of the long-term effects of early intellectual deprivation, but it is an excellent test of the effects of early deprivation of a one-to-one relationship with a mother or caretaker. (Recall that the staff were discouraged from showing interest in any one child, and each child had large numbers of caretakers.) This study is a good test of the deprivation of a mother figure because the babies were not deprived in other respects, and the study was unusual in assessing the impact of institutionalization and later adoption on emotional as well as intellectual development.

Tizard's findings with respect to intellectual development can be compared with the findings of Dennis and Kagan. Children who left the institution between 2 and 4 years went from slightly below to above average (mean IQ 115) if adopted, but stayed average if restored to their own families. These results held at both 4 and 8 years, at which age the pattern for school results was the same. Thus it is clear that there need be no long-term deleterious effects on intellectual development of not having a mother figure during infancy so long as an otherwise sufficiently stimulating environment is provided.

The adopted children fared better than those who were restored to their mothers, although both had had similar experiences in their first 2 years. The adopted had better intellectual development and were more cooperative in the testing situation, and more of them concentrated well (66%, compared with 27% of the restored children). These differences in test-taking behaviors undoubtedly account for at least part of the difference in intellectual performance, because it takes concentration and cooperativeness to do one's best on a test.

These findings show that later environment also affects IQ. The parents of these two groups differed in many ways. The adoptive parents were anxious to have

a child and many had waited a long time to adopt. They were generally very accepting of their children, even when teachers saw the children as problems. Mothers of restored children were conflicted about them, as was evidenced by their having left the babies in the orphanage. They often had had other children, were living with men who were not the subject child's father, were less well-off financially than the adoptive parents, and were less likely to read to, play with, or provide many toys for their children. Thus the restored children were likely to enter new, intact families with younger children and less optimal environments. Adopted children entered more emotionally accepting and intellectually stimulating environments. After several years in these environments, the adopted children both approached intellectual tasks in a more positive fashion and performed better on them. Because the two groups were similar in intellectual performance when they left the institution, these differences must be attributed to their later environments.

Conclusions about those who were adopted or restored to their natural parents between the ages of 4½ and 7 years (five adopted and four restored children) are speculative because of the small number of such children. Nevertheless, the findings are intriguing because of their fit with the Dennis data. (Dennis's subjects all showed IQ improvements and Tizard's did not, but that is likely to be because Dennis's children started their home lives with low IQs, whereas Tizard's were average.) Unlike the earlier-adopted children, only one of Tizard's later-adopted children increased in IQ from 4 years (before leaving the institution) to 8 years, and the others, if anything, declined. (Of the restored children, two stayed the same and two declined.) Thus the children adopted later did not show the intellectual improvement of those adopted earlier. The major difference between the results of the two studies is that the age at which growth in mental age shifted from greater than average to average was 2 years earlier for the children in Dennis's study. The most likely interpretation is that the more severe the deprivation, the earlier the age after which a normal family life will not suffice to overcome the effects.

It was noted in connection with the Dennis study that improvement might have been greater for later adoptees had their environments been optimal. Tizard noted that the environments of later-adopted children might have been less optimal than those of the earlier-adopted children. First, later adoptees were in school, and so had less time to experience one-to-one stimulation from their parents. Second, their parents did not expect their children to excel in school, and thus they may not have pushed them to do their best or may have created conditions for a self-fulfilling prophecy of low average performance. Tizard did not argue that the children were beyond a stage at which the mother's influence could make a difference. Rather, she argued that, assuming the child to be equally vulnerable, the environment of the later-adopted children was not as facilitative as it would have been had they been adopted earlier.

Let us summarize the findings on the effects of early deprivation on intellectual development: Early deprivation of sensory-perceptual-intellectual stimulation alone (Kagan's Guatemalan babies), and combined with maternal deprivation (Dennis's Crèche babies), caused severe intellectual retardation. In either case, if the subsequent environments were reasonably stimulating, the babies' mental development became normal. Early deprivation of a mother figure resulted in essentially normal intellectual performance *if* sensory-perceptual-intellectual stimulation was adequate. Whether the early deprivation effects were completely overcome depended in part on the age at which the environment was changed and in part on the quality of the subsequent environment. What has been most surprising to many people is that the effects of even 2 years of severe deprivation can be overcome. Thus it is clear that infancy is not a critical period for permanent effects on intellectual development. There may be a critical period that starts somewhere between 1 and 2 or after 2 years, but the data are also consistent with the hypothesis that it is the duration of the deprivation, and not the timing, that produces effects that seem irreversible.

Long-Term Effects on Social and Emotional Development

As noted earlier, Tizard's (1977) is one of the few systematic studies of the effects of early deprivation on the later social and emotional development of humans. Tizard gathered four kinds of systematic data at 4½ and 8 years: children's initial responses to the psychologist (prior to being tested), children's behaviors during testing (assessed by the tester), parents' reports of children's behavior problems and attachment, and teachers' reports of children's behavior problems. For example, parents were asked a series of questions about specific behaviors, such as "Will he sit still through a meal?" and "Has he woken in the night for the past four weeks?" Asking specific questions rather than general questions such as "Is he restless?" is a good method to minimize bias in mothers' reports.[5] The responses of the parents were then categorized as

reflecting severe, moderate, or negligible problems in each area. For example, a child who awoke and called out at least three times a week was rated as having severe sleep problems.

This discussion will concentrate on the results for the 24 early-adopted children, because they experienced the more optimal postinfancy environment and should have experienced the strongest recovery. In general, they did not show evidence of emotional disturbance. In fact, at age 4½, they showed fewer problems than the home-reared working-class controls, which might be attributable to the social class differences. At 8 years the adoptive children seemed very similar to a middle-class control group in terms of behavior problems. The only consistent problems adoptive parents reported were that the children tended to be overly friendly to strangers and overly seeking of attention at both 4½ and 8 years. Of the 20 children studied at 8 years, 6 appeared to have significant problems. Parents reported that 2 were "too good" (overinhibited), 3 were impulsive and had to be watched, and 1 had temper tantrums. Of the 6 who had been described as difficult while in the orphanage, 3 showed great improvement at 4½ years, but all 6 still exhibited more problems than the others at 8 years.

Teachers had much more negative impressions of the adopted children at 8 years than the parents did. On a scale of behavior problems (the Rutter B scale, on which a score of 9 or greater is believed to indicate a need for special help; Rutter, 1979), the average score for the adopted children was 10. The mean for classmates who served as controls was 3, and that for the original working-class control sample was 5. Some of the specific problems noted by teachers were that the children were restless, fidgety, quarrelsome, disobedient, lying, attention seeking, and resentful or aggressive when corrected. Tizard noted that the parents and teachers generally agreed on the behaviors that the children exhibited, even though they disagreed on whether the children had problems. The data suggest that excessive attention seeking may have created the school problems, because such needs would be more difficult to meet in school than at home. If so, the children's subsequent frustration could well lead to fidgeting, quarreling with other children, and so forth. Indeed, several mothers noted that the schools were unable to cope with their children's attention seeking, while they, the mothers,

---

5. Development of these specific questions ideally should be guided by theory to minimize researcher bias in choice of items or their interpretation.

found it little bother (and hence may not have tried to correct it).

The most crucial of the social-emotional measures for the critical periods hypothesis, as seen by Freud, Erikson, Bowlby, Ainsworth, and others, is attachment. These children had had very little opportunity to form close attachments to any adults in their first years, and at 2 years they responded indiscriminately to familiar adults. There was no standard measure of attachment in 4-year-olds, so Tizard used parental reports. To try to find out whether these children had specific affectionate relationships with one or both parents, Tizard asked the parents whether the child preferred being put to bed or comforted when ill by one or both parents rather than by a less familiar person. Half preferred to be put to bed by a parent and more than 70% preferred to be comforted by a parent, but they were much more likely than controls to allow a stranger to put them to bed. (The preference numbers are comparable to those of the working-class home-reared group.) Of the 24 mothers, 20 were absolutely convinced that their adopted children were deeply attached to them. Adoptive parents often spontaneously commented that their children were exceptionally affectionate, most to anyone they knew well, and 4 to strangers as well. This could reflect shallow and indiscriminate affections, a stereotype about institutionalized children.[6] Alternatively, this general affectionate tendency could reflect the children's experience in an institution where all adults were friendly, helpful, and to be trusted, and they simply generalized this to the outside world.

By 8 years of age, the adopted children were more discriminating in their affection. Only 1 of the 20 tested was affectionate with strangers, and only 4 did not seem deeply attached to their mothers, by their mothers' reports. Of these 4, 3 were the ones whose mothers had expressed the same doubts when the children were 4. Far from fitting the stereotype that adopted children are shallow and flat emotionally, 3 of these 4 children seemed hostile to their parents. Reservations about their children's attachment occurred in 3 of the 30 mothers of the home-reared children as well. Thus insecure attachment would seem to be only 20% among the adopted group and 10% among the home reared.

Teachers reported that the adopted children were not liked by their peers and were frequently quarrelsome. However, their problems seemed limited to those with their age-mates, inasmuch as they often formed good relations with their younger and older siblings. This is the reverse of the pattern of the home-reared children, who frequently had problems relating to their siblings but got along well with their age-mates at school. The reasons for these differences would make a fruitful area of study.

Thus most of the adopted children appeared to have been able to establish strong, personal ties to their new parents and siblings. They had more difficulty with relationships in school, both with their teachers, who found them more difficult to handle than other children, and with their peers. But they performed well academically.

The description of the children restored to their mothers was similar to that of the adopted children, but whenever they differed, the restored group was worse. For example, 44% of restored children, but only 28% of adopted and none of the control children, were described as very restless. For the most persistent problem, attention seeking from both strangers and teachers, 78% of the restored children, 61% of the adopted, and 7% of the controls were so described.

Another study of infants adopted from a high-quality institution that concentrated on long-range effects on social and emotional development as measured by personality tests was also a study of the effects of multiple mothering (Gardner et al., 1961). Infants who had lived in a home management house run by home economics students as part of their university training and who were exposed to a new group of "mothers" every few days were studied. Like Tizard's subjects, these infants had no opportunity to form intense attachments to any specific persons, although presumably they received optimal care in other ways. These children had generally been adopted at an early age (about 1 year). To determine whether they had suffered lasting emotional harm, they were followed up when they were from 8 to 17 years old. Due to the wide age span, the controls were selected from the same schools as adoptees and matched for sex, age, and intelligence. Batteries of personality tests were administered. The home economics residents, who had many loving caretakers in their first year but no one-to-one relationship with a mother figure, did not differ from the controls in terms of personality processes, frustration tolerance, anxiety levels, personal or social adjustments, or school achievement. These results corroborate Tizard's findings of minimal emotional differences between home-reared babies and babies

---

6. It is interesting that more recent Greek data show that young infants who had attachment figures in an orphanage began to form new attachment to adoptive mothers within 2 weeks and did not show indiscriminate attention seeking, detachment, or other negative behaviors sometimes thought typical of institutional babies (Dontas et al., 1985).

reared for their first 1 or 2 years in quality institutions in which one-to-one relationships were discouraged. Indeed, they extend those findings to cover infants raised with many short-lived close relationships.

In conclusion, it is clear from Tizard's study that most children deprived of a mother figure in infancy, when given parents who care a lot and work hard to give love, affection, and a good environment to their children, become attached. Therefore, it seems that the dire predictions made by Freud and others of later inability to love as a result of early deprivation of a primary love object are wrong. Tizard's adopted children were not so difficult that their adopted parents found them problems to raise. In the eyes of the adopted parents, the children were turning out quite nicely, and there was no clear evidence for major personality problems. Gardner and colleagues' (1961) adopted subjects did not differ from controls on personality tests. Nevertheless, it is impossible to conclude that these children suffered no long-term effects, primarily because the teachers' ratings of the 8-year-olds in Tizard's study judged about half of the adopted children to be greater problems than their classmates and to have difficulties with their peers. It is possible that adoption by 2 years of age is more deleterious than by 1 year, because Tizard's study found some negative results and Gardner et al.'s did not. It is also possible that the care of young women who were not discouraged from having warm relations with their charges provided a better base for emotional growth for the infants in the latter study. It is impossible to be sure, however, because the dependent measures used in the two studies were entirely different.

Tizard's study also showed clearly the importance of later child rearing. Whenever the two groups of previously institutionalized children differed, the children restored to their natural parents were consistently worse off than the adopted children. We can only speculate about what the crucial differences were. These environments differed on emotional, economic, and intellectual dimensions. Adoptive parents (including fathers) tended to be more accepting and less ambivalent toward their children, and provided more enriching experiences. All of these kinds of differences are likely to be important.

Multiple Mothering

The question of harmful effects of multiple mothering has been extremely controversial, because of the strong theoretical support given by Freud and his followers to the widespread belief that all infants ought to be cared for by their own biological mothers. The effects found in early studies of institutionalization were interpreted as being due to the absence of a mother, even though children in those institutions also suffered many other deprivations—of fathers, toys, sensory and perceptual stimulation, attention, and even exercise. So powerful has this belief system been that babies were removed from home economics "homes" (such as that studied by Gardner et al., 1961). Even the Harlow studies on the effects of various rearing conditions in monkeys have been (wrongly) interpreted as demonstrating the need for a full-time, real-life mother. Authors of popular and professional articles and books long assumed that all children have the inalienable right to the total attention of their mothers for at least 3 years, after which that attention may have to be shared with a new baby, a process that may be repeated in another few years.

The strength of this belief system is surprising, considering how really rare (over the course of history and range of cultures) the nuclear family with mother as full-time caregiver is. The nuclear family with a nonworking mother became the norm in Western societies only after urbanization and the increased mobility of modern times, and it is the norm only for part of that culture. The poor have never had this option, and the rich in many times and places have placed their children in the primary care of nursemaids or governesses.[7] In many other cultures, children are routinely left in the care of relatives (adults or children) or other members of the community while the mother works (see the data on attachment to child caretakers reported in Chapter 12).

The traditional Freudian view that all children must establish an exclusive love relationship with their mothers actually includes several hypotheses. In this chapter, two aspects of this view will be discussed: (a) Do babies deprived of any deep attachment suffer irreversible effects from such deprivation? (b) Should babies experience one deep relationship rather than several attachments? The research on institutionalization is relevant to the first question. Three tentative conclusions can be summarized based on that research:

(1) Infants who form no single intense relationship during infancy but are not otherwise deprived are neither permanently retarded nor seriously dis-

---

7. An excellent description of the effects of wet-nurses on the roles of both women and children and the abuse of children in earlier times, including during the Industrial Revolution, is included in Piers (1978).

turbed, although some may suffer some emotional consequences even if subsequently placed in good homes (Dennis, 1973; Gardner et al., 1961; Jaffee & Fanshel, 1970; Tizard, 1977).

(2) It is possible for people to form deep, meaningful relationships with significant others even if their early prototypical mother-infant relationships were not formed during the hypothetically critical period of infancy (Gardner et al., 1961; Jaffee & Fanshel, 1970; Tizard, 1977).

(3) The presence of a biological mother is not sufficient to overcome intellectual deficit if the environment is restrictive (Kagan, 1976b).

The research clearly provides no positive support for the Freudian notion of the crucial role of an exclusive strong attachment to mother, although arguments softening or eliminating the negative impact on Freudian theory can be found.

This section addresses the question of whether attachment to several figures does any harm. According to Freudian theory, the mother-infant relationship must be primary. Secondary attachments to other people are fine so long as they do not diffuse the all-important primary relationship. In this view, mothers who share the caregiving role put their babies at risk. Research is available on two natural situations relevant to this issue: studies of other cultures in which multiple mothering is the norm, and studies of infant day care in the United States in which infants spend full days in day-care centers.

Studies of multiple mothering in which the biological mother is one of the "mothers" also allow us to address other questions of concern to mothers of all sorts. Can both mothers and substitute caregivers provide a secure base for exploration? Do infants come to prefer the mother or the caregiver? Is it important that the caregivers be stable or will changing caregivers do just as well? What sorts of multiple rearing environments are best? All of these questions are of crucial importance in the United States today, because, like it or not, many infants are being reared by multiple caretakers. As of 1976, U.S. Department of Labor statistics showed that 46% of children in the United States had working mothers, including 37% of children under 5 years of age; these figures are, of course, even greater today. Many mothers work because of economic necessity, and many work because they expect to be happier (and also more successful parents) if they pursue careers. The extent of the practice makes it crucial to find out whether children are adversely affected and, if so, what forms of care can avoid adverse effects. Two forms of communal rearing as well as day care are explored below.

COMMUNAL REARING

The Israeli kibbutz started as a largely agricultural collective settlement, begun by Zionists long before the state of Israel was established. Thus some kibbutzim (plural of *kibbutz*) have existed over several generations. Although kibbutzim vary, and some are now manufacturing or service industry oriented (within the kibbutz itself), a general characterization of the care of children can be made. Communal care begins at 4 days of age, when babies are transferred from the hospital to an infant house under the care of a professional caretaker called a metapelet (plural, metaplot). The mother, who has a 6-week maternity leave, may care for her baby as much as she wants, although in many kibbutzim all babies sleep in the infant house. After 6 weeks the mother gradually resumes her normal kibbutz duties and the metapelet takes over the child care (Figure 13.2). At around 3-4 months of age a group of infants are put under the care of a second metapelet, who remains their primary caregiver until the children enter preschool. The mother assumes a regular work load (7-8 hours a day), and the metapelet assumes responsibility for the child. Even though the metapelet has responsibility during this first year of life, the mother spends twice as much time with the baby as the metapelet (Gewirtz & Gewirtz, 1968). The mother's time with her infant gradually diminishes until, by 1½ years, the child spends only a few hours a day visiting with his or her parents.

The relative roles of the parents and of the metaplot are clearly defined. The parents are to be "friends," and the metaplot are to care for and socialize the children. The metaplot are to train the children to eat by themselves, to wash and dress themselves, to eliminate in the toilet; they are to answer the children's questions about sex, to define limits for their aggressive behaviors, and to place demands on them in all spheres of activity. Physical punishment is taboo; the primary forms of discipline are explanation, isolation from the group, or both. Children themselves also contribute directly to their peers' socialization. They directly imitate the metaplot's admonishments and also sometimes invent their own wordings for sanctions. They also sometimes use the physical punishment that metaplot avoid (Faigin, 1958).

Kibbutz rearing has no negative influence on motoric or mental development. Kohen-Raz (1968) conducted an extensive and well-controlled study of 130 communally raised kibbutz infants, 152 infants reared in private homes, and 79 raised in institutions. The infants ranged from 1 to 27 months of age. Although the educational levels of the parents of home-reared infants were higher than those of the kibbutz parents, the difference probably reflected the social structure of the kibbutz rather than the abilities of the parents. There were also no differences in ethnic origins between these groups. In contrast, the institutionalized children presumably came from a lower socioeconomic stratum, although records on them were not available.

The kibbutz babies came from 21 kibbutzim selected as a representative sample of all those in which infants lived in separate infant houses. (Size and age of kibbutz, geographic area, and the four major political movements were all proportionally represented, so that the results could be generalized to all kibbutz-reared infants who live in separate infant houses.)

Home-reared babies were chosen at random from about 670 infants living in Jerusalem and Rehovoth. The institutionalized babies were selected from the total infant population in five baby homes located in Jerusalem, Tel Aviv, and Haifa. A shortage of such babies, plus epidemics current at the time of the study, made a truly representative group of institutionalized babies unachievable. Babies with known problems were excluded.

All babies were evaluated by the Bayley scales in their natural surroundings by a highly trained group of examiners with the participation of mothers or caretakers. Both kibbutz- and home-reared infants tended to score above the U.S. norms on the mental scales. This was to be expected, because of the parents' educational and social levels. Kibbutz infants surpassed home-reared babies in the earlier months, but this difference tended to disappear with age. The institutionalized babies were inferior to the other groups and to the U.S. norms. Motor scores did not vary as much as the mental scales did; institutionalized babies were motorically retarded at all ages prior to 15 months (except for the 10-month sample), but had caught up at 18, 24, and 27 months.

The relation of mental development to a number of environmental and family background variables was assessed where these were known. A few findings of special relevance are worth mention here. There was no relation between the frequency of caretaker changes and the DQ. There was a tendency for male infants from private homes where the mothers worked (most in full-time jobs) to have higher DQs than those whose mothers stayed home. (Other evidence in the discussion of day care below suggests that multiple mothering can in some circumstances help intellectual development.) There was also a tendency in the kibbutz group for firstborn infants to score higher than later-borns (see also Gewirtz & Gewirtz, 1965), which

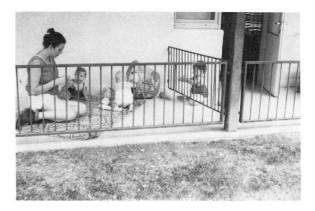

Figure 13.2. Toddlers and their metapelet on the playpen porch of a kibbutz. Note the child from the neighboring group trying to interact. (Photograph courtesy of Jeannette Stone.)

Bayley (1965) reported for home-reared subjects in the United States.

Certainly these data show that the separation of infants from mothers for large parts of the day and night and their collective education by other female adults and with other infants do not adversely affect their motor or mental development. Hence these findings with kibbutz children confirm the findings in the studies of institutionalization. A single female caretaker in the first 2 years of life (the exact time that has often been supposed to be most important) is not a prerequisite of normal intellectual development.

Social development is, as noted previously, difficult to measure. In infants the major measure used is attachment. By that measure, kibbutz-reared infants are clearly attached to their mothers. Early studies showed few differences in any of their attachment behaviors (protest, proximity behaviors, distance-attention behaviors) from those of home-reared U.S. infants (Levy-Shiff, 1983; Maccoby & Feldman, 1972). Fox (1977) found that kibbutz babies showed greater attachment to their mothers than to their metaplot as judged from reunion behaviors.

While there are more insecurely attached kibbutz infants, the meaning of this for later social-emotional development is unclear. Oppenheim et al. (1988) found that social-emotional development at age 5 was not affected by infant-mother attachment classification. In contrast, infant-father and infant-metaplot attachment was. Infants judged secure in these relationships were later more socially competent than C (resistant) infants. Those secure with their fathers were more ego resilient and field independent than Cs, and those secure with their metaplot were more empathic and less ego controlled than Cs. These findings are more like those for attachment to mother in U.S. studies.

In most studies, multiple mothering does not disrupt attachment to mother, even when someone else has the major responsibility for child rearing and socialization. The studies cited above all included kibbutz babies older than 1½, when the mothers no longer saw them for more than 3 hours a day. Why is so little time effective in eliciting attachment? The quality of the time parents and infants spend together may be more important than the quantity. Schaffer and Emerson (1964), in their study of family-reared Scottish infants, found that those babies who spent the most time with their mothers were not necessarily the most attached. Rather, how the mother acted—how much time she spent playing with her infant and how responsive she was—was related to the intensity of attachment. In the kibbutz, parent-child time is considered very important, and parents are freed of all other responsibilities for that period. Their job is to be friends with their children, thus the amount of play and emotional support is likely to be very high. Indeed, older kibbutz children (10-14-year-olds) report more support (nurturance, help with homework, consistency of expectations, encouragement of autonomy) and less discipline, particularly physical punishment and strictness, than do home-reared children (Avgar et al., 1977).

A second factor that may be important is that the mother and father are the stable adults in the infant's life. Although in theory an infant should have only one metapelet from the age of 3 or 4 months until preschool, in actuality infants have many more because of high turnover. In Fox's (1977) study, he tried to limit his sample to children whose metaplot had been with them for more than 4 months, but he had to relax that criterion on occasion.

Both quality of time and stability may well be important. At this time it is possible only to guess why babies attach to their mothers as well as or better than they do to their metaplot, but that they do so is a strong and replicated finding. Furthermore, there are analogous findings with day-care babies in the United States.

Relatively little evidence on other aspects of social and emotional development is available. Faigin (1958) conducted 6 months of extensive observations of 2- and 3-year-olds at two kibbutzim with different philosophies. She described the frequent events and activities and made systematic observations of several categories of aggression and dependency, two categories of behaviors that were popular subjects of

study when learning theory dominated child psychology. Aggression included physical actions with intent to hurt and instrumental physical aggression (designed to achieve a goal such as getting a toy or attention), defense, and verbal aggression. Dependency included crying, affection to adults and peers, instrumental dependency (asking help to achieve a goal), displaying achievements, and thumb sucking. Recall that crying and affection are also included in attachment measures. Here they may have a different meaning, because the children were older (in most cultures separation fears are waning by 2 years) and were observed in everyday, uncontrolled situations rather than in a specific stress situation such as Ainsworth's.

Faigin unfortunately did not include a control group of nonkibbutz children, so it is impossible to ascribe any of her findings to communal child rearing. Nevertheless, as a description of the behaviors of preschoolers in a kibbutz, certain of her findings are enlightening.

Aggression was well within normal limits. Half of the 31 children in the two kibbutzim showed no more than one instance of physical aggression in an average 15-minute period. There were large individual differences in the amount of physical aggression, with several children being very aggressive. The worst, a 2-year-old, had 20 instances of physical aggression in an average 15 minutes. Although sampling problems make it difficult to know how unusual this was, it is clear that individuality was not eliminated by regimentation of the kibbutz, as was predicted by many detractors.

Verbal aggression was nonexistent. This is surprising, because verbal aggression is often more frequent than physical aggression in studies of nursery schools in the United States. The difference, however, may be the result of age differences or of general differences between Israel and the United States in socialization practices, rather than of communal rearing. The kibbutz children in this study were younger than most children in U.S. nursery school samples at that time and may be have been less verbally adept. They may also have experienced more tolerance for physical aggression and less tolerance for verbal aggression.

Overall, dependency responses were about three times as frequent as aggressive responses—an average of more than 30 responses per child in an hour. This frequency of dependency responses does not appear unusually high, particularly because they included both crying and affectionate responses. Responses to other children showed that for the youngest children aggressive responses were more frequent than affectionate responses (the only dependency behavior toward children that was measured). They were approximately equal for older children. In sum, Faigin's exploratory study failed to show any major disturbance in the development of aggression or dependency, although its methodological limitations make it impossible to draw firm conclusions.

The studies of kibbutz-reared infants suggest that they behave much like those reared in family homes, but that does not tell us whether there are long-term negative consequences of kibbutz rearing. Kibbutz children have been shown to be more cooperative in school (Hertz-Lazarowitz et al., 1989) and not to have a higher incidence of psychiatric problems. Problems such as thumb sucking appear to be more frequent among kibbutz children than in the Israeli population at large, but eating problems, male homosexuality, and juvenile delinquency are less frequent in kibbutzniks (Kaffman, 1965; Nagler, 1963). Differences in emotionality that are not maladaptive enough to be considered pathological could exist, but these are difficult to measure. Unfortunately, many studies designed to get at them have used clinical interviews or projective tests that may be vulnerable to investigator bias. Indeed, the conclusions from these studies have been as varied as the theoretical biases of the researchers (Bettelheim, 1969; Handel, 1961; Kardiner, 1954; Pelled, 1964; Rabin, 1957, 1958, 1961; Spiro, 1958). Considered as a whole, these studies have failed to show consistent findings of inferior or changed emotional structure expected from Freudian theory (e.g., diluted or flat affective relationships, disturbed Oedipal resolution). Even those who have reached negative conclusions about communal child rearing grudgingly admit that kibbutz members do all right in life. For example, Kardiner (1954) concluded that kibbutz members are well controlled, a state they achieve by repressing envy and greed and by exhibiting high self-criticism and social vigilance.[8] Failing to find the gross distortions in positive affect, high anxiety, rage, and insecure relationships with others that he expected, he concluded that the feelings were present but repressed, rather than that his hypotheses were wrong. In an extensive study of adolescents using projective techniques (Rorschach, Sentence Completion, and Thematic Apperception Test), Rabin (1961) found that kibbutz adolescents were at least as well adjusted as family-reared Israelis, and perhaps more spontaneous. Kibbutzniks were equally positive toward their parents, had less conflict with them, and involved them less in their fantasies.

The above summary of these older studies of children raised in kibbutzim and followed into childhood and adolescence is important because of more recent

findings on differences in attachment. Although there are some differences from family-reared children, kibbutzniks do not seem to be at a major disadvantage from partial maternal deprivation (or from having multiple mothers, whichever way one looks at it). Most show strong and normal attachment to their mothers and to their metaplot, and they appear to end up as emotionally normal children, adolescents, and adults. Indeed, as adults, they have contributed a greater proportion of military and civilian leaders to Israeli society than any other group.

Kibbutzim are unusual environments in ways other than their communal child-rearing system. They are socialistic and communal in all aspects of living, and their inhabitants now constitute a decreasing proportion (decreasing from 2%) of the Israeli population. They grew from ideological fervor, rather than from societal evolution. It is impossible to determine whether the outcomes for their children are the result of communal child rearing or other differences between the kibbutz and other Israeli environments. In a study of children's emotional attitudes toward their parents and others, Avgar et al. (1977), compared kibbutz children with children on moshavim, which are cooperative agricultural settlements based on family structures, rather than communal child rearing. Moshav children were more like children of kibbutzim than they were like family-reared urban Israeli children. This suggests that the similarities between kibbutzim and moshavim, such as being cooperative, rural, and in agricultural settings, are responsible for some differences between these children and those in the family-reared sample.[9]

Another multiple-mothering situation is found among the Kikuyu of Kenya. In this culture some babies are raised primarily by their mothers, whereas others are shared between mothers and one or more other caretakers, most often older sisters; thus this culture provides a contrast between single and multiple mothering within the same cultural context (the same village). Leiderman and Leiderman (1974) measured attachment and cognitive development in the third and fourth quarters of the first year of life among the Kikuyu. The infants in both groups were clearly attached to their mothers as measured by both positive

---

8. *Repression* is a Freudian term that means that unacceptable feelings are not acknowledged consciously or directly in behavior, but that these feelings come out in hidden, distorted ways.

9. For a more comprehensive review of issues of socialization and development from the cross-cultural perspectives provided in Israel, see Greenbaum and Kugelmass (1980).

affective responses and protest at separation. They were also attached to their caretakers. Attachment, as measured by the babies' positive affective behaviors, was equally strong to mothers and caretakers. As judged by protest at separation, the caretakers became secure bases later than the mothers did, but they nevertheless became secure bases by the end of the first year. This difference seems reasonable because the mothers generally spent much more time with the baby for the first 6 months of life (see the discussion on caretaker attachment in Chapter 12).

The only evidence for any difference between single- and multiple-mothering groups was that multiply mothered babies were more apprehensive of strangers than were the singly mothered babies. Similar apprehension toward or lack of cooperation with strangers has been found in kibbutz babies (Levy-Shiff, 1983; Maccoby & Feldman, 1972) and in Guatemalan infants from a village (San Marcos) with little variety of experience (Kagan, 1976a). Leiderman and Leiderman raise the possibility that such apprehension may be a more sensitive measure of insecurity than babies' behaviors in the more familiar situation of the going and coming of mother or caretaker (i.e., the Strange Situation). Maccoby and Feldman (1972) do not attribute the apprehension to general insecurity (remember the arguments for this position in Chapter 12), but rather suggest that the kibbutz babies were more afraid of strangers simply because they saw fewer in their world than did family-reared children. This may also be true of the Kikuyu children and of the Guatemalans from San Marcos. Kikuyu mothers who were primary caretakers took care of their babies more than 75% of the time. It is likely that when these mothers left their babies, they left them with various strangers. Those with secondary caretakers were probably left with those familiar caretakers and not with strangers. Institutionalized children also have few opportunities to meet strangers outside the context of caretaker adults.

The strongest difference between singly and multiply mothered babies in the Kikuyu was in cognitive development. Multiply mothered babies were *advanced* relative to singly mothered babies, but the effect was significant only for the economically poorest in the group. It appears that caregivers provide some perceptual and cognitive stimulation to poor babies that their mothers are too busy or too preoccupied to

provide. This supports research findings with babies in the United States that show that infants from economically disadvantaged homes are particularly vulnerable to environmental effects (for example, Hess, 1970) and that good infant day care provides enhanced cognitive development for babies from lower-class homes (see, for example, Caldwell, 1964, 1974), an issue that will be discussed later.

DAY CARE

Issues related to day care are of enormous importance, given the number of infants in some form of nonmaternal care. In the United States, close to 53% of women with infants under 3 years of age were employed in 1988 (U.S. Department of Labor, 1989). One would have hoped that professional inquiry could have provided a great deal of clarification of the advantages and disadvantages of day care over the last 5 or 10 years, but, unfortunately, this is not the case. It is clear that day care, if reasonably good, does no harm to and may help cognitive development. However, the research focus has moved from this issue to another question: Does it affect emotional behavior or damage attachment relations? This debate is highly active.[10] Researchers cannot even agree on whether *day care* is two words, one word, or a hyphenated word (in this volume, the noun is two words; the attributive form is hyphenated).

Day care can be described as the U.S. version of polymatric rearing (rearing by more than one mother) and is more similar to the Kikuyu system than to the kibbutz. Typically, American children live with their mothers and, when the mothers must be away at work, are taken to alternative caretakers, cared for in their homes by alternative caretakers, or taken to day-care centers. Research has so far been concerned primarily with day-care centers, and little is known about the effects of being cared for by relatives, being cared for by paid caregivers in the home, or being in family day care (in which a small number of children are cared for in the home of an alternative caregiver).

Even though this discussion will be restricted to day-care centers, that still leaves a wide range of settings. Comparing different day-care centers is sometimes like comparing apples and oranges. Child:caregiver ratios vary, the training of caregivers varies, the stability of the groups providing care varies, policies with respect to encouraging specific attachments vary, and the aims and curricula (nature and variety of activities) vary.[11] Furthermore, the relation of the family to the center, the reasons the parents chose day care, the family's fit to the aims of the center, the consistency between day-care

---

10. A 1990 book is titled *Infant Day Care: The Current Debate* (Fox & Fein, 1990).

11. For an excellent overview of the problems in doing day-care research, see Seitz (1982).

and family practices, and the nature and extent of family support provided by the center vary. Researchers are just beginning to include some of these variables in their studies.

Most research is limited in applicability by having been done in centers set up to provide models of good infant day care. They typically have low child:caregiver ratios and programs designed to foster development. Studies of this type of center have consistently shown no negative effects on intellectual development, even for infants in day care from early infancy (for reviews, see Ricciuti, 1976; Scarr et al., 1990).

Cognitive Enhancement

Far from producing retardation, model day care often has positive, though modest, effects on intellectual development. These are sometimes dramatic when day care provides experiences lacking at home. For example, in one program greater effects were found for more disadvantaged (black) children than for more advantaged (white) children (Robinson & Robinson, 1971; Robinson et al., 1979). This stemmed partly from the fact that intellectual performance of the no-day-care controls decreased in their second year of life. This strongly suggests that day care in this case was providing experiences that non-day-care disadvantaged children did not get. In a study by Kagan et al. (1978), Chinese-American infants, many of whose families were not English speaking, scored higher on a test of basic language concepts at 29 months of age than their home-reared controls. Similar results have been found in several other studies as well (Garber & Heber, 1981; Golden et al., 1978; Heber et al., 1972; Lally, 1973, 1974; McCartney et al., 1985; Ramey & Haskins, 1981; Ramey & Smith, 1976). Intentional communicative behaviors were enhanced by day-care intervention in a low-SES sample (O'Connell & Farran, 1982). In addition, it appears that center care is more advantageous than other types of care settings (Clarke-Stewart, 1984; Howes & Rubenstein, 1981; Rubenstein et al., 1981).

The facilitation of intellectual development for day-care infants typically does not appear until the infants are 18 to 24 months of age (see, e.g., Beller et al., 1981; Fowler & Kahn, 1974, 1975; Heber et al., 1972; Ramey & Smith, 1976; Robinson & Robinson, 1971). This consistent finding parallels findings from the studies of institutionalized infants that found that intellectual deprivation during the first 2 years is reversible. It is not clear whether the effects are cumulative—that is, whether it takes 2 years of day care to produce the positive effects. As a supplement to chil-

dren's home environments, it might only be necessary or even helpful to place children in day care between 1 and 2 years of age. But, since most research shows that starting day care in infancy is not harmful to children's intellectual development, there is no need to wait until then.

The gains in IQ from day-care programs typically disappear by 5 years of age (see Clarke-Stewart & Fein, 1983). However, long-term effects are found on other measures of cognitive competence (not repeating grades or being in special education), as well as being less likely to have behavior problems (e.g., Darlington et al., 1980; Lazar & Darlington, 1982; Schweinhart & Weikart, 1980).

In terms of multiple mothering, these studies of model day-care facilities lead to exactly the same conclusion as those reached in the studies of orphanage, kibbutz, and Kikuyu children: Multiple mothering can be at least as adequate a situation for intellectual development as exclusive care by the mother alone. Because the findings from research using several different operational definitions of multiple mothering are consistent, confidence in the validity of the outcomes is high.

Although the research using model day-care centers is informative, the conclusions cannot be generalized to more typical day-care settings, which often have much higher child:caregiver ratios and often do not have programs designed to promote intellectual development. Comparable research on such all-too-typical day-care settings is rare (but see Vandell et al., 1988) and yields conflicting conclusions.

Cognitive Disadvantage

Methodologically flawed studies of day-care centers with high numbers of children per caretaker show lowered intellectual functioning. In a study of all children in a parish (county) in Bermuda, black children in day-care centers with large groups had lower IQs at 2 years. White children did not show intellectual deficits (Schwarz et al., 1981). Group size and amount of time spent in care were two factors correlated with IQ in the Bermuda study. Caucasian children in the same model day-care setting as the Chinese-Americans cited earlier scored lower than home-reared controls (Kagan et al., 1978).

Emotional Development

Emotional development is the area of greatest concern to psychoanalytically oriented pediatricians, psychiatrists, and psychologists, who expect emotional disturbances to result from nonmaternal care and for it to show up first in mother-infant relationships. The original study that sparked concern with negative effects of day care on attachment came from that tradition (Blehar, 1974).

Several attempts to replicate Blehar's (1974) findings failed to show negative effects (Kagan et al., 1978; Moskowitz et al., 1977; Portnoy & Simmons, 1978). The general finding of these studies was of no or very small differences between day-care and home-reared infants, some of which favored day care over exclusive home rearing (for reviews of the early studies, see Belsky & Steinberg, 1978). Recent evidence suggests that children who start day care prior to 2 years and who spend full-time in good centers are advantaged in terms of social-emotional development (Field, 1991). The more months the children in Field's (1991) sample spent in such care, the greater the number of friends and extracurricular activities they had in second grade, the higher their parents rated them on emotional well-being and assertiveness, and the lower their parents rated them on aggression ($r = -.57$). Also, the longer the time in day care, the less depressed their self-drawings were scored ($r = -.80$). The positive correlations ranged from .38 to .48, which are certainly high for such a time span.

The methodological problems referred to in discussing the effects on cognitive development are exacerbated when discussing effects on emotional development or attachment. Here the problems of the influence of the broader family context are crucial, and these are only beginning to be addressed. They are particularly important in view of the fact that infants are rarely randomly assigned to day care or home care. Questions concerning the emotional quality (as opposed to physical quality or child:caregiver ratio) of day care, an important variable, are virtually unaddressed. Only a few studies have been undertaken to explore the effects of day care on social relationships with peers. And the limitation of most studies to Strange Situation behaviors, which are a very limited set from the whole realm of emotional and interactive behaviors, makes the generalizability of any conclusions tenuous (see, e.g., Fein & Fox, 1988; Lamb & Sternberg, 1990). All of these problems must be borne in mind when looking at the following review of the literature.

The Kagan et al. (1978) study, conducted in a center designed to be a model for good day care, used a variety of measures of emotional development over substantial time periods (observations of the children interacting with other children at 13, 20, and 29 months of age, mothers' judgments, and frequent measures of separation anxiety). The researchers found

no strong differences between day-care and home-reared babies. They did find differences between Chinese and Caucasian children, thus emphasizing the importance of total family context. There were no differences between day-care and home-reared infants in disobedience or aggression, and the two groups were similar in emotional development except that day-care infants were less shy and more patient with strange adults.

Black infants cared for in day-care centers that were not models were consistently less responsive and less communicative than home-reared infants, although the size of these effects were small (Schwarz et al., 1981). The characteristics of the different day-care situations that were related to these measures were as follows: amount of time spent at the center (a variable Schwartz, 1983, also found related to negative behaviors at 18 months in the Strange Situation), size of the group, and child:caregiver ratio. Thus these data suggest that emotional development is likely to be somewhat negatively affected by day-care settings when the centers are inadequate.

Starting in the mid-1980s, probably as an outgrowth of the increasing interest in attachment theory, a series of reports, both professional and popular, suggested that early nonparental care might adversely affect infant-parent attachment and related development (Belsky, 1986, 1988b, 1989). Belsky (1988b) cited a figure of 41% insecure attachments for those cared for out of the home and 26% for those cared for in the home, provoking a series of rebuttals and reanalyses of the data. The latter suggested that the group differences were only half as large as Belsky had reported (only 8-9% more insecurely attached among day-care infants).

In a recoding of the data from a number of the studies, no significant differences were found in attachment overall, nor did the age of the infants (under or over 15 months) or whether they spent more or less than 20 hours per week in day care make a difference (Lamb et al., 1992). Belsky (1988a) noted that the evidence was somewhat inconsistent, but made a case for extensive infant day care being associated with insecure attachment during infancy and with more aggression and noncompliance in preschool and early school years. However, children who had earlier been in day care have also been found to be more cooperative in school (Fuchs et al., 1989). More than 20 hours per week in day care led to slightly more cases of insecure attachment in one study (Belsky & Rovine, 1988), but not in a recent study (Caldera, 1991). Compliance was greater for those full-time in either day or home care and lower for those in part-time day care. For boys in the Belsky and Rovine (1988) study, the insecurity was with the father as well as the mother. Similarly, Chase-Lansdale and Owen (1987) found a higher proportion of insecure attachments to fathers for boys in families where the mother was employed, but Easterbrooks and Goldberg (1985) did not.

A series of criticisms mixed with suggestions for needed work and alternative interpretations appeared in the same issue of *Early Child Research Quarterly* as Belsky's (1988a) article (Clarke-Stewart, 1988; Fein & Fox, 1988; Richter & Zahn-Waxler, 1988; R. Thompson, 1988). Clarke-Stewart (1988, 1989) agrees that studies show that infants whose mothers work full-time during their first year are more likely than those whose mothers work part-time or not at all to be classified as insecurely attached. However, the differences are small and do not necessarily reflect emotional maladjustment, and interpretations of the data as effects of variables other than day care are more plausible. Some authors have gone so far as to state that no research in any country supports the idea that infants under 3 years old are better off at home with mom (Melhuish & Moss, 1990).

It has been pointed out that the Strange Situation was developed with infants who were not receiving outside care and hence may not be a valid measure for infants reared under other conditions (e.g., see Clarke-Stewart, 1989). The robustness of similar classifications in most cultures or settings (see Chapter 12) casts some doubt on this challenge. However, there are some data supporting its validity. Maternal responsiveness, supposedly a key ingredient in secure attachment, was found by Jaeger et al. (1991) to be related to attachment ratings at 18 months only if the mothers were not employed. In the same sample, Q-set, but not Strange Situation, ratings of attachment were related to ego resiliency and sociability (r=.53 and .52) at 34 to 75 months.

Nonetheless, there is some indication that under certain circumstances, day-care or nonmaternal-care infants might be negatively affected. We might also note that under some circumstances infants might be negatively affected by home rearing. Infants from some homes are likely to be better off in at least moderately good day-care centers. Some infants are likely to be more vulnerable than others. Relatively little research has focused on circumstances that might negatively influence the day-care experience, such as the age at which day care is entered; the home environment, including the quality of the relationship between mother and infant; the quality of attachment of infants to day-care workers; the stability of the caregivers; and the congruence of the child-rearing practices of the caregivers and the parents. Some of the evidence that exists is considered below.

Age at Which Day Care Is Started

One focus of research has been on when, within the period of infancy, it is best to start infants in day care (Ricciuti, 1974, 1976; Ricciuti & Poresky, 1973; Willis & Ricciuti, 1974). Not surprisingly, infants who enter day care at the height of the so-called stranger anxiety period (7-12 months) may have more difficulty adjusting than those who enter either earlier or later. Whether such infants suffer a disruption in attachment or any long-term effects of this initial disturbance is not known. Caldera (1991) found that the age at which 14-month-olds had entered day care was not related to either attachment or compliance. In a study by Portnoy and Simmons (1978), 3- to 4-year-olds who had experienced day care in infancy did not differ in attachment to their mothers from children who had stayed at home.

Children who stayed at home, in the care of a sitter, starting at least 4 months prior to their first birthdays, had higher-than-usual numbers of avoidantly attached infants at 12 to 13 months, but only if they were first-borns and their mothers worked full-time (Barglow et al., 1987). The authors' interpretation of this finding is that routine, daily separations from the mother increase avoidant attachment (although 53% in their study were securely attached). The results differ from those of a study in which infants were taken to family day-care homes (Chase-Lansdale & Owen, 1987). Different from the speculations of Barglow et al. is my speculation that being left in one's normal environment daily by one's mother may have different effects than being taken to a new environment. The environmental differences might serve as cues for adaptations to dealing with a different caregiver, and the presence of peers may greatly cushion the force of the effects of "being left."[12]

Belsky's arguments have focused on ill effects of day care in the first year, when the supposedly crucial mother-infant attachment is being formed. But entering day care after the first year, or after attachment has been formed, has also been shown to have adverse effects, depending on the quality of care and the family environment (Howes, 1990). In a study by Bates et al. (1991), extensive day care between 2 and 4 years (as re-

---

12. Perhaps you have had the experience as an older child or adolescent of noting that you react differently to having your parents leave you than to your leaving your parents.

called by parents) was related to aggression at age 5, but not day care in the first year. For a small group of poor children randomly assigned to an intervention day-care center or comparison, attendance at day care in the first year was not related to more problems in school at age 8, and neither was insecure attachment at age 1; day care and attachment did not interact (Burchinal & Bryant, 1991). The Bates et al. (1991) study had a large and highly varied sample in which SES and parental discipline were important predictors of adjustment outcomes (focused on aggression and assessed by teachers, peers, and observers). Day care accounted for 1-2% of the variance after controlling for SES. Both entering day care early and attending for long hours have been related to being seen as different on some behaviors, but the direction of the differences has been divided between those thought to be desirable and those thought undesirable (Volling et al., 1990).

Home Environment/Maternal Characteristics and Effects of Day Care

Attention is beginning to be paid to the mediating factors in effects of day care, as many critics have requested. Older studies found that day-care children whose mothers were more involved with them explored a strange situation more freely (were more securely attached?) (Farran & Ramey, 1977; Hock, 1976; Ross et al., 1975).

Recently, paternal involvement in child rearing, marital relationships, and maternal characteristics have been identified as contributing to the attachment relations between working mothers and their infants (Sachere, 1990). Characteristics of the mother predicted both attachment and compliance in the Caldera (1991) study. Infants whose mothers were sensitive/responsive and who had high self-esteem were apt to be rated as securely attached. Those whose mothers gave a lot of praise, but few directives, and who were not sensitive/responsive were apt to be compliant, and high SES predicted low compliance. Volling et al. (1990) found that children from controlling and rigidly structured families were far more likely to be distractible and aggressive in day care.

Maternal separation anxiety (reflected in overt behaviors or tension) when leaving the child in day care or with caretakers may be a major factor in the child's reaction, but it has received very little attention. One study examined both parental and infant behaviors on leave-taking and reunion, both at the start of the year and later (Field et al., 1984). Toddlers showed more negative behaviors than infants or preschoolers, and their mothers showed more hovering and sneaking out

of the room than did those of preschoolers (signs of the mothers' insecurity?). Children dropped off by their mothers showed more attention getting and crying than those dropped off by their fathers. In the second semester, infants and parents both showed increased clinging and hovering. The reunion behaviors at the end of the day were primarily positive and were a function of developmental age. Girls were more likely than boys to continue play during reunion, but also reached out to the parent more. Children picked up by fathers more often continued to play. The greater amount of attention getting and crying with mothers than fathers might reflect the infants' sense of the mothers' societally induced insecurity about leaving their children in day care (see Sachere, 1990). A possible support for that idea is reported by Easterbrooks and Goldberg (1985), who found that 26% of employed mothers in their sample, but only 4% of their husbands, saw the mother's employment as detrimental to the mother-infant relation. This is despite the fact that almost two-thirds of both parents in this middle-class sample had expected it to be, and the fact that there was *no* significant relation of maternal employment to attachment classification either to mother or father for either boys or girls. Higher maternal separation anxiety was related to planning not to work, and actual employment led to its decline. Low self-esteem was related to higher anxiety, and anxiety was higher for 3- than for 9-month-olds and higher for sons than for daughters (McBride & Belsky, 1988). Mothers of securely attached infants were likely to be moderate in their level of separation anxiety. The complex relations between types of anxiety and attachment led the authors to suggest that the effects of day care on children "may be more a function of maternal and family processes than of the child-care experience itself."

Mother's self-esteem has been found to be related to secure attachment (Caldera, 1991). The mother's role satisfaction has been shown to be more predictive of preschool sociability and compliance (for boys, not girls) than her employment status, which we can assume to be associated with day care (Kuzela et al., 1991). Role satisfaction may be an *outcome* of satisfactory attachment—not, as some have thought, a cause of it (Hahn et al., 1991). This is congruent with the finding that employment preferences (not employment) are important for understanding how women balance career and motherhood (DeMeis et al., 1986).

Wachs (1989) has recently taken a sophisticated approach to characterizing the home environment that offers hope of more meaningful dimensions for study in relation to child outcomes and effects of day care on infants. This approach serves to clarify relations between physical and social environments. It would be valuable if Wachs would also work on a similar characterization of day-care environments.

The Effects of Caregivers

If day-care children become attached to their caregivers, does this attachment compete with or dilute their attachment to their mothers? Does the stability of the caregiver influence the outcome? Does inconsistency between the kind of care given by the caregiver and by the parents disrupt the emotional development of the child?

Day-care babies do form attachments to caregivers, as discussed in Chapter 12. More than 50% of 2-year-olds show signs of contentment and pleasure such as waving and smiling when left with caregivers (King & Perrin, 1987). They generally prefer their caregivers to strangers, but they prefer their mothers to their caregivers (e.g., Cummings, 1980; Farran & Ramey, 1977; Kagan et al., 1978; Ricciuti, 1974; Ricciuti & Poresky, 1973). This was found even in a sample in which most of the infants lived in extended families and usually went from the day-care center to relatives or neighbors because their mothers were not at home at night (Farran & Ramey, 1977). These findings seem similar to those reported in comparisons of kibbutz infants' attachments for mothers versus metaplot. Secure attachment to caregivers is enhanced both by a good infant:caregiver ratio and by the total group's not being too large (Allhusen & Cochran, 1991).

The other questions have received little study. The importance of stability of caregivers has rarely been experimentally studied. Cummings (1980) examined differences between infants with stable and nonstable caregivers. The latter were not strangers (the child had experience with them for at least 1 month), but stable caregivers had worked with the experimental children at least 100 hours more than the unstable caregivers. In the Strange Situation both kinds of caregivers were preferred to strangers, with no preference between them. However, children preferred to be left with the stable caregiver when their mothers dropped them at the day-care center. In the Kagan et al. (1978) setting, all caregivers were stable by Cummings's criteria but each infant was given a primary caregiver. Over the course of their experience (the first 29 months of life) the children would run to the primary caregiver for comfort and help first, and to secondary personnel if the primary person was not available. A recent study was made of ethnically heterogeneous sixth-grade children who had highly educated parents with dual ca-

reers (Field, 1991). Those who had started full-time day care prior to age 2 and who had attended a variety of quality day-care centers, and thus lacked stability in both caregivers and locale, were rated by their teachers as higher in emotional well-being, attractiveness, and assertiveness the longer they had been in day care. The length of time they had been in day care was also positively related to their showing more physical affection with peers, being placed in the gifted program, and getting good math grades. Even over this long time span the correlations ranged from .29 to .49.

With the exception of Field's (1991) work, the studies mentioned above do not address the most crucial question of whether there are any long-term deleterious effects of instability of caregivers. Such studies are sorely needed, because many day-care centers have rapid turnover of staff, and some are set up to minimize the development of child-caregiver attachments. More and more experts today recommend stable caregivers, so that the children have a base of security and consistency of caregiving. The Cummings study provides limited support for this opinion, because the children were less stressed when they were left at the day-care center in the hands of a stable caregiver.

The evidence from other settings is also tenuous. It appears that kibbutzim often have high metaplot turnover, yet kibbutzniks grow up to be normal. Tizard's institutionalized children experienced systematic attempts to prevent attachment. They were able to form attachments later, although they apparently suffered some emotional sequelae. The infants reared in home management houses, which had perhaps the least stable sets of caretakers, had no long-range personality defects (Gardner et al., 1961). Our best guess, then, on the basis of woefully inadequate evidence, is that high turnover in caregivers is not a major detriment to the development of children, but that some stability is desirable, at least in the short run.

Consistency Between Parents and Caregivers. Consistency of child-rearing techniques of parents and caretakers has been very little studied. One of the most popular beliefs in child rearing is that children need consistency. Consistent feedback from the environment is necessary for learning, and inconsistency has been suggested as the cause of various sorts of psychopathology. Inconsistency is often blamed for deleterious effects of disadvantaged homes. Parents frequently complain about the "reentry" problems created by the inconsistency between their care and that provided by grandparents. And frequently the two parents have inconsistent views of child rearing. There is little direct evidence on these topics generally and certainly not on the degree of inconsistency that exists between parents and day-care personnel, parents and family day-care providers, or kibbutz parents and metaplot. It has been shown that for infants in centers with less adequate infant:caregiver ratios, continuity of care in the same center is more important than that of the individual caregiver (Allhusen & Cochran, 1991). It is likely, however, that unless parents make an effort to find a caretaker who shares their child-rearing philosophy, child-rearing techniques are bound to vary as a function of philosophy, as well as of differing roles.

A clear case of inconsistency occurred in the study where Chinese babies were being raised in traditional Chinese families but attended a Western-style day-care center (Kagan et al., 1978). The researchers gathered impressionistic evidence with respect to the infants' behaviors in these two diverse settings during their frequent parent-teacher interchange sessions. They found that the children evidently conformed to each of the two settings. At home the Chinese children were as quiet and nonassertive as their siblings, but they were more outgoing and "American" in day care. The American children, particularly those of the middle class, were seen by their parents to be much better behaved and more compliant at day care than at home. Thus it appears that even very young children can respond appropriately to two different rearing environments and thrive in both.[13] There is a clear need for much more research in this area, research in which differences and inconsistencies in rearing are more precisely analyzed and infants' responses are more closely and systematically measured.

Within-Group Differences

More studies that look at the within-group variations, as opposed to mean differences between groups with varied day-care experiences, may teach us more about many of the factors that may mediate effects of day care. One recent study looked at consistency between children's behaviors (as perceived by their mothers) and the mothers' ratings of what behaviors were most important to them (and similarly for the

child and caretaker) (Volling et al., 1990). The more sociable children were good fits with both their mothers' and their caregivers' important qualities. Difficult children were poorer fits with their home environment, and aggressive children were poorer fits with their caretaking environment. Statistical analyses showed that child-care experience (quality not measured) explained no significant amount of variance in child behaviors. Rather, 17% of the variance in being seen by mother as a difficult child and 14% of the variance in the amount of aggression were explained by the goodness of fit. As seen by the caregiver, day-care experience did not contribute significantly to variance, but goodness of fit accounted for 15% of sociability and 18% of aggression.

EPILOGUE

This analysis of the effects of multiple mothering has consistently led to the conclusion that there are very few negative outcomes if a baby has more than one caregiver, so long as the alternative care is good. This review also suggests that a caregiver who is a stable, though not always present, individual in the baby's life is important. Babies seem always to prefer those most stable caregivers, their mothers, and the most negative outcomes from multiple mothering were found in one of the studies in which the children were denied any stable caregiver.

One topic that needs a good deal more research is that of different effects for boys than for girls. Several studies have found differences, always in the direction of boys being more disadvantaged. Allhusen and Cochran (1991) found that not only were girls more securely attached to caregivers, but that care providers for girls were more effective than those for boys, a variable that deserves more attention.

It is interesting, in light of the evidence presented above, to consider the state of expert advice in this area. Etaugh (1980) reviewed the child-care books and articles that appeared in leading women's magazines from 1956 to 1976 for what they had to say on the effects of day care.[14] It was possible to divide the evaluations into three categories: harmful, not harmful or beneficial, and mixed. The last category included articles that endorsed part-time employment for mothers who wished to work or advocated that good day-care programs should be established for mothers who must work.

What is the tally of these views over the years? From 1956 to 1959 little appeared on the topic. There was one article in each category, and the principal parenting book (Dr. Spock's 1946 edition of *Baby and Child*

---

13. Anecdotally, I note that my children were able to behave in ways that suited their grandparents when staying with them, and in ways that suited us when with us. However, their behavior became disorganized when the three generations were under one roof for a time.

14. Only three magazines have shown a sustained interest in this topic (*Ladies' Home Journal, Redbook,* and *Parents*), and they account for 28 of the 31 articles found in the seven magazines. Today, for good or ill, the media are more attentive to the topic.

Care) was negative. The distribution for the decade of the 1960s and for 1970-1976 is shown in Table 13.2. It documents a marked shift toward a more positive view of day care. Nevertheless, there were still plenty of negative opinions, particularly in books. Spock's 1970 articles in *Redbook* were still highly negative. The third edition of his *Baby and Child Care* (1976) did a major turnaround and stressed the responsibilities of both parents for both child care and careers. Salk (1974), another pediatrician, took a dim view of working mothers or day care for infants. So did a number of psychologists, some based on psychoanalytic precepts and some on arguments for the necessity of maternal stimulation and provision of attachment. Brazelton (1974), in a book excerpted in popular magazines, argued that separation from parents affects children adversely in unobservable ways that cannot be measured. His position at that time appeared to rule out the relevance of scientific data altogether. He did console parents or reduce their guilt by allowing for the possibility that a good, nurturant day-care center might compensate for some of the damage. Recently he has softened his stand still further and has been a strong advocate for establishing day-care centers and standards for them.

This brief review shows that prior to the mid-1970s, parents reading books and articles were likely to be advised that putting infants into day care was harmful. Such advice contrasted sharply with the available evidence. This contrast between expert advice and evidence is, unfortunately, still common. Again, in the late 1980s and early 1990s, parents have been faced with the same sort of scare literature in the popular press, much of it based on the testimony of good developmental psychologists before Congress. (I recommend the reading of "Facts, Fantasies and the Future of Child Care in the United States," by Scarr et al., 1990, cited earlier, as an antidote for the scare literature. Day care and its related social policy issues are discussed by Zigler & Gordon, 1982; a different view is offered by Sroufe, 1988. The issue of *Early Childhood Research Quarterly* in which Sroufe's article appears is devoted entirely to articles on infant day care.) In areas as emotionally charged as the day-care debate, parents need to be cautious or appropriately skeptical about expert advice (on both sides of the issue). They should investigate available evidence themselves, attending to its relevance to their family, their projected form of care, and their child, rather than rely on the nonagreeing experts.

Table 13.2

Attitudes Toward Day Care Expressed in Books and Articles, 1960-1976

	Positive	*Negative*	*Mixed*
1960-1969			
books	1	10	2
articles	9	6	3
1970-1976			
books	8	10	8
articles	11	4	0

SOURCE: Based on data reported by Etaugh (1980).

Preventing or Overcoming Deprivation Effects Through Intervention Programs

Much of the previous discussion has focused on deprivation, actual or potential, but the twin topic of enrichment has never been far away. Indeed, intervention studies with both institutionalized and poverty-level infants and the possible good effects of day care have been mentioned. Some of these studies provide examples of preventive intervention, where an enrichment program was introduced to a population of infants who would be expected to suffer deprivation effects if no one intervened. The studies measured whether such deprivation effects were thereby prevented. The outcomes of the two types of preventive interventions already discussed are summarized below, followed by discussion of a type of preventive intervention program in which the primary target of the intervention is the mother (or day-care provider) or the caregiver-infant pair. Researchers hoped that these programs would have longer-lasting effects, because, if caregivers can be taught how to interact with babies successfully, then the improved environment should continue to have effects on the target children and their siblings when the intervention is over.

Finally, intervention programs that provide experiences to children who have already developed deprivation effects will be discussed. The adoption studies were of this type, because children were removed from deprived environments and put into more advantageous ones. When effects remain after adoption, as Dennis (1973) found in the intellectual achievement of children adopted after 2 years of age, adoption studies cannot answer the question of whether such effects could be eliminated. To do that, intervention studies that provide experiences not necessarily provided by the normal environment are needed. Optimal experiences might overcome deprivation in situations where normal environments cannot. This kind of research is particularly germane to the question of whether the effects of critical periods are permanent. Most available research on this question has used animals as subjects.

PREVENTIVE INTERVENTION PROGRAMS WITH HUMANS

There have been remarkably successful intervention programs to deal with the deprivation experienced by institutionalized infants. Institutions that focused on providing enrichment experiences were successful in preventing retardation. Model day-care programs designed to provide enrichment also prevented intellectual retardation. Because so many successful projects used such varied interventions, it is safe to conclude that the details of enrichment activities are not crucial, as long as there are enough active and involved caregivers to give such experiences.

The recent trend in intervention programs is to focus on training the caregivers. Some programs train mothers and others train day-care providers. Three of the first kind and one of the second are described here to give a flavor of the kinds of intervention provided and their effectiveness.

The first set of studies was spurred by a program of the U.S. government, the Parent-Child Development Project (for summaries, see Andrews, 1981; Andrews et al., 1982), which sponsored multidimensional programs that intervened with low-income parents of infants between birth and 3 years. Three such programs were started in 1970-1971, in Birmingham, Alabama; Houston, Texas; and New Orleans, Louisiana. In Birmingham and New Orleans, families began the program when the infants were 2 and 3 months old, respectively, and in Houston when the infant was 1 year old. The Houston program had less disadvantaged participants. All three programs focused on the parents, but varied in the extent to which the infants themselves were incorporated into the project, from Birmingham, in which the training focused on mother-child dyads, to New Orleans, in which the infants were not directly involved.

Positive maternal behaviors (e.g., giving emotional support, asking questions, and interfering less) increased for all three programs, but these effects were found only after 2 years in the Birmingham and New Orleans programs and after 3 years in the Houston program. Only the New Orleans program evaluated effects on mothers' negative behaviors toward their children and found a decrease of borderline significance ($p<.06$). Thus it appears easier to increase mothers' positive behaviors than to decrease their negative ones.

The intervention children in all three studies had higher IQs at 3 years than their controls, and again at 4 years, a year after completion of the program. It seems that mothers can be taught skills while their babies are small that will influence their children's intellectual development.

Beller et al. (1981) began a similar intervention study designed to help day-care providers. The goal was to change the providers' orientation from that of custodial caretakers to one of active participants in the development of their charges. The researchers taught the caregivers through workshops and interactional modeling sessions in a naturalistic setting. Caregivers kept charts of behavioral development to make them more aware of development and more sensitive to the progress of their charges, and to enable them to provide appropriate educational activities, using the children's strengths to develop their weak points. For one group of children caregiver intervention began when the children were from 4 to 7 months old; for a second group, when they were 14-17 months old. For both, it ended 6 months later.

Training changed behaviors in the specific situations trained: feeding, diapering, and toileting. Caregivers became more communicative and attentive, provided more opportunities for the children to learn, intruded less into the children's ongoing behavior, and adapted more to the children's needs. These changes had positive effects on independence in body care, awareness of surroundings, socioemotional development, play activities, speech, cognition, and motor functioning. Changes were always greater in the older group, and only they had higher DQs than the control infants at the end of the study. The finding of larger effects with toddlers is consistent with the research on model day-care centers. Whether the changes in caregiver behaviors generalized beyond the specific situations must be determined by future analysis.

As was true in the maternal intervention program, negative caretaker behaviors were not changed. Trained caregivers did not change in their communication of negative feelings or in exerting pressure or criticism, and this was paralleled by the data showing that the experimental children exhibited as much stress as control children.

These studies corroborate one of the most widely believed hypotheses about infant development, that how caregivers act makes a difference in how infants behave and develop. They make the hypothesis more specific, in that provision of more information about the nature of infants and training of specific skills were major components of all programs. In all programs caregivers became more positive, attentive, and cognitively enriching, but, in studies that measured them, did not change negative behaviors. It may be that intervention programs provide mothers with skills that promote positive behaviors in their babies, and hence the mothers are able to enjoy the babies' company more fully. These skills may not change the ways in which they experience negative emotions or communicate negative messages to their babies. These negative behaviors may require their own specific interventions.

THERAPEUTIC INTERVENTIONS WITH ANIMALS

Intervention studies with infrahuman animals are possible, because rearing intelligent mammals under conditions of severe deprivation produces profound effects on social and emotional development (see Harlow & Harlow, 1962, 1965). The effects of such deprivation and the interventions designed to overcome them are described in turn below.

Experimental animals who are isolated are typically raised in solitary cages with no direct contact with either humans or other animals. They have no toys or other objects of amusement. Their sensory environments are limited to the sights of their four walls and the muted sounds of the laboratory (e.g., other animals, human keepers, scraping of food and water dishes). Animals kept in these isolation conditions for long enough periods become very peculiar. For example, dogs demonstrate greatly heightened diffuse activity, diminished social capacity, a tendency to epilepticlike seizures, and a curious apparent insensitivity to pain. For example, they might repeatedly approach and touch a lighted match with only generalized excitement, not the normal obvious signs of distress (Melzak & Scott, 1957). W. R. Thompson (1955) summarized such dogs' behaviors as appearing to reflect retarded development, because when full grown they showed the excitability and diffuseness typical of puppies.

Similar effects are found in some species of monkeys, including the rhesus. Isolated monkeys sit immobile in their cages or pace in circles with stereotyped gestures or clasp their heads in their arms and rock for long periods of time. They aggress against themselves, especially when approached by humans, and they do not exhibit appropriate social aggression when they encounter age-mates. They exhibit avoidance and fear of both normal and unusual environmental stimuli (including others of their own species, humans, masks, and toys). When they reach sexual maturity, they are unable to mate. They seem interested, approach the opposite sex, and show parts of the sexual pattern, but only rarely succeed in mating if given extensive sup-

port from experienced animals and the help of humans. Interestingly, isolation has little effect on rhesus' intellectual abilities, although they are not always able to exhibit their potential. The strength of the isolation effects depends on both the duration and the timing of the isolation, which supports a critical period hypothesis. It appears that 12 months of isolation produces more severe effects than 6 months (Rowland, 1964). Isolation effects occur only if the monkeys are isolated from birth; if they are first allowed to develop social affections and then isolated, the effects are far less marked (Clark, 1968; Harlow & Novak, 1973; Harlow & Suomi, 1971).

Similarly, the isolation of puppies from other dogs and humans produces abnormal social behaviors and even learning deficits in ways that support a critical period hypothesis (Scott, 1958; Scott & Marston, 1950; Scott et al., 1973; for a review, see Scott, 1967). Furthermore, in dogs the effects of isolation and of treatments depend on genetic factors, that is, on the breed of dog (Fuller & Clark, 1966).

Attempts to overcome isolation effects have been instituted with both dogs and rhesus monkeys. Such research has the potential to test the critical periods hypothesis, which predicts that recovery from early isolation should be impossible. Furthermore, discovering what works and what does not work to overcome isolation effects reveals something about the nature of the deprivation.

Fear plays an important role in producing and maintaining isolation effects. Fuller and Scott (1967) found that if puppies reared in isolation were tranquilized, they approached harmless objects (such as the human experimenters they earlier had avoided) and they could learn mazes they had been unable to do prior to the use of tranquilizers. After the effects of the tranquilizers wore off, the puppies were still willing to approach harmless objects. These studies are impressive in showing that a relatively brief experience after the so-called critical period for socialization could eliminate its deleterious effects. Second, because the effect of the intervention was to allow the animals to deal with the environmental stimuli in a calm state, it suggests that fear or excitement prevented the isolates from being able to process stimuli accurately. Thus it is possible to infer that what happens during isolation is that animals develop abnormal fear responses to almost all stimuli. This highlights one of the purported roles of attachment figures, to provide a secure base from which the young can explore without the interference of fear (see Chapter 12).

Another area of research on overcoming deprivation effects involves rhesus monkeys. Although several therapeutic attempts failed, Harlow and his collaborators found a therapy that worked. Isolate monkeys exposed to younger (3-month-old) monkeys for 1-2 hours several days a week for 6 months showed virtually complete recovery (Suomi & Harlow, 1972); 12-month isolates showed remarkable recovery in social situations and improved in the appropriateness of their behaviors while alone, although not all their peculiar behaviors disappeared (Novak & Harlow, 1975). Younger peers may be effective therapy agents because they repeatedly initiate social contact and do so without aggression. They were successful at such attempts because the isolates were immobile and withdrawn. The persistence of the therapists eventually paid off, reciprocal relationships were established, and the isolates' self-directed activities (such as huddling and rocking) decreased. A second advantage of immature peers was that their social patterns were simple at the beginning of therapy and their play became more complex as they grew older, which set the stage for the development of more complex social interactions as the therapy progressed.

Thus again there is little evidence for a strict critical period because the isolation effects were largely reversible. A sensitive period hypothesis is still viable, however, because timing is important. After 6 months of total isolation, exposing isolates to socially competent age-mates does not overcome the negative effects, but exposure to younger monkeys does (Harlow et al., 1965). Isolation effects do not develop if monkeys are raised with same-age peers for the first 6 months.

Although it is dangerous to generalize from dogs and rhesus monkeys to humans, the information gathered from these species suggests possible interventions to try with humans: (a) Take great care to ameliorate children's fear responses; (b) provide a persistent, actively initiating, and reliable love object (something Tizard's, 1977, adoptive parents may have done); and (c) match the emotional and intellectual capabilities of the child with the demands of the environment (a notion that Hunt repeatedly suggested). Younger peers often provide just such an environment for older children and might, under carefully supervised circumstances, be helpful.

Biology and the Effects of Experience

Unlike many topics in infant research, those discussed in this chapter have been studied extensively and ingeniously with humans. The two strategies of "natural experiments" and intervention experiments have provided a rather clear picture of the effects of

deprivation and intervention. The focus here is on research with humans when possible, but research with humans has different practical and ethical limitations than does animal research. I would therefore like to report on a few classic studies with laboratory animals that either corroborate the conclusions reached from studying humans or make points that research with humans has as yet been unable to make.

PHYSIOLOGICAL/ANATOMIC EFFECTS OF EARLY EXPERIENCE

Rosenzweig and his collaborators produced a body of research that examined effects of enrichment and deprivation on brain growth. Their impoverished rat pups were less stimulated than the worst orphanage groups, except that they could eat and drink whenever they wanted and as much as they wanted. They were in individual cages, could not see or touch other rats, and were in quiet, dimly lit rooms. Each impoverished rat pup had a littermate who lived in an enriched environment. The enriched rats lived in a large cage with 10 or 12 other pups and a new selection of toys (e.g., ladders, wheels, boxes, and platforms) each day (see Figure 13.3). They were taken daily in groups of 5 or 6 for half-hour exploratory sessions in a larger field with barriers that changed daily. After 30 days, formal training in mazes (what might be called "cognitively enriched day care") was given. It was found that the cortex of the brain weighed more in 101 (of 130 pairs) of the enriched pups than in the impoverished littermates (in contrast to their body weights, which were lower). The ratio of cortex weight to total brain weight was also higher in the enriched littermates for 115 of the 130 pairs. Actually, Bennett and colleagues were able to affect the size of different portions of the brain according to the particular types of enrichment provided (see Bennett, Diamond, Krech, and Rosenzweig, in a series of studies and publications cited in Diamond, 1988; Rosenzweig, 1966). In addition to the brain weight differences, this group has been able to demonstrate biochemical differences (Bennett et al., 1964; Bennett & Rosenzweig, 1971; Diamond, 1988). (An excellent recent summary can be found in Diamond's book *Enriching Heredity: The Impact of the Environment on the Anatomy of the Brain*, 1988. No knowledge of technical language is needed to understand Chapters 9, "Learning and Behavior," and 10, "The Significance of Enrichment.")

The researchers cited above, and others, have gone on to show that brain structure is altered by environmental differences. The numbers and branching of dendritic spines (Globus et al., 1973; Greenough &

Volkmar, 1973) and the number and thickness of synapses in the cerebral cortex of rats are affected by the environments (enriched, impoverished, or standard rat colony) in which they have lived (Diamond, 1988; Diamond et al., 1975). Such effects have also been demonstrated in other rodents (Rosenzweig & Bennett, 1978). Brain structure and dendritic branching depend not only on environmental rearing conditions, but on other biological factors, such as nutrition (Carughi et al., 1989). Rats suckled by malnourished dams given both nutritional rehabilitation and an enriched environment showed greatly enhanced dendritic branching and thickness of the occipital cortex, but environment did not affect those that continued to be malnourished. This may have a message for us with respect to enrichment programs for children who are and continue to be malnourished. The message is two-way, in that we know from human studies that psychosocial intervention makes nutritional supplementation more effective (e.g., Super et al., 1990).

Environmental enrichment affects the results of brain lesions. It both aids the recovery of learning capacity and affects the actual brain measures (Will et al., 1976, 1977). Their original studies exposed rat pups to the different environments starting at weaning, when some assume their brains are at an initial critical or sensitive period for stimulation, but the researchers felt that they would be more plastic. Adult rats exposed for the same length of time (80 days) to the same enriched conditions in later studies showed the same increased brain growth (Rosenzweig, 1983). However, a recent review concluded that cortical lesions do produce different anatomical and behavioral effects depending on the age at which the brain is damaged (Kolb, 1989). This review makes the point that learned behaviors are the ones usually tested in work in this area, and that they may show better recovery than so-called species-specific behaviors (e.g., mating, nesting). Recent work has identified a protein that appears to be responsible for the plasticity in brain development (Aoki & Siekevitz, 1988).

All of these animal studies suggest considerable plasticity of both brain development and behavior. They also suggest that the growth, structure, and biochemistry of the brain are affected by environmental manipulations, and that these effects are not limited to early critical periods of development or to intact organisms. The results are congruent with the human adoption studies, and, together, they argue against the hypothesis that the effects of early damage or environmental deprivation are irreversible. Both human and animal studies support the view that even late intervention can sometimes be successful.

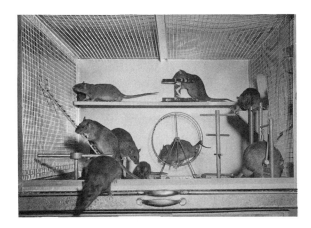

Figure 13.3. The enriched environment of the rats raised by Rosenzweig. (Photograph courtesy of Mark R. Rosenzweig.)

Environmental differences included both physical and social differences. Human studies have focused on social environment to the near exclusion of physical or inanimate aspects of the environment (see MacPhee et al., 1984; Wohlwill & Heft, 1987). However, HOME measures some aspects of physical environment and has been correlated with later outcomes for infants as in some of the studies of prematures (see Chapter 2). Wachs (1990), using the Purdue Home Stimulation Inventory, has shown that the physical environment is related to several aspects of play behavior in 1-year-olds, including social mastery in free play, after controlling for social environment. The reverse is not true. Social environment was not related to these behaviors after controlling for physical environment.

INTERACTION OF EFFECTS OF EXPERIENCE WITH CHARACTERISTICS OF THE ORGANISM

Most of the research discussed in this chapter has ignored the problem of individual differences. The issues have been stated in terms of the general case; for example, does institutionalization affect infants? Even when individual differences were obtained (e.g., the 4 of Tizard's 24 adopted babies who did not attach to their adopted parents), the reasons for the different outcomes were not explored. Failure to study individual differences masks a very large source of influence on outcomes. The same environmental event or situation is not likely to affect each and every infant to the same degree or in the same way. Studies with laboratory animals have explored individual differences operationalized as genetic differences (that is, strain or breed differences). These studies found interactions between the environmental manipulation and the genetic constitution of the individual (or group) exposed. Thus they established that, at least in some restricted circumstances (genetically based individual differences in infrahuman animals), a particular environmental event affects different individuals in different ways.

Cooper and Zubek (1958) explored the influence of enrichment and deprivation on rats of varying genetic potential for learning. They bred rats to be good or poor at running mazes (considered a standard test of rat intelligence; see Figure 13.4). After many generations, when the brightest rat in the maze-dull group was poorer at running mazes than the dullest rat in the maze-bright group, rat pups from each group were subjected to one of three rearing conditions: normal laboratory environment, deprived environment, or enriched environment. They were then tested for the number of trials it took them to learn a maze. The results are reproduced in Table 13.3. Notice that any general statement about the effects of enriched or deprived environments would be misleading. An enriched environment improved performance of maze-dull rats, compared with a normal or restricted environment, and made them like the maze-bright rats reared in a normal environment. An enriched environment had no significant effect on maze-bright rats. This is similar to the lack of improvement shown by middle-class children in a good day-care program in which disadvantaged children improved. However, a restricted environment affected the learning ability of maze-bright rats who had the same number of errors as the maze-dull rats. Differences between rats with different genetic potentials were maximized in the normal laboratory environment and minimized in both enriched and deprived environments. A normal environment permitted maze-bright rats to reach their genetic potential, whereas maze-dull rats reached theirs only in an enriched environment.

This finding that extra stimulation does not enhance the performance of some animals brings us to a caveat: More is not always better, and can even be detrimental (Gardner et al., 1984; see also Brownell & Strauss, 1984; Strauss & Brownell, 1984). Stimulation needs to be geared to the current status of the organism to which it is directed. In the enrichment studies done with prematures (see Chapter 2), this was not always the case. Optimal levels of stimulation depend on total levels that include both internal and external stimulation, and hence differ for different babies and at different times. An example is that full-term, healthy newborns who received multimodal stimulation in a hammock during sleep periods had less mature orien-

Table 13.3

Mean Errors on Running a Maze for Rats of Varying Genetic Potential and Subjected to Different Rearing Environments

Genetic Potential	Rearing Environment		
	Restricted	Normal	Enriched
Maze-bright	169	117	111
Maze-dull	169	164	119

tation, motor, and state regulation behaviors on the NBAS than controls (Koniak-Griffin & Ludington-Hoe, 1987). However, the quantity of stimulation was related to favorable maternal perceptions of infant behavior.

It is dangerous to attempt to draw precise conclusions about the effects of the interaction between environment and genetics on learning ability in human babies on the basis of a rat study. Nevertheless, the study is important in that it suggests that the abilities and characteristics children bring to their environments influence what they get out of those environments. Wachs (1987) corroborated the finding from Schaffer's early work that active children may be less dependent on their environments than inactive children in developing mastery behaviors. He also found that difficult children were more influenced by their environments than easy children, and that boys are more influenced than girls, and often in different ways. Furthermore, the research on genetic influences on IQ later in childhood demonstrates consistently that there are genetic differences in intellectual potential that interact with environment.

Interaction of environmental and genetic differences has also been studied in relation to social and emotional development using groups with different genetic constitutions (different strains of rats, or breeds of dogs). Although we do not know the nature of the genetic differences, we can be certain that there were some, because strains and breeds are highly inbred.

Maternal stress during pregnancy in rats affects the behavior of the offspring (see Chapter 4). W. R. Thompson (1955) found offspring of stressed mothers to be more "emotional" (to defecate more and to explore less in an open field). But some efforts to replicate these findings have failed and some have succeeded. The crucial determinant of positive findings is the particular strain of rats used (Joffe, 1969). In short, the effect of a prenatal environmental event on rats depends on the genotype of the rat that is exposed to it.

Second, the effect of particular disciplinary techniques on the behavior of dogs depends on their breed characteristics. In a study by Freedman (1958), four breeds of dogs (Shetland sheepdogs, wirehaired fox terriers, beagles, and basenjis) had litters that were divided into two pairs based on similarity (both physical and behavioral). Each pair member was assigned to either indulgent or disciplined rearing, and had two 15-minute interactions with a single human caretaker daily from their third to eighth week. Indulged puppies were encouraged in any activity they initiated and were never punished; disciplined pups were at first restrained in the experimenter's lap and later trained to sit, stay, come on command, and finally to follow on a leash. All were then tested for 8 days for obedience to the command to not eat meat in their room. The adult rearer spent 3 minutes swatting them and shouting "No!" each time they attempted to eat. The dogs were then left alone and watched through a one-way mirror to see whether they started to eat in the next 10 minutes, and, if so, how soon.

To all intents and purposes the rearing made no long-term difference to either the Shetland sheepdogs or the basenjis. After the first few days, basenjis all ate within 3 minutes of being left, but no Shetland sheepdog ate in the 10 minutes after being left. Thus these two breeds behaved very differently and their behavior was dependent more on breed than on rearing. The fox terriers waited longer to eat than did the beagles, but, unlike the sheepdogs and basenjis, these breeds showed differences based on rearing. Indulged dogs waited longer to eat than did disciplined dogs. Thus breed affected both obedience and effectiveness of rearing conditions. One breed (Shetlands) was obedient regardless of rearing, one (basenjis) was disobedient regardless of rearing, and the other two were obedient only when indulgently reared.

Our third example involves breed differences in the effects of social isolation. Pigtailed macaque monkeys did not develop the isolate syndrome (withdrawn, personally bizarre, abnormal in social, sexual, and exploratory behavior) to the extent described for rhesus monkeys (Harlow et al., 1965; Sackett et al., 1976). They were not deficient in exploratory behavior, and they showed some positive social behaviors when placed with socially normal age-mates after rearing in isolation. Nevertheless, compared with normally reared controls, they had deficits similar to, but less serious than, those found for the rhesus. Crab-eating, pigtailed, and rhesus macaques all showed different behaviors during isolation and were differently affected in their postrearing social interactions (Sackett et al., 1981). Not only did rearing in isolation produce

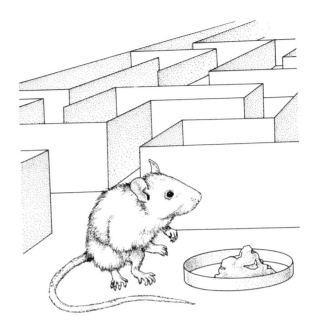

Figure 13.4. A rat in a maze.

markedly varied amounts of isolate syndrome behaviors among the different species, but the amount of isolate syndrome behavior did not predict the degree of exploratory behavior or even the degree of positive social behavior.

These examples make it very clear that in both intellectual and social-emotional development the influence of the environment depends on the strain studied. Although there is no comparable evidence with humans, it seems likely that individual differences exert at least as great an influence on the effects of various environments on human babies.

Summary

In the 1940s Spitz documented that children in orphanages failed to thrive and were retarded. Both then and for a considerable period of time thereafter it was thought that these conditions were due to a lack of mothering. Several lines of research have shown this view to be wrong. First, in institutions that typically produced retardation, providing additional perceptual and intellectual stimulation or additional opportunities for exercise of motor capacities, or both, did a great deal to lessen the retardation normally found in old-fashioned orphanages. Stimulation in a particular mode fosters development in that mode (for example, vocal stimulation facilitates vocal behaviors), but it is not known whether certain kinds of stimulation facilitate in nonspecific ways. Further, the amount of time devoted to extra stimulation does not have to be large. Second, children in orphanages with low child:caregiver ratios and enrichment programs exhibited normal intelligence and generally good emotional development. And third, Guatemalan infants who spend their first year of life in cognitively impoverished environments suffered retardation despite unimpaired relationships with their mothers. Thus effects of institutionalization result from inadequate stimulation of infants' developing cognitive abilities, and not from lack of a mother or from institutionalization as such.

Because for many years infancy was thought to be a critical period for development of both intellectual and social-emotional functioning, institutionalization effects were thought to be permanent. Studies that followed the development of children after they left the deprived environments of institutions and moved into more normal and stimulating environments demonstrated that such effects are not irreversible. Dennis's study of the Crèche children adopted at different ages showed that those adopted by 2 years of age had no lasting deficits. Children who were severely deprived for longer than the first 2 years did not entirely make up for their earlier deficits, although they developed at a normal rate after being adopted. It is impossible to determine from these data whether the permanent deficits occurred because the children were deprived for such a long time, or whether the postinfancy period is a crucial time for intellectual development. Also unanswered is the question of whether special enrichment for them or training for their adoptive parents could erase the deficits found among those adopted after 2 years of age. These conclusions from Dennis's research were confirmed by the later research of Kagan and of Tizard. Evidence concerning subsequent social-emotional development after early deprivation is more difficult to obtain because of the paucity of adequate measures. Available research indicates that there are no startling negative effects. Tizard's findings suggest that adopted children have good relationships with their parents and with their siblings, but are more likely to have difficulties with school peers and teachers. Gardner and colleagues found no personality deficits as measured by standard personality tests.

The next question explored was, Are multiple mothers harmful in situations in which infants are able to form specific attachments to their own mothers? Such situations occur in cultures that practice communal child rearing and, to a lesser extent, in day care in the United States. Infants develop strong, specific attachments to both their mothers and their alternative caretakers, but their attachments are stronger to their mothers. There is little reliable evidence for any resulting important difficulties in social-emotional development.

Many of the studies of day care are of centers designed to maximize development. In such centers, intellectual development may be superior to that of home-reared infants for children from disadvantaged backgrounds. It is fairly easy to design or to select day-care centers that promote intellectual development. The specifics of the program do not seem to be crucial; if there is a focus on fostering development and providing stimulating experiences, children develop well. It is more difficult to specify what promotes social-emotional development. Although there is little evidence, it may be less disruptive to provide children with stability in their caregivers. With respect to consistency of caregiving between home and center, the limited research suggests that children can easily deal with inconsistencies.

The research that led to enrichment programs in orphanages and in model day-care programs demonstrated that it is both possible and feasible to provide programs that prevent intellectual retardation in children who might otherwise suffer such effects. Recent programs that focused on intervening with caregivers have been successful in teaching caregivers about children, in training caregivers in specific skills, and in increasing caregivers' positive behaviors, but not in decreasing their negative behaviors. Such changes have demonstrable effects on children's development. In both day-care and home intervention studies, the interventions appear to be more effective in the second year of life. This may be because effects are cumulative (they take 2 years to work) or because shorter interventions at later ages are more effective.

The research on therapeutic intervention with infrahuman animals indicates that deprivation effects on social-emotional development can be overcome with appropriate experiences. This makes it clear that a critical periods hypothesis is not viable and that even a sensitive periods hypothesis may not be sufficient to explain subsequent plasticity. This research also suggests the need in such interventions (a) to overcome fear so that the animals can learn to cope, (b) to provide social interaction in a context that is safe for the deprived animal, and (c) to match the environmental demands with the animals' capabilities, moving gradually from simpler to more complex situations.

The last section of the chapter reviewed research with animals that further elucidated the mechanisms of deprivation and intervention. First, studies of the effects of enrichment and deprivation on brain development in rats demonstrate that enriched experiences stimulate the brain's growth and its structural development, but that such growth, as measured by current biochemical means, is no greater during infancy than in adulthood. This suggests that these effects do not operate by a critical periods mechanism. Second, the animal research makes it quite clear that genetic differences produce large individual differences in susceptibility to particular environmental experiences.

References

ALLHUSEN, V. D., & Cochran, M. M. (1991, April). *Infants' attachment behaviors with their day care providers.* Paper presented at the meeting of the Society for Research in Child Development, Seattle.

ANDREWS, S. R. (1981). Mother-infant interaction and child development: Findings from an experimental study of parent-child programs. In M. J. Begab, H. Garber, & H. C. Haywood (Eds.), *Psychosocial influences in retarded performance: Strategies for improving competence* (Vol. 2, pp. 245-256). Baltimore: University Park Press.

ANDREWS, S. R., Blumenthal, J. B., Johnson, D. L., Kahn, A. J., Ferguson, C. J., Laseter, T. M., Malone, P. E., & Wallace, D. B. (1982). The skills of mothering: A study of parent child development centers. *Monographs of the Society for Research in Child Development, 47*(6, Serial No. 198).

AOKI, C., & Siekevitz, P. (1988, December). Plasticity in brain development. *Scientific American,* pp. 56-64.

ATKIN, R., Bray, R., Davison, M., Herberger, S., Humphreys, L., & Selzer, V. (1977). Cross-lagged panel analysis of sixteen cognitive measures at four grade levels. *Child Development, 48,* 944-952.

AVGAR, A., Bronfenbrenner, U., & Henderson, C. R., Jr. (1977). Socialization practices of parents, teachers, and peers in Israel: Kibbutz, moshav, and city. *Child Development, 48,* 1219-1227.

BADGER, E. (1973). *Mother's guide to early learning.* Paoli, PA: McGraw-Hill.

BADGER, E. (1977). The infant stimulation/mother training project. In B. Caldwell & D. Stedman (Eds.), *Infant education: A guide for helping handicapped children in the first three years.* New York: Walker.

BARGLOW, P., Vaughn, B. E., & Molitor, N. (1987). Effects of maternal absence due to employment on the quality of infant-mother attachment in a low risk sample. *Child Development, 58,* 945-954.

BATES, J. E., Marvinney, D., Bennett, D. S., Dodge, K. A., Kelly, T., & Pettit, G. S. (1991, April). *Children's daycare history and kindergarten adjustment.* Paper presented at the meeting of the Society for Research in Child Development, Seattle.

BAYLEY, N. (1965). Comparisons of mental and motor test scores for ages 1-15 months by sex, birth order, race, geographical location, and education of parents. *Child Development, 36,* 379-412.

BELLER, E. K., Laewen, H., & Stahnke, M. (1981). A model of infant education in day care. In M. J. Begab, H. Gardner, & H. C. Haywood (Eds.), *Psychosocial influences in retarded performance: Strategies for improving competence* (Vol. 2).

Baltimore: University Park Press.

BELSKY, J. (1986). Infant day care: A cause for concern? *Zero to Three, 6,* 1-9.

BELSKY, J. (1988a). The "effects" of infant day care reconsidered. *Early Childhood Research Quarterly, 3,* 235-272.

BELSKY, J. (1988b). Infant day care and socioemotional development: The United States. *Journal of Child Psychology and Psychiatry and Allied Disciplines, 29,* 397-406.

BELSKY, J. (1989). Infant-parent attachment and day care: In defense of the strange situation. In J. Lande, S. Scarr, & N. Gunzenhauser (Eds.), *Caring for children: Challenge to America* (pp. 23-48). Hillsdale, NJ: Lawrence Erlbaum.

BELSKY, J., & Rovine, M. J. (1988). Nonmaternal care in the first year of life and the security of infant-parent attachment. *Child Development, 59,* 157-167.

BELSKY, J., & Steinberg, L. D. (1978). The effects of day care: A critical review. *Child Development, 49,* 929-949.

BENNETT, E. L., Diamond, M. C., Krech, D., & Rosenzweig, M. R. (1964). Chemical and anatomical plasticity of the brain. *Science, 146,* 610-619.

BENNETT, E. L., & Rosenzweig, M. R. (1971). Chemical alterations produced in brain by environment and training. In A. Lajtha (Ed.), *Handbook of neurochemistry* (Vol. 6). New York: Plenum.

BETTELHEIM, B. (1969). *The children of the dream.* New York: Macmillan.

BLEHAR, M. C. (1974). Anxious attachment and defensive reaction associated with day care. *Child Development, 45,* 683-692.

BRAZELTON, T. B. (1974). *Toddlers and parents.* New York: Delacorte.

BROUSSARD, M., & Décarie, G. (1971). The effects of three kinds of perceptual-social stimulation on the development of institutionalized infants: Preliminary report of a longitudinal study. *Early Child Development and Care, 1,* 111-130.

BROWNELL, C. A., & Strauss, M. S. (1984). Infant stimulation and development: Conceptual and empirical considerations. In Infant intervention programs: Truths and untruths [Special issue]. *Journal of Children in Contemporary Society, 17,* 108-130.

BURCHINAL, M. R., & Bryant, D. M. (1991, April). *Infant-mother attachment, infant daycare, and school-aged classroom behaviors.* Paper presented at the meeting of the Society for Research in Child Development, Seattle.

CALDERA, Y. M. (1991, April). *Infant daycare and maternal characteristics as predictors of attachment and compliance in toddlers.* Paper presented at the meeting of the Society for Research in Child Development, Seattle.

CALDWELL, B. M. (1964). The effects of infant care. In M. L. Hoffman (Ed.), *Review of child development research* (Vol. 1). New York: Russell Sage Foundation.

CALDWELL, B. M. (1974). A decade of early intervention programs: What we have learned. *American Journal of Orthopsychiatry, 44,* 491-496.

CARUGHI, A., Carpenter, K. J., & Diamond, M. C. (1989). Effect of environmental enrichment during nutritional rehabilitation on body growth, blood parameters and cerebral cortical development of rats. *Journal of Nutrition, 119,* 2005-2016.

CHASE-LANSDALE, P. L., & Owen, M. T. (1987). Maternal employment in a family context: Effects on infant-mother and infant-father attachments. *Child Development, 58,* 1505-1512.

CLARK, D. L. (1968). *Immediate and delayed effects of early, intermediate, and late social isolation in the rhesus monkey.* Unpublished doctoral dissertation, University of Wisconsin—Madison.

CLARK, E. A., & Hanisee, J. (1982). Intellectual and adaptive performance of Asian children in adoptive American settings. *Developmental Psychology, 18,* 595-599.

CLARKE-STEWART, K. A. (1973). Interactions between mothers and their young children: Characteristics and consequences. *Monographs of the Society for Research in Child Development, 38*(6-7, Serial No. 153).

CLARKE-STEWART, K. A. (1984). Predicting child development from day care forms and features: The Chicago study. In D. Phillips (Ed.), *Predictors of quality child care* (Research Monograph No. 1). Washington, DC: National Association for the Education of Young Children.

CLARKE-STEWART, K. A. (1988). The "effects" of infant day care reconsidered: Risks for parents, children and researchers. *Early Childhood Research Quarterly, 3,* 293-318.

CLARKE-STEWART, K. A. (1989). Infant day care: Maligned or malignant? *American Psychologist, 44,* 266-273.

CLARKE-STEWART, K. A., & Fein, G. G. (1983). Early childhood programs. In P. H. Mussen (Ed.), *Handbook of child psychology* (Vol. 2, 4th ed., pp. 917-999). New York: John Wiley.

COOPER, R. M., & Zubek, J. P. (1958). Effects of enriched and restricted early environments on the learning ability of bright and dull rats. *Canadian Journal of Psychology, 12,* 159-164.

CUMMINGS, E. M. (1980). Caregiver stability and day care. *Developmental Psychology, 16,* 31-37.

DARLINGTON, R. B., Royce, J. M., Snipper, A. S., Murray, H. W., & Lazar, I. (1980). Preschool programs and the later school competence of children from low-income families. *Science, 208,* 202-204.

DeMEIS, D. K., Hock, E., & McBride, S. L. (1986). The balance of employment and motherhood: Longitudinal study of mothers' feeling about separation from their first-born infants. *Developmental Psychology, 5,* 627-632.

DENNIS, W. (1960). Causes of retardation among institutional children: Iran. *Journal of Genetic Psychology, 96,* 47-59.

DENNIS, W. (1973). *Children of the Crèche.* New York: Appleton-Century-Crofts.

DIAMOND, M. C. (1988). *Enriching heredity: The impact of the environment on the anatomy of the brain.* New York: Free Press.

DIAMOND, M. C., Lindner, B., Johnson, R., Bennett, E. L., & Rosenzweig, M. R. (1975). Differences in occipital cortical synapses from environmentally enriched, impoverished, and standard colony rats. *Journal of Neuroscience Research, 1,* 109-119.

DONTAS, C., Maratos, O., Fafoutis, M., & Karangelis, A. (1985). Early social development in institutionally reared Greek infants: Attachment and peer interaction. *Monographs of the Society for Research in Child Development, 50,* 136-146.

EASTERBROOKS, M. A., & Goldberg, W. A. (1985). Effects of early maternal employment on toddlers, mothers and fathers. *Developmental Psychology, 21,* 774-783.

EPSTEIN, H. T. (1974a). Phrenoblysis: Special brain and mind growth periods: I. Human brain and skull development. *Developmental Psychobiology, 7,* 207-216.

EPSTEIN, H. T. (1974b). Phrenoblysis: Special brain and mind growth periods: II. Human mental development. *Developmental Psychobiology, 7,* 217-224.

ETAUGH, C. (1980). Effects of nonmaternal care on children: Research evidence and popular views. *American Psychologist, 35,* 309-319.

FAIGIN, H. (1958). Social behavior of young children in the kibbutz. *Journal of Abnormal and Social Psychology, 56,* 117-129.

FARRAN, D., & Ramey, C. (1977). Infant day care and attachment behaviors toward mothers and teachers. *Child Development, 48,* 1112-1116.

FEIN, G. G., & Fox, N. (1988). Infant day care: A special issue. *Early Childhood Research Quarterly, 3,* 227-234.

FIELD, T. (1991). Quality infant day-care and grade school behavior and performance. *Child Development, 62,* 863-870.

FIELD, T., Gewirtz, J. L., Cohen, D., Garcia, R., Greenberg, R., & Collins, K. (1984). Leave takings and reunions of infants, toddlers, preschoolers and their parents. *Child Development, 55,* 628-635.

FOWLER, W., & Kahn, N. (1974, December). *The development of a prototype infant and child day care center in metropolitan Toronto* (Year III Progress Report). Unpublished manuscript.

FOWLER, W., & Kahn, N. (1975, December). *The development of a prototype infant and child day care center in metropolitan Toronto* (Year IV Progress Report). Unpublished manuscript.

FOX, N. (1977). Attachment of kibbutz infants to mother and metapelet. *Child Development, 48,* 1228-1239.

FOX, N., & Fein, G. G. (Eds.). (1990). *Infant day care: The current debate.* Norwood, NJ: Ablex.

FREEDMAN, D. G. (1958). Constitutional and environmental interactions in rearing of four breeds of dogs. *Science, 127,* 585-586.

FULLER, J. L., & Clark, L. D. (1966). Genetic and treatment factors modifying the postisolation syndrome in dogs. *Journal of Comparative and Physiological Psychology, 61,* 251-257.

FULLER, J. L., & Scott, J. P. (1967). Experiential deprivation and later behavior. *Science, 158,* 1648-1652.

GARBER, H., & Heber, R. (1981). The efficacy of early intervention with family rehabilitation. In M. J. Begab, H. C. Haywood, & H. L. Garber (Eds.), *Psychosocial influences in retarded performance: Strategies for improving competence* (Vol. 2, pp. 71-88). Baltimore: University Park Press.

GARDNER, D. B., Hawkes, G. R., & Burchinal, L. G. (1961). Noncontinuous mothering in infancy and development in later childhood. *Child Development, 32,* 225-234.

GARDNER, D. B., & Swiger, M. K. (1958). Developmental status of two groups of infants released for adoption. *Child Development, 29,* 521-530.

GARDNER, J. M., Karmel, B. Z., & Dowd, J. M. (1985). Relationship of infant psychobiological development to infant intervention programs. In Infant intervention programs: Truths and untruths [Special issue]. *Journal of Children in Contemporary Society, 17,* 93-108.

GEWIRTZ, H. B., & Gewirtz, J. L. (1968). Visiting and caretaking patterns for kibbutz infants: Age and sex trends. *American Journal of Orthopsychiatry, 38,* 427-443.

GEWIRTZ, J. L., & Gewirtz, H. B. (1965). Stimulus conditions, infant behaviors, and social learning in four Israeli child-rearing environments: A preliminary report illustrating differences in environment and behavior between the "only" and the "youngest" child. In B. M. Foss (Ed.), *Determinants of infant behavior* (Vol. 3). New York: John Wiley.

GLOBUS, A., Rosenzweig, M. R., Bennett, E. L., & Diamond, M. C. (1973). Effects of differential experience on dendritic spine counts. *Journal of Physiological and Comparative Psychology, 82,* 175-181.

GOLDEN, M., Rosenbluth, L., Grossi, M., Policare, H., Freeman, H., & Brownlee, E. (1978). *The New York City infant day care study.* New York: Medical and Health Research Association of New York City.

GOLDFARB, W. (1945a). Effects of psychological deprivation in infancy and subsequent stimulation. *American Journal of Psychiatry, 102,* 18-33.

GOLDFARB, W. (1945b). Psychological privation in infancy and subsequent adjustment. *American Journal of Orthopsychiatry, 15,* 247-255.

GOLDFARB, W. (1955). Emotional and intellectual consequences of psychological deprivation in infancy: A re-evaluation. In E. H. Kockhand & J. Zubin (Eds.), *Psychopathology of childhood.* New York: Grune & Stratton.

GREENBAUM, C. W., & Kugelmass, S. (1980). Human development and socialization in cross-cultural perspective: Issues arising from research in Israel. In N. Warren (Ed.), *Studies in cross-cultural psychology* (Vol. 2). London: Academic Press.

GREENOUGH, W. T., & Volkmar, F. R. (1973). Pattern of dendritic branching in occipital cortex of rats reared in complex environments. *Experimental Neurology, 40,* 491-504.

HAHN, N. B., Jaeger, E., & Weinraub, M. (1991, April). *Maternal employment and infant attachment: Is maternal responsiveness the missing link?* Paper presented at the meeting of the Society for Research in Child Development, Seattle.

HANDEL, A. (1961). Self-concept of the kibbutz adolescent [in Hebrew]. *Megamot, 11,* 142-159. (Abstract from Rabin, A. I., 1971. *Kibbutz studies.* East Lansing: Michigan State University Press)

HARLOW, H. F., Dodsworth, R. O., & Harlow, M. K. (1965). Total social isolation in monkeys. *Proceedings of the National Academy of Sciences, 54,* 90-96.

HARLOW, H. F., & Harlow, M. K. (1962). Social deprivation in monkeys. *Scientific American, 207,* 136-146.

HARLOW, H. F., & Harlow, M. K. (1965). The affectional systems. In A. M. Schrier, H. F. Harlow, & F. Stollnitz (Eds.), *Behavior of nonhuman primates* (Vol. 2). New York: Academic Press.

HARLOW, H. F., & Novak, M. A. (1973). Psychopathological perspectives. *Perspectives in Biology and Medicine, 16,* 461-478.

HARLOW, H. F., & Suomi, S. J. (1971). Production of depressive behaviors in young monkeys. *Journal of Autism and Childhood Schizophrenia, 1,* 246-255.

HEBER, R., Garber, H., Harrington, S., Hoffman, C., & Falender, C. (1972). *Rehabilitation of families at risk for mental retardation* (Progress Report). Madison: University of Wisconsin, Rehabilitation & Training Center.

HERTZ-LAZAROWITZ, R., Fuchs, I., Sharabany, R., & Eisenberg, N. (1989). Students' interactive and noninteractive behaviors in the classroom: A comparison between two types of classrooms in the city and the kibbutz in Israel. *Contemporary Educational Psychology, 14,* 22-32.

HESS, R. D. (1970). Social class and ethnic influences on socialization. In P. Mussen (Ed.), *Carmichael's manual of child psychology* (Vol. 2, 3rd ed., pp. 457-557). New York: John Wiley.

HOCK, E. (1976). *Alternative approaches to child rearing and their effects on the mother-infant relationship* (Final Report, Grant No. OCD-490). Washington, DC: U.S. Department of Health, Education and Welfare, Office of Child Development.

HOWES, C. (1990). Can the age of entry into child care and the quality of child care predict adjustment in kindergarten? *Developmental Psychology, 26,* 292-303.

HOWES, C., & Rubenstein, J. L. (1981). Toddler peer behavior in two types of day care. *Infant Behavior and Development, 4,* 387-393.

HUNT, J. M. (1981). *Language acquisition and experience: Tehran.* Unpublished manuscript, University of Illinois, Urbana.

HUNT, J. M. (1982). Facilitating the development of social competence and language skill. In L. A. Bond & J. M. Jaffe (Eds.), *Facilitating infant and early childhood development.* Hanover, NH: University Press of New England.

HUNT, J. M., Mohandessi, K., Ghodessi, M., & Akiyama, M. (1976). The psychological development of orphanage-reared infants: Interventions with outcomes (Tehran). *Genetic Psychology Monographs, 94,* 177-226.

HUNT, J. M., Paraskevopoulos, J., Schickedanz, D., & Uzgiris, I. C. (1975). Variations in the mean ages of achieving object permanence under diverse conditions of rearing. In B. L. Friedlander, G. M. Sterrir, & G. E. Kirk (Eds.), *The exceptional infant: Vol. 3. Assessment and intervention.* New York: Brunner/Mazel.

JAEGER, E., Kuzela, A., & Weinraub, M. (1991, April). *Attachment security and maternal employment revisited: Validity issues concerning the Strange Situation and the Attachment Q-set.* Paper presented at the meeting of the Society for Research in Child Development, Seattle.

JAFFEE, B., & Fanshel, D. (1970). *How they fared in adoption: A follow-up study.* New York: Columbia University Press.

JOFFE, J. M. (1969). *Prenatal determinants of behavior.* Oxford: Pergamon.

KAFFMAN, M. (1965). A comparison of psychopathology: Israeli children from kibbutz and from urban surroundings. *American Journal of Orthopsychiatry, 35,* 509-520.

KAGAN, J. (1976a). Emergent themes in human development. *American Scientist, 64,* 186-196.

KAGAN, J. (1976b). Resilience and continuity in psychological development. In A. M. Clarke & A. D. B. Clarke (Eds.), *Early experience: Myth and evidence* (pp. 97-121). New York: Free Press.

KAGAN, J., Kearsley, R. B., & Zelazo, P. R. (1978). *Infancy: Its place in human development.* Cambridge, MA: Harvard University Press.

KARDINER, A. (1954). The roads to suspicion, rage, apathy, and societal disintegration. In I. Galdson (Ed.), *Beyond the germ theory.* New York: Health Education Council.

KING, M. A., & Perrin, M. S. (1987). Arrival time behavior of two-year-olds in child care. *Child and Youth Care Quarterly, 16,* 235-240.

KOHEN-RAZ, R. (1968). Mental and motor development of kibbutz, institutionalized, and home reared infants in Israel. *Child Development, 39,* 488-504.

KOLB, B. (1989). Brain development, plasticity, and behavior. *American Psychologist, 44,* 1203-1212.

KONIAK-GRIFFIN, D., & Ludington-Hoe, S. M. (1987). Paradoxical effects of stimulation on normal neonates. *Infant Behavior and Development, 10,* 261-277.

KUZELA, A. L., Hahn, N. B., & Weinraub, M. (1991, April). *Maternal employment status and maternal role satisfaction as predictors of preschool adjustment.* Paper presented at the meeting of the Society for Research in Child Development, Seattle.

LALLY, R. (1973). *The Family Development Research Program* (Progress Report). Syracuse, NY: Syracuse University.

LALLY, R. (1974). *The Family Development Research Program* (Progress Report). Syracuse, NY: Syracuse University.

LAMB, M. E., & Sternberg, K. J. (1990). Do we really know how day care affects children? *Journal of Applied Developmental Psychology, 11*, 351-379.

LAMB, M. E., Sternberg, K. J., & Prodromidis, M. (1992). Nonmaternal care and the security of infant-mother attachment: A reanalysis of the data. *Infant Behavior and Development, 15*, 71-83.

LAZAR, I., & Darlington, R. B. (1982). Lasting effects of an early education. *Monographs of the Society for Research in Child Development, 47*(2-3, Serial No. 195).

LEIDERMAN, P. H., & Leiderman, G. F. (1974). Affective and cognitive consequences of polymatric infant care in the East African Highlands. In A. D. Pick (Ed.), *Minnesota Symposia on Child Psychology* (Vol. 8, pp. 81-110). Minneapolis: University of Minnesota Press.

LEVENSTEIN, P. (1977). The mother-child home program. In M. C. Day & R. K. Parker (Eds.), *The preschool in action: Exploring early childhood programs* (2nd ed., pp. 27-49). Boston: Allyn & Bacon.

LEVENSTEIN, P., Kochman, A., & Roth, B. (1973). From laboratory to real world: Service and delivery of the mother-child home program. *American Journal of Orthopsychiatry, 43*, 72-78.

LEVENSTEIN, P., Kochman, A., Roth, B., & Sunley, R. (1968). Stimulation of verbal interaction between disadvantaged mothers and children. *American Journal of Orthopsychiatry, 43*, 116-121.

LEVY-SHIFF, R. (1983). Adaptation and competence in early childhood: Communally raised kibbutz children versus family raised children in the city. *Child Development, 54*, 1606-1614.

LONGSTRETH, L. E. (1981). Revisiting Skeels' final study: A critique. *Developmental Psychology, 17*, 620-625.

MACCOBY, E., & Feldman, S. S. (1972). Mother-attachment and stranger-reactions in the third year of life. *Monographs of the Society for Research in Child Development, 37*(1, Serial No. 146).

MacPHEE, D., Ramey, C., & Yeates, K. (1984). Home environment and early cognitive development. In A. Gottfried (Ed.), *Home environment and early cognitive development: Longitudinal research* (pp. 343-370). New York: Academic Press.

McBRIDE, S., & Belsky, J. (1988). Characteristics, determinants, and consequences of maternal separation anxiety. *Developmental Psychology, 24*, 407-414.

McCARTNEY, K., Scarr, S., Phillips, D., & Grajek, S. (1985). Day care as intervention. *Journal of Applied Developmental Psychology, 6*, 247-260.

MELHUISH, E. C., & Moss, H. A. (1990). *Day care for young children: International perspectives*. London: Routledge, Chapman & Hall.

MELZAK, R., & Scott, T. H. (1957). The effects of early experience on the response to pain. *Journal of Comparative and Physiological Psychology, 50*, 155-161.

MOSKOWITZ, D., Schwarz, J., & Corsini, D. (1977). Initiating day care at three years of age: Effects on attachment. *Child Development, 48*, 1271-1276.

NAGLER, S. (1963). Clinical observations on kibbutz children. *Israeli Annals of Psychiatry and Related Disciplines, 1*, 201-216.

NOVAK, M. A., & Harlow, H. F. (1975). Social recovery of monkeys isolated for the first year of life: I. Rehabilitation and therapy. *Developmental Psychology, 11*, 453-465.

O'CONNELL, J. C., & Farran, D. C. (1982). Effects of day-care experience on the use of intentional communicative behaviors in a sample of socioeconomically depressed infants. *Developmental Psychology, 18*, 22-29.

OPPENHEIM, D., Sagi, A., & Lamb, M. E. (1988). Classifications of infant-adult attachment on Israeli kibbutzim in the first year of life and their relation to socio-emotional development four years later. *Developmental Psychology, 24*, 427-433.

PARASKEVOPOULOS, J., & Hunt, J. M. (1971). Object construction and imitation under differing conditions of rearing. *Journal of Genetic Psychology, 119*, 301-321.

PELLED, N. (1964). On the formation of object-relations and identifications of the kibbutz child. *Israeli Annals of Psychiatry and Allied Disciplines, 2*, 144-161.

PIERS, M. (1978). *Infanticide: Past and present*. New York: W. W. Norton.

PORTNOY, F., & Simmons, C. (1978). Day care and attachment. *Child Development, 49*, 239-242.

RABIN, A. I. (1957). Personality maturity of kibbutz (Israeli collective settlement) and non-kibbutz children as reflected in Rorschach. *Journal of Projective Techniques, 21*, 148-153.

RABIN, A. I. (1958). Some psychosexual differences between kibbutz and non-kibbutz Israeli boys. *Journal of Projective Techniques, 22*, 328-332.

RABIN, A. I. (1961). Kibbutz adolescents. *American Journal of Orthopsychiatry, 31*, 493-504.

RAMEY, C. T., & Haskins, R. (1981). The causes and treatment of school failure: Insights from the Carolina Abecedarian Project. In M. J. Begab, H. C. Haywood, & H. L. Garber (Eds.), *Psychosocial influences in retarded performance: Strategies for improving competence*. Baltimore: University Park Press.

RAMEY, C. T., & Smith, B. (1976). Assessing the intellectual consequences of early intervention with high-risk infants. *American Journal of Mental Deficiency, 81*, 318-324.

RICCIUTI, H. N. (1974). Fear and the development of social attachments in the first year of life. In M. Lewis & L. A. Rosenblum (Eds.), *The origins of fear* (pp. 73-106). New York: John Wiley.

RICCIUTI, H. N. (1976, October). *Effects of infant day care experience on behavior and development: Research and implications for social policy*. Review prepared for the Office of the Assistant Secretary for Planning and Evaluation, U.S. Department of Health, Education and Welfare.

RICCIUTI, H. N., & Poresky, R. (1973, March). *Development of attachment to caregivers in an infant nursery during the first year of life*. Paper presented at the biennial meeting of the Society for Research in Child Development, Philadelphia.

RICHTER, J. E., & Zahn-Waxler, C. (1988). The infant day care controversy: Current status and future directions. *Early Childhood Research Quarterly, 3*, 319-336.

ROBINSON, H. B., & Robinson, N. M. (1971). Longitudinal development of very young children in a comprehensive day care program: The first two years. *Child Development, 42*, 1673-1683.

ROBINSON, N. M., Robinson, H. B., Darling, M. A., & Holm, G. (1979). *A world of children: Daycare and preschool institutions*. Belmont, CA: Brooks/Cole.

ROSENZWEIG, M. R. (1966). Environmental complexity, cerebral change, and behavior. *American Psychologist, 21*, 321-332.

ROSENZWEIG, M. R. (1983, August). *Experience, memory and the brain*. Paper presented at the annual meeting of the American Psychological Association, Anaheim, CA.

ROSENZWEIG, M. R., & Bennett, E. L. (1978). Experiential influences on brain anatomy and brain chemistry in rodents. In G. Gottlieb (Ed.), *Studies in the development of behavior and the nervous system: Vol. 4. Early influences*. New York: Academic Press.

ROSS, G., Kagan, J., Zelazo, P., & Kotelchuk, M. (1975). Separation protest in infants in home and laboratory. *Developmental Psychology, 11*, 256-257.

ROWLAND, G. L. (1964). *The effects of total isolation upon the learning and social behavior of rhesus monkeys*. Unpublished doctoral dissertation, University of Wisconsin—Madison.

RUBENSTEIN, J. L., Howes, C., & Boyle, P. (1981). A two-year follow-up of infants in community-based day care. *Journal of Child Psychology and Psychiatry and Allied Disciplines, 22*, 209-218.

RUTTER, M. (1979). Maternal deprivation 1972-1978: New findings, new concepts, new approaches. *Child Development, 50*, 283-305.

SACHERE, K. (1990). Attachment between working mothers and their infants: The influence of family processes. *American Journal of Orthopsychiatry, 60*, 19-34.

SACKETT, G. P., Holm, R. A., & Ruppenthal, G. C. (1976). Social isolation rearing: Species differences in behavior of macaque monkeys. *Developmental Psychology, 12*, 283-288.

SACKETT, G. P., Ruppenthal, G. C., Fahrenbruch, C. E., Hold, R. A., & Greenough, W. T. (1981). Social isolation rearing effects in monkeys vary with genotype. *Developmental Psychology, 17*, 313-318.

SALK, L. (1974). *Preparing for parenthood*. New York: David McKay.

SCARR, S., Phillips, D., & McCartney, K. (1990). Facts, fantasies and the future of child care in the United States. *Psychological Science, 1*, 26-35.

SCARR, S., & Weinberg, R. A. (1976). IQ test performance of black children adopted by white families. *American Psychologist, 10*, 726-739.

SCHAFFER, H. R., & Emerson, P. E. (1964). The development of social attachments in infancy. *Monographs of the Society for Research in Child Development, 29*(3, Serial No. 94).

SCHWARTZ, P. (1983). Length of day-care attendance and attachment behavior in eighteen-month-old infants. *Child Development, 54*, 1073-1078.

SCHWARZ, J. C., Scarr, S. W., Caparulo, B., Furrow, D., McCartney, K., Billington, R., Phillips, D., & Hindy, C. (1981, August). *Center, sitter, and home day care before age two: A report on the first Bermuda infant care study*. Paper presented at the annual meeting of the American Psychological Association, Los Angeles.

SCHWEINHART, L. J., & Weikart, D. P. (1980). Young children grow up: The effects of the Perry Preschool Program on youths through age 15. *Monographs of the High Scope Educational Research Foundation, 3*.

SCOTT, J. P. (1958). Critical periods in the development of social behavior in puppies. *Psychosomatic Medicine, 20*, 42-54.

SCOTT, J. P. (1967). The development of social motivation. In D. Levine (Ed.), *Nebraska Symposium on Motivation* (Vol. 15, pp. 111-132). Lincoln: University of Nebraska Press.

SCOTT, J. P., & Marston, M. (1950). Critical periods affecting the development of normal and maladjustive social behavior of puppies. *Journal of Genetic Psychology, 77*, 25-60.

SCOTT, J. P., Stewart, J. M., & DeGhett, V. J. (1973). Separation in infant dogs: Emotional response and motivational consequences. In J. P. Scott & E. C. Senay (Eds.), *Separation and depression: Clinical and research aspects* (pp. 3-32). Washington, DC: American Association for the Advancement of Science.

SEITZ, V. (1982). A methodological comment on the problem of infant day care. In E. F. Zigler & E. W. Gordon (Eds.), *Day care: Scientific and social policy issues* (pp. 243-251). Boston: Auburn House.

SKEELS, H. M. (1936). The mental development of children in foster homes. *Pedagogical Seminar and Journal of Genetic Psychology, 49*, 91-106.

SKEELS, H. M. (1966). Adult status of children with contrasting early life experiences. *Monographs of the Society for Research in Child Development, 31*(3).

SKEELS, H. M., & Dye, H. B. (1939). A study of the effects of differential stimulation of mentally retarded children. *Proceedings of the American Association on Mental Deficiency, 44*, 114-136.

SKODAK, M. (1939). Children in foster homes: A study of mental development. *University of Iowa Studies in Child Welfare, 16*(1).

SKODAK, M., & Skeels, H. M. (1945). A follow-up study of children in adoptive homes. *Journal of Genetic Psychology, 66*, 21-58.

SKODAK, M., & Skeels, H. M. (1949). A follow-up study of one hundred adopted children. *Journal of Genetic Psychology, 75*, 85-125.

SPIRO, M. E. (1958). *Children of the kibbutz*. Cambridge, MA: Harvard University Press.

SPITZ, R. A. (1945). Hospitalism: An inquiry into the genesis of psychiatric conditions in early childhood. In R. S. Eissler (Ed.), *Psychoanalytic study of the child*. New Haven, CT: Yale University Press.

SPITZ, R. A. (1946). Hospitalism: A follow up report. *Psychoanalytic Study of the Child, 2*, 113-118.

SPOCK, B. J. (1946). *Baby and child care*. New York: Simon & Schuster.

SPOCK, B. J. (1976). *Baby and child care* (3rd ed.). New York: Pocket Books.

SROUFE, L. A. (1988). A developmental perspective on day care. *Early Childhood Research Quarterly, 3*, 283-291.

STRAUSS, M. S., & Brownell, C. A. (1984). A commentary on infant stimulation and intervention. In Infant intervention programs: Truths and untruths [Special issue]. *Journal of Children in Contemporary Society, 17*, 133-139.

SUOMI, S. J., & Harlow, H. F. (1972). Rehabilitation of isolate-reared monkeys. *Developmental Psychology, 6*, 487-496.

SUPER, C. M., Herrera, M. G., & Mora, J. O. (1990). Long-term effects of food supplementation and psychosocial intervention on the physical growth of Colombian infants at risk of malnutrition. *Child Development, 61*, 29-49.

THOMPSON, R. (1988). The effects of infant day-care through the prism of attachment theory: A critical reappraisal. *Early Childhood Research Quarterly, 3*, 273-282.

THOMPSON, W. R. (1955). Early environment: Its importance for later behavior. In P. H. Hoch & J. Zubin (Eds.), *Psychopathology of childhood*. New York: Grune & Stratton.

TIZARD, B. (1977). *Adoption: A second chance*. New York: Free Press.

U.S. Department of Labor. (1989). *Facts on working women* (Publication No. 89-3). Washington, DC: Government

Printing Office.

VANDELL, D. L., Henderson, V. K., & Wilson, K. S. (1988). A longitudinal study of children with day-care experiences of varying quality. *Child Development, 59*, 1286-1292.

VOLLING, B., Braungart, J., Nuss, J., & Feagans, L. (1990, April). *The effects of infant day care on children's social behavior: An examination of within-group differences.* Paper presented at the International Conference on Infant Studies, Montreal.

WACHS, T. D. (1987). Specificity of environmental action as manifest in environmental correlates of infant's mastery motivation. *Developmental Psychology, 23,* 782-790.

WACHS, T. D. (1989). The nature of physical microenvironment: An expanded classification system. *Merrill-Palmer Quarterly, 35,* 399-419.

WACHS, T. D. (1990). Must the physical environment be mediated by the social environment in order to influence development? A further test. *Journal of Applied Developmental Psychology, 11,* 163-178.

WHITE, B. L., & Watts, J. (1973). *Experience and environment: Major influences on the development of the young child* (Vol. 1). Englewood Cliffs, NJ: Prentice-Hall.

WILL, B. E., Rosenzweig, M. R., & Bennett, E. L. (1976). Effects of differential environments on recovery from neonatal brain lesions, measured by problem solving scores and brain dimensions. *Physiology and Behavior, 16,* 603-611.

WILL, B. E., Rosenzweig, M. R., Bennett, E. L., Hebert, M., & Morimoto, H. (1977). Relatively brief environmental enrichment aids recovery of learning capacity and alters brain measures after postweaning brain lesions in rats. *Journal of Comparative and Physiological Psychology, 91,* 33-50.

WILLIS, A., & Ricciuti, H. N. (1974, January). *Longitudinal observations of infants' daily arrivals at a day care center* (Tech. Rep.). Ithaca, NY: Cornell University.

WOHLWILL, J., & Heft, A. (1987). The physical environment and development of the child. In D. Stokels & I. Altman (Eds.), *Handbook of environmental psychology* (pp. 281-328). New York: John Wiley.

ZIGLER, E. F., & Gordon, E. W. (Eds.). (1982). *Day care: Scientific and social policy issues.* Boston: Auburn House.

Author Index

Subject Index

aversive reactions to, 253
blood type and, 81
inborn errors of metabolism and, 59
representation of, 77(fig.)
rubella and, 96
Amnion, amniotic sac, 21, 23
Amniotomy, 164
Amphetamine, 124
Ampicillin, 109
Analog study, 472
Androgen, 33, 34, 70
Androgenic, 106
Anencephalics, 82, 214, 312
Anesthesia, 157
dangers of, 163
epidural, 154, 156
general, 162-163
regional, 160-162
Aneuploid, 61
Anger, 254
cries and, 222, 224
exposure to, 221
facial expressions and, 220
Animals
observations of, 37
therapeutic interventions with, 529-530
A-not-B error, 412-413
Anoxia, 41, 150
altitude and, 104
assessing, 331
delivery and, 151-152, 173
delivery pain and, 163
intrauterine growth retardation and, 95, 104
sitting-up deliveries and, 173
Antibiotics, 96, 109, 133
Anticipation, 400
Anticonvulsants, 108
Antidepressants, 109
Antiepileptic drugs, 108
Anxiety
delivery and, 157, 163
prenatal exposure to, 129-131
Apathy, newborns and, 326
Apgar, 161
Aphasics, 447
APIB (Assessment of Preterm Infants' Behavior), 335-336
Apnea, 46, 343
Arbitrariness, language and, 431
Aromatic solvents, 109
Arousal, laughter and, 232-233
Asian flu, 133
Asphyxia, 152, 226
Aspirin, 105, 107-108, 133
Assessment of Preterm Infants' Behavior (APIB), 335-336
Assimilation, 392
Association areas, development of, 310
Associationist theory, 390-391
Associative learning, 415
Associative memory, 412-413

Astigmatism, 273n.6
Attachment, 458-477
across life span, 474
action-initiation phase, 460
adoption and, 514
biological mechanism and, 465
day care and, 522-523, 525-526
defining, 461-464
father and, 486
functions of, 464-468
history and theories of, 458-459
institutionalization and, 509
locomotor period and, 465-467
long-term consequences of, 468-469
mothers' role in development of, 469-475
multiple mothering and, 517-518, 519-520
other cultures, 475-477
peer relations and, 490
playmates and, 467
quality of, 463-464
security of, 468-469, 473-474, 481
social development and, 458-477
stability of, 462-463
stages in, 459-461
Attachment Q-set, 467
Attention, 205-207, 235, 331
development and, 206-207
IQ and, 357
joint, 450
orientation response and, 355
predicting cognitive development and, 358-359
Attentional deficits, 45
Attention getting, 206, 223
Attention holding, 206
Audition, 259-267
complexity and, 263-265
continuity of stimulation, 266
localization and, 261-263
loudness and, 261
newborns and, 260-261
pitch and, 263-266
See also Auditory system; Hearing impaired
Auditory brain stem responses (ABRs), 267
Auditory discrimination, brain hemispheres and, 445
Auditory evoked potentials, 260
Auditory localization, 394
Auditory stimulation, 5, 335
attending, 206
feeding and, 480
laughter and, 232
reaching and, 324
smiles and, 231
state changes, 209
stopping cries and, 227
visual stimuli and, 290-291
Auditory system
affective development and, 252

myelination, 35
speech detectors, 436
Auditory system fibers, 310
Autism
fragile X and, 72
rubella and, 95
Autonomic nervous system, 222
cries and, 222, 223
sleep and, 356
Autosomal, 72
Autosomal chromosomes, abnormalities of, 60-67
Autosomal pairs, 58
Autosomal recessive trait, 78
Avoidance
looming and, 286
visual cliff and, 289
Avoidant, 463
Axons, 35, 36

Babbling, 430, 432-434, 436
Babkin reflex, 361
Baby biographies, 4-9
Baby's day, states and, 208-210
Bag of waters, 23
Balance, 315
Balanced polymorphic system, 78-79
Barbiturates, 157, 160, 162
Barr body, 68, 84
Base rate, 70
Battered prematures, 180
Bayley Motor Scale, 313, 320, 334, 340-342, 517
Behavior
alcohol use and, 112-113
assessing meaning of, 6
genetic variances, 3, 59
intentional, 399
prenatal development and, 37
See also Behavior problems
Behavioral development, physical growth and, 306
Behavioral study of infants, 4-9
Behavioral teratology, 94, 132
Behavioral tests, 327-330
Behavior problems
difficultness and, 236
Down syndrome and, 66
early deprivation and, 513-514
smoking and, 117
weaning and, 219
Benzoic acid, 107
Beta thalassemia, 80
Between groups design, 14
Biased samples, 12
Bilirubin, 41, 42, 80, 214-215
Binet-Simon, 340
Binocular acuity, 273
Binocular disparity, 283
Binocular field, 268
Binocular perception, 286
Biological factors

About the Authors

Judy F. Rosenblith taught for 19 years at Wheaton College, where she is Professor Emerita. She has also held teaching positions at Simmons College, Harvard University, and Brown University, as well as research appointments at Harvard Medical School (Head, Laboratory of Human Development, Massachusetts General Hospital) and Brown University (1961-1975). She is senior editor of *The Causes of Behavior: Readings in Child Development and Educational Psychology* (three editions). Her most recent book chapter is a biography and summary of the accomplishments of Pauline S. Sears in *Women in Psychology* (1990). She has held various editorial posts and has written a number of book reviews for *Contemporary Psychology*, for which she has served as Consulting Editor. She has 25 publications in the field of newborn testing and relations between newborn behavior and later developmental outcomes. She is a member and former Secretary of the Society for Research in Child Development and a Fellow of the American Psychological Association, and is active on various committees and task forces. She is a past member of the Maternal and Child Health Research Advisory Committee of the National Institute of Child Health and Human Development. She is the mother of two and the grandmother of three, ages 2-22.

Paula N. Menyuk is a Professor in the Language, Literacy and Cultural Studies Program at the School of Education, and in the Applied Linguistics Program in the Graduate School of Arts and Sciences at Boston University. She obtained her A.B. in speech sciences at New York University and her Ed.M. in speech pathology and audiology at Boston University. With a predoctoral fellowship from NIMH, she studied psychology at Radcliffe College, linguistics at MIT, and communication disorders at Boston University. She obtained a D.Ed. at Boston University. She has published numerous articles and four books on the subjects of language development in normally developing children and in those with handicapping conditions. Her latest book is a text titled *Language Development: Knowledge and Use* (1988). She is currently conducting research on the effects of middle ear disease (chronic otitis media) on language development, on the effects of language disorder on reading, and on the role of metalinguistic processing in oral and written language development. She serves as a member on the Advisory Board of the National Institute of Deafness and Other Communication Disorders, a new institute of the National Institutes of Health, and as a member of the Social and Behavioral Sciences Review Committee of the National Foundation March of Dimes for Birth Defects.

Judith E. Sims-Knight is Professor of Psychology at the University of Massachusetts, Dartmouth. She earned her B.A. at Brown University, her M.A. at City University of New York, and her Ph.D. in Child Psychology at the University of Minnesota. She taught at Florida Atlantic University and Wheaton College before going to UMass Dartmouth. Throughout her career her central research concerns have been the intellectual development of children of all ages. Her research has ranged widely across these areas, including developmental studies of memory, problem solving, visual representation, logical reasoning, and mathematical thinking. With her husband, Raymond Knight, she has studied cognitive processes in schizophrenics and developmental antecedents of sexual aggression. Currently she has become interested in the cognitive processes underlying computer use and is studying how adolescents solve computer problems. Dr. Sims-Knight coauthored the first version of this text with Dr. Rosenblith.